Miller's Nursing for Wellness in Older Adults

SECOND AUSTRALIAN AND NEW ZEALAND EDITION

Sharyn Hunter, RN, BSc(Hons), PhD
Grad Cert Workplace Assessment
Grad Cert Tertiary Teaching
Grad Cert Advanced Practice (Aged Care)
School of Nursing and Midwifery, Faculty of Health
The University of Newcastle (Callaghan Campus)
Newcastle, New South Wales

Original US edition by

Carol A. Miller, MSN, RN-BC, AHN-BC
Gerontological Clinical Nurse Specialist and Nurse Case Manager
Care & Counseling, Miller/Wetzler Associates, Cleveland, Ohio
Clinical Faculty, Frances Payne Bolton School of Nursing
Case Western Reserve University, Cleveland, Ohio

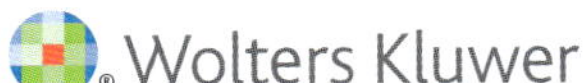

Philadelphia • Baltimore • New York • London
Buenos Aires • Hong Kong • Sydney • Tokyo

Wolters Kluwer Health
Two Commerce Square, 2001 Market Street, Philadelphia, PA 19103

Publisher: Julie Stegman
Product Manager: Caroline Hunter
Editor: Karen Enkelaar, Do Write
Proofreader: Karen Enkelaar, Do Write
Indexer: Puddingburn Publishing Services
Typesetter: Aptara, Inc.
Cover design: XouCreative
Printer: RR Donnelley, Shenzhen, China

National Library of Australia Cataloguing-in-Publication entry
Creator: Hunter, Sharyn, author.
Title: Nursing for wellness in older adults/by Sharyn Hunter.
Edition: Second edition.
ISBN: 9781922228758 (paperback) 9781922228765 (ebook: epub)
Notes: Includes bibliographical references and index.
Subjects: Geriatric nursing–Australia–Textbooks.
Nursing–Australia–Textbooks.
Older people–Care.
Other Creators/Contributors: Miller, Carol A. Nursing for wellness in older adults.
Dewey Number: 618.970231

RRS1710

Reviewers

Judith ANDERSON **RN MHSM MN BN PhD**
Senior Lecturer, School of Nursing
Midwifery and Indigenous Health
Charles Sturt University, Bathurst, New South Wales

Jean BOOTH **RN DipAppSc BHSc MHSc PhD**
Aged Care Consultant

Marguerite BRAMBLE **RN BN(Hons) BEc GCert(StratMkt) GCert(ResearchMgt)**
Project Manager
NHMRC Paro Research Project/Adjunct Senior Lecturer
Griffith University/University of Tasmania
Brisbane, Queensland/Launceston, Tasmania

Angela CASEY **RN ICUCert GDipAppSc(AdvN) MEd(Lead&Mgt)**
Lecturer in Nursing, School of Nursing and Midwifery
La Trobe University, Melbourne, Victoria

Leah EAST **RN BN(Hons) GCertAP Cert(Reprod&SexHN) PhD**
Senior Lecturer, School of Nursing and Midwifery
Faculty of Health, Deakin University, Geelong, Victoria

Lisa HEE **BN GDipGerN MEd(ProfPrac) MMgt(AgedCare)**
Lecturer, School of Nursing
Queensland University of Technology
Kelvin Grove, Queensland

Eleanor HORTON **BHScN MHScN AdvDipN PhD**
Senior Lecturer, School of Nursing and Midwifery
University of the Sunshine Coast
Maroochydore, Queensland

Paul McDONALD **RN BHScN MN(Clin) MPET**
Lecturer, School of Nursing
Midwifery and Paramedicine
Australian Catholic University
North Sydney, New South Wales

Michael J. McGIVERN **RMN RGN BN DipHEd NCAET CertMgt(HServ) PGDipHSc(AN) DipCDM(PrimCare)**
Nursing Lecturer, NorthTec School of Nursing
Whangarei, Northland, New Zealand

Molly PAGE **RN MN**
Lecturer, Health Faculty
Bachelor of Nursing Programme
Whitireia Community Polytechnic
Porirua, New Zealand

Wendy PENNEY **RN MN PhD**
Head of School, Nursing Midwifery and Healthcare
Federation University, Ballarat, Victoria

Vivien RODGERS **RN BA BN GDipGN MN(DocCandidate)**
Lecturer, School of Nursing, Massey University
Palmerston North, New Zealand

Monica SCHOCH **BN(Hons) MN**
Lecturer in Nursing, School of Nursing and Midwifery
Deakin University, Geelong, Victoria

Caroline VAFEAS **RN MA BSc(Hons) PhD**
Senior Lecturer, School of Nursing & Midwifery
Edith Cowan University, Joondalup, Western Australia

Claudia VIRDUN **BN(Hons) MSc(AdvProfHCarePrac[CancerCare]) PhD Candidate(PalCare)**
Lecturer, Faculty of Health
Sydney University of Technology, Sydney
New South Wales

Cecilia YEBOAH **RN RM MN PhD**
Lecturer/International Academic Advisor—Nursing
School of Nursing
Midwifery and Paramedicine
Australian Catholic University
Melbourne, Victoria

Preface

BACKGROUND

The population of older adults is increasing and so is their use of health services. These trends are posing a challenge for health services across the globe. As nurses are the primary healthcarers of older adults, it is evident that nurses require skills and knowledge to meet the care needs of the older adult. Knowledge about the ageing process and risk factors for physical, cognitive and psychosocial decline of older adults is fundamental knowledge required by all nurses and not specialist knowledge required by some.

Historically heathcare systems have viewed ageing negatively, but this is changing. The trends already mentioned have compelled health services to change to a more positive approach. There is an increasing focus on "wellness" and health when caring for older adults. Healthy ageing describes the ongoing activities an older adult undertakes to reduce the risk of illness and disease and to maintain their physical, cognitive and mental health. It also includes the activities an older adult undertakes in response to an illness or disease that supports optimal recovery.

Nurses are required to deliver care that supports wellness outcomes and healthy ageing. Nurses do this by providing information to older adults about their health, and working with them so they can optimise the ageing experience. When nurses use a healthy-ageing approach, the assessment of older adults' health and ageing, especially from a person-centred perspective, is critical. Person-centred care addresses the body–mind–spirit interconnectedness of each older adult, emphasises the person, and recognises that wellness encompasses more than physiological functioning.

It is the intent of the Australian and New Zealand edition of *Nursing for Wellness in Older Adults* to provide nursing students with learning materials to assist them with developing their knowledge, skills, behaviours and attitudes that are aligned with older–person-centred care and which emphasise wellness outcomes and support healthy ageing.

ORGANISATION

Nursing for Wellness in Older Adults has 29 chapters, organised into five parts. Chapters in Parts 1 and 2 introduce topics relevant to ageing, wellness, older adults, and the role of nurses in promoting wellness in older adults. Chapters in Parts 3 and 4 are organised around the Functional Consequences Theory of Nursing Older Adults, so each facet of physiological or psychosocial function is presented according to age-related changes, risk factors, functional consequences, nursing assessment, nursing issues, wellness outcomes, nursing interventions and the evaluation of nursing care. The three chapters in Part 5 help nurses provide holistic care for older adults during illness.

The intent of Part 1, older adults and wellness (Chapters 1–4), is to help nurses apply a wellness philosophy to their care of older adults. Chapters 1 and 2 integrate the concepts of wellness and ageing and provide an overview of the characteristics and diversity of older adults. Chapter 3 explicates the Functional Consequences Theory, which is applied throughout this text as a framework for wellness-oriented nursing care of older adults. Chapter 4 provides an overview of theories that are pertinent to ageing well.

Part 2, nursing considerations for older adults (Chapters 5–10), discusses nurses' roles while addressing the unique challenges of caring for older adults and emphasising health promotion in relation to older adults. Roles for nurses working with older adults are described in relation to the care settings that comprise the continuum of care for older adults. This section also covers the complex topics of assessment, medications, and legal and ethical concerns, because nurses address these aspects of care with the majority of the older adults for whom they provide care. Elder abuse and neglect also are addressed in this section because nurses need to be aware of these concerns when caring for older adults.

Part 3, promoting wellness in psychosocial function (Chapters 11–15), extensively reviews cognitive and psychosocial function and provides guidelines for a comprehensive nursing assessment of psychosocial function, with emphasis on healthy older adults. In addition, this part covers delirium, dementia and depression, which are three of the most commonly occurring pathological conditions that have serious psychosocial consequences for older adults.

Part 4, promoting wellness in physical function (Chapters 16–26), includes chapters that address each of the following specific aspects of functioning in older adults: hearing, vision, digestion and nutrition, urinary function, cardiovascular function, respiratory function, mobility and safety, integument, sleep and rest, thermoregulation and sexual function. Selected common pathological conditions also are addressed in these chapters when these conditions affect a particular aspect of functioning in older adults.

The information provided in Part 5, promoting wellness in all stages of health and illness (Chapters 27–29), has been considerably expanded in the second edition and addresses topics of caring for older adults during illness or pain and when they are at the end of life.

PEDAGOGICAL FEATURES

- **Learning objectives** help the reader identify important chapter content and focus their reading.
- **Key points** listed at the beginning of the chapter and bolded in the text highlight important vocabulary.
- **Theory illustrations** at the beginning of each chapter on specific aspects of functioning present an overview of the Functional Consequences Theory, which follows a **nursing clinical reasoning approach**.
- **Icons** identify the five major components of the Functional Consequences Theory:

 Age-related changes

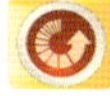 Risk factors

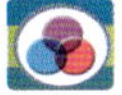 Functional consequences

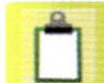 Nursing assessment

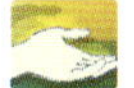 Nursing interventions

- Unfolding case studies provide real-life examples of the effects of age-related changes and risk factors, beginning in young-old adulthood and continuing through all the stages of later adulthood. **Thinking points** after each segment of the case assist the student in applying the content of the chapter to the case example. Many chapters include a concluding **Case study** with a sample **Nursing care plan**.
- **Chapter highlights** in an easy-to-read bulleted format facilitate review of the material.
- **Critical thinking exercises**, listed at the end of each chapter help readers to gain insight and develop problem-solving skills through purposeful, goal-directed thinking.
- **References** give readers additional information about the most up-to-date research that supports evidence-based practice.

Practice-oriented features

- **Evidence-based practice** boxes are included in clinically oriented chapters to summarise guidelines for research-based care of older adults.
- **Wellness opportunities** are sprinkled throughout the clinically oriented chapters to draw attention to ways in which nurses can promote wellness during the usual course of their care activities.
- **A student's perspective** provides reality-based stories, written by nursing students, which illustrate the application of wellness concepts in clinical practice.
- **A nurse's perspective** provides insights into the roles of nurses who work with older adults to promote nursing students' understanding of these roles.
- **Cultural considerations** boxes help the reader to appreciate cultural differences that may influence his or her approach to a patient, resident or client.
- **Diversity notes** give brief information about differences among specific groups; for example, men and women.
- **Assessment boxes** provide the reader with specific approaches for nursing assessment. Commonly used assessment tools are described (and, in many cases, illustrated).
- **Interventions boxes** provide succinct guides for nursing interventions, with a strong focus on health promotion. Guides for "best practice" in nursing interventions are given. Many of the interventions boxes can be used as tools for teaching older adults and their caregivers/carers about how to improve functional abilities.
- **Resources sections** direct the reader to sources for clinical tools, evidence-based practice and health education.

TEACHING AND LEARNING PACKAGE

Instructor resources

Tools to assist you with teaching your course are available upon adoption of this text at the text's accompanying website located on thePoint at http://thepoint.lww.com.

- **PowerPoint Presentations** provide an easy way for you to integrate the textbook with your students' classroom experience, either via slide shows or handouts. Multiple-choice and True/False questions are integrated into the presentations to promote class participation.
- **Multiple-choice questions** help you assess your students' understanding of the course material.
- **An image bank** contains illustrations from the book in formats suitable for printing and incorporating into PowerPoint presentations and Internet sites.
- **Multi-media progressive case study** can be used as a class activity or group assignment.
- Access to all student resources.

SUMMARY

Providing wellness-oriented nursing care for older adults is an opportunity to care for people who are striving to meet the challenge of remaining well while coping with age-related changes and risk factors that affect their functioning and quality of life. The goal of *Nursing for Wellness in Older Adults* is to provide nursing students with an evidenced based approach to assisting older adults in meeting the many challenges of older adulthood in positive and creative ways.

SHARYN HUNTER, RN, BSc(Hons), PhD
Grad Cert Workplace Assessment, Grad Cert Tertiary Teaching, Grad Cert Advanced Practice (Aged Care)

Acknowledgements

The adaptation of Carol Miller's original version of *Nursing for Wellness in the Older Adults* has been a collaborative effort between myself and many others. I would like to acknowledge all of those people who helped make this text a reality.

I thank Carol Miller for agreeing to this adaptation. I am reminded of a saying when I reflect on Carol's contribution to this text: "We are like dwarfs standing on the shoulders of giants." I have been able to build on her exceptional work to create an innovative text appropriate for nursing students in Australia and New Zealand.

I want to extend my sincerest appreciation to several staff at Wolters Kluwer who assisted with the text's development and production. To Caroline Hunter and Karen Enkelaar, thank you for your support and patience on the journey to complete this edition.

Closer to home: to my husband, who provided unconditional support during the many months when I was completely absorbed in writing; to my puppy dogs who provided the much needed companionship while I separated myself from the world to write; and to my retired neighbours for their continued interest and encouragement while I was writing.

Finally, thank you to the older adults and their families whom I have encountered while nursing: you have facilitated my development and understanding of ageing, which has been integral to writing this edition.

Sharyn Hunter

Contents

CHAPTER 13

Cognitive and psychosocial assessment 242

CHAPTER 14

Impaired cognition: Delirium and dementia 274

CHAPTER 15

Impaired cognition: Depression 310

PART 

Promoting wellness in physical function 335

CHAPTER 16

Hearing 335

CHAPTER 17

Vision 358

CHAPTER 18

Digestion, nutrition and hydration 384

Assessment, intervention and evidence-based practice boxes

Assessment boxes

Safety and functioning

Medicines

Psychosocial assessment

Impaired cognitive function

Impaired affective function

Hearing

Vision

Digestion, nutrition and hydration

Urinary function

Cardiovascular function

Respiratory function

Mobility and safety

Integument

Sleep and rest

Thermoregulation

Sexual function

Illness

Interventions boxes

Health promotion

Medicines

Cognitive function

Psychosocial function

Psychosocial assessment

Impaired cognitive function

Impaired affective function

Hearing

Vision

Digestion, nutrition and hydration

Urinary function

Cardiovascular function

Respiratory function

Mobility and safety

Integument

Sleep and rest

Thermoregulation

Sexual function

Illness

Pain

End of life

Evidence-based practice boxes

PART 1

OLDER ADULTS AND WELLNESS

Chapter 1

Seeing older adults through the eyes of wellness

By Carol Miller and Sharyn Hunter

LEARNING OBJECTIVES

After reading this chapter, you should be able to:

1. Describe the relationship between ageing and wellness.
2. Define healthy ageing from several perspectives.
3. Identify barriers to and opportunities for nurses to promote wellness in older adults.
4. Recognise the effects of ageism and attitudes about ageing.
5. Identify myths that affect nursing care of older adults.
6. Describe demographic, health and socioeconomic characteristics of older adults in Australia and New Zealand.
7. Discuss the trends for older adults as givers and recipients of care.
8. Describe the global aspects of ageing.

KEY POINTS

age attribution
ageism
ageing
ageing anxiety
anti-ageing
baby boomers
carer/caregiver burden
chronological age
comorbidities
functional age
healthy ageing
high-level wellness
informal caregiver
old-old
perceived age
sandwich generation
skipped-generation households
subjective age

Despite the common perception that older adulthood is an extended period of declining health and functioning, conceptualisations of ageing are broadening. Currently most gerontologists and many older adults themselves view ageing as a complex process that includes both losses and gains. This perspective is consistent with the broadening base of knowledge about ways in which older adults can age well. It also is consistent with a bio-psycho-social-emotional-spiritual perspective on ageing, which addresses all aspects of ageing, with particular attention to increasing diversity of older adults as a group and respect for the unique characteristics of each older person. Although knowledge about all aspects of ageing—ranging from healthy ageing to frail elders—is evolving rapidly, many gaps still exist. Because many challenges of older adulthood involve health and functioning, older adults need accurate information, not only about normal ageing but also about interventions to promote wellness. Nurses are in ideal positions to work with older adults and teach them about health while ageing, and empower them to implement problem-solving strategies directed towards achieving and maintaining a high level of functioning and a good quality of life.

The intent of this nursing text is to provide comprehensive and research-based information so that nurses can distinguish between the changes associated with normal ageing and those that result from other factors. In addition, the text provides tools and guides for nursing assessment, interventions and health education in relation to all aspects of physical and psychosocial functioning. Nurses can use this information to promote wellness—which includes improved health, functioning and quality of life—for the older adults for whom they provide care.

This chapter provides an overview of concepts related to ageing and wellness and presents information about myths and information about older adults in the Australia and New Zealand in terms of demographic, health, socioeconomic characteristics, and trends in caring. Lastly, it presents a brief overview of ageing worldwide to provide a broader perspective.

RELATIONSHIP BETWEEN AGEING AND WELLNESS

If asked to define *ageing and wellness*, most people associate wellness with peak achievement in younger adulthood and ageing with declining health that eventually leads to death. This description of wellness does not address well-being of the body, mind and spirit. Similarly, many definitions of human ageing focus narrowly on physical health and functioning rather than holistically—and accurately—on humans as complex bio-psycho-social-spiritual individuals.

Definitions of ageing

Gerontologists and lay people define ageing from many perspectives. Objectively, **ageing** is a universal process that begins at birth; in this context, it applies equally to young and old people. Subjectively, however, ageing is typically associated with being "old" or reaching "older adulthood", and people define ageing in terms of personal meaning and experience.

Children usually do not view themselves as ageing, but they delight in announcing how old they are and they anticipate birthdays with great enthusiasm. They view their birthdays as positive events that will permit them to enjoy additional opportunities and responsibilities. Likewise, adolescents view ageing as the mechanism that allows them to participate legally in important activities such as driving and voting. In contrast, adults tend to view "old age" as something to be avoided and they are likely to define the onset of older adulthood as a decade beyond their current age.

The term **subjective age** (also referred to as *feel age*) is used to describe someone's perception of his or her age. Studies have found that older people judge the onset of both middle and older age as occurring at a later chronological age than do younger people (Musaiger & D'Souza, 2009; Prevc & Doupona, 2009). Nurses often observe this phenomenon when they hear people whose chronological age is 75 years, 80 years or older, refer to "old people" as if they were a group older than and distinct from themselves.

Since the 1980s gerontologists have used the concept of **perceived age**—which is another person's estimated age of someone based on appearances—in many studies, including several large longitudinal studies. These studies have confirmed that perceived age correlates very closely with health and is a strong predictor of survival, especially for people aged 70 years and older (Christensen, Thinggaard et al., 2009).

Objectively, people define **chronological age** as the length of time that has passed since birth. Western culture is particularly fascinated by numbers, quantities and relative values that can be measured. Among the questions frequently asked and answered are *How much? How far? How often?* and *How old?* Our fascination with age is particularly evident in newspaper articles, which invariably state the age of the subjects, regardless of the relevance of age to the topic. In addition to being easily measured, another advantage of chronological age is that it serves as an objective basis for social organisation. For example, societies establish chronological age criteria for certain activities, such as education, voting, driving, marriage, employment, alcohol consumption, military service, and the collection of retirement benefits. To participate legally in these activities, people must provide documentation of a certain chronological age.

During the 1960s, gerontologists viewed 65 years of age as an acceptable chronological criterion for ageing. This is consistent with the accepted definition in Australia and New Zealand that "the aged" are 65 and over. The Productivity Commission (PC) refers to those aged 65 and over as "older", while those who are aged over 85 years are the "**old old**" (2005, p. xvi). However, in recent decades, gerontologists agree that ageing is too complex to be defined only by one's birth date. From both scientific and humanistic perspectives, a person's chronological age is relatively insignificant because there is no biological measurement that applies to everyone at a specific age. Consequently, gerontologists have commonly divided older adulthood into subgroups, such as young-old, middle-old, old-old, and oldest-old. As one of the first gerontologists to challenge the original criterion stated:

> *We have used sixty-five as the economic marker, then as the social and psychological marker, of old age. A set of stereotypes has grown up that older persons are sick, poor, enfeebled, isolated, and desolated. While these stereotypes have been greatly overdrawn even for the old old, they have become uncritically attached to the whole group over sixty-five. (Neugarten, 1978, pp. 47–48)*

The trend in gerontology to divide old age into chronological subcategories is an improvement over the categorisation of all people older than 65 years as one homogeneous group, but it has the disadvantage of creating additional stereotypes and age biases. For example, if a chronologically old-old person needs a complicated or expensive medical treatment to maintain or potentially improve his or her health status, such treatment may be denied or withheld based on advanced age. More recently, there is increasing recognition that decisions about treatment approaches should be based on broad evidence-based criteria, especially for those people who are chronologically categorised as old-old (Lerolle et al., 2010; Wilson, Thurston & Lichlyter, 2010). For healthcare providers whose practice focuses on older adults, as well as for most older adults, the important indicators of age are:

- Physiological health
- Psychological well-being
- Socioeconomic factors
- Ability to function and participate in desirable activities.

Based on this understanding of ageing, gerontologists have used the term **functional age** for several decades. This concept is associated with a shift in emphasis from chronological factors to such factors as whether individuals can contribute to society and benefit others and themselves.

Functional age is a concept that is used worldwide, but its definition varies according to different cultural contexts. For example, industrialised societies may associate functional age with self-sufficiency and physiological function, whereas other cultures might associate it more closely with social or psychological function than with physiological function.

One advantage of functional definitions of age over chronological definitions is that the former are associated with higher levels of well-being and with more positive attitudes about ageing. From a holistic perspective, the concept of functional age provides a more rational basis for care than the measurement of how many years have passed since the person was born. Thus, the question *How functional?* is more relevant than *How old?* Even more relevant for promoting wellness in older adults are such questions as:

- How well do you feel?
- What goals do you have for improving your level of wellness?
- Is there anything that you would like to do that you cannot do?
- What goals do you have for improving your quality of life?

In this text, the term *older adult* applies to individuals experiencing the cumulative effects of age-related changes and risk factors that affect their health and functioning (refer to Chapter 3 for further definition and discussion). From a holistic perspective, this conceptualisation addresses all aspects of bio-psycho-social-spiritual health and functioning, as discussed in the next section in relation to healthy ageing.

Wellness and older adults

The concept of wellness came to public attention in the early 1960s when Halbert L. Dunn, MD, PhD, retired from his formal public health career and became a "lecturer and consultant in high-level wellness work" (Dunn, 1961, p. 244). Dunn believed that education at all points in a person's life was the key to high-level wellness, and he developed a series of radio talks with the theme "High-Level Wellness for Man and Society".

He defined **high-level wellness** as an "integrated method of functioning that is oriented towards maximising each person's potential, while maintaining a continuum of balance and purposeful direction within the person's environment" (Dunn, 1961, pp. 4–5). He also addressed stereotypes about ageing and emphasised that "healthy maturity" is characterised not only by physical decline but also by wisdom. He discussed the relationship between mind, body and spirit and stressed the importance of older adults having a purpose in life, communicating with others, maintaining personal dignity, and contributing to society (Dunn, 1961). He proposed that all healthcare workers should foster a sense of value and dignity for older adults by directing interventions towards improved health and functioning (Dunn, 1958). Dunn described the role of healthcare professionals with regard to older adults as follows (1958, p. 51):

> *The later years of life will come to be more widely regarded as years of opportunity for older people and for society if, in addition to prevention, care, and various health-related activities, direct attention is devoted to the promotion of high-level wellness. This will require a major reorientation.*

Descriptions of wellness while ageing

For several decades research has focused on identifying the most agreed-upon components of ageing well. However, there are a number of terms that are used to describe ageing well and these include successful ageing, healthy ageing, positive ageing and active ageing (National Ageing Research Institute [NARI] and Council on the Ageing [COTA], 2012). Each term describes ageing well differently, yet all agree that it involves more than just physical or functional health (p. 1). The following are some current terms and definitions in common use:

- *Successful ageing* "is the avoidance of disease and disability, the maintenance of high physical and cognitive function, and sustained engagement in social and productive activities" (Rowe & Kahn, 1997).
- *Successful ageing* "is the adaptation of one's remaining capacities and the compensation for limitations" (Baltes & Catstensen, 1996).
- *Healthy ageing* refers to activities and behaviours that aim to reduce the risk of illness and disease, and increase physical, emotional and mental health during the ageing process (Australian Institute of Health and Welfare [AIHW], 2010).
- *Positive ageing* "embraces a number of factors, including health, financial security, independence, self-fulfilment, community attitudes, personal safety and security, and the physical environment" (New Zealand Ministry of Social Policy, 2001).
- *Active ageing* "is the process of optimising opportunities for health, participation and security in order to enhance quality of life of each older age group" (World Health Organization, 2002).

In 2013, several gerontologists commented on differing views of ageing well (Flatt, Settersten, Ponsaran et al., 2013). They stated, "The idea that one can 'succeed' at ageing, and that some strategies and interventions might increase that success, has reached a position of near ubiquity within today."

In this text book the term **healthy ageing** has been adopted and refers to activities and behaviours that aim to reduce the risk of illness and disease, and increase physical, psychological and spiritual health while ageing. The healthy ageing process encourages older adults to apply adaptive processes to preserve their well-being and transcend limitations associated with ageing, diseases

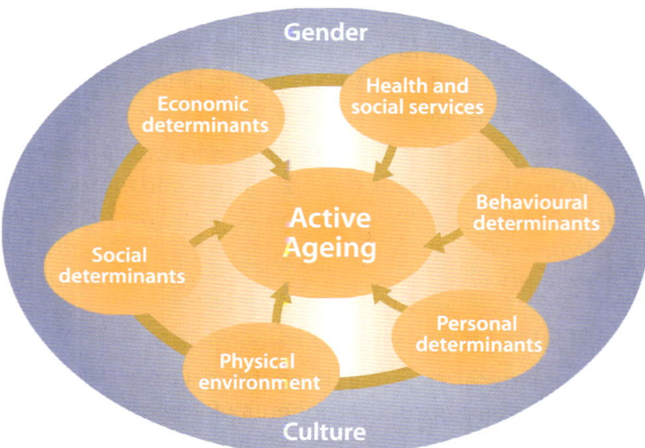

FIGURE 1-1 The World Health Organization's Active Ageing Model. (World Health Organization. [2002]. Active ageing: A policy framework [Fig. 8: The determinants of active ageing, p. 18.] Geneva: Author. Copyright WHO 2002. Available 16 March 2015 at www.who.int/ageing/publications/active_ageing/en.)

and functional limitations (Woods, Cochrane, LaCroix et al., 2012).

Many studies have explored healthy ageing in older adults and found a number of factors associated with it, including:

- All or most ethnic groups identified longevity, leisure, spirituality, social involvement, continuous learning, and good physical and cognitive health as essential aspects of ageing well (Laditka et al., 2009)
- Having a sense of purpose in life (Boyle et al., 2009; Gruenewald et al., 2009)
- Leisure activities, psychosocial support, functional capacity, health and perceived well-being, and family and social relationships and engagement were important (Bowling, 2009; Chaves et al., 2009)
- Older adults in Brazil viewed old age as a time for experiencing new possibilities and felt that being healthy was essential for keeping their autonomy (Silva & Boemer, 2009).

These studies support the international model of healthy ageing (referred to as active ageing) developed by the World Health Organization (WHO) (2002). This model proposes that many elements or determinants influence the health of the older adult (see Figure 1-1). In particular this model identifies the key role that culture and gender have in influencing the other determinants, which "... shapes the way in which we age..." (WHO, 2002, p. 20). Further, this model supports the importance of being holistic or person centred when nursing older adults for wellness.

Barriers to ageing well

Research as well as expert opinion supports the concept of wellness when ageing being achievable and desirable. However, barriers remain that limit wellness when ageing and these include:

- Older adults may be pessimistic about their ability to improve their health and functioning.
- Survival needs and a multitude of health problems may take precedence over the "luxury" of being able to focus on wellness and quality of life.
- Despite the purported emphasis on wellness and health promotion, healthcare environments have in the past focused more on treating disease than on preventing illness and addressing whole-person needs.
- Older adults and healthcare providers can mistakenly attribute symptoms to ageing rather than identify and address the contributing factors that are reversible and treatable.
- Healthcare providers might not believe older adults are capable of learning and implementing health-promoting behaviours that are inherent in wellness-oriented care.

Because many of these barriers arise from myths, misperceptions and lack of knowledge, accurate information about older adults and the relationship between ageing and wellness is an indispensable tool for addressing these barriers.

Wellness and nursing care of older adults

Nurses have many opportunities to promote wellness for older adults through actions that are integral to person-centred care. A major focus of a "wellness approach" to older adult healthcare is addressing the body–mind–spirit interconnectedness of each older adult as a unique and respected individual. This requires that nurses assess each older adult in the full context of his or her personal history and current situation. Based on this person-centred assessment, nurses identify realistic wellness outcomes and plan interventions directed towards improved functioning, quality of life, and health. This approach may seem challenging—or even impossible—for older adults who are seriously or terminally ill, or for those who have overwhelming chronic conditions. However, even when there are serious physical challenges, nurses need to recognise that they can implement interventions directed towards improved physical comfort and psychological and spiritual growth. Some nursing actions that promote wellness for older adults are:

- Addressing the body–mind–spirit interrelatedness of each older adult
- Identifying and challenging ageist attitudes (including their own), especially those that interfere with optimal healthcare
- Assessing each older adult from a person-centred perspective
- Incorporating wellness nursing care as a routine part of care
- Planning for wellness outcomes that are directed towards improved functioning, quality of life and health
- Using nursing interventions to address the factors that interfere with optimal functioning (including lack of accurate information about ageing)

- Recognising each older adult's potential for improved health and functioning as well as psychological and spiritual growth
- Working with older adults to increase their level of knowledge and abilities about self-care behaviours that improve health and functioning (including carers of dependent older adults)
- Promoting wellness for carers and other people who care for older adults (including self-care for nurses).

McMahon and Fleury published a concept analysis of wellness related to nursing care of older adults and stated (2012, p. 49):

> *Wellness coexists across all functional and health statuses... In its current state of development within nursing, wellness has the potential to provide nurses with tools to foster being well and living values among older adults by addressing their strengths and promoting growth while simultaneously addressing their changing and diverse needs.*

A student's perspective

My interview with Mr H. was an enlightening experience. I was able to learn a great deal about the time period in which this man grew up. Also, it was eye opening to see how healthy a man of 84 years could be. His health reinforced what we are learning. He does have diabetes, but he still is independent. He can still drive and get around. Negative attitudes that I have heard about older people were defeated by this man. Reading about ageing in a book is one thing, but actually interacting with older people and learning first hand is much better.

Jordan S.

ATTITUDES TOWARDS AGEING

Images of and attitudes towards ageing arise from long-term patterns of falsely attributing pathological conditions and undesirable characteristics to normal ageing. In reality, most older adults function independently and report high levels of satisfaction with their health and quality of life, even with their high prevalence of chronic conditions. Historically, societal attitudes towards ageing have ranged from respect and veneration to fear of ageing, and the idealisation of youth. The pendulum is slowly swinging again towards positive attitudes towards ageing and older adulthood. This shift is attributable to the increasing emphasis on ageing well and the emergence of accurate information about the difference between ageing and disease. Despite this focus on healthy ageing, the care of older adults continues to be influenced by long-standing negative attitudes towards ageing that are held by society as well as healthcare professionals. Thus, an important part of nursing is to recognise the effects of ageism and address attitudes that can interfere with holistic care of older adults.

Ageism

The term *ageism* was coined by Robert Butler in 1968 and was first used the next year in *The gerontologist* (Butler, 1969). With the publication of Butler's Pulitzer Prize-winning book *Why survive? Being old in America* (1975), *ageism* became an accepted new word in the English language. Butler defines **ageism** as "the prejudices and stereotypes that are applied to older people sheerly on the basis of their age... Ageism, like racism and sexism, is a way of pigeonholing people and not allowing them to be individuals with unique ways of living their lives" (Butler, Lewis & Sunderland, 1991, p. 243).

A review of ageism among younger and older adults proposed that younger adults develop ageist attitudes to protect themselves from death anxiety because they associate death with ageing. In contrast, older adults develop ageist attitudes because of negative stereotypes about their own group (Bodner, 2009). Common manifestations of ageism include negative stereotypes of social isolation, psychological rigidity, asexual behaviour, lack of creativity, physical and mental decline, and economic and familial burden. For example, a review of 262 articles published in the *Economist* between 1997 and 2008 found that 64% portrayed an ageist view of older people being a burden on society (Martin, Williams & O'Neill, 2009).

In the late 1960s, Erdman Palmore and other researchers concluded that between 1950 and 1970, the effects of ageism diminished more slowly than those of racism (Palmore, 2005). Based on his research, Palmore developed two versions of a 25-item Facts on Ageing Quiz, as indirect measures of ageism. These quizzes have been used in hundreds of studies and classrooms and consistently show more negative bias than positive bias towards older adults (Palmore, 2005).

Palmore later developed a 20-item Ageism Survey to measure directly older adults' experiences of ageism (Figure 1-2). Studies using this survey have found that most respondents frequently experienced ageism (Palmore, 2005). For example, one study of 247 community-dwelling adults between the ages of 60 and 92 years found that 84% of the participants said they had experienced at least one type of ageism, with the most common forms being jokes and greeting cards that poked fun at older people (McGuire, Klein & Chen, 2008).

Although ageism is not unique to Australia and New Zealand, it does not exist in all cultures. Ageism has developed and grown as a result of dominant cultural beliefs and trends, such as the glorification of youth, the perception of the individual as autonomous, and the equating of human worth with economic worth. Contrasting cultural perspectives on independence versus interdependence is another factor that can account for differences in attitudes about ageing (Plath, 2009). For example, the Japanese acceptance of interdependence, which is rooted in the Confucian precept, results in adult children respecting and supporting their parents and this has been shown to assist

The Ageism Survey

Please put a number in the blank that shows how often you have experienced that event: Never = 0; Once = 1; More than once = 2. ("Age" means older age.)

____ 1. I was told a joke that pokes fun at old people.
____ 2. I was sent a birthday card that pokes fun at old people.
____ 3. I was ignored or not taken seriously because of my age.
____ 4. I was called an insulting name related to my age.
____ 5. I was partronized or "talked down to" because of my age.
____ 6. I was refused rental housing because of my age.
____ 7. I had difficulty getting a loan because of my age.
____ 8. I was denied a position of leadership because of my age.
____ 9. I was rejected as unattractive because of my age.
____ 10. I was treated with less dignity and respect because of my age.
____ 11. A waiter or waitress ignored me because of my age.
____ 12. A doctor or nurse assumed my ailments were caused by my age.
____ 13. I was denied medical treatment because of my age.
____ 14. I was denied employment because of my age.
____ 15. I was denied promotion because of my age.
____ 16. Someone assumed I could not hear well because of my age.
____ 17. Someone assumed I could not understand because of my age.
____ 18. Someone told me, "You're too old for that."
____ 19. My house was vandalized because of my age.
____ 20. I was victimized by a criminal because of my age.

Please write in your age: ____

Please check: Male ____ Female ____

What is the highest grade in school that you completed? __________

FIGURE 1-2 The Ageism Survey is being used to measure the prevalence and identify types of ageism. (Used with permission from Palmore, E. [2000]. *The Ageism Survey*. Durham, NC: Duke Center for the Study of Aging.)

the older adult with maintaining their functional health (Levy & Leifhelt-Limson, 2009). A potentially positive outcome of the increasing cultural diversity in the Australia and New Zealand is that the dominant cultural values that foster ageism may be challenged by cultural values of other groups. See Cultural considerations 1-1 for a summary of various cultural perspectives on older adults. Chapter 2 further discusses cultural diversity and older adults living in Australia and New Zealand.

Effects of ageism

In recent years, gerontologists have identified some of the specific effects of negative attitudes and stereotypes on older adults. A review of studies found the following serious negative consequences of ageism (North & Fiske, 2012):

- In medical care: older people often receive less aggressive treatment for common ailments, which are dismissed as a natural part of ageing.
- In the workplace: older job applicants are rated less positively than younger ones, even when they are similarly qualified and despite considerable research showing that job performance does not decrease in older adults.
- In residential aged care and home settings: elder abuse and neglect is underreported. One study found that women, but not men, associated older age identities with pessimistic outlooks about their own cognitive ageing (Schafer & Shippee, 2010).
- In media: older adults are underrepresented and stereotyped.

Another outcome of ageism is **ageing anxiety**, which is experienced by people of all ages as fears and worries about detrimental effects associated with older adulthood (e.g. social losses, financial insecurity, changes in appearance, and declines in health and functioning). One study found that ageing anxiety about loss of attractiveness was higher among women who are younger, white, employed, heterosexual, separated or divorced and less financially independent (Barrett & Robbins, 2008). Ageing anxiety is reinforced by negative stereotypes of older adults and the associated fear that these problems are likely to occur in one's own later life. In contrast, people who have accurate information about ageing and positive experiences with older adults are less likely to have ageing anxiety.

One aspect of ageism that is particularly relevant to providing care for older adults is related to **age attribution**, which is the tendency to attribute problems to the ageing process rather than to pathological and potentially treatable conditions. For example, the phrase "senior moment" has been used since the mid-1990s to describe a lapse in memory. Because age attribution can have the effect of a self-fulfilling prophecy, healthcare professionals need to be cognisant of messages they give to older adults. Negative effects of age attribution include worse

CULTURAL CONSIDERATIONS 1-1
Cultural perspectives on older people and family caregiving relationships

Chinese
- Traditional Chinese values place family and society above the individual.
- Older people are highly respected and honoured.
- Multigenerational households are common.

Filipinos
- Respect for older people is a cornerstone of Filipino values demonstrated by deference in verbal and non-verbal communication.
- Children (especially the oldest daughter) are expected to care for parents to repay their debt of gratitude (*utang na loob*).

Germans
- Close intergenerational relationships are maintained by first- and second-generation Germans, but family mobility may affect this.
- Children are expected to help their parents stay in their own homes as long as possible.
- Because German Baptists view family relationships as reciprocal throughout life, grandparents usually live with their children or move from child to child.

Greeks
- Elderly women have higher status and more power within the family than younger women do and are expected to live with or near adult children, especially daughters.

Indigenous Australians*
- Older people are highly respected.
- The traditional value of caring by the family continues.
- People who are part of the older person's kinship network have the responsibility for providing care, and they may be extended family or a distant relative of the older person.
- The Indigenous community is also considered a source of support.

Japanese
- Older people are highly respected and those who are able help in caring for children and grandchildren.
- Older people commonly maintain separate households; when they need help, the eldest son's family is expected to care for them at home.

Koreans
- Caring for elderly kin is a family duty that is associated with respect for older people and family bonds inherent in Confucianism
- Grandparents frequently provide care for grandchildren; older people are welcome to live with family during times of need.

Māori†
- Family members, or *whānau*, are at the centre of caregiving relationships. Carers can be *whānau, whakapapa whānau*, or others with a family-like commitment, *kaupapa whānau*.
- Usually the eldest daughter, or one who is not partnered, cares for older Māori.

Pacific people‡
- Extended families are important and embrace connectedness, duty, obligation and mutual benefit.
- Generally prefer family to care for their elders as they are often uncomfortable sharing problems outside the family.

Russians
- Older people are highly respected and remain close to their children.
- Even if older people do not live with their children, they are expected to help raise grandchildren and participate in decision making.

Vietnamese
- They believe that the more one respects the elderly, the greater one's chance is of reaching old age.
- Young adults are expected to assume full responsibility for caring for older people at home.

Sources: Lipson, J. G. & Dibble, L. (2005). *Culture & clinical care*. San Francisco: UCSF Nursing Press.
*McGrath, P. (2008). Family care giving for Aboriginal peoples during end of life: Findings from the Northern Territory. *Journal of Rural and Tropical Public Health, 7*, 1–10; †Collins, A. & Wilson, G. (2008). Māori and informal caregiving: A background paper prepared for the National Health Committee; ‡Medical Council of New Zealand. (2010). Best health outcomes for Pacific peoples: Practice implications. Accessed at www.mcnz.org.nz/assets/News-and-Publications/Statements/Best-health-outcomes-for-Pacific-Peoples.pdf.

physical functioning, delayed treatment for health problems, and an increased risk of mortality (Levy, Ashman & Slade, 2009). One study found that exposure to images associated with healthy ageing had a more positive effect on older adults, as compared with younger adults (Lineweaver, Berger & Hertzog, 2009).

When older adults or healthcare professionals falsely attribute symptoms of pathological conditions to normal ageing, they are likely to overlook treatable conditions, and significant harm can result from this negligence. An important responsibility of gerontological nurses is to be knowledgeable about the differences between age-related changes and pathological conditions, so appropriate nursing interventions can be initiated. An essential first step in planning interventions, especially health-promotion interventions, is to identify those factors that are not inherent consequences of ageing. Throughout this text, emphasis is placed on differentiating between age-related changes, which cannot be modified, and those factors that can be addressed through interventions. Chapter 3 describes a nursing model for this approach to promoting wellness for older adults.

Another consequence of ageism is the emergence of the **anti-ageing** movement, which has been promoted since the early 1990s. The anti-ageing movement views ageing as a process that can be stopped and the life-span as something that can be extended for up to 200 years. Anti-ageing interventions include exercise and lifestyle modifications, but there also is strong emphasis on dietary supplements and other products that have not been proved effective. A main criticism is that the anti-ageing movement is directed more towards selling products than towards the advancement of sound scientific evidence. One gerontologist concluded that anti-ageing concepts are based on an understanding of ageing as a bodily failure, which can be counteracted only when scientists no longer hold ageist preconceptions that are embedded in a wider ageist culture (Vincent, 2008).

Addressing attitudes of nurses and other healthcare workers

Negative attitudes about ageing that are held by healthcare workers can negatively affect the care older adults receive. Although studies have found that nurses and nursing students hold negative attitudes about caring for older adults, these attitudes are improving because of a broader base of evidential information in nursing education (Baumbusch, Dahlke & Phinney, 2012; Eymard & Douglas, 2012). Healthcare workers are likely to be influenced not only by ageism in society but also by their own experiences in healthcare, which often are with those older adults who are the most impaired and in need of interventions. It is important, therefore, that healthcare workers in all clinical settings recognise that most older adults are healthy and functional and strive towards improved levels of wellness and functioning.

Attitudes are changed through education, but changing attitudes requires first recognising their existence. Because ageism is subtle but pervasive in Western societies, nurses first need to become aware of the attitudes they hold towards older adults. The first critical thinking exercise at the end of this chapter suggests ways of becoming aware of one's own attitudes about older adults. Another way of improving negative attitudes about older adults is to listen carefully to them as they talk about beliefs, values, hopes and experiences that are integral to their self-identities. Nurses have daily opportunities to learn about ageing and older adulthood simply by listening to the older adults for whom they provide care. In addition, nurses can equip themselves with accurate information about the older adult population. Such information may be the most effective antidote to negative attitudes resulting from misunderstandings or myths. The next sections address myths about ageing by providing an accurate snapshot of older adults living in Australia and New Zealand.

A student's perspective

I personally have ageing anxiety. After working at a residential aged care facility for the past year and a half, I have seen some pretty tragic and depressing events happen in the lives of these residents. Many of these residents tell me they do not know why God has kept them around this long. But listening to the stories of others has given me hope. I found it very encouraging to see the older people taking exercise classes and enjoying the discussions they were a part of. I would imagine that it would be tempting to give up when the mental or physical functioning is not what it used to be, but some of the people gave me hope for ageing. They make me want to be a stronger person even now at the age of 20 years. They seem to have so much passion and intensity to their lives. Not only can they serve to encourage people in their younger years to continually embrace life, but I hope other older people can be encouraged that they do not have to let go of their dreams just because they are ageing. You can age healthily, as these people have, by living life to its fullest and persevering to keep your individuality and talents alive.

Jessica S.

DEBUNKING MYTHS: UNDERSTANDING REALITIES ABOUT OLDER ADULTS IN AUSTRALIA AND NEW ZEALAND

As a consequence of ageism and negative attitudes about ageing, many myths and negative stereotypes about older adults have been perpetuated, especially with regard to aspects of health and functioning. These myths and stereotypes can be particularly detrimental when healthcare providers lack accurate information on which to base their decisions or actions about older adults, because misconceptions lead to suboptimal goals for care. At best, older adults do not experience the benefits of wellness-focused care; at worst, they experience unnecessary decline.

This chapter provides information about characteristics of the older adult population, while Chapter 2 extends this overview by addressing the cultural diversity of older adults. Aspects of functioning by older people can be significantly affected by myths and misunderstandings about ageing. Table 1-1 lists some of the myths and misperceptions about ageing commonly held by older adults and healthcare professionals. The related realities about each aspect of health and functioning also are identified, along with a reference to the chapter that provides accurate information to dispel the myths.

The characteristics of the older adult population in Australia and New Zealand summarised in this section are based on census data and other reliable sources; however, this information can reflect only trends and compilations. The intent is to provide an overview of population demographics and characteristics of older adults that are most pertinent to caring for older adults to achieve wellness outcomes and health. Nurses need to keep in mind that older adults are a highly diverse group and this general information does not necessarily apply to every older individual. Boxes 1-1 and 1-2 provide a snapshot of the characteristics of older adults living in Australia and New Zealand.

TABLE 1-1 Myths and realities of ageing

Myth	Reality
Older adulthood is something to be dreaded because it represents disability and death.	Most older adults live independently, have high levels of self-reported health, and are ageing successfully. *(Chapter 1)*
People consider themselves "old" on their 65th birthday.	People usually feel old based on their health and function, rather than on their chronological age. *(Chapter 1)*
Gerontologists have discovered that, by the age of 75 years, people are quite homogeneous as a group.	The more gerontologists learn about ageing, the more they realise that, with increased age, people become more diverse, and individuals become less like their age peers. *(Chapters 1, 2, and 4)*
Ageism is a natural part of all societies.	Ageism is more common in industrialised societies and is highly influenced by stereotypes and cultural values. *(Chapter 1)*
Gerontologists have recently discovered a theory that explains biological ageing.	Theories about biological ageing continue to evolve, and there is little agreement on any one theory. *(Chapter 4)*
In today's society, families no longer care for older people.	Eighty per cent of the care of older adults is provided by their families. *(Chapter 1)*
As people grow older, it is natural for them to want to withdraw from society.	Because older people are unique individuals, each of them responds differently to society. *(Chapter 4)*
By the age of 70 years, an individual's psychological growth is complete.	People never lose their capacity for psychological growth. *(Chapters 4 and 12)*
Increased disability in older people is attributable to age-related changes alone.	Although age-related changes increase one's vulnerability to functional impairments, the disabilities are attributable to such risk factors as diseases and adverse medication effects. *(Chapter 3)*
Health-promotion efforts are not beneficial to older adults who have two or more chronic conditions.	Research has debunked the myths that prevention is not effective after the onset of chronic illness. *(Chapter 5)*
About 20% of people aged 65 years and older live in nursing homes as long-term residents.	Between 4% and 5% of older adults live in a long-term residential care facility at any time. *(Chapters 1 and 6)*
Widowhood and other life events have been found to have a consistently negative impact on older people.	No one life event affects all older people negatively. The most important consideration governing the impact of an event is its unique meaning for the individual. *(Chapter 12)*
In old age, there is an inevitable decline in all intellectual abilities.	A few areas of cognitive ability decline in healthy older adults but other areas show improvement. *(Chapter 11)*
Older adults cannot learn complex new skills.	Older adults are capable of learning new things, but the speed with which they process information slows down with age. *(Chapter 11)*
Constipation develops primarily because of age-related changes.	Constipation is attributable primarily to risk factors, such as restricted activity and poor dietary habits. *(Chapter 18)*
Urinary incontinence is a normal consequence of ageing that is best managed by using incontinence products.	In most cases, underlying causes of urinary incontinence can be addressed and a variety of self-care methods can be initiated. *(Chapter 19)*
Skin wrinkles can be prevented by using oils and lotions.	The best way to prevent skin wrinkles is to avoid exposure to ultraviolet light. *(Chapter 23)*
Older people are less sexually active primarily because they lose the ability to enjoy sex.	Declines in sexual activity in older people are primarily because of such risk factors as diseases, adverse medication effects, and loss of partner. *(Chapter 26)*
Healthcare professionals readily recognise adverse medication effects in older adults.	Adverse medication effects are often overlooked in older adults because they are mistakenly attributed to ageing or pathological conditions. *(Chapter 8)*
Some degree of "senility" is normal in very old people.	"Senility" is an inaccurate term used to refer to dementing conditions, which are always caused by pathological changes. *(Chapter 14)*
Most old people are depressed and should be allowed to withdraw from society.	About one-third of older people exhibit depressive symptoms; however, depression is a very treatable condition at any age. *(Chapter 15)*

Demographics of ageing

Australia's and New Zealand's life expectancy has continually increased over the last 100 years, resulting in an increased population of people living beyond retirement (AIHW, 2013; Statistics New Zealand, 2007). The proportion of those aged 65 years and over in the 2010 Australian population and the 2013 New Zealand population was approximately 14% (AIHW, 2013; Statistics New Zealand, 2014).

Discussions about current demographic trends in Australia and New Zealand inevitably focus on the so-called **baby boomers**, which is the large group of people born between 1946 and 1964. This group began turning 65 in 2011, and they will bring about major demographic changes. Some statistics are summarised in Table 1-2 and Figures 1-3 and 1-4. Projected trends are based on forecasts about a variety of factors that will affect the morbidity and

BOX 1-1
A snapshot of older adults living in Australia

- Over 3.2 million Australians (14% of the population) are aged 65 years or over; 54% are female.
- Less than 1% are of Aboriginal or Torres Strait Islander origin, and 36% were born overseas.
- More than 94% live in private homes or self-care accommodation.
- One per cent are participating in formal education.
- Twelve per cent are employed, with 53% of these working part time.
- Thirty-one per cent participate in voluntary work.
- Twenty per cent are carers.
- Two-thirds of those living in private households rate their own health as good or better.
- Fifty-three per cent have some form of disability, and 20% have a severe or profound disability.
- Seventy-eight per cent receive the Age Pension or means-tested income support administered through the Department of Veterans' Affairs, and 59% receive a full-rate pension.

Source: Australian Institute of Health and Welfare. (2013). *Australia's welfare 2013*. Australia's welfare no. 11. Cat. no. AUS 174. Canberra: Author.

BOX 1-2
A snapshot of older adults living in New Zealand

- Approximately 0.65 million (14% of the population) are aged 65 years and over.
- Females have a longer life expectancy, living about four more years than males.
- Most older adults live with their spouse, alone or in non-private settings such as retirement homes.
- Home ownership increases with age, with about 80% of 70 to 74 year olds owning or partly owning the dwelling in which they live.
- Older adults experienced about one-third of the total health loss despite being 14% of the population.
- Forty-five per cent have some form of disability.
- One-third of older adults with a disability live alone.
- Approximately 22% of older adults were employed in 2013, while only 11.4% were employed in 2001.
- Older adults have lower than average incomes than younger adults.

Source: Statistics New Zealand. (2013a). Census QuickStats about national highlights. Available from www.stats.govt.nz; New Zealand Ministry of Health. (2011). *Tatau Kura Tangata: Health of older Māori chart book 2011*. Wellington: Author.

TABLE 1-2 Statistics in brief: Changing demographics of ageing in Australia and New Zealand

Demographics	Australia			New Zealand		
Median age of population	*Period*		*Age (years)*	*Period*		*Age (years)*
	1989		31.8	1971		26
	2009		36.9	2005		36
	2014		37.3	2013		38
	2056		41.9–45.2	2045		45
Life expectancy at 65 years	*Period*	*Female (years)*	*Male (years)*	*Period*	*Female (years)*	*Male (years)*
	1970–72	15.9	12.2	1950–52	14.8	12.8
	2005–07	21.8	18.7	1990–92	18.5	14.8
	2009–11	22.0	19.1	2005–07	20.6	18.0
				2010–12	21.2	18.8
Actual percentage of population aged 65+ years	*Period*	*%*	*No. people (million)*	*Period*	*%*	*No. people (million)*
	1971	8.3	1.1	1960s	8.0	
	2011	14.0	3.2	2005	12.1	0.50
				2006	12.3	
				2013	14.0	0.607
Projected percentage of population that will be aged 65+ years	2051	26.0	6.3	2032	22.0	1.37
				2041	32.0	1.81
85+ age group as a percentage of people aged 65 years and over		*Period*	*%*		*Period*	*%*
	Actual	2001	9	Actual	2005	11
	Projected	2021	13	Projected	2051	25
		2051	20			
Estimated number of centenarians	*Period*		*No. people*	Over 100 years not available		
	1971		200	*Period*	*No. people 90+ years*	
	2007		2800	2011	26,000	
	2014		4000			
	Projected			Projected		
	2056		71,200	2051	49,000	

Source: Australian Bureau of Statistics. (2008). *Population projections, Australia, 2006 to 2101*; New Zealand Ministry of Health. (2007). *Older people's health chart book 2006*; Statistics New Zealand. (2007). *New Zealand's 65+ population: A statistical volume 2007*; Statistics New Zealand (2013a). Census QuickStats about national highlights. Available from www.stats.govt.nz; Australian Bureau Statistics. (2014). Ageing population. From *Australian demographic statistics, June 2014*. Cat. no. 3101.0. Canberra: Author. Accessed March 2015 at www.abs.gov.au/ausstats/abs@.nsf/0/1CD2B1952AFC5E7ACA257298000F2E76?OpenDocument.

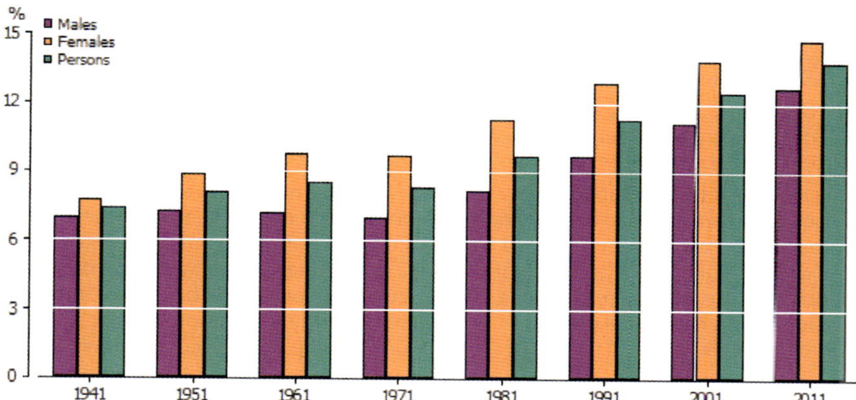

FIGURE 1-3 Older adults as a proportion of the total population, 1941–2011. (Australian Bureau Statistics. [2012]. Who are Australia's older people? From *Reflecting a nation: Stories from the 2011 census 2012–2013*. Cat. no. 2071.0. Canberra: Author. Accessed March 2015 at www.abs.gov.au/ausstats/abs@.nsf/lookup/2071.0main+features752012-2013. Permission to reproduce granted under a Creative Commons Attribution 2.5 Australia licence.)

mortality of people who are baby boomers, as well as generations who are not yet born. The most commonly cited projections are based on the assumption that the pace of improvements in mortality will be slowing down. More information about other population trends such as greater cultural diversity and increased life expectancy is described in Chapters 2 and 4, respectively.

Health characteristics

Most older adults living today in Australia and New Zealand are generally healthier than previous generations. Although the major focus of health characteristics of older adults is about chronic conditions and levels of functioning, many studies show that the prevalence of disability among older adults has decreased during the past few decades, despite the increasing in the prevalence of chronic conditions among middle-aged and older adults. These improvements are attributed to advances in medical care, improved socioeconomic conditions, and increased use of technology that helps maintain independence.

Some older adults do require care and support, and this is more common with advancing age, particularly the 85 years and over group, and when the person has a number of multiple chronic conditions, termed **comorbidity**. Questions have been raised about whether the increasing prevalence of chronic conditions among the baby boomer generation will eventually result in poorer health outcomes as they get older (Martin, Williams & O'Neill, 2009).

The greatest concern about the ageing population is the increasing number of older adults who are 85+ years, the "old old" group. Although levels of disability have been shown to be associated with ageing, they are the highest for the 85+ group. Healthcare providers are preparing for an increased demand on healthcare services over the next three decades.

The Australian and New Zealand Governments also recognise healthy ageing as a national health and research priority because of its association with improved quality of life, reduction in care requirements, and a reduced burden on society. Healthcare providers are encouraged to provide services that support the health of the older adult, irrespective of their age or level of morbidity. Healthcare services do this by:

- Focusing on the prevention of the disabling consequences of chronic illnesses
- Working with adults, both younger and older, to increase their understanding of and capacity to perform self-care practices
- Supporting optimal functioning and quality of life.

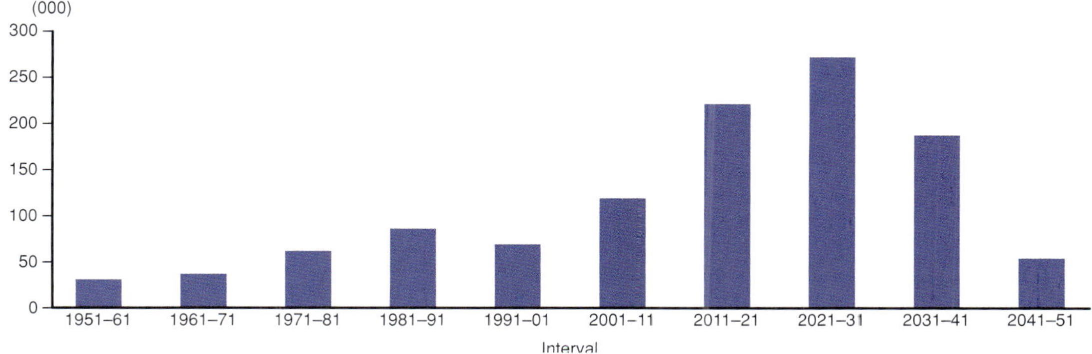

FIGURE 1-4 Growth in 65+ population for New Zealand by 10-year intervals, 1951–2051. (Statistics New Zealand. [2007]. *New Zealand's 65+ population: A statistical volume*. Wellington: Author.)

TABLE 1-3 Statistics in brief: Health characteristics of people ages 65+ years in Australia and New Zealand

Health characteristics	Australia	New Zealand
Percentage living in private households report on general health	• 76% of adults aged 65–74 and • 65% of adults aged 75+ reported health as good, very good or excellent	46% of adults reported health as good, very good or excellent
Percentage needing help with personal care	54% have some form of disability 20% of older Australians had a severe or profound level of disability (i.e. need help with self-care, mobility, communication); of those, 58% were aged 85+ 75% of long-term residential care had high-care needs	45% have some form of disability *Mobility* (includes people who have difficulty with or cannot walk): 18.8% *Agility* (includes people who have difficulty with or cannot: bend over to pick something off the floor; dress or undress themselves; cut their own toe nails; grasp or handle small objects such as scissors; reach in any direction; cut their own food; or get themselves into and out of bed): 6.7%
Body weight	Overweight/obese: *Years* / *F* / *M* 65–74 / 69.5% / 79.9% 75+ / 67.0% / 68.7%	Overweight/obese: *Years* / *F* / *M* 50–64 / 61% / 76% 85+ / 41% / 50%
Number of 65+ age group with chronic conditions	Five or more chronic conditions: *Years* / *F* / *M* 65–74 / 49.3% / 49.1% 75–85 / 59.7% / 52.6% 85+ / 71.1% / 68.0%	One to three chronic conditions: *Years* / *F* / *M* 65–74 / 64% / 70% 75–85 / 62% / 70% 85+ / 63% / 74%
Chronic conditions prevalent in the 65+ age group	**Australia and New Zealand** Circulatory diseases—CVD and CVA Cancer Dementia Osteoarthritis Respiratory conditions Type 2 diabetes	Osteoporosis Partial deafness Cataracts

Note: The SF-36 is a questionnaire for measuring self-reported physical and mental health status, available from QualityMetric via www.sf-36.org.
Source: Australian Bureau of Statistics. (2006a). *Health of older people in Australia: A snapshot, 2004–05*; Australian Institute of Health and Welfare. (2010). *Australia's health*; New Zealand Ministry of Health. (2007). *Older people's health chart book 2006*; New Zealand Ministry of Health. (2011). *Tatau Kura Tangata: Health of older Māori chart book 2011*; Statistics New Zealand. (2013b). New Zealand General Social Survey 2012. Accessed March 2015 at www.stats.govt.nz/browse_for_stats/people_and_communities/Households/nzgss_HOTP2012.aspx.

Table 1-3 summarises statistics describing the health characteristics of older adults in Australia and New Zealand. A similar profile is observed for older adults in both countries, where most report good health but approximately half have some form of disability. Nearly half of the older adults live with a number of chronic conditions and 20% have difficulty with a core activity; both of which increase significantly after 85 years. Figure 1-5 demonstrates that, as Australians age, so does the level of severe disability. Figure 1-6 describes the current level of disability for older

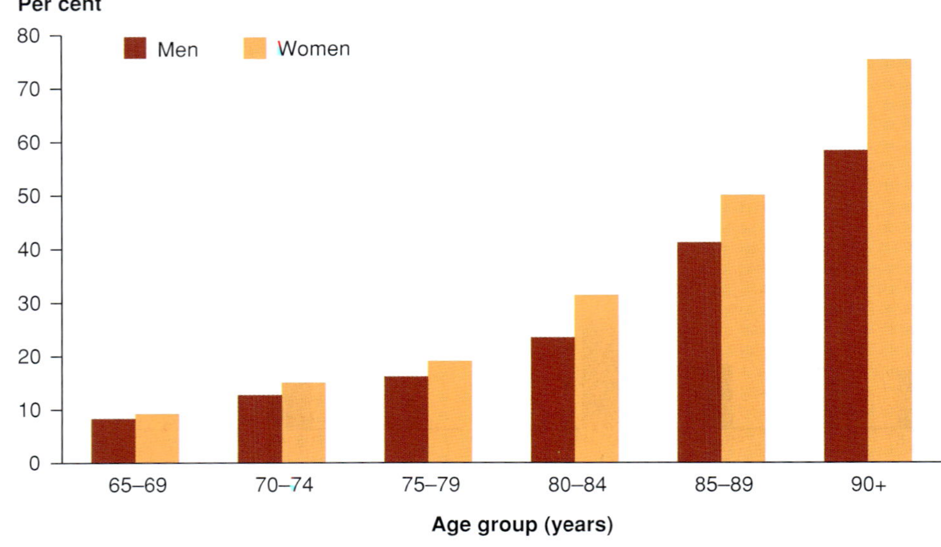

FIGURE 1-5 Older Australians with severe or profound core activity limitation, 2009. (Australian Institute of Health and Welfare. [2013]. *Australia's welfare 2013*. Australia's welfare series no. 11. Cat. no. AUS 174. Canberra: Author. Permission to reproduce granted under a Creative Commons BY 3.0 [CC BY 3.0] licence.)

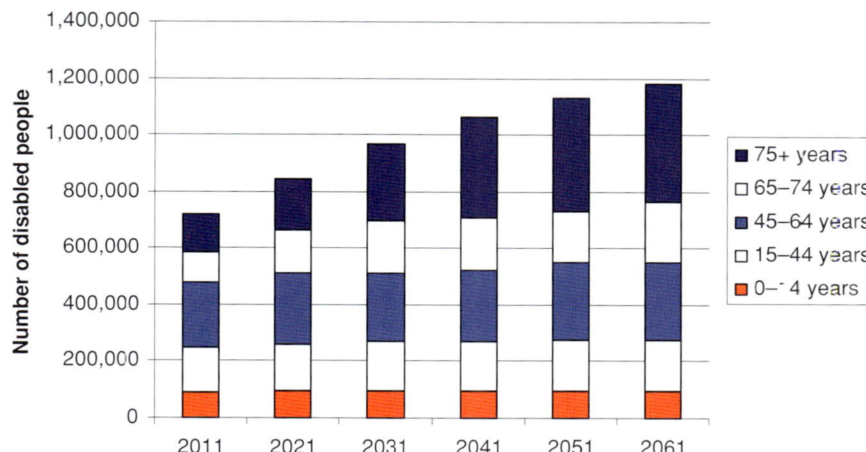

FIGURE 1-6 Projection of number of disabled people living in New Zealand by age. (New Zealand Ministry of Social Development. [2012]. New Zealanders: Getting older, doing more. Briefing for the incoming Minister. Accessed March 2015 via www.msd.govt.nz.)

people living in New Zealand and the increases expected in future years. It has been identified in recent years that health disparities exist among groups of older minority groups in Australia and New Zealand, and this is further discussed in Chapter 2. Chapter 4 provides more information about life expectancy and ethnic ty.

Socioeconomic characteristics

Socioeconomic characteristics that most commonly affect health of older adults include income, education and occupation, and combinations of these aspects. In particular, poverty and a lower educational level can affect ageing well because these factors are associated with an earlier onset of disease and mortality (Crimmins, Kim & Seeman, 2009).

In recent decades, the overall poverty rate for older adults has been declining, but this does not mean that all older people are economically better off today than they were 40 years ago. Statistics should be viewed cautiously about poverty and be interpreted in relation to a broader perspective on the economic conditions of older adults in Australia and New Zealand. Many older adults in Australia and New Zealand rely on a government benefit or pension as income, which they are entitled to receive once they have retired. This benefit is means tested. Many older adults own a home and have other assets, ensuring an adequate level of economic well-being despite being reliant on the government benefit. In New Zealand in 2006 the median income for older adults was approximately 30% lower than all New Zealanders; but despite this, it was reported that older New Zealanders have low hardship rates (4%) compared with the whole population (13%) (Perry, 2008). Australia has a similar situation, where only 4% of older adults reported they had a cash flow problem in the last 12 months, compared with 25% of people aged 18–44, and 17% of those aged 45–64 (AIHW, 2013).

Older adults have a wide range of financial resources, which varies significantly according to ethnicity, gender and living arrangements. Studies found that older women are more likely to be poor than older men, and poverty is more common among women aged 75 years and older, and those who are widowed or living alone (Gornick, Sierminska & Smeeding, 2009). Marital status affects other aspects of older adults' lives in many ways, including economic resources, living arrangements, and availability of a carer for those who are dependent. Table 1-4 summarises statistics about socioeconomic characteristics of older adults in Australia and New Zealand.

Living arrangements of older adults

Living arrangements for older adults are influenced by such factors as health, marital status, family relationships, and socioeconomic conditions. Despite the common misconception that most older adults live in nursing homes, the majority of older Australians and New Zealanders (approximately 94%) live in the community (AIHW, 2013). Approximately 6% of older adults live in long-term residential care. The proportion of older adults who live in the community does decrease with age; but even so, most people 85 years and over still live at home. In Australia approximately 93% of older adults live in private dwellings, with 71% owning their home; 7% had a mortgage; and ; 5% were renting (AIHW, 2013). Only 25% live alone and, of these, 51% are over 85 years and are women. Seven per cent of older Australians are homeless and the majority are men; however, it is expected that the proportion of older adults who own their own home will decline in the future.

In New Zealand approximately 76% of older adults live in owner-occupied dwellings (NZMOH, 2011, p. 18). About 20% of older women and 25% of older men do not live in their own homes. About 2% are considered to live in a home that is overcrowded. Older men are more likely to live alone as they get older, especially between the ages of 75 and 90, while the number of females living alone continues to increase until approximately 85 years. Figures 1-7 and 1-8 describe the living arrangements of older adults in Australia and New Zealand.

TABLE 1-4 Statistics in brief: Socioeconomic characteristics of adults 65 years and over

Socioeconomic characteristics of people aged 65+ years	Australia	New Zealand
Education	Higher School (Year 12 or equivalent): 65–74 23% 75–84 19% 85+ 15% High School (Year 10 or equivalent): 65–74 24% 75–84 17% 85+ 14% Did not go to school: 65–74 2% 75–84 2% 85+ 2%	School Leaving Certificate (Level 2 or higher): 39.9% for females and 52.7% for males Degree: 65–69 1.7% (7300) 75–79 0.9% (3800) 85–89 0.3% (1100)
Financial status	11% employed 53% working part time 78% receive Age Pension Smaller number self-funded retirees Home ownership: • 86% for couples • 69% for single people 3% of couple households and 6% of lone-person households had a cash-flow problem in 2006	18% are employed mostly part time 82% are not in the labour force Of these 98.0% receive New Zealand Superannuation (NZS): • 40% sole form of income • 20% receive 85% of NZS Home ownership: 75% females 80% males Live in overcrowded conditions: • 2.1% males • 2.4% females 4% had high hardship rates
Marital status	65+ years: Married 57% Widowed 26% Divorced 10% Never married 7% 85+ years: Widowed 77% women; 34% men	Never married 4% Married (not separated) 53% Separated 2% Divorced 7% Widowed 28% Not included elsewhere 6%
Volunteering	31% volunteered in the last 12 months (2010) 55% of these volunteered at least fortnightly	Approx. 35% volunteered in the last 12 months (2009)

Source: Australian Bureau of Statistics. (2006b). *Census 2006*; Australian Institute of Health and Welfare. (2010). *Australia's health*; Statistics New Zealand. (2007). *New Zealand's 65+ population: A statistical volume 2007*; New Zealand Ministry of Health. (2007). *Older people's health chart book 2006.*

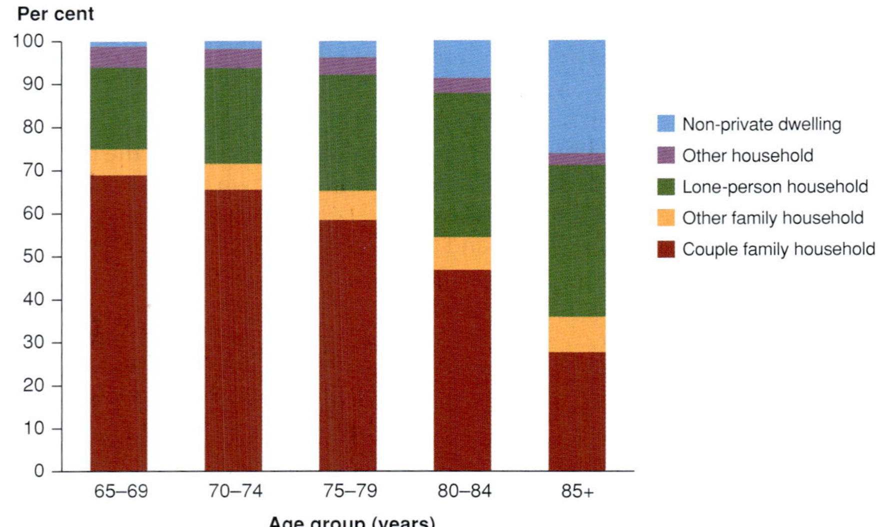

FIGURE 1-7 Living arrangements of older people by age in Australia. (Australian Institute of Health and Welfare. [2013]. *Australia's welfare 2013*. Australia's welfare series no. 11. Cat. no. AUS 174. Canberra: Author. Permission to reproduce granted under a Creative Commons BY 3.0 [CC BY 3.0] licence.)

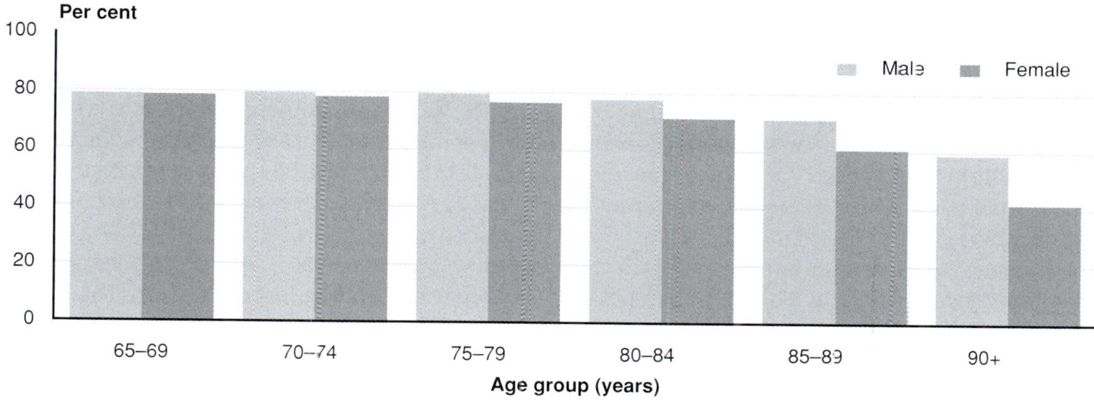

FIGURE 1-8 Percentage of older adults who own or partly own their own home in New Zealand by age and sex. (Statistics New Zealand. [2007]. *New Zealand's 65+ population: A statistical volume*. Wellington: Author.)

Many older adults who live in independent settings receive significant levels of assistance from family members, as discussed in the following sections on caregiving. Many also receive significant levels of support from a broad range of community-based services and agencies. Older adults have an increasingly wide range of community care options that address the needs of the growing number of older adults who require daily assistance but not full-time care. Further discussion about care options for older people occurs in Chapter 6.

Because the range of community-based services is rapidly increasing, decisions about staying in one's own home or moving to another type of facility are becoming more complex. Although nurses may not be familiar with all care options in their communities, at a minimum, they need to know about the various types of facilities that are commonly available. Moreover, nurses are responsible for suggesting referrals to social service agencies and offices on ageing so that older adults and their families can find additional information.

OLDER ADULTS AND CARING

Major demographic trends in Australia and New Zealand have brought about important changes in family relationships in recent decades. Trends towards improved health and increased longevity for older adults have occurred in parallel with trends towards increased diversity of family constellations among all generations. Concurrent with these trends, the prevalence of dementia and other chronic conditions that lead to functional decline has led to increased demands for family caregiving. On the other side of the coin, societal changes have led to increased demands for grandparents to assume roles of caregiving for dependent younger generations. This section discusses implications of these shifting demographics in relation to their influence on care of older adults.

Trends in caregiving

The increasing numbers of middle-aged adults who simultaneously juggle the demands of caring for older and younger generations are referred to as the **sandwich generation**. Responsibilities of middle-aged adults with parents who depend on them for care (i.e. the sandwich generation) are described demographically by the parent support ratio.

Demographics such as these have influenced patterns of family caregiving, particularly for women. The mid-1980s, for example, marked the beginning of an era in which the average woman in the Australia and New Zealand spent more time caring for her parents than for her children. Despite the emphasis on women as carers/caregivers for older adults, it is important to recognise that about one-quarter of caregivers are men. However, studies show that female caregivers are more likely to care than male caregivers (PC, 2011; New Zealand Ministry of Social Development [NZMSD], 2008).

Since the pre-industrial period, nuclear family living arrangements have been predominant in developed countries. Typically, younger family members establish separate households after marriage, and older family members attempt to maintain independent households for as long as possible. For much of Australia's and New Zealand's history, the "ideal" relationship between older and younger generations in families has been to be far enough away to preserve independent lifestyles but close enough for social support and emotional connectedness. Moreover, this kind of family relationship provides for meeting occasional caregiving needs of family members while allowing for the maintenance of differing lifestyles for both younger and older generations. These family relationships are based on the principle of reciprocity across generations, characterised by mutual assistance and extensive exchanges among kin. The current trend in Australia and New Zealand is that caregiving needs of elders are met primarily by spouses and secondarily by adult children, especially daughters and unmarried children.

In recent years, increased rates of divorce and remarriage among younger generations have resulted in the proliferation of varieties of blended families across several generations. In addition, increased rates of remarriage among older adults who are widowed or divorced have led to increasing numbers of later-life blended families. One consequence of these trends is that family dynamics can become quite complex, particularly when adult stepchildren assume new roles as carers or decision makers for dependent older adults. For example, adult children may share caregiving and decision-making responsibilities regarding their impaired parent with a parent's spouse whom they hardly know. Similarly, adult children may assist their parent with caregiving or decision making about a step-parent whom they are just getting to know. Relationships among blended families usually are complicated by concerns regarding financial resources and questions about inheritance.

Expectations and attitudes about caregiving practices have also changed due to societal trends that affect relationships between older adults and their families. In the early 1900s, for example, the tradition of deep involvement in generational assistance, reinforced by strong family and ethnic values, was dominant. By the mid-1960s, trends were shifting towards a tradition of individualistic values and lifestyles, due in part to the proliferation of public support and services for older adults. Another major influence on trends has been the increasing numbers of women who have careers independent of their roles in families, which can lead to conflict between the younger generation of adult children and older family members who expect care. Even with complex and evolving social and demographic trends, studies consistently show that the of care older dependent adults is provided by family members and other "informal" sources. The term **informal caregiver** refers to the provision of non-professional or unpaid assistance to a family member or friend to support the person in a community setting.

In Australia, 83% of the older adults who receive assistance in the community have care provided by informal carers (AIHW, 2011), although 47% of older people who receive assistance do so from both informal and formal carers. It has been estimated that over 500,000 (20%) of older Australians who provide informal care to older adults with a disability are family or friends (AIHW, 2013). About 77% of primary carers are older adults; they are the main person responsible for meeting most of the care needs of the older adult. Partners comprise 45% of all informal carers of older adults (PC, 2011). If informal care delivered to Australians, including the older adults, was replaced by paid carers, it is estimated that the cost would be over $40 billion a year (PC, 2011, p. 18). Of concern is the increasing number of adults aged 85+ years who are primary carers (AIHW, 2013).

In New Zealand, 25% of those aged between 65 and 74 are cared for by an informal carer, and this increases to 85% in the 85+ age group (Office for Disability Issues and Statistics New Zealand, 2009). Eleven per cent of people aged between 65 and 84 care for their older spouse and this reduces to 4% in the 85+ group. The New Zealand Carers' Strategy Action Plan is available in New Zealand to improve support for carers (NZMSD, 2014). The Strategy has four guiding principles, to "... recognise diversity; be proactive; enable carers and be inclusive" (p. 9). The Strategy and an updated guide for carers (NZMSD, 2013) can be accessed via www.msd.govt.nz.

Studies indicate that family carer-support delays or prevents the use of long-term residential care facilities, and also accounts for fewer days in acute care settings (Houser & Gibson, 2008). Spousal and filial responsibilities are traditions that have directed family caregiving in Australia and New Zealand for centuries, and this continues, even though the specific dynamics of the care are changing. Cultural considerations 1-1 summarises some cultural perspectives related to older adults and family caregiving.

Older adults as recipients and givers of care

Although much of the literature related to care of older adults focuses on middle-aged women who care for dependent older adults, many older adults themselves are carers. Many studies focus on **caregiver burden**, which refers to the stresses and negative consequences associated with caregiving. These studies include middle-aged and older adult carers, and many of the studies focus on care provided to people living with dementia in community settings.

Some of the most consistent findings are that people who provide care for adult family members who are chronically ill experience many negative effects, including higher levels of stress, anxiety, depression, poor mental and physical health, and lower levels of social interaction and quality of life (Berg & Woods, 2009; Chang, Chiou & Chen, 2010; Ho et al., 2009). Although fewer studies have focused on positive effects of being a carer, most carers experience a mixture of negative and positive consequences. Benefits or gains identified in studies centre on such themes as learning new skills; feeling needed, useful and fulfilled; and adding a sense of purpose or meaning to one's life (Koerner, Kenyon & Shirai, 2009; Okamoto et al., 2009). Additional information about carers is discussed in Chapter 14 because many of the studies focus on caregiving in relation to people with dementia.

Grandparents raising grandchildren

Older adults are increasingly involved in the care of their grandchildren. Older adults in Australia provide care on a regular basis to 937,000 (26%) children aged 12 years or under (AIHW, 2013). Another phenomenon currently being experienced is the dramatic increase in the number of children younger than 18 years living in households maintained by a grandparent with no parent present. These households are referred to as **skipped-generation households**. In New Zealand, 33% of the children had been living with the grandparents for 10 years or longer, 49% from 6 to 9 years, and 18% between 4 and 5 years (Grandparents Raising Grandchildren Trust, 2009). Support for grandparents is available through the organisation Grandparents Raising Grandchildren (GRG) Trust, contacted on 0800 472 637, extension 1 for GRG enquiries.

In Australia 19% of children receive regular care from their grandparents (AIHW, 2013). Households in which children are being raised by both their parents and grandparents are called three-generation, shared-care households. In both countries the percentage of older adults and children in these two situations is increasing significantly and there are major implications for children, grandparents and society. Common reasons for grandparent custody include child abuse; teen pregnancy; parental abuse of drugs or alcohol; and death, disability, mental illness or incarceration of adult parents.

Some studies have found positive effects of becoming a custodial grandparent; however, more studies have documented negative effects (Namkung, 2010). Rewards of grandparent caregiving include role enhancement, sense of purpose in life, motivation to keep physically active, close relationships with younger generations, and satisfaction with maintaining family well-being. Negative consequences include significant stresses, role overload, social isolation, detrimental effects on health, and increased likelihood of being poor. Specifically, studies have found that custodial grandparents were more likely to report more functional limitations, poorer self-rated health, increased prevalence of chronic disease, more depressive symptoms, and lower levels of life satisfaction than non-carers (Namkung, 2010).

OLDER ADULTS IN THE WORLD

This chapter presents characteristics of older adults living in Australia and New Zealand that are pertinent to nursing, but it would be incomplete without a brief perspective on global aspects of ageing because the world's population is now ageing at an unprecedented rate. Declines in fertility rates and improvements in health and life expectancy that occurred during the 20th century has resulted in significant increases in the number and proportion of older adults in most of the world. Even more significantly, projections for 2050 indicate continued increases in all groups of older adults, compared with much lower increases in younger age groups, as illustrated in Figure 1-9. Much of the information about global ageing discusses differences between *developed* countries and *developing* countries because of significantly different conditions that affect population ageing in these two types of countries. Organisations such as census bureaus, the United Nations and

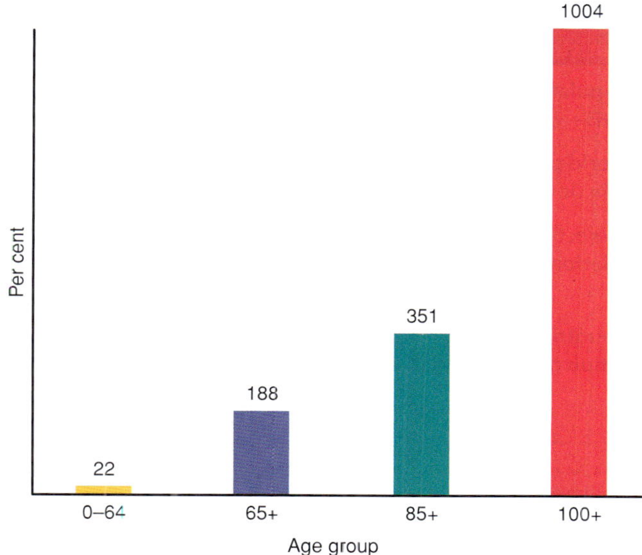

FIGURE 1-9 Percentage change in the world's population by age: 2010–2050. (Adapted from National Institute on Aging. [2011]. Global health and aging. Bethesda, MD: Author. Accessed March 2015 at www.nia.nih.gov/research/publication/global-health-and-aging/living-longer *Source:* United Nations. [2010]. *World population prospects: The 2010 revision*. New York: Author. Available March 2015 via http://esa.un.org/unpd/wpp.)

the World Health Organizations, use these terms to differentiate between countries according to level of development. Although there are no universally accepted standards for classifying countries as more or less developed, commonly used criteria include life expectancy, literacy rate, and per capita income.

The United Nations classifies Japan, Australia, New Zealand and all nations in Europe and North America as developed nations, and all other nations of the world as developing nations. World population trends show that the most developed nations have the highest percentages of older adults and the highest median age and some may have more grandparents than young children by 2050. However, many of the developing countries are experiencing more recent and rapid declines in fertility rates, so the proportion of older adults in developing countries is expected to increase significantly during the next decades (Kinsella & He, 2009). Figure 1-9 and Box 1-3 summarise demographic information about global ageing.

Challenges of an ageing population

As the population ages an increased burden is placed on the healthcare system to deliver services. The major challenges experienced with this increasing burden are to ensure an adequate workforce that is appropriately skilled, and the availability of suitable services for supporting those ageing. The information presented in this chapter demonstrates that older adults living in Australia and New Zealand are living longer but many are not ageing well.

BOX 1-3
Statistics in brief: Global ageing

Population changes: People aged 65+ worldwide	• 2008 • 2040	7% 14%
World population aged 65+ living in developing countries	• 2008 • 2040	62% 76%
Projected increase in world population between 2003 and 2040	• Age 80+ • Age 65+ • All ages	233% 160% 33%
Countries with highest proportion of people aged 65+	• Japan • Italy • Germany • Greece	21.6% 20.0% 20.0% 19.1%

Source: U.S. Census Bureau. (2009). *An aging world.* Washington, DC: U.S. Government Printing Office.

With increasing age and levels of disease, there is increasing prevalence of disability and need for healthcare services. There are also increasing levels of diversity in the older adult group, and this is further discussed in Chapter 2.

In order to address these challenges, governments in both Australia and New Zealand, not to mention globally, recognise that one solution is to support the health of older adults irrespective of their age, level of disability or diversity. By adopting this strategy, healthcare providers can support older adults to live longer and improve their quality of life, thereby reducing the burden of the healthcare system. Research has demonstrated that the decline associated with ageing can be slowed and managed.

Currently older adults in Australia and New Zealand have the potential to live longer and live better than before. Nurses and other healthcare providers have a key role in achieving this vision. This textbook focuses on providing nurses with information to support the healthy ageing of older adults. It provides a framework utilising ageing and wellness concepts, as well as the contemporary processes of nursing. The framework is described in Chapter 3, and provides a person-centred approach to facilitate working with older adults and their families to achieve health while ageing. Within this text, many nursing interventions are presented that improve an older adult's safety, function, quality of life and health.

CHAPTER HIGHLIGHTS

Relationship between wellness and ageing

- Definitions of ageing can be understood in terms of chronological age, age identity or functional age. Addressing functional age is most appropriate in wellness-oriented nursing care.
- There are many terms that refer to wellness while ageing, and this text has adopted the term *healthy ageing*.
- Healthcare professionals have recognised the importance of incorporating wellness goals in their care of older adults; however, there are many conceptual and practical barriers.
- Barriers to promoting wellness in older adults include older adults' negative attitudes about being able to improve, the existence of more serious or pressing health concerns, the focus of healthcare environments on disease treatment rather than prevention or health promotion, the false attribution of symptoms of pathological conditions to normal ageing processes, and the belief that older adults are not capable of learning and implementing health-promoting behaviours inherent in wellness-oriented care.
- Rather than having a narrow focus on physical health and functioning, wellness-focused nursing considers the older adult's physical, mental, social and spiritual well-being.

Attitudes towards ageing

- Negative images of ageing and ageism are pervasive in modern societies and can have a negative impact on care provided to older adults, especially when healthcare providers—including nurses—base their care on myths and inaccurate information.
- Nurses need to identify myths about older adults (Figure 1-2), examine attitudes towards ageing (including their own), and use accurate information as an antidote so they can provide wellness-oriented care for older adults (Table 1-1).
- Cultural perspectives have a significant influence on attitudes about ageing, older adults, and family caregiving relationships (Cultural considerations 1-1).

Debunking myths: Understanding realities about older adults in Australia and New Zealand

- The older adult population in Australia and New Zealand is increasing, living longer, and reflecting greater diversity (Boxes 1-1 & 1-2; Figures 1-3 to 1-6; Tables 1-2 & 1-3).
- Despite a high prevalence of chronic illnesses, many older adults report good-to-excellent health (Table 1-3).
- Socioeconomic characteristics and living arrangements of older adults vary significantly among subgroups (Table 1-4 & Figures 1-7 & 1-8).
- The current trend in Australia and New Zealand is that the caregiving needs of elders are met primarily by spouses and secondarily by adult children, especially daughters and unmarried children.
- Older adults are increasingly responsible for caring for their grandchildren. Some may be responsible for raising grandchildren in skipped-generation households.

Older adults in the world

- Populations in both developed and developing countries are ageing (Box 1-3, Figure 1-9)

CRITICAL THINKING EXERCISES

1. Increase your awareness of attitudes towards ageing and older adults through the following exercises:
   - During the next 2 weeks, as you go about your usual activities, keep a small notebook handy and jot down examples of images of older adults whom you see or hear in the following media: newspapers, magazines, Internet, television, greeting cards and social conversations. Note whether the images convey a neutral, positive or negative image.
   - During the next 2 weeks, pay attention to your thoughts and conversations about older adults and identify the perceptions you hold, the terms you use, and the images you convey.
   - Rephrase each of the 20 questions in the Ageism Survey (Figure 1-2) to ask yourself how often you have done any of those activities in the past few months (e.g. "How often did I tell a joke that pokes fun at old people?").
   - Ask an older relative, friend or acquaintance to fill out the Ageism Survey and discuss his or her experiences.
2. Define old age and ageing from each of the following perspectives: chronological age, age identity, and functional age.
3. Use the Internet to explore one of the sources listed in the following resources section and explore additional information about demographic trends and characteristics of older adults in Australia and New Zealand.
4. Use the Internet to explore sources listed in the resources section for information about global ageing to find out more information about demographic trends in developed and developing nations.

RESOURCES

For an extensive range of additional resources to enhance teaching and learning and to facilitate understanding of this chapter, please see the text's accompanying website located on thePoint at http://thepoint.lww.com.

Characteristics of older adults in Australia and New Zealand

Australian Bureau of Statistics, health of older people: www.abs.gov.au/ausstats/abs@.nsf/mf/4833.0.55.001

Australian Bureau of Statistics, 2011 census data: www.abs.gov.au/ausstats/abs@.nsf/Lookup/2071.0main+features752012-2013

Australian Government Department of Health and Ageing: www.health.gov.au

Australian Institute of Health and Welfare: http://aihw.gov.au/ageing-disability-and-carers

New Zealand Ministry of Health: www.health.govt.nz

New Zealand Ministry of Social Development: www.msd.govt.nz/what-we-can-do/seniorcitizens/positive-ageing/trends/index.html

Statistics New Zealand: www.stats.govt.nz/browse_for_stats/people_and_communities/older_people.aspx

Global ageing

U.S. Census Bureau, *An aging world*: www.census.gov/prod/2001pubs/p95-01-1.pdf

Global Action on Aging: http://globalaging.org

International Research Centre for Healthy Ageing and Longevity (IRCHAL): http://irchal.org

United Nations, global ageing 1950–2050: www.un.org/esa/population/publications/worldageing19502050

United Nations, Department of Economic and Social Affairs, Population Division: www.un.org/en/development/desa/population/theme/ageing/index.shtml

World Health Organization, ageing: www.who.int/topics/ageing/en

REFERENCES

Australian Bureau of Statistics. (2006a). *Health of older people in Australia: A snapshot, 2004–05*. Cat. no. 4833.0.55.001. Canberra: Author.

Australian Bureau of Statistics. (2006b). *Census 2006*. Canberra: Author.

Australian Bureau of Statistics. (2008). *Population projections, Australia, 2006 to 2101*. Cat. no. 3222.0. Canberra: Author.

Australian Bureau Statistics (ABS). (2012). Who are Australia's older people? From *Reflecting a nation: Stories from the 2011 census*. Cat. no. 2071.0. Canberra: Author. Accessed March 2015 at www.abs.gov.au/ausstats/abs@.nsf/lookup/2071.0main+features752012-2013.

Australian Bureau Statistics (ABS). (2014). Ageing population. From *Australian demographic statistics, June 2014*. Cat. no. 3101.0. Canberra: Author. Accessed March 2015 at www.abs.gov.au/ausstats/abs@.nsf/0/1CD2B1952AFC5E7ACA257298000F2E76?OpenDocument.

Australian Institute of Health and Welfare (AIHW). (2010). *Australia's health 2010*. Accessed March 2015 at www.aihw.gov.au/publication-detail/?id=6442468376.

Australian Institute of Health and Welfare (AIHW). (2013). *Australia's welfare 2013*. Australia's welfare series no. 11. Cat. no. AUS 174. Canberra: Author.

Baltes, M. M. & Carstensen, L. L. (1996). The process of successful ageing. *Ageing and Society, 16*, 397–422.

Barrett, A. E. & Robbins, C. (2008). The multiple sources of women's aging anxiety and their relationship with psychological distress. *Journal of Aging and Health, 20*(1), 32–65.

Baumbusch, J., Dahlke, S. & Phinney, A. (2012). Nursing students' knowledge and beliefs about care of older adults in a shifting context of nursing education. *Journal of Advances in Nursing, 68*(11), 2550–2558.

Berg, J. A. & Woods, N. F. (2009). Global women's health: A spotlight on caregiving. *Nursing Clinics of North America, 44*, 375–384.

Bodner, E. (2009). On the origins of ageism among older and younger adults. *International Psychogeriatrics, 21*(6), 1003–1014.

Bowling, A. (2009). Perceptions of active ageing in Britain: Divergences between minority ethnic and whole population samples. *Age and Ageing, 38,* 703–710.

Boyle, P. A., Barnes, L. L., Buchman, A. S., Bennett, D. A. & Rush Alzheimer's Disease Center & Departments of Behavioral Sciences and Neurological Sciences. (2009). Purpose in life is associated with mortality among community-dwelling older persons. *Psychosomatic Medicine, 71*(5), 574–579.

Butler, R. N. (1969). Ageism: Another form of bigotry. *Gerontologist, 9,* 243–246.

Butler, R. N., Lewis, M. I. & Sunderland, T. (1991). *Aging and mental health* (4th ed.). New York, NY: Merrill/Macmillan.

Chang, H.-Y., Chiou, C.-J. & Chen, N.-S. (2010). Impact of mental health and caregiver burden on family caregivers' physical health. *Archives of Gerontology and Geriatrics, 50,* 267–271.

Chaves, M. L., Camozzato, A. L., Eizirik, C. L. & Kaye, J. (2009). Predictors of normal and successful aging among urban-dwelling elderly Brazilians. *Journal of Gerontology: Psychological Sciences, 64B*(5), 596–602.

Christensen, K., Thinggaard, M., McGue, M., Rexbye, H., Hjelmborg, J. V. B., Aviv, A., . . . Vaupel, J. W. (2009). Christmas 2009: Young and old; Perceived age as clinically useful biomarker of ageing: Cohort study. *British Medical Journal, 339,* b5262. Accessible via doi:http://dx.doi.org/10.1136/bmj.b5262.

Collins, A. & Wilson, G. (2008). Māori and informal caregiving: A background paper prepared for the National Health Committee. Viewed March 2015 via www.nhc.health.govt.nz/resources/publications/m%C4%81ori-and-informal-caregiving-background-paper-prepared-national-health.

Crimmins, E. M., Kim, J. K. & Seeman, T. E. (2009). Poverty and biological risk: The earlier "aging" of the poor. *Journal of Gerontology Series: A Biological Sciences and Medical Sciences, 64*(A), 286–292.

Dunn, H. L. (1958). Significance of levels of wellness in aging. *Geriatrics, 13*(1), 51–57.

Dunn, H. L. (1961). *High-level wellness.* Arlington, VA: R.W. Beatty.

Eymard, A. S. & Douglas, D. H. (2012). Ageism among health care providers and interventions to improve their attitudes toward older adults: An integrative review. *Journal of Gerontological Nursing, 38*(5), 26–35.

Flatt, M. A., Settersten, R. A., Ponsaran, R. et al. (2013). Are "Anti-Aging Medicine" and "Successful Aging" two sides of the same coin? Views of anti-aging practitioners. *Journals of Gerontology: Psychological Sciences and Social Sciences, 68*(6), 944–955.

Gornick, J. C., Sierminska, E. & Smeeding, T. M. (2009). The income and wealth packages of older women in cross-national perspective. *Journal of Gerontology: Social Sciences, 64B*(3), 402–414.

Grandparents Raising Grandchildren Trust. (2009). The healing power of grandparents. Media release 9.09.09. Accessed March 2015 at www.raisinggrandchildren.org.nz/Media-Release-9.09.09.html.

Gruenewald, T. L., Karlamangla, A. S., Greendale, G. A., Singer, B. H. & Seeman, T. E. (2009). Increased mortality risk in older adults with persistently low or declining feelings of usefulness to others. *Journal of Aging and Health, 21*(2), 398–425.

Ho, S. C., Chan, A., Woo, J., Chong, P. & Sham, A. (2009). Impact of caregiving on health and quality of life: A comparative population-based study of caregivers for elderly persons and noncaregivers. *Journal of Gerontology Series A: Biological Sciences and Medical Sciences, 64A*(8), 873–879.

Houser, A. & Gibson, M. J. (2008). *Valuing the invaluable: The economic value of family caregiving* (2008 update). Washington DC: AARP Public Policy Institute.

Kinsella, K. & He, W. (2009). *An aging world: 2008* (U.S. Census Bureau, International Population Reports, P95—09-1). Washington, DC: Government Printing Office.

Koerner, S. S., Kenyon, D. Y. B. & Shirai, Y. (2009). Caregiving for elder relatives: Which caregivers experience personal benefits/gains? *Archives of Gerontology and Geriatrics, 48,* 238–245.

Laditka, S. B., Corwin, S. J., Laditka, J. N., Liu, R., Tseng, W., Wu, B., . . . Ivey, S. L. (2009). Attitudes about aging well among a diverse group of older Americans: Implications for promoting cognitive health. *Gerontologist, 49*(S1), S30–S39.

Lerolle, N., Trinquart, L., Bornstain, C., Tadie, J. M., Imbert, A., Diehl, J. L., . . . Guérot E. (2010). Increased intensity of treatment and decreased mortality in elderly patients in an intensive care unit over a decade. *Critical Care Medicine, 38*(1), 59–64.

Levy, B. R., Ashman, O. & Slade, M. D. (2009). Age attributions and aging health: Contrast between the United States and Japan. *Journal of Gerontology: Psychological Sciences, 64B*(3), 335–338.

Levy, B. R. & Leifheit-Limson, E. (2009). The stereotype-matching effect: Greater influence on functioning when age stereotypes correspond to outcomes. *Psychology and Aging, 24*(1), 230–233.

Lineweaver, T. T., Berger, A. K. & Hertzog, C. (2009). Expectations about memory change across the life span are impacted by aging stereotypes. *Psychology and Aging, 24*(1), 169–176.

Lipson, J. G. & Dibble, L. (2005). *Culture & clinical care.* San Francisco: UCSF Nursing Press.

Martin, R., Williams, C. & O'Neill, D. (2009). Retrospective analysis of attitudes to ageing in the *Economist:* Apocalyptic demography for opinion formers? *British Medical Journal, 339,* b4914. Available March 2015 via doi:http://dx.doi.org/10.1136/bmj.b4914.

McGrath, P. (2008). Family care giving for Aboriginal peoples during end of life: Findings from the Northern Territory. *Journal of Rural and Tropical Public Health, 7,* 1–10.

McGuire, S. L., Klein, D. A. & Chen, S. L. (2008). Ageism revisited: A study measuring ageism in East Tennessee, USA. *Nursing and Health Sciences, 10*(1), 11–16.

McMahon, S. & Fleury, J. (2012). Wellness in older adults: A concept analysis. *Nursing Forum, 47*(1), 39–49.

Medical Council of New Zealand. (2010). Best health outcomes for Pacific peoples: Practice implications. Accessed at www.mcnz.org.nz/assets/News-and-Publications/Statements/Best-health-outcomes-for-Pacific-Peoples.pdf.

Musaiger, A. O. & D'Souza, R. (2009). Role of age and gender in the perception of aging: A community-based survey in Kuwait. *Archives of Gerontology and Geriatrics, 48*(2009), 50–57.

Namkung, E. H. (2010). Grandparents raising grandchildren: Ethnic and household differences in health and service use. Paper presented at the Society for Social Work and Research, 14th Annual Conference, San Francisco.

National Ageing Research Institute (NARI) and Council on the Ageing (COTA). (2012). *Healthy ageing: A literature review.* Melbourne: Victorian State Department of Health.

National Institute on Aging. (2011). *Global health and aging.* Bethesda, MD: Author. Accessed March 2015 at www.nia.nih.gov/research/publication/global-health-and-aging/living-longer.

Neugarten, B. L. (1978). The rise of the young-old. In R. Gross, B. Gross & S. Seidman (Eds), *The new old: Struggling for decent aging* (pp. 47–49). Garden City, NY: Anchor Press/Doubleday.

New Zealand Ministry of Health (NZMOH). (2007). *Older people's health chart book 2006.* Wellington: Author. Accessed March 2015 at www.health.govt.nz/publication/older-peoples-health-chart-book-2006.

New Zealand Ministry of Health (NZMOH). (2011). *Tatau Kura Tangata: Health of older Māori chart book 2011.* Wellington: Author. Accessed March 2015 at www.health.govt.nz/publication/tatau-kura-tangata-health-older-maori-chart-book-2011.

New Zealand Ministry of Social Development. (2008). New Zealand Living Standards Survey. Accessed March 2015 at www.msd.govt.nz/about-msd-and-our-work/publications-resources/monitoring/living-standards/living-standards-2008.html.

New Zealand Ministry of Social Development. (2012). New Zealanders: Getting older, doing more. Briefing for the incoming Minister. Accessed March 2015 at www.msd.govt.nz/about-msd-and-our-work/publications-resources/corporate/briefing-incoming-minister/2012-briefing-papers.html.

New Zealand Ministry of Social Development. (2013). A guide for carers/He Aratohu mā ngā Kaitiaki. Accessed April 2015 via www.msd.govt.nz/about-msd-and-our-work/work-programmes/policy-development/carers-strategy.

New Zealand Ministry of Social Development. (2014). New Zealand Carers' Strategy Action Plan, 2014 to 2018. Wellington: Author. Available March 2015 at www.msd.govt.nz/about-msd-and-our-work/work-programmes/policy-development/carers-strategy.

New Zealand Ministry of Social Policy. (2001). The New Zealand Positive Ageing Strategy: Towards a Society for All Ages. Wellington: Author. Accessed March 2015 www.ifa-fiv.org/wp-content/uploads/2012/11/060_NZ-Positive-Ageing-Strategy.pdf.

North, M. S. & Fiske, S. T. (2012). An inconvenienced youth? Ageism and its potential intergenerational roots. *Psychology Bulletin, 138*(5), 982–997.

Office for Disability Issues and Statistics New Zealand. (2009). *Disability and informal care in New Zealand in 2006: Results from the New Zealand Disability Survey.* Wellington: Author. Retrievable March 2015 from www.stats.govt.nz/browse_for_stats/health/disabilities/disability-and-informal-care-in-nz-in-2006.aspx.

Okamoto, K., Momose, Y., Fujino, A. & Osawa, Y. (2009). Life worth living for caregiving and caregiver burden among Japanese caregivers of the disabled elderly in Japan. *Archives of Gerontology and Geriatrics, 48,* 10–13.

Palmore, E. (2000). *The Ageism Survey.* Durham, NC: Duke Center for the Study of Aging.

Palmore, E. (2005). Three decades of research on ageism. *Generations, 29*(3), 87–90.

Perry, B. (2008). *Household incomes in New Zealand: Trends in indicators of inequality and hardship 1982 to 2007.* Wellington: Ministry of Social Development. Available March 2015 via www.msd.govt.nz/about-msd-and-our-work/publications-resources/monitoring/household-incomes.

Plath, D. (2009). International policy perspectives on independence in old age. *Journal of Aging and Social Policy, 21*(2), 209–223.

Prevc, F. & Doupona, T. M. (2009). Age identity, social influence and socialization through physical activity in elderly people living in a nursing home. *Collegium Antropologicum, 33*(4), 1107–1114.

Productivity Commission (PC). (2005). Economic Implications of an Ageing Australia: Research Report. Canberra: Commonwealth of Australia.

Productivity Commission (PC). (2011). Caring for Older Australians: Inquiry Report No. 53. Canberra: Author.

Rowe, J. W. & Kahn, R. L. (1997). Successful aging. *Gerontologist, 37,* 433–440.

Schafer, M. H. & Shippee, T. P. (2010). Age identity, gender, and perceptions of decline: Does feeling older lead to pessimistic dispositions about cognitive aging? *Journals of Gerontology Series B, 65B*(1), 91–96.

Silva, M. G. & Boemer, M. R. (2009). The experience of aging: A phenomenological perspective. *Revista Latino-Americana de Enfermagem, 17*(3), 380–386.

Statistics New Zealand. (2007). *New Zealand's 65+ population: A statistical volume 2007.* Accessible March 2015 via www.stats.govt.nz/browse_for_stats/people_and_communities/older_people/new-zealands-65-plus-population.aspx.

Statistics New Zealand. (2013a). Census QuickStats about national highlights. Accessed March 2015 via www.stats.govt.nz.

Statistics New Zealand. (2013b). New Zealand General Social Survey 2012. Accessed March 2015 at www.stats.govt.nz/browse_for_stats/people_and_communities/Households/nzgss_HOTP2012.aspx.

Statistics New Zealand. (2014). *Population projections tables*. Accessed March 2015 at www.stats.govt.nz/tools_and_services/nzdotstat/tables-by-subject/population-projections-tables.aspx#national.

U.S. Census Bureau. (2009). *An aging world*. Washington, DC: U.S. Government Printing Office.

United Nations. (2010). *World population prospects: The 2010 revision*. New York: Author.

Vincent, J. A. (2008). The cultural construction old as a biological phenomenon: Science and anti-aging technologies. *Journal of Aging Studies, 22*(2008), 331–339.

Wilson, D. M., Thurston, A. & Lichlyter, B. (2010). Should the oldest-old be admitted to the intensive care unit and receive advanced life-supporting care? *Critical Care Medicine, 38*(1), 303–304.

Woods, N. F., Cochrane, B. B., LaCroix, A. Z. et al. (2012). Toward a positive aging phenotype for older women: Observations from the Women's Health Initiative. *Journals of Gerontology: Biological Sciences and Medical Sciences, 67*(11), 1191–1196.

World Health Organization. (2002). Active ageing: A policy framework. Geneva: Author.

Chapter 2

Addressing diversity of older adults

By Carol Miller and Sharyn Hunter

LEARNING OBJECTIVES

After reading this chapter, you should be able to:

1. Understand that the diversity of older adults living in Australia and New Zealand is increasing.
2. Discuss the importance of providing culturally and linguistically competent safe care for older adults.
3. Perform a cultural self-assessment.
4. Describe three major health belief systems that influence cultural perspectives on health and wellness.
5. Describe the characteristics and health inequalities that affect older adults of different ethnic groups living in Australia and New Zealand.
6. Identify sources of information that nurses can use to improve cultural competence and safety.

KEY POINTS

culturally and linguistically diverse (CALD)
cultural competence
cultural safety
health belief system
health disparities
health literacy
linguistic competence

The increasing diversity that is characteristic of all age groups in Australia and New Zealand affects almost every facet of healthcare, because cultural background significantly influences values, communication, health beliefs, health-related behaviours and many other aspects of daily life. Nurses who care for older adults from culturally diverse backgrounds need to recognise that seven or more decades of cultural influences significantly affect their patients' health beliefs and behaviours, as well as their relationships with healthcare providers and their receptivity to interventions.

It is beyond the scope of this text to present all the data and address all the implications related to cultural diversity of older adults. This chapter also only discusses the concepts of cultural competence and cultural safety as they relate to the nursing care of older adults. Other nursing resources are available that address these concepts more thoroughly and their relationship with nursing. The intent of this chapter is to discuss major implications of the increasing diversity of the older population in relation to the nursing care. This chapter provides an overview of diverse groups of older adults in Australia and New Zealand; however, as with any information related to cultural diversity, it is imperative to recognise that, at best, the overviews provide basic statistics about particular groups. Each group is composed of many individuals and each individual has some characteristics that are common to the group and many that are not. Because overviews do not apply to all individuals within the group, nurses need to avoid stereotypes and generalisations because they care for individual older adults.

CULTURAL DIVERSITY IN AUSTRALIA AND NEW ZEALAND

As discussed in Chapter 1, remarkable changes have occurred in the age-related demographics of all countries because of increased life expectancy among most groups and decreased fertility rates among many groups. At the same time that the trend towards population ageing has been occurring worldwide, a trend towards increasing ethnic diversity has been occurring in Australia and New Zealand, attributable largely to post-war immigration patterns. Both countries have Indigenous ethnic groups, who are also addressed in this chapter. Information about the increasing diversity of the older adult population is provided in the overview of cultural and ethnic groups of older adults in Australia and New Zealand, and older adults in other diverse groups sections.

Those older adults born overseas from non-English-speaking countries are described as being a **culturally and linguistically diverse (CALD)** group. In 2011 in Australia, 36% of older adults were born overseas (Australian Bureau of Statistics [ABS], 2012). CALD older people were most commonly born in Italy, Greece, Germany, the Netherlands and China.

Figure 2-1 lists the percentage of overseas born and describes the country's ageing profile. The Italian population has one of the oldest population profiles, while the Vietnamese have the youngest age profile. Overall, those born overseas have an older age structure than people born in Australia (Khoo, 2012). The next two decades will produce changes in this profile as the number of overseas-born older adults from Europe will decrease and those from an Asian background increase (Productivity Commission [PC], 2011). Australia's population of older people from CALD backgrounds is expected to increase by over 40% between 2011 and 2026, in line with the overall increase in the older population (PC, 2011, p. 246).

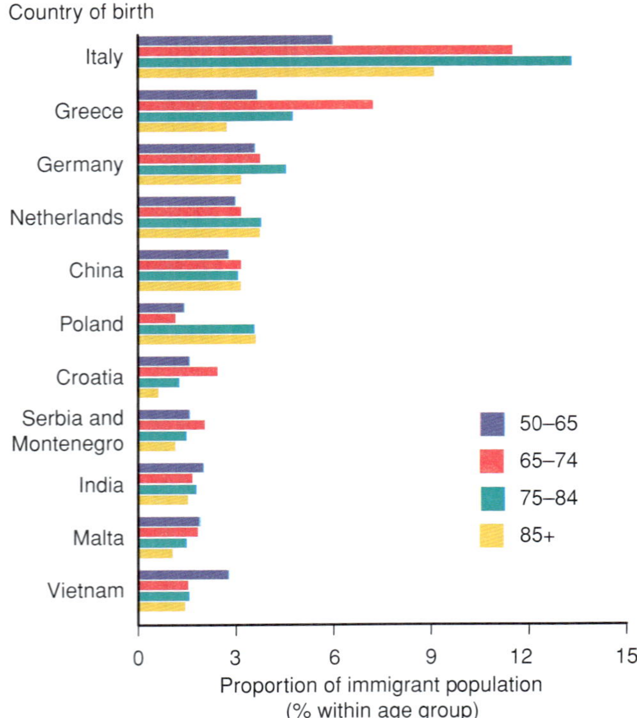

FIGURE 2-1 Percentage of overseas-born Australians by country of birth and age group for 2006. (Australian Institute of Health and Welfare. [2007]. *Older Australia at a glance* [4th ed.]. Cat. no. AGE 52. Canberra: Author. Viewed 19 March 2015 at www.aihw.gov.au/publication-detail/?id=6442468045. Permission granted under a Creative Commons BY 3.0 [CC BY 3.0] licence.)

The ageing profile of Indigenous Australians is also expected to change. In 2006, only 1% of Indigenous people was 75 years or over, while non-Indigenous Australians aged 75 or over consisted of 6.3% of the total population. It is expected that, with population growth and improvements in life expectancy (see later section on Indigenous Australians), the proportion of older Indigenous Australians will grow more quickly than the total number of older people in Australia. For instance, an increase in life expectancy at birth by 5 years would see the older Indigenous population (aged 55 years and over) more than double by 2021 (PC, 2011, p. 49).

In New Zealand in 2006 there were 27% of people aged 65 years and over who were born overseas (Statistics New Zealand, 2007). Most (55%) were born in the U.K. or Ireland. Another 15,400 were born in Asia (mainly China, India and South-East Asia); 12,000 in the Pacific Islands; 12,000 in north-western Europe and about 6400 in Australia. The European group is the largest group of overseas-born older adults (15.2%) and "...this is over three times the corresponding proportion for Māori, Pacific and Asian populations, which all had a figure of less than 5%" (p. 37). Figure 2-2 lists the actual and projected ethnic share of New Zealand's population for the 65+ age group.

It is expected that the proportion of all CALD groups who are older (that is, the Māori, Pacific and Asian groups) will increase in the future (Statistics New Zealand, 2007, pp. 37–38):

> *Among ethnic minorities, the increase in 65+ populations will be largest for the Asian population (409%), from 11,000 in 2001 to 56,000 in 2021. Over the same period, the Pacific peoples aged 65+ years are projected to increase by over 180% to 26,000. The European 65+ population will grow by 63% by 2021, when they will make up 22% of all European residents in New Zealand.*

Māori and Pacific peoples were less likely to rate their health as excellent or very good (54% and 55%, respectively)

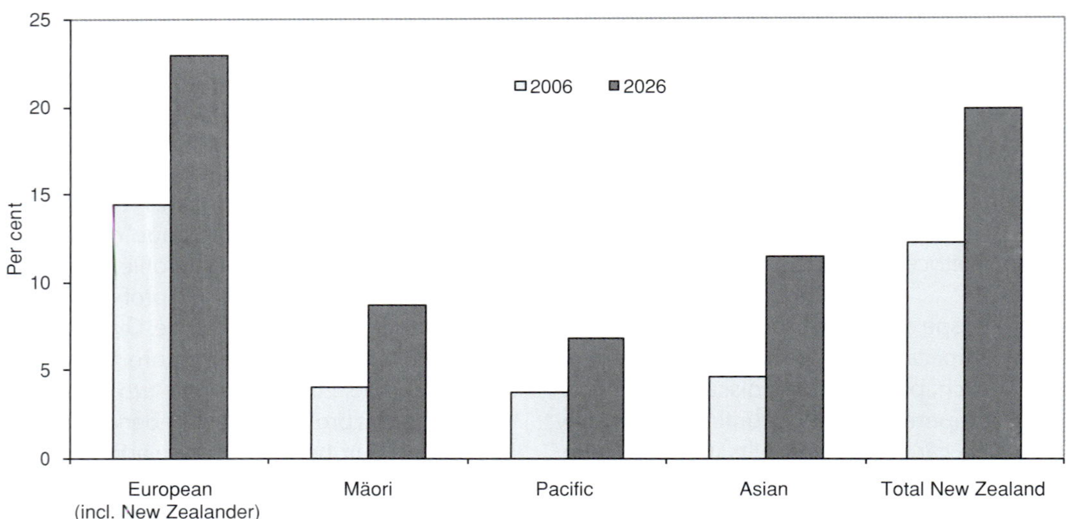

FIGURE 2-2 Ethnic share of New Zealand's recent and estimated population for the 65+ age group for the years 2006 and 2026. (Statistics New Zealand. [2009]. *Ageing of ethnic groups [structural change and the 65+ population articles]*. Wellington: Author.)

than Europeans (62%) or Asians (60%) (Statistics New Zealand, 2013). There is increasing attention to additional variables besides race and ethnicity that affect health. A recent review of studies emphasises that lower socioeconomic position—as measured by income, gender, and minority status—is "an overriding determinant of health status and health disparities" because it is associated with increased exposure to stress and decreased utilisation of important social supports (Lincoln, 2014). Another emerging focus of gerontology is on unique needs of other diverse groups of older adults, including lesbian, gay, bisexual and transgender (LGBT), and those who are homeless or live in rural areas. Current emphasis is on identifying interrelationships between health and minority status, whether that is based on gender, ethnicity, citizenship, religion, socioeconomic status or other factors (Abdou, 2014).

It is important to recognise that any defined group also includes many subgroups. Thus, definitions of groups and subgroups vary depending on the census definitions and other classifications available when data were collected or cited in research. Again, it is imperative to keep in mind that even the best evidence-based information does not address individual differences and that each person has unique characteristics that are not representative of any particular cultural group. The increasing diversity that is characteristic of the Australian and New Zealand population is also reflected in the healthcare workforce. This is especially noticeable in nursing staff, including nursing assistants, who provide care for older adults in community and long-term residential care settings. In home care settings, care is often provided by caregivers who might not have learned to speak English fluently. In these situations, communication barriers between care providers and care recipients are challenges that need to be addressed. It is important to recognise that cultural diversity in healthcare settings encompasses a wide range of situations, and each situation requires a high degree of **cultural competence** and **cultural safety** on the part of the healthcare provider.

HEALTH DISPARITIES

Cultural characteristics have been identified as a factor that may affect an individual's health. In recent years there has been increasing awareness of major health disparities, with much data pointing towards lower levels of health and functioning in groups of non-white older adults. **Health disparities** are defined as significant differences with regard to the rates of disease incidence, prevalence, morbidity, mortality or life expectancy between one population and another. Although some health disparities arise from biocultural factors, such as a genetic disposition to certain cancers, most are associated with sociocultural factors, such as low income and education. A common theme is that health disparities are especially pronounced for diseases that can be prevented through health promotion interventions, such as preventive care and patient teaching. In recent years in both Australia and New Zealand it has been recognised that all medical practitioners, nurses and allied health professionals must be aware of healthcare disparities and address them at the level of the individual.

Information about health disparities is not intended to reinforce stereotypes; rather, a major purpose is to be aware of risk factors based on race or ethnicity. Another major clinical implication is that health promotion interventions, such as teaching about prevention and early detection of certain conditions, are particularly important when caring for older adults who are members of a minority group. In addition to race and ethnic factors, a lower level of health literacy is a major risk for health disparities, as discussed in the following section.

Despite the increasing emphasis on eliminating health inequalities, they still exist in a number of the CALD older population groups in Australia and New Zealand. Although there is progress in some areas, there are still many gaps to be filled. For instance, there continues to be longevity gap between Indigenous people in Australia and New Zealand and non-Indigenous people (further discussion in the section on Indigenous people).

HEALTH LITERACY

Health literacy is increasingly recognised by healthcare practitioners and policy makers as a major determinant of health outcomes and a measure of quality of care. Definitions widely used during the past three decades all include the straightforward idea "that health literacy involves the need for people to understand information that helps them maintain good health" (Institute of Medicine, 2013, p. 1). "The concept of health literacy is broader than the ability to read labels, fill in forms and follow instructions. It also encompasses the ability to access health information and interpret conflicting advice critically, navigate the healthcare system, and communicate effectively on health-related matters" (Australian Institute Health and Welfare [AIHW], 2012, p. 182).

In Australia results from a national survey about heath literacy show that about 83% of older Australians (aged 65–74) did not have an adequate level of health literacy (ABS, 2009). Although data about cultural groups is limited, higher health literacy levels were found in those who were employed, had higher levels of formal education, great community participation or who spoke English as a first language. In New Zealand it has been identified that Māori and non-Māori people across all age groups have poor health literacy, and those aged 50–65 years have significantly lower health literacy than most other younger age groups (New Zealand Ministry of Health [NZMOH], 2010).

The factors identified that increase the risk for low health literacy include poverty, lower levels of education, and minority group membership. Reviews of studies (e.g. Cloonan, Wood & Riley, 2013; Nemmers, Jorge & Leahy, 2013) find that low health literacy is associated with the following negative outcomes related to individual health and increased healthcare costs:

- Increased hospitalisations, visits to emergency rooms, and re-admissions within 30 days of discharge
- Decreased use of preventive services such as immunisations and cancer screenings
- Shorter life expectancy
- Increased prevalence of multiple chronic diseases
- Poor access to healthcare
- Decreased adherence to prescribed medication regimen
- Lower levels of self-reported functional status and physical and mental health
- Decreased ability to self-manage chronic conditions.

Current national initiatives are identifying and implementing evidence-based approaches to assessment of and interventions for health literacy. These include a 2009 report from the National Health and Hospitals Reform Commission, which identified improving health literacy as a national health reform direction for Australia (NHHRC, 2009). A key recommendation from this report relevant to older adults was to "...improve access to evidence-based, consumer-friendly information that supports people in better understanding their health and making decisions" (AIHW, 2012, p. 182). In New Zealand the Ministry of Health (2012) has developed the resource, Rauemi Atawhai—A guide to developing health education resources in New Zealand, to assist health services produce health education material that is easy to understand and to support improved health literacy. This resource has six guiding principles:

1. Be prepared
2. Be clear on your audience and your key messages
3. Be open
4. Be relationship focused
5. Be accountable
6. Test, test and test again with your audience and stakeholders. (NZMOH, 2012, p. 3)

Because these initiatives relate to health promotion, Chapter 5 discusses health literacy in the context of health promotion for older adults.

CULTURAL COMPETENCE

Since the 1950s, transcultural nursing (i.e. the provision of nursing care across cultural boundaries) has focused on the comparative study of different cultural groups. Although transcultural nursing is an important specialisation, the demographic trend towards ever-expanding diversity requires that *all* healthcare professionals are culturally competent. Every nurse–person/patient encounter involves some degree of cultural differences because of the unique values and characteristics of each individual. Even when two people have similar cultural backgrounds, each one experiences and expresses cultural factors in a unique way. Consequently, nurses and nursing organisations are among the groups that are taking action to ensure the provision of culturally competent care.

Within Australia and New Zealand, the national governments and nursing bodies have mandated the delivery of culturally safe and competent nursing care (Nursing and Midwifery Board of Australia [NMBA], 2011; Nursing Council of New Zealand [NCNZ], 2011). In Australia, cultural competence has been defined as "...a set of congruent behaviours, attitudes and policies that come together in a system, agency or among professionals and enable that system, agency or those professions to work effectively in cross-cultural situations" (National Health and Medical Research Council [NHMRC], 2006, p. 7). The Nursing Council of New Zealand, responsible for the regulation of nursing in New Zealand, requires nurses to practise in a culturally safe manner. Cultural safety is defined as:

> *The effective nursing practice of a person or family from another culture, and is determined by that person or family. Culture includes, but is not restricted to, age or generation; gender; sexual orientation; occupation and socioeconomic status; ethnic origin or migrant experience; religious or spiritual belief; and disability. The nurse delivering the nursing service will have undertaken a process of reflection on his or her own cultural identity and will recognise the impact that his or her personal culture has on his or her professional practice. Unsafe cultural practice comprises any action which diminishes, demeans or disempowers the cultural identity and well-being of an individual. (NCNZ, 2011, p. 7)*

Cultural safety empowers those who are receiving nursing services to comment on nursing care and participate in achieving wellness. In Australia the term *cultural competence* encompasses cultural safety (Nash, Meiklejohn & Sacre, 2006). For nurses to be culturally competent and safe they must have an understanding of their own culture, their beliefs and values, and how these influence their nursing practice. Nurses also require an understanding of the historical, social and political influences on the health of the CALD groups. This understanding enables nurses to deliver culturally competent and safe care. However, a limitation of this chapter is that it focuses on presenting information about the diversity of older adults living in Australia and New Zealand and their health, and does not address the historical or political influences. Other resources should be accessed to obtain this understanding. When nurses are using any source of information, it is imperative to recognise that these resources can describe general characteristics of a particular group, but they cannot describe the unique way in which each individual is a member of the group. These generalisations can be detrimental if they lead to stereotypical perceptions rather than provide a compilation of information that may be applicable to individuals within the group. As already stated, all healthcare providers need to recognise that the culture of each individual is based on his or her membership in many groups and is internalised in a unique and personal way. Thus, nurses need to be knowledgeable about different cultural groups, but they need to use this information as a backdrop for exploring the ways in which individuals identify with the characteristics of the various cultural groups to which they belong. This is achieved by communicating a non-judgemental attitude and asking open-ended questions to elicit information about each person's life experiences and cultural influences, as discussed in Chapter 13.

In this text, culturally specific information pertinent to nursing care of older adults is discussed in the following sections of this chapter and highlighted in other chapters in featured cultural considerations boxes and diversity notes. Nurses are encouraged to supplement this information by reading journals and other references. In addition, many of the organisations listed at the end of other chapters provide culturally appropriate educational materials and resources in languages other than English. These materials can be important resources for health promotion interventions and are usually available at little or no cost. In addition, all healthcare professionals are encouraged to contact local organisations to obtain culturally specific information about groups who reside in their local area.

Performing a cultural self-assessment

Nursing texts emphasise that individual cultural competence is an ongoing process, rather than an end point, in which the nurse continuously strives to work effectively within the cultural context of the individual, family or community (Andrews, 2012a). This process is often described as a progression from judgemental attitudes and practices to positive approaches. For example, Purnell (2013) describes a continuum that begins with being unconsciously incompetent, which is being unaware that one is lacking knowledge about another culture. When the person becomes aware of this knowledge gap, he or she is consciously incompetent and takes actions to learn about the cultural group. The next stage of being consciously competent involves learning about the other culture, verifying generalisations, and providing culturally specific interventions. In the final stage, the care provider is unconsciously competent and automatically provides culturally congruent care to clients and patients of diverse cultures.

Although it is difficult for healthcare professionals to achieve high levels of cultural competency in relation to a broad spectrum of different ethnic/cultural groups, they are expected to achieve cultural competency in relation to the specific cultural groups for whom they provide care. Moreover, they are expected to be non-judgemental and avoid stereotyping by recognising the extent to which cultural views and practices influence their own attitudes and perceptions, as well as the care they provide. This can be achieved through a cultural self-assessment, which is an awareness-raising tool for gaining insight into the health-related values, beliefs, attitudes and practices that one holds (Andrews, 2012a). Box 2-1 describes a cultural self-assessment that is particularly applicable for nurses caring for older adults. It is important to recognise that people can internalise social stigma and prejudices that apply to members of one's own groups. Thus, the self-assessment includes questions to increase one's awareness of internalised stigma.

BOX 2-1
Cultural self-assessment for nurses working with older adults

What self-identity influences my world view?
- With what sociocultural and religious groups do I most closely identify?
- What does it mean to belong to these groups?
- Is there any stigma associated with any of these groups?
- What negative and positive images are associated with these groups?
- What do I like and dislike about these groups and my sociocultural identity?

How has my cultural background influenced me?
- How has (does) the society in which I grew up (currently live in) influenced the dominant values that I now hold?
- What is my perception of concepts such as time, work, leisure, health, family and relationships?
- How do my perceptions differ from those of people who come from different cultural backgrounds?

What is my attitude towards older adults who
- Are immigrants?
- Have difficulty with the English language?
- Have difficulty communicating?
- Have a cultural background different from my own?
- Look or act like the stereotype of people who are gay, lesbian or transgender?

What are my attitudes about and experiences with health practices that differ from my own?
- Do (did) members of my family have healthcare practices that differ(ed) from conventional Western medicine practices (e.g. herbs, poultices, folk remedies)?
- Do (did) they consult with folk, Indigenous, religious or spiritual healers?
- How do I feel about alternative or complementary healthcare practices for myself and for older adults?

How well do I communicate and understand?
- What do I do and how do I feel when I have difficulty understanding people whose accents and primary language are different from my own?
- What have I learned about myself because of this self-assessment?

A student's perspective

After completing the cultural assessment, I learned that I do not have a thorough grasp on my own culture. We learned in class that nurses must be aware and knowledgeable about their own culture before they can relate to their patients. I have not gotten that one under wraps yet. Doing the cultural assessment does make me aware of biases. I do feel uncomfortable thinking about immigrants, in that, I do not know who I define as immigrants or where I believe they come from. I also tend to imagine "we are all the same" when in reality all cultures are very different in positive ways, and to generalise is to say that the things that make cultures different are unimportant, when that is not true.

Doing this assessment is only the first step; I must continue to question what I believe, where I come from, and who I relate to. Then I can help my patients.

Erin H.

A student's perspective

I came from a highly educated, Christian, Caucasian family and this affects how I see the world, both consciously and unconsciously. Education is a very important part of my life. My Christian upbringing makes me value honesty, justice, compassion and forgiveness. I was raised to have an open mind and not judge people until I got to know them. I think that has been the most important idea that I live my life around.

I get very frustrated when I don't understand people because of their heavy accent or inability to speak English. I think it is important to take into consideration other's beliefs and incorporate them as best as you can into their care. I am sure I will continue to discover my true values and beliefs as I grow in nursing. I think it is a good idea to keep reviewing my own cultural beliefs so that I become aware of them and how they affect my practice.

Sarah L.

BOX 2-2
Guidelines for using interpreters

Before the interaction

- Whenever possible, use the services of a professional interpreter. Avoid using visitors or staff from auxiliary services unless permission to do so has been obtained from both the older adult and the interpreter.
- Be certain that the correct language and dialect have been identified before arranging for an interpreter. For example, does the person speak Cantonese or Mandarin Chinese?
- If an interpreter for the primary language is unavailable, determine whether the older adult speaks other languages. For example, many older adults from Vietnam and some African nations are also fluent in French.
- Be aware of age, gender and socioeconomic class considerations in selecting an interpreter. In general, it is best to use an interpreter who is the same gender and of the same approximate age and socioeconomic class as the older adult.
- Organise your thoughts and plan ahead to ensure that the most important topics are covered.
- Allow sufficient time for the interaction and expect that it will take longer than an interaction with an older adult for whom English is the primary language.

During the interaction

- Review the importance of confidentiality.
- Talk to the older adult, not the interpreter.
- Talk about only one topic at a time.
- Use short sentences and simple vocabulary.
- Use the active voice. Avoid vague modifiers.
- Avoid professional jargon, idioms and slang.
- Be aware that many words do not translate into another language. For instance, the English word depression has no equivalent in many Asian and other languages.

Linguistic competence in care of older adults

Linguistic competence, which refers to healthcare services that are respectful of and responsive to a person's linguistic needs, is a part of cultural competence. This concept is important for nurses because they work with older adults whose primary language differs from their own. Immigrants who come to Australia or New Zealand as adults may be particularly disadvantaged because they may not have the same opportunities to learn English as do school-age children. Even when older adults are able to speak English, the high prevalence of low levels of health literacy can have negative health effects (Cordasco et al., 2009). The challenge of communicating with people who do not speak the same language or dialect is magnified when the person also has dementia or sensory impairments, as is often the case in long-term residential care settings. Even if the older adults had achieved English competency since immigration, if they experience cognitive impairment, acute or progressive, they can revert back to their "mother tongue". This reversion poses a challenge for nurses involved in their care.

An excellent evidence-based protocol has been developed for nurses, called Interpreter Facilitation for Individuals with Limited English Proficiency, which provides comprehensive guidelines to facilitate the effective use of language interpretation services with older adults who have limited English proficiency (Enslein et al., 2002). Nurses need to be aware of interpreter resources available in all acute healthcare settings. All of the states within Australia and the District Health Boards in New Zealand have policies that direct the use of interpreters and outline the responsibilities of healthcare providers when using interpreters. Australia has a Centre for Cultural Diversity in Ageing that has many multilingual resources (e.g. communication cards) available at www.culturaldiversity.com.au. In Australia, an Aboriginal and Torres Strait Islander Liaison Service is available in the public hospitals to assist with communication. In New Zealand, a Māori liaison team can assist with communication with older Māori while they are in hospital. Box 2-2 summarises guidelines for using interpreters in healthcare settings with older adults.

CULTURAL PERSPECTIVES ON WELLNESS

As discussed in Chapter 1, nurses have numerous opportunities to promote wellness for older adults, even under the most challenging of circumstances, through holistic nursing interventions to improve physical comfort and psychological and spiritual growth. To achieve this, nurses need to have a good understanding of the meaning of health and wellness to each individual older adult. Nurses can explore this with older adults by asking such questions as "What does it mean to you to be healthy?" or "How do you achieve wellness in your life?" If appropriate, nurses can explore this topic from the perspective of cultural diversity with a question such as "I'm interested in knowing more about how Chinese people view wellness. Can you tell me your thoughts about this?"

Healthcare practices and beliefs of individuals are strongly influenced by the **health belief system** (defined as the health-related attitudes, beliefs and practices) of one's cultural group. Andrews (2012b) described three major health belief systems that underpin health beliefs and health-related behaviours of individuals, as summarised in Cultural considerations 2-1. It is important to recognise that many people integrate beliefs from two or all of these paradigms, but some people are firmly entrenched in one health belief system.

Examples relevant to one ethnic group, Māori, are contained in Box 2-3. It shows there are three health models that express the views Māori have about health, and all are based on wellness and a holistic approach. It has been observed by Māori that the health beliefs held by Western cultures lack *taha wairua* or the spiritual dimension (NZMOH, 2014a).

Nurses need to be aware of the health beliefs that influence the older adults so they can adapt their interventions accordingly. For example, people who adhere to the holistic paradigm described in Cultural considerations 2-1 may view their condition as an imbalance between "hot" and "cold" energies and request a particular food or herbal remedy for restoring balance.

Another focus of research about older adults is the influence of religion and spirituality on health and well-being, but very few of the studies address non-Christian faith traditions or spiritual practices outside of religion. A recent review found that higher levels of life satisfaction and well-being are reported by older adults who have a belief in the efficacy of prayer and are affiliated with a religion (Chatters, Nguyen & Taylor, 2014).

CULTURAL CONSIDERATIONS 2-1
Major health belief systems

Magico-religious paradigm

- Supernatural forces dominate the fate of the world and all those in it depend on the actions of supernatural forces (e.g. God, gods).
- Origins of illness include sorcery, breach of a taboo, intrusion of a disease object, intrusion of a disease-causing spirit, and loss of soul.
- Illness is initiated by a supernatural agent with or without justification, or by a person who practices sorcery or engages the services of sorcerers.
- Health is a gift or reward given as a sign of God's blessing and goodwill.
- Health and illness belong first to the community and then to the individual, so there is a strong sense of community.
- Common among Indigenous Australians and Middle Eastern groups.

Holistic paradigm

- Forces of nature must be kept in balance or harmony.
- Human life is only one aspect of nature and a part of the general order of the universe.
- The whole person is viewed in the context of the total environment.
- Disease is caused by an imbalance or disharmony between the human, geophysical and metaphysical forces of the universe.
- Illness is not an intruding agent but is a natural part of life's rhythmic course; health and illness are both natural parts of a continuum.
- Diseases of civilisation (e.g. unemployment, discrimination, ghettos, suicide) are just much illnesses as are biomedical diseases.
- Health and healing reflect the quality of wholeness associated with healthy functioning and well-being.
- Common among Māori, Pacific people, Asians and Indians.

Scientific (biomedical) paradigm

- Life is controlled by a series of physical and biochemical processes that can be studied and manipulated by humans.
- Principles of determinism: a cause-and-effect relationship exists for all natural phenomena.
- Principles of mechanism: life processes can be controlled through mechanical, genetic and other engineered interventions.
- Principles of reductionism: all life can be reduced or divided into smaller parts (e.g. the mind and body are two distinct entities).
- Disease is a breakdown of the human machine as a result of stress, internal damages, or external trauma or invasion.
- Health is the absence of disease.
- Common among most Western cultures.

Source: Andrews, M. M. (2012b). The influence of cultural and health belief systems on health care practices. In M. M. Andrews & J. S. Boyle. *Transcultural concepts in nursing care* (pp. 73–88). Philadelphia, PA: Lippincott Williams & Wilkins; New Zealand Ministry of Health. (2014a). Māori health models. Accessed at www.health.govt.nz/our-work/populations/maori-health/maori-health-models; Poroch, N., Arabena, K., Tongs, J., Larkin, S., Fisher, J. & Henderson, G. (2009). Spirituality and Aboriginal People's social and emotional wel being: A review. Discussion paper no. 11. Darwin: Cooperative Research Centre for Aboriginal Health; Medical Council of New Zealand. (2010). Best health outcomes for Pacific peoples: Practice implications. Accessed via www.mcnz.org.nz.

BOX 2-3
Māori health models

Te Whare Tapa Whā

The four cornerstones of Māori health are *whānau* (family health), *tinana* (physical health), *hinengaro* (mental health) and *wairua* (spiritual health).

Te Wheke

This model of health is based on *Te Wheke*, the octopus. The head of the octopus represents *te whānau* (family), the eyes of the octopus as *waiora* (total well-being for the individual and family), and each of the eight tentacles representing a specific dimension of health:

- *Wairuatanga:* spirituality
- *Hinengaro:* mind
- *Taha tinana:* physical wellbeing
- *Whanaungatanga:* extended family
- *Mauri:* life force in people and objects
- *Mana ake:* unique identity of individuals and family
- *Hā a koro ma, a kui ma:* breath of life from forbearers
- *Whatumanawa:* open and healthy expression of emotion

Te Pae Mahutonga

Te Pae Mahutonga (Southern Cross Star Constellation) is a health promotion and the model has:

- Four central stars of the Southern Cross, representing four key tasks of health promotion:
  - *Mauriora* (cultural identity)
  - *Waiora* (physical environment)
  - *Toiora* (healthy lifestyles)
  - *Te Oranga* (participation in society)
- Two pointers, representing *Ngā Manukura* (community leadership) and *Te Mana Whakahaere* (autonomy).

Source: New Zealand Ministry of Health. (2014a). Māori health models. Accessed March 2015 via www.health.govt.nz.

OVERVIEW OF CULTURAL AND ETHNIC GROUPS OF OLDER ADULTS IN AUSTRALIA AND NEW ZEALAND

To provide culturally competent care, nurses need to learn about the cultural groups in the populations they are nursing. Researchers are increasingly addressing interrelationships among race, ethnicity, ageing and health. More recently, nonprofit organisations and gerontologists are addressing the ageing-related concerns of other diverse groups such as rural, homeless and incarcerated older adults.

Information about the cultural and ethnic groups of older adults in Australia and New Zealand is presented in the following sections. Although progress has been made in research relating to diverse groups of older adults, many subgroups continue to be lumped together. It is important to realise that conclusions from studies may not apply to all the subgroups that are categorised as one. Nurses can use this information to learn about the cultural traditions of the people they are nursing, as stated earlier, and must be careful not to generalise or stereotype on the basis of a person's race or ethnicity.

Indigenous people

This section provides a description the demographics, health determinants, health status and care utilisation of older Indigenous people in Australia and New Zealand.

Indigenous Australians

The number of older Indigenous Australians 65 years and over is increasing and they comprise 0.7% of the total population (ABS, 2012). In 2011, 3.4% of the total Indigenous population were 65 years and over, while the non-Indigenous of a similar age were 14.2% of the total population (AIHW, 2014). Figure 2-3 shows the age and sex profile of Indigenous versus non-Indigenous Australians. Overall Indigenous Australians are a younger population group compared with the non-Indigenous. Indigenous Australians have a much lower life expectancy at birth (approximately 11 years less for males and 10 years less for females) than for the total population. However, as Indigenous Australians get older this difference in life expectancy between Indigenous and non-Indigenous becomes smaller. It has been estimated that the life expectancy difference is reduced to 5 years for females and 7 years for males for Indigenous Australians 65 and over (AIHW, 2007). Because of the life expectancy gap, the small population of Indigenous people over 65 and their high levels of disability, the older Indigenous Australian statistics usually include all those who are aged 50 years and over (AIHW, 2007).

Fewer Indigenous people report "very good" or "excellent" health than non-Indigenous Australians, and the greatest reported difference between these two population groups is from the older age groups (Australian Health Ministers' Advisory Council [AHMAC], 2012). Indigenous people also have higher rates of disability across all age groups than non-Indigenous people (see Figure 2-4). The difference is greatest between ages 59 years and 74 years, where double the number of Indigenous Australians required help with self-care, mobility and communication (core activities).

Indigenous people mainly live in metropolitan areas (34%) and regional areas (43%), while the remainder live in remote areas and very remote areas (AHMAC, 2015). However, one-third of Indigenous people aged 45 years and older who live in a very remote area were reported not to speak English well or at all.

Indigenous Australians are at higher risk of poor health because of such factors as poor nutrition and housing, and lower education levels (AHMAC, 2012). Older Indigenous Australians have higher rates of smoking, higher BMIs and lower levels of physical activity than non-Indigenous (Thomson et al., 2010). Diabetes, COPD and hypertension are more prevalent among Indigenous Australians than among non-Indigenous Australians (AIHW, 2011). The proportion of Indigenous people with end-stage renal disease (ESRD) at ages 45 to 54 years is about the same as non-Indigenous people at 65 years and over (Thomson et al., 2010). Tuberculosis has a higher prevalence in older Indigenous Australians and hospitalisation rates are

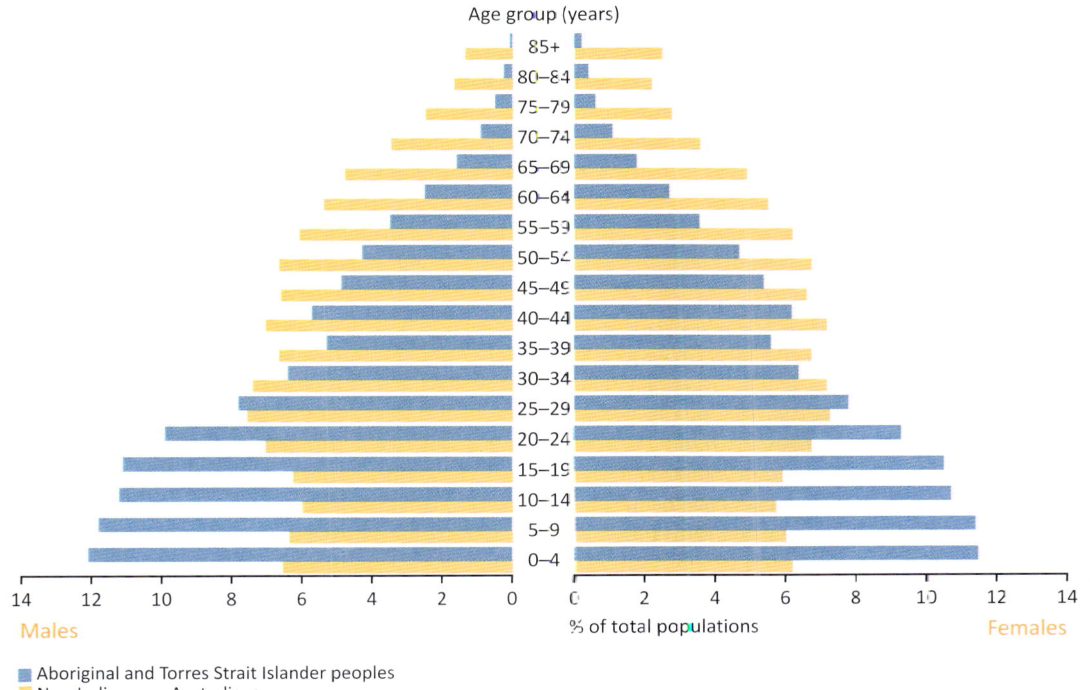

FIGURE 2-3 Age and sex profiles of Indigenous and non-Indigenous Australians, 2014 (projections). (Australian Health Ministers' Advisory Council. [2015]. *Aboriginal and Torres Strait Islander health performance framework, 2014 report* [Fig. 19, p. 17]. Canberra: Author. Permission granted under the Creative Commons Attribution 3.0 Australia Licence.)

much higher (AIHW, 2011). Hospitalisations for chronic disease in Indigenous people aged 55 years and over were higher than non-Indigenous people (AHMAC, 2012).

Generally, the use of community-based care by Indigenous Australians is higher than those of non-Indigenous Australians. Access by Indigenous Australians in remote and very remote areas is restricted because of the limited availability of community services. A unique strategy, the National Aboriginal and Torres Strait Islander Flexible Aged Care Program, has been developed by the Australian Government. This program is not a part of the Australian aged care system and therefore it is not required to comply with the *Aged Care Act 1997* (Cth). This enables the program flexibility to deliver care culturally appropriate for older Indigenous Australians. About 200 services deliver care in rural and remote areas (PC, 2011, p. 145). Older Indigenous people also use residential aged care at higher rates than non-Indigenous Australians.

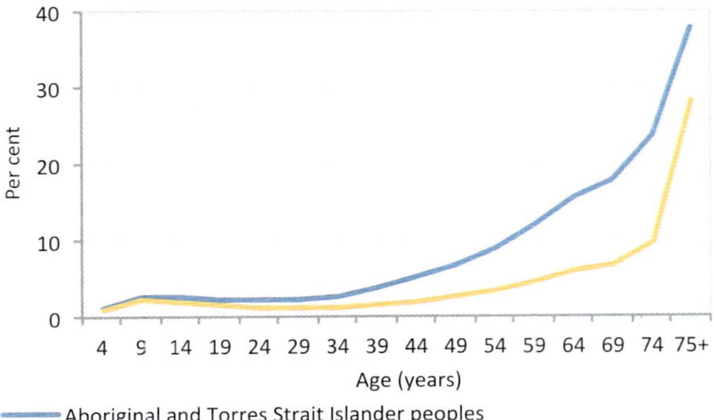

FIGURE 2-4 Proportion of persons with a core activity need for assistance by Indigenous status and aged group, 2006. (ABS and AIHW analysis of 2006 census data. In Australian Health Ministers' Advisory Council [AHMAC]. [2012]. *Aboriginal and Torres Strait Islander health performance framework, 2012 report* [Fig. 54, p. 46]. Canberra: Author.)

Improving the health status and reducing the difference in life expectancy of Indigenous Australians are the greatest challenges faced by the healthcare system in Australia. "Closing the Gap" is a state government and Australian Government initiative that aims to reduce Indigenous Australians' disadvantage in areas of education, early childhood development, health and employment (Thomson et al., 2010, p. 50).

When working with older Indigenous Australians, nurses must recognise and respond appropriately to five key domains of health and well-being that are important to this group: the spiritual, cultural, social, psychological and physical domains (de Crespigny, cited in Lewis & Foley, 2014, p. 168). Nurses must also understand that involving family has been identified as a key factor when facilitating the health of Indigenous people. Engaging with families in a culturally competent way is recommended to improve health literacy and reduce health disparities (AHMAC, 2012). Nurses may suggest that the older Indigenous person "…be visited by a trusted Elder from their community or a Traditional Healer…" so that they can address the spiritual, cultural and social needs (de Crespigny, 2014, p. 168).

CASE STUDY ONE

Mrs Irvin is a 62-year-old Indigenous woman who lives with her daughter and son-in-law. Mrs Irvin believes that health is closely linked with being in harmony with the environment, family members and supernatural forces. She regularly attends Indigenous healing ceremonies. Mrs Irvin has had diabetes and hypertension for several years, and is about 10 kilograms over her ideal weight. She receives medical care at the Indigenous Health Service, where you are the nurse. During a recent visit you found Mrs Irvin's blood pressure was 164/98 mm Hg; her random blood sugar level as measured on the glucometer was 10 mmol/L. You know from previous visits that Mrs Irvin does not want to take any prescription medications because she thinks they are not in harmony with spiritual forces. When you explain that both her blood sugar and blood pressure are high, she promises you that she will visit a traditional healer. You know from your experience with the Indigenous Health Service that nurses have been successful in persuading Indigenous people to perform physical exercise if it is viewed in a larger cultural context. For example, when the nurse consulted an Elder in developing an exercise program, the Indigenous people at a community health centre were receptive to incorporating mild aerobic exercise into their daily routines in the form of traditional dance movements.

Thinking points

- What cultural factors are likely to influence Mrs Irvin's understanding of diabetes and hypertension?
- How would you use metaphors and cultural knowledge to help Mrs Irvin understand her diabetes and hypertension?
- What questions would you ask Mrs Irvin to identify teaching strategies and other interventions that might be successful with regard to her diabetes and hypertension?
- What strategies are likely to be successful in implementing dietary and lifestyle interventions for Mrs Irvin?
- What steps would you take to improve your cultural competence in working with Mrs Irvin?

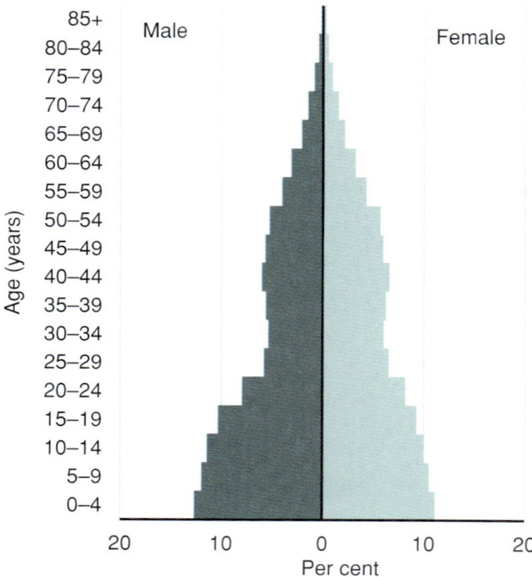

FIGURE 2-5 Age distribution of the Māori population in New Zealand, by gender, 2013. (Statistics New Zealand [2014]. Census QuickStats about culture and identity. Accessed via www.stats.govt.nz. Permission granted under the Creative Commons Attribution 3.0 New Zealand licence.)

Māori

Approximately 1.2 million people (30%) aged 50 years or above were recorded in 2006, and 6.8% of this age group were Māori (NZMOH, 2011a). The proportion of Māori aged 65 years and over was only 0.57% of the total population. Figure 2-5 shows the age distribution of the Māori by gender for 2013. The Māori are a much younger population group than the non-Māori. However the proportion of Māori aged 65 years and over has increased from 4.1% in 2006 to 5.4% in 2013 (Statistics New Zealand, 2014). Between 2005 and 2007, life expectancy at birth was 8.6 years less for Māori males and 7.9 years less for Māori females than non-Māori (New Zealand Ministry of Social Development, 2010).

Like the Indigenous Australians, Māori have a life expectancy gap, a smaller proportion of the population of Indigenous people over 65 years, and higher levels of disability as they age (NZMOH, 2011a). Consequently, older Māori statistics usually include all those who are aged 50 years and over. It is expected that between 2011 and 2026, the older Māori population will increase by 7%, while the older non-Māori population will increase only by 3.3%. It has been forecasted that the Māori will make up 9.5% of the older population in New Zealand by 2026.

Older Māori were less advantaged across all the socio-economic indicators that were surveyed in the 2006 census than older non-Māori (NZMOH, 2011a). Older Māori compared with non-Māori are four times more likely to live in the most deprived areas. Older Māori have significantly lower health literacy skills than non-Māori, and this contributes to a reduced ability to make informed and appropriate health decisions. The prevalence of smoking is significantly higher for Māori females in the 50–64 years group compared with non-Māori females of the same age. Older Māori are significantly more likely to be overweight or obese.

Overall older Māori and non-Māori have similar utilisation rates of medical practitioners in general practice (NZMOH, 2011a). Older Māori also report going to a Māori primary healthcare provider first when feeling unwell or injured. However, evidence suggests that older Māori had significantly higher "deaths from those conditions for which variation in mortality rates (over time and across populations) reflects variation in the coverage and quality of healthcare delivered to individuals" than older non-Māori (p. 58). More information about the health of older Māori is contained in the *Tatau Kura Tangata: Health of older Māori chart book 2011*, available via www.health.govt.nz.

Improving the health status of older Māori is one of the greatest challenges faced by the healthcare system in

New Zealand (NZMOH, 2011a). "Māori health and disability providers that are owned and governed by Māori are a distinctive feature of the New Zealand health sector and play a crucial role in developing health services that work for Māori" (p. 2). These services provide a range of healthcare, which is delivered in a way that empowers Māori to become active participants in their healthcare. A resource, Statement on best practices when providing care to Māori patients and their *whānau*, produced by the Medical Council of New Zealand (2006), provides an understanding of what is required by health professionals when working with this population group and it is available via www.mcnz.org.au.

The NCNZ (2011) provides guidelines for nurses for cultural safety, the *Treaty of Waitangi*, and Māori health. When interacting with older Māori, nurses must:

- Acknowledge and respect the diversity of worldviews that might exist among Māori consumers or health services
- Understand the historical processes and social, economic and political power relationships that have contributed to the current status of Māori health
- Embody the principle of the *Treaty of Waitangi*, now integral to the Public Health and Disability Act (2000)
- Reflect the values inherent in *Kawa Whakaruruhau*.

(Topia, cited in Lewis & Foley, 2014, p. 184)

Other ethnic groups

Australia

Older adults born overseas in non-English-speaking countries (CALD) are a diverse group and each CALD population has a unique set of health characteristics and issues. Of the 36% of older Australians born overseas in 2011, 14% were from English-speaking countries and 22% from other countries (AIHW, 2013). Most, 73%, were originally from Europe. This population group has an older age structure, with 18% aged 65 years and over, whereas of the Australian born, 12% were aged 65 years and over.

Figure 2-6 shows the number of older adults by age, sex and cultural and linguistic background. Older people of Italian and Greek origin are the two largest groups of CALD older people. These two groups and other CALD older people are more likely to live with a spouse and family than other Australians. Evidence available suggests that CALD older people tend to have higher life expectancies than those older immigrants from English-speaking countries, and are higher than in their country of origin. It has been hypothesised that the "healthy migrant" effect (migration selected on health) is the reason for this difference. People from countries such as Vietnam and China have particularly high life expectancies (AIHW, 2007). Older people from Lebanon, Turkey and Vietnam have lower social and economic well-being than other CALD older people and other older Australians (Khoo, 2012). The CALD older people from Malaysia, Singapore, Hong Kong, India and Sri Lanka usually have good English-language skills, education and better incomes than other older people from Asia.

CALD older people generally have lower rates of death for some causes of death than other older Australians (AIHW, 2010). However, the death rates were higher for diabetes among those people born in Greece, Italy, Lebanon and Poland and higher for coronary heart disease for those born in Poland (p. 271). Many CALD older people are more involved with their families than other older Australians (Khoo, 2012). They generally participate less in paid employment and volunteering. There is evidence that they access some health services less than other Australians. For instance, CALD females aged between 50 and 69 years were less likely to participate in breast screening (45%) than other females (59%) (AIHW, 2011).

It has been reported that older CALD are more likely to need assistance with core activities—25% CALD versus 17% other Australians (AIHW, 2013). They are also more likely to

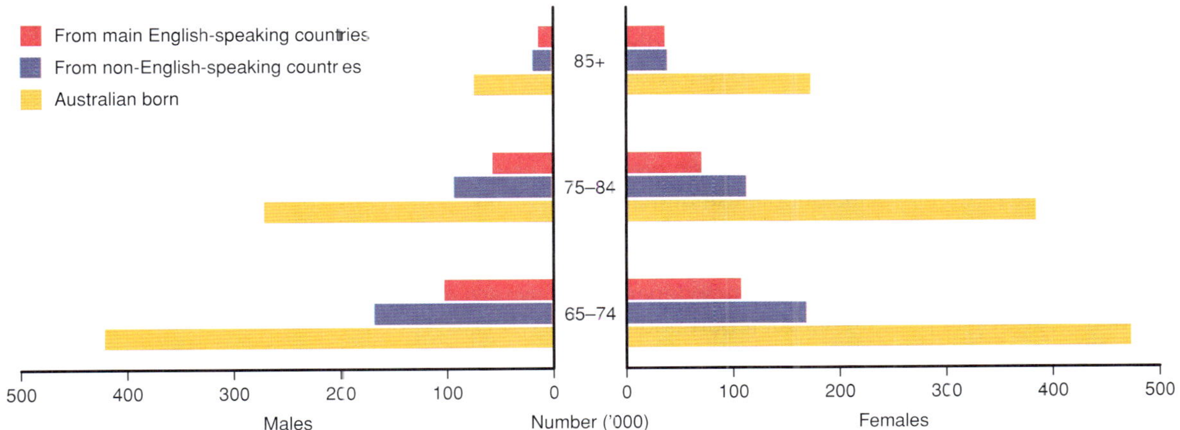

FIGURE 2-6 Older Australians by age, sex and cultural and linguistic background, 30 June 2006. (Australian Institute of Health and Welfare. [2007]. *Older Australia at a glance* [4th ed.]. Cat. no. AGE 52. Canberra: Author. Permission granted under a Creative Commons BY 3.0 [CC BY 3.0] licence.)

use home-based rather than residential care services (AIHW, 2007). Community aged care services have been successful in providing services to CALD who are older in Australia. This may be because of "… cultural preferences and practices concerning family and home-based care, their English language proficiency and the availability of residential care which is considered to be culturally appropriate" (AIHW, 2007, p. 147). CALD people who are older enter long-term residential care at much higher dependency levels than other Australians.

In Australia, two services developed to assist the delivery of culturally appropriate care to older people from CALD backgrounds are the Community Partners Program (CPP), and the Partners in Culturally Appropriate Care Program (PICAC) (PC, 2011).

New Zealand

The two largest groups of CALD older people in New Zealand, besides Māori, are Pacific and Asian people. The Pacific population group as a whole has a much younger age structure than the total population, and only 4% of Pacific people were aged over 65 years, compared with 12% of the total population in the 2006 census (NZMOH, 2014b).

Overall, older Pacific people have a lower life expectancy than any other ethnic groups, excluding Māori (NZMOH, 2011b). Their social and economic well-being is low, where nearly one-third live in severe hardship compared with 8% of the total population. Only 1% of older Pacific people report enjoying "very good living standards". They are also less likely to own their own homes (26% compared with 55% nationally) and more likely to live in overcrowded households. They also have high levels of risk factors for disease. The prevalence of smoking and obesity is high among the Pacific people, approximately 31% and 65%, respectively (New Zealand Ministry of Social Development, 2010).

The poor social and economic well-being and risk factors for disease of the Pacific people contribute to their poor health status (NZMOH, 2011b). The older Pacific people have higher rates of chronic diseases, leading to higher mortality and morbidity. Cardiovascular disease, stroke and cancer are the major causes of death. The prevalence of diabetes is approximately three times higher for Pacific people than other New Zealanders. Despite the high prevalence of chronic diseases, the Pacific people use primary and preventative health care services less than other New Zealanders.

Pacific people have higher rates of emergency department attendances and GP appointments but report poorer outcomes and receive fewer referrals for the management of chronic diseases. A number of barriers have been identified for Pacific people in accessing primary and other healthcare services (Medical Council of New Zealand, 2010). A resource, Best health outcomes for Pacific peoples: Practice implications, provides and understanding of what is required by health professionals when working with this population group. It is available at www.mcnz.org.au.

The health of the older Asian ethnic group, which includes Chinese, Indian and other Asians, across a range of health characteristics has been shown to be of an equitable standard to other New Zealanders (NZMOH, 2007). Some of these characteristics for older Asians include the following (NZMOH, 2006):

- Most indicators of the health of the older Asian ethnic group, particularly the Chinese, are excellent.
- The deprivation distribution is similar to the total New Zealand population.
- They are more likely to have higher educational qualifications than the average New Zealander.
- The prevalence of smoking (13%) and obesity (12%) is lower than the Pacific people and Māori.
- English is not an issue for the Indian group.
- The health status, especially of the Chinese group, is higher than would be expected given their socioeconomic position.

However, there are some inequalities for older Asians. These include:

- The incomes of Asian New Zealanders are lower than those of the total population.
- English language is an issue for some Chinese and the other-Asians group.
- There is a high prevalence of obesity, type 2 diabetes and cardiovascular disease among the Indian ethnic group.

There are differences in health service use between older Asians and others. For instance, older Asians are significantly less likely to have visited a medical practitioner in the last 12 months than New Zealand Europeans (NZMOH, 2007). Women of this group also have lower levels of mammography and cervical screening when compared with New Zealand European women.

CASE STUDY TWO

Mrs Chan is a 76-year-old Chinese widow who lives in a city apartment. She has lived within the same 1-kilometre radius since her parents brought her to the city from Mainland China when she was 14 years old. All three of her children are married; two live about an hour away, and the other one lives in another state. Although she can speak and read English, she prefers to use her native Chinese dialect, and all of her reading materials are in Chinese. She completed a high-school education in Chinatown and married a Chinese immigrant when she was 19 years old. She served as her husband's primary caregiver after he developed lung cancer several years ago until his death last year.

Mrs Chan has hypertension, arthritis and coronary artery disease. Mrs Chan sees a local herbalist every few weeks to obtain the herbal medicines that will keep her yin and yang energies in balance, and she chooses foods according to their yin and yang characteristics. She periodically has acupuncture treatments when her arthritis bothers her. Although Mrs Chan believes she can control her heart problem and high blood pressure with herbs and diet, she takes her two medications as prescribed because the nurse at the medical clinic has emphasised that these pills are essential for keeping her energy in balance.

Mrs Chan recently had a stroke and received medical treatment and rehabilitation services. She is being discharged to her apartment with a referral for community nursing. Discharge orders also include the need to instruct Mrs Chan in a low-sodium diet. In addition to having some aphasia and left-sided paralysis, Mrs Chan has some residual memory impairment from the stroke. Before discharge from the rehabilitation program, she said she would not need any home health-aide assistance because she expected that her daughter and daughter-in-law would take turns coming over every day and that they would take care of her. You are the nurse assigned to do the initial assessment and your visit is scheduled for the day after discharge when the daughter-in-law will be there.

Thinking points

- What cultural factors might influence Mrs Chan's acceptance of you and of home care services in general?
- What would you do to gain cultural competence to work more effectively with Mrs Chan?
- What are your specific healthcare concerns for Mrs Chan, and what strategies would you use to develop an effective and acceptable care plan?

OLDER ADULTS IN OTHER DIVERSE GROUPS

It is important to recognise that the concept of cultural competence encompasses all groups of people, including one's own group, because people can be influenced by internalised stigma. As already discussed, nurses need to periodically perform a cultural self-assessment and learn about other cultural groups. Some cultural differences are quite obvious (e.g. people with differently coloured skin or a different spoken language), but many differences are subtle, not noticed, or even purposefully hidden (e.g. sexual orientation, religious affiliations). Nurses need to learn about groups of older adults who may be less visible and smaller in numbers but with unique needs. In recent years, gerontologists are identifying the needs of some of these groups, such as those considered rural or homeless. Other groups, such as those who are discriminated against because of sexual orientation, are advocating on their own behalf to identify and address their unique needs. Information about some of these groups is discussed in this section, and nurses are encouraged to use the resources listed at the end of this chapter to learn more about these and other groups.

Older adults in rural areas

Although significant local differences exist among rural areas, some common characteristics and needs have been identified. Populations in rural regions in Australia, including older adults, tend to be poorer and less educated and have worse health outcomes than their urban counterparts (AIHW, 2007). The 2006 census older adults were mostly living in large cities, 35% regional areas, and 1% in remote communities (p. 150). In addition, the number of older adults in rural areas is rising (PC, 2011).

Health status is poorer and life expectancy is also lower for rural older adults (AIHW, 2007). Older adults in regional and "... remote areas are more likely to be smokers, to drink alcohol in hazardous quantities, to be overweight or obese, and to be physically inactive" (p. 150). Rural older adults have limited transportation options and less access to healthcare services, including meal and social programs, because of isolation. It is expected that there will be an increased demand in rural areas for healthcare service by older adults (PC, 2011).

Homeless older adults

The category of "older homeless" typically extends downwards to the age of 50 years because homeless people have significant health problems and other characteristics typically associated with older chronological age. Increased homelessness among older adults is associated with increased poverty rates among certain segments and declining availability of affordable housing. Homeless people 65 years old and older are entitled to health services provided by the government but, in many instances, they do not feel empowered to access services or do not realise they need care (PC, 2011). Approximately 6200 homeless older adults aged over 65 years were identified in the Australian 2011 census and account for 6% of the homeless population in Australia (AIHW, 2013).

Health disparities among homeless older adults include significantly higher mortality rates, higher levels of disability, higher overall rates of chronic and mental illnesses, and high rates of geriatric syndromes (e.g. falls, frailty, major depression, urinary incontinence, and cognitive and sensory impairment) (Brown, Kiely, Bharel et al., 2013; Hearth Inc., 2011). Since the mid 1980s, social service and healthcare providers have recognised the need to provide rehabilitative services to address health, social and behavioural problems of homeless older adults, in addition to addressing their basic needs for food and shelter.

Lesbian, gay, bisexual, and transgender older adults

Lesbian, gay, bisexual, and transgender (LGBT) older adults have been called "the invisible elderly" and nurses are increasingly recognising the need to identify and address the unique needs of these diverse groups (Hardacher, Rubinstein, Hotton et al., 2013; Jablonski, Vance & Beattie et al., 2013). The acronym LGBT is an umbrella term that includes three groups whose sexual orientation is not heterosexual (lesbian, gay or bisexual), and several groups whose gender identity and/or gender expression differs from the sex they were assigned at birth (e.g. transgender, cross-dressers). Although sexual orientation and gender identity are distinct entities, these subgroups share a common bond of being viewed outside the norms of sexual expression and identity and they all experience similar societal stigma, isolation, stereotypes and prejudices. Surveys estimate that about 2% of adults age 50 years and older self-identify as lesbian, gay or bisexual, and that this population will double between 2000 and 2030 (Fredriksen-Goldensen, 2011). Despite the relatively small numbers and invisibility of LGBT older adults, there is growing recognition of the unique barriers, challenges and disparities that affect these groups, as indicated by such recent developments as:

- The American Society on Aging, the Gerontological Society of America and other major professional organisations supporting research, education and training related to LGBT older adults.
- The Australian Government releasing the National Lesbian, Gay, Bisexual, Transgender and Intersex Ageing and Aged Care Strategy in 2012, the first national strategy in the world to focus on the needs of LGBT elders, available via www.dss.gov.au.
- The establishment in Australia of the Rainbow Tick program, which is a process where healthcare services in Victoria can be accredited because they are able to meet LGBT needs, available via Gay and Lesbian Health at www.glhv.org.au.
- In New Zealand the release of the Silver Rainbow kit: Caring for lesbian, gay and bisexual (LGB) residents in aged residential care, prepared in collaboration by the School of Nursing at the University of Auckland. These guidelines for care staff, which provide best practice information for rest homes and the community, are available via the university at www.tamaki.auckland.ac.nz.

These initiatives and reports universally identify a need for more evidence-based recommendations addressing health-related needs of subgroups that are currently under the umbrella term of LGBT. The little research that has been done on LGBT older adults has focused disproportionately on whites, lesbians and gay men, with very limited attention to bisexual, transgender, racial/ethnic minorities, or those who are 85 years and older (Institute of Medicine, 2011). Consequently, it is imperative to keep in mind that conclusions about LGBT older adults are based on limited research and do not necessarily apply to individuals or even subgroups within the larger group.

A common bond among different subgroups of LGBT individuals is their experiences of various levels and types of stigma, but this varies significantly because vastly different sociopolitical forces shape each age group. Cohorts of LGBT older adults older than 70 years entered into young adulthood at a time when homosexuality was considered a crime or a mental illness. This group of older adults has lived through unique experiences, including a lifelong process of coming out, marginalisation inside and outside the LGBT community, multidimensional effects of the HIV/AIDS epidemic, and LGBT pride and resilience (Institute of Medicine, 2011; Van Wagenen, Driskell & Bradford, 2013). Among the subgroups included in LGBT, transgender older adults are the ones who experience the most stigma, victimisation, discrimination and misunderstandings (Fredriksen-Goldensen et al., 2013; Institute of Medicine, 2011).

Many LGBT people experience their sexual orientation along a continuum and they do not necessarily live as either heterosexual or gay/lesbian during their entire adult lives. Moreover, 70% of transgender older adults report that they delayed gender transition treatments to avoid discrimination in employment (Grant, Mottet, Tanis et al., 2011). Thus, it is important to recognise that older LGBT individuals vary widely not only in the length of time they have identified themselves as such but also in the ways in which they have addressed their sexual identities.

Some LGBT have biological, adopted or step children, grandchildren or great grandchildren, and very close relationships with their families. Other LGBT older adults have no biological family—or have been rejected by their families—but they have strong bonds with their "family of choice". This extended network of family and friends often becomes the caregivers for older LGBT who need assistance, but all people involved in these situations face social, economic and legal challenges that do not affect heterosexuals. Older LGBT vary greatly in their intimate relationships and many have had or continue to have monogamous, committed partnerships. However, these relationships are not universally associated with the same legal standing as traditional heterosexual marriages. An important aspect of providing culturally competent care for LGBT older adults is using gender-neutral terminology in reference to intimate or partner relationships, which is a topic discussed in Chapter 26. Some LGBT older adults, especially couples in committed long-term relationships, live very comfortably; however, others do not. An absence of studies on LGBT groups is considered one of the most pronounced gaps in health-disparities research, and consequently it has become a research priority. Some recent information is available, as in the following examples:

- Lesbian, bisexual and gay adults aged 50 years and older have a higher risk of disability, poor mental health, smoking and excessive drinking.
- Bisexual men aged 50 years and older have a higher rate of diabetes and a lower rate of being tested for HIV than gay men.
- Transgender adults aged 50 years and older are at significantly higher risk for poor physical health, increased functional impairment, perceived stress, and depressive symptoms.
- Lifetime victimisation and financial barriers to healthcare are factors that significantly and independently

contribute to health disparities among lesbian, gay and bisexual older adults. (Fredriksen-Goldensen et al., 2012)

Despite the prominence of health disparities and other issues that affect LGBT older adults, there is much evidence pointing toward resilience and strengths. On a positive note, many older adults who identify as lesbian, gay, bisexual or transgender report that their experiences prepare them for ageing by helping them overcome adversity. Strengths identified in a study of more than 1200 LGBT older adults included being more accepting of others, not taking anything for granted, being more resilient, having greater inner strength, having greater self-reliance, having a chosen family, and being more careful about legal and financial matters (Institute of Medicine, 2011).

CHAPTER HIGHLIGHTS

Cultural diversity in Australia and New Zealand

- The populations of Australia and New Zealand, including older adults, are increasing in diversity (Figures 2-1 & 2-2).

Health disparities

- Members of ethnic groups experience many health inequalities, and these have significant implications for older adults.

Health literacy

- Health literacy is a major determinant of health outcomes and a measure of quality of care.
- Lower health literacy has been reported for some diverse groups of older adults in Australia and New Zealand.

Cultural competence and cultural safety

- All nurses are expected to develop cultural competence and cultural safety by assessing their own attitudes (Box 2-1) and learning about culturally diverse groups.
- All healthcare providers need to be linguistically competent and be able to use resources to address needs of people who are not proficient in English (Box 2-2).

Cultural perspectives on wellness

- Nurses need to explore what health and wellness mean to individual older adults.
- Definitions of health and wellness are embedded in the three major health belief systems (Cultural considerations 2-1).

Overview of cultural groups of older adults in Australia and New Zealand

- Both Australia and New Zealand have many CALD groups (Figure 2-6). Both countries have an Indigenous population: Indigenous Australians and Māori (Figures 2-3 & 2-5).
- Nurses can develop cultural safety and competence by educating themselves about the cultural traditions of the older adults in their geographical areas.
- Characteristics of some of these groups are summarised, but it is important to recognise that the larger groups are composed of many subgroups and there is great diversity within them.

Older adults in other diverse groups

- Researchers and non-profit organisations are identifying and addressing the unique needs of other diverse groups, including rural, homeless and LGBT older adults.

CRITICAL THINKING EXERCISES

1. Complete the cultural self-assessment in Box 2-1 and think about whether you have internalised any stigma or prejudices about any of the cultural groups to which you belong.
2. Reflect on your encounters during the past few weeks with people who differ from you culturally. Make a list of the obvious differences and another list of differences that you may not have recognised but most likely existed (e.g. you most likely interacted with someone who was LGBT). Ask yourself how accepting and non-judgemental you feel about these people.
3. Identify one culturally diverse group that you are likely to work within your current geographic area. Contact the agencies and organisations that serve these groups to find out what services they offer; ask about unique healthcare issues affecting these particular groups.
4. Go to the Internet site of a culturally specific organisation listed in the resources section and find information that you might use if you were presenting a health education program to a group of older adults who are of a particular cultural background (e.g. Chinese). Think about how the health promotion materials for a specific cultural group differ to those that have been developed for the Western culture.
5. Think of the various settings in which you work with older adults and describe what you would do or whom you would call if you needed to communicate with a person who did not speak English.

RESOURCES

For an extensive range of additional resources to enhance teaching and learning and to facilitate understanding of this chapter, please see the text's accompanying website located on thePoint at http://thepoint.lww.com.

Aboriginal Health & Medical Research Council of New South Wales (AH&MRC): www.ahmrc.org.au

Australian Indigenous Health*InfoNet:* www.healthinfonet.ecu.edu.au

Australian Institute of Health and Welfare: http://aihw.gov.au

Centre for Cultural Diversity in Ageing (Australia): www.culturaldiversity.com.au
Centre for Culture, Ethnicity and Health: www.ceh.org.au
Directory on Cultural Diversity (New Zealand): www.decisionmaker.co.nz
Gay and Lesbian Health Victoria: www.glhv.org.au
Māori Health: www.maorihealth.govt.nz
Ministry of Pacific Island Affairs: www.minpac.govt.nz
New Zealand Ministry of Health: www.health.govt.nz
Nursing Council of New Zealand (NCNZa): www.nursingcouncil.org.nz/About-us/Treaty-of-Waitangi
Nursing Council of New Zealand (NCNZb): www.nursingcouncil.org.nz/Nurses/Code-of-Conduct
Office of Ethnic Affairs, ethnic communities: http://ethniccommunities.govt.nz
Pacific Peoples Health: www.pacificpeopleshealth.co.nz
Te Puni Kōkiri (Ministry of Māori Development): www.tpk.govt.nz

REFERENCES

Abdou, C. M. (2014). Minority aging before birth and beyond: Life span and intergenerational adaptation through positive resources. In K. E. Whitfield & T. A. Baker (Eds), *Handbook of minority aging* (pp. 9–24). New York, NY: Springer.

Andrews, M. M. (2012a). Culturally competent nursing care. In M. M. Andrews & J. S. Boyle (Eds), *Transcultural concepts in nursing care* (6th ed., pp. 17–37). Philadelphia, PA: Lippincott Williams & Wilkins.

Andrews, M. M. (2012b). The influence of cultural and health belief systems on health care practices. In M. M. Andrews & J. S. Boyle (Eds), *Transcultural concepts in nursing care* (6th ed., pp. 73–88). Philadelphia, PA: Lippincott Williams & Wilkins.

Australian Bureau of Statistics (ABS). (2009). Health literacy. Accessed March 2015 at www.abs.gov.au/AUSSTATS/abs@.nsf/Lookup/4102.0Main+Features20June+2009.

Australian Bureau of Statistics (ABS). (2012). Who are Australia's older people? From *Reflecting a nation: Stories from the 2011 census*. Cat. no. 2071.0. Canberra: Author. Accessed March 2015 at www.abs.gov.au/ausstats/abs@.nsf/lookup/2071.0main+features752012-2013.

Australian Health Ministers' Advisory Council (AHMAC). (2012). *Aboriginal and Torres Strait Islander health performance framework, 2012 report*. Canberra: Author.

Australian Health Ministers' Advisory Council (AHMAC). (2015). *Aboriginal and Torres Strait Islander health performance framework, 2014 report* (pp. 16–17). Canberra: Author. Viewed June 2015 via www.dpmc.gov.au/indigenous-affairs/publication/hpf.

Australian Institute of Health and Welfare (AIHW). (2007). *Older Australia at a glance* (4th ed.). Cat. no. AGE 52. Canberra: Author. Retrieved March 2015 from www.aihw.gov.au/publication-detail/?id=6442468045.

Australian Institute of Health and Welfare (AIHW). (2010). *Australia's health 2010*. Health series no. 12. Cat. no. AUS 122. Canberra: Author. Retrieved from www.aihw.gov.au/publication-detail/?id=6442468376.

Australian Institute of Health and Welfare (AIHW). (2011). *Australia's welfare 2011*. Welfare series no. 10. Cat. no. AUS 145. Canberra: Author. Retrieved from http://aihw.gov.au/publication-detail/?id=10737420536.

Australian Institute of Health and Welfare (AIHW). (2012). *Australia's health* 2012. Accessed March 2015 at www.aihw.gov.au/WorkArea/DownloadAsset.aspx?id=10737422169.

Australian Institute of Health and Welfare (AIHW). (2013). *Australia's welfare 2013*. Welfare series no.11. Cat. no. AUS 174. Canberra: Author.

Australian Institute of Health and Welfare (AIHW). (2014). *Australia's health 2014*. Health series no. 14. Cat. no. AUS 178. Canberra: Author.

Brown, R. T., Kiely, D. K., Bharel, M., et al. (2013). Factors associated with geriatric syndromes in older homeless adults. *Journal of Health Care for Poor and Underserved, 24*(2), 456–468.

Chatters, L. M., Nguyen, A. W. & Taylor, R. J. (2014). Religion and spirituality among older African Americans. In K. E. Whitfield & T. A. Baker (Eds), *Handbook of minority aging* (pp. 47–64). New York, NY: Springer.

Cloonan, P., Wood, J. & Riley, J. B. (2013). Reducing 30-day readmissions: Health literacy strategies. *Journal of Nursing Administration, 43*(7/8), 382–387.

Cordasco, K. M., Asch, S. M., Franco, I. & Mangione, C. M. (2009). Health literacy and English language comprehension among elderly inpatients at an urban safety-net hospital. *Journal of Health and Human Services Administration, 32*(1), 30–50.

De Crespigny, C. (2014). Assessment in Aboriginal and Torres Strait Islander communities. In Lewis, P. & Foley, D. (Eds), *Weber & Kelly's health assessment in nursing* (2nd Australian and New Zealand ed.). Sydney: Lippincott Williams & Wilkins.

Enslein, J., Tripp-Reimer, T., Kelley, L. S., Choi, E. & McCarty, L. (2002). Interpreter facilitation for individuals with limited English proficiency. *Journal of Gerontological Nursing, 28*(7), 5–11.

Fredriksen-Goldensen, K. I. (2011). Resilience and disparities among lesbian, gay, bisexual, and transgender older adults. *Public Policy and Aging Report, 21*(3), 3–7.

Fredriksen-Goldensen, K. I., Cook-Daniels, L., Kim, H-J. et al. (2013). Physical and mental health of transgender older adults: An at-risk and underserved population. *Gerontologist, 54*(3), 488–500.

Fredriksen-Goldensen, K. I., Emlet, C. A., Kim, H-J. et al. (2012). Physical and mental health of lesbian, gay male, and bisexual (LGB) older adults: The role of key health indicators and risk and protective factors. *Gerontologist, 53*(4), 664–675.

Fredriksen-Goldensen, K. I., Kim, H-J., Barkan, S. E. et al. (2013). Health disparities among lesbian, gay, and bisexual older adults: Results from a population-based study. *American Journal of Public Health, 103*(10), 1802–1809.

Grant, J. M., Mottet, L. A., Tanis, J. et al. (2011). *Injustice at every turn: A report of the National Transgender Discrimination Survey*. Washington, DC: National Center for Tansgender Equality and National Gay and Lesbian Task Force.

Hardacher, C. T., Rubinstein, B., Hotton, A. et al. (2013). Adding silver to the rainbow: The development of the nurses' health education about LGBT elders cultural competency curriculum. *Journal of Nursing Management, 22*(2), 257–266.

Hearth Inc. (2011). Ending homelessness among older adults and elders through permanent supportive housing. Available March 2015 via http://hearthinc.squarespace.com/publications.

Institute of Medicine. (2011). *Health of lesbian, gay, bisexual, and transgender people: Building a foundation for better understanding*. Washington, DC: National Academies Press.

Institute of Medicine. (2013). *Health literacy: Improving health, health systems, and health policy around the world*. Workshop summary. Washington, DC: National Academies Press.

Jablonski, R. A., Vance, D. E. & Beattie, E. (2013). The invisible elderly: Lesbian, gay, bisexual, and transgender older adults. *Journal of Gerontological Nursing, 39*(11), 46–52.

Khoo, S.-E. (2012). Ethnic disparities in social and economic well-being of the immigrant aged in Australia. *Journal of Population Research, 29*(2), 119–140. Accessed March 2015 at http://link.springer.com/article/10.1007%2Fs12546-012-9080-y.

Lincoln, K. D. (2014). Social relationships and health among minority older adults. In K. E. Whitfield & T. A Baker (Eds), *Handbook of minority aging* (pp. 25–46). New York, NY: Springer.

Medical Council of New Zealand. (2006). Statement on best practices when providing care to Māori patients and their *whānau*. Accessed March 2015 at www.mcnz.org.nz/assets/News-and-Publications/Statements/Statement-on-best-practices-when-providing-care-to-Maori-patients-and-their-whanau.pdf.

Medical Council of New Zealand. (2010). Best health outcomes for Pacific peoples: Practice implications. Accessed March 2015 at www.mcnz.org.nz.

Nash, R., Meiklejohn, B. & Sacre, S. (2006). The Yapunyah Project: Embedding Aboriginal and Torres Strait Islander perspectives in the nursing curriculum. *Contemporary Nurse, 22*(2), 296–316.

National Health and Hospitals Reform Commission (NHHRC). (2009). A healthier future for all Australians: Final report of the National Health and Hospitals Reform Commission—June 2009. Canberra: Commonwealth of Australia.

National Health and Medical Research Council (NHMRC). (2006). *Cultural competency in health: A guide for policy, partnerships and participation*. Canberra: Author. Accessed March 2015 at www.nhmrc.gov.au/_files_nhmrc/publications/attachments/hp19.pdf.

Nemmers, T. M., Jorge, M. & Leahy, T. (2013). Health literacy and aging. *Topics in Geriatric Rehabilitation, 29*(2), 79–88.

New Zealand Ministry of Health (NZMOH). (2006). *Asian health chart book 2006*. Wellington: Author. Accessed March 2015 at www.health.govt.nz/publication/asian-health-chart-book-2006.

New Zealand Ministry of Health (NZMOH). (2007). *Older people's health chart book 2006*. Wellington: Author. Accessed March 2015 at www.health.govt.nz/publication/older-peoples-health-chart-book-2006.

New Zealand Ministry of Health (NZMOH). (2010). *Kōrero Mārama: Health literacy and Māori: Results from the 2006 Adult Literacy and Life Skills Survey*. Wellington: Author.

New Zealand Ministry of Health (NZMOH). (2011a). *Tatau Kura Tangata: Health of older Māori chart book 2011*. Wellington: Author. Accessed March 2015 at www.health.govt.nz/publication/tatau-kura-tangata-health-older-maori-chart-book-2011.

New Zealand Ministry of Health (NZMOH). (2011b). Pacific people's health. Accessed March 2015 via www.stats.govt.nz.

New Zealand Ministry of Health (NZMOH). (2012). Rauemi Atawhai: A guide to developing health education resources in New Zealand. Wellington: Author.

New Zealand Ministry of Health (NZMOH). (2014a). Māori health models. Accessed March 2015 at www.health.govt.nz/our-work/populations/maori-health/maori-health-models.

New Zealand Ministry of Health (NZMOH). (2014b). Tagata Pasifika in New Zealand. Accessed March 2015 at www.health.govt.nz/our-work/populations/pacific-health/tagata-pasifika-new-zealand.

New Zealand Ministry of Social Development. (2010). *The social report 2010: Health*. Accessed March 2015 at www.socialreport.msd.govt.nz/health.

Nursing and Midwifery Board of Australia (NMBA). (2011). Code of Ethics for Nurses. Melbourne: Author. Accessed March 2015 via www.nursingmidwiferyboard.gov.au.

Nursing Council of New Zealand (NCNZ). (2011). Guidelines for cultural safety, the Treaty of Waitangi and Māori health in nursing education and practice. Wellington: Author. Accessed March 2015 via www.nursingcouncil.org.nz.

Poroch, N., Arabena, K., Tongs, J., Larkin, S., Fisher, J. & Henderson, G. (2009). Spirituality and Aboriginal People's social and emotional wellbeing: A review. Discussion paper no. 11. Darwin: Cooperative Research Centre for Aboriginal Health.

Productivity Commission (PC). (2011). Caring for older Australians. Inquiry report no. 53. Canberra: Author. Accessed March 2015 at www.pc.gov.au/__data/assets/pdf_file/0016/110932/aged-care-overview-booklet.pdf.

Purnell, L. D. (2013). *Transcultural health care: A culturally competent approach*. Philadelphia, PA: F. A. Davis.

Statistics New Zealand. (2007). *New Zealand's 65+ population: A statistical volume 2007*. Wellington: Author. Accessed March 2015 via www.stats.govt.nz.

Statistics New Zealand. (2009). *Ageing of ethnic groups (structural change and the 65+ population articles)*. Wellington: Author.

Statistics New Zealand. (2013). New Zealand General Social Survey: 2012. Accessed March 2015 via www.stats.govt.nz.

Statistics New Zealand. (2014). Census QuickStats about culture and identity. Accessed March 2015 via www.stats.govt.nz.

Thomson, N., MacRae, A,. Burns, J., Catto, M., Debuyst, O., Krom, I., Midford, R., Potter, C., Ride. K., Stumpers, S. & Urquhart, B. (2010). Overview of Australian Indigenous health status, April 2010. Perth, WA: Australian Indigenous Health*InfoNet*.

Topia, H. (2014). Assessment in Māori communities. In Lewis, P. & Foley, D. (Eds), *Weber & Kelly's health assessment in nursing* (2nd Australian and New Zealand ed.). Sydney: Lippincott Williams & Wilkins.

Van Wagenen, A., Driskell, J. & Bradford, J. (2013). "I'm still raring to go": Successful aging among lesbian, gay bisexual, and transgender older adults. *Journal of Aging Studies, 27*, 1014.

Chapter 3

Applying a nursing model for promoting wellness in older adults

By Carol Miller and Sharyn Hunter

LEARNING OBJECTIVES

After reading this chapter, you should be able to:

1. Discuss the concepts that underpin the Functional Consequences Theory for older adults.
2. Define concepts of age-related changes, risk factors and functional consequences as they relate to the nursing care of older adults.
3. Describe the domains of nursing (i.e. person, nursing, health and environment) in the context of the Functional Consequences Theory.
4. Apply the Functional Consequences Theory to the practice of nursing to promote wellness in older adults.

KEY POINTS

age-related changes	nursing
environment	older adult
Functional Consequences Theory for Promoting Wellness in Older Adults	person
	person-centred care
	risk factors
health	wellness outcomes

As discussed in Chapter 1, myths about ageing are insidious and pervasive in society and form the foundation of ageism, which has serious detrimental effects on older adults. Nurses are influenced not only by societal myths and ageist attitudes but also by their experiences with older adults in healthcare settings, which often reinforce the perception that older adults are frail, confused, depressed and dependent. These attitudes can lead to a sense of pessimism—or even hopelessness—regarding caring for older adults. Fortunately, knowledge can be an effective antidote to ageism, and the theoretical base of information about ageing has expanded exponentially during the past half-century (as discussed in Chapter 4). Research-based information enables healthcare providers to differentiate between age-related changes that are inevitable, and factors that can be addressed or even prevented. Chapters in this text provide research-based information about age-related changes and other factors affecting a particular aspect of functioning, with emphasis on the changes and risks that nurses can address. Nurses can apply this information to promote wellness for older adults by identifying ways of improving functioning and quality of life.

Theories about ageing and older adults attempt to answer questions about why and how people age, and they provide a base for identifying the risk factors that healthcare providers can address. However, they do not address *nursing* care of older adults, as does a *nursing theory* that explains relationships among the core concepts of person, nursing, health and environment. Discipline-specific nursing theories guide nursing care and are essential to promoting wellness for older adults. A recent review of the literature identified major gaps in evidence-based information to help nurses intentionally promote wellness (Strout, 2012). The **Functional Consequences Theory for Promoting Wellness in Older Adults**, which is delineated in this chapter and used throughout this text, provides a framework that nurses can use to promote wellness and improve functioning and quality of life for older adults.

A NURSING THEORY FOR WELLNESS-FOCUSED CARE OF OLDER ADULTS

During the 1980s, a model for nursing older adults was developed by C. A. Miller (1990). Since its inception, this model has emphasised the significant role of nurses in using health education interventions to promote optimal health, functioning and quality of life for older adults. The model is called the Functional Consequences Theory for Promoting Wellness in Older Adults. The model reflects and incorporates the understanding of wellness that is evolving as an integral aspect of healthcare. Nurses can apply this model in any situation in which a goal of nursing care is to promote wellness for older adults. The theory was developed to explain questions, such as "*What is unique about promoting wellness for older adults?*" and "*How can nurses address unique wellness needs of older adults?*"

The purpose of nursing theories is to describe, explain, predict or prescribe nursing care based on scientific evidence. Since the time of Florence Nightingale, nurses have developed theories that address the relationships among the domains of person, nursing, health and environment. In recent years, nursing theories are increasingly focusing on models that connect the work of theorists, researchers and practitioners (Marrs & Lowry, 2009). The Functional Consequences Theory (FCT) is based on a combination of research on ageing and health and Miller's four decades of providing nursing care for older adults. It also draws on theories that emphasise concepts related to wellness, health promotion and person-centred nursing. When it is applied in this text to specific aspects of functioning, it incorporates the currently available evidence-based practice. Thus nurses can use this theory as a framework for promoting wellness in older adults because it provides evidence-based information about factors that affect health and quality of life for older adults. The fundamental principles upon which the Functional Consequences Theory is based are:

- Person-centred nursing care, which encompasses individualistic and holistic approaches, is situated at the core of the FCT. FCT addresses the body–mind–spirit interconnectedness of each older adult, emphasises the person and recognises that wellness encompasses more than physiological functioning and that it is unique for each older adult.
- Although age-related changes are inevitable, many issues affecting older adults are caused by risk factors, which are usually diseases.
- Older adults experience *negative functional consequences* because of a combination of age-related changes and other factors that increase the risk.
- Interventions can be directed towards alleviating or modifying the negative functional consequences of other factors.
- Nurses can promote wellness in older adults through *health promotion interventions* and other nursing actions that address the negative functional consequences.
- Nursing interventions result in positive functional consequences, also called **wellness outcomes**, which enable older people to function at their highest level despite the presence of age-related changes and other factors.

This theoretical framework, shown in Figure 3-1, can be illustrated by the following example.

Example of the theory related to an older person's vision

Because of age-related visual changes, older adults experience an increased sensitivity to glare and have difficulty seeing clearly when they face bright lights or when lights reflect off shiny surfaces. For instance, it is difficult to see clearly when driving towards increased sunlight or reading shopping mall maps that are enclosed in glass cases.

In addition to this age-related change, older adults are likely to have disease-related conditions, such as cataracts, that further interfere with their visual abilities. In addition, environmental factors such as bright lights, highly polished floors, and white or glossy paint, can intensify glare. These age-related changes and risk factors can interfere with vision to the extent that older adults stop performing activities or might perform them unsafely. To counteract these functional consequences, the older person or a nurse can initiate any of the following interventions, which are discussed further in Chapter 17:

- Wearing sunglasses and using glare-reducing glasses (self-care)
- Addressing environmental conditions by using adequate non-glare lighting (self-care)
- Obtaining periodic evaluations from an ophthalmologist (self-care)
- Teaching about the use of sunglasses and glare-reducing glasses (nursing intervention)
- Teaching about environmental modifications (nursing intervention)
- Taking actions to avoid glare (e.g. not standing in front of a bright window when talking with an older adult) (nursing intervention)
- Teaching older adults about the importance of having their eyes evaluated at least annually for treatable conditions (nursing interventions).

Wellness outcomes resulting from these interventions include improved safety, function and quality of life. The terms teach/teaching are clarified in Chapter 5.

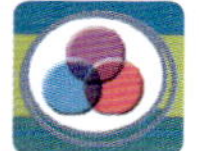

CONCEPTS UNDERLYING THE FUNCTIONAL CONSEQUENCES THEORY

The Functional Consequences Theory draws from theories that are pertinent to ageing, older adults, nursing and **person-centred care**. The nursing domain concepts of person, environment, health and nursing are linked together specifically in relation to older adults. However, before discussing these domain concepts, the concepts of functional consequences, age-related changes and the other factors that increase the risk (referred to as risk factors in the Functional Consequences Theory) are explained. Box 3-1 summarises the key concepts in the Functional Consequences Theory for Promoting Wellness in Older Adults.

Functional consequences

Functional consequences are the observable effects of actions, risk factors and age-related changes that influence the quality of life or day-to-day activities of older adults. Actions include, but are not limited to, purposeful interventions initiated either by older adults or by nurses and other carers. Risk factors can originate in the environment or arise from physiological and psychosocial influences. Functional consequences are *negative* when they interfere with a person's level of function or quality of life or increase a person's dependency. Conversely, they are *positive* when they facilitate the highest level of performance and the least amount of dependency.

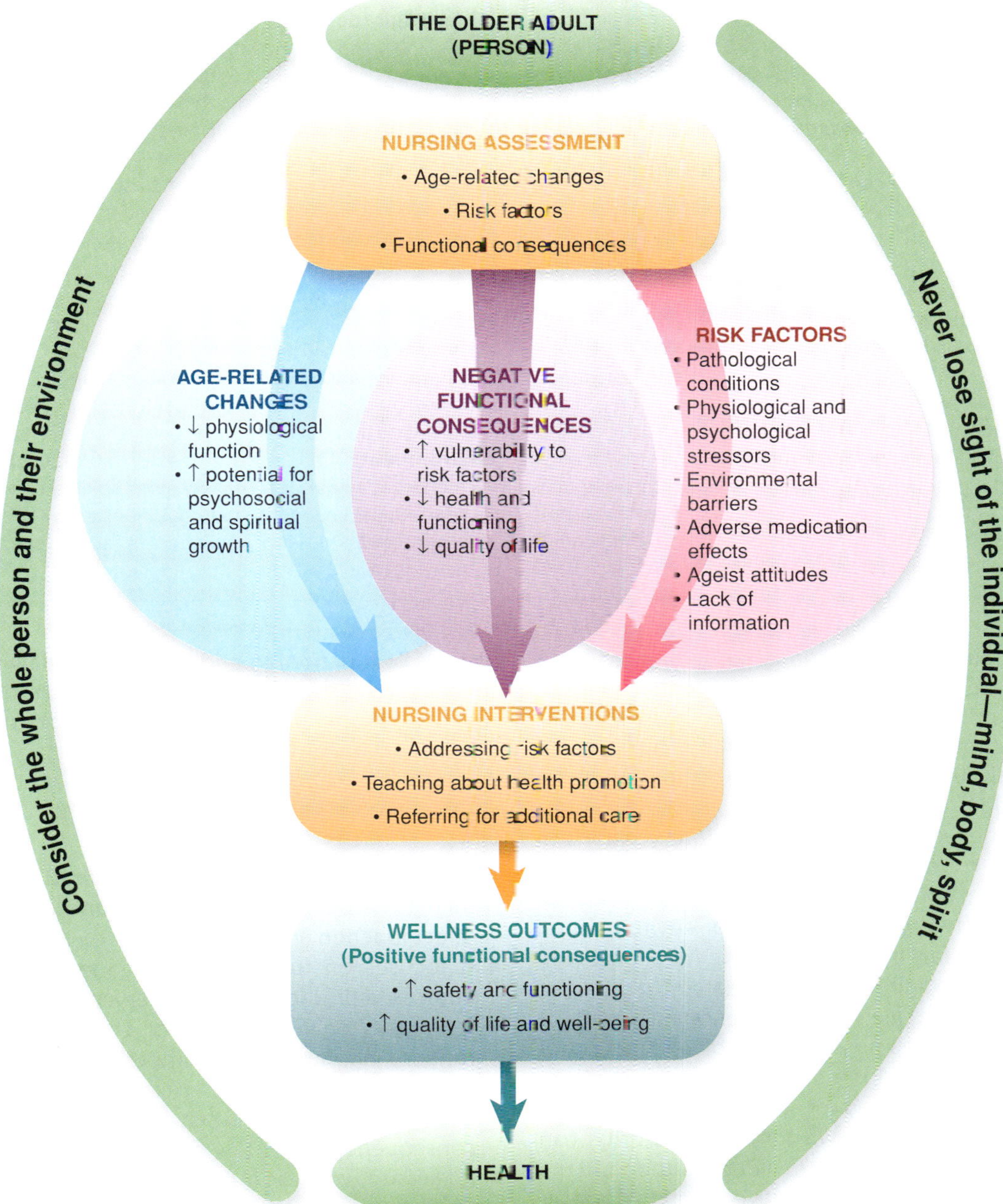

FIGURE 3-1 The Functional Consequences Theory for Promoting Wellness in Older Adults. Age-related changes and risk factors combine to cause negative functional consequences. Nurses holistically assess older adults and initiate interventions to counteract or minimise negative functional consequences. Nursing actions result in wellness outcomes.

Negative functional consequences typically occur because of a combination of age-related changes and risk factors, as illustrated in the earlier example of impaired visual performance. They also may be caused by interventions, in which case the interventions become risk factors. For example, constipation resulting from the use of an analgesic medication is an example of a negative functional consequence caused by an intervention. In this case, the medication is both an intervention for pain and a risk factor for impaired bowel function.

Positive functional consequences can result from automatic actions or purposeful interventions. Often, older

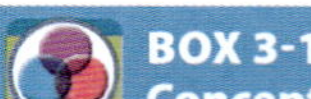

BOX 3-1
Concepts in the functional consequences theory for promoting wellness in older adults

Functional consequences: Observable effects of actions, risk factors and age-related changes that influence the quality of life or day-to-day activities of older adults. The effects relate to all levels of functioning, including body, mind and spirit.

- ***Negative functional consequences:*** Those that interfere with the older adult's functioning or quality of life.
- ***Positive functional consequences:*** Those that facilitate the highest level of functioning, the least dependency, and the best quality of life. When positive functional consequences are the result of nursing interventions, they are called **wellness outcomes**.

Age-related changes: Inevitable, progressive and irreversible changes that occur during later adulthood and are independent of extrinsic or pathological conditions. On the physiological level, these changes are typically degenerative; however, on psychological and spiritual levels, they include potential for growth.

Risk factors: Conditions that increase the vulnerability of older adults to negative functional consequences. Common sources of risk factors include diseases, environment, lifestyle, support systems, psychosocial circumstances, adverse medication effects, and attitudes based on lack of knowledge.

Older adult (person): A complex and unique individual whose functioning and well-being are influenced by the acquisition of age-related changes and risk factors. When risk factors cause the older adult to be dependent on others for daily needs, their carers/caregivers are considered an integral focus of nursing care.

Nursing: The focus of nursing care is to minimise the negative effects of age-related changes and risk factors and to promote wellness outcomes. Goals are achieved through the nursing process, with particular emphasis on health promotion and other nursing interventions that address the negative functional consequences.

Health: The ability of older adults to function at their highest capacity, despite the presence of age-related changes and risk factors. It is not limited to physiological function and encompasses psychosocial and spiritual function. Thus, it addresses well-being and quality of life as defined by each older adult.

Environment: The context and external conditions, including carers, that influence the body, mind, spirit and functioning of older adults. Environmental conditions are risk factors when they interfere with function, and they are interventions when they enhance function.

adults bring about positive functional consequences when they compensate for age-related changes with or without conscious intent. For example, an older person might increase the amount of light for reading or begin using sunglasses without realising that these actions are compensating for age-related changes.

At other times, older adults initiate interventions in response to a recognised need. In the example cited earlier, improved function would likely result from purposeful interventions, such as cataract surgery or environmental modifications. In a few instances, positive functional consequences are caused directly by age-related changes. For example, a woman may view the postmenopausal inability to become pregnant as a positive effect of ageing. Consequently, sexual relationships may become more satisfying in later adulthood. Similarly, positive functional consequences, such as increased wisdom and maturity, can result from psychological growth in older adulthood. In the context of the nursing process, positive functional consequences are called *wellness outcomes* because they result from purposeful nursing interventions.

The concept of functional consequences draws on concepts and research regarding functional assessment, which focuses on a person's ability to perform activities of daily living (ADLs) that affect survival and quality of life, as discussed in Chapter 7. From a research perspective, functional assessment provides a framework for research and a method for planning health services for dependent people. From a clinical perspective, healthcare practitioners view the multidimensional functional assessment as an important component in the care of older people. Evidence-based tools are widely available for assessing specific aspects of functioning and activities of daily living, and there is strong support for using these tools in clinical settings. Although the Functional Consequences Theory draws on concepts related to functional assessment, its scope is much broader. The Functional Consequences Theory differs from functional assessment in the following ways:

- It distinguishes between age-related changes that increase a person's vulnerability and risk factors that affect function and quality of life.
- It focuses on functional consequences that can be addressed through nursing interventions.
- It focuses on assessment of conditions that affect functioning, rather than simply identifying a person's functional level.
- It leads to interventions that address negative functional consequences.
- It leads to wellness outcomes, such as improved functioning and quality of life.

Many standardised and easy-to-use assessment tools are available for use in clinical settings, and those that are most pertinent to nursing care of older adults are cited in clinically oriented chapters of this text. In addition, all clinically oriented chapters contain comprehensive assessment and intervention boxes that apply evidence-based information to a wellness-oriented approach to nursing care of older adults.

Age-related changes and risk factors

A unique challenge of caring for older adults is the need to differentiate between age-related changes and risk factors, because the interventions for age-related changes differ from those for risk factors. Age-related changes cannot be reversed or altered, but it is possible to compensate for their effects so that wellness outcomes are achieved. By contrast, risk factors can be modified or eliminated to improve functioning and quality of life for older adults. See the following student's perspective.

A student's perspective

Most older adults live outside nursing homes and are actively involved in maintaining their independence and functional abilities as much as possible. Because of my recent experience in acute care, it is very easy for me to assume that all older adults have many underlying chronic diseases and do very little to comply with their medical therapies. It does help to separate what is a part of the ageing process from what is part of a chronic condition, since problems resulting from chronic conditions may be receptive to medical and nursing interventions.

Darris C

In the Functional Consequences Theory, **age-related changes** are the inherent physiological processes that increase the vulnerability of older people to the detrimental effects of risk factors. However, from a body–mind–spirit perspective, age-related changes are not limited to physiological aspects but include potential for increased cognitive, emotional and spiritual development. Thus, nurses holistically focus on the whole person by identifying age-related changes that can be strengthened to improve the older adult's ability to adapt to physiological decline. For example, nurses can work with older adults to strengthen their coping skills, as discussed in Chapter 12. In addition, nurses have many opportunities to build on the wisdom of older adults, especially their "everyday problem-solving" skills (as discussed in Chapter 11) by teaching about interventions to address risk factors.

The definition of age-related changes in the context of the Functional Consequences Theory draws primarily on research on ageing. Biological theories can help differentiate between age-related and disease-related processes; usually, however, there is some overlap among these processes, as discussed in Chapter 4. In addition to biological theories of ageing, other theories about ageing and older adulthood can shed light on age-related changes that contribute to the ability of older adults to respond to the challenges of ageing. Chapters in Parts 3 and 4 of this text discuss research on age-related changes pertinent to specific aspects of functioning.

Risk factors are the conditions that are likely to occur in older adults and have a significant detrimental effect on their health and functioning. Risk factors commonly arise from environments, acute and chronic conditions or diseases, psychosocial conditions, or adverse medication effects. Although many risk factors also occur in younger adults, they are more likely to have serious functional consequences in older adults because of the following characteristics:

- They are cumulative and progressive (e.g. long-term effects of smoking, obesity, inadequate exercise or poor dietary habits).
- The effects are exacerbated by age-related changes (e.g. effects of arthritis are exacerbated by diminished muscle strength).
- The effects may be mistakenly viewed as age-related changes rather than reversible and treatable conditions (e.g. mental changes from adverse medication effects may be attributed to normal ageing or dementia).
- They would not have negative functional consequences in a younger person (e.g. glare or background noise would not affect the vision or hearing of someone who is not experiencing age-related sensory changes).

Researchers and healthcare providers commonly address risk factors in relation to prevention and treatment of medical conditions. For example, evidence-based practice emphasises weighing the probable risks versus benefits for pharmacological or surgical treatments. Similarly, researchers are focusing on identifying factors that increase the chance of developing conditions, such as heart disease, so these risks can be addressed through health promotion interventions.

Nurses incorporate the concept of risk factors in many aspects of care delivery. For example, many nursing issues, interventions and outcomes address the control, identification and detection of risk. In particular, nurses identify risk factors that they can address through health promotion interventions. For example, from a perspective, nurses routinely assess for risks associated with stress, smoking, obesity, poor nutrition and inadequate physical activity.

A unique aspect of caring for older adults is the need to assess for risk factors associated with myths or ageist attitudes that can affect interventions. For example, if urinary incontinence is mistakenly attributed to "normal" ageing, then the older adult will not receive appropriate evaluation and interventions. Environmental risks are also particularly pertinent to older adults because additional risk factors such as sensory, mobility or cognitive impairments can compromise their safety and functioning. Risk factors are a major focus of the Functional Consequences Theory because nurses have numerous opportunities for promoting wellness by identifying and addressing the many modifiable factors that affect functioning and quality of life for older adults.

NURSING DOMAIN CONCEPTS

Person (older adult)

In the Functional Consequences Theory, the concept of **person** applies specifically to older adults. The holistic approach of the theory considers each **older adult** as a complex and unique individual whose functioning and well-being is influenced by many internal and external factors. Further, older adults are viewed not simply according to chronological criteria. From this perspective, an older adult is characterised by the acquisition of physiological and psychosocial characteristics that are associated with increasing maturity. *Physiological characteristics* include slowing down of physiological processes, compromised ability to respond to physiological stress, and increased vulnerability to pathological conditions and other risk factors. *Psychosocial characteristics* include an increased potential for psychosocial strengths, such as wisdom and creativity, and the potential for advanced levels of personal and spiritual growth.

Because ageing is a complex and gradual process involving all aspects of body, mind and spirit, a person does not suddenly become an older adult at a particular chronological age. Rather, people who live long enough recognise at some point that they have reached a stage of life that society categorises as older adulthood. When they reach this point, they may or may not identify with social labels such as elder, senior, or older adult. Although this concept has the distinct disadvantage of being difficult to measure, it has the advantage of accurately reflecting the realities of older adulthood as a continuum within the life-course continuum. Because people become more heterogeneous rather than homogeneous as they age, any definition of the older adult must, by its nature, be broad. In the context of the Functional Consequences Theory, an individual is an older adult when he or she manifests several or many functional consequences attributable to age-related changes alone, or to age-related changes in combination with risk factors. Stated simply, the accumulation of age-related functional consequences defines someone as an older adult. Moreover, because ageing involves many gradual, interacting and cumulative processes, each older adult experiences his or her own unique continuum. This concept is applied in the progressive case examples in the chapters of Parts 3 and 4 of this text, which illustrate the progression of one person from young–old, to old–old, as he or she is affected by functional consequences pertinent to a particular aspect of functioning.

The older adult is further conceptualised in the context of his or her relationships with others, because a person is not an isolated entity but a dynamic being who continually influences, and is influenced by, the environment and other people. This context is particularly important for older adults because, the more functionally impaired a person is, the more important are support resources and environmental factors.

When functional consequences accumulate to the extent that the older adult is very dependent on others for daily needs, nurses shift their primary focus to working with carers to identify and implement interventions. Even for older adults who do not rely on others for assistance, this context is important because older people have a long history of interpersonal relationships that influence their health behaviours and well-being. Thus, nurses assess and address the needs of older adults in the context of their relationships.

Although no characteristics apply universally to all older adults, the cumulative effects of ageing affect them all and they are all vulnerable to the effects of risk factors. Nurses need to be knowledgeable about the facts and myths about normal ageing so that they can implement interventions to address negative functional consequences. Moreover, nurses need to assess each older adult's unique response to the effects of ageing and risk factors to implement appropriate interventions to improve function and quality of life. The Functional Consequences Theory emphasises the importance of identifying and respecting the unique characteristics of each older adult that affect his or her functioning and well-being. This viewpoint is consistent with nursing theories that focus on the need to relate to person in the context of their unique lived experiences, rather than simply as members of a cultural group (Doane & Varcoe, 2009).

Nursing

The conceptualisation of **nursing** in the Functional Consequences Theory draws on many nursing theorists, and these are described in Box 3-2. In addition to drawing on many nursing theories, the concept of nursing in the Functional Consequences Theory embraces the concept of person-centred care. With person-centred care, the older adult is at the centre of their own care and it is about partnership between the health providers and the older adult. Therefore it is essential for nurses to get to know the person and this can be achieved through nursing assessments. See Box 3-3 for principles of person-centred care.

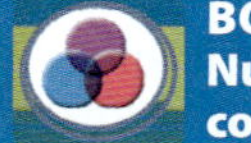

BOX 3-2
Nursing theories that support the conceptualisation of nursing

Florence Nightingale: Nurses foster an environment conducive to healing and health promotion

Virginia Henderson: Nurses provide assistance with daily activities to help gain independence as rapidly as possible

Modelling and Role-Modelling Theory: Nursing is an interactive, interpersonal process that nurtures strengths to achieve a state of perceived holistic health

Imogene King: Nurse and person interact to achieve a specific health-related goal

Jean Watson: Nursing consists of knowledge, thought, values, philosophy, commitment, and action with passion in human care transactions

Martha Rogers: Nurses promote person–environment interactions for unitary human beings

Margaret Newman: Nursing is the act of assisting people to use their power to evolve towards higher levels of consciousness

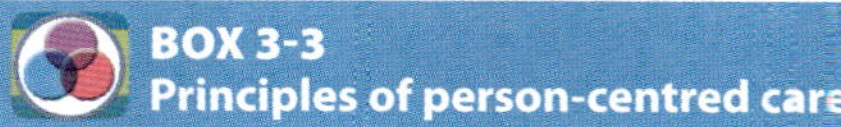

BOX 3-3
Principles of person-centred care

These principles include:

1. Getting to know the older adult as a person by using a holistic approach as well as an individual approach
2. Sharing of power and responsibility with the older adult because they are at the centre of care and an expert in their own health, sharing decision making and information
3. Accessibility and flexibility (of health provision)
4. Coordination and integration (consideration of the whole experience from the point of view of the service user)
5. Having an environment that supports person-centred care (supportive of staff working in a person-centred way and easy for the older adults to navigate) (p. 1)

Source: Victorian Government Department of Human Services. (2011). *What is person-centred healthcare? A literature review*. Melbourne: Author. Viewed March 2015 via www.health.vic.gov.au/older/publications.htm.

Health

The Functional Consequences Theory defines **health** as the ability of older adults to function at their highest capacity, despite the presence of age-related changes and risk factors. It encompasses psychosocial as well as physiological function, including well-being and quality of life as defined by each older adult. In this model, health is individually determined, based on the functional capacities that are perceived as important by that person. For example, one person might define the desired level of function as a capacity for intimate relationships, whereas another might define it as being able to perform aerobic exercise for half an hour daily.

Some definitions of health that support the conceptualisation of health in the Functional Consequences Theory are described in Box 3-4. Wellness is a closely related concept used throughout this book in reference to outcomes that address the person's highest potential for well-being. In recent years, nurse researchers have focused on identifying components of wellness in relation to care of older adults. A concept analysis of wellness in older adults by McMahon and Fleury (2012) concluded that scholars agree that wellness in not dependent on states of health or illness. They synthesised a collective description of wellness as it relates to older adults as "a purposeful process of individual growth, integration of experience, and meaningful connection with others, reflecting personally valued goals and strengths, and resulting in being well and living values" (McMahon & Fleury, 2012, p. 48). This evidence-based conclusion is consistent with the concept of health in the Functional Consequences Theory as it is applied in this text.

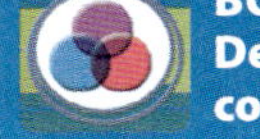

BOX 3-4
Definitions of health that support the conceptualisation of health

To be healthy is:

Florence Nightingale: To be well, but to be able to use well every power we have

Imogene King: A dynamic life experience involving continuous adjustment to stressors through optimum use of one's resources to achieve maximum potential for daily living

Calista Roy: A state and process of being and becoming integrated and whole

Jean Watson: Unity and harmony within the mind, body and soul; congruence between the self as perceived and the self as experienced

Margaret Newman: Expanding one's consciousness; an evolving pattern of the whole of life

Rosemarie Parse: A way of being in the world; the living of day-to-day ways of being

Madeleine Leininger: A state of well-being that is culturally constituted, defined, valued and practised by individuals or groups that enables them to function in their daily lives

Environment

In the Functional Consequences Theory, **environment** is a broad concept that includes all aspects of the context in which the care is provided; for dependent older adults, the environment also includes their carers. Some aspects of the conceptualisation may seem to be contradictory because the environment can be a source of both negative functional consequences and wellness outcomes. For example, the environment is a risk factor when it interferes with functioning (e.g. glare or poor lighting), but it also can facilitate wellness outcomes when it is used to improve functioning (e.g. grab bars, or brighter, non-glare lighting).

The following are some definitions of environment from nursing theories that are pertinent to the Functional Consequences Theory and these are described in Box 3-5. Since the 1970s, gerontologists have studied the influence of the environment on functioning of older adults. For example, the Person–Environment Fit Theory (discussed in Chapter 4) focuses on the interrelationship between the individual person and his or her environment. This theory is used to study the effects of environments (e.g. homes,

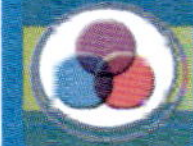

BOX 3-5
Definitions of environment from nursing theories pertinent to the Functional Consequences Theory

A healthy environment is:

Florence Nightingale: Essential for healing and includes specific aspects such as noise level, cleanliness and nutritious food

Madeleine Leininger: The totality of an event, situation or particular experience that gives meaning to human expressions, interpretations and social interactions in certain physical, ecological, socio-political and cultural settings

Imogene King: The background for human interactions, which is both internal and external to the individual

Margaret Newman: All internal and external factors of influences that surround the person or system

Calista Roy: All conditions, circumstances and influences that surround and affect the development and behaviour of humans

neighbourhoods) on many aspects of functioning and quality of life for older adults and people with mobility limitations (Greenfield, 2012; Rosenberg, Huang, Simonovich et al., 2013). Some of the questions addressed by gerontologists as well as nurses are as follows:

- How does the environment affect the older adult's level of functioning?
- How does the environment affect the older adult's quality of life?
- Is the environment comfortable for the older adult?
- Is the environment a source of risks that interfere with functioning and well-being of the older adult (e.g. does it increase the risk for falls?)?
- How can the environment be adapted to improve functioning for the older adult?

Throughout this text, the Functional Consequences Theory provides a framework for addressing such questions as an integral part of the nursing assessment and interventions for specific aspects of functioning.

A student's perspective

Today I cared for Lorna, who has had two previous cerebrovascular accidents, with the second one leading to left-sided hemiplegia. As I was caring for her I noticed a few things in her room that may have significance for her. First, I noted that she had poles both by her bed and in the bathroom; both were bolted to the ceiling and the floor. These poles made it easier for Lorna to stand on her own with little assistance from anyone else. I feel that these make her more independent and help her use the strong side of her body.

Lorna also had a divided box, with different kinds of tea in each section. I feel that this is significant to her because she is able to have the type of tea she likes whenever she wants it. It allows her to make choices each day and provides one of the comforts of "home". A third item was a triangle pillow that she sleeps on rather than a regular one. This is significant because it allows her to breathe better in the night or whenever she is sleeping. Because Lorna has chronic obstructive pulmonary disease, it is hard for her to breathe.

Kelly Z.

APPLYING THE THEORY TO PROMOTE WELLNESS IN OLDER ADULTS

In the context of the Functional Consequences Theory (FCT), nurses direct their care towards addressing age-related changes and risk factors, and promoting wellness outcomes for older adults. Nurses apply the FCT to assess age-related changes and risk factors that lead to the identification of nursing issues. Next nurses set goals to achieve wellness outcomes, implement nursing interventions, and evaluate the effectiveness of their interventions. One focus of nursing care is on educating older adults and the carers of dependent older adults about interventions that will eliminate risk factors or minimise their effects. The educational aspects are particularly important when older adults are influenced by myths and misunderstandings about age-related changes. For example, nurses can provide information about the difference between normal ageing changes and risk factors to an older person who believes that functional impairments are a necessary consequence of old age, and identify ways of minimising the effects of risk factors and compensating for the effects of age-related changes.

When using the FCT, the focus and goals of care will vary in different settings. For acute care, the focus is initially on treatment of pathological conditions that create serious risks; goals include helping vulnerable older adults recover from illness and maintain or improve their level of functioning. However, the nurse in acute care must also have an understanding of age-related changes and risk factors, and incorporate this understanding where appropriate into the care of the older adult. For instance, when an older person is admitted to hospital with the diagnosis of pneumonia, nurses would address issues related to pneumonia. But, because care is person centred, nurses understand there might be other issues relating to ageing and other risk factors that require assessment and care; for example, exploration of the issue of falls risk. The Functional Consequences Theory is also relevant to rehabilitation settings, where the focus is on preventing negative functional consequences and promoting wellness outcomes so that the older adult can return to prior levels of function (Gouveia, Jardim & Martins, 2011). For long-term residential care, the primary focus is on the multiple risk factors and the functional consequences. Here the goals can include maintaining functioning and, most importantly, quality of life.

In home and other community settings, the focus is on short- and long-term goals aimed at both the age-related changes and risk factors; the goals include improving or preventing decline in functioning and addressing quality of life.

In long-term residential care, the home and other community settings, older adults will also receive end-of-life care. In this instance, the primary focus is on the functional consequences and risk factors; goals are created to achieve the wellness outcomes of comfort and quality of life.

Irrespective of the setting, nurses can incorporate wellness outcomes to address each older adult's personal aspirations towards well-being of body, mind and spirit. Examples of goals and interventions that achieve wellness outcomes are delineated in all the clinically orientated chapters of this text.

Providing nursing care for older adults is both challenging and rewarding, despite the common misconception that it is futile and discouraging. Although nursing care of older adults is often associated with limited goals, a holistic perspective focuses on the potential of every person to experience wellness by achieving higher levels of psychological or spiritual functioning. Even older adults who have dementia (and other progressive conditions that can profoundly affect psychological function) may have potential for spiritual growth in ways that are not always observable or measurable.

The Functional Consequences Theory helps nurses see older adults as more than an accumulation of age-related physiological changes and pathological conditions leading to diminished functioning. Thus, it provides a framework for promoting wellness because it addresses the whole-person needs of the older adult and his or her relationships with self, others and the environment. It reminds nurses to identify strengths and potentials in relation not only to physical aspects of functioning, but also to psychological and spiritual well-being. Moreover, it leads to nursing interventions directed towards achieving wellness outcomes, such as improved quality of life for older adults.

CHAPTER HIGHLIGHTS

A nursing theory for wellness-focused care of older adults

- The Functional Consequences Theory explains the unique relationships among the concepts of person, health, nursing and environment in the context of promoting wellness for older adults.

Concepts underlying the Functional Consequences Theory

- Combinations of age-related changes and risk factors increase the vulnerability of older people to negative functional consequences, which interfere with the person's level of functioning or quality of life.
- Nurses assess the age-related changes, risk factors and functional consequences, with particular emphasis on identifying the factors that can be addressed through nursing interventions.
- Wellness outcomes enable older adults to function at their highest level despite the presence of age-related changes and risk factors.

Applying the theory to promote wellness in older adults

- Nurses can incorporate wellness outcomes to address each older adult's personal aspirations for well-being of body, mind and spirit.
- Nurses educate older adults and carers about interventions to minimise risk factors or their effects.
- Providing nursing care for older adults is rewarding when approached from a person-centred perspective using the FCT so that opportunities for wellness in physical, psychological and spiritual aspects of function are realised.

CRITICAL THINKING EXERCISES

Bring to your mind a vivid image of an older friend, relative or patient who is at least 80 years old, and apply the following questions to one obvious functional consequence (e.g. impaired mobility). Develop an opportunity to talk with that person about what you have learned about the Functional Consequences Theory for Promoting Wellness in Older Adults and use Figure 3-1 as a basis for discussion.

1. What age-related changes and risk factors interact to contribute to this functional consequence?
2. What environmental conditions either improve or interfere with the affected aspect of functioning?
3. How can you use your nursing knowledge to improve health and quality of life in relation to that aspect of functioning?

RESOURCES

For an extensive range of additional resources to enhance teaching and learning and to facilitate understanding of this chapter, please see the text's accompanying website located on thePoint at http://thepoint.lww.com.

Clinical tools

Hartford Institute for Geriatric Nursing, ConsultGeriRN.org: http://consultgerirn.org/resources
Assessment tools *Try This®* series and *How to Try This* resources (tools and resources for achieving the best practices in the care of older adults)

Evidence-based practice

Boltz, M., Capezuti, E., Fulmer, T. & Zwicker D. (Eds). (2012). *Evidence-based geriatric nursing protocols for best practice* (4th ed.). New York: Springer.
Hartford Institute for Geriatric Nursing: http://hartfordign.org
Joanna Briggs Institute: http://connect.jbiconnectplus.org
National Guideline Clearinghouse: www.guideline.gov

REFERENCES

Doane, G. W. & Varcoe, C. (2009). Toward compassionate action: Pragmatism and inseparability of theory/practice. In P. G. Reed & N. B. Crawford Shearer (Eds), *Perspectives on nursing theory* (5th ed., pp. 111–121). Philadelphia, PA: Wolters Kluwer Health/Lippincott Williams & Wilkins.
Gouveia, B. F., Jardim, H. & Martins, M. M. (2011). Foundation of gerontological rehabilitation nursing: Applicability of the Functional Consequences Theory. *Referencia [Suppl.], 1*(4), 475.
Greenfield, E. A. (2012). Using ecological frameworks to advance a field of research, practice, and policy on aging-in-place initiatives. *Gerontologist, 52*(1), 1–12.
Marrs J. & Lowry, L. W. (2009). Nursing theory and practice: Connecting the dots. In P. G. Reed & N. B. Crawford Shearer (Eds), *Perspectives on nursing theory* (5th ed.,

pp. 3–12). Philadelphia, PA: Wolters Kluwer Health/ Lippincott Williams & Wilkins.

McMahon, S. & Fleury, J. (2012). Wellness in older adults: A concept analysis. *Nursing Forum, 47*(1), 39–50.

Miller, C. A. (1990). *Nursing care of older adults: Theory and practice.* Glenview, IL: Scott, Forsman/Little, Brown Higher Education.

Rosenberg, D. E., Huang, D. L., Simonovich, S. D. et al. (2013). Outdoor built environment barriers and facilitators to activity among midlife and older adults with mobility disabilities. *Gerontologist, 53*(2), 268–279.

Strout, K. (2012). Wellness promotion and the Institute of Medicine's Future of Nursing Report. *Holistic Nursing Practice, 26*(3), 129–136.

Victorian Government Department of Human Services. (2011). What is person-centred healthcare? A literature review. Melbourne: Author. Viewed March 2015 via www.health.vic.gov.au/older/publications.htm.

Chapter 4

Theoretical perspectives on ageing well

By Carol Miller and Sharyn Hunter

LEARNING OBJECTIVES

After reading this chapter, you should be able to:

1. Describe theoretical perspectives on the relationships among ageing, disease, health and quality of life.
2. Discuss pertinent concepts from biological theories of ageing and their relevance to nursing care of older adults.
3. Discuss pertinent concepts from sociocultural theories of ageing and their relevance to nursing care of older adults.
4. Discuss pertinent concepts from psychological theories of ageing and their relevance to nursing care of older adults.

KEY POINTS

active life expectancy
activity theory
age stratification theory
compression of morbidity
cross-linkage theory
disengagement theory
free radical theory
gerotranscendence
human needs theory
immunosenescence theories
kilojoule restriction theory
life expectancy
lifespan
person–environment fit theory
program theory
rectangularisation of the curve
selection, optimisation and compensation
senescence
socioemotional selectivity theory
strength and vulnerability integration theory
subculture theory
wear-and-tear theory

People have always looked for answers to such universal questions as *How long can we live? Why do we age?* and *How can we prevent the unwanted effects of ageing?* Since early times, scientists and philosophers have tried to answer these questions from various perspectives using biological, sociological and psychological theories. As knowledge about unique and variable aspects of ageing expanded, it became evident that ageing is multidimensional and requires a multidisciplinary approach. Now a dominant question is *How can we live both long and well?* and the concept of ageing well is prominent in studies.

As discussed in Chapter 1, several terms to describe ageing well appear in the literature. Fernandez-Ballesteros et al. (2013) suggest the terms describe various elements of ageing well. For instance, the term *active ageing* emphasises a high level of physical and cognitive functioning and positive affect and control, while the term *healthy ageing* emphasises the minimisation of illness and disease and the maintenance of activities of daily living. Despite this diversity there is consensus that ageing well is achievable and that strategies and actions can facilitate this process.

This chapter discusses theoretical perspectives pertinent to ageing well and applies this information to nursing care of older adults.

HOW CAN WE LIVE LONG AND WELL?

Questions about how long we can live are addressed by measuring lifespan, life expectancy, and morbidity and mortality rates. The more important questions about how we can live both long and well are addressed by exploring the relationships among ageing, health and disease, as is the current focus of gerontological research. For the past several decades, gerontological research has increasingly focused on identifying ways to delay the effects of ageing and maintain high levels of functioning and quality of life. This more optimistic approach is attributable to the large group of adults who are currently turning 65—the so-called Baby Boomers—who view themselves as ageing better than the way previous generations aged or are ageing (Madden & Cloyes, 2012). Gerontologists currently are exploring answers to such questions as *What is usual or normal ageing?* and *What differentiates healthy ageing from pathological ageing?* They are intensely investigating this complex topic. For example, recently many countries have significantly increased funding for projects investigating factors that influence healthy ageing (Willcox, Suzuki, Donlon et al., 2013).

Lifespan and life expectancy

Two measures that gerontologists use to address questions about how long we can live are lifespan and life expectancy. **Lifespan**, defined as the maximum survival potential for a member of a species, is relatively stable as evident by the barely perceptible extensions that occur over the evolutionary timescale. The human lifespan is about 110 to 115 years, with only 1 of 5 million people living beyond 110 years in industrialised nations and far fewer in less developed countries (Andersen, Sebastiani, Dworkis et al., 2012). Jeanne Calment lived for 122 years and 165 days and is verified to be the longest living human. A link to an excellent video about Jeanne Calment is provided in the resources at the end of this chapter.

Life expectancy is the predictable length of time that one is expected to live from a specific point in time, such as birth or age 65. In contrast to the relatively stable time frame for lifespan, life expectancy at birth has increased from since 1900. During the past century humans have gained more years of average life expectancy at birth than in the last 10,000 years (Caruso, Passarino, Puca et al., 2012). The dramatic increase in life expectancy at birth is due largely to improved infant and child mortality and control of communicable disease. This is illustrated by the following statistics: in 1900, about 40% of babies born in Western countries were expected to live past age 65, today 88% of babies born in those same countries will live beyond age 65 (Caruso, Passarino, Puca et al., 2012). It is also interesting to note that between 1994 and 2012 the estimated prevalence of centenarians in developed nations has doubled from 1 in 10,000 people to 1 in 5000 (Sebastiani & Perls, 2012). Because of these changes in life expectancy trends, centenarians are now the fastest growing demographic group worldwide, with projections that their numbers will more than quintuple between 2005 and 2030 (Willcox, Willcox & Poon, 2010).

In Australia and New Zealand, life expectancies continue to increase. Figure 4-1 further illustrates the changing life expectancies at birth for Australians and New Zealanders, from 1960 to 2009. Current life expectancies for both countries are listed in Box 4-1. In contrast, the life expectancies for the Indigenous peoples of both countries are less. Figure 4-2 compares the life expectancy estimates of Indigenous people for Australia, New Zealand, Canada and the U.S. This figure demonstrates that the life expectancy of Indigenous Australians was lowest of all four Indigenous groups in 1982, and has improved little since.

BOX 4-1
Life expectancies at different ages for Australians and New Zealanders

Australia

At birth in 2012	Males 79.9 years Females 84.3 years
At the age of 65 in 2012	Men are expected to live to 84.1 years (an additional 19.1 years after 65 years) Women are expected to live to 87 years (an additional 22.0 years after 65 years)

New Zealand

At birth during 2010–2012	Males 79.3 years Females 83 years
At the age of 65 during 2010–2012	Men are expected to live to 73.8 years (an additional 18.8 years after 65 years) Women are expected to live to 86.2 years (an additional 21.2 years after 65 years)

Sources: Australian Institute of Health and Welfare. (2014). *Australia's health 2014.* Australia's health series no. 14. Cat. no. AUS 178. Canberra: Author; Statistics New Zealand. (2013). *New Zealand period life tables.* Accessed March 2015 via www.stats.govt.nz/browse_for_stats/health/life_expectancy.aspx.

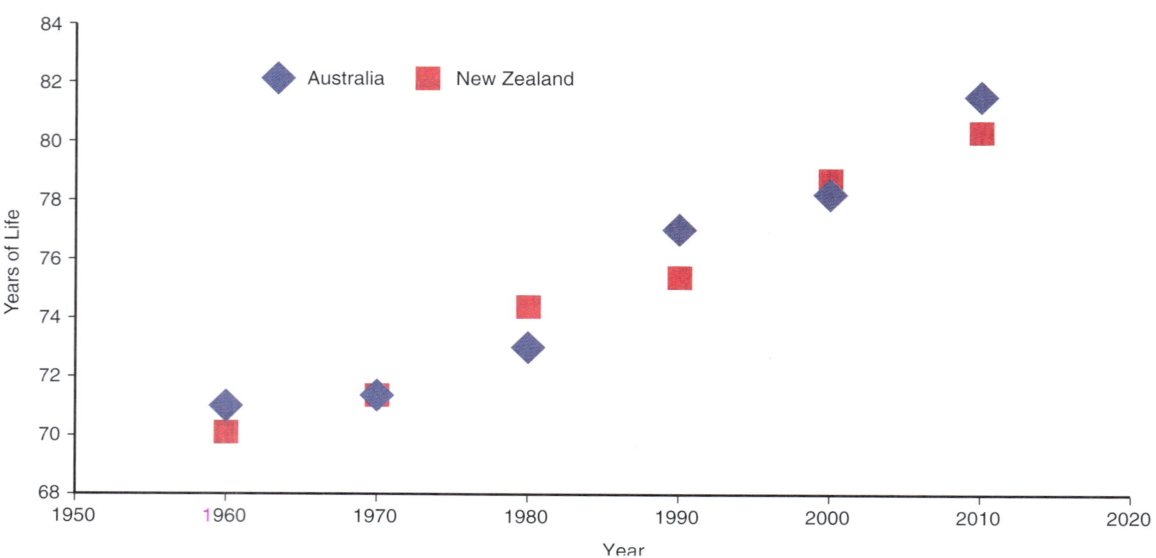

FIGURE 4-1 The World's, Australia's and New Zealand's life expectancies at birth from 1960 to 2012. (World Bank. [2012]. Australia and New Zealand data. In *Life expectancies at birth, total (years).* Accessed March 2015 via http://data.worldbank.org/indicator/spdynle00.in.)

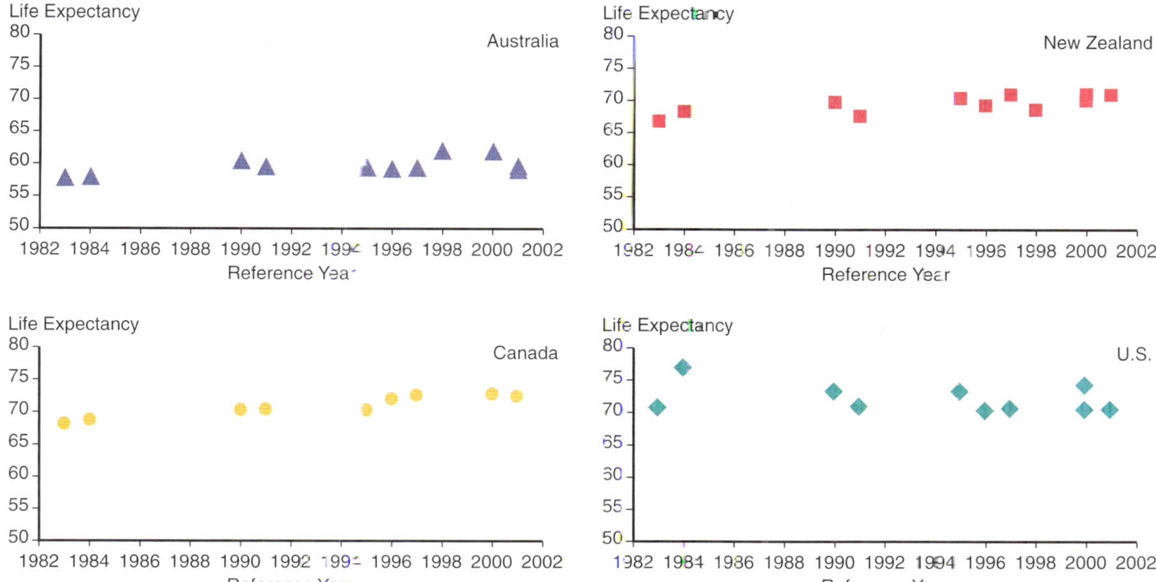

FIGURE 4-2 Life expectancy estimates of Indigenous people in Australia, New Zealand, Canada and the U.S. (AIHW. [2011]. *Comparing life expectancy of Indigenous people in Australia, New Zealand, Canada and the United States: Conceptual, methodological and data issues*. Cat. no. IHW 47. Canberra: Author. Permission granted under a Creative Commons BY 3.0 [CC-BY 3.0] licence).

In New Zealand, Indigenous people's life expectancy has improved but remains significantly less than other New Zealanders (Statistics New Zealand, 2013).

DIVERSITY NOTE

Indigenous Australians have the greatest life expectancy gap between themselves and the non-Indigenous population, and between Indigenous people in New Zealand, Canada and the U.S. (Australian Institute of Health and Welfare [AIHW], 2011).

Rectangularisation of the curve and compression of morbidity

Despite the remarkable changes, life expectancy at birth will be limited to about 90 years because major causes of death—represented by mortality rates—cannot be eliminated (Carnes, Olshansky & Hayflick, 2013). Mortality rates are graphically represented in a survivorship curve, which illustrates the changes occurring in death rates over different periods of time. The vertical axis designates the percentage of survivors, whereas the horizontal axis represents the age of survivorship. Since the 1980s, the rate of increase in average longevity has continued to rise, but the pace of increase has slowed down. This change in pace has resulted in the squaring of the human survival curve, meaning that life expectancy has not been prolonged as significantly after the age of 75 or 80 years. This **rectangularisation of the curve** is attributed to changes in survival caused by various significant factors occurring at different points in time (see Figure 4-3).

The first major change, during the age of pestilence and famine, resulted from improved housing and sanitation, and the second major change was brought about by the advent of immunisation programs and other advances in public health practices during the age of pandemics. The third major change, which occurred between 1960 and 1980, is attributable to biomedical breakthroughs such as organ transplants, heart–lung machines and cancer treatments. Recently, gerontologists have identified a fourth stage—the age of delayed degenerative diseases—characterised by the later onset of death from diseases that cause disability and chronic illness. Although it is clear that increased life expectancy involves a longer time in chronic illness, it is less clear whether this is necessarily associated with a longer time in a state of disability. Thus, the focus of geriatric research and practice shifted from an emphasis on disease processes per se to an emphasis on the functional losses that are of key importance to older people.

James Fries, a physician, first brought attention to this concern in an article on the **compression of morbidity**, in which he argued that the onset of significant illness could be postponed, but that one's life expectancy could not be extended to the same extent. Consequently, disease, disability and functional decline are "compressed" into a period averaging 3 to 5 years before death. Fries and Crapo emphasised that preventive approaches must be directed towards preserving health by postponing the onset of chronic illnesses (Fries & Crapo, 1981). Results of population studies and ongoing longitudinal studies that began in 1984 and 1986 support this theory, confirming that health promotion interventions such as exercise and risk reduction

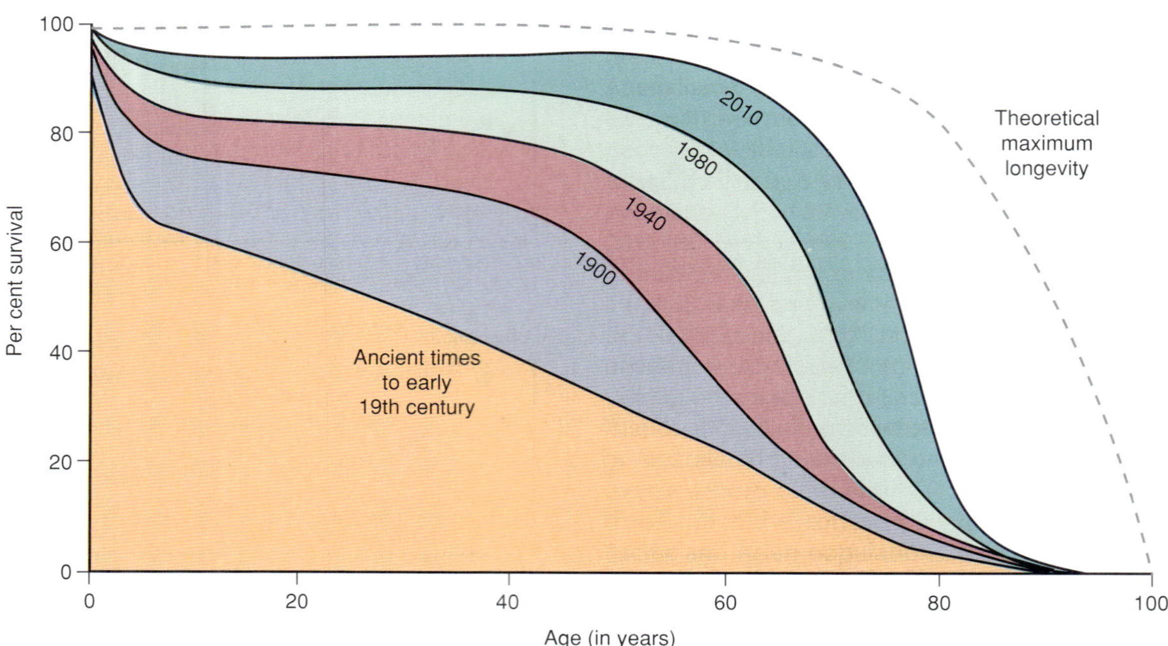

FIGURE 4-3 Changes in survivorship rates from ancient times to the theoretical maximum longevity. (Adapted with permission from Strehler, B. L. [1975]. Implications of aging research for society. *Proceedings of the Federation of American Societies for Experimental Biology*, *34*, 6.)

behaviours can postpone disability by 10 to 16 years compared with control or high-risk groups (Fries, 2012).

Active life expectancy

Spurred partly by Fries' compression of morbidity hypothesis, gerontologists developed the concept of **active life expectancy**, which is measured on a continuum ranging from inability to perform activities of daily living to full independent functioning, as an indicator of quality of life during later adulthood. Gerontologists emphasise that the goal of science, medicine and gerontology should be the extension of healthy lifespan through research on health promotion interventions rather than disease-oriented mechanisms (Carnes & Witten, 2013; Rattan, 2013).

Since the 1980s, gerontologists have analysed longitudinal data about functional disability (i.e. loss of various self-maintenance functions) in both the U.S. and developed countries as a reliable measure of health status and quality-of-life issues. Most, but not all, studies indicate that younger cohorts of older adults (i.e. those people turning 65 more recently) are living longer with less disability (Hung, Ross, Boockvar et al., 2011; Manton, Gu & Lowrimore, 2008). One analysis of data concluded that more recent cohorts are likely to experience a decade free of disability, with increased disability being associated with stroke, arthritis, diabetes and hip fracture (Taylor & Lynch, 2011).

Improvements in the level of functioning are attributed to such factors as a more educated population of older adults, and environments and medical interventions that improve function and accessibility. Continuation of this trend towards improved functioning depends on the degree to which individuals engage in healthy behaviours, such as those related to weight, nutrition, physical activity and smoking cessation (Wolinsky, Bentler, Hockenberry et al., 2011). Currently, there is growing concern that this trend towards improved functioning during later life will not continue, or that it may even be reversed, due to increasing prevalence of obesity and low levels of physical activity (Antonucci et al., 2012; Lowry, Vallejo & Studenski, 2012).

Relationships among ageing, disease and death

Whether age-associated diseases are inevitable is an important question related to living both long and well. The noted gerontologist Leonard Hayflick described the complex relationship between ageing and disease as analogous to the "weak links" in automobiles. According to his analogy, both humans and particular makes and models of cars are characterised by weak links that increase the probability of component failure. For cheap cars, the "mean time to failure" is 4 or 5 years; while for developed countries it is about 76 years. The weakest links for people in developed countries are the vascular system and the cells in which cancer commonly occurs. As Hayflick (2001–2002) stated, "The ageing process increases vulnerability to the pathologies that become the leading causes of death" (p. 21).

Theories about **senescence**, defined as the post-reproductive period leading to increased probability of death, address questions about the relationships between ageing and death. Kohn (1982) proposed a senescence theory based on post mortem studies of 200 people who died at the age of 85 years or older. Kohn compared findings from autopsies with the listed cause of death and found that at least 26% of the subjects had no disease process that would be a cause of death. Kohn concluded that, had the same degree of disease occurred in middle-aged people, the condition would not have been fatal. Thus, he concluded that ageing itself was the actual cause of death in a large fraction of the aged population (Kohn, 1982). Kohn further suggested that, when death in older people cannot be ascribed to a disease process that would cause death in middle-aged people, the cause of death should be listed on the death certificate as senescence.

Studies of older adults who are healthy and long-lived

Studies of long-lived people who are healthy and functional explore the most important question of all: *How can we live a life that is not only long but also functional, productive and satisfying?* This question is particularly relevant to the growing attention to adding quality, not just quantity, to life. The first study of "extreme longevity" was the Okinawa Centenarian Study, which began in 1975, and since then more than a dozen major longitudinal studies have been ongoing worldwide for a decade or more (Willcox, Willcox & Poon, 2010). As these studies progressed, they also included "exceptional survivors" or "supercentenarians", defined as the oldest-old population who are 110 years or older. For example, the New England Centenarian Study in the U.S. currently has the largest sample in the world, with about 107 supercentenarians and about 1600 centenarians as study participants in 2014 (New England Centenarian Study, 2014). Another source, the Supercentenarian Research Foundation (see the resources section), maintains a list of age-validated supercentenarians. People who survive to 100 years and older are a heterogeneous group with a wide range of health and socioeconomic characteristics. Most centenarians experience good health and relatively good functioning until their mid-90s or later because they have escaped common pathologies such as stroke, cancer and myocardial infarction (Andersen, Sebastiani, Dworkis et al., 2012; Vacante, D'Agata, Motta et al., 2012). Common health characteristics of the New England Centenarian Study (2014) include the following:

- Lean or healthy body mass index
- No history of smoking
- High levels of cognitive functioning
- Better than average ability to handle stress
- Family history of exceptional longevity.

Variables commonly identified as predictors of healthy longevity include nutritional patterns with a high intake of plant-based foods (i.e. fruits, vegetables, nuts), high levels of physical activity, and strong social networks (Davinelli, Willcox & Scapagnini, 2012). Psychosocial variables found in centenarians include maintaining strong interests, feeling satisfied with life, and being resilient in the face of stress (Hutnik, Smith & Koch, 2012).

HOW DO WE EXPLAIN BIOLOGICAL AGEING?

Biological theories of ageing address questions about the basic ageing processes that affect all living organisms. These theories answer such questions as *How do cells age?* and *What triggers the process of ageing?* Biological ageing is the gradual and progressive decline in physiological functioning that occurs throughout adulthood and ends in death. It is important to recognise that each biological theory of ageing attempts to explain a specific aspect of ageing from a particular perspective. As such, each theory provides a narrow lens through which biological ageing can be viewed, but they do not provide a broad vision.

Overview of and conclusions about biological theories

Biological theories provide insight into the inevitable consequences of normal ageing as well as the increased susceptibility of older adults to diseases. In addition, these theories attempt to identify the factors that can predict long as well as healthy lives. Hundreds of biological theories of ageing have been proposed during the past several centuries, and some have been disproved, whereas others continue to provide groundwork for gerontologists today. Table 4-1 summarises some commonly cited theories of ageing that have laid the groundwork for studies of biological ageing.

Much of the current research on biological ageing has evolved since the 1990s as an outcome of major advances in genetic science. Studies of twins and families confirm that genetic factors account for about 25% of a person's life expectancy, with environmental factors during the prenatal time and early life accounting for another 25% of variability, and life circumstances during adulthood accounting for the other 50% (Caruso, Passarino, Puca et al., 2012; Melzer, Pilling, Fellows et al., 2013). Current studies indicate that the genetic effect on longevity is due to modest effects of many genes interacting, with some genes increasing one's susceptibility to age-related disease and early death and other genes slowing the ageing process and leading to a longer life (Murabito, Yuan & Lunetta, 2012).

Since the early 2000s, when the Human Genome Project mapped the location of each human gene, gerontologists have access to a wealth of data that is improving our understanding of genetic factors that influence ageing. In particular, gerontologists are applying information from

TABLE 4-1 Biological theories of ageing

Theory	Description
Wear-and-tear theory	A human body is like a machine: It functions well for a certain time and broken parts can be fixed or replaced, but eventually it stops working because of accumulated effects of wear and tear. Longevity is affected by the genetic components as well as by the care provided. For humans, the wearing-out process is exacerbated by harmful factors, such as stress, disease, smoking, poor diet and alcohol abuse.
Free radical theory	Free radicals are ionised oxygen molecules that are highly unstable because they have an extra electron. They are waste products of metabolism and they can damage cells. Healthy bodies have protective mechanisms that can remove and repair damaged cells; however, these mechanisms become less effective with increased age and cellular damage becomes cumulative.
Immunosenescence theories	Immunosenescence, which is an age-related decline of the immune system, increases the susceptibility of older people to diseases such as cancer and infections. The immune system may even attack healthy cells, leading to autoimmune conditions, such as rheumatoid arthritis.
Cross-linkage theory	Biochemical processes create linkages, or connections, between structures that normally are separated. This causes a build-up of collagen-like substances that leads to failure of tissues and organs.
Program theory	The lifespan of each animal species is predetermined by a genetic program, which allows for a maximum of about 110 years in humans. Abnormal cells, such as cancer cells, are not subject to this predictable program and can proliferate an indefinite number of times.
Kilojoule/calorie restriction theory	Numerous animal studies have found that reducing kilojoule intake by 30% to 40% without causing malnutrition results in enhanced ability to protect cells, increased resistance to stress, and overall longer and healthier life expectancy. However, to date, this research has not been applied to humans.

the Human Genome Project to address questions about the relationship among health, diseases and long life. For example, Bloss, Pawlikowska and Schork (2011) proposed the following explanations about the relationship between longevity and genetic factors:

1. An individual does not possess disease-predisposing genetic variations, and therefore does not develop life-threatening diseases to the same extent as others.
2. A person lives in a health-enhancing environment and/or engages in healthy behaviours.
3. An individual possesses disease-predisposing genetic variations or lives in an unhealthy environment, but also possesses "protective" genetic variations that mitigate detrimental effects.
4. A person has a combination of these factors.

Recent studies of genome sequences indicate that centenarians would be in the 3rd category; that is, they have genetic variants associated with increased risk for age-related disease (e.g. stroke, cancer, heart disease), but they also have high numbers of genetic variants associated with longevity (Sebastiani, Bae, Sun et al., 2013; Sebastiani, Riva, Montano et al., 2012).

In conclusion, all biological theories of ageing recognise that ageing is a multidimensional process that is directly influenced by many interacting factors. Moreover, because of the great variability among people—which increases with ageing—no single theory can explain the complex phenomenon of ageing that involves many processes and mechanisms. Although no one theory can explain biological ageing, these theories lead to the following conclusions:

- Biological ageing affects all living organisms.
- Biological ageing is natural, inevitable, irreversible and progressive with time.
- The course of ageing varies from individual to individual.
- The rate of ageing for different organs and tissues varies within individuals.
- Biological ageing is an intrinsic process that is independent of external factors but is strongly influenced by non-biological factors.
- Biological ageing processes are different from pathological processes.
- Biological ageing increases a person's vulnerability to disease.

A student's perspective

One thing I feel I did well during my first week of providing patient care was seeing my patient for the person that she is and not just as a set of problems that needed caring for. I can understand how difficult it may be in today's healthcare settings to stop for a minute and really "see" the patient. When I cared for Mrs S., I was able to look past the wrinkles and white hair and see the spunky spirit that she really is. It is easy to just categorise someone in your mind as old, senile or dependent. One very important lesson that I will take with me for the rest of my career is that you cannot categorise someone because everyone is so different. It's amazing what you can discover if you actually take the time to see people for who they truly are. Taking care of a person holistically means taking care of them physically, psychologically and spiritually as well.

Sarah L.

Relevance to nurses

A primary role of nurses is to help older adults identify and address the modifiable factors that can lead to diseases, disability and death, as well as those health-promoting factors that can contribute to a longer and healthier life. Thus nurses need to understand not only the relationship between ageing and disease but also what "causes" healthy ageing and longevity. Biological theories of ageing shed light on the differences between age-related changes and the risk factors that affect the health and functioning of older adults. Nurses then can use this knowledge to implement interventions that promote wellness and a higher level of functioning.

Biological theories of ageing also are applicable to attitudes of healthcare professionals about ageing. If, for example, healthcare providers hold the perspective of "what do you expect; you're old", reversible disease conditions may go untreated. Similarly, if healthcare providers subscribe to the theory that ageing is an ultimately fatal disease, their attitude may reflect a hopelessness that pervades their care for older patients. Biological theories of ageing can be used to point out that such fatalistic perspectives are outdated. Nurses can base their care on a holistic perspective and use studies of healthy and functional oldest-old people to identify health promotion interventions that will improve quality of life for older adults. Nurses often are in positions to serve as teachers and advocates for older adults whose care might be based on an outdated or narrow approach that incorrectly equates ageing and disease. The Functional Consequences Theory for Promoting Wellness in Older Adults (discussed in Chapter 3) provides a framework for a holistic approach that identifies the risk factors and covers those that are modifiable in older adults. This text addresses each aspect of functioning from this perspective, with emphasis on those factors that nurses can address through health promotion interventions.

Biological theories highlight the need for health promotion interventions to prevent disease conditions and minimise the negative effects of ageing. However, these theories do not address the significant influence of nursing, medical and psychosocial interventions that can improve a person's functioning and life expectancy. From a broader perspective, ageing is more than an unrelenting progression of cellular deterioration. Survival to old age is an accomplishment that denotes strong will and the ability to adapt. As emphasised throughout this text, older adulthood is a dynamic part of the lifespan continuum and has the potential to be a most rewarding part of the life cycle, during which one experiences personal growth and self-understanding, fulfilment of potential, and the ability to establish clear priorities. These aspects of ageing are addressed in the following sections, which describe sociocultural and psychological theories of ageing.

CASE STUDY

Imagine you are 72 years old and your mother and father are 96 and 95 years old, respectively, and they live in a unit located in a village with a long-term residential care facility. You have a brother who died last year at the age of 70 years and you have a sister who is 69 years old. You have two children, three grandchildren, and two great-grandchildren. Your mother is moderately obese and has osteoarthritis, hypertension glaucoma and type 2 diabetes. Functionally, she uses a walker, needs help with getting in and out of the bathtub, and has some trouble reading but can see well enough to watch television and get around familiar environments. Your father has hypertension, osteoarthritis and a recent diagnosis of prostate cancer. Functionally, he is independent in his basic activities of daily living but is quite hearing impaired. Both of your parents have some memory impairment, but have support from several community services, which help with their needs for meals, medication administration, and reminders about other instrumental activities of daily living. They also are able to access help from the residential care facility in an emergency.

Thinking points

- Using the concepts of rectangularisation of the curve and compression of morbidity, what would you expect the health, functioning and life expectancy to be for each of the five generations in your family?
- Pick a biological theory of ageing that you think is applicable for your family and use it to explain to your great-grandchildren why their great-great grandparents are still living.
- Pick a theory about the relationships among age, disease and death or a theory about active life expectancy and functional health and use it to respond to your mother's statement, "I'm 96 years old—what does it matter if I follow a diabetic diet? If the sugar hasn't killed me so far, then eating two donuts this morning isn't going to kill me. It's old age that will take me, not my diet."
- Pick a theory about the relationships among age, disease and death or a theory about active life expectancy and functional health and use it to respond to your father's declaration that "Of course I have prostate cancer! I'm 95 years old!"
- What perspectives on ageing would you want your father's primary care provider to use in addressing your father's prostate cancer?

SOCIOCULTURAL PERSPECTIVES ON AGEING

Sociocultural theories of ageing attempt to explain the interrelationship between older adults and the societies and environments in which they live. Early sociocultural theories viewed older adults in the context of societal problems, but more recent theories explore the complex interrelationship between older people and their personal, cultural, physical, political and socioeconomic environments. The following sections present a sampling of the widely recognised sociocultural theories of ageing.

Disengagement theory

Disengagement theory, the first sociological theory of ageing, proposed that a society and older people engage in a mutually beneficial process of reciprocal withdrawal to maintain social equilibrium (Cumming & Henry, 1961). This process occurs systematically and inevitably and is governed by society's needs, which override individual needs. Moreover, older people desire this withdrawal and are happy when it occurs. As the number, nature and diversity of the older person's social contacts diminish, disengagement becomes a circular process that further limits opportunities for interaction. This theory challenged traditional beliefs about the relationship between a person and society and it stimulated much discussion and controversy, but it is no longer viewed as credible.

Activity theory

During the early 1970s, social gerontologists built upon the work of Havighurst and Albrecht (1953), which emphasised the relationship between successful ageing and keeping active, and proposed the **activity theory**. The activity theory postulates that older people remain socially and psychologically fit if they remain actively engaged in life. For example, one's self-concept is affirmed through activities associated with various roles, and the loss of roles in old age negatively affects life satisfaction. Support for this theory comes from many studies finding that volunteer activities and altruistic attitudes improve life satisfaction, positive affect and quality of life for older adults (Cattan, Hogg & Hardill, 2011; Kahana, Bhatta, Lovegreen et al., 2013). This theory underlies many current theories about successful ageing, which recognise that later life can be a time of engagement, contribution and well-being (Johnson & Mutchler, 2014).

A student's perspective

I think that over the past few weeks, I have really been able to see that it doesn't matter if a person is 90 or 50 or 5; they have a story, a family, a life. They have values and friends and things that are important to them. I think that this is what I will take away from this experience the most. I will try to remember in my nursing career that each patient has a story and that I will be a better nurse if I take the time to find out that story and connect with my patients, no matter what age they are.

Erika B.

Subculture and age stratification theories

The **subculture theory**, first proposed by Rose in the early 1960s, states that old people, as a group, have their own norms, expectations, beliefs and habits; therefore, they have their own subculture (Rose, 1965). The theory also maintains that older people are less well integrated into the larger society and interact more among themselves, compared with people from other age groups. Moreover, the theory holds that the formation of an aged subculture is primarily a response to the loss of status resulting from old age, which is so negative that people do not want to be viewed as old. In the aged subculture, individual status is based on health and mobility, rather than on the occupational, educational or economic achievements that were previously important. Rose (1965) envisioned that one outcome of the aged subculture would be the development of an ageing group consciousness that would serve to improve the self-image of older people and change the negative cultural definition of ageing.

The aged subculture constitutes a minority group that can organise and make public demands. For instance, Age Concern New Zealand and the COTA groups in Australia are two organisations that are socially important for the aged subgroup. When considered along with the activity theory, the subculture theory supports the perspective that there is a strong relationship between peer group participation and the adjustment process of ageing.

The **age stratification theory**, first proposed by Riley, Johnson and Foner (1972), addresses the interdependencies between age as an element of the social structure, and the ageing of people and cohorts as a social process. This theory emphasises the following concepts:

- People pass through society in cohorts that are ageing socially, biologically and psychologically.
- New cohorts are continually being born and each experiences a unique sense of history.
- A society can be divided into various strata according to age and roles.
- Society itself is continually changing, as are the people and their roles in each age stratum.
- A dynamic interplay exists between individual ageing and social change.
- Thus, ageing people and the larger society are constantly influencing each other and changing both the cohorts and the society.

Based on this theory, older adults will always be viewed as an "out-group" that is subject to ageist attitudes, despite the fact that ageism is the one form of discrimination that allows the "non-old" to discriminate against their "future selves" (Jonson, 2013).

Person–environment fit theory

The **person–environment fit theory** considers the interrelationships between personal competence and the environment (Lawton, 1982). According to this theory, personal competence involves the following factors that collectively contribute to a person's functional ability: ego strength, motor skills, biological health, cognitive capacity and sensory–perceptual capacity. The environment is viewed in terms of its potential for eliciting a behavioural response from the person. Lawton asserts that for each person's level of competence there is also a level of environmental demand, or environmental press, which is most advantageous to that person's function. People who function at relatively lower levels of competence can tolerate only low levels of environmental press, whereas people who function at higher levels of competence can tolerate increased environmental demands. An often-quoted correlate is that the more impaired the person, the greater the impact of the environment. This theory is often used in planning appropriate environments for older adults with disabilities.

Emerging sociocultural theories

A current focus of sociocultural theories is on issues that are associated with the increasing diversity of older adults in many developed counties. For example, in response to the increasing numbers of minorities in many nations there is much current focus on how culture influences various aspects of caregiving (Knight & Losada, 2011). Another currently emerging focus is on identifying sociocultural factors, such as inequities in social and economic resources, which contribute to the racial and ethnic disparities in health among older adults (Keith, 2014). Current theories also address questions about the effects of education and other sociocultural factors that affect mortality and longevity differences across racial and ethnic groups (Hummer, Melvin, Sheehan et al., 2014). A third evolving trend is the development of feminist gerontology, which examines ageing from perspectives specific to the experiences of older women. These types of theories address gender inequalities with regard to care roles, diseases (e.g. cardiovascular disease) and economic status (Meyer & Parker, 2011).

Relevance of sociocultural theories of ageing to nurses

Sociocultural theories of ageing help nurses view older adults in relation to society and environments. Thus, these perspectives contribute to a better understanding of such influences as culture, family, education, community, ascribed roles, cohort effects, home and living settings, and personal and political economics. These theories remind healthcare practitioners that there are patterns of similar responses among cohorts, but within those larger patterns, each person is unique. Some older people achieve their identity in a subculture; others may define successful ageing in relation to their activities, and still others may find new roles in society.

Sociocultural perspectives encourage nurses to consider not only the cultural needs of individual older adults but also the role of culture in shaping societal attitudes about ageing. Feminist-based theories provide a broad and holistic understanding of the needs of older adults as well as their families and carers. Information about diverse aspects of ageing such as cultural or gender differences is discussed throughout this text, and pertinent information gleaned from studies appears in the diversity notes. Theories about person–environment interactions are stimulating interest in broadening the environments of institutional settings to include pets and intergenerational activities.

In addition, these theories emphasise the importance of assessing both environmental and psychosocial factors that influence the functioning of an older person. Concepts from the person–environment fit theory help nurses appreciate the importance of environmental adaptations as interventions to improve functional status, especially when working with dependent older adults. Lawton's theory also suggests that, when an older person has difficulty coping, interventions can be directed towards improving personal competency or decreasing environmental demands, or both. Some of the risk factors discussed throughout this text identify environmental factors that interfere with the health and functioning of older adults. Similarly, many of the nursing interventions discussed identify ways of modifying the environment to improve the functioning of older adults.

CASE STUDY

Imagine you are 76 years old and have been retired for 10 years. Create an image of yourself at that age, making sure you incorporate some changes that are likely to occur as you grow older. Describe the people who are an active part of your relationships during a typical month. Describe the activities you would engage in during a typical week for each of the following aspects of your life: leisure activity, physical activity, intellectual stimulation, emotional growth, social interaction and spiritual nurturing. Are you active in any volunteer organisations? What would your health and functioning be and where would you be living? Based on the image of yourself at 76 years old that you just created, answer the following questions.

Thinking points

- How could you apply the activity theory to your life, as it compares with your life at your present age?
- Would any of the concepts in the subculture or age stratification theories explain your activities and relationships?
- How would the person–environment fit theory explain the relationship between you and your environment?

PSYCHOLOGICAL PERSPECTIVES ON AGEING

Psychological theories of ageing focus on the psychological factors that affect health, longevity and quality of life. These theories are especially relevant to psychosocial aspects of ageing because they address variables such as learning, memory, emotions, intelligence and motivation. The following sections review some of the major psychological theories of ageing. In addition, relevant psychological theories about cognitive function, stress, and coping and depression are discussed in Chapters 11, 12 and 15, respectively.

Human needs theory

Maslow's hierarchy of needs framework forms the basis of the **human needs theory**, one of the psychological theories that gerontologists use to address the concepts of motivation and human needs. According to Maslow's (1954) theory, the five categories of basic human needs, ordered from lowest to highest, are physiological needs, safety and security needs, love and belongingness, self-esteem and self-actualisation. The attainment of lower-level needs takes priority over higher-level needs; self-actualisation can occur only when lower-level needs are met to some degree. People continually move between the levels but always strive towards higher levels. This theory is particularly applicable to older adults because Maslow describes self-actualised people as fully mature humans who possess such desirable traits as autonomy, creativity, independence and positive interpersonal relationships.

Life-course and personality development theories

Two closely related types of psychological theories of ageing are personality development theories, which identify personality types as predictive forces of successful or unsuccessful ageing, and life-course theories, which address old age within the context of the life cycle. Carl Jung's (1960) personality development theory categorises personalities as either extroverted and oriented towards the external world, or introverted and oriented towards subjective experiences. A balance between the two orientations, both of which are present to some degree in all people, is essential for mental health. Jung further theorised that people tend to be more extroverted in their younger years because of the nature of the demands and responsibilities associated with family and social roles. As these demands change and diminish, beginning around the age of 40 years, people become more introverted. Jung (1954) describes later adulthood as a period of taking stock, a time during which a person looks backwards rather than forwards and is responsible for devoting serious attention to self. Successful ageing, according to Jung's theory, depends on accepting one's diminishing capacity and increasing the number of losses.

Erik Erikson's (1963) original theory about the eight stages of life has been used widely in relation to older adulthood. Erikson defines the stages of life as trust versus mistrust, autonomy versus shame and doubt, initiative versus guilt, industry versus inferiority, identity versus identity diffusion, intimacy versus self-absorption, generativity versus stagnation, and ego integrity versus despair. Each of these stages presents the person with certain conflicting tendencies that must be balanced before he or she can move successfully from that stage. As in other life-course theories, how one stage is mastered lays the groundwork for successful or unsuccessful mastery of the next stage. In works published between 1950 and 1966, Erikson emphasised the life course from childhood to young adulthood; in later publications, however, he reconsidered the meaning of these stages. In 1982, when he was 80 years old, Erikson described the task of old age as balancing the search for integrity and wholeness with a sense of despair. He believed that the successful accomplishment of this task, achieved primarily through life-review activities, would result in wisdom. Erikson's conceptualisation of continuing development throughout adulthood is cited as "seminal" work underlying current gerontological research (Kivnick & Wells, 2014).

Peck (1968) expanded Erikson's original theory and divided the eighth stage—ego integrity versus despair—into additional stages occurring during middle age and old age. The stages described by Peck as specific to old age are ego differentiation versus work-role preoccupation, body transcendence versus body preoccupation, and ego transcendence versus ego preoccupation.

Some life-course theories concentrate on middle or later adulthood and address tasks of late life such as the following:

- Adjusting to decreasing physical strength and health
- Coping with physical changes of ageing
- Adjusting to retirement and reduced income
- Adjusting to the death of a spouse
- Redirecting energy to new roles and activities, such as retirement, widowhood and grandparenting
- Establishing an explicit association with one's age group
- Adapting to social roles in a flexible way
- Establishing satisfactory physical living arrangements
- Accepting one's own life
- Developing a point of view about death.

A current focus of life-course theories is on "human potential stages", with emphasis on the "ever extant potential for growth that occurred not in spite of old age but because of it" (Agronin, 2013).

Psychological theories of ageing well

Psychological theories of ageing address questions such as *How is emotional well-being maintained during older adulthood? Does psychological well-being differ in younger and older adults?* and, perhaps most importantly, *How do people define and achieve "healthy ageing"?*

Many studies found an "unexpected positive relationship between ageing and happiness"—a phenomenon that is referred to as "the paradox of well-being" because ageist stereotypes portray older adulthood as a time of loss and sadness (Carstensen, Turan, Scheibe et al., 2011; Gana, Bailly, Saada et al., 2013). Four psychological theories of ageing that help explain this finding are: selection, optimisation and compensation; socioemotional selectivity; gerotranscendence; and strength and vulnerability integration.

The theory of **selection, optimisation and compensation** has been proposed to explain healthy ageing based on a dynamic model of development as a continuous process of specialisation and loss (Baltes & Carstensen, 1996; Zarit, 2009). According to this theory, older adults *select* certain goals and tasks while disengaging from other goals; they *optimise* necessary resources to achieve these goals; and they *compensate* by establishing new resources to substitute for lowered or lost abilities and skills (Rohr & Lang, 2009). Morley (2009) describes the following examples of well-known people who illustrate this theory:

- Grandma Moses became a famous painter of miniatures after arthritis limited her ability to make quilts.
- Monet invented modern impressionism when his eyesight was clouded by cataracts.
- Renoir held his paintbrush in his clenched fist after he developed arthritis.
- Maurice Ravel composed his famous *Bolero* after he developed dementia.

Researchers have used this theory extensively to explain aspects of ageing well such as coping with stress, managing careers and recovering from stroke (Donnellan & O'Neill, 2013; Unson & Richardson, 2013).

The **socioemotional selectivity theory** has been proposed to explain emotional well-being during older adulthood. This theory proposes that in contrast to younger adults, who view time as unconstrained, older adults recognise that their time is limited, so they focus on emotional goals rather than on knowledge-seeking goals (Kryla-Lighthall & Mather, 2009). Studies using this theory found that, when compared with younger adults, older adults found more meaning in life because they had less time in which to fulfil their goals (Hicks, Trent, Davis et al., 2012). Another study supporting both the socioemotional selectivity theory and the selection, optimisation and compensation theory found that older adults reported more goals focused on the present, emotions, generativity and prevention of loss, and fewer goals focusing on the future or knowledge acquisition (Penningroth & Scott, 2012).

The theory of **gerotranscendence** was proposed in the early 1990s by Lars Tornstam (1994) and has become widely recognised in Sweden and other Scandinavian countries. This theory proposes that human ageing is a process of shifting from a rational and materialistic metaperspective to a more cosmic and transcendent vision. This shift includes the following aspects (Tornstam, 1996):

- Decreased self-centeredness
- Less concern with body and material things
- Decreased fear of death
- Discovery of hidden aspects of self
- Increased altruism
- Increased time spent in meditation and solitude
- Decreased interest in superfluous social interaction
- Urge to abandon roles
- Increased understanding of moral ambiguity
- Increased feelings of cosmic union with the universe
- Increased feelings of affinity with past and coming generations
- A redefinition of one's perception of time, space and objects.

Recent studies based on this theory indicate that gerotranscendence (i.e. a shift from a materialistic and rational vision to a more cosmic and transcendent one) may explain successful ageing, or psychological well-being, to counteract a negative influence of functional decline in people who are 90 years and older (Gondo, Nakagawa & Masui, 2013). A longitudinal study found that gerotranscendence was higher among older adults who experienced more negative life events (Read, Braam, Lyyra et al., 2013).

The **strength and vulnerability integration theory** posits that older adults experience age-related gains as well as losses in emotion-related processes, but overall they maintain a relatively positive level of emotional experience (Charles, 2011). Strengths of older adults include improved abilities to (1) direct emotional attention away from negative stimuli, (2) appraise situations, and (3) remember experiences more positively. Age-related vulnerabilities are defined as diminished physiological ability to respond to high levels of stress. This theory is relatively new, but one study found that it is a useful model for understanding age-related patterns in emotional experiences of people diagnosed with colorectal cancer (Hart & Charles, 2013).

A student's perspective

My comfort level at the nursing home increases each and every week, and I find myself enjoying my time there more and more. Today there was a children's program in the dining room for all the residents. It was very cute. The kids were great, and most of the residents expressed true appreciation and enjoyment while the kids visited. For instance, my patient Mr B. was chatting with a young boy and his mother. As the boy got more and more involved in the conversation, Mr B.'s attitude changed completely; he became so happy and engaged with the young boy. I had seen Mr B. smile a couple of times before, but not to the extent of how he smiled and laughed with the little one. After the boy left, Mr B. told me that the boy reminded him of his own grandson, whom he doesn't get to see very much. I think it brought Mr B. joy and a sense of comfort because he felt like he was with his family. Personally, I was quite touched. Sometimes, everyone gets so caught up in current tasks or problems, when really at the end of the day it comes down to making people smile and helping them to enjoy life to the best of one's abilities.

Caitlin B.

Relevance of psychological theories of ageing to nurses

In caring for older adults, nurses can use psychological theories of ageing as a framework for addressing certain issues, such as response to losses and continued emotional development. Maslow's hierarchy of needs framework is useful for conceptualising the nature of interventions in institutional or home settings. For instance, if older adults are unable to purchase food, they are unlikely to feel secure. Likewise, if older adults feel insecure about being able to meet their shelter needs, they are unlikely to have a sense of trust. However, older adults who have already met their lower-level needs can be encouraged to focus on higher-level achievements such as self-actualisation.

In addition, psychological theories imply that devoting some time and energy to life review and self-understanding can be beneficial for older adults. Nurses can facilitate this process by asking sensitive questions and by listening attentively to older adults as they share information about their past. Reminiscence is a positive experience that is essential for continued psychological development, and it can be promoted by nurses on either an individual or group basis.

Life-course models can help nurses identify those areas of personality that are likely to change and those that are more likely to remain stable. Nurses have used lifespan theories to develop a multidisciplinary theory of thriving (Haight et al., 2002). This model proposes that thriving is achieved when there is concordance between the person and the human and non-human environment; that is, when these three elements are mutually engaged, supportive and harmonious. In contrast, failure to thrive is the result of discordance among these three elements, causing a failure of engagement and mutual support and disharmony (Haight et al., 2002). In addition to these implications, nurses consider implications regarding specific aspects such as cognitive function and coping responses (see Chapters 11 and 12) in the context of psychological theories of ageing.

CASE STUDY

Imagine, again, that you are 76 years old and add the following information to the description of yourself that you created for the discussion of sociocultural theories. Describe your personality, including but not limiting, the following characteristics: emotional stability, adjustments to losses, contentedness with life, optimism versus pessimism, engagement in activities versus withdrawal from activities, and feelings of self-efficacy versus feelings of powerlessness. Describe your beliefs about your gender-specific roles (i.e. those aspects of roles that are defined by you being a woman or a man). Based on this image of yourself at 76 years old, answer the following questions.

Thinking points

- Where do you think you would be in Maslow's or Erikson's stages, and how would you have moved between the levels in the past decades?
- What aspects of your lifestyle at 87 years old could be explained by the gerotranscendence theory?
- How would any concepts in the personality development theories apply to you?
- Based on your own experiences, how has your perception of ageing changed over time?

A HOLISTIC PERSPECTIVE ON AGEING AND WELLNESS

From a holistic perspective—the one that is most pertinent to promoting wellness—it is necessary to consider the body–mind–spirit interconnectedness of each older adult for whom nurses provide care. Thus, questions about how we can live long and well must be answered in the context of the interplay among the many factors that influence health and ageing. This requires an integrated perspective on ageing, an avoidance of stereotypes, and a commitment to identifying the factors that most directly affect—both negatively and positively—the health and quality of life for each unique older adult. Current theories point to the following determinants of living long and well:

- Inherit good genes
- Avoid oxidative damage (e.g. from tobacco, environmental conditions)
- Protect from oxidative damage with antioxidants from natural sources (e.g. fruits and vegetables)
- Maintain optimal weight
- Engage in physical exercise
- Engage in meaningful social interactions
- Develop close personal relationships
- Maintain a sense of spiritual connectedness
- Reject ageist stereotypes.

The Functional Consequences Theory for Promoting Wellness presented in Chapter 3 provides a nursing framework for addressing the factors that affect the health and functioning of older adults. Although it is beyond the scope of any nursing text to address all aspects of body–mind–spirit interconnectedness, nurses can use the functional consequences perspective, in conjunction with information from theories discussed in this chapter, to help older adults answer their own questions about ageing. When older adults express resignation in the "What-do-you-expect-you're-old?" outlook, nurses can rephrase that viewpoint and ask "So, what *do* you expect because you are older?" or "What *will* you expect when you are older?" Nurses can challenge ageist stereotypes and approach the question from a holistic perspective that acknowledges the interconnectedness among one's body, one's mind and one's spirit. From this point of view, nurses can emphasise that even though some degenerative changes affect one's body with increasing age, one's mind and spirit can continue to thrive and even improve.

Because self-responsibility is an essential component of wellness, nurses can ask older adults to identify for themselves those factors that most significantly influence their health and functioning and can focus care on those aspects within the scope of nursing. Nurses also need to avoid communicating ageist stereotypes, which requires that we examine our own attitudes about ageing and make sure that our nursing care of older adults is based on accurate, theory-based information. Nurses can check their attitudes about their own ageing and periodically ask, *What do I expect (or wish) for my own wellness when I am older tomorrow?... a week from now?... a month from now?... a year?... 10 years?... 20 years?* Even more importantly, ask, *What am I doing today that will affect how well I am ageing tomorrow?... 10 years from now?* If we acknowledge that no matter what else is happening, we are ageing biologically, we are likely to pay careful attention to health-related behaviours that affect how well we age. Likewise, if we approach our care of older adults holistically, we will be able to identify interventions that promote wellness of body, mind and spirit.

CHAPTER HIGHLIGHTS

How can we live long and well? (Figures 4-1, 4-2 and 4-3; Box 4-1)

- Gerontologists develop theories to answer questions about how and why we age. From a holistic perspective, the most important question is, *How can we live a life that is both long and healthy?* Nurses address this question by promoting wellness and facilitating optimal level of functioning for older adults.
- The rectangularisation of the curve illustrates the changes in survivorship and life expectancy that have been occurring in developed countries.
- The compression of morbidity describes the phenomenon of postponing disability until the last years before death.
- Studies of people who are healthy and long-lived provide insights into characteristics of healthy ageing.

How do we explain biological ageing?

- Biological theories of ageing address questions about inevitable consequences of normal ageing.
- Examples of biological theories of ageing are wear and tear, free radical, immunosenescence, cross-linkage, program and kilojoule restriction.
- Nurses can apply information about biological theories of ageing to teach older adults about health promotion interventions.

Sociocultural perspectives on ageing

- Sociocultural theories of ageing attempt to explain how a society influences its old people and how old people influence their society.
- Sociocultural theories include disengagement, activity, subculture, age stratification and person–environment fit theories.
- Nurses can apply information from sociocultural theories to holistically address the multidimensional needs of older adults.

Psychological perspectives on ageing

- Psychological theories of ageing provide a framework for addressing certain psychosocial issues that are common among older adults (e.g. responses to losses and continued emotional development).
- Maslow's human needs theories and the theories of Jung, Erikson and Peck underlie many psychological theories of ageing.
- Gerontologists are especially interested in theories of successful ageing, such as selection, optimisation and compensation; socioemotional selectivity; gerotranscendence; and strength and vulnerability integration.
- Psychological theories of ageing help nurses address the psychosocial needs of older adults.

A holistic perspective on ageing and wellness

- Nurses can use theories of ageing developed by other disciplines in conjunction with the Functional Consequences Theory (see Chapter 3) to develop and implement a holistic approach to promoting wellness in older adults.

CRITICAL THINKING EXERCISES

You are assessing an 81-year-old woman who is being admitted to the hospital with heart failure for the third time in the past 2 years. She does not have any cognitive impairment and she lives alone in her own home. When you ask her why she came to the hospital, she states, "I'm 81 years old, you know. Isn't that a good enough reason to be sick? Don't you think you'll be in the hospital when you're my age?"

1. How do you respond to her?
2. What additional assessment information would you want?
3. What health teaching would you think about incorporating into your care plan?

RESOURCES

For an extensive range of additional resources to enhance teaching and learning and to facilitate understanding of this chapter, please see the text's accompanying website located on thePoint at http://thepoint.lww.com.

Age Concern New Zealand: www.ageconcern.org.nz
Ageing Research Online (Australia): www.aro.gov.au
American Federation for Aging Research: http://afar.org
COTA Australia: www.cota.org.au
Gerontology Research Group: www.grg.org
Health Direct Australia, seniors' health: www.healthdirect.gov.au/seniors-health
Jeanne Calment video: www.youtube.com/watch?v=u5XDuyE8SD8&feature=related
National Ageing Research Institute Ltd (NARI) (Australia): www.mednwh.unimelb.edu.au
National Institute on Aging Information Center: www.nia.nih.gov/health
New Zealand Institute for Research on Ageing: http://ips.ac.nz/Ageing/Index.html
Supercentenarian Research Foundation: http://supercentenarian-research-foundation.org

REFERENCES

Agronin, M. E. (2013). From Cicero to Cohen: Developmental theories of aging, from antiquity to the present. *Gerontologist, 54*(1), 30–39.

Andersen, S. L., Sebastiani, P., Dworkis, D. A. et al. (2012). Health span approximates life span among many supercentenarians: Compression of morbidity at the approximate limit of lifespan. *Journals of Gerontology: Biological Sciences and Medical Sciences, 67*(4), 395–405.

Antonucci, T. C., Ashton-Miller, J. A., Brant, J. et al. (2012). The right to move: A multidisciplinary lifespan conceptual framework. *Current Gerontology and Geriatrics Research*. Article ID 873937. Available at http://dx.doi.org/10.1155/2012/873937.

Australian Institute Health and Welfare (AIHW). (2011). *Comparing life expectancy of Indigenous people in Australia, New Zealand, Canada and the United States: Conceptual, methodological and data issues*. Cat. no. IHW 47. Canberra: AIHW. Retrieved 11 January 2015 from www.aihw.gov.au/WorkArea/DownloadAsset.aspx?id=10737418932.

Australian Institute of Health and Welfare. (2014). *Australia's health 2014*. Australia's health series no. 14. Cat. no. AUS 178. Canberra: Author.

Baltes, M. M. & Carstensen, L. L. (1996). The process of successful ageing. *Ageing and Society, 16*, 397–422.

Bloss, C. S., Pawlikowska, L. & Schork, N. J. (2011). Contemporary human genetic strategies in aging research. *Ageing Research Review, 10*(2), 191–200.

Carnes, B. A. & Witten, T. M. (2013). How long must humans live? *Journals of Gerontology: Biological Sciences and Medical Sciences*, *69*(8), 965–970.

Carnes, B. A., Olshansky, S. J. & Hayflick, L. (2013). Can human biology allow most of us to become centenarians? *Journals of Gerontology: Biological Sciences and Medical Sciences, 68*(2), 136–142.

Carstensen, L. L., Turan, B., Scheibe, S. et al. (2011). Emotional experience improves with age: Evidence based on over 10 years of experience sampling. *Psychology of Aging, 26*(1), 21–33.

Caruso, C., Passarino, G., Puca, A. et al. (2012). "Positive biology": The centenarian lesson. *Causes of Immunity & Ageing, 9*(5). Available March 2015 at www.immunityageing.com/content/9/1/5.

Cattan, M., Hogg, E. & Hardill, I. (2011). Improving quality of life in ageing populations: What can volunteering do? *Maturitas, 70*(4), 428–432.

Charles, S. T. (2011). Emotional experience and regulation in later life. In K. W. Schaie & S. L. Willis (Eds), *Handbook of the psychology of aging* (7th ed., pp. 295–310). New York: Elsevier.

Cumming, E. & Henry, W. (1961). *Growing old: The process of disengagement*. New York: Basic Books.

Davinelli, S., Willcox, C. & Scapagnini, G. (2012). Extending healthy ageing: Nutrient sensitive pathway and centenarian population. *Immunity & Ageing, 9*(9). Available March 2015 at www.immunityageing.com/content/9/1/9.

Donnellan, C. & O'Neill, D. (2013). Baltes' SOC model of successful ageing as a potential framework for stroke rehabilitation. *Disability and Rehabilitation, 36*(5), 424–429.

Erikson, E. H. (1963). *Childhood and society* (2nd ed.). New York: W. W. Norton.

Fernandez-Ballesteros, R., Molina, M. A., Schettini, R. et al., (2013). The semantic network of aging well. *Annual Review of Gerontology and Geriatrics, 33*, 79–107.

Fries, J. F. (2012). The theory and practice of active aging. *Current Gerontology and Geriatrics Research*. Article ID 420637. Available at http://dx.doi.org/10.1155/2012/420637.

Fries, J. F. & Crapo, L. M. (1981). *Vitality and aging: Implications of the rectangularization of the curve*. San Francisco, CA: W. H. Freeman.

Gana, K., Bailly, N., Saada, Y. et al. (2013). Does life satisfaction change in old age: Results from an 8-year longitudinal study. *Journals of Gerontology: Psychological Sciences and Social Sciences, 68*(4), 540–552.

Gondo, Y., Nakagawa, T. & Masui, Y. (2013). A new concept of successful aging in the oldest old. *Annual Review of Gerontology and Geriatrics, 33*, 109–132.

Haight, B. K., Barba B. E., Tesh, A. S. & Courts, N. F. (2002). Thriving: A life span theory. *Journal of Gerontological Nursing, 28*(3), 14–22.

Hart, S. L. & Charles, S. T. (2013). Age-related patterns in negative affect and appraisals about colorectal cancer over time. *Health Psychology, 32*(3), 302–310.

Havighurst, R. J. & Albrecht, R. (1953). *Older people*. New York: Longmans, Green.

Hayflick, L. (2001–2002). Anti-aging medicine hype, hope, and reality. *Generations, 20*, 20–26.

Hicks, J. A., Trent, J., Davis, W. E. et al. (2012). Positive affect, meaning in life, and future time perspective: An application of socioemotional selectivity theory. *Psychology and Aging, 27*(1), 181–189.

Hummer, R. A., Melvin, J. E., Sheehan, C. M. et al. (2014). Race/ethnicity, morality, and longevity. In K. E. Whitfield & T. A. Baker (Eds), *Handbook of minority aging* (pp. 11–129). New York: Springer.

Hung, W. W., Ross, J. S., Boockvar, S. et al. (2011). Recent trends in chronic disease, impairment and disability among older adults in the United States. *BMC Geriatrics, 11*, 47. Available March 2015 at www.biomedcentral.com/1471-2318/11/47.

Hutnik, N., Smith, P. & Koch, T. (2012). What does it feel like to be 100? Socio-emotional aspects of well-being in the stories of 16 centenarians living in the United Kingdom. *Aging & Mental Health, 16*(7), 811–816.

Johnson, K. J. & Mutchler, J. E. (2014). The emergence of a positive gerontology: From disengagement to social involvement. *Gerontologist, 54*(1), 93–100.

Jonson, H. (2013). We will be different? Ageism and the temporal construction of old age. *Gerontologist, 53*(2), 198–204.

Jung, C. G. (1954). Marriage as a psychological relationship. In W. McGuire, H. Reed, M. Fordham & G. Adler (Eds) (R. F. C. Hull, trans.), *Collected works: The development of personality* (Vol. 17). New York: Pantheon Books.

Jung, C. G. (1960). The stages of life. In W. McGuire, H. Reed, M. Fordham & G. Adler (Eds) (R. F. C. Hull, trans.), *Collected works: The structure and dynamics of the psyche* (Vol. 8, pp. 387–403). New York: Pantheon Books.

Kahana, E., Bhatta, T., Lovegreen, L. D. et al. (2013). Altruism, helping, and volunteering: Pathways to well-being in late life. *Aging & Mental Health, 25*(1), 159–187.

Keith, V. M. (2014). Stress, discrimination, and coping in late life. In K. E. Whitfield & T. A. Baker (Eds), *Handbook of minority aging* (pp. 65–84). New York: Springer.

Kivnick, H. Q. & Wells, C. K. (2014). Untapped richness in Erik H. Erikson's Rootstock. *Gerontologist, 54*(1), 40–50

Knight, B. G. & Losada, A. (2011). Family caregiving for cognitively or physically frail older adults: Theory, research, and practice. In K. W. Schaie & S. L. Willis (Eds), *Handbook of the psychology of aging* (7th ed., pp. 353–365). New York: Elsevier.

Kohn, R. R. (1982). Cause of death in very old people. *Journal of the American Medical Association, 247*, 2793–2797

Kryla-Lighthall, N. & Mather, M. (2009). The role of cognitive control in older adults' emotional well-being. In V. L. Bengston, M. Silverstein, N. M. Putney & D. Gans (Eds), *Handbook of theories of aging* (2nd ed., pp. 323–344). New York: Springer.

Lawton, M. P. (1982). Competence, environmental press, and the adaptation of older people. In M. P. Lawton, P. G. Windley & T. O. Byerts (Eds), *Aging and the environment: Theoretical approaches* (pp. 33–59). New York: Springer.

Lowry, K. A., Vallejo, A. N. & Studenski, S. A. (2012). Successful aging as a continuum of functional independence: Lessons from physical disability models of aging. *Aging and Disease, 3*(1), 5–15.

Madden, C. L. & Cloyes, K. G. (2012). The discourse of aging. *Advances in Nursing Science, 35*(3), 264–272.

Manton, K. G., Gu, X. & Lowrimore, G. R. (2008). Cohort changes in active life expectancy in the U.S. elderly population: Experience from the 1982–2004 National Long-Term Care Survey. *Journal of Gerontology: Social Sciences, 63B*(5), S269–S281.

Maslow, A. H. (1954). *Motivation and personality*. New York: Harper & Row.

Mehta, N. K., Sudharsanan, N. & Elo, I. T. (2014). Race/Ethnicity and disability among older Americans. In K. E. Whitfield & T. A. Baker (Eds), *Handbook of minority aging* (pp. 13 –161). New York: Springer.

Melzer, D., Pilling, L. C., Fellows, A. D. et al. (2013). Gene expression biomarkers and longevity. *Annual Review of Gerontology and Geriatrics, 3*, 233–258.

Meyer, M. H. & Parker, W. M. (2011). Gender, aging, and social policy. In L. George (Ed.), *Handbook of aging and the social sciences* (7th ed., pp. 323–335). New York: Elsevier.

Morley, J. E. (2009). Successful aging or aging successfully. *Journal of the American Medical Directors Association, 10*(2), 85–86.

Murabito, J. M., Yuan, R. & Lunetta, K. L. (2012). The search for longevity and healthy aging genes: Insights from epidemiological studies and samples of long-lived individuals. *Journals of Gerontology: Biological Sciences and Medical Sciences, 67*(5), 470–479.

New England Centenarian Study. (2014). Why study centenarians? An overview. Available March 2015 at www.bumc.bu.edu/centenarian/overview.

Peck, R. C. (1968). Psychological developments in the second half of life. In B. L. Neugarten (Ed.), *Middle age and aging* (pp. 88–92). Chicago, IL: University of Chicago Press.

Penningroth, S. L. & Scott, W. D. (2012). Age-related differences in goals: Testing predictions from selection, optimization, and compensation theory and socioemotional selectivity theory. *International Journal of Aging and Human Development, 74*(2), 87–111.

Rattan, S. (2013). Healthy aging, but what is health? *Biogerontology, 14*(6), 673–677.

Read, S., Braam, A. W., Lyyra, T. M. et al. (2013). Do negative life events promote gerotranscendence in the second half of life? *Aging & Mental Health, 18*(1), 117–124.

Riley, M. W., Johnson, M. & Foner, A. (1972). *Aging and society*. Vol. 3: A sociology of age stratification. New York: Russell Sage Foundation.

Rohr, M. K. & Lang, F. R. (2009). Aging well together—A mini review. *Gerontology, 55*, 333–343.

Rose, A. M. (1965). The subculture of the aging: A framework for research in social gerontology. In A. M. Rose & W. Peterson (Eds), *Older people and their social worlds*. Philadelphia, PA: F. A. Davis.

Sebastiani, P., Bae, H., Sun, F. X. et al. (2013). Meta-analysis of genetic variants associated with human exceptional longevity. *Aging, 5*(9), 653–661.

Sebastiani, P. & Perls, T. (2012). The genetics of extreme longevity: Lessons from the New England Centenarian Study. *Frontiers in Genetics*. Article ID 277. doi:10.3389/fgene.2012.00277.

Sebastiani, P., Riva, A., Montano, M. et al. (2012). Whole genome sequences of a male and female supercentenarian, ages greater than 114 years. *Frontiers in Genetics*. Article ID PMC3262222. doi:10.3389/fgene.2011.00090.

Statistics New Zealand. (2013). *New Zealand period life tables*. Accessed March 2015 via www.stats.govt.nz/browse_for_stats/health/life_expectancy.aspx.

Strehler, B. L. (1975). Implications of aging research for society. *Proceedings of the Federation of American Societies for Experimental Biology, 34*, 6.

Taylor, M. G. & Lynch, S. M. (2011). Cohort differences and chronic disease profiles of differential disability trajectories. *Journals of Gerontology: Psychological Sciences and Social Sciences, 66*(6), 729–738.

Tornstam, L. (1994). Gerotranscendence: A theoretical and empirical exploration. In L. E. Thomas & S. A. Eisenhandler (Eds), *Aging and the religious dimension*. Westport, CT: Greenwood.

Tornstam, L. (1996). Gerotranscendence: A theory about maturing into old age. *Journal of Aging & Identity, 1*, 37–50.

Unson, C. & Richardson, M. (2013). Insights into the experiences of older workers and change: Through the lens of selection, optimization, and compensation. *Gerontologist, 5*(3), 484–494.

Vacante, M., D'Agata, V., Motta, M. et al. (2012). Centenarians and supercentenarians: A black swan. Emerging social, medical and surgical problems. *BMC Surgery, 12*(Suppl. 1), S36.

Willcox, B. J., Suzuki, M., Donlon, T. A. et al. (2013). Optimizing human health span and lifespan. *Annual Review of Gerontology and Geriatrics, 3*, 136–170.

Willcox, D. C., Willcox, B. J. & Poon, L. W. (2010). Centenarian studies: Important contributors to our understanding of the aging process and longevity. *Current Gerontology and Geriatrics Research.* Article ID 484529. Available at http://dx.doi.org/10.1155/2010/484529.

Wolinsky, F. D., Bentler, S. E., Hockenberry, M. P. et al. (2011). Long-term declines in ADLs, IADLs, and mobility among older Medicare beneficiaries. *BMC Geriatrics, 11*, 43.

World Bank. (2012). Australia and New Zealand data. In *Life expectancies at birth, total (years)*. Accessed March 2015 via http://data.worldbank.org/indicator/SP.DYN.LE00.IN.

Zarit, S. H. (2009). A good old age: Theories of mental health and aging. In V. L. Bengston, M. Silverstein, N. M. Putney & D. Gans (Eds), *Handbook of theories of aging* (2nd ed., pp. 675–691). New York: Springer.

PART 2

NURSING CONSIDERATIONS FOR OLDER ADULTS

Chapter 5

Nursing older adults and the promotion of wellness

By Carol Miller and Sharyn Hunter

LEARNING OBJECTIVES

After reading this chapter, you should be able to:

1. Discuss the importance of nurses requiring the skills and knowledge to meet the healthcare needs of older adults.
2. Describe the scope of gerontology and geriatrics.
3. Discuss the difference in the practice of gerontological advanced practice nurses as opposed to other nurses who work with older adults.
4. Identify and use resources for improving competence in the care of older adults.
5. Describe health promotion programs and interventions that support the wellness of older adults.
6. Identify and use resources for evidence-based health promotion programs for older adults.

KEY POINTS

geriatrics
gerontology
gerontological nursing
health
health promotion
health-related quality of life
Stages of Change Model or Transtheoretical Model of Change (TTM)
teaching
wellness

What emerges from the information in Part 1 is an image of older adults as a diverse group of individuals from varied socio-cultural backgrounds who are more heterogeneous than homogeneous. What is becoming clear is that, even among the same-age cohorts, as people age, they become less and less like others of the same age. Indeed, the most universal characteristic of increasing age is increasing individuality and diversity.

Because the provision of healthcare and other services to this population is so complicated, several branches of science have evolved to address the unique issues related to ageing and older adults. In recent years there has been increasing attention to the importance of all nurses becoming competent in addressing the unique healthcare needs of older adults and applying evidence-based guidelines to nursing practice. There also has been increasing attention of the importance of **health promotion** interventions and the roles of nurses in promoting **wellness**.

NURSING OLDER ADULTS

Chapter 1 highlighted the issue of the increasing population of older adults who have high levels of morbidity. Although older adults comprise approximately 14.7% of the total population, they account for nearly 48% of hospital discharges in Australia (Australian Institute Health and Welfare [AIHW], 2013). Figure 5-1 further supports the increased use of hospital care by older Australian adults, illustrating the number of days that older people were patients in hospital.

In New Zealand there are approximately 14.5% of older adults and they account for 30% of the discharges (New Zealand Ministry of Health [NZMOH], 2012a). Figure 5-2 demonstrates the increased use of hospitals by older adults in New Zealand.

These trends pose a challenge for the healthcare systems in both countries. As nurses are the primary healthcarers of older adults, it is evident that all nurses require skills and knowledge to meet the healthcare needs of the older adult. Knowledge about the ageing process and risk factors for the physical, cognitive and psychosocial decline of older adults is fundamental knowledge required by all nurses and not specialist knowledge required by geronto-

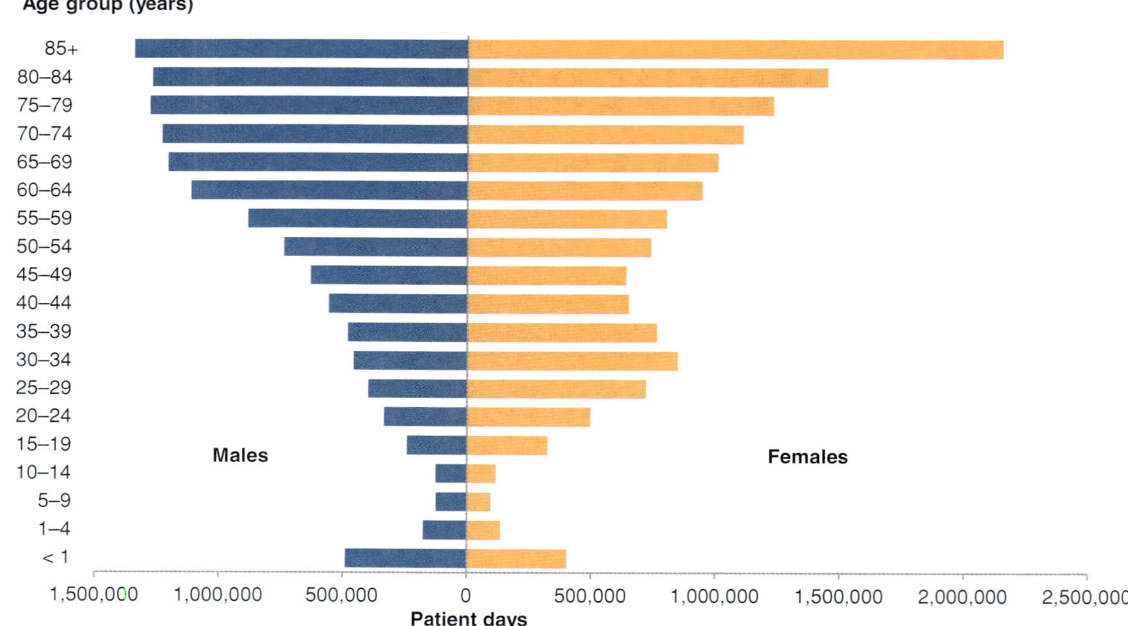

FIGURE 5-1 Patient days by sex and age group for all Australian hospitals, 2011–2012. (Australian Institute of Health and Welfare. [2013]. *Australian hospital statistics 2011–12* [Fig. 7.5, p. 121]. Cat. no. HSE 134. Canberra: Author. Permission granted under a Creative Commons BY 3.0 [CC-BY 3.0] licence.)

logical nurses. Nurses require the skills to assess older adults comprehensively and provide in-depth prevention and wellness promotion services.

The concurrent emphasis on the need to improve the quality and cost of healthcare for the growing number of older adults has stimulated the development of new models of care. Most of these models include innovative and expanded roles for nurses. These models and the associated roles for nurses who work with older adults are described in detail in Chapter 6. The remainder of this section focuses on recent developments related to gerontological advanced practice nurses.

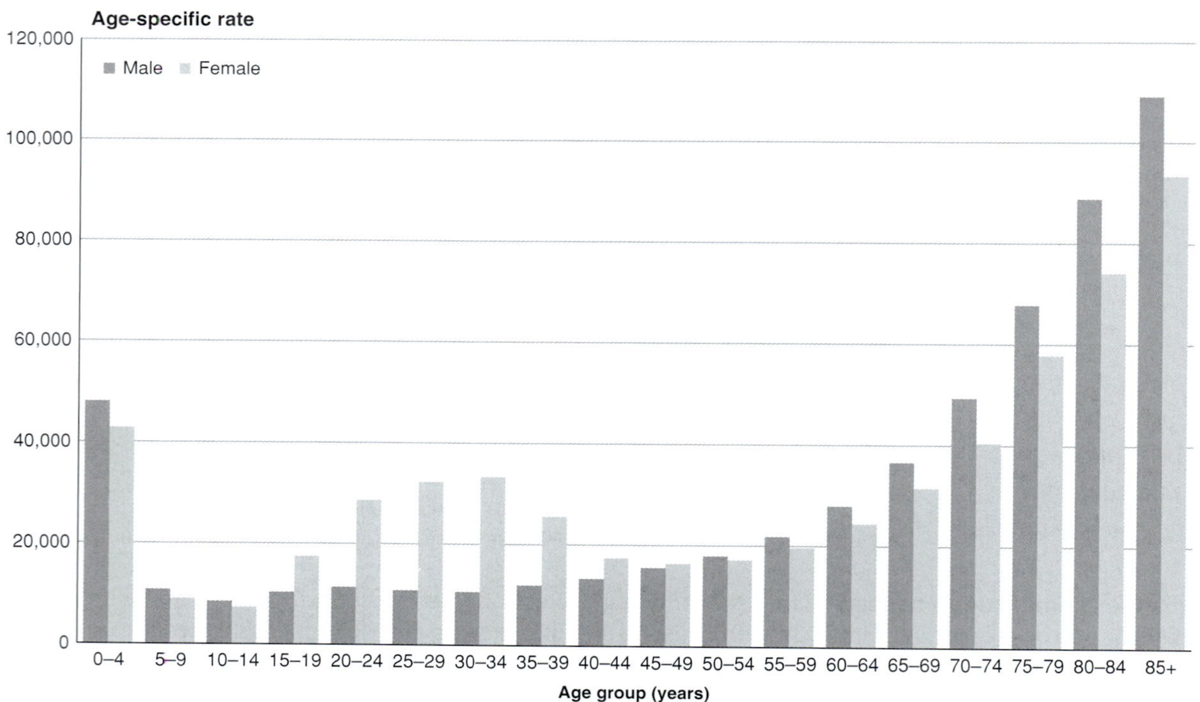

FIGURE 5-2 Publicly funded New Zealand hospital discharge rates by age group and sex for 2011/12. (New Zealand Ministry of Health. [2012b]. *Hospital events 2011/12*. Wellington: Author.)

Gerontology is the study of ageing and older adults. Gerontology was first recognised as a specialty in the mid 1940s with the establishment of the Gerontological Society of America and the publication of the first issue of the *Journal of Gerontology*. Since its inception, gerontology has addressed problems that "transcend the knowledge and methods of any one discipline or profession" (Frank, 1946, p. 1).

Gerontology continues to be multidisciplinary and is a specialised area within various disciplines, such as nursing, psychology, social work, and certain allied health professions. In the early decades of gerontology, researchers and practitioners focused on problems of ageing and older adults; but in recent decades, the focus shifted to an emphasis on healthy and successful ageing.

In addition to focusing on healthy ageing, gerontologists are addressing the increasing diversity among older people, including the increased complexity of caring for older adults in healthcare settings. Consequently, the healthcare specialties of geriatric medicine and **gerontological nursing** have emerged. **Geriatrics** is associated with the diseases and disabilities of old people, and geriatric medicine is a subspecialty of internal medicine or family practice that focuses on the medical problems of older people. The American Geriatrics Society was established in 1942 and, in its first publication *Geriatrics*, the editor called for physicians to "alleviate the inevitable deficiencies and limitations inherent in growing old" (Touhy, 1946, p. 17). In 1953, the society changed the name of its journal to the *Journal of the American Geriatrics Society* and broadened its focus to address various issues that affect the **health** and functioning of older adults. These changes reflected the shift in geriatrics from medically oriented care to care that is more preventive—a shift in emphasis from curing, to caring. Consistent with this shift in orientation, the current foci of geriatrics include quality-of-life issues, interventions to maintain optimal functioning, and health promotion as a means of delaying the onset of disability.

Although nurses first recognised the importance of addressing the unique nursing needs of older adults in the early 1900s, geriatric nursing was not considered a subspecialty until the 1960s. By the mid 1970s the American Nurses Association (ANA) advocated using the term *gerontological nursing*, instead of *geriatric nursing*, to reflect more accurately the broader scope of nursing care rather than a focus on disease conditions. Since the 1990s, gerontological nursing has been recognised both as a specialty and as an essential and integral component of adult nursing.

In America gerontological nursing is a well-developed speciality and certification in gerontological nursing has been available since 1974. In Australia and New Zealand there is no register of gerontological nurses, and qualifications are not recognised formally by professional nursing organisations. However, there is a strong demand by registered nurses for post-graduate qualifications in gerontological nursing. Increasing numbers of registered nurses with these qualifications are being recruited to new-speciality advanced nursing roles, focusing on older adults. A number of advanced nursing practice roles in gerontology have evolved since the turn of the century.

In New Zealand the Ministry of Health has adopted an innovative strategy where they showcase nursing older adults. District Health Boards across New Zealand share their development in this area of practice using videos, case studies and stories to describe the roles and the support and training that are available for nurses working in all areas of aged care. These descriptions can be accessed at www.health.govt.nz/publication/showcasing-aged-care-nursing, or alternatively found by searching aged care nursing on the New Zealand Ministry of Health website.

A gerontological advanced practice nurse is a registered nurse who holds a degree higher than an undergraduate qualification and demonstrates clinical expertise in the care of older adults. Categories include gerontological nurse practitioners, gerontological clinical nurse consultants, and gerontological clinical nurse specialists. These nurses have advanced clinical knowledge, skills and care planning, and have an ability to assume responsibility and accountability for the care of the older adult. Roles of advanced practice nurses include teacher, researcher, consultant, administrator, expert clinician, independent practitioner, care/case manager, individual/group counsellor, and multidisciplinary team member/leader. Advanced practice nurses often manage acute and chronic conditions of older adults in their roles as primary care practitioners. It is anticipated that nurses with gerontological specialisation will continue to be in demand because of the growing requirements for healthcare by older adults. Gerontological nurses also strive to improve current nursing practice and the future healthcare for older adults by participating in the generation, testing, utilisation and evaluation of research findings. An important role for advanced practice nurses with clinical expertise in gerontology is to examine evidence from systematic literature reviews so that the best approaches for older adult care are developed. Increasingly advanced practice nurses are being recruited into long-term residential care facilities to enable the delivery of evidence-based care through direct care and support of care staff.

A gerontological nurse's perspective

Our job is to deal with those really difficult situations in the community where people are hanging on at home, but they are on the edge and going to hospital a lot and have many functional issues. We also work with and support staff in residential aged care facilities, because they are pretty isolated. We have developed care guides covering the basics of looking after older people… The people in residential facilities have big needs. Everything is under huge pressure so we are trying to look at ways to provide support… We are doing high-quality, good work that is making a difference and the data shows that.

Dr Michal Boyd, nurse practitioner (NP), aged care primary health

Source: New Zealand Ministry of Health, Nursing Council of New Zealand, DHBNZ & NPAC-NZ. (2009). *Nurse Practitioners: A healthy future for New Zealand* (pp. 42–43). Wellington: New Zealand Ministry of Health.

Nurse competencies and older adults

There has been much development and increased availability of knowledge about the healthcare of older adults over the last two decades. Since the early 1990s, a number of organisations have demonstrated a major commitment to improving the nursing care of older adults by increasing nursing knowledge and evidence-based clinical practice.

In the U.S. in 1992, the John A. Hartford Foundation funded a major initiative called the Nurses Improving Care to the Hospitalized Elderly (NICHE). The NICHE program is ongoing and includes more than 225 hospitals nationwide. It has been shown to improve quality of care for older adults as well as job satisfaction for nurses. Studies of outcomes at NICHE hospitals have demonstrated improvements in clinical care, cost effectiveness, nursing knowledge, and nurse perceptions of the nursing practice environment and quality of care for older adults (Boltz et al., 2008).

In 2007, the Hartford Foundation collaborated with the *American Journal of Nursing* to develop and promulgate a series of 28 cost-free online articles and corresponding videos that nurses and nursing students can use to improve their care of older adults. The Hartford Foundation for Geriatric Nursing also offers many cost-free resources that specifically address evidence-based nursing care of older adults (available at http://consultgerirn.org/resources).

Since the early 2000s, the Joanna Briggs Institute in Australia has produced a number of resources about evidence-based care for older adults. Most of the Joanna Briggs Institute resources, and resources from the *Cochrane Review* database, are available only through memberships; however, many guidelines are accessible through non-profit agencies, educational institutions and government agencies (e.g. the National Guideline Clearinghouse). Clinically oriented chapters in this text include evidence-based practice, summarising pertinent evidence-based protocols. In addition, the resources sections towards the end of each chapter provide information about weblinks for evidence-based guidelines and clinical practice tools.

Another way of improving nurse competencies in the care of older adults is through continuing education programs. Palmer et al. (2008) describe the use of clinical simulations for nursing older people. These peer-reviewed simulations focus on caring for older adults who experience a sudden change in health status, an exacerbation of a chronic condition, or a sentinel event such as a fall. Evaluations found that nurses enjoyed using the simulation, reported increased clinical competency, and significantly increased their knowledge (Kowlowitz et al., 2009).

Many new roles for advanced practice nurses in gerontology have developed in healthcare systems, which support the development of nurse competencies in the care of older adults. These nurses are responsible for the coaching of nursing staff and the implementation of evidence-based practice about older adults into the healthcare system.

A nurse's perspective

My role as the clinical nurse consultant (CNC) for the acute care of older people is to facilitate the development of knowledge and skills of nurses caring for older people. Some ways I achieve this include formal education programs, participation in research projects, and reviews of clinical practice in the individual care environments. Assisting and encouraging nurses to reflect on practice in relation to person-centred care and evidence-based practice is another way I work with nurses to improve the care of the older person.

Deb

HEALTH, WELLNESS AND PROMOTION OF HEALTH

Nurses often use the terms *health* and *wellness* interchangeably because of the shifting paradigm from the traditional health–illness continuum to a whole-person model and person-centred care. This paradigm shift is evident in holistic nursing definitions of health and wellness. For example, a holistic nursing definition of health is "an individually defined state or process in which the individual (nurse, client, family, group, or community) experiences a sense of well-being, harmony, and unity such that subjective experiences about health, health beliefs, and values are honoured; a process of becoming an expanded consciousness" (Mariano, 2013, p. 60). Similarly, a holistic nursing definition of wellness is "integrated, congruent functioning aimed toward reaching one's highest potential" (Mariano, 2013, p. 61). In this text, *health* is defined as the ability of older adults to function at their highest capacity despite the presence of age-related changes and risk factors, whereas *wellness* is an outcome (also called a positive functional consequence) for older adults whose well-being and quality of life is improved through nursing interventions. The growing emphasis on wellness recognises the importance of health promotion and broadens the focus on self-responsibility.

HEALTH PROMOTION FOR OLDER ADULTS

Health promotion refers to programs or interventions that focus on behaviour changes directed towards improved health and well-being of individuals, groups, communities and nations in relation to their environments. Traditionally, health promotion programs emphasised disease prevention (i.e. risk reduction) and health maintenance (i.e. sustaining a neutral state of health), but more recently health promotion also emphasises personal responsibility for health and self-care actions to achieve high-level wellness. Based on this broader approach, promoting wellness for older adults inherently involves helping older adults incorporate health-enhancing behaviours into their daily lives. The scope of health promotion interventions for older adults includes all the following aspects:

- Regularly engaging in several types of physical exercise
- Assuring optimal nutritional intake and avoiding foods associated with risk for disease
- Engaging in recommended screening and preventive services, such as blood pressure checks and vaccinations
- Using stress-reduction methods, such as meditation and relaxation
- Fostering healthy relationships with others
- Engaging in self-wellness actions (e.g. getting adequate rest and sleep, taking time for enjoyable activities alone or with others)
- Attending to spiritual growth
- Engaging in holistic wellness practices (e.g. yoga, tai chi).

In addition, promoting discussions about advance care planning is a topic currently receiving attention as an aspect of health behaviour change (Centers for Disease Control and Prevention, 2014; Fried, Redding, O'Leary et al., 2012).

Because of the importance of reducing healthcare costs and improving quality of care, health promotion programs increasingly focus on evidence-based interventions to prevent, detect and manage conditions that are leading causes of death and disability (e.g. cardiovascular disease, cancer, stroke). Another focus of health promotion for older adults is on effective management, including self-management, of chronic conditions such as diabetes, which occur more commonly among older adults and affect independent functioning and quality of life.

In addition to having an impact on cost of care, health promotion can have a positive effect on quality of life. A commonly cited goal of gerontological health care is to *add life to years, not just more years to life,* which is synonymous with improved quality of life. Currently, there is increasing attention to improved **health-related quality of life** as an outcome of health promotion interventions related to specific conditions. For example, a study of visually impaired older adults with comorbidities found that the health promotion intervention of a referral for visual rehabilitation services could have a beneficial effect on their health-related quality of life (van Nispen et al., 2009). Many advocacy groups are emphasising the need to focus more on health promotion and disease prevention in any health system. An emerging emphasis with regard to health promotion for older adults is on preventing "bounce-back" hospital admissions (i.e. re-admission shortly after discharge from a hospital).

Even though health promotion interventions are cost-effective ways of preventing disease and disability and improving functioning and quality of life for older adults, older adults as a group receive fewer prevention and screening services than other populations. This is due to such misperceptions as (1) older adults are less responsive to health promotion interventions, and (2) preventive services are less effective after the onset of chronic illness. In reality health promotion is essential for older adults precisely because they have more chronic conditions, have complex healthcare needs, and use considerably more healthcare services than younger adults. In addition, longitudinal studies show that, even after the age of 75 or 80 years, health-promoting interventions for older adults are effective for improving functioning and quality of life and increasing life expectancy (Gustafsson, Wilhelmson, Eklund et al., 2012; Pascucci, Chu, Leasure, 2012; Rizzuto, Orsini, Qui et al., 2012).

A student's perspective

On our first day at the facility, we interviewed Terri, the registered nurse who oversees all the clinical care. She has been a nurse for about 15 years and she was very animated and passionate about her job. Throughout her years as a nurse, she has worked in such settings as hospitals, the ICU, and now in long-term residential care. She did not think she would ever work in a long-term residential care facility.

Terri talked about some of the different ways the staff promotes wellness for residents, including things such as quality of life activities that include health and fitness programs, special outings, and cultural events to enhance a resident's mind, body and spirit. They strive to help the residents keep their independence as long as possible and I really enjoyed that aspect of their care.

Molly D.

In reality, health promotion is essential for older adults precisely because they have more chronic conditions, have complex healthcare needs, and use considerably more healthcare services than younger adults.

Health promotion initiatives for older adults

Both the Australian and New Zealand Governments have developed healthy ageing strategies (see Box 5-1) that promote the health of older adults.

The Australian Government is currently in the midst of reforming care for older adults to improve access to quality aged care services. In 2012 implementation of the "Living Longer Living Better" package of reform began. The changes presented aim "…to give older people more choice, easier access and better care" (Australian Government Department of Social Services, 2015, paragraph 4). In New Zealand the government has developed a Positive Ageing Strategy with the following vision:

> *Our vision is for a society where people can age positively, where older people are highly valued and where they are recognised as an integral part of families and communities. New Zealand will be a positive place in which to age when older people can say that they live in a society that values them, acknowledges their contributions and encourages their participation.* (New Zealand Ministry of Social Development, 2013, p. 4)

The two major goals of health promotion initiatives are increasing quality and years of healthy life, and eliminating health disparities. For older adults, the first goal is associated

BOX 5-1
National health initiatives and resources important to older adults about healthy ageing

Australia

- Ageing Research Online provides access to information about ageing: www.aro.gov.au
- Australian Government Department Social Services. Aged Care Reform: www.dss.gov.au/our-responsibilities/ageing-and-aged-care/aged-care-reform
- Australian Indigenous Health*InfoNet* provides information and resources about Indigenous older people's health: www.healthinfonet.ecu.edu.au/population-groups/older-people
- Australian Institute of Health and Welfare provides statistics on healthy ageing: www.aihw.gov.au/statistics-on-healthy-ageing
- Health Promotion Service for Older People provides information for older people about healthy ageing: www.cpsa.org.au
- National Ageing Institute of Research (NARI) provides information about health promotion research for older people: www.mednwh.unimelb.edu.au
- National Seniors Productive Ageing Centre (NSPAC) supports research and provides information about productive ageing: www.productiveageing.com.au

New Zealand

- Age Concern provides information and resources about healthy ageing: www.ageconcern.org.nz
- Agewell, Healthy Promotion for Older People provides information and resources about healthy ageing: www.agewell.org.nz
- enliven ageing, Positive Ageing Services: www.enlivenconnect.co.nz/node/440
- Office for Senior Citizens provides information about the New Zealand Government's Positive Ageing Strategy: www.osc.govt.nz/positive-ageing-strategy

Other sources

- Centers for Disease Control and Prevention (CDC) provide quality information and resources about healthy ageing: www.cdc.gov/aging

with preventing chronic illness as well as exacerbations of existing illnesses. The second goal addresses health disparities that disproportionately affect specific older populations. Programs being implemented through national initiatives are summarised in Box 5-1, along with weblink information about the governments' policies, programs and related resources that are useful for nurses about healthy ageing and health promotion. One Australian initiative resulting from research on the healthy ageing of Australians is the development and implementation of the online Healthy Ageing Quiz (National Ageing Research Institute, 2010). The quiz is proving to be a valid and reliable assessment tool that assists people who are ageing to increase their awareness and knowledge about ageing and health (Cyarto et al., 2013).

Types of health promotion interventions for older adults

Interventions to promote physical and psychosocial well-being include screening programs, risk-reduction interventions, environmental modifications, and health education. This section reviews these types of programs in relation to promoting wellness for older adults. All clinically oriented chapters of this text emphasise health promotion because this is a central focus of the Functional Consequences Model for Promoting Wellness. Nursing interventions are directed towards improved health, functioning and quality of life for older adults, with emphasis on working with older adults and their carers/caregivers about health-promoting activities.

Screening programs

Screening programs are an essential component of disease prevention because they may detect serious and progressive conditions as early as possible. The National Guideline Clearinghouse publishes numerous evidence-based recommendations for screening related to conditions such as glaucoma, diabetes, hypertension, hyperlipidaemia, osteoporosis, hypothyroidism and many types of cancer. Recommendations focus on conditions that can be accurately detected and effectively treated before they progress to a serious or fatal stage. Cost effectiveness of a screening test is determined according to criteria such as its ability to detect a condition or risk factor at an early stage and without excessive false-positive or false-negative results. Another criterion for recommending a screening test is that early intervention must be superior to waiting until signs or symptoms of disease are present.

A consideration that is particularly pertinent to older adults is the increasing attention to age-based recommendations. For example, screening recommendations for breast, colon, prostate and cervical cancer are often based on predictions of life expectancy and health status. This is consistent with the current focus on increasing years of healthy living rather than on simply extending the quantity of life. Although the intent of these recommendations is to target those older adults who are most likely to benefit, this does not always happen. One study found that many older women in poor health were screened for cancer, whereas many of those in good health did not receive recommended screenings (Schonberg, Leveille & Marcantonio, 2008). Another consideration related to screening programs for older adults is the need to address health beliefs that are likely to influence participation.

Many organisations disseminate guidelines for health promotion interventions, and they are not always in agreement, especially with regard to recommendations for older adults. Box 5-2 summarises some of the more widely agreed upon guidelines for use when educating older adults about health promotion interventions.

Risk-reduction interventions

Risk-reduction interventions, which are based on an assessment of the risk for developing a particular condition, are directed towards reducing the chance of developing that condition. Some risk-reduction interventions (e.g. vaccinations) are applicable to all older adults, and other

BOX 5-2
Guidelines for prevention and health promotion interventions for older adults

Immunisations

For all older adults

- **Tetanus-diphtheria** booster shot every 10 years
- **Influenza** annually at beginning of influenza season
- **Pneumovax** once after age 65 years; booster after 5 years if initial vaccination was before age 65 years or if other risk factors are present

For at-risk older adults

- **Hepatitis A and B**
- **Measles, mumps, rubella** if evidence of lack of immunity and significant risk for exposure
- **Varicella** if evidence of lack of immunity and significant risk for exposure

Screening

For all older adults

- **Blood pressure** checks at least annually, more frequently if range is 130–139 mm Hg systolic or 85–90 mm Hg diastolic or if other risk factors are present (e.g. diabetes)
- **Serum cholesterol** every 5 years, more frequently in people with risk such as personal or family history of cardiovascular disease
- **Faecal occult blood and rectal examination** every 2 years
- **Visual acuity and glaucoma screening** annually
- **Breast examination:** self-examination monthly, annually by medical practitioner

For women

- **Pap smear and pelvic examination:** Between 18 and 70 years for a Pap smear every 2 years
- **Mammogram** every 2 years between 50 and 69 years

For men

- **Digital rectal examination** annually

For at-risk older adults

- **Blood glucose level**
- **Thyroid function**
- **Heart function (electrocardiography)**
- **Bone density**
- **Mental status assessment**
- **Screening for dementia, depression, substance abuse**
- **Urinary incontinence assessment**
- **Functional assessment**
- **Screening for adverse medication effects and drug interactions**
- **Skin cancer assessment**
- **Fall risk assessment**
- **Pressure ulcer assessment**
- **Elder abuse or neglect assessment**

For men

- **Prostate-specific antigen (PSA) blood test**

Health promotion counselling

For all older adults (unless contraindicated)

- **Exercise:** at least 30 minutes of moderate-intensity physical activity daily
- **Nutrition:** adequate intake of all vitamins and minerals, especially calcium, vitamin D and antioxidants
- **Dental care and prophylaxis:** every 6 months
- **Protective measures:** seat belts, sunscreens, smoke detectors, fall risk prevention

For older adults if applicable

- **Smoking cessation**
- **Substance abuse cessation**
- **Weight loss**
- **Dietary supplements**

interventions vary according to specific risk factors and the health level of an older person. Risk assessment tools have been developed for various conditions pertinent to older adults, including falls, incontinence, heart disease, pressure ulcers, and elder abuse and neglect. These tools often include a rating scale to identify people who are most likely to develop a particular condition so that healthcare professionals can plan and implement preventive interventions for them. These tools also serve to identify risk factors that can be addressed through preventive interventions.

However, even without formal assessment tools, health-care professionals can usually identify risk factors that can be addressed to prevent disease or disability. Priority usually is given to reducing the risk factors that are most dominant or likely to have the most serious negative consequences. For example, health promotion interventions for a relatively healthy older adult with a history of hypertension, hypercholesterolaemia, and family history of heart attacks would address risk factors for heart disease. Health promotion interventions for a frail older adult who is in a skilled care unit and who is recovering from a fractured hip would focus on risk for falls.

For all older adults, risk-reduction interventions include lifestyle factors, such as weight management, optimal nutrition, adequate physical activity, sufficient sleep, avoidance of second-hand smoke, and appropriate stress-relieving techniques. Smoking cessation is a risk-reduction activity for all people who smoke. Health promotion activities to reduce risk may also include the use of over-the-counter medications (e.g. low-dose aspirin), nutritional supplements (e.g. vitamins), and complementary and alternative therapies (e.g. yoga).

Some risk-reduction interventions are recommended for all, or most, older adults. For example, for many years, vaccinations for influenza, pneumonia and tetanus have been routinely recommended for all older adults.

Environmental modifications

Environmental modifications are health promotion activities when they reduce risks or improve a person's level of functioning. The Functional Consequences Model for Promoting Wellness addresses environmental modifications as health promotion interventions in relation to many aspects of functioning in the clinically oriented chapters of this text. For example, environmental modifications can be effective health promotion interventions when their implementation reduces fall risks (Chapter 22), improves hearing and vision (Chapters 16 & 17), and prevents urinary incontinence (Chapter 19).

Health education

Health education is an essential component of health promotion because it focuses on working with people to encourage them to engage in self-care activities that are preventive and wellness enhancing. In this text the terms teach or teaching are used to describe this intervention (see below). For example, a randomised trial found that tailored health-education materials were effective in improving self-care behaviours of adults at risk for skin cancer (Glanz, Schoenfeld & Steffan, 2010). Similarly, an educational intervention to improve recognition of heart attack and stroke symptoms was directed towards improving the ability of older adults to seek immediate medical attention when appropriate (Bell et al., 2009).

Nurses incorporate health education not only in relation to specific conditions but also in relation to lifestyle factors that affect health and functioning. For example, engaging in regular exercise is a major focus of health education because lack of physical activity is well recognised as a risk factor that contributes to numerous unhealthy conditions. Additional topics of health education that are important for all adults are nutrition, dental care, and avoidance of smoking and second-hand smoke (see Chapters 18 & 21). As discussed in Chapter 2, nurses must have an understanding of the person's health literacy before teaching can begin. Cultural considerations, in relation to health education discussed in Chapter 2, must also be incorporated. Clinically oriented chapters of this text contain intervention boxes with guidelines for teaching older adults and their carers about specific aspects of health and functioning (refer to the list at the end of the table of contents in the front of this book).

Teaching

Throughout this text the words teach and teaching are used frequently to describe the interventions that nurses undertake when providing health education. **Teaching** occurs when the older adult and their carers become active participants in health education. The nurse works with older adults and their carers, and empowers them to implement strategies directed towards achieving the wellness outcomes of safety, improved functioning and quality of life (Kemppainen, Tossavainen & Turunen, 2012). When the nurse is participating in health education they assume the roles of resource person and enabler.

Examples of health promotion interventions for older adults

Because of the national healthy ageing strategies there is an increasing amount of resources to research and develop health promotion interventions for older adults. Table 5-1 lists some examples of and references for evidence-based programs that have been successfully implemented for older adults.

The current evidence supports unquestionably the need for increased physical activity for older adults such that physical activity has emerged as the most widely heralded health promotion intervention today. In recent years there is increasing emphasis on the premise that moderate-intensity

TABLE 5-1 Examples of health promotion programs for older adults

Example	Reference
Mobile Smoking Cessation Program: a pilot program in which trained counsellors provide group health education, individual counselling, and a 4-week supply of nicotine replacement therapy for elderly Chinese smokers in Hong Kong	Abdullah et al., 2008
Enhance Fitness: an evidence-based community exercise program to promote adherence among ethnic older adults	Chiang, Seman, Belza & Tsai, 2008
Resources and Activities for Life Long Independence: an evidence-based exercise program that uses behavioural principles to improve physical activity in people with mild cognitive impairment	Logsdon, McCurry, Pike & Teri, 2009
Demonstration project that used patient education, individualised coaching, and doctor care management to reduce decline in physical functioning during the 22-month study period	Meng et al., 2009
Wellness Tour: A health promotion program of AARP and Walgreens that uses nine buses staffed by trained medical personnel to make 2000 stops in 300 cities to provide 1.3 million free screenings for cholesterol, blood pressure, bone density, glucose levels, waist circumference, and body mass index; educational materials to promote self-responsibility for health	Novelli, 2009
Lifestyle Interventions and Independence for Elders Pilot: a 10-week group-mediated behavioural program that improved functional status of participants and enhanced long-term rates of adherence	Rejeski et al., 2009
Sickness Prevention Achieved through Regional Collaboration (SPARC): a program that provided immunisations and screening for cancer and cardiovascular disease in collaboration with area agencies on ageing	Shenson, Benson & Harris, 2008
Experience Corps: a program that used a high-intensity senior volunteer program as a health promotion intervention to improve physical activity in high-risk older adults	Tan et al., 2009
Active for Life: an initiative that evaluated two evidence-based behavioural programs to increase physical activity in almost 2000 older adults from nine community-based organisations	Wilcox, Dowda et al., 2009

physical activity can improve overall health and quality of life and lower the risk for disease. Numerous studies have found that adequate exercise decreases the risks for stroke, obesity, osteoporosis, sarcopenia, type 2 diabetes, loss of function, and some forms of cancer (Blair & Morris, 2009; Elsawy & Higgins, 2010). Some recent studies about physical activity and older adults are as follows:

- In a sample of 884 adults aged 65 years and older, leisure-time walking was associated with many positive health outcomes, including the prevention of cognitive decline (Prohaska et al., 2009).
- A study of 846 people aged 66 to 98 years at death found that physical activity in middle and later life lowered the risk for dementia, impaired mobility, and the need for inpatient or long-term residential aged care (Bonsdorff et al., 2009).
- A longitudinal study of 2205 men indicated that increased physical activity during middle age was associated with reduced mortality to the same level as that associated with smoking cessation (Byberg et al., 2009).
- A meta-analysis found that increased physical activity was associated with modest improvements in quality of life among adults with chronic illnesses (Conn, Hafdahl & Brown, 2009).
- A pilot study of 102 sedentary adults aged 70 to 89 years who were at increased risk for cognitive disability showed a positive association between moderate-intensity physical activity and improved cognitive function (Williamson et al., 2009).
- A randomised trial of 544 older adults found some statistically significant benefits of participating in a multiple-component physical activity program with regard to self-efficacy, exercise participation, adherence in the face of barriers, and increased upper and lower body strength (Hughes et al., 2009).
- Four controlled trials were conducted to assess whether a program reduced falls and injuries in older people living in the community living in New Zealand. Here 1016 women and men aged between 65 and 97 participated in the study. "Overall the effect of the exercise program was a 35% reduction in the number of falls and a 35% reduction in the number of fall-related injuries" (Otago Medical School, 2003, p. 9).
- A *Cochrane Review* about the effects of interventions to reduce the incidence of falls in older people living in the community concluded that exercise interventions reduce risk and rate of falls (Gillespie et al., 2009).

Despite the wealth of undisputed evidence about the beneficial effects of physical activity for older adults, many older adults in Australia and New Zealand do not engage in exercise regularly (see Box 5-3).

Nurses take many roles in promoting physical activity for older adults; in particular, teaching older adults about the health benefits of physical activity. It also is important to teach about the latest recommendations for type, frequency, duration and intensity of physical activity. Nurses also assess for and address other factors that positively or negatively influence an older adult to participate in regular physical activity. Nurses can use Box 5-4 and Figure 5-3 to teach older adults about recommended exercises. In both Australia and New Zealand there are guidelines available, based on evidence, about physical activity and older adults:

- Brown, W. J., Moorhead, G. E. and Marshall, A. L. (2005). Choose health: Be active. A physical activity guide for older Australians. Canberra: Commonwealth of Australia and the Repatriation Commission. Accessible via www.healthyactive.gov.au
- Australian and New Zealand Society for Geriatric Medicine. (2013). Exercise guidelines for older adults. Available via www.anzsgm.org
- New Zealand Ministry of Health. (2013). New Zealand guidelines on physical activity for older people (aged 65 years and over). Accessible via www.health.govt.nz.

BOX 5-3
Exercise and older adults in Australia and New Zealand

Australia

- 56.9% of people aged 75 years and over report being sedentary and 25.8% doing low levels of exercise

New Zealand

- 34.2% of people age 75 years and over report being sedentary
- In this age group almost 10% more women (37.9%) than men (29.2) report being sedentary

Source: Australian Bureau of Statistics (ABS). (2013). Exercise. *Profiles of health, Australia 2011–13*. Accessed February 2015 at www.abs.gov.au/ausstats/abs@.nsf/Lookup/4338.0main+features112011-13; New Zealand Ministry of Health. (2012b). *The health of New Zealand adults 2011/12: Key findings of the New Zealand Health Survey*. Wellington: Author.

MODELS OF BEHAVIOUR CHANGE FOR HEALTH PROMOTION

Health promotion interventions for preventing disease often require changing from detrimental health-related behaviours to those that enhance wellness. Even after people adopt new behaviours, they need to maintain these healthier behaviours and not revert to unhealthy ones. The more ingrained and rewarding or pleasurable the behaviours that must be changed, the more difficult it is to refrain from these activities. Some unhealthy behaviours, such as cigarette smoking, have a strong addictive component that increases the difficulty of behaviour change. Similarly, the more comfortable a person is with the absence of healthy behaviours, such as physical activity, the more difficult it will be to develop healthier behaviours.

Initiation and maintenance of healthy behaviours involve both motivation and action steps. The role of healthcare professionals in health promotion interventions is to lead and support the older person in replacing unhealthy behaviours with health-promoting behaviours. The Stages of Change

BOX 5-4
Health education about types of exercise

Type	Definition	Benefits	Intensity	Frequency
Aerobic (e.g. brisk walking, jogging, walking up stairs)	Activity that requires the body to use oxygen to produce the energy necessary for the activity	Lowers blood pressure, strengthens heart muscle, improves lipids and triglycerides, diminishes blood glucose, decreases intra-abdominal fat, decreases risk for cardiovascular disease, improves self-esteem, relieves symptoms of anxiety and depression	Identify your target heart rate by subtracting your age in years from 220 (this is the maximum heart rate) and multiplying by 0.65	2.5 hours weekly of moderate intensity OR 1.25 hours weekly of vigorous intensity (in episodes of at least 10 minutes)
Strength or resistance training (stretch bands, weights, strap-on sandbags, bicep curls, bench presses)	Performance of muscle contractions against a resistance that is greater than usual for that muscle; slow and controlled movements of major muscle groups such as arms, back, hips, chest and shoulders, with exhalation during exertion and inhalation during return to the starting position	Improves balance and diminishes risk for falls, strengthens musculoskeletal system, improves function and independence, decreases risk for osteoporosis, favourably modifies risk factors for cardiovascular disease and type 2 diabetes	You should be able to repeat the movement 8 consecutive times, but not more than 12 times, before experiencing significant muscle fatigue	8–10 different sets of exercises working all major muscle groups, each repeated 8–12 times, several days a week
Stretching (e.g. yoga, range-of- motion exercises)	Activity that improves body flexibility	Increases flexibility, reduces muscle soreness, improves performance of daily activities	Stretch muscle groups, but not to the point of pain, and hold for 10–30 seconds	Repeat each stretch at least 4 times, a minimum of 2–4 times weekly

Notes: Physical activity is any skeletal muscle activity that causes energy expenditure. Exercise refers to structured and repetitive body movements performed with the goal of attaining physical fitness.

Model (also called the **Transtheoretical Model [TTM]**) has been widely used by healthcare professionals to explain stages of behaviour change. During the last three decades, the Stages of Change model has been used successfully in programs for stress management, sun exposure, smoking cessation, medication compliance, alcohol and drug cessation, diet and weight control, and screening for cancers. As the name implies, the Stages of Change model describes five specific stages through which a person progresses in accomplishing behaviour changes (Table 5-1). A description of each stage follows as well as an example of an interaction between a practice nurse and an older client for each stage.

In the first stage, *precontemplation,* the person is unaware of the problem, is in denial of the need for change, or is resistant to change. At this stage, the person has no intention of changing his or her behaviours within the next 6 months. Appropriate health promotion interventions for a person in this stage include providing information about the problem behaviour and providing unconditional encouragement for thinking about behaviour change. When working with an older adult in this stage, nurses can offer information, discuss their own beliefs, and help the person identify the personal benefits of the health-promoting behaviours. The nurse also can acknowledge the person's perspective and point out the negative consequences of current behaviours. Here is a discussion example where an older person has been referred to the practice nurse from the medical practitioner after a regular blood test showed a low level of vitamin D:

Nurse: Are you aware that women after menopause are at increased risk of developing brittle bones or osteoporosis and that this increases your risk of breaking a bone?

Older person: I have seen some advertisements on the TV but I thought it didn't apply to me as I eat dairy.

Nurse: That is a great start but there are other risk factors, including low vitamin D, low levels of exercise and many others. The doctor has found in your recent blood tests that your vitamin D level is low.

Older person: Really! I rarely go out into the sun but I thought I was doing the right thing, you know, taking care of my skin. You also mentioned exercise. I think I exercise enough. I have slowed down but I still manage to do the housework every day.

Nurse: We now know that you need to spend some time in the sunlight to ensure we have adequate vitamin D levels. Here is some information from Osteoporosis Australia about this. It also contains some information about exercise levels as well.

Older person: Okay, I'll take a look.

The second stage, *contemplation,* is characterised by an intention to change in the foreseeable future, based on some acknowledgement of the negative consequences

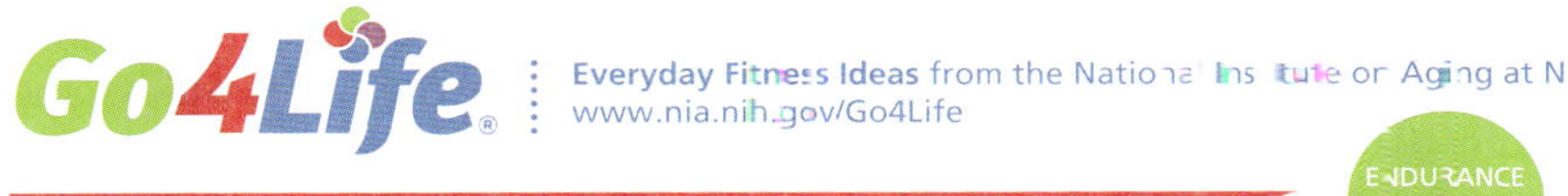

Include All 4 Types of Exercise

ENDURANCE STRENGTH FLEXIBILITY BALANCE

Exercise generally falls into four main types: endurance, strength, balance, and flexibility.

Some activities fit into more than one type of exercise; for example, some endurance activities help build strength, and some flexibility exercises also improve balance. Be creative and choose exercises from each of the four types to see the benefits!

Endurance. Activities that increase your heart rate and breathing for an extended period of time, such as walking, jogging, swimming, dancing, yard work, climbing stairs.
BENEFITS: Everyday activities, like gardening or shopping, become easier to do.
HOW MUCH & HOW OFTEN: Build up to at least 30 minutes of moderate-intensity endurance activity on most or all days of the week.

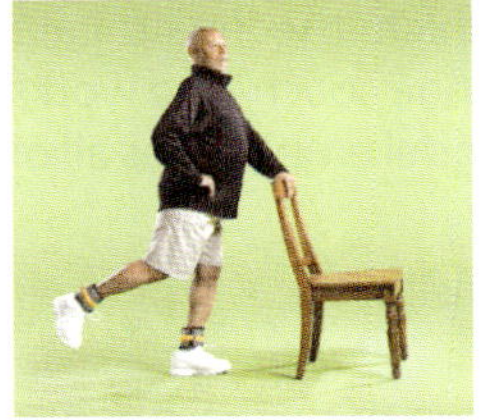

Strength. Activities that increase your muscle strength, such as using resistance bands or small weights (even cans of food) to strengthen groups of muscles.
BENEFITS: Improve ability to do everyday and enjoyable activities and remain independent.
HOW MUCH & HOW OFTEN: Aim for a 30-minute session two or more days a week and include all major muscle groups.

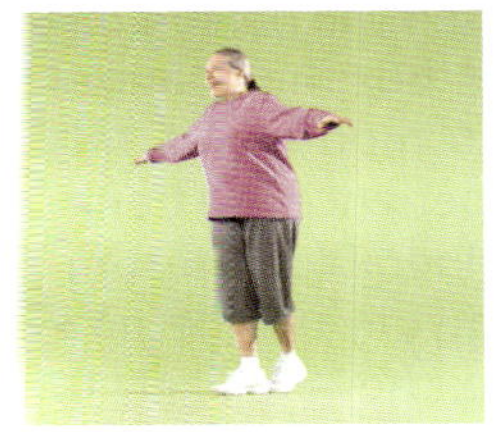

Balance. Activities that improve your balance, such as tai chi, standing on one foot, heel-to-toe walking.
BENEFITS: Help prevent falls and improve safety when performing activities such as standing on tiptoe to reach for objects on high shelves.
HOW MUCH & HOW OFTEN: Do these often, anywhere and anytime; be sure to use a wall or sturdy object for support as needed for safety.

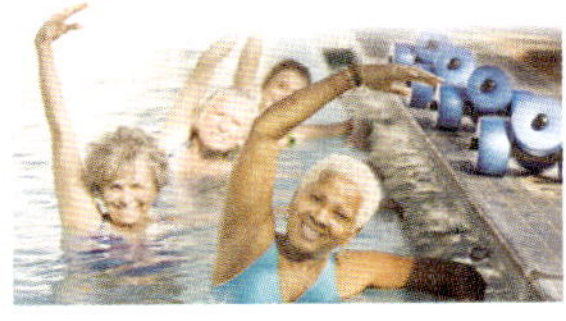

Flexibility. Activities that stretch groups of muscles, or shoulder and upper arm stretches.
BENEFITS: Give you more freedom of movement for daily activities, such as getting dressed.
HOW MUCH & HOW OFTEN: Stretch a group of muscles as far as possible without pain, hold the position for 10 to 30 seconds, relax, breathe, then repeat 3 to 5 times.

FIGURE 5-3 Example of an educational handout about recommended types of exercise for older adults. (Adapted from Everyday fitness ideas from the National Institute on Ageing at NIH. Accessible via http://go4life.nia.nih.gov.)

of current behaviours and positive consequences of different behaviours. The person is likely to ask questions and to seek information about the short- and long-term risks and benefits of various behaviours. He or she is likely to be ambivalent about giving up a rewarding activity or taking on an activity that is viewed as difficult or less enjoyable. During this stage, the nurse can help the person see that the benefits outweigh the disadvantages, even though the person may not experience the benefits immediately. Appropriate health promotion interventions for this stage include providing additional information about the risks and benefits and exploring with the person how he or she can begin establishing personal goals for a healthier lifestyle. Interventions also include increasing the person's sense of self-efficacy by helping the person to see himself or herself practising these new behaviours. When working with an older adult in this stage it is helpful to express confidence in the person's ability to develop health-promoting behaviours. Continuing with the example:

Nurse: Have you had a chance to read the information I gave to you about osteoporosis?

Older person: Yes, I did. It says I need to spend 10 minutes a day outside, but I don't like going out into the sun. I find it hurts my eyes and gives me a headache.

Nurse: Okay. Spending 10 minutes in sunlight does not mean the whole body needs to be in the sun. It is recommended that at least your arms are exposed, or legs. So you could sit with your head in the shade and your legs and some of your arms in the sun.

Stage three, the *preparation* stage, is characterised by some ambivalence about the unhealthy behaviour but a stronger inclination to change to healthier behaviours. The person acknowledges the need for change, expresses serious intent to adopt the healthier behaviours within the next month, and begins to identify strategies for implementing them. During this stage, people usually benefit from support from family and friends, and they are likely to state their intentions and seek help from others in accomplishing their goals. Nurses can support and provide positive reinforcement for the person's intent to change; they also can point out the progress that the person already has made in developing an action plan. An important role for nurses is to assist with developing a plan and identifying the person's goals and small-step strategies to achieve them. Although discussing the barriers to changing behaviours might be necessary, it is important to focus on the benefits of the new behaviour. Planning strategies for dealing with anticipated difficulties in implementing the plan is also helpful. Continuing with the example:

Nurse: Having you tried sitting out in the sun since we last met?
Older person: Yes, I did it one day but I found my eyes still hurt.
Nurse: Okay. Do you think wearing sunglasses might help with your eyes?
Older person: Yes, I see. Why didn't I think of wearing sunglasses? I only think of them when I'm in the car. Okay, I'll give them a go.

Action, the fourth stage, occurs when the person has already made the behaviour change, but the changes have been practised for less than 6 months. At this stage, people usually do not fully experience the benefits of the new behaviour and are vulnerable to resuming prior unhealthy behaviours or giving up the new healthy behaviours. At the same time, they are likely to have high levels of self-efficacy and to feel good about the progress they have made. Health promotion interventions during this stage are directed towards reinforcing the progress that has been made as well as towards identifying barriers to continuing the healthy behaviours. Nurses can help the older adult identify motivators, establish a reward system, and plan strategies for overcoming the identified obstacles. They also can ask about support from friends and family and help the person identify ways of extending their support system if necessary. Continuing with the example:

Nurse: So how is the sun-sitting going?
Older person: Yes, I have been doing it most days and the sunglasses have worked.
Nurse: That's great. Now, at your next visit, I will organise the doctor to take a blood test and measure your vitamin D level.

Stage five, *maintenance,* occurs when the person has continued the healthy behaviours for 6 months or longer. By this time, the person is experiencing positive effects of the healthier behaviour and the risk of relapse is less. During this stage, levels of self-efficacy are usually high and the person is motivated to maintain the healthier lifestyle. Because the person has less need for external support, the role of nurse diminishes. Health promotion interventions during this stage include reinforcement of progress and positive feedback about the healthier behaviours. In addition, the nurse can ask about any difficulties in maintaining the progress and help the person identify strategies to overcome any difficulties. Continuing with the example:

Nurse: Since your last visit, are you still keeping up with the sun-sitting?
Older person: I am. I found I was getting bored doing it, though. But now my hubby is sitting with me and we have a cuppa together.
Nurse: That's great you have been able to make it part of your life. I am sure that your blood test today will show an improvement in your vitamin D level.

Models of behaviour change that have been developed more recently are based on a positive approach and build on the person's strengths. *Motivational interviewing* is an example of a positive model in which the healthcare professional assumes the role of a "change coach" and works in partnership with the person. This model emphasises all of the following:

- Personal autonomy and self-responsibility
- Capacity rather than incapacity
- Actions to facilitate change, rather than reasons for avoiding change
- Communication techniques of affirmation, summarising, reflective listening, open-ended questions, and avoiding argumentation or direct persuasion
- Discussion about the person's awareness of the problem, main concerns, intention to change, and confidence about changing
- Exploration of goals and the costs and benefits of changing versus not changing
- Communicating empathy, caring and a genuine interest in the person's perspective.

Although the full use of motivational interviewing requires extensive training, nurses can apply a brief form to health promotion interventions (Noordam et al., 2013; Stawnychy, Creber, Riegel et al., 2014).

Appreciative inquiry is another positive model that has recently been applied to promoting behaviour change in healthcare settings. This model replaces deficit thinking with possibility thinking and uses a set of questions to appreciate and value the best of what is, to envision a future of what might be, and to dialogue about and create what will be. The process is divided into four steps, designated as discover, dream, design and delivery. Moore and Charvat (2007) propose that nurses use the appreciative inquiry approach to explore the person's experiences of what works or has worked to promote health, as in the following questions for each of the four steps:

- *Discover:* Describe a time when you had an exceptionally healthy lifestyle and consider the following questions: What did you appreciate about the experience? How did

BOX 5-5
Communication techniques for encouraging behaviour change

Self-efficacy: increasing the older adult's confidence in accomplishing the desired behaviour

- "You deserve a lot of credit for losing those first 2 kilograms. Sometimes those are the hardest ones to lose, so you can be confident that you can keep making progress, kilo by kilo."
- "Think about a time when you were successful in the face of a challenge, even though you weren't confident."
- "Describe a personal characteristic that helps you accomplish your goals."

Values clarification: helping older adults identify values in order to reconcile differences between expectations and behaviours

- "People often have mixed feelings about changing behaviours. For example, you know that being overweight increases the risks to your health, but at the same time, you enjoy eating. Let's talk about the ways in which your health is important to you."
- "It sounds like you have a conflict between believing that getting more exercise is good for your health and believing that you have time for this. Let's talk about how you can use your time to support your health."

Consciousness raising: increasing the older adult's awareness about risks that are identified objectively (e.g. elevated blood pressure or abnormal laboratory values for lipids) but are not associated with immediate symptoms

- "Your blood pressure has been around 156/90 for several weeks lately. Are you aware that the ideal range is below 120/80?"
- "Your weight has been increasing during the last 3 years and it is at the point that you are at an increased risk for diabetes, especially because you also have high blood pressure."

Restructuring: using positive thinking to focus on ways of overcoming barriers

- "I know it's hard to get outside in the winter, so let's try to identify some ways of getting more exercise indoors during your usual activities. For instance, are there times that you could walk in shopping malls or even around your house?"
- "You've identified several barriers to achieving your goal. Can you pick the one that is the easiest to tackle and we'll see if we can find some ways to overcome it. I know that one of your strengths is facing your challenges, so let's look at one of those challenges and come up with a strategy that might work for you."

Focusing on benefits (also called reinforcing rewards): immediately and frequently reinforcing benefits, which are classified as tangible, social or self-generated

- "Describe how you felt the last time you were at your ideal body weight."
- "Can you identify a healthy reward for engaging in physical activity, for example, by treating yourself to fresh fruit after you come back from the park?"
- "Let's talk about the benefits of quitting smoking. For example, within a day of quitting you've already decreased your risk for heart attack. Can you think of another benefit?"

Strengthening social support: involving family and friends in healthy behaviours

- "That's an excellent idea to walk with your friend for a half-hour right after you both come back from the lunch program at the senior centre."
- "When your grandchildren visit, would it be feasible to take them to the park or a playground?"

Adapted from C. A. Miller. (2013). *Fast facts for health promotion in nursing: Promoting wellness in a nutshell*. Used with permission from Springer Publishing Company.

you make this happen? What people or situational factors supported this positive experience?

- *Dream:* Imagine you are so physically active that you feel very fit and healthy and consider the following questions: What would you feel like on a daily basis? What would you be doing? How would you look? What would you be doing for exercise? How do you think it would help your heart?
- *Design:* What could you do now to be more in charge of your own health and care? Who would you go to for help?
- *Delivery:* What are we going to do to start this process?

Through this interaction the nurse and older adult engage in a cooperative search for strengths, passions and life-giving forces, so the person is open to new possibilities.

Nurses can apply principles from these models as they work with older adults to promote healthy behaviours related to nutrition, physical activity, weight management and other lifestyle factors that increase the risk for disease and affect the person's health and functioning. Nurses also have applied principles of appreciative inquiry to develop a transitional care coaching intervention to improve care for chronically ill medical inpatients when they are discharged from hospital to home (Scala & Costa, 2014). Although most nurses are not professional health coaches, all nurses can incorporate communication techniques for encouraging behaviour change such as the following: self-efficacy, values clarification, consciousness raising, restructuring, focusing on benefits, and strengthening social support. Box 5-5 briefly describes these interventions and provides examples of communication techniques that can be used to help older adults increase healthy behaviours or decrease those that endanger their health.

CASE STUDY

Mrs Hapfau is 72 years old and visits the local medical centre. Once a month she comes to see you, the practice nurse, to have her blood pressure checked. Mrs Hapfau takes medication for high blood pressure and has expressed concern about heart disease. When you discuss risk factors for heart disease with Mrs Hapfau, she says that she would like to incorporate more physical activity into her daily life, as long as it doesn't worsen her arthritis. She agrees to begin meeting with you regularly to develop a plan. Table 5-2 shows how you might apply the transtheoretical model to your work with Mrs Hapfau.

TABLE 5-2 Applying the transtheoretical model to Mrs Hapfau

Stage	Nurse	Mrs Hapfau
I: Precontemplation		
Assessment	"I know you're concerned about preventing heart disease because you've talked with me about your high blood pressure and you pay attention to avoiding high-fat foods. How do you think you rate on a scale of 1 to 10, with 1 being the lowest level and 10 being the best, in level of physical activity for preventing heart disease?"	"I would rate myself about 10. I take the dog out for a 5-minute walk every morning. My friend says we don't need more than 10 minutes of walking a day after we're 70 years old."
Intervention	"Did you know that there is extremely good evidence that 30 minutes of physical activity every day—even if it's not done all at once—is a good measure for protecting against heart disease? Would you be willing to read this pamphlet from the Heart Foundation and let me know what you think when I see you again next week?"	"I've seen that before, but I'll try to read it this week if I have a chance."
II: Contemplation		
Assessment	"Now that you've had a chance to read that brochure, what's your understanding of the role of physical activity in preventing heart problems?"	"I think the Heart Foundation is on an exercise kick—they must think we all want to participate in marathons! Maybe they have a point about walking more than 15 minutes a day, but don't they realise that those of us who are in our 70s have a lot of problems walking? Most of us have arthritis. I think that brochure was written for people in their 20s, but on the other hand, maybe they do know what they're talking about."
Intervention	"From what I know, the Heart Foundation focuses on helping people prevent heart disease through healthy habits. They strongly urge everyone to do physical exercise for 30 minutes every day to keep the heart healthy. Many studies of people of all ages support this recommendation. You already walk 5 minutes with your dog every day, so you've gotten a good start on daily exercise. I bet your dog would love to go just a little further each day and you would be quite capable of increasing your walk by just a little bit."	"Well, the dog is getting pretty fat, and it would probably do her good to get out for another walk in the evening. But it's hard enough for me to get out once a day with the weather as cold as it is right now. With my arthritis, I think I should wait a couple of months until the weather is warmer."
III: Preparation		
Assessment	"Since we met a couple of months ago, what are your current thoughts about increasing your walking?"	"I've been doing a lot of thinking about what we discussed, and now that spring is finally here, I think it's time to increase my walking time by a little bit each day. I just hope my arthritis doesn't get worse if I walk more."
Intervention	"So, have you thought of a plan that might work for you? Can you identify people who might be helpful in supporting your efforts?"	"Well, to begin with, I thought I could walk for 10 minutes every morning instead of 5—my dog sure would like that. I could increase that by 5 minutes every few weeks until I get up to 30 minutes a day. I've told my daughter that I'm trying to do more walking, and she said she might come over and walk with me and the dog on Saturdays. I do worry about my arthritis, though."
IV: Action		
Assessment	"It's so good to hear that you've been increasing your walking time for 3 months now. Congratulations on getting up to 30 minutes a day. How are you feeling about that?"	"My dog sure likes it, but I'm not sure that it's doing any good for me. I guess it feels good to pay attention to my health, but I haven't noticed that I'm feeling any better physically—at least not yet. My daughter came with me for the first few weeks and that was a good chance to see her, but she hasn't been coming for the last 3 weeks."

TABLE 5-2 Applying the transtheoretical model to Mrs Hapfau (*continued*)

Stage	Nurse	Mrs Hapfau
Intervention	"You deserve a lot of credit for accomplishing your goal—do you give yourself any rewards? It sounds as though you're disappointed that your daughter stopped walking with you—is there anyone else who might walk with you?"	"I guess I do deserve some credit—I did buy myself a new pair of walking shoes last week. A neighbour lady has talked to me about my walking and she said she'd like to get out there and join me, but I didn't encourage that because I thought my daughter would be coming with me. Maybe I'll invite her along—she could use the exercise, too."
V: Maintenance		
Assessment	"Congratulations on walking for 30 minutes every day for 7 months—that's quite an accomplishment and a nice gift for yourself and your health. You also deserve credit for getting your neighbour to join you at least a couple of days a week. Are you concerned about any temptations to cut down on your walking routine?"	"Thanks for the encouragement—my neighbour says she appreciates me inviting her along, and I enjoy the chance to keep up on neighbourhood happenings by chatting with her when we walk. I am a little concerned about keeping up with the walking during the winter. I don't even take the dog out when it rains."
Intervention	"Have you thought about walking in the mall when the weather is bad? I'm not sure if you can take the dog along, but the mall opens every day an hour before the stores open so that walkers can come. I understand there's quite a group that walks there in the mornings."	"That sounds like a good idea—my neighbour mentioned that we might go there in bad weather. I think I'll try that out—maybe if we went to the mall, I could get my daughter to meet me there on Saturdays."

Thinking points about Mrs Hapfau's situation and behavioural changes for health promotion

Precontemplation stage

- From a health promotion perspective, how would you assess Mrs Hapfau's understanding of the role of exercise in prevention of heart disease? What misconceptions would you want to address?
- What are the goals of your teaching interventions at this stage?

Contemplation stage

- How would you assess Mrs Hapfau's perception of the advantages and disadvantages of increased levels of exercise?
- What are the goals of your teaching interventions at this stage?
- What additional teaching points would you incorporate in your health promotion interventions at this time?

Preparation stage

- What additional assessment questions would you ask Mrs Hapfau?
- What are the goals of your teaching interventions at this stage?
- What additional teaching points would you incorporate, particularly with regard to Mrs Hapfau's concerns about her arthritis?

Action stage

- What concerns would you have about Mrs Hapfau during this stage, and what additional questions would you ask?
- What additional teaching points would you make?

Maintenance stage

- What additional assessment questions would you be able to ask Mrs Hapfau?
- What additional teaching points would you make?

CHAPTER HIGHLIGHTS

Nursing older adults

- Nurses are the primary health carers of older adults.
- Nurses require skills and knowledge to meet the healthcare needs of the older adult.
- Nurses require the skills to assess older adults comprehensively and provide in-depth prevention and wellness promotion services.
- Nurses have many resources for information about evidence-based practice and improving care with regard to older adults.
- Gerontology and geriatrics are areas of professional specialisation that have evolved since the mid 1940s to address the unique needs of older adults.
- These specialties initially focused on problems associated with ageing, but the current focus is on quality-of-life issues and promoting optimal health and functioning.
- Gerontological nursing was first recognised as a nursing specialty during the 1960s and it continues to develop. Innovative models of care have paved the way for many roles for gerontological nurses, including opportunities for advanced practice nurses.

Health, wellness and health promotion

- Nurses have important roles in health promotion interventions, which are essential for preventing chronic conditions, reducing mortality and improving quality of life for older adults (Box 5-1).

- Many major national initiatives focus on health promotion for older adults and provide valuable resources that nurses can use (Box 5-1).
- Types of health promotion interventions applicable to older adults include screening programs, risk-reduction interventions, environmental modifications and health education to promote good health practices (Table 5-1, Box 5-2).
- Nurses have important roles in teaching older adults about the benefits of physical activity and promoting exercise (Box 5-4; Figure 5-3).

Models of behavioural change for health promotion

- The Stages of Change model has been used to address disease prevention and health promotion interventions that require a change in health-related behaviours (Table 5-2).
- Positive models of behaviour change include motivational interviewing and appreciative inquiry.
- Nurses can incorporate communication techniques to address all the following: self-efficacy, values clarification, consciousness raising, restructuring, focusing on benefits, and strengthening social support (Box 5-5).

CRITICAL THINKING EXERCISES

1. You are discussing with your fellow students the choices you will be making about a practice area after graduation. You tell them that you are planning to specialise in gerontological nursing, and they challenge your decision with statements such as "You'll be bored to death taking care of old fogies. Why don't you specialise in something exciting like trauma care? Besides, there's not much to do about the conditions of older folks, and what's the challenge in taking care of people who aren't going to get better?" How do you respond to these statements?
2. Identify one health-related behaviour that you would like to change in your life (e.g. smoking cessation, increased level of exercise, decreased dietary fat intake) and develop a care plan for your behaviour change using the TTM of health promotion (as in the case study).

RESOURCES

For an extensive range of additional resources to enhance teaching and learning and to facilitate understanding of this chapter, please see the text's accompanying website located on thePoint at http://thepoint.lww.com.

Clinical tools

Hartford Institute for Geriatric Nursing, ConsultGeriRN.org: http://consultgerirn.org/resources
Assessment tools *Try This*® series and *How to Try This* resources
General assessment series:

- *Try This*, issue 21: Immunizations for older adults. S. Greenberg (2012).
- *Try This*, issue 27: General screening recommendations for chronic disease and risk factors in older adults. K. T. Hall. (2010).

Evidence-based practice

National Guideline Clearinghouse: www.guideline.gov
Search for:

- Guidelines, by organisations, and practice guidelines from numerous professional organisations from many countries, with delineation of level of evidence to support recommendations.
- Guideline syntheses for topics such as Alzheimer's disease.
- Guidelines in progress, updated protocols related to clinical practice guidelines such as Management of hip fractures in the elderly (American Academy of Orthopaedic Surgeons) and Prevention of type 2 diabetes evidence-based nutrition practice guideline (Academy of Nutrition and Dietetics).

Hartford Institute for Geriatric Nursing, ConsultGeriRN.org: http://consultgerirn.org/resources

- *Try This* series of best practice assessment tools (all updated or developed during or after 2007).
- *How to Try This* series of 58 cost-free and web-based videos and articles (developed and published between 2007 and 2014), illustrating application of geriatric assessment tools.
- Protocols from *Evidence-based geriatric nursing protocols for best practice* (4th ed.), by M. Boltz, E. Capezuti, T. Fulmer & D. Zwicker (Eds). (2012). New York: Springer.

Joanna Brigs Institute: http://connect.jbiconnectplus.org

- Evidence-based summaries.

Recommended practices for nursing older adults

College of Nurses Aotearoa New Zealand, older person nursing: www.nurse.org.nz/elder-person-nursing.html
Hartford Institute for Geriatric Nursing: http://hartfordign.org
Australian College of Nursing, Australia: www.acn.edu.au/search/node/aged%20care
New Zealand Ministry of Health, Showcasing aged care nursing: www.health.govt.nz/publication/showcasing-aged-care-nursing

Health promotion materials

Age Concern New Zealand: www.ageconcern.org.nz
Age Positive: http://humanrights.gov.au/age-positive
Age Well, health promotion for older people in New Zealand: www.agewell.org.nz
myaged*care* (Australian Government Department of Social Services portal): www.myagedcare.gov.au/healthy-and-active-living
National Institute on Aging: www.nia.nih.gov
National Seniors Productive Ageing Centre, Australia: www.productiveageing.com.au
Office of Disease Prevention and Health Promotion: http://odphp.osophs.dhhs.gov/resources.asp
Seniors Online: www.seniorsonline.vic.gov.au

REFERENCES

Abdullah, A. S. M., Lam, T. H., Chan, S. K., Leung, G. M., Chi, I., Ho, W. W. & Chan, S. S. (2008). Effectiveness of a mobile smoking cessation service in reaching elderly smokers and predictors of quitting. *BMC Geriatrics, 8*(25), 1–9.

Australian Bureau of Statistics (ABS). (2013). Exercise. *Profiles of health, Australia 2011–13*. Accessed February 2015 at www.abs.gov.au/ausstats/abs@.nsf/Lookup/4338.0main+features112011-13.

Australian and New Zealand Society for Geriatric Medicine. (2013). Exercise guidelines for older adults. Sydney: Author.

Australian Government Department of Social Services. (2015). Ageing and aged care: Age care reform. Accessed February 2015 at www.dss.gov.au/our-responsibilities/ageing-and-aged-care/aged-care-reform.

Australian Institute of Health and Welfare (AIHW). (2013). *Australian hospital statistics 2011–12*. Cat. no. HSE 134. Canberra: Author.

Bell, M., Lommel, T., Fischer, J. G., Lee, J. S., Reddy, S. & Johnson, M. A. (2009). Improved recognition of heart attack and stroke symptoms after a community-based intervention for older adults, Georgia, 2006–2007. *Preventing Chronic Disease, 6*(2), 1–11.

Blair, S. N. & Morris, J. N. (2009). Healthy hearts—and the universal benefits of being physically active: Physical activity and health. *Annals of Epidemiology, 19*, 253–256.

Boltz, M., Capezuti, E., Bowar-Ferres, S., Norman, R., Secic, M., Kim, H., ... Fulmer, T. (2008). Changes in geriatric care environment associated with NICHE (Nurses Improving Care for Health System Elders). *Geriatric Nursing, 29*(3), 176–185.

Bonsdorff, von M. B., Rantanen, T., Leinonen, R., Kujala, U. M., Törmäkangas, T., Manty, M. & Heikkinen, E. (2009). Physical activity history and end-of-life hospital and long-term care. *Journal of Gerontology Medical Sciences 64A*, 778–784.

Brown, W. J., Moorhead, G. E. & Marshall, A. L. (2005). Choose health: Be active. A physical activity guide for older Australians. Canberra: Commonwealth of Australia and the Repatriation Commission.

Byberg, L., Melhus, H., Gedeborg, R., Sundström, J., Ahlbom, A., Zethelius, B., ... Michaëlsson, K. (2009). Total mortality after changes in leisure time physical activity in 50 year old men: 35 year follow-up of population based cohort. *British Medical Journal, 338*, 1–8.

Centers for Disease Control and Prevention. (2014). Advance care planning: Ensuring your wishes are known and honored if you are unable to speak for yourself. Viewed March 2015 at www.cdc.gov/aging/pdf/advanced-care-planning-critical-issue-brief.pdf.

Chiang, K. C., Seman, L., Belza, B. & Tsai, J. H. C. (2008). "It is our exercise family": Experiences of ethnic older adults in a group-based exercise program. *Preventing Chronic Disease, 5*(1), 1–12.

Conn, V. S., Hafdahl, A. R. & Brown, L. M. (2009). Meta-analysis of quality-of-life outcomes from physical activity interventions. *Nursing Research, 58*, 175–183.

Cyarto, C., Dow, B., Vrantsidis, F. & Meyer, C. (2012). Promoting healthy ageing: Development of the Healthy Ageing Quiz. *Australasian Journal on Ageing, 32*(1), 15–20.

Elsawy, B. & Higgins, D. O. (2010). Physical activity guidelines for older adults. *American Family Physician, 81*(1), 55–59.

Frank, L. K. (1946). Gerontology. *Journal of Gerontology, 1*(1), 1–11.

Fried, T. R., Redding, C. A., O'Leary, J. et al. (2012). Promoting advance care planning as health behavior change. *Patient Education and Counseling, 86*(1), 25–32.

Gillespie, L. D., Robertson, M. C., Gillespie, W. J., Lamb, S. E., Gates, S., Cumming, R. G. & Rowe, B. H. (2009). Interventions for preventing falls in older people living in the community. *Cochrane Database of Systematic Reviews*, 2. Art. no. CD007146. doi:10.1002/14651858.CD007146.pub3.

Glanz, K., Schoenfeld, E. R. & Steffen, A. (2010). A randomized trial of tailored skin cancer prevention messages for adults: Project SCAPE. *American Journal of Public Health, 100*, 735–741.

Gustafsson, S., Wilhelmson, K., Eklund, K. et al. (2012). Health-promoting interventions for persons aged 80 and older are successful in the short term: Results from the randomized and three-armed Elderly Persons in the Risk Zone study. *Journal of the American Geriatrics Society, 60*(3), 447–454.

Hughes, S. L., Seymour, R. B., Campbell, R. T., Whitelaw, N. & Bazzarre, T. (2009). Best-practice physical activity programs for older adults: Findings from the National Impact Study. *American Journal of Public Health, 99*, 362–368.

Kemppainen, V., Tossavainen, K. & Turunen, H. (2012). Nurses' roles in health promotion practice: An integrative review. *Health Promotion International, 28*(4), 490–501.

Kowlowitz, V., Davenport, C. S. & Palmer, M. H. (2009). Development and dissemination of web-based clinical simulations for continuing geriatric nursing education. *Journal of Geriatric Nursing, 35*(4), 37–43.

Logsdon, R. G., McCurry, S. M., Pike, K. C. & Teri, L. (2009). Making physical activity accessible to older adults with memory loss: A feasibility study. *Gerontologist, 51*, S94–S99.

Mariano, C. (2013). Holistic nursing: Scope and standards of practice. In B. M. Dossey & L. Keegan (Eds), *Holistic nursing: A handbook for practice* (6th ed., pp. 59–83). Boston, MA: Jones and Bartlett.

Meng, H., Wamsley, B., Liebel, D., Dixon, D., Eggert, G. & Van Nostrand, V. (2009). Urban–rural differences in the effect of a Medicare health promotion and disease self-management program on physical function and health care expenditures. *Gerontologist, 49*(3), 407–417.

Miller, C. A. (2013). *Fast facts for health promotion in nursing: Promoting wellness in a nutshell*. New York: Springer.

Moore, S. M. & Charvat, J. (2007). Promoting health behavior change using appreciative inquiry: Moving from deficit models to affirmation models of care. *Family & Community Health Nursing, 30*(15 Suppl. 1), S64–S74.

National Ageing Research Institute. (2010). Healthy Ageing Quiz: Practical tips for ageing well. Canberra: Australian Government Department of Health.

New Zealand Ministry of Health. (2012a). *Hospital events 2008/09 and 2009/10*. Wellington: Author.

New Zealand Ministry of Health. (2012b). *The health of New Zealand adults 2011/12: Key findings of the New Zealand Health Survey*. Wellington: Author.

New Zealand Ministry of Health. (2013). Guidelines on physical activity for older people (aged 65 years and over). Wellington: Author.

New Zealand Ministry of Health, Nursing Council of New Zealand, DHBNZ & NPAC-NZ. (2009). *Nurse practitioners: A healthy future for New Zealand* (pp. 42–43). Wellington: New Zealand Ministry of Health.

New Zealand Ministry of Social Development. (2013). Older New Zealanders: Healthy, independent, connected and respected. Accessed March 2015 at www.msd.govt.nz/what-we-can-do/seniorcitizens/positive-ageing/connected.

Nguyen, H. Q., Ackermann, R. T., Maciejewski, M., Berke, E., Patrick, M., Williams, B. & LoGerfo, J. P. (2008). Managed-Medicare health club benefit and reduced health care costs among older adults. *Preventing Chronic Disease, 5*(1), 1–10.

Noordam, J., de Vet, E., van der Weijden, T. et al. (2013). Motivational interviewing within the different stages of change: An analysis of practice nurse–patient consultations aimed at promoting a healthier lifestyle. *Social Sciences & Medicine, 87*, 60–67.

Novelli, B. (2009). Health care reform hinges on private-sector collaboration. *Preventing Chronic Disease, 6*(2), A74.

Otago Medical School. (2003). Otago exercise programme to prevent falls in older adults: A home-based, individually tailored strength and balance retraining programme. Viewed March 2015 at www.acc.co.nz/PRD_EXT_CSMP/groups/external_providers/documents/publications_promotion/prd_ctrb118334.pdf.

Palmer, M. H., Kowlowitz, V., Campbell, J., Carr, C., Dillon, R. Durham, C. F., ... Rasin, J. (2008). Using clinical simulations in geriatric nursing continuing education. *Nursing Outlook*, 56, 159–166.

Pascucci, M. A., Chu, N. & Leasure, A. R. (2012). Health promotion for the oldest of old people. *Nursing Older People, 24*(3), 22–28.

Prochaska, T. R., Eisenstein, A. R., Satariano, W. A., Hunter, R., Bayles, C. M., Kurtovich, E., ... Ivey, S. L. (2009). Walking and the preservation of cognitive function in older populations. *Gerontologist, 49*, S86–S93.

Rejeski, W. J., Marsh, A. P., Chmelo, E., Prescott, A. J., Dobrosielski, M., Walkup, M. P., ... Kritchevsky, S. (2009). The lifestyle interventions and independence for elderly pilot (LIFE-P): 2-year follow-up. *Journal of Gerontology: Medical Sciences, 64A*, 462–467.

Rizzuto, D., Orsini, N., Qui, C. et al. (2012). Lifestyle, social factors, and survival after age 75: Population based study. *British Medical Journal, 345*, e5568.

Scala, E. & Costa, L. (2014). Using appreciative inquiry during care transitions. *Journal of Nursing Care Quality, 29*(1), 44–50.

Schonberg, M. A., Leveille, S. G. & Marcantonio, E. R. (2008). Preventive health care among older women: Missed opportunities and poor targeting. *American Journal of Medicine, 121*, 974–981.

Shenson, D., Benson, W. & Harris, A. C. (2008). Expanding the delivery of clinical preventive services through community collaboration: The SPARC model. *Preventing Chronic Disease, 5*(1), 1–7.

Stawnychy, M., Creber, R. M. & Riegel, B. (2014). Using brief motivational interviewing to address the complex needs of a challenging patient with heart failure. *Journal of Cardiovascular Nursing*, 29(5), E1–E6.

Tan, E. J., Rebok G. W., Yu, Q., Frangakis, C. E., Carlson, M. C., Wang, T., ... Fried, L. P. (2009). The long-term relationship between high-intensity volunteering and physical activity among older African American women. *Journal of Gerontology: Social Sciences, 64B*, 304–311.

Touhy, E. L. (1946). Geriatrics: The general setting. *Geriatrics: Official Journal of the American Geriatrics Society, 1*(1), 17–20.

Van Nispen, R. M., de Boer, M. R., Hoeijmakers, G. J., Ringens, P. J. & van Rens, G. (2009). Co-morbidity and visual acuity are risk factors for health-related quality of life decline: Five-month follow-up EQ-5D data of visually impaired older patients. *Health and Quality of Life Outcomes, 7*(18), 1–9.

Wilcox, S., Dowda, M., Dunn, A., Ory, M. G., Rheaume, C. & King, A. C. (2009). Predictors of increased physical activity in active for life program. *Preventing Chronic Disease, 6*(1), 1–6.

Williamson, J. D., Espeland, M., Kritchevsky, S. B., Newman, A. B., King, A. C., Pahor, M., ... Miller, M. E. (2009). Changes in cognitive function in a randomized trial of physical activity: Results of the Lifestyle Interventions and Independence for Elders Pilot Study. *Journal of Gerontology: Medical Sciences, 64A*, 688–694.

Chapter 6
Continuum of care for older adults

By Carol Miller and Sharyn Hunter

LEARNING OBJECTIVES

After reading this chapter, you should be able to:

1. Describe the policy, structure and services that are included in a continuum of care for older adults in Australia and New Zealand.
2. Describe sources of payment for healthcare services for older adults.
3. Describe the types of long-term residential care available, including newer models of care.
4. Describe the types of community care services available for older adults, and explain how people obtain these services, including adult day centres, respite services, health promotion programs, and other care programs.
5. Discuss ways in which each of the following programs facilitates the coordination of care: chronic care models and case management services.
6. Describe the characteristics of several models of acute care programs for older adults.
7. Discuss the roles of nurses caring for older adults in long-term residential care community settings and acute care.

KEY POINTS

acute care for elders units (ACE)
adult day centres
Aged Care Act 1997
ageing-in-place
case management services
continuum of care
culture change movement
Eden Alternative
hospital-at-home model
home-based care
long term care
long-term residential care
rest homes
respite care
small-house nursing home
subacute care units
telehealth
transitional care
transitional care units (TCUs)

Since the late 1960s the specialised needs of the older person has been recognised and healthcare organisations have developed care services to address these needs. This has resulted in the development of a **continuum of care** for older adults aimed at promoting health and reducing the impact of illness.

These services have led to the expansion and emergence of new roles for nurses caring for older adults. Most nurses today are caring for older adults. In Australia it has been reported that approximately "two-thirds of adult patients in a general hospital are 65 or over, and up to a third of them are likely to have dementia", suggesting that "…nurses are, by default, aged care nurses" (Bail & Draper, 2011, pp. 24 & 25).

This chapter presents an overview of the continuum of healthcare services available for older adults that began decades ago and continues to evolve today. It also discusses the roles of nurses working with older adults in these services.

DEVELOPMENT OF A CONTINUUM OF CARE FOR OLDER ADULTS

A confusing array of terms related to healthcare services and settings for older adults has evolved over several decades. For example, such phrases as **long-term care**, continuum of care, and **ageing-in-place** are used to refer to various models without standards that define the types of care.

Recent developments with regard to chronic care models and care facilities have added to the confusion. For example, some ageing-in-place or continuing care programs require that residents move to a new location within a larger facility or group of facilities when their needs change. Gerontologists and healthcare practitioners have raised concerns about the application of this concept in these settings, because within-facility transitions may be disruptive to the residents' social interaction, sense of home, and sense of autonomy (Shippee, 2009). Box 6-1 describes pertinent care terms, and the following sections describe the variety of settings and models that address unique and complex needs of older adults. In addition to describing settings where older adults receive care, the sections focus on pertinent issues that are currently being addressed to improve the quality of healthcare for older adults. Unique roles for nurses in various settings are also described.

Healthcare services for older adults arose from an increased concern about health expenditure, and from a raised awareness of the importance of meeting the complex care needs of the older adult in a way that addresses both quality-of-life issues and financial concerns.

BOX 6-1
Terms describing models of care for older adults

Long-term residential care: In the 1960s this term referred to nursing homes, which were the only place of care for people with long-term disabilities who could no longer manage in their own home. Although the term is still strongly associated with care provided in institutional settings, long-term care services are provided in community settings such as homes and apartments.

Ageing-in-place: A range of services provided in one setting to address different levels of care as the needs of the older adult change. This concept initially referred to supporting people in their own homes, but it has expanded to include institutional settings that provide a wide range of services.

Continuum of care: Programs that provide comprehensive, coordinated and multidisciplinary services (e.g. primary and preventive care, acute care, transitional care, rehabilitation services, long-term care, respite care, social services, home healthcare, adult day centres, and care management services).

BOX 6-2
Objectives of Australia's Aged Care System

The objectives set out in the *Aged Care Act 1997* include:

- Promoting high quality care and accommodation
- Protecting the health and well-being of care recipients
- Helping recipients of aged care enjoy the same rights as all other people in Australia
- Ensuring that aged care is accessible and affordable for people who require it
- Planning effectively for the delivery of aged care services
- Ensuring that aged care services and funding are targeted towards people and areas with the greatest need
- Encouraging services that are diverse, flexible and responsive to individual needs
- Providing funding that takes account of the quality, type and level of care
- Providing respite for families and others who care for older people, and
- Promoting "ageing in place"; that is, helping older people stay where they want to live, by linking care and support services. (paragraph 8)

Source: Australian Government Department of Social Services. (2015). Guides to social policy law: Guide to aged care law. Accessed April 2015 at http://guides.dss.gov.au/guide-aged-care-law.

OVERVIEW OF CARE SERVICES FOR OLDER PEOPLE IN AUSTRALIA AND NEW ZEALAND

Australia

The current system of care for older Australians is a nationalised, complex, comprehensive system that is continually undergoing review to meet the changing demands for services (Productivity Commission [PC], 2011). The main regulator, funder and provider of aged care services for older adults is the Australian Government. The system is referred to as the Australian Aged Care System. It is regulated by legislation, the ***Aged Care Act 1997*** (Cth), and other subordinate (emerging) legislation from the Aged Care Act; for example, the Quality of Care Principles 2014. The Australian Government "...aims to ensure that all frail older Australians have timely access to appropriate care and support services as they age...through a safe and secure Aged Care System" (PC, 2011, p. xxvii). A number of objectives set out in the *Aged Care Act 1997* are listed in Box 6-2.

Australia is currently preparing major revisions to the national Aged Care System. The Productivity Commission report (2011), Caring for Older Australians, provided the recommendations for reform. The Living Longer Living Better aged-care reform package was developed in response by the Australian Government and it provides a program of reforms to be enacted over 10 years, commencing in 2012.

There are two major components of the Australian Aged Care System, *long-term residential care* and *community care*. Access to both types of service requires an assessment by an organisation within the system known as the Aged Care Assessment Team (ACAT), which applies in all states except Victoria, where it is referred to as the Aged Care Assessment Service (ACAS). The role of the ACAT is to assess the older adult's needs and determine the services appropriate for the person and, because of this role, the ACAT is commonly known as the "Gatekeeper" of the Australian Aged Care System. Currently in development is a National Screening and Assessment Tool (2015), which will be used by ACAT in the future to screen and assess older adults' needs regarding community and longer-term residential care.

Prior to July 2014 there were two types of long-term residential care facilities, low and high care, but now there is only one, referred to as aged care homes. Community aged care services have also recently been changed to a Home Care Packages Program. Since the introduction of the Home Care Packages Program a new approach, the Consumer-Directed Care approach (CDC), has been implemented. This approach:

> *...allows people to have greater choice and control over the care and support services they receive, to the extent that they are capable and wish to do so. The concept of "choice" in CDC varies, and can include allowing people to make choices about the types of care services and benefits they access, the delivery of those services and benefits, or choice of service provider. (PC, 2011, p. xvii)*

The CDC approach encourages older adults to have greater control over their lives by increased participation in making decisions about care in an endeavour to increase the level of independence and wellness of the older adult.

All services within the Australian Aged Care System must undergo external review to assess standards of care and operation to receive funding, and the organisation responsible for this is the Australian Aged Care Quality Agency. *Accreditation* is the process that assesses standards of care that occurs in residential care facilities and these standards are contained in the Quality of Care Principles 2014. There are four Standards:

- Standard one—Management systems, staffing and organisational development
- Standard two—Health and personal care
- Standard three—Care recipient lifestyle
- Standard four—Physical environment and safe systems.

The Home Care Package services undergo a process of *quality review* and these standards are also contained in the Quality of Care Principles 2014. There are three Standards:

- Standard one—Effective management
- Standard two—Appropriate access and service delivery
- Standard three—Service user rights and responsibilities.

There are two other important components of the Australian Aged Care system. My Aged Care is a portal (myaged*care*) created to be an entry point for service providers and older adults and their carers to the Australian Aged Care System. Currently it provides relevant and comprehensive information about aged care, but it is anticipated that myaged*care* will continue to evolve to enable the collection of older adults' information so it can be shared between services to facilitate service provision. Finally, there is an Aged Care Complaints Scheme, a free service for any member of the community, to lodge any concerns about the quality of care or services being delivered to older adults receiving services delivered within the Australian Aged Care System. These components as well as others are discussed in the appropriate subsequent sections. Box 6-3 provides a summary of the major components of the Australian Aged Care System.

New Zealand

A major reform in the delivery of healthcare to older adults in New Zealand occurred in 2002 when the Health of Older People Strategy was developed to implement the objectives of the New Zealand Positive Ageing Strategy 2001. The Health of Older People Strategy proposed an integrated approach to health and support services responsive to older adults' healthcare needs. "The purpose of the Health of Older People Information Strategic Plan is to improve health outcomes for older people by ensuring that access to quality information is available to older people, their family, *whānau* and carers and health and disability support service providers, funders, planners and policy makers in a timely manner for effective and efficient health decision making" (New Zealand Ministry of Health [NZMOH], 2006, p. 4). This strategy has encouraged focus on the older adult as the centre of care and the development of seamless services across a variety of hospitals, primary healthcare services, and other community health services.

Although the New Zealand Ministry of Health has the primary responsibility for regulating and funding healthcare, the 21 District Health Boards (DHBs) across New Zealand are responsible for managing all aspects of healthcare in their district. This includes the hospitals, long-term residential care (known as **rest homes**) and community care services (Office of the Auditor-General, 2011).

BOX 6-3
Summary of the major components of the Australian Aged Care System

My Aged Care (the aged care gateway website, myaged*care*) assists older adults, their families and carers to access aged care information and services

Aged Care Assessment Teams (ACAT) are the gatekeepers of the Australian Government's aged care services. ACATs complete a nationalised process of assessment to determine appropriate care services for the older adults

Residential care	In aged care homes: • One type of care home, and • The Aged Care Funding Instrument (ACFI) are used to determine funding for different levels of care needs in long-term residential care
Community aged care services	Home care programs enable: • Increasing levels of care—Levels 1 to 4, and • Delivery of a range of services, including basic care, clinical and other services Commonwealth Home Support Program (to be implemented in 2015) is an entry level to home care services and includes four programs: • Commonwealth Home and Community Care (HACC) Program • National Respite for Carers Program (NRCP) • Day Therapy Centres (DTC) • Program Assistance with Care and Housing for the Aged (ACHA) Program
Australian Aged Care Quality Agency	• Monitors the quality of community and long-term residential care services • Accredits long-term residential care facilities
Transition Care Program	Provides care assistance moving from hospital to home or to an aged care home
Aged Care Complaints Scheme	Enables concerns to be lodged about the quality of care or services

The DHBs deliver services for older adults to support them to continue to live at home and be responsive to their changing needs. DHBs ensure these services are provided in a consistent and integrated manner and are coordinated with other health services. DHBs also fund private organisations to deliver services for older adults. DHBs provide funds for rest home care for older adults who are eligible for a government subsidy. When this occurs, a contract must be entered into by the rest homes and the funding DHB.

For older adults to access home-based services, respite care, or long-term residential care funded by the DHBs, they are required to have had a *needs assessment* performed by a Needs Assessment and Service Coordination (NSCA) agency, which is a part of the DHBs (NZMOH, 2011a). The NSCA assesses older adults and determines their level of need for a service. In New Zealand there are several types of long-term residential care delivered and this is discussed in the later section describing the types of long-term residential care services. Residential care facilities must be certified by the NZMOH to receive government funds for operation. To be certified, the residential care facilities are audited every 1 to 4 years for safe and appropriate care that meets the standards described in the Health and Disability Services (Safety) Act 2001 (NZMOH, 2012). There are 50 standards that can be assessed in an audit.

The NZMOH has set standards for the appropriateness and range of home-based services, but there are no compulsory standards about the quality or level of services. Standards New Zealand produced a standard that can be applied to home-based support services, the *Home and community support sector standard*, NZS 8158:2012. Unlike Australia there is little national monitoring of these services. It has been noted that there is difficulty with the determination of the consistency and equity of service delivery. Home-based community services that are funded by the DHBs for older adults are: home help; stand alone day care; stand alone dementia day care; and day care in a residential facility.

The DHBs are also involved with Primary Health Organisations (PHOs) established throughout the country in 2002 (Ashton, 2005). PHOs are funded by DHBs and are required to be non-profit and responsive to their communities' needs. PHOs consist of general practitioners (GPs), primary care nurses and other primary healthcare providers. They provide comprehensive preventive and treatment services and are responsible for the primary healthcare of those who receive care. To receive care from a PHO, people must be enrolled in the organisation. The PHOs are an integral part of the New Zealand Government's system of care for older adults in New Zealand.

Unlike Australia, New Zealand does not have a centralised mechanism of complaints. Complaints related to long-term residential care can be referred to three agencies: District health boards (DHBs), the New Zealand Ministry of Health, and the Health and Disability Commissioner. The Health and Disability Advocacy Service is a service that assists with information about making a complaint regarding any health and disability service.

PAYING FOR HEALTH SERVICES FOR OLDER ADULTS

In Australia and New Zealand, services for the older adult are mostly funded from the money collected by the national taxation system. It is a goal of both countries to continue to provide affordable care services for all older adults. Despite large contributions made by the Australian and New Zealand Governments to provide services for older adults, contributions by individuals are still required. However, these vary, depending on income assessment and service delivered. Further discussion about the costs of specific services is contained in the later relevant sections. As the costs of services are continually revised, nurses are able to access up-to-date information from myaged*care* (Australia) and the Ministry of Health (New Zealand).

Despite the complexity of healthcare services for older adults, nurses need to know enough about the most common sources of payment for health services so they can understand and address some of the barriers to and challenges of implementing nursing care plans and discharge plans. For example, knowing if the older adult is receiving a pension as opposed to a self-funded retiree enables the nurse to make referrals for different types of care services. The self-funded retiree may be able to access private services rather than wait for publicly funded services to become available. Nurses are encouraged to keep up to date about major sources of healthcare coverage for older adults.

TYPES OF LONG-TERM RESIDENTAL CARE SERVICES

In Australia, aged care homes, and in New Zealand, rest homes, refer to **long-term residential care** settings for older adults who need assistance with daily living activities (ADLs). The care recipients are called *residents* rather than *patients* because the facility is considered to be their home. In Australia, higher levels of long-term residential care include nursing services for older people who need assistance with many ADLs. Higher level care covers such services as nursing care, other complex care, equipment to assist with mobility, medical management and therapy services. Lower levels of care include accommodation and related everyday living support (meals, laundry, cleaning), as well as some personal care services. *Personal care services* can include assistance with bathing, toileting, eating, dressing, mobility, managing incontinence, community rehabilitation support, assistance in obtaining health and therapy services, and support for people with cognitive impairments (PC, 2011, p. 25).

The Australian Government provides long-term residential care services with operational funding called the Residential Aged Care Subsidy, which focuses on residents' care needs. The Aged Care Funding Instrument (ACFI) is the tool used to allocate the funding. The ACFI consists of 12 questions about care that require a rating of A, B, C or D. The rating then determines the care subsidy for each resident in the facility. There are three components of care assessed by the ACFI:

- Activities of Daily Living (ratings on Nutrition, Mobility, Personal Hygiene, Toileting and Continence questions are utilised to determine the level of the basic subsidy)
- Behaviour Supplement (ratings on Cognitive Skills, Wandering, Verbal Behaviour, Physical Behaviour and Depression questions are utilised to determine the behaviour supplement)
- Complex Health Care Supplement (ratings on Medication and Complex Health Care Procedure questions are utilised to determine the complex healthcare supplement). (Australian Government Department of Social Services, 2014a, p. 2)

Older Australians are required to contribute to the costs of their long-term residential care. Contributions include "…basic daily fees, income tested fees, total asset tested accommodation payments, extra service fees and additional services fees" (PC, 2011, p. 30). Also in Australia, medication costs are in addition to the residential care costs, and it is usual for the general practitioners to bulk bill the resident for medical services so that the older adult does not incur an additional cost.

In New Zealand, rest homes provide residential care for older adults with lower level care needs. Long-term hospital care in a rest home provides higher levels of care. Higher care exists when there is 24-hour care that is supervised by nurses. All rest homes and residential care hospitals provide "…accommodation, food, laundry, nursing services, continence products, equipment for mobility and personal care, and divisional care" (NZMOH, 2012, p. 20). Unlike Australia, the rest home covers the cost of prescribed medicines and general practitioner visits.

In New Zealand the federal government provides financial assistance to older adults in long-term residential care by the provision of a Residential Care Subsidy (NZMOH, 2012). Eligibility for this subsidy is determined by a financial means assessment. The older adult must still contribute to the cost of residential care but the subsidy "will make up the difference between what the older adults pays as set by the financial means assessment and the price of care that is agreed between the residential care facility and the DHB" (p. 17).

In both Australia and New Zealand long-term residential care also includes dementia-specific units that provide care for older adults who have a diagnosis of dementia. In Australia dementia care units provide care for those with high or low care needs. In New Zealand dementia care units provide the same type of services as rest homes but care is provided in a secure environment, while those who have a very high level of dementia or challenging behaviours are cared for in a psycho-geriatric care unit. In both type of units, staff members with qualifications and experience in relation to dementia are employed to provide special care.

Admission to long-term residential care

Gerontologists have identified the reasons older people are admitted to nursing homes for long-term care. These admissions commonly occur after a period of gradual decline in functioning because of a chronic condition, such as dementia. Studies indicate that more severe functional limitations, cognitive impairment, and problematic behaviours in people with dementia are predictors of admission to nursing facilities for long-term care (Cho, Zarit & Chiriboga, 2009). Additional factors that increase the likelihood of being admitted to a nursing home include female sex, living alone, advanced age, and low socioeconomic status (Martikainen et al., 2009). It is recognised that admission to long-term residential care is determined not only by the person's level of functioning but also by the availability of capable and willing carers/caregivers. Thus, many older people move to residential care not because their condition has changed significantly, but because there has been a change in the availability or abilities of the carer.

As mentioned previously, to gain admission into long-term residential care in Australia the older adult must be assessed by ACAT. At present (2015), the ACAT completes an Aged Care Client Record (ACCR), which then determines the older adult has care needs that are appropriate for long-term residential care. In New Zealand the NSCA completes the interRAI assessment tool for residential care to determine admission to long-term residential care (see also Chapters 7 and 9). Information about the assessment process in Australia and New Zealand can be found via the interRAI Coordinating Centre at http://interrai-au.org. In New Zealand, admission assessment support is available via findaresthome.co.nz.

Trends in long-term residential aged care

In recent decades, changes in healthcare services for older adults have significantly influenced long-term residential care. Approximately 6% of older adults live in residential care in Australia and New Zealand, and the majority of these people are over 80 (approximately 75%) (Statistics New Zealand, 2007; PC, 2011). In both Australia and New Zealand there has been a steady increase in the proportion of residents being classified as needing higher levels of care. Between 1998 and 2008 in Australia, the number of residents classified as high care on admission rose from 58% to 70% (PC, 2011, p. 27). A longitudinal study in New Zealand showed an increased level of dependency in long-term residential care from 1988 to 2008 (Boyd, Broad, Kerse et al., 2011).

Also in New Zealand, spending on home-based support services has been steadily increasing, with a 70% increase during the 4 years leading up to 2008–2009. By comparison, spending for residential care in the same period rose by only 35%. In Australia in 2014 there were approximately 66,000 home care packages delivered by about 2212 home care services (Australian Government Department of Social Services [DSS], 2014b) and the intention is to increase the number of Home Care Packages to 100,000 by 2017.

These statistics reflect the following major trends in healthcare for older adults in Australia and New Zealand:

- An increasing dependency of residents in long-term residential care
- Increasing availability and use of community **home-based care** services that substitute for long-term residential care.

These trends have developed because of the successful implementation of community care programs for older adults. More people are receiving care in the community and, when older adults are transferred to long-term residential care, they are increasingly more dependent, with higher care needs.

Roles for nurses in long-term residential care

Nurses have always assumed strong leadership roles in long-term residential care and opportunities for role expansion have accompanied the increasing complexity of care of the residents. Also, because of the focus on improved quality of care in long-term residential care, nurses have many opportunities to implement innovative changes in delivery of care. Registered nurses provide direct care, but they are accountable for all nursing components of care (Burger et al., 2009; Hunter & Levett-Jones, 2010). Registered nurses now spend less time in direct care and more time supervising and documenting the care given (Hunter & Levett-Jones, 2010).

Common roles for registered nurses in long-term residential care settings include team leader, nursing supervisor, director of nursing, and assistant director of nursing. Nurses also have very strong roles in the education of the other care team members. Nurses have developed a model for teaching other carers how to implement a restorative approach to change the way in which care is provided in long-term residential care (Resnick et al., 2009). A nurse-led state-wide initiative to improve care in long-term residential care resulted in improvements in all of the following quality indicators: falls, weight loss, pressure ulcers and bedfast status (Rantz et al., 2009).

Since the introduction of accreditation (Australia) and certification (New Zealand), roles have opened up for advanced practice gerontological nurses. In New Zealand the Ministry of Health (2014) has showcased nurses working in different roles in long-term residential care by video presentations of five case studies showing a range of initiatives in Canterbury, Wellington, Taranaki, Waitemata and Counties Manukau.

In addition to direct care of residents, advanced practice nurses may provide staff education, assist with program development, act as consultants in planning and implementing care, establish support groups for clients and families, and act as advocates for clients and their families. Additional details about the roles available for advance practice nurses are discussed in Chapter 5.

Newer models of long-term residential care

During the past two decades, healthcare consumers, providers and organisations have increasingly focused on concerns about quality of care and quality of life for people who need long-term care. At the same time, there has been increasing concern about the cost of care in traditional long-term residential care settings (formerly known as nursing homes) and an associated interest in developing lower cost and better-quality alternatives. Because of these concerns, a new era in long-term residential care has evolved. It is referred to as the **culture change movement**.

A student's perspective

This week in the nursing home, I found it was important to listen to Mrs R. while allowing her to make her limitations known to me. I asked if she needed help, and didn't just provide it. I paid close attention to her body language and non-verbal communication. After finding her fast asleep sitting up during breakfast, I woke her and allowed her to tell me what was next. She determined that going to the bathroom and then getting washed would be best.

After she was ready, I helped her down to the beauty salon to get her hair done, which is something she does every Friday afternoon. It can be easy to fall into the patient care aspect of a nursing home where you expect them to be on a schedule; however, you have to treat it as their home and allow them to pick and choose their activities and rest periods.

Jillian B.

The Pioneer Network in Long-Term Care—which is considered the umbrella organisation of the culture change movement—has evolved since 1997 from a landmark meeting of pioneers across the U.S., which had the goal of changing the philosophy of care in nursing homes (White-Chou et al., 2009). The Pioneer Network identifies 13 core values that focus on individualised and holistic care; optimal use of all aspects of the physical, organisational and psychological–social–spiritual environment; and ongoing growth and continuous quality improvement. Two of the most widely implemented models of care that are part of the Pioneer Network are the Eden Alternative and the Green House Project. These models of care have been embraced by Australian and New Zealand long-term residential care providers.

The **Eden Alternative**® is a model developed in the mid-1990s by William Thomas, MD, with the intent of creating small-group neighbourhoods of residents to combat boredom, loneliness, helplessness and lack of meaning that are common in traditional nursing homes. The Eden Alternative is a comprehensive program of transforming the organisational culture as well as the physical, spiritual, psychosocial and interpersonal environments of a facility. An essential component is the systematic introduction of pets, plants and children to create a home-like setting and improve the quality of life of residents. In addition, the Eden Alternative incorporates strategies to engage and empower staff in bringing about the environmental change. Residential aged care facilities that adopt this comprehensive model and pledge to abide by Eden Principles are listed in the Eden Registry. Outcomes of this model that have been identified in studies include enhanced staff retention, increased satisfaction of staff and residents, and reduction in the number of medications and infections (Bowers et al., 2009). There are many Eden Alternative facilities in both Australia and New Zealand, with 36 noted in 2011 (Brownie, 2011). Nurses can find additional information about this model and about Eden facilities in Australia and New Zealand at www.edeninoznz.com.au.

The Green House Project, described as a **small-house nursing home**, has also been promoted by William Thomas, MD, who is the founder of the Eden Alternative and a major leader in the Pioneer Network. The first project opened in 2003 and consisted of four self-contained Green Houses that operated under the licence of a sponsoring nursing home in Tupelo, Missouri. Green Houses typically house seven to 12 residents in a home that blends in with neighbouring houses. These small-house nursing homes provide a full range of licensed and certified nursing home services to older people with high levels of disability including those associated with dementia, in a normal household setting.

The Green House approach emphasises relationships and meaning-making in any interventions for dementia-related behavioural disturbances. A study of the first 2 years of this model found that residents experienced better outcomes on many dimensions of quality of life and had no declines in health outcomes (Kane & Cutler, 2008). Researchers also have found that families were more satisfied with the care and their own experiences, appreciated increased autonomy and enhanced privacy for the residents, and had no greater family burden (Lum et al., 2008–2009). Overall, early studies of the small-house model identified many benefits for cognitively impaired older adults as well as improved job satisfaction for nurses who work in an environment that promotes holistic and person-centred care (Rabig, 2009). Three organisations, one in Australia and two in New Zealand, have created Green Houses. They are Embracia in Australia, and the Rangiura Trust Board, Putaruru and Enliven Presbyterian Support Central (PSC) in Wellington, New Zealand.

Roles for nurses in newer models of care

These changes pose many challenges and opportunities for nurses working in long-term residential care. Newer models of care involve philosophical and organisational changes that affect all staff. For example, the Green House model conceptualises nurses and other professionals as members of a visiting clinical support team that order and supervise care within their area of professional practice. Nurses do not supervise the direct-care staff, but they often assume administrative and consultative roles. Burger et al. (2009) identified a number of opportunities that are pertinent to nurses who work in long-term residential care when they are experiencing culture change, and these are as follows:

- The goals and philosophy of culture change are highly compatible with those of nursing because both support and incorporate resident-directed care.
- Intense nursing participation is essential for providing coordinated, evidence-based clinical nursing care in the context of a resident (person)-centred philosophy of care.
- Nurses need to be care-team leaders and role models so they can foster and promote a team approach in which direct-care staff are involved in decision making.
- Nurses need to be involved in the decision making about culture change to facilitate its implementation.
- Nurse managers also need to have both clinical and management skills in the decentralised models and they may be unprepared for this role.

COMMUNITY CARE SERVICES

Older adults and other dependent populations have always received much of their healthcare at home, and visiting nurse services have existed since the late 1800s. As mentioned, since 1997 in Australia, and at the turn of the century in New Zealand, there has been an increasing focus on the funding and delivery of community care services for older adults.

A wide spectrum of long-term home care services is becoming increasingly available for the older adults who need home care. At one end of the spectrum is non-skilled care provided by companions and home healthcare workers. The most common services provided are meal preparation, light housekeeping, assistance with personal care, accompaniment to medical appointments, and grocery shopping. These services can be supplemented by community-based services such as home-delivered meals and community nursing services. The frequency of services ranges from a couple of hours per week to several hours per day. A nurse may be involved in assessing the client and supervising the services.

In Australian the community care programs of Community Aged Care Packages (CACPs), Extended Aged Care at Home (EACH) packages, and the Extended Aged Care and

Home Dementia (EACHD) packages are being phased out and the new system of home care is called the Home Care Packages. Their support to people includes (DSS, 2014b):

- Home Care Level 1—basic care needs
- Home Care Level 2—low level care needs
- Home Care Level 3—intermediate care needs
- Home Care Level 4—high care needs.

To obtain these services the ACAT currently completes an Aged Care Client Record (ACCR), which then determines the level of home service the older adult requires. In the later half of 2015 another change is expected in the community aged care system with the establishment of a national Commonwealth Home Support program, which combines other community support services, including the:

- Existing Commonwealth Home and Community Care program for older people
- National Respite for Carers program (see the section on respite services for further discussion)
- Day Therapy Centres program (see the section on adult day centres for further discussion)
- Assistance with Care and Housing for the Aged program.

The Home and Community Care Program (HACC) delivers a low level of home care. HACC was previously controlled by the state governments of Australia and serviced both older adults (about 70% of the users) and those with disability. Since 2012 the responsibility of this service has been transferred to the Australian Government and from 2015 the service will deliver only to older adults. Assessment tools currently being used are the HACC, Australian Community Care Needs Assessment (ACCNA) and the Carer Eligibility and Needs Assessment (CENA). These and other national tools are listed under the Centre for Health Service Development (CHDS) in New South Wales via http://ahsri.uow.edu.au/screening. The Assistance with Care and Housing for the Aged (ACHA) program was created for older adults who are at risk of becoming homeless as they get older. Older adults are required also to contribute to the cost of community services they receive. They will be required to pay a basic daily fee and an income-tested care fee (DSS, 2014c).

In New Zealand community services for older adults may include "...personal care—getting out of bed, showering, dressing, medication management, equipment to help with your safety at home; household support—cleaning, meal preparation; [and] carer support—help for the person who lives with you and/or looks after you for 4 hours or more each day and specialist services if required" (NZMOH, 2011a, p. 9). For home care, older New Zealanders are assessed to establish their eligibility for subsidised services. Only those older adults with a Community Service Card are able to receive help with housework, while all older adults who require assistance with activities of daily living are eligible. During assessment the DBH will visit the home and complete the interRAI™ Home Care (HC) Assessment Form. Support with the eligibility assessment process is available via www.findaresthome.co.nz. Box 6-4 lists the types of home care services that are available in New Zealand.

BOX 6-4
Home care services in New Zealand

Domestic assistance

- Basic home cleaning and laundry
- Meal preparation and grocery shopping

Personal care

- Assistance with bathing, dressing, toileting
- Help with mobility, eating and drinking

Community and social interaction

- Visitor services

Community nursing

- Medication and wound management
- Bladder and bowel care

Complex personal care

- Supervision of chronic conditions, including type 2 diabetes and dementia
- End-of-life care
- Medication management

Source: Adapted from Find A Rest Home.co.nz. (2015). Home care: What home care services are available? Accessed March 2015 at www.findaresthome.co.nz/process/S04a-information-about-home-care.htm.

Nurses may also be responsible for case managing the care of the older adult in community programs and providing care education to the older adult and their carers. Recipients of care include older people who are able to manage most of their daily care at some level of independence and people who are dependent in many functional areas and receive help from families and friends to supplement the care services.

Assisted-living facilities

In addition to the models described in this chapter, older adults may receive a range of healthcare services in retirement communities. Retirement communities or villages are usually independent community-based housing options and maybe stand alone or be co-located with a residential care facility. However, some of these villages have evolved to provide care in serviced apartments and this type of care is referred to as *assisted living*. With assisted living, services are available on a user-pays basis and are not subsided by the government. These services may include:

- Meals provided in a dining area or delivered to the unit
- Assistance with daily living activities
- Cleaning services
- Support with emergency call systems
- Transportation
- Medication management. (Your Life Choices, 2015)

Further assistance can be provided if required by government-funded community services, as discussed in the previous section. In both Australia and New Zealand there is legislation that regulates the operation of the retirement villages. In Australia the retirement living sector has doubled to 5.3% in 2010 (PC, 2011, p. 29). It has been projected that this could increase to 8% by 2025.

Other community services for older adults

Public and private agencies have provided many types of community support resources for older adults for decades, and the range of these services is continually broadening. Older adults and their caregivers often are not aware of the great variety of services available to meet the health needs of older adults in their own homes. Even when they are aware of the availability of such services, they may not know the eligibility criteria for publicly funded services to which they are entitled. Also, if community-based services are not culturally relevant, older adults or their families may not use them, even when they are aware of their existence. Because the use of these resources may improve the health, functioning and quality of life of the older adult, nurses need to address any lack of information about these services. Also, nurses need to assess barriers to the use of community services, as discussed in Chapter 13.

Adult day centres

Adult day centres have become a major community-based resource for the care of dependent older adults. These centres provide structured social and recreational activities for functionally impaired older people in a group setting. In addition to group social activities, adult day centres provide meals and any of the following services: transportation, assistance with personal care and medication, physiotherapy, occupational and speech therapy, and podiatry. Adult day centres generally provide supervised care on weekdays, including therapies, social interaction and other unstructured activities.

Participants in adult day centres usually are impaired to the point that they need supervision or assistance in several functional areas. Most participants are cognitively impaired, but depression and physical disabilities are also common conditions among adult day centre participants. Participants typically live with a family member, but some live independently. The goals of these programs are to maintain or improve the functional abilities of impaired older people; delay or prevent the need for institutional care; provide relief for carers of dependent older adults; and improve the quality of life for impaired older adults and their carers. Researchers have found that adult day centres improve the quality of life for participants and are an important source of support for carers (Molzahn, Gallagher & McNulty, 2009).

Adult day centre programs are publicly funded and only a small cost is incurred by the older adult. Most adult day centres are located nearby or even within a residential care facility.

Health promotion programs

There is a growing emphasis on health promotion in Australia and New Zealand, and health promotion services for older adults are emerging. As policy directions support the development of these services, it is anticipated that continued growth in these types of programs will occur.

An example of an Australian health promotion is the Healthy at Home program in New South Wales, which focuses on preventing hospital admissions. This program provides community support and clinical care to older adults who have been identified as at risk of decline that would lead to a hospital admission. Also available nationally in Australia is the 75+ years Health Assessment (Australian Government Department of Health, 2014). This assessment is funded by the federal government and is conducted by the older adult's general practitioner. However, the completion of the assessment is usually performed by the practice nurse on behalf of the general practitioner. This assessment identifies health issues and preventable conditions and develops interventions that address both the improvement in health and/or the quality of life of the older adult.

In New Zealand there is an organisation, Age Well, which has a website dedicated to the health promotion of older adults (www.agewell.org.nz). Other New Zealand initiatives, funded by the Accident Compensation Corporation, are falls prevention groups that focus on exercise and education for older adults who have fallen or are identified at risk (Office of Senior Citizens, 2013).

Increasingly, such organised group activities as senior programs frequently take place in or are sponsored by community-based senior centres that exist in almost every community. Hospitals and other healthcare institutions are becoming more involved in providing this kind of program and are employing nurses to address the needs of older adults in the community. Senior centres and healthcare agencies often co-sponsor programs to address specific health issues such as diabetes, cholesterol or blood pressure. These programs provide a valuable health promotion service for older adults.

Roles for nurses in community care services

Community care services for older adults provide many opportunities for innovative roles for nurses in various settings. In addition to the usual responsibilities related to assessment and interventions, nurses often have primary responsibility for the coordination of care, referrals for additional services, and the organisation and management of programs. Community care relies heavily on the contribution of family carers, so home and community care nurses direct their interventions as much towards the caregivers of dependent older people as towards the older people themselves.

A characteristic of nursing roles in community settings is that nurses typically work in collegial relationships with other members of a multidisciplinary team, including primary care providers, psychiatrists, social workers, physical therapists and other healthcare providers to address the needs of older adults as well as their carers. Nurses also work closely with community-based services providers, many of whom have little or no formal training in professional disciplines. For example, nurses need to maintain good communication and relationships with people who work in many community settings. Nurses assume responsibility for training volunteers and for teaching service providers about many health-related needs of older adults.

One challenge for nurses in home and community settings is to keep up to date with technological advances that are increasingly an integral part of healthcare services. In addition to the increasing use of electronic medical records, technological advances have significantly influenced the availability of new communication systems commonly used in home care. **Telehealth** (also called telemedicine) is the use of audio, video and Internet-based devices to collect and transmit information regarding patient assessment through physiological monitors connected to a computer in the home. Assessment data are then sent through a telephone connection to a nurse or other healthcare professional who verbally communicates with the patient to obtain additional information. Some systems use videophones to allow for visual as well as audio communication. One current focus of telehealth is the management of arrhythmias through the use of telemonitors that can send electrocardiogram information to a call centre, where a healthcare professional is alerted to potential problems (Bayne & Boling, 2009). In addition to collecting assessment information, telehealth technology is used to share information, review care plans, and introduce patient teaching materials. Telehealth is particularly useful in rural and remote areas where physical access to health professionals is limited.

A nurse's perspective

We each find our place as nurses. For some this means an ICU; for others, paediatrics. I found my place in a context that allowed me to be comfortable with my values and interests, and this was as a community nurse.

To be invited into the homes of older people, to see their lives unfold as you travel through their home, allows a connection that values each person as a unique member of their community and family. Most have battled with major health issues or an injury and yet, underneath, they still have a love of life. They live on and want to be part of the world. You are privileged as they share their life story with you, introduce you to family members, and work with you to stay well. You are a team, and your relationship develops over time and to a depth that allows you to truly understand what it is to have lived through time and to now be old. They gently tell you what it is to live with illness or disease, and what it is to be resilient, to battle on. They understand the world in ways that I do not, but can come to understand as we share time together.

Jenny D.

RESPITE SERVICES

Respite care refers to any service whose primary goal is to relieve caregivers periodically from the stress of their usual caregiving responsibilities. Gerontologists first used this term in the late 1970s because of the recognition that carers had substantial risk of developing social isolation, clinical depression, psychological distress and other problems directly related to the burden of caregiving. As such, respite services are provided for people who are living in a home setting and are being cared for by family members or other unpaid help. The goals of respite services include improved well-being for caregivers and delayed institutionalisation of dependent older people. Types of respite services include:

- Care from a few hours each week to overnight in the older adult's home
- A day care centre, either full- or half-day care
- Residential care for several weeks.

In Australia a component of the Aged Care System, the National Respite for Carers Program (NRCP), provides information about respite and coordinates the organisation, purchase and management of all aspects of respite care. The Australian Government does contribute to the cost of respite services, but older adults are required to pay a fee, dependent on their income.

In New Zealand a Carer Support Subsidy, funded by a DHB, provides funding to assist with the costs of respite so the carers are supported in their caregiving role. The Carer Support Subsidy can be used for respite in-home, residential care, or day care (NZMOH, 2011a).

ACUTE CARE SERVICES

Acute care settings are an important part of the continuum of care because of the complexity of care associated with illnesses in older adults (detailed in Chapter 27). In response to the increasing recognition of the need for specialised services for older adults, many acute care settings have implemented innovative models of care, as discussed in the following sections.

Specialised geriatric acute care units

Comprehensive geriatric assessment units provide multidisciplinary assessment and care planning for frail older adults during their acute hospital admission. These units are becoming more common and are known as **acute care for elders (ACE)** units.

The underlying premise for all types of ACEs is that older adults have complex and unique needs that can be addressed by a specially trained multidisciplinary team to prevent functional decline during hospitalisation. A meta-analysis of 11 studies of ACE units showed that, compared with patients who receive usual hospital care, those who receive care in ACE units had an 18% reduction in functional decline and a better chance of living at home after discharge

(Baztan et al., 2009). In addition to these benefits, studies found that ACE units could reduce the length of hospital stay (Zelada, Salinas & Baztan, 2009).

Key elements of ACE units are interdisciplinary team management, patient(person)-centred nursing care, early discharge planning, a specially adapted physical environment, and assessment and interventions for common geriatric syndromes (e.g. mobility, fall risk, self-care, skin integrity, continence, confusion, depression and anxiety). In addition to nurses, the healthcare teams in ACE units typically include a geriatrician, pharmacist, social worker, various rehabilitation therapists (e.g. speech, physical or occupational therapists), and mental health professionals (e.g. psychologists or psychiatrists). Some teams also include music, activity or horticultural therapists.

Nurses in any acute care setting can identify risk factors for functional decline by using the Hospital Admission Risk Profile (HARP) clinical tool, listed in the resources section towards the end of this chapter.

Subacute care units

Subacute care units are another development within acute care settings that address medically complex needs of hospitalised older adults. These programs provide nursing and other care services for people who need comprehensive rehabilitation after such major health-altering episodes as a stroke or cardiac or orthopaedic surgery.

Two common types of subacute care units are rehabilitation and transitional care units. Rehabilitation units, unlike transitional care units, are usually not older-person specific. **Transitional care units (TCUs)** were introduced during the last decade and are part of the Australian Aged Care System. The aim of a TCU is to improve the functional ability of the older person to a level that allows for safe discharge home. Although not a rehabilitation unit, the older adults' independence is encouraged and therapies are available to assist with recovery. See the section on transitional care models for a continuing discussion about TCUs.

Other inpatient services

A number of other acute care services have developed in response to the increasing demand by older adults. The goal of these services is to ensure that all of the older adult's healthcare needs are identified and strategies are developed to manage these needs. Many acute hospitals have an Aged Service Emergency Team (ASET) or similar, where the team is responsible for developing a plan of care for older adults as they transition from the emergency department. Advanced practice nurses are essential members of this team. Another role for nurses that has evolved in some acute care services is the management of older adults from residential aged care presenting to emergency departments. This service is led by nurses and provides specialist assessment, coordination, care provision and treatment of the older adult.

Transitional care models

The concept of **transitional care** was introduced during the 1990s in reference to specialised subacute care units in hospitals. The term is now applied to a range of services and settings designed to promote the safe and timely movement of people through various care settings (Naylor & Keating, 2008). A main goal of transitional care is to provide coordination and continuity of healthcare across different settings (Graham, Ivey & Neuhauser, 2009).

Transitional care from acute care settings has gained much attention in recent years because of increasing concerns about frequent hospital re-admissions soon after discharge among older adults. A survey of healthcare systems in eight developed countries found that hospital re-admission rates within a short time after discharge were problematic in all countries, and this was interpreted as a health risk related to inadequate care during hospital stays and transitions to home (Schoen et al., 2009). Studies have confirmed that many of the re-hospitalisations could be prevented if systems were in place to address the underlying issues that contribute to re-admissions (Greenwald & Jack, 2009). Studies have also found that the two most common problems during transitions are medication discrepancies and a lack of continuity of care (Boling, 2009).

One service that has developed to improve transitions is the role of a liaison nurse (may be referred to as a case manager), an advanced practice nursing role. Here the nurse is responsible for the coordination of the process of long-term residential care placement or community services. These nurses work with the care team in the acute care unit to assess an older adult's care needs and liaise with all those involved in caring for the older adult to ensure a safe and seamless transition to residential care.

The Australian Aged Care System delivers transitional care through the Transition Care Program (TCP), and it can be delivered in transitional care units (TCUs), or long-term residential care or as a home-based service. The TCP has been designed to limit extended hospital stays and premature admission to residential care. TCUs, although located in a hospital, are funded and regulated by the Australian Aged Care System and not by the state or territory governments, whose role is to regulate the hospital system. Eligibility for admission to the Transition Care Program is assessed by ACAT. This service is available for a period up to 12 weeks and, within this time, the older adult is expected to maintain or improve their functional and health status. In New Zealand one DHB (2012) has introduced an Enhanced Intermediate Care Assessment and Treatment Team (EICATT) program into residential care (NZMOH, 2014). This program transfers older adults from hospital to a rest home in New Plymouth for rehabilitation before returning home.

Other types of transitional care service are available in Australia. These are not a part of the Australian Aged Care System but are available to people (mostly older adults) being discharged from public hospitals and who require immediate access to services for a safe return home from hospital. The required care may be clinical and/or non-clinical is usually case managed and available for a period of several weeks from the time of discharge. An example of this type of service is ComPacks, a transitional care service that delivers personal care, domestic assistance, transport and social support for people discharged from public hospitals in New South Wales. In New Zealand community rehabilitation teams are increasingly being used to help older adults transition safely from hospital to home and prevent transfer to a long-term residential care (Office for Senior Citizens, 2013).

Nurses have developed an easy-to-use and evidence-based screening tool called the Transitional Care Model (TCM): Hospital Discharge Screening Criteria for High Risk Older Adults, which is used to identify older adults who are at risk for poorly managed transitions. Studies demonstrate that the use of this tool by nurses resulted in improved patient outcomes and substantial decreases in healthcare costs (Bixby & Naylor, 2009). The tool is available as part of the *Try This* series, sourced from the Hartford Institute for Geriatric Nursing and it is listed as a clinical tool at the end of this chapter. Nurses are encouraged to use this tool to identify older adults who need special attention for transitional care interventions. Nurses can make sure that older adults/families have information about all the following: presenting-problem and final diagnoses; discharge medications (including schedule, purpose and cautions for each) and changes from pre-admission; follow-up appointments; any anticipated problems and suggested interventions; a 24-hour, 7-day call-back number; and all relevant care providers (Podrazik & Whelan, 2008).

Outpatient services

Outpatient services are another example of subacute care. Outpatient clinics are a common type of outpatient service that provide multidisciplinary and consultative assistance for all people. However, the following types of clinics mostly serve older adults: complex wound care; pain management; falls and mobility; diabetes; memory; continence; osteoarthritis; and management of complex respiratory care. Memory clinics and falls and mobility clinics focus on assessing difficulties and risks and develop a care plan that best supports healthy ageing. The rehabilitation clinic focuses on delivering care to restore optimal function and independence. Nurses are involved in all of these clinics and assist with assessment and management of care.

Hospital-at-home model

The **hospital-at-home model** was introduced in Europe during the 1990s as a cost-cutting measure in response to the increasing demand for hospital admissions. These multidisciplinary programs provide a specific service that requires active participation by healthcare professionals for a limited time.

Types of hospital-at-home models include those that facilitate early discharge from the acute care setting and those that substitute entirely for an inpatient admission. Conditions that are addressed through these models include cellulitis, pneumonia, infusion therapy, post-surgical care, chronic heart failure and chronic obstructive pulmonary disease. An analysis of ten randomised trials found that at 3 months there was no significant difference in mortality for people who received care at home, but at 6 months the mortality rate was significantly lower for those people (Shepperd et al., 2009). Additional findings of Shepperd and colleagues were that these programs were less expensive than admission and people reported more satisfaction.

Another study of four hospital-at-home programs found that participants experienced modest improvements in their activities of daily living (ADL), whereas patients who received hospital care for the same problems experienced a decline in ADL (Leff, 2009).

Roles for nurses in acute care services

As acute care settings have implemented services to address the unique needs of hospitalised older people, new roles have emerged for nurses. Advanced practice gerontological nursing roles are continuing to develop. These nurses are likely to serve as consultants and role

A nurse's perspective

As the dementia/delirium clinical nurse consultant, the majority of people whom I assess are older adults in the hospital setting. I see people on both medical and surgical units. Some are unwell with infections or exacerbations of their chronic conditions; others have had a fall and injured themselves. Approximately 33% of older adults admitted to hospital will have delirium on admission and about 50% of older postoperative hip fracture patients will develop delirium. Part of my role is to assess for signs of delirium and to develop and implement a plan of care for the older person with delirium. The focus of this plan is to maintain the safety and functionality of the older person. In my role I offer the family or carer education and support regarding dementia and delirium.

Often the team needs to meet with the family to develop a discharge plan. This may be the first time the family has been told that their loved one has dementia. I refer families to the Dementia Advisory Service for ongoing support. This role also has an education component and I facilitate dementia education for staff members throughout the year. The more the staff understands about dementia and delirium, the easier the caring for the person with these issues will be.

Behaviour management planning is not to be overlooked. There is usually a reason an older person with dementia or delirium does something out of the ordinary. Most of the time, in my experience, the behaviour is due to a need that has not been met. My job is to be the detective and discover the need, have it met, and de-escalate the situation.

Fran D.

models for other nurses and often assist in developing and implementing evidence-based care services and policies and procedures for hospitalised older adults.

MODELS ADDRESSING THE COORDINATION OF CARE

Consumer demand for community-based programs and persistent increases in the cost of care have stimulated the development of new models of care coordination.

Chronic care models

There is widespread awareness that medical care for people with advanced chronic conditions drives most healthcare costs. Moreover, many older adults with functional limitations and high chronic illness burden have preventable hospitalisations and receive fragmented care that is not person centred (Boling, 2009). Thus, governments and healthcare planners and providers have developed innovative and cost-effective models of care that address the needs of people with chronic medical conditions. One example is the Connecting Care (Severe Chronic Disease Management) Program in New South Wales, which provides a coordinated approach to chronic disease management. Nurses in this program are involved in the identification, assessment, monitoring, planning and coordination of care. They also encourage and support self-care management. In New Zealand in 2012 the Diabetes Care Improvement Packages (DCIP) were introduced. The DCIP encourages healthcare providers "…to develop a tailored approach to managing diabetes", based on the older adult's needs (Office for Senior Citizens, 2013, p. 13).

Case management services

As the range of services for older adults has expanded and healthcare needs have become more complex, the identification of appropriate services and coordination of care has become more necessary and more challenging. Although family members sometimes take on these tasks, they may not be prepared to assume this challenge or might not have the time or availability to do so. Two societal trends that have affected the ability and availability of families to manage the care of the older person are the entry of more women into the paid workforce, and the across-country, or even international, mobility of adult children away from their hometowns. These factors, along with the significant increase in the number of people aged 85 years and older, have led to the need for independent, community-based professional geriatric care management services.

Case management services are provided within an organisational context as part of a broader institution-based program. Hospitals and other healthcare organisations use case managers to make sure people receive the most appropriate and cost-effective services. Case management services also are usually provided as an integral part of comprehensive models to facilitate the coordination and continuity of care. One study found that case management services in comprehensive models were highly valued by older people and their caregivers for improving access to healthcare, increasing psychosocial support, and improving communication with healthcare professionals (Sheaff et al., 2009). A review of studies on case management services found that there should be more priority given to implementing case management programs that focus on patient advocacy and that nurses have important roles in developing these programs (Oeseburg et al., 2009).

An example of this type of service in New Zealand occurs within Integrated Family Health Centres, where nurses act as case managers for people with chronic conditions (NZMOH, 2011b). In Australia there is the Hospital Admission Risk Program (HARP), which is state-government funded, with no or small user contribution. This service provides support for people with chronic and complex diseases using a case-managed approach. A comprehensive care needs assessment and care plan is developed with the client, their family, other community services, healthcare professionals and medical practitioners. These two examples of case management services help reduce the demand for emergency and inpatient hospital care by better managing chronic conditions and minimising acute illness episodes.

CHAPTER HIGHLIGHTS

Development of a continuum of care for older adults

- Many new models of care have emerged to address the diverse healthcare needs of older adults. Such terms as ageing-in-place, continuum of care and long-term care are used to describe the focus of various settings of care for older adults (Box 6-1).

Overview of care services for older people in Australia and New Zealand

- Australia has a nationalised, complex and comprehensive aged care system, which is continually being revised to meet changing demands for services. The Australian Government is the main regulator, funder and provider of long-term residential and community aged care services.
- New Zealand does not have a specific aged care system; however, District Health Boards (DHBs) have an integral role in the funding of long-term residential and community aged care.

Paying for health care services for older adults

- In Australia and New Zealand services for older adults are mostly funded from the national taxation system as well as some means-tested contributions from the consumer.

Types of long-term residential settings

- Residential aged care facilities are licensed residential institutional settings that provide a combination of nursing and personal care services for long-term residents.
- The reasons older adults need long-term residential care usually involve a combination of a gradual decline in functioning due to chronic conditions and a lack of carers who can provide the care at home.
- In recent decades the level of dependency in long-term residential care residents has increased, and dementia care units have been established to meet the needs of those living with dementia.
- Nurses in long-term residential care settings also often assume teaching and leadership roles.
- Newer models of long-term residential care have the goal of transforming the philosophy and practice in residential care facilities to emphasise resident- or person-centred care.
- The Pioneer Network in Long-Term Care promotes the development of culture change models, such as the Eden Alternative and the Green House Project.
- Newer models of care associated present many challenges as well as opportunities for nurses.

Community care services for older adults: Home-based care

- Because of many changes in healthcare trends during the past four decades, different types of home care services have emerged to address different needs: low and increasing levels of care services.
- Long-term home care includes a wide spectrum of services, ranging from non-skilled care such as meal preparation and grocery shopping, to hands-on nursing care.
- People obtain home care services through formal sources, such as community care organisations, or informal sources, including independent carers, and family and friends.

Community care services for older adults: Other community-based services for older adults

- A wide variety of community-based services are available through public and private agencies.
- Adult day centres provide structured activities for functionally impaired older people in a group setting.
- The primary goal of respite services is to relieve caregivers periodically from the stress of their usual caregiving responsibilities.
- Health promotion programs provide organised screening and health education services in community settings.
- Nurses have many opportunities for innovative roles in establishing and implementing programs to address health-related needs of older adults in community settings.

Models addressing coordination of care

- Chronic care models are currently being developed and promoted as cost-effective models of care that address the needs of people with chronic medical conditions.
- Case management services involve comprehensive assessment, care planning, implementation, monitoring and reassessment to address immediate and long-term needs of older adults.
- Case management services are provided to ensure that older adults receive the most appropriate and cost-effective services.

Acute care settings

- Acute care for elders (ACE) units address the complex needs of hospitalised older adults though multidisciplinary assessments and interventions.
- Subacute care units address the medically complex needs of hospitalised older adults.
- The hospital-at-home model provides cost-effective care for older adults with complex medical needs that can be addressed in a home setting.
- Transitional care is a term used in relation to models that provide coordination and continuity when people move from one setting to another.

CRITICAL THINKING EXERCISES

1. Mrs Sim is 84 years old and was recently diagnosed with dementia. She is able to care for herself as long as someone reminds her to eat her meals and take her medications. Two months ago, she began living with her daughter, who works part time, and the other days she cares for her grandchildren. Two days a week, Mrs Sim's daughter takes her to an adult day centre at 8.30 a.m. and Mrs Sim returns home using the centre's bus. What types of additional services might Mrs Sim's daughter need to use?
2. Mrs Frank is a patient in a rehabilitation unit where you work. She had been living alone in her own home before being admitted to the hospital with a fractured hip 4 weeks ago. She has regained much of her independence and walks with a walker and a one-person assist. She expects to ambulate independently, using a walker, within 2 weeks, at which time she expects to return to her own home. She asks you what kind of services would be available in her home. What additional information would you want to know before you answered her questions? What information would you give to her? What suggestions would you make?
3. Your grandmother, who is 72 years old, states she "should be thinking about moving into a residential care facility as it is all getting too much for me". She currently lives alone, with no services. What questions would you ask? What information would you provide? What suggestions would you make?

RESOURCES

For an extensive range of additional resources to enhance teaching and learning and to facilitate understanding of this chapter, please see the text's accompanying website located on thePoint at http://thepoint.lww.com.

Clinical tools

Hartford Institute for Geriatric Nursing, ConsultGeriRN.org: http://consultgerirn.org/resources

Assessment tools *Try This*® series and *How to Try This* resources

General assessment series:

- *Try This*, issue 24: The Hospital Admission Risk Profile (HARP). Graf, C. (2008). *Best Practices in Nursing Care to Older Adults.*
- *How to Try This* (article): The Hospital Admission Risk Profile. Graf, C. (2008). *American Journal of Nursing, 108*(8), 62–71.
- *How to Try This* (video): The Hospital Admission Risk Profile (HARP).
- *Try This*, issue 26: The Transitional Care Model (TCM): Hospital Discharge Screening Criteria for High Risk Older Adults. Bixby, B. (2009). *Best Practices in Nursing Care to Older Adults.*

Hartford Geriatric Nursing Initiative (HGNI)

- Preparing the Nursing Profession to Care for the Growing Number of Older Adults: http://consultgerirn.org/resources/hartford_geriatric_nursing_initiative_hgni

Nurses Improving Care for Healthsystem Elders (NICHE)

- Geriatric Registered Nurse Model: www.nicheprogram.org/models_of_care

Health education

Age Concern New Zealand: www.ageconcern.org.nz

Australian Government's guide to aged care law: http://guides.dss.gov.au/guide-aged-care-law

Centre for Health Service Development (CHSD), for HACC, ACCNA, CENA, etc., tools: http://ahsri.uow.edu.au/screening

Eldernet New Zealand: www.eldernet.co.nz

Health Direct Australia, seniors' health: www.healthdirect.gov.au/seniors-health

interRAI Coordinating Centre, Australia and New Zealand: http://interrai-au.org

myaged*care* Australia: www.myagedcare.gov.au

National Institute on Aging (U.S.): www.nia.nih.gov

New Zealand Ministry of Health, older people's health data and statistics: www.health.govt.nz

Office for Senior Citizens New Zealand: www.osc.govt.nz

Paying for healthcare services, New Zealand: www.newzealandnow.govt.nz/living-in-nz/healthcare/paying-for-healthcare services

Pioneer Network (Eden Alternative and Green House Project): www.pioneernetwork.net

Productivity Commission Australia: www.pc.gov.au

Seniorline New Zealand, helping older people navigate the health system: www.adhb.govt.nz/SeniorLine

REFERENCES

Ashton, T. (2005). Recent developments in the funding and organisation of the New Zealand health system. *Australia and New Zealand Health Policy, 2*, 9.

Australian Government Department of Social Services (DSS). (2014a). Aged Care Funding Instrument (ACFI) user guide. Accessed March 2015 at via www.dss.gov.au.

Australian Government Department of Social Services (DSS). (2014b). Home care packages. Available March 2015 via www.dss.gov.au.

Australian Government Department of Social Services (DSS). (2014c). Ageing and aged care. Accessed March 2015 via www.dss.gov.au.

Australian Government Department of Social Services. (2015). Guides to social policy law: Guide to aged care law. Accessed April 2015 at http://guides.dss.gov.au/guide-aged-care-law.

Australian Government Department of Health (AGDH). (2014 update). Health assessment for people aged 75 years and older. Accessed March 2015 via www.health.gov.au.

Bail, K. & Draper, B. (2011). The blurring lines between acute and aged care. *Nursing Review*, 24 & 25.

Bayne, C. G. & Boling, P. A. (2009). New diagnostic and information technology for mobile medical care. *Clinics in Geriatric Medicine, 25*, 93–107.

Baztan, J. J., Suarez-Garcia, F. M., Lopez-Arrieta, J., Rodrigues-Manas, L. & Rodrigues-Artalejo, F. (2009). Effectiveness of acute geriatric units on functional decline, living at home, and case fatality among older patients admitted to hospital for acute medical disorders: Meta-analysis. *British Medical Journal, 338*, b50.

Bixby, M. B. & Naylor, M. D. (2009). The Transitional Care Model (TCM): Hospital discharge screening criteria for high risk older adults. *Try This* series, issue 26. *Best Practices in Nursing Care to Older Adults*. Hartford Institute for Geriatric Nursing. Retrieved from http://consultgerirn/resources.

Boling, P. A. (2009). Care transitions and home health care. *Clinics in Geriatric Medicine, 25*, 135–148.

Bowers, E., Nolet, K., Roberts, T. & Edmond, S. (2009). Implementing change in long-term care: A practical guide to transformation. Canberra: Commonwealth Fund. Retrieved from www.commonwealthfund.org/Content/Innovations/Tools/2009/Apr/Implementing-change.

Boyd, M., Broad, J. B., Kerse, N., et al. (2011). Twenty-year trends in dependency in residential aged care in Auckland, New Zealand: A descriptive study. *Journal* of the American Medical Directors Association, 12(7), 535–540.

Brownie, S. (2011). A culture change in aged care: The Eden Alternative™. *Australian Journal of Advanced Nursing, 29*(1), 63–68.

Burger, S. G., Kantor, B., Mezey, M., Mitty, E., Kluger, M., Algase, D., … Rader, J. (2009). Nurses' involvement in nursing home culture change: Overcoming barriers, advancing opportunities. The Hartford Institute for Geriatric Nursing Coalition for Geriatric Nursing Organizations & Pioneer Network. Available March 2015 via http://hartfordign.org.

Cho, S., Zarit, S. H. & Chiriboga, D. A. (2009). Wives and daughters: The differential role of day care use in the nursing home placement of cognitively impaired family members. *Gerontologist, 49*, 57–67.

Find A Rest Home.co.nz. (2015). Home care: What home care services are available? Accessed March 2015 at www.findaresthome.co.nz/process/S04a-information-about-home-care.htm.

Graham, C. L., Ivey, S. L. & Neuhauser, L. (2009). From hospital to home: Assessing the transitional care needs of vulnerable seniors. *Gerontologist, 49*, 23–33.

Greenwald, J. L. & Jack, B. W. (2009). Preventing the preventable: Reducing rehospitalizations through coordinated, patient-centered discharge processes. *Professional Case Management, 14*, 135–140.

Hunter, S. & Levett-Jones, T. (2010). The practice of nurses working with older people in long-term care: An Australian perspective. *Journal of Clinical Nursing, 19*(3–4), 527–536.

interRAI Australia. (2011). interRAI Coordinating Centre, Australia and New Zealand. Viewed March 2015 at http://interrai-au.org.

Kane, R. A. & Cutler, L. J. (2008). Sustainability and expansion of small-house nursing homes: Lessons from the Green Houses® in Tupelo, MS. Minnesota, MN: Division of Health Policy and Management, School of Public Health, University of Minnesota. Viewed March 2015 via www.hpm.umn.edu.

Leff, B. (2009). Comparison of functional outcomes associated with hospital at home care and traditional acute hospital care. *Journal of the American Geriatrics Society, 57*, 273–278.

Lum, T. Y., Kane, R. A., Cutler, L. J. & Yu, T. C. (2008–2009). Effects of Green House nursing homes on residents' families. *Health Care Financing Review, 20*, 35–51.

Martikainen, P., Moustgaard, H., Murphy, M., Einiö, E. K., Koskinen, S., Martelin, T. & Noro, A. (2009). Gender, living arrangements, and social circumstances as determinants of entry into and exit from long-term institutional care at older ages: A 6-year follow-up study of older Finns. *Gerontologist, 49*, 34–45.

Molzahn, A. E., Gallagher, E. & McNulty, V. (2009). Quality of life associated with adult day centers. *Journal of Gerontological Nursing, 35*(8), 37–46.

Naylor, M. & Keating, S. A. (2008). Transitional care: Moving patients from one care setting to another. *American Journal of Nursing, 108*, 58S–63S.

New Zealand Ministry of Health (NZMOH). (2006). Health of Older People Information Strategic Plan: Directions to 2010 and Beyond. Wellington: Author. Accessed March 2015 via www.health.govt.nz.

New Zealand Ministry of Health (NZMOH). (2011a). Needs assessment and support services for older people: What you need to know. Accessed March 2015 via www.health.govt.nz.

New Zealand Ministry of Health (NZMOH). (2011b). Better, sooner, more convenient primary health care. Accessed March 2015 via www.health.govt.nz.

New Zealand Ministry of Health (NZMOH). (2012). Long-term residential care for older people: What you need to know. Accessed March 2015 via www.health.govt.nz.

New Zealand Ministry of Health (NZMOH). (2014). *Showcasing aged-care nursing*. Wellington: Author.

Oeseburg, B., Wynia, K., Middel, B. & Reijneveld, S. A. (2009). Effects of case management for frail older people or those with chronic illness. *Nursing Research, 58*, 201–210.

Office for Senior Citizens. (2013). Older New Zealanders: Healthy, independent, connected and respected. Accessed March 2015 via www.msd.govt.nz.

Office of the Auditor-General. (2011). Home-based support services for older people. Accessed March 2015 at www.oag.govt.nz/2011/home-based-support.

Podrazik, P. M. & Whelan, C. T. (2008). Acute hospital care for the elderly patient: Its impact on clinical and hospital systems of care. *Medical Clinics of North America, 92*, 387–406.

Productivity Commission (PC). (2011). Caring for Older Australians. Inquiry Report No. 53. Canberra: Author. Available March 2015 via www.pc.gov.au.

Rabig, J. (2009). Home again: Small houses for individuals with cognitive impairment. *Journal of Gerontological Nursing, 35*(8), 10–15.

Rantz, M. J., Cheshire, D., Flesner, M., Petroski, G. F., Hicks, L., Alexander, G., … Thomas, S. (2009). Helping nursing homes "at risk" for quality problems: A statewide evaluation. *Geriatric Nursing, 30*, 238–249.

Resnick, B., Gruber-Baldini, A. L., Galik, E., Pretzer-Aboff, I., Russ, K., Hebel, J. R. & Zimmerman, S. (2009). Changing philosophy in long-term care: Testing of the restorative care intervention. *Gerontologist, 49*, 175–184.

Schoen, C., Osborn, R., How, S. K., Doty, M. M. & Peugh, J. (2009). Experiences of patients with complex health care needs in eight countries. *Health Affairs (Millwood), 28*(1), w1–w16.

Sheaff, R., Boaden, R., Sargent, P., Pickard, S., Gravelle, H. & Roland, M. (2009). Impacts of case management for frail elderly people: A qualitative study. *Journal of Health Services Research Policy, 14*, 88–95.

Shepperd, S., Doll, H., Angus, R. M., Clarke, M. J., Iliffe, S., Kalra, L., … Wilson, A. D. (2009). Avoiding hospital admission through provision of hospital care at home: A systematic review and meta-analysis of individual patient data. *Canadian Medical Association Journal, 180*, 175–182.

Shippee, T. P. (2009). "But I am not moving": Residents' perspectives on transitions within a continuing care retirement community. *Gerontologist, 49*, 418–427.

Standards New Zealand. (2012). *Home and community support sector standard*: NZS 8158 2012. Accessed March 2015 via www.standards.co.nz.

Statistics New Zealand. (2007). *New Zealand's 65+ population: A statistical volume 2007*. Accessed March 2015 via www.stats.govt.nz.

White-Chou, E. G., Graves, W. J., Godfrey, S. M., Bonner, A. & Sloane, P. (2009). Beyond the medical model: The culture change revolution in long-term care. *Journal of the American Medical Directors Association, 10*, 370–378.

Your Life Choices. (2015). Assisted living. Accessed March 2015 at www.yourlifechoices.com.au/aged-care/what-is-aged-care/assisted-living.

Zelada, M. A., Salinas, R. & Baztan, J. J. (2009). Reduction of functional deterioration during hospitalization in an acute geriatric unit. *Archives of Gerontology and Geriatrics, 48*, 35–39.

Chapter 7

Assessment of health and functioning

By Carol Miller and Sharyn Hunter

LEARNING OBJECTIVES

After reading this chapter, you should be able to:

1. Discuss factors that contribute to the complexity of assessing older adults.
2. Use basic nursing assessment and functional assessment tools.
3. Describe how the older adult's environment, use of adaptive and assistive devices, and cognitive abilities can affect functioning.
4. Discuss nursing roles related to function-focused care and comprehensive geriatric assessments.
5. Assess safety of older adults in their home settings.
6. Explain how nurses can assess and address concerns about safe driving by older adults.

KEY POINTS

activities of daily living (ADLs)
Aged Care Funding Instrument (ACFI)
complexity of assessing health in older adults
comprehensive geriatric assessment
everyday competence
functional assessment
function-focused care
instrumental activities of daily living (IADLs)
inter Resident Assessment Instrument (interRAI)
Minimum Data Set (MDS) for Resident Assessment and Care Screening
nursing assessment tools
safe driving

The assessment of the health and functioning of older adults is an essential and complex component of nursing care. This chapter discusses the general approach to assessing the older adult's health and functioning and provides tools for functional assessment. In addition, this chapter concludes with an example of how nurses assess an older adult's health and functioning in relation to their ability to drive a motor vehicle. Driving is a major safety concern, with implications for society and individual older adults.

HEALTH ASSESSMENT OF OLDER ADULTS

A major challenge when nursing older adults is the **complexity of assessing health in older adults**, especially from a comprehensive, and person-centred perspective. The assessment of an older adult would:

- Focus on the whole person
- Occur through a relationship of trust between the nurse and the person
- Be approached through an understanding of the older adult's history
- Be based on the person's understanding and values about their health, and
- Take into account the older adult's capabilities. (Ford & McCormack, 2000)

Several factors contribute to the complexity of assessing the health and functioning of older adults:

- Older adults commonly have one or more chronic conditions in addition to any acute health conditions for which they are being assessed. These conditions often interact, causing older adults' health to fluctuate unpredictably.
- Manifestations of illness, even acute illness, tend to be obscure and less predictable in older adults than in younger adults. For example, in older adults, one of the most common manifestations of illness or an adverse medication effect is a change in behaviour or mental status.
- For any one manifestation of illness in an older adult, there are usually several possible explanations. For example, changes in function can be caused by a combination of several of the following conditions: acute illness, psychosocial factors, environmental conditions, age-related changes, a new chronic illness, an existing chronic illness, or an adverse effect of medication(s) or other treatments.
- Treatments are often directed towards the symptoms, while the source of a problem is obscure and unresolved. This approach can mask the underlying problem even further and cause additional complications (e.g. when adverse medication effects are not recognised as such and are treated with additional medications).
- Cognitive impairments can make it difficult for older adults to report accurately or describe a physiological problem and there may be few or no reliable sources of information.
- In many cases, by the time illness in an older adult is detected and addressed, the underlying physiological disturbance is in an advanced stage, and additional complications have developed.
- Myths and misunderstandings can lead healthcare providers, family members or older adults to falsely attribute treatable conditions to ageing.

The aim of an assessment is to identify all needs for care and support of the older person. Because of all of the factors identified above, nurses must take a detective-like approach to assessing older adults. This approach requires nurses to assess all aspects of the person's body, mind and spirit to look for clues—which are usually many and complicated and range from subtle to obvious—to the underlying causes of changes in health or functioning. Nurses will enquire into physiological functioning, growth and development, family relationships, social networks, spiritual and other interests. All the information obtained is critical to the development of an individualised person-centred plan of care that enhances personal health status and quality of life.

The Functional Consequences Model for Promoting Wellness in Older Adults is described in Chapter 3 and is applied to specific aspects of functioning throughout this text. Nurses can use these detailed guides to assess older adults holistically and to plan and implement nursing interventions towards wellness (refer to the lists of boxes and tables at the beginning of the text). Nurses also can refer to information in Chapter 27 about unique and atypical manifestations of illness in older adults.

Clinically oriented chapters of this text also include information about normal age-related variations that nurses need to consider when assessing specific aspects of health and functioning. It is necessary for nurses to have knowledge about age-related variations in laboratory values to complete a nursing assessment. Table 7-1 lists the variations in laboratory values that occur with ageing.

COMPREHENSIVE AND NURSING ASSESSMENT TOOLS

Comprehensive assessment models

As gerontologists and healthcare providers began addressing the complexity of care for older adults, they recognised the need for assessment models that were more comprehensive than those that focused specifically on particular aspects of health or functioning (refer to Chapter 6 for a description of these programs). Thus, in the early 1980s, standardised tools for **comprehensive geriatric assessments** were developed, but they were not widely implemented at that time.

During the last decade it has been recognised that comprehensive and integrated assessment processes are essential for older adults, to promote healthy ageing and improve the effectiveness of the delivery of healthcare. Comprehensive assessments for older adults include:

- Standardised assessment and screening tools
- Standard methods of both collecting and reporting information
- Assessment of the areas of personal care, social participation, safety, health status and functional abilities
- Assessment of the carers/caregivers
- A management plan that would be developed with the older adult and their carers following assessment, and
- Effective interventions and regular follow-up.

(New Zealand Ministry of Health and New Zealand Guidelines Group [NZMOH & NZGG], 2003, p. xvii)

A number of comprehensive geriatric assessments have been developed in Australia, New Zealand and in the U.S. In the U.S. all Medicaid- and Medicare-funded long-term residential care facilities use a standardised assessment form as part of the effort to improve quality of care through regulation and inspections. This form, known as the **Minimum Data Set (MDS) for Resident Assessment and Care Screening**, includes several hundred items that document 18 areas of functioning, such as the medical, mental and social characteristics of nursing home residents. A major advantage of the MDS is that it requires nursing staff to assess the health and functional status of each older resident on admission to identify problems and strengths, and to reassess every 3 months and document any changes (Shin & Scherer, 2009). The MDS has been successful in improving care and has resulted in other gerontological healthcare settings using it. A community version of the MDS (MDS-HC) has been developed and, in Italy, the MDS-HC is used as an integral part of community-based team assessment and care management services, and this has led to a reduced rate of admissions to hospitals and other healthcare facilities (Wieland & Ferrucci, 2008).

The MDS has been internationally recognised and both the long-term residential care and home care versions have been translated, validated and implemented in many countries, including Canada, Australia, and Asian and European countries. Gerontologists have cited the MDS as a prototype assessment instrument that has established a new philosophy and approach to the care of older adults and which has laid the groundwork for evidence-based geriatric assessment and management (Bernabei et al., 2008).

In Australia and New Zealand, a component of the MDS, the **inter Resident Assessment Instrument** (interRAI), is being used (interRAI Australia, 2011). The interRAI comprises a suite of instruments that can be used in the assessment and care of older adults. These include assessments in acute care, community care and long-term residential care, for low and high levels of care. These instruments have been modified for the Australian and New Zealand healthcare contexts. In Australia the interRAI is being used in several community-based services in Victoria and hospitals in Queensland, but in only one large provider of long-term residential care. The use of the interRAI is more widespread in New Zealand, where it is used for community and long-term residential care assessments (National Health IT Board, 2015). The data from the interRAI in New Zealand is being used to compare information across services and facilities to encourage "best care practices". New Zealand has a national guideline that directs the comprehensive assessment processes of older people (NZMOH & NZGG, 2003), of which the interRAI is an integral part. This guideline also recommends appropriate

TABLE 7-1 Age-related variations in laboratory values

Test values	Age-related changes	Considerations
Serum		
Albumin, 32–45 g/L	Younger than age 65: higher in men Older than age 65: equal levels that then decrease at same rate	Increased dietary protein intake needed in older patients if liver function is normal; oedema: a sign of low albumin level
Alkaline phosphatase • Men: 53–128 u/L • Women: 42–90 u/L	Increases	May reflect liver function decline or vitamin D malabsorption and bone demineralisation
Beta globulin, 0.8–2.5 mg/L	Increases slightly	Increases in response to decrease in albumin if liver function is normal; increased dietary protein intake needed
Blood urea nitrogen, 2.9–8.2 mmol/L	Increases	Slight increase acceptable in absence of stressors, such as infection or surgery
Cholesterol, <4.0 mmol/L	Men: increases to age 50, then decreases Women: lower than men until age 50, increases to age 70, then decreases	Rise in cholesterol level (and increased cardiovascular risk) in women as a result of postmenopausal oestrogen decline; dietary changes, weight loss and exercise needed
Creatine kinase, 44–150 umol/L	Increases slightly	May reflect decreasing muscle mass and liver function
Creatinine • Female: 50–110 umol/L • Male: 60–120 umol/L	Increases in men	Important factor to prevent toxicity when giving drugs excreted in urine
Creatinine clearance, 104–125 mL/min	Men: decreases; formula: (140 – age) × kg body weight/72 × serum creatinine Women: 85% of men's rate	Reflects reduced glomerular filtration rate; important factor to prevent toxicity when giving drugs excreted in urine
Glucose tolerance test • Fasting: <6.1 mmol/L • After 2 hours: <11.0 mmol/L	Rises faster in first 2 hours, then drops to baseline more slowly	Reflects declining pancreatic insulin supply and release and diminishing body mass for glucose uptake. (Rapid rise can quickly trigger hyperosmolar hyperglycaemic non-ketotic syndrome. Rapid decline can result from certain drugs, such as alcohol, beta-adrenergic blockers, and monoamine oxidase inhibitors.)
Haematocrit (per cent) • Men: 0.40–0.54 • Women: 0.37–0.47	May decrease slightly (unproven)	Reflects decreased bone marrow and haematopoiesis, increased risk of infection (because of fewer and weaker lymphocytes and immune system changes that diminish antigen–antibody response)
Haemoglobin • Men: 115–165 g/L • Women: 130–180 g/L	Men: decreases Women: unknown	Reflects decreased bone marrow, haematopoiesis, and (for men) androgen levels
High-density lipoprotein, 0.9–2.0 mmol/L	Levels higher in women than in men but equalise with age	Compliance with dietary restrictions required for accurate interpretation of test results
Lactate dehydrogenase, 110–230 u/L	Increases slightly	May reflect declining muscle mass and liver function
Leucocyte count, 4–11 × 10^9/L	Decreases	Decrease proportionate to lymphocyte count
Lymphocyte count, 1.5–4.0 × 10^9/L	Decreases	Decrease proportionate to leucocyte count
Platelet count, 150–400 × 10^9/L	Change in characteristics: decreased granular constituents, increased platelet-release factors	May reflect diminished bone marrow and increased fibrinogen levels
Potassium, 3.8–5.0 mmol/L	Increases slightly	Requires avoidance of salt substitutes composed of potassium, vigilance in reading food labels, and knowledge of hyperkalaemia's signs and symptoms
Thyroid-stimulating hormone, 0.4–5.0 mIU/L	Increases slightly	Suggests primary hypothyroidism or endemic goiter at much higher levels
Thyroxine, 9–25 pmol/L	Decreases 25%	Reflects declining thyroid function
Triglycerides, <2 mmol/L	Range widens	Suggests abnormalities at any other levels, requiring additional tests such as serum cholesterol
Triiodothyronine, 3.5–6.5 pmol/L	Decreases 25%	Reflects declining thyroid function
Urine		
Glucose, <0.003 nmol/L	Decreases slightly	May reflect renal disease or urinary tract infection (UTI); unreliable check for older diabetic people because glucosuria may not occur until plasma glucose level exceeds 16 mmol/L
Protein, 0–50 mg/L	Increases slightly	May reflect renal disease or UTI
Specific gravity, 1.002–1.030	Decreases to 1.024 by age 80	Reflects 30%–50% decrease in number of nephrons available to concentrate urine

Laboratory values that are not affected by increased age:

- Prothrombin time
- Partial thromboplastin time
- Serum chloride
- Serum carbon dioxide
- Serum acid phosphatase
- Aspartate aminotransferase
- Total serum protein

From *Handbook of geriatric nursing care* (2nd ed., Appendix B, pp. 628–629). (2003). Philadelphia, PA: Lippincott Williams & Wilkins; Australasian Society of Clinical and Experimental Pharmacologists and Toxicologists (ASCEPT), Pharmaceutical Society of Australia and Royal Australian College of General Practitioners. (2008). *Australian medicines handbook*. Adelaide, SA: Australian Medicines Handbook Pty Ltd.

and effective assessment processes for older Māori and Pacific people.

In Australia, another comprehensive evidence-based and easy-to-use system of assessment was developed to facilitate the delivery of quality care to older adults in long-term residential care facilities. The National Framework for Documenting Care in Residential Aged Care Services (NATFRAME) was developed by a national working group made up of experts in documentation and aged care. The fundamental elements of the NATFRAME include the:

- Assessment of the older adult
- Identification of the older adult's capabilities, needs or problems
- Development of interventions, actions and strategies
- Development of strategies required to meet the needs of the older adult, and
- Ongoing evaluation of the older adult's response to the care given.

(Australian Government Department of Health and Ageing [DoAH], 2005)

Originally one of the motivators for the development of the NATFRAME was to create a system that could also be used as a replacement for the funding tool used by the Australian Government for subsidising care in long-term residential care. However, in 2008, the Australian Government introduced the **Aged Care Funding Instrument (ACFI)** as a replacement (DoHA, 2010). Recently the NATFRAME has been archived but is still accessible (Australian Government Department of Social Services, 2014). See the weblinks provided at the end of the chapter.

It is important to note that the ACFI is a funding tool and not a system of evidence-based practice assessments and documentation. The ACFI does contain some evidence-based practice assessments but it does not provide a system for assessing the older adult from a person-centred perspective.

Nursing assessment tools

Since the late 1980s, the Hartford Institute for Geriatric Nursing has been in the forefront of developing, promulgating and updating evidence-based and easy-to-use **nursing assessment tools** for use in various settings. These assessment guides, which are called *Try This: Best Practices in Nursing Care to Older Adults*, and a series of cost-free online articles and corresponding videos demonstrating the application of these tools, are available online via http://consultgerirn.org/resources. These tools do not replace a comprehensive assessment but are useful for identifying specific areas to address in the care plan. Assessment tools from the Hartford Foundation and other reliable sources are listed in the clinical tools sections towards the ends of chapters in this text.

An easy-to-use tool that has been widely used since 1991 to identify common syndromes in older adults that require nursing interventions is the Fulmer SPICES, an acronym for **S**leep disorders, **P**roblems with eating or feeding, **I**ncontinence **C**onfusion, **E**vidence of falls, and **S**kin breakdown (Fulmer & Wallace, 2012). Another tool that has been developed by nurses in community settings is the functional assessment tool, SHOW ME (Narayan, Salgado & VanVoorhis, 2009). This tool can be used to assess functioning in the following areas: **S**hirt & shoes, **H**ike to bathroom, **O**rganisation and use of grooming utensils, **W**alk through home in all areas needed for ADLs/IADLs, **M**edications and **E**ating and making meals.

WELLNESS OPPORTUNITY

When assessing older adults, nurses try to identify the conditions that affect not only health status and level of functioning but also quality of life.

FUNCTIONAL ASSESSMENT OF OLDER ADULTS

A functional assessment is an integral component of a holistic assessment because an essential part of promoting wellness for older adults is identifying areas where function can be improved. **Functional assessment** refers to the measurement of a person's ability to fulfil responsibilities and perform self-care tasks. Functional assessment has its roots in the 1920s when workers' compensation programs needed to determine a cash value to impairments that affected loss of function in jobs. Initially, there were no standards for this and the determination was based solely on a doctor's opinion. When rehabilitation services were developed after World War II tools were needed to measure changes in functional abilities. Functional assessment tools measure **activities of daily living (ADLs)**, which are the tasks associated with meeting one's basic needs, and **instrumental activities of daily living (IADLs)**, which are the more complex tasks that are essential in community-living situations. See Box 7-1 for the functional assessment criteria for each of the ADLs, as well as for cognitive status.

WELLNESS OPPORTUNITY

Nurses identify factors that affect the older adult's quality of life by asking a question such as, "Are there enjoyable activities that you used to do but are no longer able to do because of health problems?"

IADLs are less important in institutional settings than they are in community settings. However, in acute care settings, an assessment of IADLs is an important consideration in discharge planning. When older adults cannot perform IADLs independently, carers often provide the assistance that enables the person to remain in a community setting. Often when older adults cannot perform IADLs and have no carer to help with the task, community resources can be organised to meet these needs. Home-delivered meals programs—Meals on Wheels, for example—might be appropriate for older adults who have difficulty with shopping or meal preparation. Community resources are effective and efficient ways of improving an older adult's ability to perform IADLs.

BOX 7-1
Criteria for assessing activities of daily living (ADLs)

Bathing
5 Unable to assist in any way
4 Able to cooperate but cannot assist
3 Able to wash hands, face and chest with supervision; needs help with completing the bath
2 Able to wash face, chest, arms and upper legs; needs help with completing the bath
1 Bathes self but requires devices (e.g. long-handled sponge)
0 Bathes self-independently

Dressing
5 Needs total assistance
4 Needs total supervision but is able to dress self if clothing articles are given one at a time or set out in the order they are needed
3 Needs reminding and encouragement and some assistance with clothing selection, but can dress with little supervision
2 Dresses self, but needs help with activities requiring fine motor skills (e.g. zippers, shoelaces)
1 Dresses self, using assistive devices (e.g. zipper pullers, long-handled shoehorn)
0 Dresses independently

Mouth care
5 Cannot perform oral hygiene and requires it to be done by others
4 Needs total supervision; needs toothpaste put on brush
3 Needs reminding and some supervision
2 Needs reminding but is otherwise independent
1 Performs oral hygiene using devices (e.g. toothbrush with built-up handle)
0 Performs oral hygiene independently

Hair care
5 Cannot perform hair care and requires it to be done by others
4 Needs total supervision
3 Needs some assistance with daily care
2 Performs daily care independently but needs assistance with washing hair
1 Performs hair care using devices (e.g. hairbrush with built-up handle)
0 Performs all hair care (including washing) independently

Dietary intake
5 Cannot prepare or obtain food; cannot feed self; nutritional requirements would not be met without total assistance
4 Needs assistance in obtaining and preparing food; needs total supervision with eating, but can feed self; nutritional requirements would not be met adequately without assistance
3 Needs assistance in tasks that involve complex skills (e.g. cutting meat, opening packages, preparing and obtaining food), but feeds self; nutritional needs would be met partially without assistance
2 Requires some assistance with obtaining and preparing food, but eats independently; would maintain adequate nutrition with encouragement or a little assistance
1 Needs assistive devices for food preparation and consumption (e.g. plate rings, rocker knife); adequately maintains nutritional requirements
0 Requires no assistance

Transfer mobility
5 Cannot transfer, except with extreme difficulty
4 Needs assistance of three people for transfers, or needs two people and a lifting device
3 Needs the assistance of two people
2 Needs the assistance of one person
1 Transfers independently with a device (e.g. sliding board)
0 Transfers independently

Ambulation
5 Completely unable to walk
4 Walks with the assistance of three people
3 Walks with the assistance of two people
2 Walks with the assistance of one person
1 Walks independently with device (e.g. walker, quad cane)
0 Walks independently

Bed mobility
5 Unable to move in bed
4 Needs the assistance of two people
3 Needs the assistance of one person
2 Needs to be encouraged and supervised
1 Moves independently with device (e.g. uses side rails or trapeze)
0 Moves independently in bed

Cognitive status
5 Has extremely poor memory function; cannot follow directions; has minimal ability to identify and express needs; requires a totally structured environment
4 Has obvious memory impairment that interferes with daily life; has poor judgement and may undertake inappropriate actions; may be aware of the deficit and, consequently, may be anxious or depressed; can participate in daily routine but needs supervision; requires a strong orientation and reminder program
3 Fluctuates between levels two and four; unpredictable on a routine basis; requires monitoring and some supervision; may engage in risky behaviours at times
2 Minimal short-term memory loss; able to perform most daily tasks with only minimal reminding or supervision; has good-to-fair judgement and occasionally needs assistance, but does not engage in any risky behaviours
1 Is dependent on self-initiated reminders and cues for daily activities
0 No observable impairment in memory; no cognitive or psychosocial impairment that interferes with daily activities

Bladder and bowel elimination
5 Consistently soils self
4 Needs supervision and assistance on a regular basis
3 Needs reminding on a regular basis
2 Generally controls elimination; has accidents no more than once a week
1 Maintains control of elimination with devices
0 Fully continent without any assistance

A student's perspective

During my first week with Mr M., I was able to sit with him while he was having breakfast, and I used this time to consider his strengths and weaknesses. While studying his interactions with others, I observed that he had difficulty being understood. He struggled to articulate his various wants and needs. This seemed to lead Mr M. being more isolated than would otherwise be the case. One of his strengths was his ability to feed himself. Initially, I had hoped to read his chart more before meeting him. However, this interaction allowed me a more accurate assessment of his abilities than what would have been recorded in his chart.

After breakfast, we returned to his room to do oral care and to shave. After this, I helped transfer Mr M. to his bed and he asked for a drink, which I gave him and he started choking. I was terrified, but fortunately I was able to get help quickly and the situation was managed and he was okay. I learned from this experience to assess the person's entire environment before addressing their needs and desires. Mr M. choked because I gave him a cup of water that was not thickened.

Kimberly S.

In recent years, healthcare practitioners have increasingly recognised the value of functional assessment, particularly with regard to chronic conditions and care of older adults. In contrast to a medical diagnosis approach, a functional assessment approach focuses on improved functioning in daily life, regardless of diagnosis. In geriatric clinical settings, there is increasing emphasis on using functional assessments as a core component of function-focused care, which is a rehabilitative approach to preventing functional decline and improving an older adult's level of functioning.

FUNCTION-FOCUSED CARE

Function-focused care, which previously was referred to as restorative care, is an approach to care that focuses both on (a) evaluating a person's underlying capability with regard to functional and physical activity, and (b) on implementing interventions to optimise and maintain functional abilities and increase physical activities (Resnick, Galik & Boltz, 2013). The philosophy of function-focused care addresses direct care issues as well as broader considerations such as environmental factors and staff training. Studies find that this approach is effective in improving outcomes for older adults with acute and chronic conditions, including trauma and dementia (Burket, Hippensteel, Penrod et al., 2013; Galik, Resnick, Hammersla et al., 2014). In addition, evidence-based practice guidelines for geriatric nursing have incorporated this approach in relation to assessment of physical function and preventing functional decline in acute care settings, as summarised in Evidence-based practice 7-1 (Boltz, Resnick & Galik, 2012; Kresevic, 2012).

EVIDENCE-BASED PRACTICE 7-1
Function-focused care and assessment of physical function

Statement of the problem

- Older adults often experience functional decline during hospitalisation and this leads to poor long-term outcomes, which include increased mortality, decreased functional recovery, and increased likelihood of being discharged to a nursing facility.
- Some functional decline that occurs during hospitalisation is progressive and irreversible, but some can be prevented or ameliorated by prompt and aggressive nursing interventions (e.g. ambulation, toileting schedules, effective communication, use of adaptive equipment, and appropriate medication regimens).
- Risk factors for functional decline during hospitalisation include pain, depression, malnutrition, decreased mobility, cognitive impairment, and adverse medication effects.
- Bed rest and lack of physical activity result in loss of muscle strength and muscle mass, altered sensory awareness, reduced appetite and thirst sensation, and decreased aerobic capacity and pulmonary ventilations.
- Interdisciplinary care plans are essential for performing functional assessments, evaluating conditions that restrict physical activity (e.g. restraints), and implementing interventions for progressive mobility.

Recommendations for assessment of physical function

- Functional assessment is a critical component of nursing care and involves assessment and documentation of (1) a person's ability to perform ADLs and IADLs, with particular attention to mobility and social activities, (2) level of assistance needed, (3) sensory function, and (4) cognitive function.
- Document baseline functional status and information about recent or progressive changes.
- Assess function at appropriate intervals to validate capacity, decline or improvement.
- Assess strengths and abilities of older adults, as well as limitations.

Recommendations for care strategies to improve functional status

- Maintain the person's daily routine as much as possible through physical activity and social interaction.
- Minimise bed rest and encourage physical activity (exercise, ambulation, range of motion).
- Avoid restraints.
- Use medication judiciously and in appropriate doses.
- Assess for and manage pain.
- Facilitate referrals for rehabilitation therapy, nutrition counselling and coaching.
- Allow flexible visitation, including pets.
- Teach older adults, families and carers about the value of independent functioning and strategies to help prevent functional decline.

Source: Boltz, M., Resnick, B. & Galik, E. (2012). Interventions to prevent functional decline in acute care settings. In M. Boltz, E. Capezuti, T. Fulmer & D. Zwicker (Eds), *Evidence-based practice protocols for best practice* (4th ed., pp. 89–121). New York: Springer; Kresevic, D. (2012). Assessment of physical function. In M. Boltz, E. Capezuti, T. Fulmer & D. Zwicker (Eds), *Evidence-based practice protocols for best practice* (4th ed., pp. 89–103). New York: Springer.

Nurses and functional assessment tools

Such functional assessment tools as the Modified Barthel's Index, the Katz Index of Independence in Activities of Daily Living scale, and the Lawton Instrumental Activities of Daily Living scale, are tools that were developed for use by health professionals. As a nurse's assessment of an older adult is person centred, this would include IADLs as well as ADLs. Nurses have adapted functional assessment tools that do this. An example of one of these tools is illustrated in Figure 7-1. This tool was developed by nurses in a geriatric rehabilitation setting and can be used to measure a person's ADLs and cognitive

	Date	PTA	ADM	DISCH		
Personal Care	*Bathing* 5 completely dependent 4 dependent with some assist 3 heavy partial 2 light partial 1 independent with devices 0 independent					
	Dressing 5 complete assist 3 partial assist 1 compensated 0 independent					
	Mouth care 5 totally unable to do 3 some assist 1 independent with device 0 independent					
	Hair care 5 completely unable 3 some assist 1 independent with device 0 independent					
	Dietary intake 5 total assist 4 assist with feeding 3 supplements 2 set up/encouragement 1 independent with device 0 independent					
Mobility	*Transfer* 5 completely unable 4 3-person/portalift 3 2-person 2 1-person 1 independent with devices 0 independent					
	Ambulation 5 completely unable 4 3-person assist 3 2-person assist 2 1-person assist 1 independent with devices 0 independent					
	Bed 5 unable to move in bed 3 needs assist 1 independent with device 0 independent					
Mental Status	*Mental* 5 totally impaired 4 assist with simple tasks 3 assist with complex tasks 2 inconsistent 1 compensated 0 no impairment					

FIGURE 7-1 Functional assessment of older adults. This form allows for recording changes over time. The three time designations indicated on the form signify the period prior to admission (PTA), the time of admission (ADM), and the day of discharge (DISCH). The unmarked columns may be used at any time after discharge, or upon readmission. (Used with permission from Fairview General Hospital, Clevelend, OH.)

	Date	PTA	ADM	DISCH		
Elimination	*Bladder* 5 completely incontinent 3 occasionally incontinent 1 continent with assist/device 0 continent/independent					
	Bowel 5 completely incontinent 3 occasionally incontinent 1 continent with assist/device 0 continent/independent					
	Assist/device codes A bedside commode B bathroom C urinal D bedpan E ostomy F incontinence pads G catheter, external H catheter, indwelling I catheter, intermittent J verbal cuing/supervision K other ________					
Instrumental Activities of Daily Living	*Meal preparation* 5 unable to do 3 assist/supervise 1 independent with resources 0 independent					
	Shopping 5 unable to do 3 assist/supervise 1 compensated 0 independent					
	Telephone 5 unable to do/doesn't have 3 assist 1 independent with device 0 independent					
	Transportation 5 completely homebound 3 assist 1 arranges own 0 independent					
	Medications 5 unable to take 3 assist 1 independent 0 doesn't use					
	Housekeeping 5 unable to do 3 assist 1 independent with resources 0 independent					
	Laundry 5 unable to do 3 assist 1 independent with resources 0 independent					
	Money management 5 unable to handle 3 assist 1 independent with resources 0 independent					
	Total points					

FIGURE 7-1 (*continued*)

status over time. An important aspect of assessment by nurses is that is it ongoing. This tool documents changes that occur over time and may assist with the identification of factors that influence functional abilities. Including cognition in the functional assessment rather than using a separate mental status assessment tool reinforces the fact that cognitive function is an integral component of ADLs. In addition, it helps to determine whether ADL impairments are attributable, at least in part, to cognitive impairments rather than primarily to physical limitations. See Box 7-2 for assessment criteria for the IADLs that are included in Figure 7-1.

The functional assessment form in Figure 7-1 demonstrates how changes recorded occur over time. An initial assessment, which is performed at the time of admission (ADM), provides information on which goals for care are

BOX 7-2
Criteria for assessing instrumental activities of daily living (IADLs)

Meal preparation
5 Unable to prepare even simple meals
4 Can assist with meal preparation
3 Prepares meals but cannot obtain groceries
2 Prepares meals with reminding or supervision
1 Prepares meals and obtains food using resources (e.g. specialised equipment, Meals on Wheels program, transportation to the grocery store)
0 Independent in obtaining and preparing food

Grocery shopping
5 Cannot participate in shopping
4 Can accompany someone else and assist with food selection
3 Can shop and select appropriate food with some supervision
2 Can shop but has difficulty obtaining transportation
1 Is able to arrange for necessary help with shopping
0 Shops independently

Telephone use
5 Cannot dial or answer the phone, or carry on a routine phone conversation
4 Can talk on the phone but cannot dial or answer it
3 Can use the phone with assistance (e.g. help in dialling)
2 Can use the phone with supervision
1 Depends on adaptive devices for telephone activities (e.g. automatic dialling system, speaker phone)
0 Independent in phone-related activities

Transportation
5 Does not leave home, even for medical care
4 Leaves home only for medical care or in rare circumstances
3 Needs assistance in arranging for transportation and needs special accommodations (e.g. wheelchair lift)
2 Needs assistance in arranging for transportation but can get in and out of cars with little or no help
1 Arranges for own transportation but depends on others for any transportation other than walking
0 Independent in travelling from one place to another (e.g. drives a car)

Medications
5 Unable to obtain or take medications without assistance or complete supervision
4 Cannot obtain medications but can take them with assistance or supervision
3 Can obtain and take medications with reminders from others or with a system set up by others
2 Can obtain and take medications with a self-initiated reminder or setup system
1 Safely takes and prepares all medications
0 Does not use medications

Housekeeping
5 Cannot perform any routine household tasks
4 Can assist with household tasks (e.g. bed making, dusting, vacuuming)
3 Can perform household tasks if supervised during the activity
2 Can perform household tasks if encouraged to do so
1 Arranges for housekeeping assistance
0 Is independent in all routine tasks

Laundry
5 Cannot perform any laundry tasks
4 Can assist with folding clothes; cannot wash or iron clothes
3 With assistance, can perform laundry tasks adequately
2 Can perform laundry tasks with supervision and reminding
1 Arranges for laundry to be done
0 Completes all laundry tasks independently

Money management
5 Unable to manage any aspect of finances
4 Can handle simple cash transactions but no other financial transactions (e.g. writing cheques)
3 Can write cheques with supervision or assistance; cannot handle any higher-level transactions (e.g. bank withdrawals)
2 Maintains chequebook, pays bills appropriately and understands currency exchanges, but needs some assistance or supervision with these tasks
1 Arranges for someone else to handle financial matters
0 Handles all finances independently

based. The form also includes a column for information about the person's reported level of function before admission, which is helpful in determining the person's potential level of function. At the time of discharge, the reassessment information enables the staff to determine whether the goals were met. In settings in which post-discharge follow-up is possible, or in settings in which the person is re-admitted at different times, the same assessment form is used to measure changes over time. Each category of activity is assigned a numeric value based on the criteria listed in Boxes 7-1 and 7-2. The numeric values are then used as a guide to measure progress towards goals as the person's level of function changes.

The functional assessment form in Figure 7-1 differs from many others in several ways. First, it allows for the measurement of changes over time. The three time designations indicated on the form signify the period prior to admission (PTA), the ADM, and the day of discharge (DISCH). The unmarked columns may be used at any time after discharge, or upon re-admission. In a rehabilitative or long-term care setting, these measurements over time are particularly helpful in evaluating progress and re-evaluating goals. Second, it includes a scale for documenting mental status because it is essential to ascertain the effects of cognition on functioning. Third, for each category, the number 1 rating is used to indicate that the person does not depend on others but depends on some adaptive device or equipment for independent function in that area. The adaptive device might be as small as a shoehorn or as complex as an electric wheelchair. The importance of this designation is that the staff is then aware that the person has compensated for a deficit, but that the compensatory mechanism must be available for the person's use.

Nurses obtain information for the functional assessment from several sources. When older adults are able to provide reliable information about their level of function before admission, the nurse obtains data for the column marked "PTA" by interviewing the person (patient/resident) within 24 hours of the admission to the care facility. When, as is often the case, older adults are not able to provide this information, the nurse interviews a family member or other person who is knowledgeable about the person's level of function before admission. Nurses directly observe the person's current level of function in performing ADLs to complete the columns marked "ADM" and "DISCH". In institutional settings, nurses must obtain much of the information on IADLs by questioning the older adult or his or her carers because many of these activities pertain only to community-based settings. The source of information is noted on the chart, and any discrepancies between objective and subjective information also are noted.

In interviewing the older adult or carer, it is important to ask for specific details about how tasks are accomplished, rather than asking open-ended questions such as "Do you have any difficulty with...?" Also, it is important to find out whether the task is meaningful to the person, rather than assuming that the person wants or needs to do the task. For example, in the IADL categories, a person who lives with other people might never have to participate in grocery shopping or money management. Therefore, assessment information, particularly regarding IADLs, must be considered in relation to the person's support system and living arrangements.

Assessing function in cognitively impaired older adults

Because cognitive status and psychosocial functioning can significantly affect one's level of functioning, it is particularly challenging to assess function in older adults who have any cognitive or psychosocial limitations (e.g. dementia, delirium, depression). Some functional assessment scales have been developed specifically for people with dementia in a variety of settings and at all levels of cognitive impairment. The assessment tools address the interplay between cognition and abilities to perform ADLs. For example, the Cleveland Scale for Activities of Daily Living (CSADL) divides each ADL into smaller components to identify specific effects of the underlying cognitive deficit. Studies have found that this instrument, illustrated in Figure 7-2, is reliable and valid as a measurement of functional deficits in people with Alzheimer's disease (Mack & Patterson, 2006).

WELLNESS OPPORTUNITY

Keep in mind that formal assessment tools fulfil requirements for documentation, but their primary purpose is to improve care and quality of life for older adults.

Assessing the use or potential use of adaptive and assistive devices

The actual or potential use of such items as mobility aids (e.g. canes, walkers, wheelchairs) and adaptive equipment (e.g. grab bars) should be assessed as factors that can significantly affect safety, functioning and quality of life for older adults. Physiotherapist, occupational and rehabilitation therapists are skilled in assessing for the use of these aids, but nurses need to be familiar with the array of adaptive and assistive devices so that they can make recommendations or facilitate referrals for further evaluation. Many innovative and inexpensive devices are available through catalogues or Internet sites and can be used to improve functioning and independence in daily activities. Additional assistive devices are illustrated and discussed in many chapters of this text (e.g. see Chapters 16, 17 & 22).

Nurses also can identify problems related to the use of assistive devices and request further evaluation by a qualified therapist. For example, nurses can assess comfort and function of wheelchairs because improper fit leads to specific problems such as those summarised in Table 7-2 (p. 115). In addition, improper wheelchair fit is likely to cause pain, fatigue, discomfort, agitation and decreased tolerance for using a wheelchair (Rader, Jones & Miller, 2000).

WELLNESS OPPORTUNITY

When assessing the impact of cognitive abilities on functioning, nurses can try to identify simple interventions, such as putting labels on drawers, which can improve the person's self-esteem by promoting independence.

ASSESSING OLDER ADULTS IN RELATION TO THEIR ENVIRONMENTS

In addition to assessing the older adult's health and functioning, nurses need to be aware of environmental factors that influence the person's safety, functioning and quality of life. Researchers and practitioners increasingly are addressing the interrelationship between people and their environments, and this is particularly pertinent to care of older adults. In the late 1990s, the term **everyday competence** was used to describe the effects of cultural, physical, cognitive, emotional, social and contextual factors on a person's daily functioning. This is particularly important to consider when assessing older adults because these factors can appreciably hinder or improve functional abilities. For example, environmental factors that significantly affect hearing, vision and mobility are discussed in Chapters 16, 17 and 22, respectively.

Assessments at the home provide an excellent base for assessing the relationship between older adults and their

CLEVELAND SCALE FOR ACTIVITIES OF DAILY LIVING (CSADL)

Name or ID of Subject ______________________ Date __ __/__ __/__ __ (mm dd yy) Rater ________

Name of Informant ______________________

Relation of Informant to Subject *(Circle one.)*
1 Spouse 4 Friend or other family
2 Child 5 Professional: ____________
3 Sibling 6 Other: ____________

Contact with Subject
1 2 days/week
2 3–4 days/week
3 5 or more days/week

Interview Type
1 Visit
2 Telephone

To administer this scale, the rater must be thoroughly familiar with the Manual, which includes the full instructions. Place rating in blank after each item number. Several items have specific rating instructions. In particular, some require special questioning if the subject is rated as dependent (rating of 1, 2, or 3).

Rating	*Meaning of Rating*
0	**Never Dependent.** [S] does this effectively, quite independently, without any direction or help.
1	**Sometimes Dependent.** [S] usually does this independently, but sometimes or in some situations [S] needs direction or help.
2	**Usually Dependent.** [S] usually requires some direction or help, but sometimes or in some situations [S] does it independently.
3	**Always Dependent.** [S] always requires direction or help. [S] never does it independently.
9	Cannot rate because of insufficient information

Bathing

1. ____ Initiates bath or shower with appropriate frequency and at appropriate times
2. ____ Prepares bath/shower (draws water of proper temperature, ensures soap and towel are present, etc.)
3. ____ Gets in and out of tub or shower
4. ____ Cleans self

Toileting

5. ____ Able to physically control timing of urination
6. ____ Able to physically control timing of bowel movements
7. ____ Recognises need to eliminate
8. ____ After toileting, cleans and re-clothes self appropriately

Personal hygiene and appearance

9. ____ Initiates personal grooming with appropriate frequency and at appropriate times
10. ____ Washes hands and face
11. ____ Brushes teeth
12. ____ Combs hair, shaves (as appropriate)

FIGURE 7-2 The Cleveland Scale for Activities of Daily Living (CSADL). This functional assessment form was specifically designed for use with people with Alzheimer's disease. (Used with permission from the University Memory and Aging Center, Case Western Reserve University, Cleveland, OH © 1994.)

Dressing

13. ____ Initiates dressing at appropriate time

14. ____ Selects clothes

15. ____ Puts on garments, footwear, etc.

16. ____ Fastens clothing (buttons, shoelaces, zippers, etc.)

Eating

17. ____ Initiates eating at appropriate times of day and with appropriate frequency

18. ____ Carries out physical acts of eating (including using utensils)

19. ____ Eats with acceptable manners, e.g. with appropriate speed, does not speak with food in mouth, etc.

20. ____ Prepares own meals (includes cooking on stove). *This item requires special questioning.*

Mobility

21. ____ Initiates actively moving about the environment, as opposed to sitting, not attempting to get about, etc.

22. ____ Actively moves about environment (with or without assisting device)

22a. Does subject have physical limitations of mobility? *(Circle one of following codes.)*

0 No physical limitations of mobility

1 Yes, there are physical limitations of mobility *(Circle all that apply.)*

Needs assistance of other persons to walk	Trouble getting in or out of bed	Other mobility problems *(describe):*
Needs cane	Trouble getting in or out of chair	
Needs walker	Trouble getting on or off toilet	
Needs wheelchair	Trouble climbing or descending stairs	

Medications

23. ____ Takes medications as scheduled and in correct dosages. *If subject has taken no medications during prior year, rate item as 9. This item requires questioning.*

Shopping

24. ____ Does necessary grocery shopping, buying appropriate items and quantities. *This item requires special questioning.*

25. ____ Does necessary clothes shopping, buying appropriate items and quantities. *This item requires special questioning.*

Travel

26. ____ Finds way about in familiar surroundings

27. ____ Orients to unfamiliar surroundings without undue difficulty

28. ____ Travels beyond walking distance (i.e. driving own vehicle or using public transportation)

29. ____ Drives motor vehicle. *This item requires special questioning.*

FIGURE 7-2 *(continued)*

Hobbies, personal interests, employment

30. _____ Initiates activities of personal interest (e.g. card playing, woodworking, others). *This item requires special questioning.*

31. _____ Carries out such activities. *This item requires special questioning.*

32. _____ Does subject work for pay? *If subject does not work because of having reached an age appropriate to retirement from his or her occupation, rate 9. This item requires special questioning.*

Housework/home maintenance (as appropriate to individual situation)

33. _____ Initiates work around house as needed. *This item requires special questioning.*

34. _____ Carries out work effectively, e.g. cleanly, neatly, accurately, efficiently. *This item requires special questioning.*

Types of work done *(Don't score, just circle)*

Dish washing	Vacuuming	Mowing lawn
Sweeping	Scrubbing floors	Gardening
Personal laundry	Small home repairs	Minor car care
Other types of work *(Describe)*:		

Telephone

35. _____ Looks up numbers

36. _____ Dials numbers

37. _____ Answers phone

38. _____ Takes messages

Money management

39. _____ Pays for purchases (selecting appropriate amount and determining correct change). *This item requires special questioning.*

40. _____ Manages financial responsibilities beyond paying for immediate purchases (e.g. paying monthly bills, managing cheque or savings account, etc.). *This item requires special questioning.*

Communication skills

41. _____ Spontaneously expresses thoughts and needs to others

42. _____ Responds accurately to spoken instructions and conversation

43. _____ Reads and understands single words and short phrases (signs, lists, etc.)

44. _____ Reads and understands complex material (books, newspapers, etc.)

45. _____ Writes short phrases (lists, brief messages)

46. _____ Writes complex material (letters, diary, etc.)

FIGURE 7-2 *(continued)*

Social behaviour

47.____ Behaves in a socially appropriate manner. Socially inappropriate beha viours encompass a wide range of behaviour, including but not limited to such things as making rude remarks, belching, touching private parts, showing little regard for personal privacy, etc. For this item, dependency refers to the extent to which other people must direct or manage the subject to ensure that he or she behaves in a socially appropriate fashion.

Other problems

48.____ Are there any situations in which patient does not behave in an independent and responsible fashion that have not been covered by these questions? *(Circle one of following codes.)*

0 No other dependent behaviours

1 Yes, there are other dependent behaviours *(Please provide details below.)*

QUALITY OF INTERVIEW (Rater's judgement)

Interview appeared valid	0
Some questions about interview, but it is probably acceptable	1
Information from interview is of doubtful validity	2

Rater should record the basis for judging the interview of questionable or doubtful validity.

Comments:

FIGURE 7-2 *(continued)*

TABLE 7-2 Negative effects of improper wheelchair fit

Seating problem	Result on body	Potential effect
Wheelchair too high	Feet do not touch the floor Unable to self-propel Pelvis moves forward	Oedema and decreased circulation in legs Decreased activity Poor sitting posture
Poor back support	Compression of trunk, chest, abdomen Sliding out of chair Increased pelvic tilt	Skin breakdown on back and sacrum Impaired gastrointestinal and respiratory function
Wheelchair too heavy	Difficulty moving chair	Decreased activity
Wheelchair too wide	Pelvic shifting laterally Forward leaning Difficulty using hand rims	Shear stress on skin Poor posture, circulation Decreased mobility
Seat not firm enough ("sling" effect)	Scoliosis Sliding out of chair	Poor posture, circulation Shear stress on skin
Footrest too high	Poor femoral support Unequal pressure distribution Increased ischial tuberosity	Poor posture Skin breakdown

From Rader, J., Jones, D. & Miller, L. (2000). The importance of individualized wheelchair seating for frail older adults. *Journal of Gerontological Nursing, 26*(11), 24–31.

environments. These assessments are essential not only for identifying fall risks (as discussed in Chapter 22) but also for identifying environmental conditions that positively or negatively affect safety, functioning and quality of life. For example, proper lighting is essential for performing enjoyable activities such as reading, playing cards and engaging in hobbies. Similarly, the ability to regulate the temperature is important not only as a safety consideration for preventing hypothermia and hyperthermia but also for comfort. During home visits, it is especially important for nurses to respect autonomy and privacy and be non-judgemental, while at the same time be able to identify all factors that affect the person's functioning and quality of life. Nurses can use Box 7-3 as a

BOX 7-3
Guidelines for assessing the safety of the environment

Illumination and colour contrast

- Is the lighting adequate but not glare producing?
- Are the light switches easy to reach and manipulate?
- Can lights be turned on before entering rooms?
- Are night lights used in appropriate places?
- Is the colour contrast adequate between objects, such as a chair and the floor?

Hazards

- Are there highly polished floors, throw rugs or other hazardous floor coverings?
- If area rugs are used, do they have a non-slip backing, and are the edges tacked to the floor?
- Are there cords, clutter or other obstacles in pathways?
- Is there a pet that is likely to be running underfoot?

Furniture

- Are chairs the right height and depth for the person?
- Do the chairs have armrests? Are all tables stable and of the appropriate height?
- Is small furniture placed well away from pathways?

Stairways

- Is lighting adequate?
- Are there light switches at the top and bottom of the stairs?
- Are there securely fastened handrails on both sides of the stairway?
- Are all the steps even?
- Are the treads non-skid?
- Should coloured tape be used to mark the edges of the steps, particularly the top and bottom steps?

Bathroom

- Are grab bars placed appropriately for the tub and toilet?
- Does the tub have skid-proof strips or a rubber mat in the bottom?
- Has the person considered using a tub seat?
- Is the height of the toilet seat appropriate?
- Has the person considered using an elevated toilet seat?
- Does the colour of the toilet seat contrast with surrounding colours?
- Is toilet paper within easy reach?

Bedroom

- Is the height of the bed appropriate?
- Is the mattress firm at the edges to provide enough support for sitting?
- If the bed has wheels, are they locked securely?
- Would full or partial side rails be a help or a hazard?
- When side rails are in the down position, are they completely out of the way?
- Is the pathway between the bedroom and bathroom clear of objects and adequately illuminated, particularly at night?
- Would a bedside commode be useful, especially at night?
- Is a light near the bed, and does the person have sufficient physical and cognitive ability to turn it on before getting out of bed?
- Is furniture positioned to allow safe use of assistive devices for ambulation?
- Is a telephone situated near the bed?

Kitchen

- Are storage areas used to the best advantage (e.g. are objects that are frequently used in the most accessible places)?
- Are appliance cords kept out of the way?
- Are non-slip mats used in front of the sink?
- Are the markings on stoves and other appliances clearly visible?
- Does the person know how to use the microwave safely?

Assistive devices

- Is a call light available, and does the person know how to use it?
- What assistive devices are used?
- Would the person benefit from any assistive devices that are not being used?
- Are assistive devices being used safely and properly, or do they present additional hazards?

Temperature

- Is the temperature of the room(s) comfortable?
- Can the person read the markings on the thermostat and adjust it appropriately?
- During cold months, is the room temperature high enough to prevent hypothermia?
- During hot weather, is the room temperature cool enough to prevent hyperthermia?

Overall safety

- How does the person obtain objects from hard-to-reach places?
- How does the person change overhead light bulbs?
- Are doorways wide enough to accommodate assistive devices?
- Do door thresholds create hazardous conditions?
- Are telephones accessible, especially for emergency calls? Would it be helpful to use a cordless portable phone?
- Would it be helpful to have some emergency call system available?
- Does the person wear sturdy shoes with non-skid soles?
- Does the person keep a list of emergency numbers by the phone?
- Does the person have an emergency exit plan in the event of fire?
- Are smoke alarms present and operational?
- Is there a carbon monoxide detector in an appropriate place (if the house has gas appliances, wood burning stoves, or another object that produces carbon monoxide)?

guide to assessing home environments for safety and optimal functioning.

WELLNESS OPPORTUNITY

In addition to assessing conditions that affect functioning, nurses pay attention to environmental factors that affect quality of life.

AN EXAMPLE OF ASSESSING AND ADDRESSING HEALTH AND FUNCTIONING: DRIVING SAFETY

The ability to drive a vehicle safely is an instrumental activity of daily living that merits special consideration when assessing older adults. Driving at an advanced age is a major focus of attention, not only for healthcare providers but also for all members of society. For example, studies have identified driving as one of the top 10 tough ethical issues associated with dementia (Dobbs, Harper & Wood, 2009).

Regardless of age, most driving-related problems arise from chronic conditions that affect cognitive abilities or neurological or musculoskeletal function. However, even healthy older adults need to compensate for age-related changes in vision and other areas of function that affect driving, as discussed in Chapter 17. The Australian and New Zealand Society for Geriatric Medicine released a position statement about driving and dementia, which describes the issues and suggested actions required when challenged with driving and the older person (Australian and New Zealand Society for Geriatric Medicine, 2009).

Older drivers who recognise changes in their abilities usually self-regulate their driving behaviour through such actions as minimising their exposure to hazardous situations by restricting when, where and under what conditions they drive. Studies have identified the following self-regulation techniques used by older drivers: trip planning, reducing mileage, and avoidance of difficult driving situations such as heavy traffic or freeway driving (Morgan et al., 2009).

Decisions about **safe driving** are very complex because they are associated with many psychosocial implications, as discussed in Chapter 12. Many studies have found that "driving retirement" is associated with many negative consequences and diminished quality of life. Specific negative consequences that are usually associated with driving cessation include decreased social contacts; decreased self-esteem; increased depressive symptoms; and loss of control, freedom, dignity and independence. However, despite the many negative consequences associated with the cessation of driving, a few positive consequences have been identified. Positive themes identified in one study included increased time with family or significant other, increased community participation, strengthened social ties, a heightened sense of personal safety, and feelings of relief.

Increasingly, nurses are among the healthcare professionals responsible for addressing concerns about driving, not only as a personal safety issue for older adults but also as a moral obligation to protect society. As with other aspects of functioning, nurses are responsible for identifying potential risk factors for unsafe driving. Moreover, nurses need to be knowledgeable about resources for assessing and addressing this risk. Because decisions about driving are multidimensional, nurses work closely with other care providers, such as doctors and social workers, to address this important issue from a broad perspective. Thus, healthcare providers facilitate referrals not only for assessments of driving but also for interventions that help people retain safe driving skills as long as possible.

Nursing assessment related to safe driving

Questions about the older person's perception of or concerns about his or her driving can be used to open the discussion of this important, but sometimes sensitive, topic. Studies indicate that most older adults, including those with mild cognitive impairment and mild dementia, have insight into their driving abilities and appropriately self-regulate by avoiding complex and risky driving situations (O'Connor, Edwards, Bannon, 2013). However, some older adults have little or no insight and adamantly insist on driving despite evidence that their driving poses serious risks to themselves and others (Wood, Lacherez & Anstey, 2013). Nurses can open the discussion by indicating that questions about driving are routinely incorporated into an assessment so that any identified safety concerns can be addressed proactively. The following questions can be used for this part of the assessment:

- Do you have any concerns about your ability to drive safely?
- Have you adjusted your driving patterns to avoid certain situations, such as driving at night, on highways, or at intersections involving right-hand turns?
- Has anyone in your family expressed concerns about your driving?
- Have you gotten lost while driving in places that are usually familiar?
- Have you been in any accidents during the past couple of years? (If yes, ask about circumstances.)
- Have you had any citations related to unsafe driving or driving under the influence?

When appropriate, nurses can use these same kinds of question to elicit assessment information from family members who are likely to have made observations and concerns.

If answers to any of these questions raise concerns about driving safety, a more comprehensive assessment is warranted, as discussed in the next section. In addition, if the older person has any condition that is associated with risks for driving (e.g. dementia, functional impairment, significant vision impairment) arrangements should be made for appropriate assessments, which usually are performed by specialised rehabilitation specialists.

WELLNESS OPPORTUNITY

Nurses can promote personal responsibility by assessing the older adult's awareness of driving issues and their willingness to address these concerns.

Nursing interventions related to safe driving

Addressing risk factors that affect driving abilities is an important health promotion activity that should be integrated into usual care for older adults, preferably before significant safety concerns arise. Geriatricians have recommended that "advance driving directives" be initiated to facilitate discussions between healthcare professionals and older drivers as a routine part of care (Betz, Lowenstein, Schwartz, 2013). Geriatricians are also recommending a comprehensive approach to "stages of driving cessation" for people with dementia, which would include individualised interventions that are optimally timed, address grief, provide carer support, maintain key relationships, and explore alternative means of transportation (Liddle, Bennett, Allen et al., 2013).

Some risks for unsafe driving can be minimised through interventions that address contributing factors such as vision impairments, hearing impairments and medication-related issues (these are discussed in Chapters 17, 16, and 8, respectively). When pathological conditions affect neuromuscular functioning, nurses may suggest a referral for physical or occupational therapy to improve particular aspects of functioning that affect driving. For example, an older person with arthritis or Parkinson's disease may benefit from working with a therapist who has additional training for driving rehabilitation. Even if the therapist does not have special training, the older adult can focus on the goal of improved safety and functioning for driving skills as part of the therapy program. Older adults may be more motivated to participate in exercises prescribed by physical or occupational therapists if they see a connection between the therapies and maintaining their safe and independent functioning.

WELLNESS OPPORTUNITY

Nurses can promote quality of life for older adults by creatively identifying appropriate and acceptable ways of improving an older adult's ability to continue driving safety.

Referrals for driving evaluation and recommendations

Families are likely to seek guidance from nurses and other healthcare professionals to address their safety concerns about the driving abilities of an older adult. One way of addressing carers' concerns about driving safety is to provide information about resources that families can use to approach this issue. Driving evaluation programs, which usually are administered by occupational therapy departments, provide recommendations related to driving and appropriate follow-up for those who can benefit from education and rehabilitation. When medically warranted, these referrals are covered by Medicare and other health insurance plans. When suggesting this referral, it is important to emphasise that the purpose is not to take away the person's driving privileges but rather it is to identify interventions to improve safety for the person and others.

Recommendations of driving evaluation programs fall within a wide range and may include modifying vehicles to compensate for physical limitations, participating in driving rehabilitation therapy, or refraining from driving or restricting driving. Examples of adaptive equipment can include pedal extenders, distance sensors, left foot accelerators, steering-wheel adaptations, touchpads to operate auxiliary controls, and spot mirrors to compensate for visual and range-of-motion deficit. Examples of recommendations related to driving restrictions are no highways, only short distances or familiar areas, only daytime or fair weather driving, and requiring the presence of a navigator.

Driving education programs are another type of resource that helps older adults recognise driving issues and improve safety. For example, some of the organisations listed in the health education about driving in the resources section provide guides for helping families to talk with older members about driving as a health issue. In addition to suggesting programs that directly address safe driving, nurses can suggest referrals to programs that provide transportation for older adults.

CHAPTER HIGHLIGHTS

Assessing health of older adults

- Assessment of older adults is a multidimensional process addressing the complex interactions among older adults, their health and all contextual factors (e.g. culture, environments, medical conditions, adverse medication effects).
- Factors that contribute to the complexity of assessing older adults include multiple interacting conditions, unique manifestations of illness, treatments that mask the underlying problem, inaccurate or inadequate sources of information, and myths and misunderstandings about ageing.
- Nurses need to be aware of age-related variations in laboratory values for older adults (Table 7-1).

Assessment tools: Comprehensive and nursing

- The Minimum Data Set (MDS) is used in long-term residential care facilities and home care agencies to document 18 areas of functioning

- In Australia and New Zealand, the MDS has been adapted and it is known as the interRAI. Currently the interRAI does not have widespread use in Australia.
- In Australia the NATFRAME provides a comprehensive framework for the assessment and care of the older adult in long-term residential care
- Evidence-based nursing assessment tools and web-based articles demonstrating the use of many of these tools are widely available (see the clinical tools in the resources section).

Functional assessment

- A functional assessment is a formal process of measuring a person's ability to fulfil responsibilities and perform self-care tasks.
- Functional assessment tools focus on the person's ability to perform ADLs and IADLs, as illustrated in Figure 7-1 and Boxes 7-1 and 7-2.

Function-focused care

- Function-focused care focuses both on evaluating a person's underlying capability with regard to functional status and physical activity and on implementing interventions to optimise and maintain functional abilities and increase physical activities (Evidence-based practice 7-1).

Nurses' functional assessment

- Nurses use functional assessment tools such as the Barthel's Index, the Katz Index, and the Lawton scale.
- Some assessment tools address the effect of cognitive impairment on ability to perform activities of daily living (Figure 7-2).
- Assessing the use of adaptive equipment and assistive devices is important for identifying factors that affect safety.
- Assessment of the home environment is important for identifying factors that affect safety, comfort, functioning and quality of life (Box 7-3).
- Nurses can suggest the use of innovative and inexpensive devices to improve functioning and promote independence.

Example of assessing health and functioning: Driving safety

- Nurses have an important role in identifying risk factors that compromise safe driving in older adults.
- Common risk factors include conditions that affect vision, cognition, motor responses and reaction time.
- Nurses incorporate questions about driving to identify the need for a more comprehensive assessment.
- Risks for unsafe driving can be minimised through interventions that address contributing factors (e.g. vision and hearing impairments, medication-related issues).
- Nurses have important roles in facilitating referrals for further evaluation or for programs related to driving safety, education and rehabilitation.

CRITICAL THINKING EXERCISES

1. Identify an older adult who has some functional impairment but no cognitive impairment and perform a functional assessment on him or her, using Figure 7-1.
2. Identify another older adult (in a clinical setting or someone you know personally) who has some functional impairment as well as some cognitive impairment, and perform a functional assessment on him or her, using Figure 7-2.
3. Identify an older adult (in a clinical setting or someone you know personally) who has risk factors that affect his or her driving safety, then explore one or more of the health education sites to find information applicable to addressing concerns about safe driving for this person.
4. View the video on monitoring functional status in hospitalised older adults, which is found at the website www.nursingcenter.com, and identify ways in which you can apply the information in clinical settings.

RESOURCES

For an extensive range of additional resources to enhance teaching and learning and to facilitate understanding of this chapter, please see the text's accompanying website located on thePoint at http://thepoint.lww.com.

Clinical tools

Hartford Institute for Geriatric Nursing, ConsultGeriRN.org: http://consultgerirn.org/resources

Assessment tools *Try This*® series and *How to Try This* resources

- *Try This*, issue 1: SPICES: an overall assessment tool for older adults. Fulmer, T. (2012). *Best Practices in Nursing Care to Older Adults.*
- *How to Try This* (article): Fulmer SPICES. Fulmer, T. (2007). *American Journal of Nursing, 107*(10), 40–48.
- *How to Try This* (video): *SPICES: An Overall Assessment Tool.*
- *Try This*, issue 2: Katz Index of Independence in Activities of Daily Living (ADL). Wallace, M. & Shelkey, M. (2012). *Best Practices in Nursing Care to Older Adults.*
- *How to Try This* (article): Monitoring functional status in hospitalized older adults. Wallace, M. & Shelkey, M. (2008). *American Journal of Nursing, 108*(4), 64–71.
- *How to Try This* (video): *Katz Index of Independence in Activities of Daily Living.*
- *Try This*, issue 23: The Lawton Instrumental Activities of Daily Living (IADL) scale. Graf, C. (2013). *Best Practices in Nursing Care to Older Adults.*
- *How to Try This* (article): The Lawton Instrumental Activities of Daily Living scale. Graf, C. (2013). *American Journal of Nursing, 108*(4), 52–62.
- *How to Try This* (video): *The Lawton Instrumental Activities of Daily Living scale.*

Australian Government Department of Social Services: www.dss.gov.au

Search for: Suggested Assessment Tools for Aged Care Funding Instrument (ACFI) (includes NATFRAME webpage archive)

Or

National Library of Australia, Welcome to NATFRAME: webarchive.nla.gov.au

Dementia Collaborative Research Centres: www.dementia-assessment.com.au

Search for: Cleveland Scale for Activities of Daily Living

interRAI Australia and New Zealand: http://interrai-au.org

Royal College of Nursing (U.K.). (2004). Nursing assessment and older people: A Royal College of Nursing toolkit. Viewed March 2015 at www.rcn.org.uk/__data/assets/pdf_file/0010/78616/002310.pdf.

Evidence-based practice

Kresevic D. M. (2012). Assessment of physical function. In M. Boltz, E. Capezuti, T. Fulmer & D. Zwicker (Eds), *Evidence-based geriatric nursing protocols for best practice* (4th ed., pp. 89–103). New York: Springer.

New Zealand Ministry of Health and New Zealand Guidelines Group. (2003). *Assessment processes for older people*. Best practice evidence-based guideline: www.health.govt.nz/publication/assessment-processes-older-people.

Health education about driving

American Geriatric Society (resources on safe driving and helping older drivers): www.americangeriatrics.org

American Occupational Therapy Association (information about driving evaluation and rehabilitation): www.aota.org/Practice/Productive-Aging/Driving.aspx

Hartford: Family Conversations with Older Drivers (to help families talk with older adults about driving safety): www.thehartford.com/your-car

NRMA Older Drivers: www.mynrma.com.au/motoring-services/education/older-drivers.htm

NZ Transport Agency, for drivers 75+: www.nzta.govt.nz/licence/renewing-replacing/over-75.html

SeniorDrivers.org (numerous reports and resources for consumers, providers and researchers on ageing and driving): http://lpp.seniordrivers.org

Transport Accident Commission (TAC), older drivers: www.tac.vic.gov.au/road-safety/safe-driving/older-drivers

REFERENCES

Australasian Society of Clinical and Experimental Pharmacologists and Toxicologists (ASCEPT), Pharmaceutical Society of Australia and Royal Australian College of General Practitioners. (2008). *Australian medicines handbook*. Adelaide, SA: Australian Medicines Handbook Pty Ltd.

Australian and New Zealand Society for Geriatric Medicine. (2009). Driving and dementia. Position statement no. 11. Viewed March 2015 at www.anzsgm.org/documents/PS11DrivingandDementiaapproved6Sep09.pdf.

Australian Government Department of Health and Ageing (DoHA). (2005). Welcome to NATFRAME. Available March 2015 via webarchive.nla.gov.au.

Australian Government Department of Health and Ageing (DoHA). (2010). New funding model for residential aged care: ACFI documents. Available March 2015 via webarchive.nla.gov.au.

Australian Government Department of Social Services. (2014). Ageing and aged care: Suggested assessment tools for Aged Care Funding Instrument (ACFI). Accessed March 2015 at www.dss.gov.au/our-responsibilities/ageing-and-aged-care/aged-care-funding/residential-care-subsidy/basic-subsidy-amount-aged-care-funding-instrument/suggested-assessment-tools-for-aged-care-funding-instrument-acfi.

Bernabei, R., Landi, F., Graziano, O., Liperoti, R. & Gambassi, G. (2008). Second and third generation assessment instruments: The birth of standardization in geriatric care. *Journal of Gerontology: Medical Sciences, 63A*, 308–313.

Betz, M. E., Lowenstein, S. R. & Schwartz, R. (2013). Older adult opinions of "advance driving directives". *Journal of Primary Care and Community Health, 4*(1), 14–27.

Boltz, M., Resnick, B. & Galik, E. (2012). Interventions to prevent functional decline in acute care settings. In M. Boltz, E. Capezuti, T. Fulmer & D. Zwicker (Eds), *Evidence-based practice protocols for best practice* (4th ed., pp. 104–121). New York: Springer.

Burket, T. L., Hippensteel, D., Penrod, J. et al. (2013). Pilot testing of the function focused care intervention on an acute care trauma unit. *Geriatric Nursing, 34*, 241–246.

Dobbs, B. M., Harper, L. A. & Wood, A. (2009). Transitioning from driving to driving cessation: The role of specialized driving cessation support groups for individuals with dementia. *Topics in Geriatric Rehabilitation, 25*, 73–86.

Ford, P. & McCormack, B. (2000). Keeping the person in the centre of nursing. *Nursing Standard, 14*, 40–44.

Fulmer, T. & Wallace, M. (2012). Fulmer SPICES: An overall assessment tool for older adults. *Try This* series. *Best practices in nursing care to older adults.* Hartford Institute for Geriatric Nursing. Available March 2015 via www.consultgerirn.org.

Galik, E., Resnick, B., Hammersla, M. et al. (2014). Optimizing function and physical activity among nursing home residents with dementia: Testing the impact of function-focused care. *Gerontologist, 54*(6), 930–943.

Handbook of geriatric nursing care (2nd ed.). (2003). Philadelphia, PA: Lippincott Williams & Wilkins.

interRAI Australia. (2011). interRAI Coordinating Centre, Australia and New Zealand. Viewed March 2015 at http://interrai-au.org.

Kresevic, D. (2012). Assessment of physical function. In M. Boltz, E. Capezuti, T. Fulmer & D. Zwicker (Eds), *Evidence-based practice protocols for best practice* (4th ed., pp. 89–103). New York: Springer.

Liddle, J., Bennett, S., Allen, S. et al. (2013). The stages of driving cessation for people with dementia: Needs and challenges. *International Psychogeriatrics, 25*(12), 2033–2046.

Mack, J. L. & Patterson, M. B. (2006). An empirical basis for domains in the analysis of dependency in the activities of daily living (ADL): Results of a confirmatory factor analysis of the Cleveland Scale for Activities of Daily Living (CSADL). *Clinical Neuropsychologist, 20*, 662–667.

Morgan, C. M., Winter, S. M., Classen, S., McCarthy, D. P. & Awadzi, K. D. (2009). Literature review on older adult gender differences for driving self-regulation and cessation. *Topics in Geriatric Rehabilitation, 25*, 99–117.

Narayan, M. C., Salgado, J. & VanVoorhis, A. (2009). SHOW ME: Enhancing OASIS functional assessment. *Home Healthcare Nurse, 27*(1), 19–23.

National Health IT Board. (2015). Comprehensive clinical assessment for aged care (interRAI). Accessed March 2015 at http://ithealthboard.health.nz/our-programmes/common-clinical-information/comprehensive-clinical-assessment-aged-care-interrai.

New Zealand Ministry of Health and New Zealand Guidelines Group (NZMOH & NZGG). (2003). *Assessment processes for older people.* Best practice evidence-based guideline. Available March 2015 at www.health.govt.nz/publication/assessment-processes-older-people.

O'Connor, M. L., Edwards, J. D. & Bannon, Y. (2013). Self-rated driving habits among older adults with clinically-defined mild cognitive impairment, clinically-defined mild cognitive impairment, clinically-defined dementia, and normal cognition. *Accident Analysis & Prevention, 61*, 197–202.

Rader, J., Jones, D. & Miller, L. (2000). The importance of individualized wheelchair seating for frail older adults. *Journal of Gerontological Nursing, 26*(11), 24–31.

Resnick, B., Galik, E. & Boltz, M. (2013). Function focused care approaches: Literature review of progress and future possibilities. *Journal of the American Medical Directors Association, 14*(5), 313–318.

Shin, J. H. & Scherer, Y. (2009). Advantages and disadvantages of using MDS data in nursing research. *Journal of Gerontological Nursing, 35*, 7–16.

Wieland, D. & Ferrucci, L. (2008). Multidimensional geriatric assessment: Back to the future. *Journal of Gerontology: Medical Sciences, 63A*, 272–274.

Wood, J. M., Lacherez, P. F. & Anstey, K. J. (2013). Not all older adults have insight into their driving abilities: Evidence from an on-road assessment and implications for policy. *Journals of Gerontology: Medical Sciences, 68*(5), 559–566.

Chapter 8

Medicines

By Carol Miller and Sharyn Hunter

LEARNING OBJECTIVES

After reading this chapter, you should be able to:

1. Examine age-related changes and risk factors that affect the action of medicines in the body and the skills involved with taking them.
2. Discuss considerations about safety and efficacy of herbs and other complementary medicines pertinent to the care of older adults.
3. Describe interactions that can occur between medications and complementary and alternative medicines.
4. Identify the adverse medication effects likely to occur in older adults.
5. Describe the purposes of a medication assessment and explain how to perform a comprehensive medication assessment.
6. Identify nursing interventions directed towards enhancing the therapeutic effectiveness of medications, reducing the risks for adverse effects and minimising the negative functional consequences of these effects.

KEY POINTS

adverse medication event
anticholinergic adverse effects
Beers Criteria
complementary and alternative medicine (CAM)
clearance rate
cytochrome P-450 enzyme system
drug-induced parkinsonism
elimination half-time
generic medications
herbs
potentially inappropriate medications
medication non-adherence
medication reconciliation
pharmacodynamics
pharmacokinetics
polypharmacy
potentially inappropriate medications
prescribing cascade
tardive dyskinesia

Although the topic of medicines and the older adult is not a distinct category of function in the same sense as physiological and psychosocial aspects of function (e.g. vision and cognition), it can be addressed from a similar perspective. This chapter presents information about age-related changes, risk factors and the functional consequences of medicines and the behaviours associated with taking them relative to older adults. Like other chapters, it addresses the role of nurses in assessing and managing medicines in the context of the functional consequences theory for promoting wellness.

INTRODUCTION TO MEDICINES

The biologically active substances that are most relevant to care of older adults are prescription and over-the-counter (OTC) medications, vitamins, minerals, and **herbs** and homeopathic remedies. Before exploring medicines using the Functional Consequences Framework, fundamental concepts about medicines and background information about herbs and homeopathy is provided to facilitate understanding.

Fundamental concepts about medications

Effects of medications in the body are usually considered in relation to **pharmacokinetics** (i.e. how the drug is absorbed, distributed, metabolised and excreted) and **pharmacodynamics** (i.e. how the body is affected by the drug at the cellular level and in relation to the target organ). Absorption refers to the passage of a medication from its site of introduction, usually the gastrointestinal tract, into the general circulation. Absorption of oral medications can be affected by diminished gastric acid, increased gastric pH, delayed gastric emptying and the presence of other substances (e.g. food, nutrients, inert ingredients of medications). Because most oral medications are absorbed by passive diffusion across the small intestine—a process that is not pH dependent—they are not usually affected by any alterations in gastric acidity. The unique chemical properties of each medication determine the degree to which it is susceptible to any gastrointestinal changes, regardless of age. For example, pH-sensitive medications, such as penicillin and ferrous sulfate, are more likely to be affected by altered gastric acid levels or by prolonged exposure to these acids because of delayed emptying.

Two measures of the efficiency of metabolism and elimination of a drug are **elimination half-time** and **clearance rate**. Elimination half-time (also called serum half-life) is the time required to decrease the drug concentration by one half of its original value. It takes five half-times to reach steady state concentrations after a drug is initiated or to completely eliminate a drug from the body after a drug is discontinued. The clearance rate measures the volume of blood from which the drug is eliminated per unit of time. An increase in serum half-time or a decrease in clearance rate may result in accumulation of the drug. The result is that the therapeutic effect is likely to be altered and the risk of adverse effects is likely to be increased.

Background information about herbs and homeopathy

Complementary and alternative medicine (CAM) is increasingly being used, especially among women, older adults and people with chronic conditions. Most studies have confirmed the increasing use of CAM during the last two decades, to the point that more than 90% of the elderly

Promoting safe and effective medication use in older adults

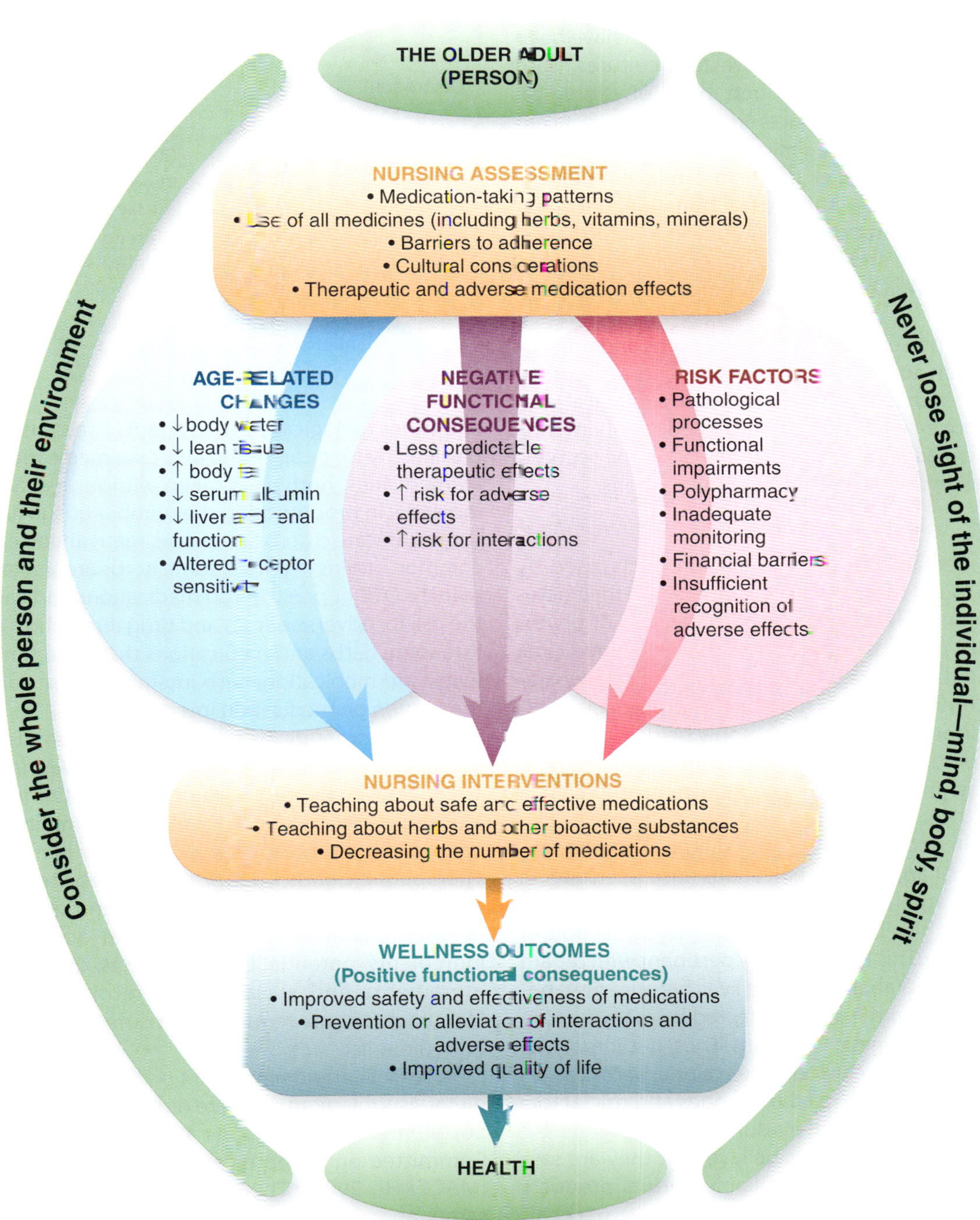

have now used CAM (Cherniack et al., 2008). All healthcare practitioners need to know what products the older person is using so they can address concerns about safety, effectiveness and potential interactions. This is particularly important with regard to such substances as herbs and other dietary supplements in relation to interactions with medications. In addition, healthcare practitioners need to be prepared to address questions the older person may ask about alternative practices, as discussed in the nursing interventions section of this chapter.

Although herbs, homeopathy and home remedies are viewed as "non-traditional" or "alternative" approaches to preventing and treating illness, these remedies have been used for centuries in many non-Western cultures. Both herbal and homeopathic products have physiological actions; however, herbal products are of particular concern because their actions can be similar to those of prescription and OTC medications. Thus, they can produce beneficial effects, adverse effects and interactions. Recently the World Health Organization (2013) published information to promote the safe and effective use of traditional medicines, called the WHO Traditional Medicine (TM) Strategy 2014–2023.

This section presents an overview of herbs and homeopathic remedies; additional aspects of herbs are discussed throughout this chapter with regard to physiological considerations, adverse effects and herb–medication interactions. Pertinent aspects also are addressed in the sections on nursing assessment and nursing interventions.

TABLE 8-1 Drugs and herbs with similar bioactivity

Drug	Herb
Aspirin	Birch bark Willow bark Wintergreen Meadowsweet
Anticoagulants	Dong quai Feverfew Garlic Ginkgo biloba Wintergreen
Caffeine	Guarana Kola nut
Ephedrine	Ephedra
Oestrogen	Black cohosh Fennel Red clover Stinging nettle
Lithium	Thyme Purslane
Monoamine oxidase inhibitors	Ginseng St John's wort Yohimbe
Nicotine	Lobelia
Calcium channel blockers	Angelica

Herbs

Herbs were perhaps the original OTC products, used by people who found these medicinal remedies in their natural environments. Herbs (also called botanicals or phytotherapies) are plant-based products that have medicinal properties. Herbs and many other pharmaceutical preparations have common origins in nature. Examples of plant-derived medications that are commonly being used today include antibiotics, anticholinergics, anticoagulants, antihypertensives, anti-neoplastic agents, aspirin and digoxin (Plotnikoff, 2010).

Information about the pharmacokinetics and pharmacodynamics that applies to medications (discussed later in the section on age-related changes that affect the action of medicines in the body) also applies to the action of herbs in the body. This is particularly pertinent with regard to herbs that are metabolised by the liver, because metabolism of substances in the liver is affected by many factors, including diet and genetic variations. Thus, it is important to keep in mind that, even when taken alone, herbs can be affected by the same age-related changes and risk factors that affect medications in older adults.

Most people who use herbs believe that they are safe because they are commonly available natural products that can be purchased without a prescription (Snyder et al., 2009). However, despite this common perception, herbs and other biologically active agents can cause problems, particularly for people who also take medications. As with all medicines, nothing is taken without risk and the risk increases in proportion to the number of substances consumed. Because herbs as well as many medications have common origins in plants, some herbs are similar in bioactivity to OTC or prescription medications and can increase the risk for adverse effects and drug interactions. Table 8-1 lists some herbs and medications that have similar bioactivity, and medication–herb interactions are addressed in the section on medication interactions.

The Therapeutic Goods Administration (TGA) is responsible for the safety and quality of CAM in Australia. The Australian Regulatory Guidelines for Complementary Medicines (ARGCM) (2014) provide information about the control of herbal substances, which can be found via the Therapeutic Goods Administration website at www.tga.gov.au. Herbs are tested for safety and quality and the labels include reliable information about additional ingredients, potential harmful effects, quantity of active ingredients and suitability of form for human use. Manufacturers are required to ensure the accuracy of the ingredient list.

In New Zealand most CAM products are marketed as dietary supplements and are regulated under the Dietary Supplements Regulations 1985 (Ministerial Advisory Committee on Complementary and Alternative Health [MACCAH], 2004). There is also no assessment of the safety and quality of these substances before they are marketed. Currently there is no systematic reporting of problems relating to the safety or quality of these substances. When adverse effects are noted, these are reported to MedSafe.

Herbal substances may have adverse effects, and the risk for adverse effects is increased for people with certain conditions, such as a history of stroke, glaucoma, diabetes, hypertension, heart disease, thyroid disorder and any disorder requiring anticoagulation therapy. Another concern is that herbs and other dietary supplements have the potential for interactions with other drugs. Types of medications most likely to interact with herbal products include antidepressants, sedative–hypnotics and drugs with a narrow therapeutic range (e.g. digoxin and theophylline). There also is increasing concern about the effects of herbs during periods of physiological stress. For example, because surgical care can be complicated by effects of herbs that interfere with coagulation or prolong the effects of anaesthetics or cause electrolyte disturbances, surgeons generally recommend that all herbs and supplements be discontinued at least 2 weeks prior to surgery when possible (Barnett, 2009). Some of the more serious effects of herbs (listed in Table 8-2) include altered liver function, electrolyte imbalance, elevated blood pressure, diminished blood-clotting mechanisms and alterations of the heart rate and rhythm. Less serious adverse effects include nausea, vomiting and other gastrointestinal symptoms from oral preparations, especially if they are taken with medications that have similar adverse effects. Table 8-3 lists some of the herbs more commonly used by older adults.

TABLE 8-2 Potential adverse effects of some herbs

Herb	Potential effect
Black cohosh	Bradycardia, hypotension, joint pains
Bloodroot	Bradycardia, arrhythmia, dizziness, impaired vision, intense thirst
Boneset	Liver toxicity, cognitive changes, respiratory problems
Coltsfoot	Fever, liver toxicity
Dandelion	Interactions with diuretics, increased concentration of lithium or potassium
Ephedra	Anxiety, dizziness, insomnia, tachycardia, hypertension
Feverfew	Interference with blood clotting mechanisms
Garlic	Hypotension, inhibition of blood clotting, potentiation of antidiabetic drugs
Ginseng	Anxiety, insomnia, hypertension, tachycardia, asthma attacks, postmenopausal bleeding
Ginkgo biloba	Increased anticoagulation
Goldenseal	Vasoconstriction
Guar gum	Hypoglycaemia
Hawthorn	Hypotension
Hops, skullcap, valerian	Drowsiness, potentiation of anti-anxiety or sedative medications
Kava	Damage to the eyes, skin, liver and spinal cord from long-term use
Liquorice	Hypokalaemia, hypernatraemia
Lobelia	Hearing and vision problems
Motherwort	Increased anticoagulation
Nettle	Hypokalaemia
Senna	Potentiation of digoxin
Yohimbe	Anxiety, tachycardia, hypertension, cognitive changes

Homeopathic remedies

Three concepts are crucial to understanding homeopathy, as a German physician, Samuel Hahnemann, initially proposed it two centuries ago. First, there is the law of similars, or "like cures like". According to this concept, homeopathy treats an illness by stimulating the body's self-healing abilities through the use of a small amount of a substance similar to that which caused the illness. For example, quinine can produce symptoms of malaria in a healthy person and it can cure malaria when administered in minute doses. The second key concept is that the more a substance is diluted, the more potent it becomes. Based on this concept, homeopathic remedies are diluted repeatedly and each dilution is vigorously shaken to increase its potency. The third concept is that illnesses are highly individualised and, therefore, the treatment must be individualised. Based on this principle, homeopathic practitioners focus on treating the person, not the disease, and they spend considerable time interviewing and assessing the person before prescribing a homeopathic remedy. Homeopathy is widely used in India, Russia, Mexico and European countries and it is gaining acceptance in Australia and New Zealand as a safe alternative to conventional medicine.

Homeopathic remedies are now also available for self-treatment and few are available through medical practitioners. Homeopathic remedies are regulated by the TGA in Australia as OTC products, while they are not regulated in New Zealand. Remedies come in a variety of single-substance or combination forms, including powders, wafers, small tablets and alcohol-based liquids. Over-the-counter homeopathic products are too weak to cause adverse effects and there are very few precautions, interactions or contraindications that apply to these products. People who are taking homeopathic remedies are advised to limit the amount taken and the length of time they are consumed. Other precautions include avoiding food, caffeine, beverages, toothpaste and mouthwashes for 15 to 60 minutes before and after taking the substance. Also, oils of camphor, eucalyptus and peppermint should be avoided during homeopathic treatments. Information about homeopathic remedies and homeopathic practitioners can be obtained from the National Center for Complementary and Integrative Health (U.S.) and the National Institute of Complementary Medicine (Australia) (see health education in the resources section).

TABLE 8-3 Selected herbs: Indications, actions and cautions

Herb	Uses	Actions and precautions
Bilberry	The German E Commission approves bilberry for acute non-specific diarrhoea and topical treatment of mild inflammation of the mouth, throat and oral mucosa. Concentrated extracts are used for retinopathy (diabetic and hypertensive), venous insufficiency and varicose veins.	High doses may inhibit platelet aggregation; monitor anticoagulants if patient is taking larger dosages. Avoid in patients with haemorrhagic disorders.
Black cohosh	The German E Commission approves preparations of fresh or dried rhizome for menopausal symptoms (hot flushes, night sweats, sleep disturbances, irritability).	Monitor liver function every 6 months because of possible hepatotoxicity. Several NIH clinical trials are in progress that may answer the question of whether long-term use of black cohosh causes endometrial hyperplasia.
Cat's claw	Osteoarthritis of the knee and rheumatoid arthritis.	Avoid in patients with organ transplants, lymphocytosis or autoimmune disease. Use with caution with antiplatelet therapy, hypertensive medication, and medications that suppress immune response. Inhibits chromosome P-450 CYP3A4 enzyme in vitro. May dilate peripheral blood vessels and increase heart rate.
Chamomile	The German E Commission approves chamomile for inflammation of GI tract and GI spasms. Topical preparation use includes inflammation of skin and mucous membranes and bacterial skin diseases.	Contraindicated with allergy to chamomile. No herb–drug interactions reported in the literature.
Cranberry	Effective in the propholaxis of UTI.	Not effective in treating a UTI.
Echinacea	The German E Commission approves for supportive therapy for colds and infections of the respiratory and urinary tract.	Caution when coadministering with drugs dependent on CYP3A or CYP1A2 for elimination. Contraindicated in progressive systemic diseases (e.g. HIV, AIDS, tuberculosis, multiple sclerosis, leukocytosis). Avoid in patients taking immunosuppressant drugs (e.g. transplant patients).
Evening primrose	Atopic dermatitis and eczema. May improve blood flow and nerve conduction deficits in diabetes.	Possible interaction with antipsychotic medications and inhibition of anticonvulsants.
Garlic	The German E Commission approves garlic use to lower cholesterol levels, prevent hardening of arteries, and treat minor respiratory infections.	Inhibits platelet aggregation; may increase risk of bleeding when taken with warfarin, aspirin or NSAIDs. Discontinue garlic supplementation 7–14 days prior to surgery, except for garlic used in cooking.
Ginger	The German E Commission approves for prevention of motion sickness. Anti-inflammatory.	Contraindicated in active gallbladder disease. Discontinue supplementation 7–14 days before surgery, except for ginger used in cooking.
Ginkgo biloba	Standardised ginkgo extract has a positive German E Commission monograph for degenerative and vascular dementia, peripheral artery occlusive disease, vertigo and tinnitus. Ginkgo leaf has a null German E Commission monograph.	American Herbal Products Association contraindicates use with monoamine oxidase (MAO) inhibitors. Potential for interaction with anticoagulant and antiplatelet medications (e.g. warfarin, aspirin). Rare case reports of spontaneous bleeding. Potential to increase blood glucose levels in type 2 diabetes. Discontinue 7–14 days before surgery.
Ginseng	The German E Commission and World Health Organization (WHO) recognise ginseng as a tonic, prophylaxis or restorative agent for invigoration during times of fatigue, exhaustion, stress and convalescence.	May cause hypoglycaemia or increase blood pressure. Avoid with MAO inhibitors. Contraindicated in acute asthma or acute infection.
Hawthorn	The German E Commission approves hawthorn leaf with flower for the treatment of congestive heart failure.	May potentiate action of digoxin and beta-blockers.

TABLE 8-3 Selected herbs: Indications, actions and cautions (*continued*)

Herb	Uses	Actions and precautions
Horse chestnut	The German E Commission approves horse chestnut for treatment of chronic venous insufficiency, night cramps and itching.	Monitor bleeding times in patients taking anticoagulants.
Kava	Used for treatment of anxiety.	May cause hepatotoxicity (leading to transplants and deaths). Has high potential for drug interactions, including decreased effectiveness of warfarin and potentiation of barbiturates.
Licorice	The German E Commission approves the use of licorice root for inflammation of the upper respiratory tract and gastric/duodenal ulcers.	Contraindicated in liver disorders, congestive heart failure or oedema. Avoid prolonged use of higher dosages. Licorice can increase blood pressure. Potential interactions with diuretics, corticosteroids and antihypertensives
Saw palmetto	The German E Commission and USP (U.S. Pharmacopoeia) recognise saw palmetto as treatment for benign prostatic hypertrophy.	No reported drug interactions.
St John's wort	The German E Commission recognises use in mild-to-moderate depressive moods, anxiety and nervousness.	Not indicated for use in severe depression. Phototoxicity is extremely rare but can occur in light-skinned people. Potential for decreased cyclosporine levels; decreased effectiveness of warfarin; possible decreased digoxin levels; reduced levels of protease inhibitors (e.g. indinavir); decreased levels of simvastatin. Avoid in patients taking multiple medications.
Valerian	Used as a mild sleep-promoting agent in nervous, restlessness, and anxiety-related sleep disturbances.	In theory, there is potential additive effect when taken with central nervous system depressants.

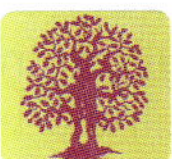

AGE-RELATED CHANGES THAT AFFECT MEDICINES IN OLDER ADULTS

Age-related changes that affect medicines in older adults are discussed in relation to those that affect the actions of the agents in the body and those that affect the skills involved with taking them. The factors that have the most significant impact on the effectiveness of medicines in older adults are not age-related changes, but risk factors, and these are considered in the section on risk factors.

Changes that affect the action of medicines in the body

An age-related decline in glomerular filtration rate, which begins in early adulthood and progresses at an annual rate of 1% to 2%, may affect the concentrations of medicines in the body, particularly those that are cleared through the kidneys. For example, diminished renal function can decrease the clearance of water-soluble medications that depend on glomerular filtration (e.g. gentamicin) or tubular secretion (e.g. penicillin) for their removal. Likewise, the consequences of diminished renal function will be greater on substances that readily reach toxic levels because they have a narrow therapeutic index (e.g. digoxin). Box 8-1 lists some medications that are likely to be affected by age-related renal changes.

An age-related decline in hepatic blood flow that begins around the age of 40 years can affect serum concentration and volume of distribution of substances that are metabolised more extensively by the liver, even in healthy older adults. This change slows down the delivery of medications that normally are rapidly metabolised. In addition to age-related changes, many other factors affect the liver metabolism of substances in people of all ages. The specific effect of age-related liver changes on the metabolism of medicines is unclear because factors such as diet, caffeine, smoking, alcohol, genetic variations and pathological conditions are likely to simultaneously affect the metabolism of substances and exert a stronger influence than any age-related factors. Box 8-1 also lists some medications whose clearance is likely to be delayed because of age-related liver changes.

In recent years there has been increasing attention paid to the role of the **cytochrome P-450 enzyme system**, which is composed of many specific enzymes responsible for the metabolism of medications and other substances, including herbs, nutrients and nicotine. The cytochrome P-450 system is particularly important with regard to interactions between herbs, medications and other substances because competition at the enzyme sites can affect clearance. Clearance of substances that depend on the cytochrome P-450 system is likely to be delayed to a small degree because of age-related

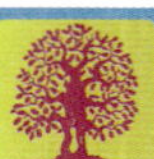

BOX 8-1
Effects of age-related changes on medication effectiveness

Decreased clearance caused by renal changes
Amantadine
Amoxicillin
Ampicillin
Atenolol
Ceftriaxone
Cephalexin
Chlorpropamide
Cimetidine
Ciprofloxacin
Colchicine
Digoxin
Enalapril
Frusemide
Hydrochlorothiazide
Lisinopril
Metformin
Ranitidine

Decreased clearance caused by hepatic changes
Amitriptyline
Barbiturates
Benzodiazepines
Codeine
Labetalol
Lignocaine
Morphine
Paracetamol
Pethidine
Phenytoin
Propranolol
Quinidine
Salicylates
Theophylline
Warfarin

Increased concentrations caused by changes in body composition
Cimetidine
Digoxin
Ethanol (alcohol)
Gentamicin
Morphine
Propranolol
Quinine
Warfarin

Decreased concentrations caused by changes in body composition
Phenobarbitone
Prazosin

Increased receptor sensitivity (increased potency)
Angiotensin-converting enzyme (ACE) inhibitors
Diazepam
Digoxin
Diltiazem
Enalapril
Felodipine
Levodopa
Lithium
Midazolam
Morphine
Temazepam
Verapamil
Warfarin

Decreased receptor sensitivity (may have delayed signs of toxicity)
Beta-blockers
Bumetanide
Dopamine
Frusemide
Propranolol

changes and to a greater degree when two or more medicines compete at these enzyme sites.

An age-related decrease in total body water and an increase in the proportion of body fat to lean body mass can alter the action of medicines in older adults. Between the ages of about 20 and 80 years, the following changes in body composition occur: body fat gradually increases by 15% to 20%, lean tissue decreases by about 20% and total body water is reduced by 10% to 15%. Because these age-related changes in body composition will affect substances according to their degree of fat or water solubility, agents that are distributed primarily in body water or lean body mass may reach higher serum concentrations in older adults and their effects may be more intense. Similarly, the serum concentration of highly fat-soluble substances, which are distributed and stored in fat tissue, may be lowered and these agents have an increased tendency to accumulate in adipose tissue. Consequently, fat-soluble substances may have a prolonged duration of action, be more erratic in their effects and have less intense immediate effects. Box 8-1 also lists some medications whose concentrations are likely to be increased or decreased because of age-related changes in body composition.

As medicines are distributed and metabolised in the body, some molecules are bound to serum albumin and other proteins, so the bound portion becomes inactive while the unbound molecules remain active. Because the unbound portion is the amount available for metabolism, tissue perfusion and renal excretion, the protein-binding capacity of an agent is an important determinant of its potential for both therapeutic and adverse effects. The degree of protein binding of each substance varies, with some medications, such as warfarin, having a protein-binding capacity of 99%. The binding capacity of substances that are highly protein bound can be influenced by diminished serum albumin levels in older adults. Additional factors that affect the degree of protein binding for any agent include the strength of the binding and the number of chemicals competing for the binding sites.

Although gerontologists disagree about the extent and cause of decreased serum albumin levels in older adults, it is generally agreed that the level diminishes by as much as 20% in the later decades of life. Diminished serum albumin levels are associated with a combination of factors, including malnutrition, pathological processes, decreased mobility and age-related liver changes. Regardless of the cause, a decrease in the serum albumin level will lead to an increased amount of the active portion of protein-bound substances. Medications that are highly protein bound, which are commonly taken by older adults, are most strongly affected. This effect is intensified when more than one protein-bound substance is consumed because the agents compete for the same sites. Medications that are most likely to have adverse effects when they are taken together or when serum albumin levels are low include aspirin, digoxin, frusemide, non-steroidal anti-inflammatory drugs (NSAIDs), hypoglycaemics, phenytoin, sertraline and sulfonamides.

Independent of any changes that affect pharmacokinetics, age-related changes in receptor sensitivity can influence pharmacodynamics and cause older adults to be more or less sensitive to particular substances. For example, an increased sensitivity of the older brain to centrally acting psychotropic medications may potentiate both the therapeutic and adverse effects of these drugs. This is particularly true for benzodiazepines, which have stronger sedative effects in older adults. Box 8-1 lists examples of drugs that have increased or decreased sensitivity in older adults. Age-related change in homeostatic mechanisms, such as thermoregulation, fluid regulation and baroreceptor control over blood pressure, also can affect pharmacodynamics. For example, inefficient fluid regulation may alter the action of medications, such as lithium, that are particularly sensitive to fluid and electrolyte balance.

Body size is an additional factor that can add to the effects of age-related changes and influence the action of medicines in the body. Because body size can affect both the therapeutic and adverse effects of substances, doses need to be adjusted for older adults who are small or have lost or are losing weight. This consideration is particularly important for older adults who are losing muscle mass or have decreased renal function.

Changes that affect behaviours related to taking medicines

For any adult, all the following factors affect the appropriate use of medicines:

- Motivation
- Knowledge about the purpose of the substance
- Cultural and psychosocial influences
- Ability to obtain correct amounts (influenced by factors such as cost, accessibility)
- Ability to distinguish the correct container
- Ability to read and comprehend directions
- Ability to hear and remember verbal instructions
- Knowledge about correct timing for consumption
- Ability to follow the correct dosage regimen
- Physical ability to remove substances from their containers and administer them
- Ability to swallow oral preparations
- Additional skills related to coordination, manual dexterity and visual acuity for substances that are administered nasally, transdermally, subcutaneously or by other methods.

Even for healthy older adults, age-related changes and functional impairments often interfere with these skills. For example, hearing or vision changes can interfere with the ability to understand instructions and read directions, especially labels on bottles. Any limitations in fine motor movement of the hands may interfere with the ability to remove lids from containers, especially when the lids are tamper resistant. Although the skills related to taking medicines are sometimes influenced by age-related changes, more often they are influenced by risk factors that commonly occur in older adults.

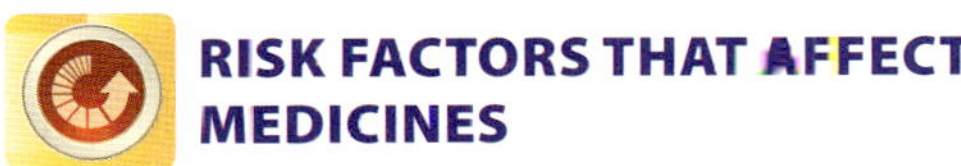

RISK FACTORS THAT AFFECT MEDICINES

By approximately age 75, even the healthiest of older adults have age-related changes that affect pharmacokinetic and pharmacodynamic processes in their bodies. Even more significant, however, are the numerous risk factors that have even greater effects on behaviours of older adults relative to taking medicines. Risk factors can be the result of the person's own attitudes, level of knowledge and socioeconomic circumstances, or they can be attributed to outside sources (e.g. medical providers).

The consumption of more than one medicine greatly increases the potential for adverse and altered therapeutic effects. Because older adults take a disproportionately greater number of medications than do younger people, they are more susceptible to adverse or altered effects. Additional risks arise from myths and misunderstandings that affect the medication consumption patterns of older adults. Finally, certain factors unrelated to age, such as weight, sex and smoking habits, combine with age-related changes and risk factors to increase further the risk of adverse and altered effects.

WELLNESS OPPORTUNITY

Nurses provide holistic care when they explore the wide range of factors that affect medicine and substance-taking behaviours.

Pathological processes and functional impairments

Because the purpose of any medication is to relieve or control symptoms, one can assume that people who take medications have at least one underlying pathological process. The increased prevalence of chronic conditions in older adults adds complexity to prescribing the safest and most appropriate medication regimen. For example, pain management for the many older adults who have both arthritis and hypertension is complicated by the common occurrence of increased blood pressure as an adverse effect of NSAIDs. Medication–disease interactions manifest themselves in any of the following ways:

- Pathological processes can exacerbate age-related changes that would otherwise have little or no impact on the medication. For example, malnutrition further decreases serum albumin, thereby increasing both the therapeutic and adverse effects of highly protein-bound medications.
- Pathological processes can also alter the therapeutic and adverse effects of substances. For instance, heart failure decreases both the metabolism and the excretion of most medications.
- Medications can cause serious adverse effects for people with pathological conditions. For example, anticholinergics may cause urinary retention in men with prostatic hyperplasia.

Pathological conditions not only influence the action of substances in the body but also contribute to nonadherence, especially in combination with functional limitations. For example, dementia can significantly affect the older adult's ability to understand directions, remember the instructions, and self-manage medication regimens. Dysphagia is an example of a physical limitation that can interfere with the ability to take substances orally.

Behaviours based on myths and misunderstandings

Myths and misunderstandings influence attitudes held by older adults, as well as their carer/caregivers, about the consumption of medicines. One attitude that can be potentially harmful for older adults is that medications, particularly OTC products, provide a "quick fix" for any uncomfortable symptom. For example, messages promoting constipation remedies can reinforce false beliefs about bowel function and could lead to laxative abuse. Although adults of any age can be influenced by these attitudes, older adults are more likely than their younger counterparts to experience the negative consequences because they are more vulnerable to adverse effects and drug interactions.

Another potentially harmful belief is that OTC preparations may be relatively safe for healthy younger adults, but they often create problems for older adults, particularly with pathological conditions and combined with other substances. For example, OTC preparations for colds and insomnia typically contain anticholinergic ingredients that are strongly associated with delirium and other serious adverse effects in older adults. In these situations, the addition of a seemingly harmless OTC product to an already complex regimen of prescription medications can be the factor that tips the scale of safety and causes a serious adverse effect, such as delirium. NSAIDs are another category of OTC drugs that commonly have serious adverse effects in older adults, either alone or with other substances (e.g. anticoagulants, prednisone). This can be especially problematic for people with hypertension because NSAIDs can increase blood pressure by causing sodium and fluid retention (Cooney & Pascuzzi, 2009). Paracetamol is another commonly used OTC product that can have serious adverse effects, including liver failure and death, when used in high doses.

Attitudes and expectations about medications as quick-fix remedies also can influence the prescribing patterns of primary care practitioners. For example, when OTC remedies are ineffective, people expect their healthcare practitioners to provide an otherwise unobtainable remedy—a prescription—for their discomfort. Sometimes, a non-pharmacological remedy is safer than and just as effective as a prescription medication, but these remedies usually demand more of the practitioner's time and some degree of motivation from the person. For example, it is easier to prescribe an antihypertensive than to advise about diet and exercise interventions. Another factor contributing to the reluctance of practitioners to suggest non-pharmacological remedies is that there are more controlled clinical trials supporting the use of medications. Sleep and anxiety complaints are examples of conditions that respond to non-pharmacological treatments, but these are often addressed by prescription medications because of the attitudes of the person or medical practitioner.

WELLNESS OPPORTUNITY

By taking time to identify an older adult's beliefs about illness and treatments (including pharmacological and non-pharmacological approaches), nurses pave the way for teaching about the safest and most effective interventions.

Communication barriers

Another factor that may contribute to an increased use of prescriptions by older adults is their own reluctance to challenge or question their medical practitioner because they perceive him or her as "all-knowing". Although the image of the infallible doctor is subsiding, older adults are still inclined to accept advice from prescribing practitioners without question.

Communication barriers and lack of confidence in one's communication skills may further inhibit someone from discussing treatment options with their healthcare practitioner. Because medical knowledge has been expanding at a tremendous pace in recent years, treatment decisions have become increasingly more complex. Consequently, older adults may hesitate to ask questions about medical decisions out of fear of appearing ignorant. Hearing and vision impairments also may interfere with person-centred discussions of a treatment plan. Other communication barriers, such as an attitude of impatience on the part of the medical practitioner, also may thwart discussion. In addition, poor command of the English language, on the part of either the older adult or the medical practitioner, can interfere with a discussion of health issues and lead to misunderstandings. Language barriers and a low education level can present major impediments to many treatment decisions, including medication adherence.

Lack of information

Despite the fact that older adults are the primary consumers of prescription and OTC medications, our knowledge about medication effects in older adults is insufficient and still in an early phase. Before the 1980s, research on the influence of age on the action of specific medications was virtually non-existent and pharmaceutical companies determined normal adult doses based on clinical trials of healthy younger men. In addition, the few studies of age-related influences on medications were cross-sectional rather than longitudinal and identified age differences rather than age-related changes. More recently, pharmaceutical companies have been required by the regulating body to include a separate geriatric-use section in drug labelling. Although some progress has been made in this area, a current concern is that evidence-based information is lacking about prescribing for older adults with multiple conditions, which is the group for whom most medications are prescribed (American Geriatrics Society, 2012a; Le Couteur et al., 2012).

Another concern is that some adverse effects and medication–medication interactions are identified only after a medication has been on the market for several years.

This is particularly important for older adults because they are most likely to have the highest risk for adverse effects and interactions. Thus, recently approved medication should be used cautiously in older adults because of the increased risk of adverse effects and unpredictable interactions.

Inappropriate prescribing practices

During the late 1980s, geriatricians began to address medication-related problems in older adults because of widespread concerns about the quantity and types of drugs prescribed for this population. The phrase "**potentially inappropriate medications**" refers to medications that pose more risks than benefits for older adults, particularly when safer alternatives exist. In 1991, an international panel of experts used consensus criteria to identify drugs that should not be used by frail older adults (Beers, Oslander, Rollingher et al., 1991). According to these explicit criteria, known as the **Beers Criteria**, medications are deemed inappropriate if they are ineffective or have poor safety profiles, or if better drugs are available (Beers, Oslander, Rollingher et al., 1991). Since the 1990s, the Beers Criteria have been updated several times. They are widely used worldwide to guide research and clinical practice.

In 2012, the American Geriatrics Society published an updated Beers Criteria list that was developed by a team of experts who used an enhanced evidence-based methodology. The updated Beers Criteria (complete title 2012 AGS Beers Criteria for Potentially Inappropriate Medication Use in Older Adults) summarise evidence-based rationales and ratings for recommendations in the following three categories (American Geriatrics Society, 2012b):

1. Potentially inappropriate medications for use in older adults by organ system/therapeutic category (e.g. anticholinergics, antithrombics, anti-infective, cardiovascular, central nervous system, endocrine, gastrointestinal and pain medications)
2. Potentially inappropriate medications for use in older adults resulting from drug effects that may exacerbate the disease or syndrome (e.g. heart failure, syncope, chronic seizures, delirium, dementia, falls/fractures, insomnia, Parkinson's disease, chronic constipation, gastric or duodenal ulcers, chronic kidney disease, urinary incontinence, and benign prostatic hyperplasia)
3. Potentially inappropriate medications that should be used cautiously in older adults (e.g. aspirin for primary prevention of cardiac events, certain antipsychotics and vasodilators).

An important theme of the Beers Criteria and other guidelines is that medications are determined to be appropriate or inappropriate in relation to the person's condition. Despite the increasing recognition of the value of the Beers Criteria, inappropriate prescribing continues to be prevalent and problematic, particularly benzodiazepines. One study found that the residents of Tasmanian long-term residential care facilities were prescribed approximately three times' higher doses of benzodiazepines than those reported in Sydney and in New Zealand (Stafford, Alswayan & Tenni, 2010). Another study of older adults discharged from intensive care units found that many of the medications were appropriate during the admission but were inappropriate following discharge (Morandi, Vasilevskis, Pandharipande et al., 2013).

The Hartford Institute for Geriatric Nursing states that the 2012 Revised Beers Criteria "should be used to inform clinical practice, evaluation, education, research, and policy to improve the safety and quality of medication prescribing for older adults" (Molony & Greenberg, 2013, p. 1). Nursing support for the 2012 Revised Beers Criteria has also been published in the *Geriatric Nursing* journal (Resnick & Fick, 2012).

WELLNESS OPPORTUNITY

Nurses have many opportunities to prevent adverse medication effects by raising questions about the use of medications that are potentially inappropriate.

Polypharmacy and inadequate monitoring of medications

There is no one definition of **polypharmacy**, but it typically refers to the use of more medications than are clinically indicated. It is important to recognise that it applies more to the appropriateness of medications than to the number of medications, and this is assessed by ensuring that the medication is not causing adverse effects and that the benefits outweigh the risks (Riker & Setter, 2012). Polypharmacy is common in older adults. One study found that nearly half of older adults living in long-term residential care facilities were taking one or more medications that are not medically necessary (Maher, Hanlon & Hajjar, 2013). An Australian survey of 4500 community-dwelling people over 50 years found that nearly 44% were taking five or more medications daily (Morgan, Williamson, Pirotta et al., 2012). Although multiple medications may be necessary for older adults with several pathological conditions, polypharmacy can lead to drug interactions and adverse medication effects.

As the number and sources of medications increase, the need for monitoring becomes more important, from the time of the initial prescription until the termination of treatment. The following risk factors could potentially interfere with medication monitoring in older adults:

- Consultations with multiple medical providers, who usually do not communicate with each other about the person's care
- Medical practitioners' lack of information about the medications obtained from a variety of sources (i.e. prescription medications offered by friends and relatives or non-prescription products such as herbs, nutritional supplements and OTC products)
- Medical practitioners' lack of information about the person's non-adherence to a treatment regimen

- A person's fear of disclosing information about home remedies or medications obtained from sources other than the prescribing medical practitioner
- A person's reluctance to disclose information about self-directed changes in the medication regimen
- An assumption by the person or medical practitioner that once most medications are started, they should be continued indefinitely
- An assumption by the person or medical practitioner that once an appropriate medication dosage is established, it will not need to be changed
- An assumption by the person or medical practitioner that a lack of adverse effects early in the course of treatment indicates that adverse effects will never occur
- Changes in the person's weight, especially weight loss, which may affect pharmacokinetic processes
- Changes in the person's daily habits (e.g. smoking, activity level or nutrient and fluid intake), which may affect pharmacokinetic processes
- Changes in the person's cognitive–emotional status, which may affect medication consumption patterns
- Changes in the person's health status, which may affect medication actions, increasing the potential for adverse effects.

Medication non-adherence

Medication non-adherence (non-compliance) refers to medication-taking patterns that differ from the prescribed pattern, including missed doses, failure to fill prescriptions or medications taken too frequently or at inappropriate times. Reviews of studies indicate that medication non-adherence occurs in about half of older adults and that half of all new medication users will fail to consume at least 80% of prescribed dose during the first year of therapy (Blackburn, Swidrovich & Lemstra, 2013; Marcum & Gellad, 2012). Medication non-adherence is associated with multiple interacting factors, including all of the following, which are consistently identified in studies: cognitive impairment, social isolation, depression, asymptomatic disease, low health literacy, adverse medication effects, long treatment duration, high number of medications or daily doses, poor communication between the person and provider, and misunderstandings about the medication or disease (Hugtenburg, Timmers, Elders et al., 2013; Lee, 2013).

Financial concerns related to prescription drugs

In recent years, attention has been paid to the increasing cost of prescription drugs, particularly for those older adults who have chronic conditions and require many medications. Despite the increasing costs, Australia and New Zealand have national systems of subsidised-medicine schemes, and both aim to provide affordable medicines. In Australia the Pharmaceutical Benefits Scheme (PBS) enables most medicines to be dispensed to all Australian residents who hold a current Medicare card at a government-subsidised price. The amount that is paid for the PBS medicine is called a co-payment. The Australian Government pays the remaining cost. In 2015, the cost of most PBS medicines was $37.70 (Australian Government Department of Health, 2015). However, there may be extra charges on some medicines or medicine brands that are not fully subsidised. An additional scheme to reduce medicine costs exists if the person has a concession card. Many older adults qualify for this service because they receive a government Aged Care Pension. In this situation the older adult pays $6.10 per dispensed PBS medicine. Another strategy that minimises the cost of medicines in Australia is the Safety Net. For concession holders, once the amount of $366.00 is reached in one year, then the person does not pay for any further PBS medicines dispensed in the same year.

In New Zealand the list of government-subsidised medicines is contained in the Pharmaceutical Schedule (Pharmac, 2014). For most prescriptions a co-payment is required of $5.00. However, there are a number of health subsidy cards for which older adults are eligible, which lowers the costs of medications (see Box 8-2).

Neither system in Australia or New Zealand covers herbal remedies, supplements that are not classified as medicines, or non-prescription medications.

> **BOX 8-2**
> **Health subsidy cards for prescription medications available in New Zealand**
>
> - A Prescription Subsidy Card (PSC) enables the cardholder and family members to pay lower government prescription charges. People can have a PSC once the family has had 20 new prescribed items in one year (1 February to 31 January), not counting prescriptions that are free.
> - A Community Services Card (CSC) may lower the cost of GP visits and prescription charges. Any family whose income before tax is less than the amount set by the Ministry of Health and who ordinarily lives in New Zealand, can have a CSC.
> - A High Use Health Card (HUHC) lowers the cost of prescribed medicines for people who have visited the doctor more than 12 times in the last 12 months. The HUHC helps people who do not have a Community Services Card, but who have high GP and prescription costs because of ongoing health problems.
>
> *Source:* Pharmac. (2014). Costs of medicines. Accessed March 2015 at www.pharmac.health.nz/medicines/medicines-information/costs-of-medicines.

Insufficient recognition of adverse medication effects

Another problem specific to older adults is that adverse effects are likely to be misinterpreted or not recognised as such because of their similarity to age-related changes or commonly occurring pathological conditions. When an older adult experiences an adverse medication reaction, two or three potential causes other than the medication

TABLE 8-4 Some adverse medication effects that may remain unrecognised in older adults

Manifestation	Medication type	Specific examples
Cognitive impairment	Antidepressants; antipsychotics; antianxiety agents; anticholinergics; hypoglycaemics; over-the-counter (OTC) cold, cough and sleeping preparations	Perphenazine, amitriptyline, chlorpromazine, diazepam, benztropine, cimetidine, digoxin, barbiturates, chlorpheniramine, diphenhydramine
Depression	Antihypertensives, antiarthritics, antianxiety agents, antipsychotics	Reserpine, clonidine, propranolol, indomethacin, haloperidol, barbiturates
Urinary incontinence	Diuretics, anticholinergics	Frusemide, doxepin, thioridazine, lorazepam
Constipation	Narcotics, antacids, antipsychotics, antidepressants	Codeine, chlorpromazine, calcium carbonate, aluminium hydroxide
Vision impairment	Digitalis, antiarthritics, phenothiazines	Digoxin, indomethacin, ibuprofen, chlorpromazine
Hearing impairment	Mycin antibiotics, salicylates, loop diuretics	Gentamicin, aspirin, frusemide, bumetanide
Postural hypotension	Antihypertensives, diuretics, antipsychotics, antidepressants	Frusemide, propranolol, chlorpromazine, imipramine, clonidine
Hypothermia	Antipsychotics, alcohol, salicylates	Haloperidol, aspirin, alcohol, fluphenazine
Sexual dysfunction	Antihypertensives, antipsychotics, antidepressants, alcohol	Timolol, clonidine, thiazides, haloperidol, amitriptyline, alcohol, cimetidine, propranolol, methyldopa
Mobility problems	Sedatives, antianxiety agents, antipsychotics, ototoxic medications	Chloral hydrate, diazepam, frusemide, gentamicin
Dry mouth	Anticholinergics, corticosteroids, bronchodilators, antihypertensives	Chlorpromazine, haloperidol, prednisone, frusemide, sertraline, theophylline
Anorexia	Digoxin, bronchodilators, antihistamines	Digoxin, theophylline, diphenhydramine
Drowsiness	Antidepressants, antipsychotics, OTC cold preparations, alcohol, barbiturates	Amitriptyline, haloperidol, chlorpheniramine
Oedema	Antiarthritics, corticosteroids, antihypertensives	Ibuprofen, indomethacin, prednisone, reserpine, methyldopa
Tremors	Antipsychotics	Haloperidol, chlorpromazine

usually can be identified, with medications being a common cause. For example, a study of older adults seeking care for urinary incontinence found that 60.5% were taking medications that potentially contributed to their symptoms, with polypharmacy being a major risk factor (Kashyap, Tu & Tannenbaum, 2013). Although adverse effects are not unique to older adults, they occur more commonly with increasing age and are more likely to be attributed erroneously to pathological conditions or age-related changes and circumstances.

The term **prescribing cascade** has been applied to the following commonly occurring scenario: an adverse drug reaction is misinterpreted as a new medical condition, a drug is prescribed for this condition, another adverse drug effect occurs, the person is again treated for the perceived additional medical condition, and the sequence perpetuates new adverse events. Table 8-4 summarises **adverse medication effects** that are likely to remain unrecognised in older adults because of their similarity to age-related changes.

WELLNESS OPPORTUNITY

Nurses promote wellness when they challenge ageist attitudes and identify adverse effects falsely attributed to ageing or pathological conditions.

MEDICATION INTERACTIONS

Medications can interact with any other biologically active substance, including other medications, herbs, nutrients, alcohol, caffeine and nicotine. These interactions occur not only with prescription medications but also with commonly used OTC products, including antacids, analgesics and remedies for coughs, colds and sleep problems. Outcomes of medication interactions with other substances include altered or erratic therapeutic effect, increased potential for adverse effects and, in rare cases, a decreased potential for adverse effects.

Medication–medication interactions

The risk of adverse effects from interactions between two or more medications increases exponentially according to the number of medications being consumed. Because older adults often take two or more medications concurrently, they are at increased risk for medication–medication interactions. Medication–medication interactions are typically caused by competitive action at binding sites, but they can be caused by any mechanism that influences the absorption, distribution, metabolism or elimination of any of the medications. The effects of medication–medication interactions include increased or decreased serum levels of

TABLE 8-5 Types and examples of medication–medication interactions

Type of interaction	Interaction example	Effect
Binding effect (e.g. an oral drug diminishes the absorption of another drug in the stomach)	Magnesium- or aluminum-containing antacids may bind with tetracycline in the stomach	Decreased effects of tetracycline
Metabolism interference effect (e.g. one drug interferes with liver metabolism of another drug)	Ciprofloxacin and anticonvulsants inhibit metabolism of warfarin	Increased effects of warfarin
Metabolism enhancing effect (e.g. one drug activates the drug-metabolising enzymes in the liver)	Phenobarbitone increases metabolism of warfarin	Decreased effects of warfarin
Elimination interference effect (e.g. one drug interferes with the renal elimination of another drug)	Frusemide can interfere with elimination of salicylates	Increased effects of salicylates
Elimination enhancement effect (e.g. renal reabsorption is blocked because of altered urinary pH)	Sodium bicarbonate can enhance excretion of lithium, tetracyclines and salicylates	Decreased effects of lithium, tetracycline, or salicylate
Competitive or displacement effect (e.g. two drugs compete at receptor sites)	Diphenhydramine may interfere with effect of cholinergic agents (e.g. tacrine, donepezil)	Decreased effects of tacrine or donepezil
Potentiating effect (e.g. two drugs produce greater effects when taken together even though they have different actions)	Paracetamol taken with codeine has a greater analgesic effect than either medication taken alone	Increased analgesic effect
Additive effect (e.g. two drugs produce greater effect because they have similar action)	Verapamil or diltiazem may have additive effect when taken with a beta-blocker	Increased effect on blood pressure

either one or both of the medications, with subsequent altered therapeutic effects and increased risk of adverse or toxic effects. Medication–medication interactions can cause serious functional consequences and are a major cause of unnecessary hospital admissions (Obreli-Neto et al., 2012).

Although it is impossible to know details about all potential medication–medication interactions, nurses can be aware of specific mechanisms that are most commonly associated with these interactions in older adults, as listed in Table 8-5, which also lists examples of each type. It is important to be aware of serious interactions that occur more frequently with certain medications. For example, warfarin requires close monitoring because serum levels are easily altered by interactions with other medications, foods and herbs.

Medications and herbs

Many medication–herb interactions have been identified in recent years because of the increased use of herbs and increased attention to interactions. Medications that are likely to be affected by herbs are warfarin, insulin, aspirin, digoxin, cyclosporin and ticlopidine (Tsai, Lin, Simon et al., 2012; Vieira & Huang, 2012). Most herb–medication interactions are mild, but a few herbs, such as St John's wort, can be sufficiently serious to endanger the person's health (Izzo, 2012). Refer to Table 8-3 for common interactions and precautions regarding herbs.

Medications and nutrients

In the context of medication–nutrient interactions, the term nutrient includes foods, beverages, enteral formulas and dietary supplements. Older adults are likely to experience medication–nutrient interactions because of a combination of age-related changes and other risk factors. For example, changes in the gastrointestinal tract can delay or diminish the absorption of medications. Another widely recognised example is the effect of grapefruit juice on increasing the bioavailability of certain drugs such as statins, benzodiazepines and calcium channel blockers (Hanley, Cancalon, Widmer et al., 2011). Clinically significant nutrient–medication interactions are likely to occur if the following medications are taken with food: bisphosphonates, levodopa, ciprofloxacin, digoxin, frusemide, glipizide, levothyroxine, metformin, metoprolol and warfarin (Anderson & Fox, 2012). Table 8.6 lists examples of nutrient–medication interactions.

Medications and alcohol

Alcohol interacts with medications in the same way as other central nervous system depressants, but health professionals do not always inquire about an older person's use of alcohol, and even when people are asked, they might not accurately acknowledge the amount of alcohol used. Alcohol is consumed not only in beverages but also in OTC preparations such as mouthwashes, vitamin and mineral tonics, and liquid cough and cold preparations.

TABLE 8-6 Medication–nutrient interactions

Effect on medication	Example of interaction effect
Delayed absorption rate, no effect on amount absorbed	Ingestion of food may delay absorption of cimetidine, digoxin and ibuprofen.
Reduced rate and amount of absorption	Calcium decreases absorption of tetracycline. A high-protein or high-fibre meal decreases absorption of levodopa. Grapefruit juice can decrease absorption of antifungals and antihistamines.
Reduced absorption because of non-nutrient components	Caffeinated tea and fibre intake interfere with iron absorption.
Increased absorption	High-fat foods increase serum levels of griseofulvin.
Decreased therapeutic effect	Vitamin K decreases the effectiveness of warfarin.
Increased rate of metabolism	A high-protein diet increases the metabolism of theophylline.
Increased concentrations and bioavailability	Potential effect of grapefruit juice and amiodarone, atorvastatin, buspirone, calcium channel blockers, carbamazepine, diazepam, lovastatin, simvastatin and triazolam.

TABLE 8-7 Medication–alcohol interactions

Type of interaction	Example of interaction effect
Altered metabolism of benzodiazepines when combined with alcohol	Increased psychomotor impairment and adverse effects
Altered metabolism of barbiturates when combined with alcohol	Central nervous system depression
Competition between alcohol and chloral hydrate at metabolic sites	Increased serum levels of alcohol and chloral hydrate
Altered metabolism of alcohol when combined with chlorpromazine	Increased serum levels of alcohol and acetaldehyde; increased psychomotor impairment
Enhanced vasodilation as a result of a combination of alcohol and nitrates	Severe hypotension and headache, enhanced absorption of glyceryl trinitrate
Altered hepatic gluconeogenesis, which influences the action of oral hypoglycaemics, as a result of alcohol	Potentiation of oral hypoglycaemics by alcohol

When taken with medications, alcohol can alter the therapeutic action of medications and increase the potential for adverse effects. Older adults might be more susceptible to medication–alcohol interactions because age-related changes in receptor sensitivity and body composition lead to higher blood-alcohol levels. Table 8-7 lists some of the medication–alcohol interactions that can occur in older adults.

DIVERSITY NOTE

Increased age and female gender are factors that increase the bioavailability of alcohol after it is consumed (Ferreira & Weems, 2008).

Medications and nicotine

Medication–nicotine interactions can be associated with tobacco smoking, smokeless tobacco and the many nicotine-based products that are increasingly being used as substitutes for smoking. Nicotine can affect medications through any of the following actions: vasoconstriction, stimulation of the central nervous system, activation of neuroendocrine pathways, increased gastric acid secretions and altered metabolism of liver enzymes. Most often the medication–nicotine interaction interferes with the therapeutic action of the medication and smokers may require higher doses of a medication than non-smokers to achieve the same therapeutic effects. Prescribing practitioners may need to adjust medication doses not only for smokers but also when the use of nicotine products is discontinued. Even a change from smoking tobacco to a nicotine product can affect some medications because hydrocarbons in tobacco smoke can affect drugs that are metabolised by the CYP-450 enzyme system. A review of studies found that dosage adjustments are clearly indicated for warfarin, olanzapine, clozapine and theophylline when a person changes smoking habits (Schaffer, Yoon & Zadezensky, 2009). This is important not only for people who voluntarily quit smoking but also for those who temporarily change smoking habits because of hospitalisation or other short-term circumstances. Table 8-8 lists some common medication–nicotine interactions.

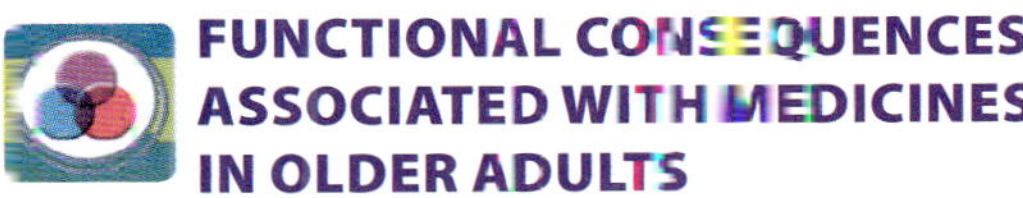

FUNCTIONAL CONSEQUENCES ASSOCIATED WITH MEDICINES IN OLDER ADULTS

The major functional consequence affecting medicines in healthy older adults who take only one substance is an increased potential for both altered therapeutic action and adverse effects. Older adults who take more than one substance or have other risk factors are likely to have additional functional consequences such as interactions with

TABLE 8-8 Medication–nicotine interactions

Effect of nicotine	Example of interaction effect
Altered metabolism	Decreased efficacy of analgesics, lorazepam, theophylline, aminophylline, beta-blockers and calcium channel blockers
Vasoconstriction	Increased peripheral ischaemic effect of beta-blockers
Central nervous system stimulation	Decreased drowsiness from benzodiazepines and phenothiazines
Stimulation of antidiuretic hormone secretion	Fluid retention, decreased effectiveness of diuretics
Activation of neuroendocrine pathways	Interacts with insulin, aggravates insulin resistance, interferes with alpha-blockers
Increase in platelet activity	Decreased anticoagulant effectiveness (heparin, warfarin); increased risk of thrombosis with oestrogen use
Increased gastric acid secretion	Decreased or negated effects of H_2 antagonists (cimetidine, famotidine, nizatidine, ranitidine)
Effect of hydrocarbons in tobacco smoke on CYP-450 enzyme system	Cessation of tobacco smoking can increase concentrations of clozapine, olanzapine, theophylline, warfarin, even when a nicotine product is initiated

other substances and a higher risk for altered therapeutic action and adverse effects. Age-related changes and risk factors also affect consumption patterns, increasing the possibility of non-adherence and its associated consequences.

Altered therapeutic effects

Age-related changes alone can alter the therapeutic action of some substances; however, most of the altered therapeutic effects that occur in older adults are caused by risk factors, such as polypharmacy. Consequently, the therapeutic effectiveness of substances is less predictable, even in healthy older adults.

The main implication is that medicines need to be monitored more closely in older adults, especially initially and when there is any change in the person's medical status or treatment regimen. Thus, the commonly accepted principle for geriatric drug prescribing is "start low and go slow".

Increased potential for adverse effects

Adverse drug events (also called adverse drug reactions or adverse medication effects) are the unintended and undesired outcomes of a medication that occur in doses normally used in humans. Consequences of adverse drug events include a decline in function, an increased risk for falls and fractures, an increased number of visits for healthcare services, admission to a hospital or prolongation of a hospital stay, and death. Up to 13% of patients taking two medications and 82% of those taking six medications experience an adverse drug event (Little & Morley, 2013). There is much agreement that adverse medication events occur commonly, have serious consequences, and frequently are avoidable. Box 8-3 lists some of the factors that can increase the risk for adverse drug events.

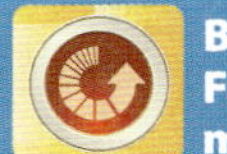

BOX 8-3
Factors that increase the risk for adverse medication effects

- Increased numbers of medications
- Frailty
- Malnourishment or dehydration
- Multiple illnesses
- An illness that interferes with cardiac, renal or hepatic function
- Cognitive impairment
- History of medication allergies or adverse effects
- Fever, which can alter the action of certain medications
- Recent change in health or functional status
- Medications in any of the following categories: anticoagulant/antiplatelet, antidiabetics, NSAIDs, central nervous system drugs

In recent years there has been increasing attention on adverse drug events as a preventable cause of hospitalisations for older adults. Medications most frequently cited as causes of emergency hospitalisations are warfarin, antiplatelet drugs and antidiabetic drugs, including insulin and oral hypoglycaemics (Budnitz, Lovegrove, Shehab et al., 2011). Attention also is focusing on adverse drug events that occur during hospitalisation. Some conditions associated with increased risk for adverse drug events during hospitalisation include renal failure, increasing number of medications, inappropriate medications, age 75 years and older, and use of central nervous system drugs and anti-infectives (Dupouy, Moulis, Tubery et al., 2013; O'Connor, Gallagher, Byrne et al., 2012).

Several aspects of adverse medication effects are particularly important for the care of older adults. As discussed in the section on risk factors, adverse effects may not be recognised as such because they are similar to the manifestations of pathological conditions or they are mistakenly attributed to ageing. Three concerns of particular importance are anticholinergic adverse effects, changes in mental status and tardive dyskinesia.

Anticholinergic adverse effects

In recent years, geriatricians have increasingly recognised that older adults are particularly susceptible to the **anticholinergic adverse effects** from medications, including some medications that are not widely recognised as having anticholinergic effects in the body. Many OTC agents commonly

BOX 8-4
Examples of medications with anticholinergic effects

Antidepressants
Amitriptyline
Imipramine
Mirtazapine
Nortriptyline
Paroxetine

Antihistamines
Diphenhydramine
Loratadine
Promethazine

Anti-parkinsonism agents
Benztropine

Antipsychotics
Chlorpromazine
Clozapine
Fluphenazine
Haloperidol
Prochlorperazine
Promethazine
Quetiapine
Risperidone

Cardiovascular agents
Captopril
Digoxin
Dipyridamole
Isosorbide dinitrate
Nifedipine

Gastrointestinal agents
Belladonna
Cimetidine
Hyoscyamine
Loperamide
Ranitidine

Urinary antispasmodics
Oxybutynin
Tolterodine

Miscellaneous agents
Amantadine
Atropine
Theophylline
Warfarin

TABLE 8-9 Mechanisms of action for mental changes caused by adverse medication effects

Mechanism of action	Examples
Anticholinergic effects	Atropine, scopolamine, antihistamines, antipsychotics, antidepressants, antispasmodics, antiparkinsonian agents
Decreased cerebral blood flow	Antihypertensives, antipsychotics
Depression of respiratory centre	Central nervous system depressants
Fluid and electrolyte alterations	Diuretics, alcohol, laxatives
Altered thermoregulation	Alcohol, psychotropics, narcotics
Acidosis	Diuretics, alcohol, nicotinic acid
Hypoglycaemia	Hypoglycaemics, alcohol, propranolol
Hormonal disturbances	Thyroid extract, corticosteroids
Depression-inducing action	Reserpine, methyldopa, indomethacin, barbiturates, fluphenazine, haloperidol, corticosteroids

used for coughs, colds and sleep problems contain anticholinergic ingredients. Anticholinergic adverse effects also can occur from systemic absorption of commonly used topical medications or ophthalmic agents (e.g. mydriatics and cycloplegics). Common types of medications with anticholinergic properties include antidepressants, antihistamines, anti-parkinsonism agents, antipsychotics, cardiovascular agents, gastrointestinal agents, and urinary antispasmodics (see Box 8-4 for examples).

Longitudinal studies have consistently identified anticholinergic agents as a causative factor for significant and long-term cognitive impairment in older adults, including delirium and mild cognitive impairment (e.g. Cai, Campbell, Khan et al., 2013; Pasina, Djade, Lucca et al., 2013; Puustinen, Nurminen, Vahlberg et al., 2012; Uusvaara, Pitkala, Kautianen et al., 2013). Another concern related to anticholinergic agents is that their pharmacological action can counteract the effects of cholinesterase inhibitors, which are prescribed as a primary treatment for dementia. The Beers Criteria and guidelines emphasise the importance of avoiding medications with anticholinergic effects because they are inappropriate for use in older adults and safer alternatives are usually available.

Altered mental status

Although medications can cause cognitive changes in anyone, older adults are at increased risk for medication-induced altered cognition because of age-related changes and risk factors. In addition, when older adults experience changes in their cognition, these changes are likely to be attributed to dementia or another pathological condition, rather than being recognised as an adverse medication effect. Nurses need to be alert to the possibility that even a simple OTC product, such as diphenhydramine, is a common cause of cognitive changes in older adults.

Delirium is an acute confusional state that can be precipitated by any medication or by medication interactions (refer to Chapter 14 for further discussion of delirium). Older adults are particularly susceptible to medication-induced delirium because of altered neurochemical activity in the brain. Moreover, some pathological conditions (e.g. dementia, dehydration, malnutrition, head injury or central nervous system infection) can increase the risk for medication-induced delirium. Even at non-toxic serum levels or at doses considered to be normal, medications can cause cognitive changes in older adults. It is important to keep in mind that medication-induced cognitive changes do not always subside immediately after the offending medication is discontinued. In some cases, it may take several weeks or even months after the medication is decreased or discontinued for cognitive function to return to the premedication level. Some medications that are likely to cause cognitive changes in older adults, as well as the mechanisms underlying these adverse actions, are listed in Table 8-9.

Tardive dyskinesia and drug-induced parkinsonism

Tardive dyskinesia refers to a constellation of rhythmic and involuntary movements of any of the following: the trunk and extremities and the jaw, lips, mouth and tongue (referred to as oro-buccal-lingual). The earliest signs are usually fine, wormlike movements of the tongue. Other early signs include chewing, grimacing, lip smacking, jaw clenching, eye blinking and side-to-side jaw movements.

Manifestations can begin as early as 3 to 6 months after the initiation of antipsychotic medications and they persist even after the causative agent is discontinued. It is considered an adverse effect of dopamine receptor-blocking agents and serotonin–noradrenaline re-uptake inhibitors (i.e. certain antipsychotics and antidepressants) (Lee, Lin, Chang et al., 2013; Waln & Jankovic, 2013). Tardive dyskinesia deserves special attention with regard to older adults because advanced age correlates with both an earlier onset and increased severity of tardive dyskinesia. Moreover, when combined with age-related changes and risk factors, tardive dyskinesia can seriously impair the older adult's ability to perform activities of daily living.

Drug-induced parkinsonism is the occurrence of Parkinson-like manifestations as an adverse medication effect. Manifestations can be reversed if the offending drug is stopped, but many times the condition is misdiagnosed as Parkinson's disease and treated inappropriately with an antiparkinsonism medication. Risk factors for development of drug-induced parkinsonism include older age, female gender, cognitive impairment, family history of Parkinson's disease, coexistence of tardive dyskinesia and taking certain medications (e.g. haloperidol, metoclopramide, risperidone, phenothiazines) (Alvarez & Evidente, 2008; Thanyi & Treadwell, 2009).

Antipsychotics in people with dementia

Antipsychotics continue to be prescribed unnecessarily, and studies continue to identify serious consequences related to antipsychotics in people living with dementia (Allen, 2012; Colloca, Tosato, Vetrano et al., 2012; Senft, 2012). The strong association between serious adverse effects and the first-generation antipsychotics (e.g. haloperidol) led to the development of second-generation (also called atypical) antipsychotics, which include risperidone, olanzapine, quetiapine, aripiprazole and ziprasidone.

During the past two decades, studies have focused on both the therapeutic effectiveness and the risk of adverse effects related to the use of atypical antipsychotics. Recent reviews have concluded that atypical antipsychotics are associated with serious adverse effects, including death, stroke, falls, delirium, hip fractures, cognitive decline, movement disorders, and these adverse effects occur in community-dwelling older adults as well as those in nursing homes (Brandt & Pyhtila, 2013; Seitz, Gill, Herrmann et al., 2013; Steinberg & Lyketsos, 2012). Because of major concerns about adverse effects, there is increasing emphasis on non-pharmacological management of neuropsychiatric symptoms in people living with dementia, as discussed in Chapter 14. Studies also confirm the need for education of nursing staff to improve knowledge, attitudes and beliefs about antipsychotic use for nursing home residents (Lemay, Mazor, Field et al., 2013).

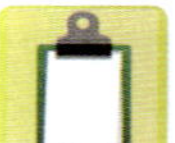

NURSING ASSESSMENT OF MEDICATION USE AND EFFECTS

Nurses assess medication regimens and medication-taking behaviours of older adults to accomplish the following:

- Determine the effectiveness of the medication regimen.
- Identify any factors that interfere with the correct regimen.
- Ascertain risks for adverse effects or altered therapeutic actions (with particular attention to older adults at increased risk).
- Detect adverse medication effects.
- Identify teaching needs with regard to medications.

During a medication assessment, nurses should clarify the prescribed medication regimen and identify the actual medication-taking behaviours so that they can assess for adherence to the treatment regimen.

Communication techniques for obtaining accurate information

Some of the many barriers to obtaining accurate information about medications and medication-taking behaviours can include time limitations, complex medication regimens and lack of a trusting relationship. Because medication assessments can be very time-consuming and because the older adult may not think of all the information during the first interview or may initially be reluctant to reveal accurate information, it may be necessary to conduct the medication assessment over the course of two or more visits. In addition, older adults may be reluctant to answer questions about their medications because they perceive this information, including information about the use of alcohol, as being very private. Many older adults have learned not to ask questions about their healthcare because they are unsure of what to ask or they falsely believe that they are not entitled to medical information. Although most older adults appreciate the opportunity to discuss medications with a nurse, they initially may hesitate to ask questions or share information. Some of this reluctance may be caused by fear of being judged, especially if the prescribed regimen is not being followed exactly or if the person uses home remedies, alternative therapies or OTC. When people do not follow the medication regimen exactly as prescribed, they are likely to recite the orders rather than describe their actual medication-taking behaviours. Another factor that contributes to this reluctance is anxiety about discussing the underlying reason for not following the regimen. For example, older adults who cannot afford medications may be embarrassed to discuss their limited finances.

Nurses can address the barriers by asking open-ended questions in a matter-of-fact way and conveying a non-judgemental attitude during the medication interview. They should also keep in mind that they need to elicit information about the use of herbs, home remedies, OTC preparations and complementary and alternative care practices. For example, "What do you do to help you sleep?" is more open-ended than "Do you take any medications for sleep?" because the latter may be interpreted only in relation to prescription medications.

Another interview technique is to use leading questions related to potential risk factors that interfere with the older person's ability to take medications accurately. For example, because the high cost of medications is a commonly acknowledged problem, nurses can ask a question such as "I know that some of these medications that are prescribed for you can be quite expensive; do you have any problems with getting them?" Similarly, asking a question such as "I know you don't drive—are you able to have your medications delivered or do you have someone who helps you get them from the pharmacy?" may elicit information about transportation barriers.

Nurses should ask additional questions about the person's ability to take his or her medications as prescribed based on specific observations. For example, if a nurse observes that a pill is very large, a question such as "Do you have any trouble swallowing these capsules?" might be appropriate. Similarly, if the nurse knows that the older adult has limited hand strength, an appropriate assessment question would be "Do you have any difficulty getting the caps off your medication bottles?" Another technique for eliciting information is to ask about the person's method of organising medications. For example, people taking medications often have a method of organising their regimen by using divided medication boxes or written charts or schedules. They usually are willing to show this organisational system to the nurse and, in fact, may be proud to discuss their method with the nurse during the medication assessment.

WELLNESS OPPORTUNITY

Nurses can build on their trusting relationship with older adults to encourage open discussion of factors that interfere with adherence to medication regimens.

Scope of a medication assessment

Medication assessments include information about all of the following:

- Prescription and OTC medications used orally and by all other routes (e.g. nasal, aural, topical, optical, injectable, dermal methods)
- Medications that are used only sporadically or as needed
- Vitamins, minerals and dietary supplements (including doses and frequency)
- Alcohol, caffeine
- Tobacco smoking, use of nicotine products (including information about recent changes)
- Home remedies and CAMs, including all herbal products and homeopathic remedies.

Information about the doses of vitamins and minerals is important because megavitamins can be harmful and even low doses can cause interactions or have adverse effects (e.g. iron or calcium carbonate can be constipating). Information about the brand names of OTC medications can help identify additives that may be causing problems or increasing the risk of altered medication action (e.g. analgesics with caffeine, antacids with lactose or bronchodilators with sulfites). Information about home remedies and complementary and alternative healthcare practices can help identify health beliefs that affect adherence and other aspects of medication-taking behaviours. Nurses also need to assess the person's understanding of the purpose of medications; doing so provides information about his or her understanding of health status and medical conditions. As with other parts of the medication assessment, it is essential to phrase questions in as open-ended and non-judgemental a manner as possible. Asking "What do you take this pill for?" with a tone of curiosity will likely elicit more information than asking questions such as, "What do you take for your heart?" or "Why do you take frusemide?"

Obtaining information about allergies and adverse reactions is essential because anyone with a history of medication-related problems will need to be closely monitored, especially if the medications being administered are similar to those that caused the reaction. Sometimes people state that they are allergic to a medication, but when they are asked about the symptoms, they describe an adverse effect, rather than an allergic reaction. Therefore, rather than simply documenting that the person is allergic to a certain medication, nurses should document the specific reaction that occurred. Nurses can use Box 8-5 as a guide to assessing medications regimens and medication-taking behaviours.

Nurses should also obtain and document information about the person's perception of and preferences for various forms of medications because this information can influence prescribing decisions, especially when there are several options that may be equally effective. Similarly, nurses should identify any cultural factors that might influence medication-taking behaviours. For example, according to some Asian traditions, illness is perceived as an imbalance of hot and cold forces. If the illness makes the body hot, then the remedy should make it cooler. Cultural considerations 8-1 lists some cultural factors that are pertinent to a medication assessment.

Another component of a comprehensive medication assessment is obtaining information about various sources of healthcare. This information is particularly important when someone receives care from more than one medical practitioner, as is often the case. Nurses can ask non-judgementally about whether the person receives care from non-Western medical practitioners, such as herbalists, spiritual healers, naturopathic practitioners or Ayurvedic doctors. Cultural considerations 8-2 summarises some culturally specific sources of healthcare and treatment modalities that older adults might use.

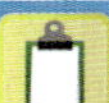

BOX 8-5
Guidelines for medication assessment

Information about the therapeutic agents

- Prescription pills, liquids, injections, eye drops, ear drops, nasal sprays, transdermal methods, and topical preparations
- Over-the-counter preparations that are used regularly or occasionally
- Vitamins, minerals and nutritional supplements
- Pattern of alcohol, caffeine or tobacco use
- Herbs and herbal preparations
- Homeopathic remedies
- Home remedies
- Sources of healthcare, including complementary and alternative practitioners.

Interview questions to assess medication-taking behaviours

- How would you describe your usual daily routine for taking medications and remedies, beginning when you get up in the morning?
- Is there anything else you do or use to treat illness or to maintain your health, such as using herbs, ointments, home remedies or nutritional supplements?
- Are you taking anyone else's medications?
- What do you do when you miss a dose of medication?
- What do you take for constipation? What do you do to help you sleep (or to alleviate any other identified problem)?
- How do you get your prescriptions filled? (Where do you get your remedies?)
- Do you have any difficulty taking your pills?
- What method do you use to keep track of your medications and remedies?
- Is there anything you do to help you remember to take your medicines or remedies at the appropriate time?

Interview questions to assess the person's understanding of the purpose of medications and other remedies

- What is this medication (or herb, etc.) for?
- For medications (or remedies) that are used as needed (PRN): How do you decide when to take this pill (or remedy)?
- What did your healthcare practitioner tell you about this medication (or herb, etc.)?
- What problems were you having when the healthcare practitioner prescribed this medication (or suggested that you use this remedy)?

Interview questions to elicit additional information

- Are there any medications or remedies you were taking at one time but are no longer taking?
- Have you ever had an allergic reaction, or any other bad reaction, to a medication or remedy? (If yes, describe what happened.)
- Where do you store your medications and remedies?

Questions and observations based on reading of prescription labels

- Who is the prescribing medical practitioner?
- If there is more than one medical practitioner, does each practitioner know all the medications that are being used?
- Are any medications the same or similar and prescribed by different medical practitioners?
- If the dates on various prescriptions are different, were the later medications supposed to be added to the medication regimen, or were they intended to replace previously prescribed medications?
- Are the date of the last refill and the number of pills in the bottle consistent with the prescribed regimen?

CULTURAL CONSIDERATIONS 8-1
Cultural considerations with regard to medication assessment and interventions

- Teaching about medications should be done in the context of culturally-based beliefs about health, illness and remedies.
- People of Vietnamese and other cultural groups may view injections as being more effective than pills, and pills as being more effective than drops.
- People of Asian, Latin and Middle Eastern heritage believe it is important to take medicine with certain foods or beverages (e.g. tea or warm water rather than cold water) to provide the necessary balance.
- Some Chinese and other Asian people may have the following preferences:
  - Balms and ointments rather than pills for local pain.
  - Teas and soups rather than antacids for indigestion.
  - Herbs rather than prescription drugs.
- The following differences in response to medications might occur:
  - Arabic people may require a lower dose of antiarrhythmics, antihypertensives, neuroleptics and psychotropics, and a higher dose of opioids.
  - Asian/Pacific people may require a lower dose of neuroleptics, antidepressants, lithium, fat-soluble medications.
- It is not unusual for Māori to use *rongoā Māori* (traditional Māori medicine) (Evans et al., 2008).
- The desire to use traditional medicines among Indigenous Australians is widespread, but because many of the plants used traditionally have not yet been studied, they should be used cautiously (Shahid et al., 2010).

Additional sources: Andrews, M. M. (2011). Cultural competence in health history and physical examination. In M. M. Andrews & J. S. Boyle. (2014). *Transcultural concepts in nursing care*. Philadelphia, PA: Lippincott Williams & Wilkins.

CULTURAL CONSIDERATIONS 8-2
Culturally specific healthcare sources and practices

Cultural group	Sources of care	Health practices
Chinese	Herbalists, acupuncturists	Herbs, food, beverages and other remedies to balance yin and yang
Christian scientists	Christian science practitioners and nurses	Medications are not used; focus is on hygiene measures
Filipino	Folk healers (*hilot*)	Prayer, exorcism, hot/cold balance
Hindu	Traditional healers (*nattuvaidhyars*)	Ayurvedic medicine (herbs and roots)
Indigenous Australians	Traditional healers	Bush medicine
Japanese	Herbalists	Herbs, prayer at temple, church or small shrines at home
Māori	Traditional healers	Traditional healing includes *mirimiri* (massage), *rongoā* (herbal treatments) and *karakia* (spiritual prayer) (New Zealand Ministry of Health, 2011)
Pacific people	Traditional healers	Traditional healing includes massage and the use herbs and food extracts (Medical Council of New Zealand, 2010)
Russians	Folk remedies	Herbal teas, sweet liquor, physical modalities (oils, ointments, enemas, mud baths)
Vietnamese	Asian physicians, folk healers, spiritual healers, magicians (sorcerers)	Herbs, acupuncture, cup suctioning, skin pinching

Additional sources: Andrews, M. M. & Boyle, J. S. (2011). *Transcultural concepts in nursing care*. Philadelphia, PA: Lippincott Williams & Wilkins; Purnell, L. D. (2014). *Guide to culturally competent health care*. Philadelphia, PA: F. A. Davis Company.

WELLNESS OPPORTUNITY

Nurses promote personal responsibility for health by encouraging discussion of various sources of care.

Observing patterns of medication use

In addition to using good communication techniques, nurses obtain essential assessment information by reviewing the person's array of medications. When nurses conduct the medication assessment in the home setting, they can ask to see all the medications that the older person uses. Direct observation of medication containers provides useful information about adherence, dates of original prescription and refills, duplication of similar medications and pharmaceutical treatments for pathological conditions. For example, if three types of antihypertensive medications have been prescribed at different times, the nurse can inquire whether the second or third medication was supposed to replace or supplement the original medication. Nurses can also assess whether the bottles contain the original medications and ask additional questions when the contents are not consistent with expectations. For example, if the label indicates that the original prescription was for 30 pills, but it has not been refilled for 1 year, the nurse might inquire about the reason. Older adults may explain that they cannot afford the prescription or they cannot manipulate the childproof lid. Another purpose for examining the medication containers is to discover information about sources of care and duplication of medications. It is not unusual to find that older people are getting prescriptions from more than one medical practitioner. Sometimes, the older person has the same or similar medications from different sources or under more than one name (e.g. generic and brand names).

Linking the medication assessment to the overall assessment

The nurse uses information from the medication interview with the overall health assessment in several ways. First, information about past and present medication patterns can provide clues to identified problems or complaints. For example, if the person complains of morning lethargy or experiences cognitive changes, the nurse can inquire about the use of medications with anticholinergic properties, including OTC products (e.g. diphenhydramine). Information about changes in health-related behaviours can also shed light on current problems, such as the recurrence of symptoms that once were controlled by medications. For example, if an insulin-dependent diabetic stopped smoking, it is important to consider whether the dose of insulin needs to be decreased. Recent medication-taking behaviours also may account for health problems that are residual or latent adverse medication effects. A common example of a residual adverse effect is the onset of diarrhoea after a course of antibiotics.

Second, nurses use the overall health assessment as a base of information to determine the expected and actual outcomes of medications. These outcomes are evaluated through subjective and objective assessment information. For example, analgesic effectiveness is measured according to the reported level of pain relief, and the effectiveness of antihypertensive medications is judged according to lowered blood pressure readings.

Third, the overall assessment, including any functional aspects, helps to anwser the question "Can the person or carers safely and effectively administer medications?" This complex question involves an assessment of all aspects of medication-taking behaviours, as described in the sections on age-related changes and risk factors. The environment also should be assessed in relation to certain conditions, such as the accessibility of water and the availability of a refrigerator (if necessary for medication storage) that can affect medication-taking behaviours. The overall assessment also might provide information about financial limitations, mobility or transportation problems that interfere with obtaining medications.

Fourth, if the home environment can be observed as part of the overall assessment, important clues to health problems and medication-taking behaviours may be disclosed. For example, observing that glyceryl trinitrate is stored on a sunny window sill may explain why the medication is not effective in relieving angina. An assessment of the home environment may lead to additional pertinent information. For example, when the nurse observes OTC preparations and remedies in the home, he or she also has the opportunity to ask about the use of these items.

Finally, the overall health assessment serves as the basis for identifying many factors that can increase the risk for non-adherence, altered therapeutic effects and adverse medication effects. For example, the nursing assessment of the older adult's cognitive abilities and abilities to perform daily activities provides valuable information about factors that can significantly influence medication-taking behaviours. Similarly, the nursing assessment of depression and other psychosocial aspects of functioning can provide important information about motivational and behavioural factors that can influence medication-taking behaviours.

Identifying adverse medication effects

The first, and sometimes most difficult, step in alleviating adverse medication effects is to recognise their existence. Because many adverse effects are subtle and superimposed on one or more symptoms of illness, they may be attributed to pathological conditions rather than to the treatment of the condition.

Nurses often are the first to recognise adverse medication effects because they generally spend more time with the person than do medical practitioners. Nurses also are more attentive to long-term monitoring of changes in day-to-day function, in contrast to the medical practitioner's focus on acute illness. Especially in long-term residential care and home settings, the nurse is the health professional most likely to notice subtle changes in function that may be attributable to adverse medication effects.

Medical practitioners may hesitate to discuss adverse medication effects with older people for any of the following reasons: (1) they may be uncertain about the potential adverse effects of a prescribed drug, especially when newer medications are prescribed; (2) they may assume that the power of suggesting possible adverse effects will become a self-fulfilling prophecy; or (3) they may fear that the older person will choose not to take the medication. The nurse can serve as an "interpreter" between the prescribing practitioner and the person by emphasising the medication's benefits as well as pointing out the problems that are most likely to arise. The nurse also can provide health education about ways to avoid adverse effects. For example, if a medication is likely to cause stomach irritation, taking the medication after meals or with milk may prevent this effect. Nurses do not automatically initiate a discussion of all the potential adverse effects of a medication, but when a change in health status is potentially related to adverse medication effects, nurses can raise that possibility.

Changes in cognition are a potentially devastating adverse medication effect that is often overlooked as such, especially when it is superimposed on existing dementia. Medication induced mental status changes (e.g. confusion, lethargy, depression or agitation) can be sudden and obvious or subtle and gradual. For example, delirium or hallucinations usually are very obvious, but they may be attributed mistakenly to pathological processes rather than to medication effects. Thus, whenever an older person experiences an alteration in mental status, medication intake must be assessed carefully. Besides considering all prescription drugs, alcohol and OTC medications (especially those with anticholinergic agents) must be considered as potential contributing factors.

When medications are a potential cause of altered mental status, consideration must be given to discontinuing or lowering the dose of the medication. Assessment also addresses the possibility that the altered mental state interferes with proper dosing (e.g. when memory impairment contributes to overdosing or under-dosing). Another aspect of assessing the relationship between cognitive changes and medications is to recognise that it may take days or even months after discontinuation of the medication before cognition returns to baseline. The resolution time depends on the particular medication involved, the length of time it was consumed and the person's general health status.

NURSING ISSUES

When the nursing assessment identifies factors that interfere with safe and accurate self-medication administration (e.g. cognitive or functional impairments affecting medication-taking ability), an applicable issue would be ineffective self-administration of medication. Related factors that might be identified include complex medication regimens, inadequate social supports, adverse effects of medication, lack of money or transportation and lack of understanding of instructions. The nursing issue of non-adherence may be appropriate in some situations, but nurses need to be sure it is not associated with a judgemental attitude on the part of the healthcare provider.

If the nursing assessment identifies adverse effects of medications, particularly those that affect one's safety or quality of life, the nurse might address the issue that is specific to the adverse effect. Examples of these include confusion, constipation, urinary incontinence, imbalanced nutrition, impaired memory, ineffective thermoregulation, sleep pattern disturbance and risk for falls because of medication-related falls and postural hypotension. These nursing issues are discussed in other chapters of this text.

WELLNESS OPPORTUNITY

Nurses can use the wellness nursing issue of readiness for enhanced self-health management when caring for older adults who are interested in addressing potential adverse effects.

GOAL PLANNING FOR WELLNESS OUTCOMES

Wellness outcomes pertinent to medications and older adults include adherence to therapeutic regimens and identification and prevention of adverse effects. Specific outcomes could include: improved adherence behaviour or health-promoting behaviours, improved knowledge about medication, improved medication response and improved self-administration of non-parenteral medication.

WELLNESS OPPORTUNITY

Participation in healthcare decisions is an outcome that is applicable when nurses empower older adults to make responsible decisions about the use of OTC products such as herbs and medications.

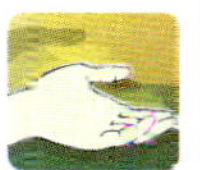

NURSING INTERVENTIONS TO PROMOTE SAFE AND EFFECTIVE MEDICATION MANAGEMENT

Promoting safe and effective medication-taking patterns in older adults is multidimensional and depends on coordinated efforts from several healthcare providers, including nurses, pharmacists and prescribing practitioners. In community settings, nurses have major roles in teaching older adults about medications and identifying interventions to support adherence to the therapeutic regimen. In all settings, nurses have major roles in preventing and identifying adverse effects. Evidence-based practice 8-1 summarises a protocol for reducing adverse drug events developed by Zwicker and Fulmer (2012). The following sections describe practical interventions that nurses can use to promote adherence, prevent adverse effects and encourage safe and effective medication-taking behaviours in older adults.

EVIDENCE-BASED PRACTICE 8-1
Reducing adverse drug events

Statement of the problem

- About 35% of older adults experience adverse drug events, with almost half of these being preventable
- Reasons for medication-related problems are: age-related physiological changes that alter the pharmacokinetics and pharmacodynamics, polypharmacy, incorrect doses of medications, inappropriate prescribing practices (e.g. the use of medications to treat symptoms that are not disease specific), adverse drug reactions and interactions, non-adherence and medication errors

Recommendations for nursing assessment

- A comprehensive medication assessment includes all the following: thorough drug history, focused questions about nicotine, alcohol, vitamins, herbs, folk remedies and all non-prescription products
- Use assessment tools to (1) evaluate ability to self-administer medications, (2) identify potential inappropriate medications and drug–drug or drug–disease interactions, (3) assess renal function (Cockroft-Gault Formula)
- Consider age-related changes in pharmacokinetics and pharmacodynamics: absorption, distribution, metabolism, clearance
- Assessment strategies: brown bag method, medication reconciliation process
  - Identify medications associated with high risk for adverse drug reactions using the Beers Criteria
  - Identify the older adult's characteristics associated with potential adverse medication effects, such as dementia, polypharmacy, renal insufficiency, multiple chronic conditions
  - Identify potential interactions with other prescriptions and with all non-prescription product.

Nursing interventions for reducing adverse drug events during and after hospitalisation

- Empower people by providing information and involving them in decisions
- Collaborate with interdisciplinary team for the following interventions: discontinuing unnecessary drugs, using safer drugs, optimising the regimen, avoiding the prescribing cascade, avoiding inappropriate medications, and using non-pharmacological approaches for symptoms
- Consider any new symptoms as a possible adverse medication effect
- Follow the prescribing principle of "start low and go slow"

Nursing interventions for reducing adverse drug events at discharge

- Use medication reconciliation during transitions in care
- Assess the person's abilities and limitations with regard to self-administration of medications
- Address adherence issues that are likely to occur
- Provide older adult and carer education about safe and effective medication management

Source: Zwicker, D. E. & Fulmer T. (2012). Reducing adverse drug events. In M. Boltz, E. Capezuti, T. Fulmer & D. Zwicker (Eds), *Evidence-based geriatric nursing protocols for best practice* (4th ed., pp. 324–362). New York: Springer.

Medication reconciliation is an evidence-based intervention that has been widely implemented in healthcare settings. Medication reconciliation is the process of identifying a person's medication errors, such as omissions, duplications, dosing errors or drug interactions during transitions in care. The three steps involved in the process are as follows: (1) verification by collecting an accurate list; (2) clarification of questions about drugs, doses, frequency and other pertinent information; and (3) reconciliation of any discrepancies or concerns by communicating with prescribing practitioners. This process is warranted because studies show that half of those hospitalised have at least one medication discrepancy on admission and that almost one-quarter experience an adverse drug event after discharge, most of which could be prevented through better communication (Cua & Kripalani, 2008). Although the initial focus of medication reconciliation was on hospital admissions and discharges, it is imperative that this process be done during any transition, even within the same facility. Important nursing interventions for a successful medication reconciliation have been described by Pincus (2013) as follows:

- Determine who administers medications.
- View all the medications.
- Be aware of medications that are commonly implicated in discrepancies (e.g. as-needed medications, medications used prophylactically during hospitalisation).
- Address the ability to get prescriptions filled.
- Address issues that affect adherence (e.g. administration difficulties).
- Allow the person to ask questions.

Clinical tools and additional information about medication reconciliation protocols are available in the resources section at the end of this chapter.

Teaching about medications and herbs

Medications are safest and most therapeutic when they are taken as prescribed and when the regimen is periodically re-evaluated for maximum effectiveness and minimal risk of adverse reactions. An effective way to initiate health education about medications is to have the person write a list of all medications and OTC agents taken and to include a history of medication allergies and adverse effects. Emphasise that this information should be available to healthcare practitioners during all interactions because it is essential that all practitioners keep track of the person's medications. This list is especially important when more than one healthcare practitioner is involved. Nurses should explain that a medication list facilitates communication and reminds the healthcare practitioner periodically to re-evaluate the medication regimen.

It is imperative to discuss each medication on the list and provide appropriate information based on assessment of the person's knowledge and understanding. Morrow and Conner-Garcia (2013) have summarised the following recommendations for communicating with older adults about medications:

- Use concrete, active and direct language with emphasis on how the medication helps the person.
- Use education materials that are concrete, matched to the person's needs, and reinforced with graphics.
- Explore the person's concerns by empathic listening.
- Verify understanding by using "teachback" techniques, such as asking older adults to state information in their own words or having them demonstrate how they can organise their medications.

Because older adults may be reluctant to question their healthcare practitioners, nurses can suggest pertinent questions for discussion with prescribing practitioners. In addition, nurses can teach older adults and their carers about obtaining medication-related information from knowledgeable sources, such as pharmacists. People need to understand that prescribing practitioners are skilled in diagnosing illnesses and deciding the most appropriate interventions, and that pharmacists are the healthcare practitioners who are most knowledgeable about the specific actions and interactions of medications. Nurses can use Box 8-6 to teach older adults about which medication questions are best answered by prescribing practitioners and which are best addressed by pharmacists.

Because good communication skills are essential to obtaining answers to the questions listed in Box 8-6, nurses can suggest ways of communicating effectively with pharmacists and other healthcare practitioners. For example, nurses can help older adults develop a list of questions about specific medications they can discuss with pharmacists or healthcare practitioners. In home settings, nurses can serve as role models of appropriate communication by calling the pharmacist or prescribing practitioner to discuss medications in the presence of the older adult or carer.

In Australia, information on registered products and adverse events is available for consumers and health professionals through the Therapeutic Goods Register at www.tga.gov.au. Information for older adults and health professionals in New Zealand can be obtained from the Medicines and Medical Devices Safety Authority (MedSafe) via www.medsafe.govt.nz.

WELLNESS OPPORTUNITY

Nurses find opportunities to empower older adults by teaching them effective ways of communicating with healthcare providers so that they can knowledgeably observe for therapeutic and adverse medication effects.

As discussed in the nursing assessment section, nurses need to ask about the use of herbs and other bioactive substances so they can observe for and teach about interactions and adverse effects, when appropriate. Although information about the use of complementary and alternative

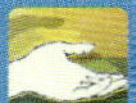

BOX 8-6
Tips on safe and effective medication use

Carry an up-to-date list of all your medications, including herbs and OTC preparations, and show the list to your medical practitioner(s).

When your medical practitioner suggests a medication, ask if there is any way to take care of the problem without medication.

Ask your medical practitioner the following questions about each new, regularly scheduled medication:

- What is the reason for taking the medication?
- How will I know if it's doing what it's meant to do?
- How soon can I expect to feel the beneficial effects?
- What will happen if I don't take it?
- How often am I supposed to take it?
- How long should I continue taking it?
- What should I do if I miss a dose?
- When will you want to see me again, and what will you want me to tell you so that you can determine whether the medication is effective?

Ask your medical practitioner the following questions at follow-up visits:

- Do I still need to take this medication?
- Can the dosage be reduced?

Ask your medical practitioner the following questions about each medication that is prescribed on an "as needed" (PRN) basis:

- What is the reason for taking the medication, and how should I determine whether I need the medication?
- How often can I take it? Is there a range of frequency?
- What is the maximum dose I can take within 24 hours?
- What should I do if the medication does not relieve the symptoms (e.g. if chest pain continues after taking several glyceryl trinitrate tablets)?

Ask your pharmacist the following questions:

- What are the generic and brand names for this medication?
- Is it likely to interact with the other medications I'm taking?
- Is it likely to interact with herbs, cigarettes, alcohol or any nutrient?
- What is the best time of day to take it?
- Does it matter if I take it before or after meals?
- Are there any side effects I should watch for?
- Is there anything I can do to minimise the risk of side effects (e.g. taking the medication with milk or meals to reduce stomach irritation)?
- Is there anything I should avoid while I'm taking this medication (e.g. milk, certain foods, driving)?
- Are there any special instructions for storing this medication?

therapies needs to be an integral part of the assessment, nurses cannot know all the details about these products. At a minimum, however, they need to know how to teach about these remedies, just as they teach about pharmacological and medical interventions. Nurses can use Box 8-7 as a tool to teach older adults about general precautions for the use of herbs and homeopathic remedies, such as being aware of potential interactions and adverse effects and making sure that all healthcare practitioners are aware of all OTC products that are used.

Another important nursing role—and a way of promoting personal responsibility—is teaching older adults

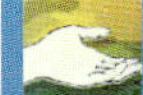

BOX 8-7
Tips on the use of herbs and homeopathic remedies

- Before treating any symptom with a non-prescription product, make sure you are not overlooking a condition that requires medical attention.
- Discuss the use of any non-prescription product with your medical provider(s).
- Be cautious about substituting herbs or any OTC product for prescribed medications.
- Seek information from objective sources and check any warnings on the label or package.
- Observe for beneficial and harmful effects.
- Report any possible side effects to your medical provider for evaluation.
- Introduce only one new substance at a time.
- Start with a low dose and increase the dose gradually.
- Doses may need to be lowered when combining two or more herbs or a herb and a medication.
- Some herbs are only for short-term use.
- Some herbs need to be taken for 1–3 months before effects are noticed (e.g. ginkgo biloba, St John's wort).
- Herbs can interact with all of the following: other herbs, food, beverages, caffeine, nutrients, prescription medications, and OTC medications.
- Some herbs are contraindicated in people with the following conditions: stroke, glaucoma, diabetes, hypertension, heart disease, thyroid disorder, and any bleeding disorder or condition requiring anticoagulation.
- Some herbs are most effective when they are taken on an empty stomach.
- Many herbs can cause gastrointestinal effects (e.g. anorexia, nausea, diarrhoea).
- Some herbs, especially those that are applied externally, can cause skin rashes.
- Herbs can cause allergic reactions.
- Some herbs are extremely toxic, or fatal, if ingested.
- A few herbs, or ingredients in herbs, can be toxic when taken in large doses or for a long time (e.g. Oregon grape, used for prostatitis, may cause heart failure).
- A few herbs are thought to be carcinogenic.
- Herbs that are used for anxiety or insomnia should not be taken before driving a car.
- Be sceptical about exaggerated claims; if it sounds too good to be true, it probably is!

and carers about reliable sources of information on which they can base decisions. For example, the U.S. National Institutes of Health established the National Center for Complementary and Integrative Health to fund research and provide evidence-based information about herbs.

Addressing factors that affect adherence

When older adults have trouble adhering to their medication regimen, nurses can work with them and their carers to identify ways to improve adherence. For example, unit-dose medication systems, which have been widely used in institutional settings, are becoming more available for use in home settings and may be helpful in improving medication adherence, especially when medication regimens are complex. A variety of simple "pill organisers" (i.e. containers with separate compartments designated for each day of the week and with one or more compartments for each day) are widely available in stores. In addition, more sophisticated devices to enhance independence and improve adherence are available and may be particularly helpful for people with cognitive or functional impairments. For example, human voice recordings, telephone–computer services and beeping watches or key chains can be used to remind the person to take medications at designated times. Medication-dispensing systems, which can be filled monthly and programmed to dispense medications at specific times, also are available. Internet sites that provide information about these more technologically advanced systems are listed in the resources section. Nurses can encourage older adults and their carers to investigate different types of devices and systems (such as those depicted in Figure 8-1) that can be used to improve medication adherence.

WELLNESS OPPORTUNITY

Nurses promote self-responsibility by addressing factors that interfere with adherence and, at the same time, supporting independence.

Even with the increased availability of prescription-drug benefits from the government, older adults and people with chronic conditions are burdened by the high and increasing cost of prescription medications. Nurses often need to address financial barriers that affect adherence to medication regimens because even a person who has an adequate income may decide that a medication is not worth the high cost, especially on an ongoing basis. Many of the newer medications are developed because they are safer or more effective than older medications; however, they usually are more expensive. Nurses can encourage older adults to be candid with their medical practitioners and ask about the availability of less costly but equally safe and effective medications.

One way of addressing high costs is to use **generic medications**, which are regulated by the TGA (Australia) and Pharmac (New Zealand). Generic medications are required to be bioequivalent (i.e. identical) to their brand-name counterparts in their dosage form, safety, purity, strength, quality, intended use, performance characteristics and route of administration. Generic drugs can be manufactured when the patent on a brand name drug expires; they become more widely available as patents

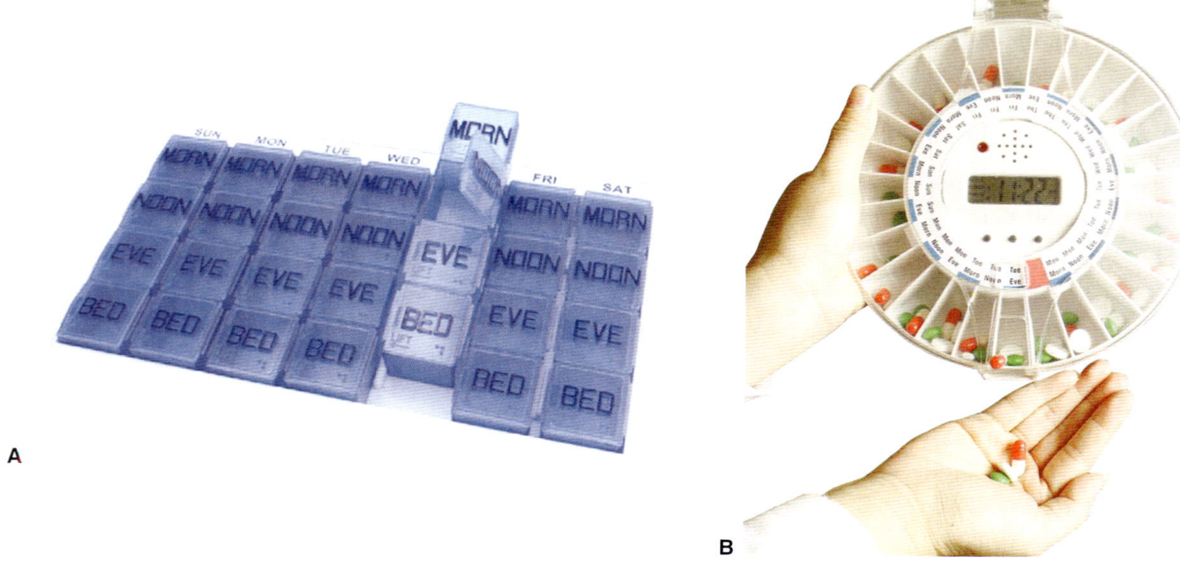

FIGURE 8-1 Examples of devices and systems designed to improve medication adherence and independence. (**A**) One of the many types of simple pill organisers available in stores. (**B**) An automatic pill dispenser with a tamper-proof locking system and an audible alarm, with 28 compartments that can be programmed for taking medications up to four times a day. (Figures A & B courtesy of ActiveForever.com.)

expire. In addition to the major cost savings of generic drugs, another important advantage is that they have a long track record of being used, so there is much information about therapeutic and adverse effects and interactions with other medicines.

In recent years, questions have been raised about the clinical equivalence of generic versus brand-name drugs, particularly with regard to those with narrow therapeutic ranges. A systematic review of 47 studies—including 38 randomised, controlled trials—confirmed that generic drugs are as safe and effective as brand-name drugs (Kesselheim et al., 2008). Studies also have confirmed that approved bioequivalence standards assure that generic drugs are therapeutically equivalent to the brand-name counterparts. Nurses can use this evidence-based information to encourage older adults to ask their prescribing practitioners about generic drugs that are appropriate for treating their conditions.

Decreasing the number of medications

Because the chance of adverse medication effects increases in proportion to the number of medications consumed, a key intervention is to decrease the number of medications to as few as possible. This intervention is important not only for preventing adverse effects but also for improving adherence (Banning, 2009). Nurses accomplish this by coordinating the efforts of the prescriber(s) to discontinue duplicate medications or medications that are no longer appropriate, and by educating the older person about the judicious use of medications that are not medically necessary. In community-based settings, nurses can teach older adults to review their medications with their medical practitioners at every visit. In community settings and long-term residential care facilities, nurses can assure that medication regimens are reviewed at least every 3 months and whenever there is a change in the person's condition. In any setting, nurses have many opportunities to raise questions about medication regimens and to communicate with prescribing practitioners about medications.

When older adults are admitted to hospital, they often are under the care of medical practitioners who were not the ones who prescribed the medications taken before the admission. Nurses usually obtain the medication history and the prescribing practitioner may automatically order the medications that are listed on the admission assessment. Because the hospital admission is an ideal time to re-evaluate the safety, efficacy and necessity of medications, nurses should ask older adults or their carers about the purpose and potential adverse effects of each medication. This assessment, which should be done with the medication reconciliation process, may provide important clues to medications or interactions that contributed to or directly caused the problem for which the person is hospitalised.

When medications are prescribed for behavioural reasons rather than for a medical condition, nurses can teach older adults and their carers about these medications and about non-pharmacological alternatives. For example, carers of people with dementia may use medications to address behaviours that might respond equally well to non-pharmacological interventions that do not have any risk of adverse effects. Once these medications are prescribed, they are likely to be used over long periods without re-evaluation. Nurses need to recognise that the efficacy may diminish (e.g. with hypnotics), the underlying reason may resolve or change (e.g. with situational anxiety) and adverse effects may develop gradually and not be recognised (e.g. with anticholinergic agents). Thus, it is imperative to review periodically all medications and to consider whether non-pharmacological approaches could be used to address the symptoms or behaviours. Behavioural problems are one example of the types of symptoms that can be managed medically, but might be managed just as well and with fewer risks, through non-pharmacological interventions. Other types of problems that can often be managed without pharmacological agents are those related to sleep, comfort, anxiety and chronic illnesses.

In community settings, it is important to make sure older adults and carers understand the appropriate use of medications that are prescribed as needed (i.e. PRN). For example, a carer of someone with dementia may be instructed to give a behaviour-modifying medication when the person becomes agitated. Although the episodes of agitation may be precipitated by environmental factors (e.g. noise or overstimulation), the carer might not realise that non-pharmacological interventions could be equally effective and carry no risk of adverse effects. In contrast to this situation, a carer may withhold medications that could improve the quality of life for the older person and for himself or herself because of misunderstandings or lack of information about the appropriate use of medications. Nurses can teach carers about non-pharmacological interventions, as well as the appropriate use of medications for behaviour management, particularly for people with dementia (discussed in Chapter 14).

In institutional settings, nurses must establish clear criteria for administering medications for behaviour management. These criteria must be based primarily on the person's needs, rather than those of the staff. As the staff members provide around-the-clock care, non-pharmacological interventions are prioritised rather than immediately turning to the use of medications.

WELLNESS OPPORTUNITY

Nurses promote wellness by talking with older adults and their carers when appropriate about choosing interventions such as relaxation techniques that can improve health and quality of life, rather than using medications.

CASE STUDY

Mrs Murray, who is 76 years old, is being discharged to her home after rehabilitation after a stroke. Residual problems from the stroke include left-sided weakness and visual–perceptual difficulties. In addition to the stroke, Mrs Murray's diagnoses include glaucoma, depression and congestive heart failure. Her medications include the following: multivitamin, one tablet daily; frusemide, 20 mg, two tablets daily; ecotrin aspirin, 81 mg daily; clopidogrel, 75 mg daily; diltiazem, 60 mg, three times daily; metoprolol tartrate, 50 mg twice daily; simvastatin, 40 mg at bedtime; sertraline, 50 mg at bedtime; and timolol, 0.25% twice daily. The hospital regimen for administering the medications is as follows:

7.30 a.m.:	Diltiazem hydrochloride 60 mg Frusemide 20 mg, 2 tablets Ecotrin asprin 81 mg Timolol, 0.25% in each eye
9.00 a.m.:	Metoprolol tartrate 50 mg
1.00 p.m.:	Multivitamin, 1 tablet Diltiazem hydrochloride 60 mg
3.30 p.m.:	Frusemide 20 mg, 2 tablets
7.30 p.m.:	Timolol, 0.25% in each eye Diltiazem hydrochloride 60 mg Clopidogrel 75 mg
9.00 p.m.:	Metoprolol tartrate 50 mg Sertraline 50 mg Simvastatin 40 mg daily

Nursing assessment

Your assessment reveals that, before her hospitalisation, Mrs Murray administered her medications independently, but the only medications she took were the eye drops, frusemide (20 mg once daily), and digoxin, which she is no longer taking. The functional assessment indicates that Mrs Murray has weakness and limited use of her left arm and hand, causing difficulty performing tasks that require fine motor movements. She has full use of her right upper extremity, and she is right-hand dominant. She ambulates independently, but slowly, with a walker. A cognitive assessment reveals that Mrs Murray is alert, oriented, and has no memory deficits; however, her abstract thinking and time perception have been impaired by the stroke. She has some expressive aphasia, but she seems to understand instructions, especially if ideas are reinforced by using concrete examples and demonstrations.

Mrs Murray expresses motivation to take her medications, but she admits to being overwhelmed by the complexity of the regimen, stating that at the hospital, they administered her medications at six different times. She is also concerned about self-administering her eye drops because she used to use her left hand to hold her eyelids open. With regard to frusemide, she says she does not like taking it twice a day because it makes her go to the bathroom too much. While at hospital, she has not had any trouble with incontinence, but she worries about what she'll do at home because there is no bathroom on the first floor. She asks whether she can take the entire dose of frusemide at night so that she will only have to get up during the night to go to the bathroom, which is located near the bedroom.

In response to your questions about medication management routines before her stroke, Mrs Murray reports using a compartmentalised medication container and taking her two medications and the eye drops after breakfast, around 9.00 a.m. She would administer the second dose of eye drops around 9.30 p.m., before getting ready for bed. She had no difficulty remembering the medications because she kept the pill container and one bottle of eye drops near the toaster, and she kept a second bottle of eye drops on her nightstand. Now, however, she expresses concern about the number of times she must take medications if the regimen remains the same as in the hospital, and she thinks she will need six pill containers but is not sure where she should put all of them. Mrs Murray also tells you that she is worried about paying for so many medications. She was taking only two generic medications and eye drops. Now that she is on so many new pills—and she knows that this will be more expensive—she needs to have her prescription drug plan reviewed and perhaps changed.

Mrs Murray lives with her husband, who is physically healthy but he has early-stage Alzheimer's disease. Their daughter lives nearby and visits two or three times weekly to assist with grocery shopping, laundry and household chores. She also provides transportation to stores and appointments.

Nursing issues

You decide on a nursing issue of non-adherence because Mrs Murray expresses a desire to take her medications, but several factors deter adherence to the current regimen. Related factors include functional impairments, complex medication regimens, negative side effects of frusemide, and concern about the cost of medications.

Nursing care plan for Mrs Murray

Goals for wellness outcomes	Nursing interventions	Nursing evaluation
Mrs Murray's medication routine will be simplified.	• Work with the pharmacist and the medical practitioner to simplify the medication regimen. • Discuss with Mrs Murray's medical practitioner the problem of the complexity of the regimen and the cost of medications. Ask Mrs Murray's medical practitioner if she can take diltiazem hydrochloride CD, 180 mg daily, rather than diltiazem hydrochloride, 60 mg, three times a day. (This will be less expensive and will eliminate two doses of medication daily.) • Ask the pharmacist about combining medications to allow twice-daily administration. • Assist Mrs Murray in establishing a routine for self-administering medications that will fit in with her usual activities. • At least 3 days before discharge from the hospital, arrange for Mrs Murray to assume responsibility for her own medication management, using pill containers that she herself fills.	• Mrs Murray follows a twice-daily medication dosing schedule.
Mrs Murray's concerns about frusemide will be addressed.	• Explain the importance of taking frusemide, as ordered, to control congestive heart failure effectively. • Suggest that Mrs Murray obtain a portable commode for use downstairs during the day.	• Mrs Murray takes frusemide as directed and does not experience any difficulty with urinary incontinence.
Mrs Murray's concerns about the cost of medications will be addressed.	• Encourage Mrs Murray to talk with her medical practitioner about her concerns over the cost of the prescribed medications. • Suggest that Mrs Murray talk with her usual pharmacist about her current prescription drug plan and ask if there might be a better plan for her.	• Mrs Murray is able to afford her prescribed medications.
A system for self-administering eye drops will be identified.	• Evaluate Mrs Murray's ability to self-administer her eye drops and to identify any assistive devices that might increase her independence and reliability in performing this task. • Have Mrs Murray practise self-administering her eye drops before she is discharged from the hospital, with staff providing whatever assistance is necessary. • Talk with Mrs Murray about the possibility of her husband assisting with the eye drop procedure if she is unable to do this independently. • Ask Mrs Murray's ophthalmologist whether the eye drop regimen can be simplified to once-daily dosing by prescribing an extended-action eye drop formula.	• Mrs Murray self-administers her eye drops or receives the assistance she needs for eye drop administration from her husband.

Thinking points

- What are the factors that influence Mrs Murray's ability to manage her medications independently?
- What additional assessment information would be helpful in establishing a plan for Mrs Murray to manage her medications independently?
- What health education would you provide to address Mrs Murray's concerns about the cost of her medications?
- What steps would you take to ensure that expected outcomes are achieved after Mrs Murray is back in her own home?

EVALUATING THE EFFECTIVENESS OF NURSING INTERVENTIONS

Nurses evaluate interventions related to medication management according to the degree to which the older adult follows a safe and effective medication regimen. This process involves an evaluation of medication-taking behaviours as well as an evaluation of the therapeutic effects of the medication. Another evaluation criterion is the extent to which negative functional consequences, such as interactions and adverse effects, are prevented, alleviated or controlled. In home settings, nurses can evaluate the effectiveness of their interventions by observing the medication-taking patterns of the older adult. In any setting, nurses can evaluate the knowledge of safe and effective use of prescription and OTC medications. Another measure of effectiveness is the degree to which barriers to adherence are eliminated or addressed.

CHAPTER HIGHLIGHTS

Introduction to medicines

- Effects of medicines in the body in relation to pharmacokinetics and pharmacodynamics
- Herbs and medications with similar bioactivity (Table 8-1)
- Potential adverse effects of herbs (Table 8-2)
- Herbs commonly used by older adults: uses, actions and precautions (Table 8-3)
- Homeopathic remedies

Age-related changes that affect medicines in older adults

- Decreased clearance due to changes in the kidneys and liver (Box 8-1)
- Metabolism by the cytochrome P-450 system
- Effects of changes in body composition (Box 8-1)
- Medications affected by serum albumin levels
- Effects of changes in receptor sensitivity (Box 8-1)
- Changes that affect medication-taking behaviours

Risk factors that affect medicines

- Pathological processes and functional impairments (e.g. medication–disease interactions, effects on the ability to take substances)
- Behaviours based on myths and misunderstandings (attitudes about and expectations for medicines)
- Communication barriers between older adults and prescribing medical practitioners
- Lack of information
- Inappropriate prescribing practices (Beers Criteria)
- Polypharmacy and inadequate monitoring
- Medication non-adherence
- Financial concerns related to prescription drugs
- Insufficient recognition of adverse effects (Table 8-4)

Medication interactions

- Medication–herb interactions (Table 8-3)
- Medication–medication interactions (Table 8-5)
- Medications and nutrients (Table 8-6)
- Medications and alcohol (Table 8-7)
- Medications and nicotine (Table 8-8)

Functional consequences associated with medicines in older adults

- Altered therapeutic effects
- Increased potential for adverse effects (Box 8-3)
- Adverse effects of anticholinergic medications (Box 8-4)
- Increased potential for altered mental status (Table 8-9)
- Increased potential for tardive dyskinesia

Nursing assessment of medication use and effects

- Communication techniques for obtaining accurate information (open-ended, non-judgemental)
- Scope of a medication assessment (all medicines, older adult's understanding of regimen, preferences) (Box 8-5)
- Cultural considerations (e.g. factors that influence medication-taking behaviours, culturally specific healthcare sources and practices) (Cultural considerations 8-1 & 8-2)
- Patterns of medication use
- Medication assessment as it relates to the overall assessment
- Factors in identifying adverse medication effects

Nursing issues

- Ineffective self-administration of medicines
- Instrumental self-care deficit: medication management
- Non-adherence
- Willingness for enhanced self-administration medication management

Goal planning for wellness outcomes

- Improved knowledge about medication
- Improved self-care management of non-parenteral medication
- Adherence behaviour

Nursing interventions to promote healthy medication-taking patterns

- Implementing evidence-based interventions (Evidence-based practice 8-1)
- Teaching about medications (Box 8-6, teaching tool)
- Teaching about herbs and other alternative substances (Box 8-7, teaching tool)
- Addressing factors that affect adherence (Figure 8-1)
- Decreasing the number of medications

Evaluating effectiveness of nursing interventions

- Medication-taking behaviours that are safe and effective
- Prevention, alleviation or control of negative functional consequences (e.g. interactions, adverse effects)

CRITICAL THINKING EXERCISES

1. You are asked to give a half-hour presentation on "Medications and Ageing" to a local senior citizens group. Describe the following:
   - What points would you cover about age-related changes?
   - How would you address the risk factors that affect medication action and medication-taking behaviours?
   - What tips would you give about taking medications?
   - What educational materials would you use?
   - How would you involve the group participants in the discussion?
2. Carefully read the interview questions in Box 8-5 and decide which questions you would use and how you would phrase the questions in your own words for each of the following situations:
   - You are doing an admission interview for a 78-year-old man who lives alone and has been admitted to the hospital for the third time in 3 months for congestive heart failure.
   - You are a community nurse visiting a recently discharged 82-year-old woman from hospital to monitor her blood pressure. You note there are lots of medications and herbal preparations placed haphazardly over the kitchen bench.
3. Carefully read the information in Boxes 8-6 and 8-7 and describe what information you would be likely to use in the following situations:
   - Discharge planning for the 78-year-old man who is described in Exercise 2, bullet 1.
   - At home with the 82-year-old woman described in Exercise 2, bullet 2.

RESOURCES

For an extensive range of additional resources to enhance teaching and learning and to facilitate understanding of this chapter, please see the text's accompanying website located on thePoint at http://thepoint.lww.com.

Clinical tools

Hartford Institute for Geriatric Nursing, ConsultGeriRN.org: http://consultgerirn.org/resources

Assessment tools *Try This*® series and *How to Try This* resources

General assessment series:

- *How to Try This*, issue 16: Beers Criteria for Potentially Inappropriate Medication Use in the Elderly, by S. L. Molony. (2013). *Best Practices in Nursing Care to Older Adults.*

Select a protocol/topic—Medications:

- Zwicker, D. (2012). Geriatric nursing protocol: Reducing adverse drug events.
- Issue 16.1: Beers Criteria for Potentially Inappropriate Medication Use in Older Adults. Part I: 2002. Criteria Independent of Diagnoses or Conditions.
- Issue 16.2: Beers Criteria for Potentially Inappropriate Medication Use in Older Adults. Part II: 2002. Criteria Considering Diagnoses or Conditions.
- *How to Try This* (article): Monitoring medication use in older adults, by S. Molony. (2009). *American Journal of Nursing, 109*(1), 68–78.
- *How to Try This* (video): *The Beers Criteria for Potentially Inappropriate Medication Use in Older Adults.*

Evidence-based practice

Zwicker, D. (2012). Reducing adverse drug events. In M. Boltz, E. Capezuti, T. Fulmer & D. Zwicker (Eds), *Evidence-based geriatric nursing protocols for best practice* (4th ed., pp. 324–362). New York: Springer.

National Guideline Clearinghouse: www.guideline.gov

Search for:

- Medication management guideline (2006, revised 2012).
- Reducing adverse drug events in older adults (2008, revised 2012).
- Improving medication management for older adult clients (2008, revised 2012).
- Substance misuse and alcohol use disorders (2008, revised 2012).

Joanna Briggs Institute: http://connect.jbiconnectplus.org

Best practice information sheets:

- Crushing and altering medication: Aged care (2014).
- Strategies to reduce medication errors with reference to older adults (2009).

Evidence-based summaries:

- Chen, Z. (2013a). Complementary therapies (aromatherapy and herbal medicine): Clinician information.
- Chen, Z. (2013b). Complementary therapies (massage, naturopathy and acupuncture): Clinician information.
- Chen, Z. (2013c). Complementary therapies: Older adults
- Sayakkara, S. M. L. (2014). Altering/crushing medication.
- Yusof, N. M., Khalil, H. & McNamara, K. (2013). Deprescribing interventions: Reducing mortality among elderly patients.

Recommended practices:

- Campbell, J. (2013). Medication management in residential aged care: Self-administration.
- Medication oral administration (including blister packs and swallowing difficulties) (2013).
- Percutaneous endoscopic gastrostomy (PEG) in aged care: Medication administration (2014).

Health education

American Botanical Council: http://abc.herbalgram.org/site/PageServer

Australian Register of Therapeutic Goods: www.ebs.tga.gov.au (go to Public TGA Information)

Herb Research Foundation (USA): www.herbs.org

Māori health, New Zealand Ministry of Health: www.health.govt.nz/our-work/populations/maori-health

Medicines and Medical Devices Safety Authority (Medsafe), New Zealand: www.medsafe.govt.nz
National Center for Complementary and Integrative Health (NCCIH) (U.S.): https://nccih.nih.gov
National Council on Aging (U.S.): www.ncoa.org
National Institute of Complementary Medicine (NICM) Australia: www.nicm.edu.au
New Zealand Natural Medicine Association (NZNMA): www.nznma.com
PHARMAC, Pharmaceutical Management Agency (New Zealand): www.pharmac.govt.nz
Therapeutic Goods Administration: www.tga.gov.au
WHO Traditional Medicine (TM) Strategy 2014–2023: http://apps.who.int/iris/bitstream/10665/92455/1/9789241506090_eng.pdf

REFERENCES

Allen, J. (2012). Avoiding overuse of antipsychotic medications. *Geriatric Nursing, 33*(4), 327–328.

Alvarez, M. V. G. & Evidente, V. G. H. (2008). Understanding drug-induced parkinsonism, separating pearls from oysters. *Neurology, 70*, e32–e34.

American Geriatrics Society. (2012a). Guiding principles for the care of older adults with multimorbidity. *Journal of the American Geriatrics Society, 60*(10), E1–E25.

American Geriatrics Society. (2012b). American Geriatrics Society Updated Beers Criteria for Potentially Inappropriate Medication Use in Older Adults. *Journal of the American Geriatrics Society, 60*(4), 616–631.

Anderson, J. K. & Fox, J. R. (2012). Potential food–drug interactions in long-term care. *Journal of Gerontological Nursing, 38*(4), 38–46.

Andrews, M. M. (2011). Cultural competence in health history and physical examination. In M. M. Andrews & J. S. Boyle (Eds), *Transcultural concepts in nursing care* (6th ed.). Philadelphia, PA: Lippincott Williams & Wilkins.

Australian Government Department of Health. (2015). 2015 PBS co-payment and safety net amounts. Viewed March 2015 at www.pbs.gov.au/info/news/2015/01/2015-pbs-co-payment-safety-net-amounts.

Banning, M. (2009). A review of interventions used to improve adherence to medication in older people. *International Journal of Nursing Studies, 46*(11), 1505–1515.

Barnett, S. R. (2009). Polypharmacy and perioperative medications in the elderly. *Anesthesiology Clinics, 27*, 377–389.

Beers, M. H., Oslander, J. G., Rollingher, J. et al. (1991). Explicit criteria for determining potentially inappropriate medications by the elderly. *Archives of Internal Medicine, 151*, 1825–1832.

Blackburn, D. F., Swidrovich, J. & Lemstra, M. (2013). Non-adherence in type 2 diabetes: Practical considerations for interpreting the literature. *Patient Preference and Adherence, 7*, 183–189.

Brandt, N. J. & Pyhtila, J. (2013). Psychopharmacological medication use among older adults with dementia in nursing homes. *Journal of Gerontological Nursing, 39*(4), 8–14.

Budnitz, D. S., Lovegrove, M. C., Shehab, N. & Chesley, C. L. (2011). Emergency hospitalizations for adverse drug events in older Americans. *New England Journal of Medicine, 365*, 2002–1012.

Cai, X., Campbell, N., Khan, B. et al. (2013). Long-term anticholinergic use and the aging brain. *Alzheimers Dementia, 9*(4), 377–385.

Cherniack, E. P., Ceron-Fuentes, J., Florez, H., Sandals, L, Rodriguzx, O. & Palacios, J. C. (2008). Influence of race and ethnicity on alternative medicine as a self-treatment preference for common medical conditions in a population of multi-ethnic urban elderly. *Complementary Therapies in Clinical Practice, 14*, 116–123.

Colloca, G., Tosato, M., Vetrano, D. L. et al. (2012). Inappropriate drugs in elderly patients with severe cognitive impairment: Results from the SHELTER Study. *PLoS One, 7*(1), e46669. Accessible via www.plosone.org.

Cooney, D. & Pascuzzi, K. (2009). Polypharmacy in the elderly: Focus on drug interactions and adherence in hypertension. *Clinical Geriatric Medicine, 25*, 221–233.

Cua, Y. M. & Kripalani, S. (2008). Medication use in the transition from hospital to home. *Annals of the Academy of Medicine, 37*(2), 136–141.

Dupouy, J., Moulis, G., Tubery, M. et al. (2013). Which adverse events are related to health care during hospitalization in elderly inpatients? *International Journal of Medical Sciences, 10*(9), 1224–1230.

Evans, D. B., McHugh, P., Shaw, J. & Wilson, C. (2008). Inpatients' use, understanding and attitudes towards traditional, complementary and alternative therapies at a provincial New Zealand hospital. *Journal of the New Zealand Medical Association, 121*(1278), 21–34.

Ferreira, M. P. & Weems, M. K. S. (2008). Alcohol consumption by aging adults in the United States: Health benefits and detriments. *Journal of the American Dietetic Association, 108*, 1668–1678.

Hanley, M. J., Cancalon, P., Widmer, W. et al. (2011). The effect of grapefruit juice on drug disposition. *Expert Opinion in Drug Metabolism & Toxicology, 7*(3), 267–286.

Hugtenburg, J. G., Timmers, L., Elders, P. et al. (2013). Definitions, variants, and causes of nonadherence with medication: A challenge for tailored interventions. *Patient Preference and Adherence, 13*(7), 675–682.

Izzo, A. A. (2012). Interactions between herbs and conventional drugs: Overview of the clinical data. *Medical Principles and Practice, 21*, 404–428.

Kashyap, M., Tu, M. & Tannenbaum, C. (2013). Prevalence of commonly prescribed medications potentially contributing to urinary symptoms in a cohort of older patients seeking care for incontinence. *BMC Geriatrics, 13*, 57. Viewed March 2015 at www.biomedcentral.com/1471-2318/13/57.

Kesselheim, A. S., Misono, A. S., Lee, J. L., Stedman, M. R., Brookhart, M. A., Choudhry, N. K. & Shrank, W. H. (2008). Clinical equivalence of generic and brand-name drugs used in cardiovascular disease: A systematic review and meta-analysis. *Journal of the American Medical Association, 300*(21), 2514–2526.

Le Couteur, D. G., McLachlan, A. J. & de Cabo, R. (2012). Aging, drugs, and drug metabolism. *Journals of Gerontology: Biological Sciences, 67*(2), 137–139.

Lee, W. K. T. (2013). Formulating medication adherence strategies using the PASSAction framework. *Canadian Pharmaceutical Journal, 146*(1), 30–32.

Lee, Y., Lin, P. Y., Chang, Y. Y. et al. (2013). Antidepressant-induced tardive syndrome: A retrospective epidemiological study. *Pharmacopsychiatry, 46*(7), 281–285.

Lemay, C. A., Mazor, K. M., Field, T. S. et al. (2013). Knowledge of and perceived need for evidence-based education about antipsychotic medications among nursing home leadership and staff. *Journal of the American Medical Directors Association, 14*(12), 895–900.

Little, M. O. & Morley, A. (2013). Reducing polypharmacy: Evidence from a simple quality improvement initiative. *Journal of the American Medical Directors Association, 14*, 152–156.

Maher, R. L., Hanlon, J. & Hajjar, E. R. (2013). Clinical consequences of polypharmacy in elderly. *Expert Opinion in Drug Safety, 13*(1), 57–65.

Marcum, Z. A. & Gellad, W. F. (2012). Medication adherence to multi-drug regimens. *Clinical Geriatric Medicine, 28*(2), 287–300.

Medical Council of New Zealand. (2010). *Best health outcomes for Pacific Peoples: Practice implications*. Wellington: Author. Available March 2015 via www.mcnz.org.nz.

Ministerial Advisory Committee on Complementary and Alternative Health (MACCAH). (2004). *Complementary and alternative medicine in New Zealand*. Wellington: Author. Accessible March 2015 via www.health.govt.nz/publication/complementary-and-alternative-health-care-new-zealand-0.

Molony, S. & Greenberg, S. A. (2013). The American Geriatrics Society Updated Beers Criteria for Potentially Inappropriate Medication Use in Older Adults. *Try This* series, issue 16 (revised 2013). *Best practices in nursing care to older adults*. Available March 2015 via www.consultgeriRN.org.

Morandi, A., Vasilevskis, E., Pandharipande, P. P. et al. (2013). Inappropriate medication prescriptions in elderly adults surviving and intensive care unit admission. *Journal of the American Geriatrics Society, 61*(7), 1128–1134.

Morgan, T. K., Williamson, M., Pirotta, M. et al. (2012). A national census of medicines use: A 24-hour snapshot of Australians aged 50 years and older. *Medical Journal of Australia, 196*(1), 50–53.

Morrow, D. G. & Conner-Garcia, T. (2013). Improving comprehension of medication information. *Journal of Gerontological Nursing, 39*(4), 22–29.

New Zealand Ministry of Health. (2011). Māori health and Rongoā Māori: Traditional Māori healing. Accessed March 2015 via www.health.govt.nz/our-work/populations/maorihealth.

O'Connor, M. N., Gallagher, P., Byrne, S. et al. (2012). Adverse drug reactions in older patients during hospitalisation: Are they predictable? *Age and Ageing, 41*(6), 771–776.

Obreli-Neto, P. R., Nobili, A., de Oliveira, B. A. et al. (2012). Adverse drug reactions caused by drug–drug interactions in elderly outpatients: A prospective study. *European Journal of Pharmacology, 68*(12), 1667–1676.

Pasina, L., Djade, C. D., Lucca, U. et al. (2013). Association of anticholinergic burden with cognitive and functional status in a cohort of hospitalized elderly. *Drugs & Aging, 30*(2), 103–112.

Pharmac. (2014). Costs of medicines. Accessed March 2015 www.pharmac.health.nz/medicines/medicines-information/costs-of-medicines.

Pincus, K. (2013). Transitional care management services. *Journal of Gerontological Nursing, 39*(10), 10–15.

Plotnikoff, G. A. (2010). Herbal medicines. In M. Snyder & R. Lindquist (Eds), *Complementary & alternative therapies in nursing* (6th ed., pp. 421–438). New York: Springer.

Purnell, L. D. (2014). *Guide to culturally competent care* (3rd ed.). Philadelphia, PA: F. A. Davis Co.

Puustinen, J., Nurminen, J., Vahlberg, T. et al. (2012). CNS medications as predictors of precipitous cognitive decline in the cognitively disabled aged: A longitudinal population-based study. *Dementia & Geriatric Cognitive Disorders, 2*, 57–68.

Resnick, B. & Fick, D. M. (2012). 2012 Beers Criteria update: How should practicing nurses use the criteria? *Geriatric Nursing, 33*(4), 253–255.

Riker, G. I. & Setter, S. M. (2012). Polypharmacy in older adults at home: What it is and what to do about it: Implications for home healthcare and hospice. *Home Healthcare Nurse, 30*(8), 474–485.

Schaffer, S. D., Yoon, S. & Zadezensky, I. (2009). A review of smoking cessation: Potentially risky effect on prescribed medications. *Journal of Clinical Nursing, 18*(11), 1533–1540.

Seitz, D. P., Gill, S. P., Herrmann, N. et al. (2013). Pharmacological treatment for neuropsychiatric symptoms of dementia in long-term care: A systematic review. *International Psychogeriatrics, 25*(2), 185–203.

Senft, D. J. (2012). Antipsychotic drug use: Understanding the recent attention and response to the increased scrutiny. *Geriatric Nursing, 33*(5), 387–390.

Shahid, S., Ryan Bleam, R., Bessarab, D. & Thompson, S. C. (2010). "If you don't believe it, it won't help you": Use of bush medicine in treating cancer among Aboriginal people in Western Australia. *Journal of Ethnobiology and Ethnomedicine, 6*(18), 1–9. Viewed March 2015 at www.biomedcentral.com/content/pdf/1746-4269-6-18.pdf.

Snyder, F. J., Dundas, M. L., Kirkpatrick, C. & Neill, K. S. (2009). Use and safety perceptions regarding herbal supplements: A study of older persons in southeast Idaho. *Journal of Nutrition for the Elderly, 28*(1), 81–95.

Stafford, A. C., Alswayan, M. S. & Tenni, P. C. (2010). Inappropriate prescribing in older residents of Australian care homes. *Journal of Clinical Pharmacy and Therapeutics, 36*, 33–44.

Steinberg, M. & Lyketsos, C. G. (2012). Atypical antipsychotic use in patients with dementia: Managing safety concerns. *American Journal of Psychiatry, 169*(9), 900–906.

Thanyi, B. & Treadwell, S. (2009). Drug induced parkinsonism: A common cause of parkinsonism in older people. *Postgraduate Medical Journal, 85*(1004), 322–326.

Tsai, H. H., Lin, H. W., Simon, P. A. et al. (2012). Evaluation of documented drug interactions and contraindications associated with herbs and dietary supplements: A systematic literature review. *International Journal of Clinical Practice, 66*(11), 1056–1078.

Uusvaara, J., Pitkala, K. H., Kautianen, H. et al. (2013). Detailed cognitive function and use of drugs with anticholinergic properties in older people: A community-based cross-sectional study. *Drugs & Aging, 30*(3), 177–182.

Vieira, M. & Huang, S.-M. (2012). Botanical-drug interactions: A scientific perspective. *Planta Medica, 78*, 1400–1415.

Waln, O. & Jankovic, J. (2013). An update on tardive dyskinesia: From phenomenology to treatment. *Tremor and other hyperkinetic movements*. Available March 2015 at http://tremorjournal.org/article/view/161.

World Health Organization (WHO). (2013). Traditional Medicine Strategy: 2014–2023. Geneva: Author. Viewed March 2015 at http://apps.who.int/iris/bitstream/10665/92455/1/9789241506090_eng.pdf.

Zwicker, D. & Fulmer, T. (2012). Reducing adverse drug events. In M. Boltz, E. Capezuti, T. Fulmer & D. Zwicker (Eds), *Evidence-based practice protocols for best practice* (4th ed., pp. 324–362). New York: Springer.

Chapter 9

Legal and ethical concerns relating to older adults

By Carol Miller and Sharyn Hunter

LEARNING OBJECTIVES

After reading this chapter, you should be able to:

1. Define the following terms: autonomy, competency and decision-making capacity.
2. Describe the following living wills/advance directives, not for resuscitation orders, Enduring Power of Attorney and Enduring Guardianship.
3. Discuss legal and ethical issues that nurses commonly address when caring for older adults.
4. Describe cultural considerations that affect autonomy, decision making and advance care directives.
5. Describe nursing responsibilities regarding advance care directives and decisions about care.

KEY POINTS

- advance care directives (ACD)
- advance care planning (ACP)
- advance directives
- artificial nutrition and hydration
- autonomy
- competency
- decision-making capacity
- Enduring Guardianship
- Enduring Power of Attorney
- executive control functions
- incompetent
- living wills
- not for resuscitation (NFR) order
- substitute decision maker
- surrogate
- values clarification

For several decades, various legislative efforts have addressed the rights of older adults and their quality of life. During the early 1980s, the state and federal governments in Australia and New Zealand began addressing issues related to vulnerable elders. In the late 1980s, legislative efforts focused on issues related to end-of-life decisions, the rights of patients and long-term care residents, and the quality of care provided. An area where nurses are commonly confronted by legal and ethical issues when caring for an older person relates to decision making. Although legislation can provide legal guidelines for issues with decision making, laws do not resolve ethical dilemmas that arise when no living will is provided, or when conflicts exist about how a living will should be interpreted or implemented. This chapter will review some of the pertinent legal and ethical issues that are relevant to the nursing care of older adults. Additional legal and ethical considerations regarding vulnerable or abused elders are addressed in Chapter 10.

AUTONOMY AND RIGHTS

Autonomy is the personal freedom to direct one's own life as long as it does not infringe on the rights of others. An autonomous person is capable of rational thought and is able to recognise the need for problem solving. The person can identify the problem, search for alternatives, and select a solution that allows their continued personal freedom, as long as it does not cause any harm to another's rights or property. People may be denied the right to autonomy if the outcome of their decisions or their lack of decision-making ability jeopardise their safety, or the rights, safety or property of others. Loss of autonomy and, therefore, loss of independence, is a very real fear among older adults. Moreover, for older adults with dementia and other conditions that affect decision-making abilities, loss of autonomy is a challenge frequently addressed by families and healthcare professionals throughout the course of the condition, which can last for many years.

Because autonomy is highly valued in many developed countries and there is no easy way to evaluate decision-making abilities—which can fluctuate from day to day—questions often arise about medical interventions and healthcare decisions. Therefore, nurses need to be familiar with legal and ethical guidelines related to competency and decision-making capacity. Nurses have a responsibility to assist older adults and their families, often as impartial mediators, when issues concerning personal autonomy arise. However, if the safety of the older person is threatened because of risky behaviours arising from impaired decision-making abilities, nurses must refer older people to the appropriate community agencies for further evaluation (see Chapter 10).

Competency

Competency is a legal term that refers to the ability to fulfil one's role and handle one's affairs in a responsible manner. All adults are presumed to be competent, and state laws designate an age of competency—usually 18 years—for participating in legally binding decisions. All adults who have not been declared **incompetent** by a judge have the legal right to make their own decisions about medical treatment and healthcare. However, families or healthcare providers often raise questions about an older person's ability to make reasonable decisions, particularly when the person is cognitively impaired.

When questions are raised about a person's ability to participate in healthcare decisions, a legally appointed, **surrogate** or **substitute decision maker**, if one has been designated, assumes decision-making responsibility.

In Australia in the absence of a substitute decision maker, or when conflicts occur among the people involved with making and implementing decisions, the Guardianship Board will be contacted to determine whether or not the person is competent. The Guardianship Board is also known by a different title, depending on its location within Australia. For instance, the Guardianship Board is located in Victoria, while the Guardianship Tribunal is in New South Wales. Often the healthcare provider, usually a medical practitioner, will contact the Guardianship Board when they are concerned that appropriate decisions are required for a person who does not seem able to make reasonable medical decisions independently. If the Guardianship Board determines that the person is incompetent (i.e. incapable of making decisions on their own behalf) the board will appoint a guardian. The Guardianship Board can also make an order for lifestyle and medical decisions and financial decisions. In New Zealand, the law about adult guardianship is regulated by the Protection of Personal and Property Rights Act 1988 (Honds, 2006). An application for guardianship is made to the Family Court. The Family Court can make similar orders as the Guardianship Boards in Australia.

Although guardianship can be revoked or reversed, the guardianship typically remains in place until the incompetent person dies. Usually, guardianship is initiated only as a last resort when there is no person who can legally qualify as a substitute decision maker. Guardianship is a drastic measure that takes away the person's rights and entails continuous monitoring. This can often be avoided if a person makes their wishes known in a comprehensive and legally binding manner, including the appointment of a substitute decision maker, before any questions arise about their mental capacities. However, in the absence of these documents, or when conflict arises about the ability of designated people to honour the person's wishes, legal and ethical issues are generally addressed by the process of guardianship.

Decision-making capacity

Decision-making capacity is a measure of a person's ability to make an informed and logical decision about a particular aspect of their healthcare. In contrast to competency—which is determined by a court of law—decision-making capacity is determined by healthcare practitioners and it relates to a single decision rather than a global determination of one's ability to manage one's own affairs (Carroll, 2010). The following abilities are widely recognised by legal and healthcare practitioners as essential components of decision-making capacity (Beattie, 2009):

- *Understanding*: Ability to comprehend information that is relevant to the decision and ability to demonstrate that comprehension
- *Appreciation*: Ability to apply the understanding to one's own situation
- *Reasoning*: Ability to use the information to consider alternatives and the associated consequences
- *Expressing a choice*: Ability to communicate the decision to others.

Nurses have a key role ensuring that older adults are provided with relevant information and in a way that enables and empowers them to make an informed decision. Another term used to describe informed decision making is *informed consent*.

When nurses are determining the decision-making capacity of older adults to make decisions, it is important to recognise the influence of differing religious and culturally-based beliefs. For example, a belief in miracles may be culturally appropriate for some people but seem to be delusional to a Western-trained care provider. Older adults are likely to have treatment preferences that are strongly based on religious or cultural beliefs and be unable to provide logical reasons for their decisions (Chettih, 2012).

An additional consideration pertinent to older adults is that determination of decision-making capacity should not be based on chronological age or a particular diagnosis. This is especially important with regard to older adults who have dementia because they may retain the ability to make safe and sufficient decisions during early stages. Moreover, people with dementia express a strong desire to remain involved in decisions about their care for as long as possible and are aware of the gradual loss of this ability as their condition progresses (Fetherstonhaugh, Tarzia & Nay, 2013). During the mild-to-moderate stages of dementia, assessment of decision-making ability is based on the person's ability to describe the importance or implications of the choice on his or her future health (Mitty & Post, 2012). As dementia progresses from early to later stages, everyday decision-making processes usually transition from supportive decision making, which involves shared decision making by the person with dementia and family carers/caregivers, to substituted decision making, which is done by family carers (Samsi & Manthorpe, 2013).

Rather than basing conclusions on a person's age or diagnosis, healthcare professionals focus on a specific situation and evaluate the person's ability to understand the issues involved, to weigh the pros and cons of choices, and to communicate about them. For example, a person with dementia may be able to decide about the appointment of a surrogate decision maker but may not be able to participate in a complex decision about medical treatment options for cancer. In this situation, it might be reasonable for the person to designate a family member to make the treatment decision.

It is important to recognise that, rather than being an "all or nothing" process, decision making typically involves considerations related to both the individual and his or her family and others whose opinions the person values. More often than not, decision making is a complex process in which information is shared between the older adult and clinicians and among family and others who are affected by the outcomes. Another consideration is that rather than being based primarily on logic and deliberation, decisions are strongly influenced by needs, values, habits, emotions and cultural factors (discussed in the section on cultural aspects of legal and ethical issues). Because the ability to value is independent of cognition, people with significant cognitive impairment—as is the case with mild-to-moderate dementia—are able to state their preferences and be involved with decisions (Smebye, Kirkevold & Engedal, 2012).

Nurses have dual roles in helping surrogate decision makers involve the older adult as much as possible and at the same time supporting shared or surrogate decision makers in assuming responsibility for decisions. This role is especially complex when decisions involve conflicting needs and values of the older adult and the carers. For example, spouses and families of people with dementia may experience conflict related to the value of caring for the person at home—a decision that involves sacrifices for the carer as well as benefits for the care recipient—and the decision to have care provided in an assisted living or nursing facility. Additional responsibilities of nurses include documenting the person's specific abilities and limitations in the care plan and ensuring that decision-making abilities are periodically re-evaluated.

It is also important to recognise that decision-making capacity can fluctuate from day to day and hour to hour and may be significantly influenced by factors that can be addressed, such as delirium, depression, polypharmacy and sleep deprivation. Thus, an important role of nurses is to promote optimal decision-making capacity by identifying and addressing the factors that influence cognitive functioning. For example, even such a relatively simple measure as ensuring that a hearing-impaired person uses his or her hearing aid may improve communication and thereby have a positive effect on decision-making abilities. Similarly, if a person with dementia has better cognitive abilities in the morning or when rested, then efforts can be made to discuss healthcare decisions during this time, rather than when the person is more confused.

The phrases decisional autonomy and executional autonomy are sometimes used in relation to decision-making capacity. *Decisional autonomy* refers to the ability and freedom to make decisions without external influence, whereas *executional autonomy* (also called executive autonomy) refers to the ability to implement the decisions. These concepts call attention to the complexity of assessing decision-making capacity and the importance of evaluating a person's ability not only to make reasonable decisions but also to carry out all of the actions necessary for implementing them. This point is particularly important in relation to people with impaired **executive control functions**, which are the cognitive skills involved in successfully planning and carrying out goal-oriented behaviour, such as self-care tasks. Conditions that are likely to cause impaired executive control functions include stroke, dementia, major depression, Parkinson's disease, traumatic brain injury, and any conditions affecting frontal lobe functioning. These situations are particularly difficult to evaluate because the person may retain the capacity to understand and make decisions (decisional autonomy) but may not have the capacity to carry them out (executional autonomy).

LIVING WILLS

Living wills are legal documents whose purpose is to allow people to specify the type of care and treatment they would want or not want if they become incapacitated as a result of terminal illness. Living wills affirm the right of a person to refuse treatment and provide an avenue for expressing wishes about preferences about pain management, organ donation, place of death, and specific treatments or care he or she would want to receive. Living wills in Australia and New Zealand are called **advance directives**.

Advance directives

Advance directives (AD) are legally binding documents that allow competent people to document what care and treatments they would or would not want to receive if they were not capable of making decisions and communicating their wishes. AD also enable people to appoint a surrogate who is a person responsible for communicating their wishes if they become incompetent or are unable to communicate them (see next section, surrogate or substitute decision maker). AD can provide instructions about treatments such as medicines and admission to the hospital. An AD provides legal assurance that the older adult's preferences will be considered when they are not capable of communicating their wishes.

Even if the document does not meet the legal requirements for an advance directive, it can used to facilitate discussion and then completion of the legally required documentation. Advance directive documents must be drawn up when the person is capable of understanding their intent, and they become effective only when the person lacks the capacity to make a particular health-related decision. Therefore, it is imperative to address advance directives before the onset of any condition, such as dementia, which can affect functioning and cognitive abilities. Studies have found that the cognitive abilities required for competent medical decision-making capacity begin to decline even during the early stages of dementia (Okonkwo et al., 2008). When the diagnosis of dementia has already been made, it is imperative that decision-making capacity be evaluated and documented specifically in relation to the task of executing advance directive documents (Mayo & Wallhagen, 2009).

In New Zealand an advance directive can be either an oral statement or a written document and all older adults have the right to make an advance directive in accordance with the New Zealand Bill of Rights Act 1990 (Wareham, McCallin & Diesfeld, 2005) and the Code of Health and Disability Services Consumers' Rights 2006 (Parliamentary Counsel Office, 2010).

In Australia an advance directive can also be referred to as an **advance care directive (ACD)**. An ACD is usually a formal written document. However, there is no legally enforceable Australia-wide definition of an ACD. Australian state and territory laws vary regarding the scope and other details of advance care directives (e.g. type of document included, or conditions under which it applies). Some states—Western Australia, Queensland, South Australia and Victoria—have specific legislation concerning ACDs, while other states and territories rely on the interpretation of common law to determine whether or not a document is a valid ACD.

In Queensland, South Australia, Tasmania, Western Australia, Victoria and the Northern Territory, ACDs are legally binding documents (Australian Government Department of Health, 2014), while New South Wales has a document called Using Advance Care Directives that guides the creation of an ACD (Advance Care Directives Working Party, 2004). When the legality of an ACD is questionable, it is recommended that if the content of the ACD is consistent and current then health professionals should follow the directions contained in the document. Box 9-1 contains recommendations for both older adults and health professionals that assist with the adherence of an ACD.

Because of the lack of uniformity and consistency across Australia, calls were made to nationalise ACD legislation. The National Framework for Advance Care Directives, published in 2011, provide guidance on policy and best practice in relation to advance care directives in an endeavour to simplify and improve ACD in Australia. It is accessible at www.health.wa.gov.au/advancecareplanning/docs/AdvanceCareDirectives2011.pdf.

Nurses need to have up-to-date information about the legal requirements for ADs, and this information is usually available in healthcare institutions. Information about ACDs for all Australian states and territories are contained at Advance Care Planning available at http://advancecareplanning.org.au. Start to Talk, available at www.start2talk.org.au, is an interactive site that enables older adults and their carers to obtain information about ACDs and share their experiences. Both Advance Care Planning and Start to Talk have resources available in different languages. In New Zealand, there is no standard format for ADs. However, there are two useful resources:

- New Zealand Medical Association
- Mental Health Commission, which provides a sample AD for people with mental illness (New Zealand Ministry Health, 2011).

In New Zealand another challenge for nurses is to incorporate the principles of the *Treaty of Waitangi* and Māori consumers' choices into their nursing practice (Wareham, McCallin & Diesfeld, 2005).

The completion of an AD is only one aspect of a process called **advance care planning (ACP)**. ACP is the process of preparing for a likely scenario near the end of life that "usually consists of assessment of, and dialogue about, a person's understanding of their medical history and condition, values, preferences and personal and family resources" (Advance Care Directives Working Party, 2004, p. 11). After completion of an AD it should be reviewed and updated periodically in keeping with medical developments and the older person's current wishes. Studies have found that older adults are generally ready and eager to discuss ADs and that the best time for doing this is during periods of relative wellness (Malcomson & Bisbee, 2009). ACP also refers to the situation when the older adult is no longer able to engage in decision making and the surrogate will collaborate with health professionals to ensure where possible that the AD is continuously upheld. Nurses as well as

BOX 9-1
Recommendations that assist with the adherence of an older adult's ACD in Australia

An ACD is likely to stand up to legal scrutiny if the following criteria are met:

- The person who created the ACD was of sound decision-making capacity when it was written.
- The document includes specific details about treatments the person would accept or refuse.
- The ACD is current and relates to the current medical problem.
- The person was not influenced by anyone when the directive was written.

A healthcare professional may be more likely to honour the terms of an ACD if:

- They are aware of its existence well in advance of its use.
- The surrogate decision-makers keep up ongoing communication with healthcare professionals about the contents of an ACD and the values and convictions behind it.
- The healthcare professional makes an effort to include discussion of advance care and treatment preferences as part of their routine.

Source: Choice (consumer advocate). (2013). Living wills. Accessed March 2015 at www.choice.com.au/reviews-and-tests/money/shopping-and-legal/legal/advance-care-directives.aspx.

BOX 9-2
Significant events that have led to advance care planning in Australia

1960s	The increasing prevalence of CPR Life-prolonging treatments are pioneered and improved The burgeoning consumer rights movement encourages patient advocacy
1970s	Most states in the U.S. ratify legislation enabling patients to record end-of-life wishes Other countries around the world also start using similar orders known as Living wills, Do Not Resuscitate (DNR) or Do Not Hospitalise (DNH) orders
1980s	Victoria, New South Wales, Queensland, Northern Territory and Tasmania enact legislation supporting advance care planning The appointment of substitute decision makers through the completion of durable Power of Attorney for healthcare forms enters U.S. legislation
1990s	South Australia enacts legislation In the U.S. a federal Self-Determination Act is passed requiring all health institutions to enquire about whether each patient has an "advance directive" and to educate and inform staff and patients about advance directives
2000s	ACT and WA enact legislation 2000—Queensland's *Guardianship and Administration Act* passed 2000—Advance Care Directives Association formed in NSW and incorporated in 2002 2004—NSW Health document Using Advance Care Directives encouraged use of common law advance directives 2006—ACT's *Powers of Attorney Act* passed, which allows an adult to give a direction about the refusal or withdrawal of medical treatment. There is no requirement for the condition to be current or terminal. It also provides for appointing an enduring power of attorney/agent for medical decisions 2008—WA's *Acts Amendment (Consent to Medical Treatment) Act* passed, which amended the *Guardianship and Administration Act 1990* to include an Advance Health Directive to refuse treatment for a current condition or terminal illness, as well as the provision to appoint an Enduring Power of Guardianship as a substitute decision maker 2009—The *Hunter and New England Area Health Service v A* case in NSW Supreme Court confirmed advance directives are legally binding in NSW U.S. federal laws include the possible withdrawal of life support 2010—A National Framework for Advance Care Directives (AHMAC) published 2012—Senate Standing Committee on Community Affairs conducts a Parliamentary Inquiry into Palliative Care in Australia 2013—Advance Care Directives to be stored on Patient Controlled Electronic Health Record (PCEHR)

Source: Advance Care Planning, Australia. (2015). A brief history of advance care planning. Accessed March 2015 at http://advancecareplanning.org.au/advance-care-planning/for-professionals/a-brief-history-of-advance-care-planning.

other health professionals have the following responsibilities in relation to ACP:

- Inform older adults of their right to refuse treatments and make healthcare decisions.
- Provide written information about the provisions for implementing advance directives.
- Ask each older adult whether an advance directive has been completed.
- Include documentation of older adults' advance directives in their medical records.
- Provide education for the staff and the community on advance directives.

Box 9-2 lists the significant events that have led to the development of ACP in Australia.

Not for resuscitation orders

A **not for resuscitation (NFR) order** is a very specific type of medical directive that may be contained in an advance directive. There is no universal term which describes the prevention of cardiopulmonary resuscitation (CPR) in situations when it is considered futile or unwanted. Other terms used are "do not resuscitate" (DNR), "do not attempt resuscitation" (DNAR) and "not for CPR". An NFR directs healthcare providers to avoid performing resuscitation if the person is not breathing and has no pulse. In Australia and New Zealand, older adults have the right to refuse medical treatments, even if it may shorten their life. The law that upholds this action in Australia is the *law of precedent*: Australian courts in recent years have reaffirmed the common law right of a competent adult to refuse medical treatment. NFR forms should be reviewed and standardised so as to be clear, uniform and consistent with the legislative framework (Levinson, Mills, Hutchinson et al., 2014). In New Zealand, the Code of Health and Disability Services Consumers' Rights 1996 (the Code) is relevant (Parliamentary Counsel Office, 2010). The Code states: "Every consumer may use an advance directive in accordance with the common law. Every consumer has the right to refuse services and to withdraw consent to services" (New Zealand Ministry of Health [NZMOH], 2014a, p. 6).

Sometimes, families, as well as carers, mistakenly associate DNR orders with directives to withhold other medical treatments. For example, they may raise questions about sending the older adult to a hospital or not requesting certain diagnostic or treatment procedures simply because a DNR order is in place. Therefore, nurses have an important role ensuring that the DNR order is understood by those involved in the care of the older adult. A procedure for implementing this request usually requires that the DNR order be formally documented by a medical practitioner.

Surrogate or substitute decision maker

A component of an AD is the appointment of a surrogate or substitute lifestyle and healthcare decision maker. This person represents the older adult during any time of incapacity and it is often considered the most important aspect of an AD. This appointment must be initiated when the older adult is competent, and it takes effect only when the person is incapacitated. The document is used with other advance directives to provide the surrogate with written guidelines stating the person's wishes on such issues as the cessation of life support. It is imperative that the surrogate has a copy of all advance directives and periodically discusses the older adult's wishes about medical treatments and end-of-life issues. Because language in AD documents can sometimes be vague, nurses should encourage older adults to discuss their wishes with their medical practitioner, other healthcare workers, and their designated surrogate before incapacity develops.

In Australia the legal term for a surrogate is different, depending on the state in which the AD is completed. In New South Wales the term **Enduring Guardianship** is used, while in some other states, for example Victoria, the surrogate is referred to as the **Enduring Power of Attorney** (medical treatment). There is a formal procedure for appointing an Enduring Guardian or Enduring Power of Attorney (Ellison et al., 2004). An appointee to an enduring guardianship is required to complete an appropriate form, and signatures of both the appointor and the appointee need to be witnessed by the same person. It important for nurses to understand the legal terminology associated with surrogates to ensure the appropriate person is consulted. Another term that nurses will encounter in Australia, which is similar to the term used for a surrogate, but is not to be confused, is the term Power of Attorney (POA). This term refers to the appointment of another person to manage financial and property matters when one is unable to do so, but it does not confer the legal authority to make health or lifestyle decisions (Ellison et al., 2004).

In New Zealand, the Protection of Personal and Property Rights Act 1988 describes the legal terms for a surrogate. A Personal Care and Welfare Enduring Power of Attorney (EPA) is the term used when "one person is appointed to make decisions about personal care and welfare on an older adult's behalf" when they are mentally incapacitated (New Zealand Ministry of Social Development, 2011, p. 1). Another type of EPA, the Property EPA, exists where another person is appointed to manage and make decisions about the older adult's property. This person has the authority to manage the property affairs while the older adult still has capacity and to continue to act if they become mentally incapacitated. Again nurses are required to understand these differences so that the appropriate person is consulted when providing care to an older person.

LEGAL ISSUES SPECIFIC TO LONG-TERM RESIDENTIAL AND COMMUNITY CARE SETTINGS

Public concern about the quality of care in long-term residential facilities during the 1970s and 1980s, the escalating costs of long-term care, and the growing numbers of older adults Australia and New Zealand resulted in a national system of aged care in both countries.

Currently in Australia national legislation directs the present system of care delivery to older adults in the community and in long-term residential care (Australian Government Department of Social Services, 2014). Significant revisions of the *Aged Care Act 1997* (Cth) occurred in 2014. This legislation has far-reaching consequences, including increased emphasis on older adults' rights and quality of life and major initiatives to improve the quality of care.

One initiative created to improve the quality of care in long-term residential care is *accreditation*. In order to receive funding from the Australian Government, long-term residential care facilities must obtain accreditation. There are four standards encompassing management, care, lifestyle, quality and safety issues, and 44 outcomes for the standards, all of which must be met to obtain accreditation. The Australian Aged Care Quality Agency, on behalf of the Australian Government, regularly conducts the process of accreditation, usually every 3 years. To achieve accreditation nurses must ensure care plans are developed and documented, provide evidence of utilisation of best practice, and continuously improve care practices.

The legislation in Australia also requires that long-term residential care facilities use the Aged Care Funding Instrument (ACFI). The ACFI is the tool used to assess the older resident's care needs and, based on this assessment, the Australian Government determines the reimbursement to the provider. A primary responsibility of nurses is to ensure that the ACFI is completed and at the appropriate time.

In Australia the Charter of Residents' Rights and Responsibilities (long-term residential care) (Australian Government Department of Health, 2015), and the Charter of Rights and Responsibilities for Community Care (Australian Government Department of Social Services, 2013), require that all recipients of aged care from Australian Government agencies are informed of their rights and that a mechanism is in place for addressing complaints if the

BOX 9-3
Charter of residents' rights in long-term residential care in Australia

Each resident of a residential care service has the right:

- to full and effective use of his or her personal, civil, legal and consumer rights
- to quality care which is appropriate to his or her needs
- to full information about his or her own state of health and about available treatments
- to be treated with dignity and respect, and to live without exploitation, abuse or neglect
- to live without discrimination or victimisation, and without being obliged to feel grateful to those providing his or her care and accommodation
- to personal privacy
- to live in a safe, secure and homelike environment, and to move freely both within and outside the residential care service without undue restriction
- to be treated and accepted as an individual, and to have his or her individual preferences taken into account and treated with respect
- to continue his or her cultural and religious practices and to retain the language of his or her choice, without discrimination
- to select and maintain social and personal relationships with any other person without fear, criticism or restriction
- to freedom of speech
- to maintain his or her personal independence, which includes a recognition of personal responsibility for his or her own actions and choices, even though some actions may involve an element of risk which the resident has the right to accept, and that should then not be used to prevent or restrict those actions
- to maintain control over, and to continue making decisions about, the personal aspects of his or her daily life, financial affairs and possessions
- to be involved in the activities, associations and friendships of his or her choice, both within and outside the residential care service
- to have access to services and activities which are available generally in the community
- to be consulted on, and to choose to have input into, decisions about the living arrangements of the residential care service;
- to have access to information about his or her rights, care, accommodation, and any other information which relates to him or her personally
- to complain and to take action to resolve disputes
- to have access to advocates and other avenues of redress and
- to be free from reprisal, or a well-founded fear of reprisal, in any form for taking action to enforce his or her rights.

Source: Australian Government Department of Social Services. (2015). Charter of Residents' Rights and Responsibilities. Viewed March 2015 at www.dss.gov.au/sites/default/files/documents/05_2014/charter_of_care_recipients_rights_responsibilities_-_residential_care_0.pdf.

older adult believes his or her rights have been compromised. Moreover, the long-term residential care facilities must post the Residents' Bill of Rights and the resources for investigating complaints in a prominent place. Box 9-3 lists the rights defined by the legislation for residents in long-term residential care in Australia.

In New South Wales in Australia is an organisation, TARS, which protects the rights of older adults who are recipients of Australian Government aged care services. TARS provides information, advice, advocacy and support to older adults and their carers to help older adults understand their rights and resolve concerns about aged care services.

In New Zealand, all hospitals and long-term residential care facilities must meet the Health and Disability Services Standards (NZMOH, 2014b) to obtain certification in order to deliver care services. The standards are part of the Health and Disability Service (Safety) Act 2001, which "… promotes the safe provision of health and disability services to the public, and enables the establishment of standards for providing health and disability services to the public safely" (p. 1). The government agency, HealthCERT, is responsible for ensuring hospitals and long-term residential care facilities meet the standards. Nurses in New Zealand must ensure that the care delivered to older adults is consistent with the Health and Disability Services Standards. Also, the nurse must ensure the appropriate interRAI assessment tool is used as a basis for planning care that addresses the changing needs of the older adult in both long-term residential and community care (New Zealand National Health IT Board, 2015).

The Code of Health and Disability Services Consumer's Rights identifies the rights of every person when receiving a health or disability service in New Zealand, including hospitals, long-term residential care and community care. Box 9-4 lists these rights.

Restraint

Since the late 1990s, government and healthcare organisations recognised that the use of physical restraints was a

BOX 9-4
Code of rights for care recipients in New Zealand

1. To be treated with respect.
2. To be treated fairly without pressure or discrimination.
3. The right to dignity and independence.
4. To receive a quality service and to be treated with care and skill.
5. To be given information that you can understand in a way that helps you communicate with the person providing the service.
6. To be given the information you need to know about your health or disability; the service being provided and the names and roles of the staff; as well as information about any tests and procedures you need and any test results. In New Zealand, people are encouraged to ask questions and to ask for more information to help them understand what is going on.
7. To make your own decision about your care, and to change your mind.
8. To have a support person with you at most times.
9. To have all these rights apply if you are asked to take part in a research study or teaching session for training staff.
10. The right to complain and have your complaint taken seriously.

Source: Health & Disability Commissioner. (2009). Your Rights (p. 2). Accessed March 2015 via www.hdc.org.nz

BOX 9-5
Different types of restraints

Physical restraint

The intentional restriction of a resident's voluntary movement or behaviour by the use of a device, or removal of mobility aids, or physical force for behavioural purposes is physical restraint. Physical restraint devices include but are not limited to:

- lap belts
- tabletops
- posey restraints or similar products
- bed rails
- chairs that are difficult to get out of such as beanbags, water chairs and deep chairs

General restraint devices include:

- bed boundary markers, to mark the edges of the bed such as mattress bumpers, rolled blankets or swimming noodles under sheets which act as a restraint if the resident cannot move past them or if they give the resident the belief that they cannot get past them
- concave mattresses
- comfort/supportive chairs that support posture and slumping but in so doing inhibit freedom of support
- chairs with deep seats
- rockers or recliners
- large pillows or bean bags on floor
- any skeletal support that restricts mobility
- lap rugs with ties
- lap sashes (waist restraints, including belts)
- hand mitts
- geri/protective chairs with tables
- wheelchair safety bars
- seat belts on chairs

High-risk restraints

- removing aids to mobility such as walking frames
- bed rails

Extreme restraint

- aversive treatment
- seclusion
- posey criss-cross vest
- leg or ankle restraint
- manacles/shackles (hard)
- soft wrist/hand restraints

Chemical restraint is the control of the person's behaviour through the intentional use of:

- prescribed medicines
- over the counter medicines and/or
- complementary alternative medicines

Chemical restraint is:

- when no medically identified condition is being treated
- where the treatment is not necessary for a condition
- to over-treat a condition

Chemical restraint includes the use of medicines when:

- the behaviour to be affected by the active ingredient does not appear to have a medical cause part of the intended pharmacological effect of the medicine is to sedate the person for convenience or for disciplinary purposes

Aversive treatment practices/punishment

An aversive practice is one that uses unpleasant physical, sensory or verbal stimuli; for example, any voice tone, command or threat that is used to limit a resident's mobility in an attempt to reduce undesired behaviour.

Aversive treatment also refers to any withholding of basic human rights or needs; for example, food, warmth, clothing, positive social interaction, a resident's goods/belongings or a favoured activity for the purpose of behaviour management or control.

Person-to-person restraint is the control of the person's behaviour through the use of:

- physical force or "hands on": no matter how gentle "hands on" is, this is a form of restraint if it limits a person's mobility
- verbal: any commands or threats that are used to limit a person's mobility
- psychological measures: any measure that creates a belief that acts to limit a person's mobility

Environmental restraint

- Environmental restraint is the restriction of movement by the person without the person's explicit and informed consent

Source: Australian Government Department of Social Services. (2012). *Decision-making tool: Supporting a restraint free environment in residential aged care* (pp. 24–26). Canberra: Author. Accessed March 2015 via www.dss.gov.au. Permission granted under a Creative Commons BY 3.0 (CC BY 3.0) licence.

major issue that was relevant to older adults in acute and long-term residential care settings. Restraint can be defined as "… any device, material or equipment attached to or near a person's body and which cannot be controlled or easily removed by the person and which deliberately prevents or is deliberately intended to prevent a person's free body movement to a position of choice and/or a person's normal access to their body" (Retsas, 1998, p. 186). Examples of all types of restraint are described in Box 9-5. In recent years, the use of restraint has been used to determine the level of quality care in long-term residential care and other healthcare settings. Major initiatives to limit or eliminate the use of any restrictive devices that infringe upon a person's rights have been introduced. Restraint has been consistently found to be associated with serious harm, including increased risks for fractures, delirium, soft tissue injury, and even death (Bradas, Sandhu & Mion, 2012). Additionally, restraints are increasing viewed as an ethical issue related to preservation of autonomy and dignity versus the person's safety and protection.

Since the introduction of accreditation (Australia) and certification (New Zealand), restraint in long-term residential care in both countries has decreased as they are required to demonstrate that its use is being reduced or minimised. Findings from Australian studies demonstrate this reduction. It was reported a decade ago that restraint use in Australian long-term residential care ranged from 12% to 47% (Joanna Briggs Institute, 2002), whereas a more recent study found the rates of 1.5% to 6.9% in four long-term residential care facilities (Courtney, O'Reilly, Edwards et al., 2010).

In New Zealand there is a standard incorporating restraint minimisation and safe practice, NZS 8134.2:2008 (Standards New Zealand, 2009), which is available to guide restraint use in long-term residential care and other healthcare settings. In Australia a comprehensive best practice guide for restraint minimisation in long-term residential care to assist with restraint reduction has been developed by the Australian Government (2012), which is called the *Decision-making tool: Supporting a restraint free environment in residential aged care*. This can be accessed at the department's ageing and aged care resources via www.dss.gov.au.

This document recommends that extreme restraints are *never* to be used in long-term residential care in Australia. It also advocates that restraints should primarily be considered a temporary solution for any behaviour of concern or other factors, but only after a comprehensive assessment has been completed, preventive strategies trialled, and reasonable alternative options exhausted. However, if restraint is considered appropriate after the comprehensive assessment then the least restrictive method is to be implemented.

The decision to restrain involves consultation between the medical practitioner, nurses, other relevant health professionals, carers and the older adult and their family (Australian and New Zealand Society for Geriatric Medicine, 2012). Those making the decision are legally accountable for the decision and the consequences. A family member or legal representative does not have the legal power to request that an older adult be restrained.

The legal requirement for consent for the use of restraint when the older person is not considered competent varies in different countries and Australian states and territories. Nurses are required to be aware of the legal requirements for consent in their context of practice. Further, it is not recommended to restrain an older adult who is not competent when they are verbally or physically objecting to restraint. If restraint is deemed necessary in these situations then it is recommended to refer to the Guardianship Board or equivalent for approval.

One study of nurses' decision-making process related to the use of physical restraints for older adults in acute care found the complex process requires that nurses obtain a good overall picture of the patient, maintain constant observations, and assess and reassess the situation (Goethals, de Casterle & Gastmans, 2013). Reducing the use of restraints for older adults requires a multi-component intervention that includes institutional policy change, staff education, consultation and availability of alternative interventions (Gulpers, Bleijlevens, Ambergen et al., 2013).

ETHICAL ISSUES COMMONLY ADDRESSED WHEN NURSING OLDER ADULTS

Ethical issues in everyday care of older adults

Although ethical issues are often associated with life-or-death situations, nurses are increasingly recognising that many daily care issues related to a person's values, preferences and quality of life involve ethical dilemmas. Nurses also deal with ethical decisions related to organisational issues such as time constraints and limitations that interfere with the provision of the best quality of care. Some questions posed by Burkhardt and Keegan (2009) in their discussion of holistic nursing ethics are as follows:

- Am I wise and courageous enough to perceive and respect others' differences and honour them as I honour my own beliefs?
- What does the person want?
- Does the person understand the choices?
- Is the person being coerced?
- What does quality of life mean for this person?
- How are others responding to the person's perceptions of quality of life?
- Does having medical technology always mean it should be used?

A process of **values clarification** is a tool that nurses can use to guide ethical decision making in everyday nursing practice. Values clarification is an ongoing process in which an individual increases their awareness of what is important and just—and why (Burkhardt & Keegan, 2009). Nurses apply this process to themselves in their professional roles and they also use it as a nursing intervention in their practice. Nurses can use values clarification to develop a "caring consciousness" that fosters a humanistic caring approach that is especially important for working with older adults (Gallagher-Lepak & Kubsch, 2009).

Ethical issues specific to long-term residential care settings

The increasing attention to quality of care in long-term care settings in recent years has led to more emphasis on autonomy, individual rights and quality of life for residents (see Chapter 6). Ethical issues are often associated with these approaches because it is not always easy to balance the needs of individual residents with those of others and the institution itself. Ethical issues also are associated with questions about safety versus freedom. For example, conflicts arise when a resident with a history of falls desires to walk freely around the facility, but staff members want to limit that person's activity to reduce the risk of falls. Additional examples of ethical decisions that nurses in long-term care settings commonly address include:

- Using restrictive measures to address concerns about safety
- Restricting cigarette smoking

- Allowing residents to refuse treatments, social activities, and food or fluid
- Providing more care assistance than necessary because it is more time-efficient for the staff
- Scheduling resident care practices for the convenience of the staff rather than according to an individual's preferences
- Accommodating residents who wish to express sexual interests and activities.

Long-term care residential settings address these ethical issues by establishing policies and procedures that are based on best practices. An important nursing responsibility is to involve residents and their substitute decision makers in developing a plan that is safe, individualised and appropriate for addressing everyday ethical issues.

Ethical issues related to artificial nutrition and hydration

Nurses frequently address ethical issues about artificial nutrition and hydration when they care for older adults who have poor nutritional intake or limited ability to chew and swallow. **Artificial nutrition and hydration (ANH)** refers to methods of bypassing the upper gastrointestinal tract to deliver nutritional substances. A percutaneous endoscopic gastrostomy (PEG) tube (sometimes referred to as a "feeding tube") is a surgically inserted tube used to deliver nutrients directly to the stomach. In addition to PEG tubes, methods of ANH include jejunostomy tubes, nasogastric tubes, hypodermoclysis (a technique used to administer fluids into the subcutaneous tissues), and total parenteral nutrition delivered through a central or peripheral vein.

Enteral nutrition has become widely recognised as a life-sustaining treatment that should be considered for people who cannot meet their nutritional needs by mouth. PEG tubes are now commonly considered in the U.S. for people with dementia when their ability to safely chew and swallow becomes compromised. Studies have found that the prevalence rate for PEG tubes in nursing home residents with advanced cognitive impairment is between 18% and 34% in the U.S. (Kuo et al., 2009). Two-thirds of long-term residents who have PEG tubes have them inserted during hospitalisation for an acute illness or for conditions such as pneumonia, dehydration and dysphagia (Kuo et al., 2009).

Because enteral feeding was becoming such a commonly used life-sustaining treatment for people with advanced dementia, many studies have addressed the safety, efficacy and outcome issues associated with this intervention. A *Cochrane Review* concluded that, despite the large number of patients receiving this intervention, there is insufficient evidence of the benefits of enteral-tube feeding for people with advanced dementia, and data are lacking on the adverse effects (Sampson, Candy & Jones, 2009). Many other studies and literature reviews conclude that the use of feeding tubes in people with advanced dementia does not result in improved outcomes, such as the prevention of aspiration pneumonia and pressure sores (Delegge, 2009). Also, the position statement of the Board of the American Geriatrics Society states that feeding tubes are unlikely to provide medical benefits or improved comfort in people living with advanced dementia. Another consideration is that people who are still able to enjoy the sensation of food are deprived of that simple pleasure when feeding tubes are used.

When people with chronically declining conditions are impaired to the extent that their nutritional status is significantly affected, they are usually in the terminal stage. There is much research to support the view that withholding artificial hydration and nutrition at this stage is not associated with suffering as long as good oral care and desired sips of water are provided. One literature review concluded that artificial nutrition and hydration did not improve comfort or meet the objectives of reducing hunger or thirst (Suter, Rogers & Strack, 2008).

In Australia and New Zealand, because of the growing evidence against the use of PEG tubes, they are not recommended for use for older adults who have advanced dementia or are very frail (Australian and New Zealand Society for Geriatric Medicine, 2012). The medical practitioner has the responsibility for making the decision to insert a PEG because it is considered a medical treatment.

Despite evidence to the contrary, families or others who make the decisions for cognitively impaired older adults may have unrealistically optimistic expectations about the benefits of PEG feeding, particularly when considerable and time-consuming assistance is required with oral hydration and nutrition, or there is a concern about hunger and discomfort. Nurses are responsible for providing up-to-date information and answering questions about the advantages and disadvantages of artificial fluid and nutrition. They can teach families that assisting with feeding and providing the benefits of social interaction and enjoyment of food may be a more compassionate approach than using feeding tubes, even if kilojoule intake is reduced. In many situations, the appropriate intervention is "comfort feeding only", which ensures the person's comfort through an individualised feeding care plan (Palecek et al., 2010). Nurses also can facilitate referrals for evaluation and treatment by a speech pathologist who can advise about swallowing and the safest and most effective ways of providing nutrients by mouth.

The nursing codes in Australia and New Zealand both emphasise respect for all persons, which includes honouring their wishes regarding treatment decisions. Nurses can use the information in Evidence-based practice 9-1 to guide decisions about AHN and alternative methods of meeting nutritional needs.

EVIDENCE-BASED PRACTICE 9-1
Key points about artificial nutrition and hydration (ANH)

Evidence-based recommendations related to the use of ANH

- The preponderance of evidence does not support the effectiveness of ANH in people with advanced dementia or other serious progressive conditions.
- ANH can be beneficial for people with a potentially reversible condition or with mechanical blockage of the upper gastrointestinal tract.
- Numerous studies have shown that tube feeding in people with serious progressive conditions does not prolong life and in fact is associated with increased risk of mortality, medical complications (including increased risk for infections), fluid overload, and skin excoriation around the tube.
- ANH does not protect against aspiration, and in some populations may increase the risk of aspiration and its complications.
- Contrary to common beliefs, ANH is associated with an increased risk of developing new pressure ulcers and slower rate of healing for existing pressure ulcers.
- Person outcomes, such as weight gain, increased kilojoule intake, or improved laboratory values are not adequate reasons for ANH in the absence of improved overall well-being.
- People with advanced illness often experience a loss of interest in eating and drinking and some may experience dysphagia; at some point most people with advanced illness will refuse food.
- Families and carers fear that when the person is undernourished experience hunger and other troublesome symptoms; however, studies show that most actively dying people do not experience hunger even if they have poor intake.
- Terminally ill persons may experience thirst or dry mouth, but these symptoms are associated with factors other than fluid intake, so ANH is unlikely to alleviate that.

Issues related to decisions about ANH

- ANH is a medical therapy that can be declined or accepted by the person's surrogate decision maker in accordance with advance directives or other indicators of the persons wishes.
- Decisions to initiate, withhold or withdraw ANH are made by the person and family with accurate and non-judgemental input from the healthcare team.
- ANH is incorporated into the person's plan only when medically appropriate and consistent with the person's beliefs.
- Healthcare providers are responsible for promoting choices, endorsing shared and informed decision making, and honouring the person's preferences.
- Perspectives of the person, family and surrogate decision makers should be assessed with cultural sensitivity by an interdisciplinary team.

Evidence-based recommendations related to care

- Nurses and all members of the healthcare team are responsible for understanding and implementing a care plan that is consistent with the previously expressed wishes of the person.
- Primary responsibilities of nurses include working with the older adult so that they understand the evidence-based information related to ANH, supporting surrogate decision makers, promoting the use of advance directives, and facilitating early discussions about goals of care and treatment choices.
- Usual care of people living with advanced dementia should include efforts to enhance oral feeding by altering the environment and creating person-centred approaches to feeding.
- Food and water offered to the person by mouth is the usual means of providing nutrition and hydration.
- Good oral care, ice chips and moistening the mouth are interventions that are likely to relieve thirst

Sources: American Geriatrics Society (2013); Australian and New Zealand Society for Geriatric Medicine (2007); Hospice and Palliative Nurses Association (2011); Teno, Gozalo, Mitchell et al. (2012).

CULTURAL ASPECTS OF LEGAL AND ETHICAL ISSUES

Religious teachings and other cultural factors have a strong influence on ethical issues, particularly with regard to advance directives and decisions about ANH and end-of-life care. Because cultural factors influence healthcare providers as well as the older adult, examining one's own biases and assuring culturally competent care (as discussed in Chapter 2) is especially important when addressing ethical issues.

A major issue with regard to ADs and decision making is that other legal requirements are strongly biased towards Anglo-centric cultures and it is important to recognise there are significant cultural differences with regard to patterns of decision making about medical interventions and healthcare services. A review of literature found that cultural groups with forms of family-centred decision making or those with less trust in healthcare professionals were less likely to have ADs than groups that valued individual autonomy (Thomas et al., 2008). For example, some families may believe that it is a sign of respect to protect an older person from the burdens of receiving information about their health status, or from making decisions about medical interventions and long-term care plans. This attitude may be in conflict with those of healthcare professionals who believe that all competent adults are entitled to information about their own health. Thus, nurses need to identify and accept individual and family decision-making preferences when they discuss ADs and other aspects of healthcare decisions.

In Australia and New Zealand, another major area of concern relative to the cultural aspects of legal and ethical issues is the need to accommodate people who do not speak English. Language barriers can significantly increase the difficulty of understanding ADs and participating in complex decisions about treatment and other aspects of care. Some states in Australia have resources available that provide ADs in different languages

- Western Australia: www.health.wa.gov.au/advancecare planning/lang/index.cfm

- South Australia: www.advancecaredirectives.sa.gov.au/information-for-you/other-lan
- New South Wales: www.swslhd.nsw.gov.au/myWishes/Further_information.html
- Victoria: www.nh.org.au/services/advance-care-planning
- Information is also available for interpreters via www.advancecaredirectives.sa.gov.au to assist them with the translation of a completed AD into English.

Even when ADs are available in the person's primary language, it is difficult to communicate the intent of these documents when there are conflicting cultural views on decisions about healthcare choices. The interventions that address language barriers are discussed in Chapter 2. At the end of this chapter are listed additional resources.

The importance of applying principles of cultural competency to all legal and ethical aspects of nursing care cannot be overemphasised, nor is this a simple process. Cultural considerations 9-1 describes characteristics of some cultural groups that potentially influence legal and ethical issues related to care of older adults This information is not

CULTURAL CONSIDERATIONS 9-1
Cultural considerations related to legal and ethical aspects of care

Cultural factors that influence ethical decision making

- The intent of advance care directives is based on Western values of individual autonomy, but many cultures believe that the fate of human beings is beyond their control.
- Values of filial piety and respect for authority of one's elders—rather than the model of individual autonomy—guide decisions about care in traditional Asian cultures.
- In collectivist cultures (e.g. the Xhosa tribe in South Africa), tribal elders make decisions about care of their members, based on distribution of human and material resources.
- Traditional Chinese and many other cultures rely on family members and their doctors to make decisions, rather than expecting to receive information and being involved in decision making.
- Ethnoreligious groups, including Jews, Muslims and Hindus, are likely to base end-of-life decisions on their beliefs on the sanctity of life.
- Religious beliefs may take precedence over scientific reasoning (e.g. opposition of blood transfusions as a life-saving measure by members of Jehovah's Witnesses).
- Some groups may prefer their own religious and spiritually based healing practices to those of scientific medicine (e.g. Christian scientists) (Pacquiao, 2008).

Cultural considerations related to ethical and legal issues in specific groups

- *Arab:* Older males assume decision-making roles; most people expect doctors to select treatments.
- *Bosnian:* Healthcare providers need to give detailed explanations of tests and procedures; trust is a major issue.
- *Chinese:* Each family has a recognised male head who has great authority and assumes all major responsibilities.
- *European:* There is great variation among families, but high value is generally placed on egalitarian relationships and decision making; advance care directives allow people to specify their wishes and designate a decision maker.
- *Filipino:* Because planning for one's death is taboo, many are adverse to discussing advance care directives or living wills.
- *German:* Extended family should be included in decision making.
- *Greek:* Older people hold positions of respect; extended nuclear family members should be included in decision making.
- *Hindu:* The patriarchal joint family, based on the notion of superiority of men over women, is the primary authority for decisions.
- *Hmong:* Traditional decision making requires that the male head of the family or clan make decisions for family members; individuals do not have the right to make their own decisions about healthcare.
- *Indigenous Australians:* Kinship systems define where an Indigenous person fits into the community, binding people together in relationships of sharing and obligation. Older Indigenous people frequently have a spokesperson who will answer some questions on behalf of the person and this may not necessarily be family members (Aboriginal Mental Health First Aid Training and Research Program, 2008).
- *Iranian:* The father and/or older male siblings have authority to make decisions for family.
- *Irish:* Families make end-of-life decisions and these are usually influenced by all the following: their definition of extraordinary means, financial considerations, quality of life, and effects on the family.
- *Italian:* Traditional families recognise the father's absolute authority and they accept his decisions as law.
- *Japanese:* Discussion of serious illness and death is taboo, so it is difficult to obtain information.
- *Jewish:* Rabbis may be included in making decisions about healthcare (e.g. organ donation or transplant).
- *Korean:* Older adults are frequently consulted on important family matters as a sign of respect for their experience.
- *Māori:* Individuals have rights of their own, but have responsibilities to the *whānau* (family). The importance of *whānau* is fundamental (NZMOH, 2012).
- *Pacific People:* Dignity is important for Pacific people. Pacific people may refuse medical treatment if they feel their dignity is threatened (Medical Council of New Zealand, 2010).
- *Russian:* It is important to ask the older adults who they want to include in medical decisions because extended family is very important.
- *Somali:* Discussing advance care directives and end-of-life care is taboo because faithful Muslins believe that Allah will determine how long a person will live; thus, these issues should be addressed indirectly.
- *Turkish:* Traditional families are patriarchal but less traditional ones are more egalitarian, so it is important to identify the family spokesperson and accept decision-making patterns without judgement.
- *Vietnamese:* Women often make family healthcare decisions.

Sources: Purnell, L. D. (2013). *Guide to culturally competent healthcare* (4th ed.). Philadelphia, PA: F. A. Davis Co.

intended to promote stereotypes, rather it is meant as a brief guide to culturally based beliefs that should be considered when developing care plans. In all situations, it is imperative to use excellent communication skills to non-judgementally assess and discuss issues related to healthcare decisions (see Chapter 2 for further guidance on culturally sensitive communication).

A student's perspective

In working with "Gigi", an 82-year-old Chinese woman, I have learned a lot about her background. She and her three brothers, two sisters and parents were all born in China.

Chinese culture emphasises respect for elders, especially the father, who is head of the family. Gigi giggles and comments, "When father said 'eat that,' we ate it, whether we liked it or not." As an adult, she worked for a time as a translator. Gigi didn't marry until she was 52. She now lives in a retirement village with her husband.

Until I learned more about her culture, I wasn't always certain she understood what was being said because she would sit with her head down and only nod, or simply say, "Yes". I now realise those behaviours are her way of showing respect to an authority figure. She seldom looks you in the eye, another form of showing respect. She is also hesitant to ask questions so as not to appear disrespectful. Gigi looks to her husband many times to make decisions for her.

Deborah L.

ROLE OF NURSES REGARDING LEGAL AND ETHICAL ISSUES

Nurses have important roles with regard to implementing advance directives and facilitating decisions about care. Although these issues are often addressed within the context of a multidisciplinary team and always with the primary care practitioner, nurses have unique and important responsibilities, which are reviewed in the following sections.

Promoting advance care planning

Advance care planning is a complex process that is much broader than simply including certain documents in the older adult's charts when they are admitted to hospitals and facilities. Rather, advance care planning describes a combination of activities that involve thinking and communicating about preferences for future care. Advance care planning is most effective when:

- It is an ongoing process that is initiated when the person is healthy as a routine part of care without distractions of other issues
- It includes learning about medical conditions that may occur, treatment options for addressing them, and thinking about relevant goals, beliefs and values related to treatment decisions
- It involves formulating and communicating about preferences with all those who will potentially be involved with decisions about the person's care (e.g. family, healthcare power of attorney, primary care practitioner, specialists)
- All relevant documents are prepared in accordance with legal requirements; and copies of all appropriate legal documents, such as ADs and NFR documents, are readily accessible to all who are involved with decisions about the person's care
- All documents are periodically reviewed and updated as necessary. (Aw, Hayhoe, Smajdor et al., 2012; Green & Levi, 2012)

Additional steps recommended for advance care planning are (1) using past experiences to clarify values, (2) verifying that surrogate decision makers understand their role, (3) deciding about the degree of leeway, if any, to give the surrogate, and (4) informing other family and friends of one's wishes (McMahan, Knight, Fried et al., 2012). Outcomes of effective advance care planning include increased feelings of autonomy, maintenance of control, increased satisfaction, improved quality of care, and reduced stress, anxiety and depression in family members (Popp e, Burleigh & Banerjee, 2013). Additional outcomes of advanced care planning related to end-of-life care are increased use of hospice, fewer in-hospital deaths, less time in the hospital during the last year, better person and family satisfaction, and improved family–provider communication (Abel, Pring, Rich et al., 2012; Bischoff, Sudore, Miao et al., 2013; Waldrop & Meeker, 2012).

Although advance care planning is commonly incorporated into usual care when people begin receiving hospice care or have been diagnosed with a serious or terminal illness, the importance of initiating the discussion when people are healthy cannot be overemphasised. For example, nurses can introduce the topic with a hypothetical question such as, "Have you designated someone to make decisions for you if you were brought to the emergency room and could not make decisions for yourself at that time?" This approach is unrelated to any diagnosis and can facilitate a transition to additional questions about advance directives.

Implementing advance directives

Evidence-based guidelines emphasise the importance of communication and education by nurses to facilitate completion of ADs and to dispel myths and misperceptions about these documents (Mitty, 2012). Legal and healthcare professionals are currently emphasising that implementation of advance directives is an ongoing process that includes working with the older adults and listening and then incorporating discussions about personal values and goals of care. Nurses can open the conversation by helping older adults and their healthcare proxies discuss what quality of life means for the older adult, the importance of preserving life, and the effects of their illness and death on others (Mitty, 2012).

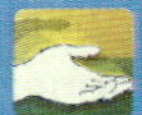

BOX 9-6
Carer wellness: Information about healthcare decisions

Advance care planning

Advance care planning is an ongoing process that involves learning about types of decisions related to healthcare, discussing these decisions with family members and healthcare providers, and making your wishes known in legal documents called advance directives.

Actions to take if you are a family carer

- Recognise that it is imperative to engage in advance care planning before any questions arise about the person's ability to express his or her wishes related to healthcare decisions.
- Explore the resources listed below to obtain information and engage in interactive educational activities related to advance care planning.
- Initiate discussions about advance directives.
- Facilitate the process of preparing appropriate documents and make sure that a healthcare power of attorney is designated.

What are advance directives?

- Advance directives are legal documents that direct decisions about medical care that is provided or withheld.
- Common types of advance directives include advance care directive and not for resuscitation
- The surrogate decision maker is extremely important. They are able to make decisions for health care decisions when someone is not able to express one's own wishes.
- Examples of medical care that are addressed in advance directives are cardiopulmonary resuscitation, ventilator use, artificial nutrition and hydration, and comfort care.

How are advance directives prepared?

- Advance directives must be prepared when the person is competent to make decisions.
- It is best to prepare advance directives before the actual need arises.
- Because requirements for advance directives are determined by each state, legally recognised documents must be obtained from each person's state of residence.
- Appropriate forms and information about preparation of advance directives are readily available from websites.
- Although advance directives do not need to be drawn up by a lawyer, if conflicts among family members are likely to arise, it may be advisable to seek legal advice.

What to do after preparing advance directives

- Make sure copies of all advance directives are readily available for healthcare providers and all those who will be involved with decision making.
- Periodically review the advance directives and update them when there are major changes in health status.
- Initially and periodically discuss the documents with anyone who will be involved with healthcare decisions.

When care is provided over long periods, documents and preferences need to be reviewed periodically and updated as appropriate and, at all times, current documents need to be included in the older adult's chart. In addition, nurses encourage people to provide copies of advance directives to their family members, designated surrogate, and anyone likely to be involved with decisions about their medical care. If written advance directives have not been completed, it is important to initiate a discussion of relevant medical care and end-of-life treatment preferences and document any statements made that express the older adult's wishes. Boxes 9-6 and 9-7 can be used as guides to communication strategies for discussing advance directives and goals of care when decisions are complex.

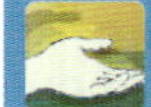

BOX 9-7
Examples of communication strategies for discussing goals of care

Questions to assess the person's understanding of the diagnosis and prognosis

- What is your understanding of what has happened?
- What have the doctors told you about your condition?
- What information would be helpful now?

Exploratory questions

- Can you explain what you mean?
- Can you talk more about your concerns?
- You indicated that you are concerned about ________. Can you tell me more about this?
- How can I be of help to you?

Questions to assess the person's supports and coping mechanisms

- How have you handled stress in the past?
- Whom can you rely on for support?
- What or who is helping you the most?
- How does your family communicate with each other?
- What are the potential areas of concern for your family?
- Is there anyone you rely on to help make important decisions?

Questions to identify the person's goals

- What do you hope for most in the next few months?
- What is important to you right now?
- Is there anything you are afraid of?

Questions for families when the person cannot make independent decisions

- Tell me about ________ so I know more about him/her.
- What was important to ________.
- What do you know about his/her wishes at the end of life from a quality-of-life point of view?

Source: Peereboom, K. & Coyle, N. (2012). Facilitating goals-of-care discussions for patients with life-limiting disease. Used with permission, Wolters Kluwer Health.

Facilitating decisions about care

Nurses play key roles not only in implementing advance directives but also in working with family members and other carers who are involved with making decisions related to care and treatment issues. Advance directives designate substitute decision makers, but the surrogates do not always have a good understanding of the person's wishes and this can be a barrier to appropriate implementation. Studies have found that family surrogates feel burdened when they need to make end-of-life decisions, and this perception of burden is compounded when they are uncertain about the older adults' preferences (Braun, Beyth, Ford & McCullough, 2008). Nurses and other healthcare professionals need to facilitate discussions about advance directives between older adults and their substitute decision makers because this can improve the chance that their preferences will be understood and honoured (Glass & Nahapetyan, 2008; Moorman & Carr, 2008). Nurses facilitate these discussions by providing accurate information on rights and statutes, addressing questions about care options, listening to the needs and concerns of all involved, attending to concerns about end-of-life care, and acting as liaisons with primary care providers when necessary.

As discussed previously, decisions about care are particularly complicated when working with older adults who have cognitive impairments. Evidence-based guidelines summarise the following nursing care strategies for healthcare decision making (Mitty & Post, 2012):

1. Communicate with the older adult, his or her family and substitute decision makers to improve their understanding of treatment options.
2. Be sensitive to racial, ethnic, religious and cultural influences with regard to care decisions, disclosure of information, and end-of-life planning.
3. Be aware of available resources for conflict resolution.
4. Assess and document the older adult's ability to state preferences, follow directions, make simple choices, and communicate consistent care wishes.
5. Assess and document fluctuations in the older adult's mental status and factors that affect it.
6. Assess the older adult's understanding, specifically in relation to a particular decision (e.g. ask them what they understand about the risks and benefits of the intervention).
7. Use appropriate decision aids.
8. Help the older adult express what he or she understands about the clinical situation and the potential outcomes.
9. Help the older adult identify who should participate in discussions and decisions.

Another important role of nurses is to involve other professionals and support resources when complex decisions must be made or when the decision makers seek additional help. In some settings, an interdisciplinary team—composed of a social worker, a religious leader, therapists, nurses and a primary care provider—may provide information and support to surrogate decision makers. Decision-making assistance from professionals may relieve families and surrogate decision makers of some of the guilt they could experience when making and implementing decisions, particularly difficult end-of-life decisions. Nurses also take a strong role in supporting and facilitating decisions about care during chronic conditions and end-of-life care. In particular, nurses provide information about the best types of services (e.g. hospice programs, palliative care) or place of care (e.g. hospital admission for nursing home residents when medical problems arise).

A model for a nurse-led intervention that is used successfully to improve surrogate decision making involves the following roles for bedside nurses in acute care settings:

1. Prepare the family to be the decision maker by educating them about the responsibilities of the surrogate.
2. Organise regular interdisciplinary meetings, including family and clinicians.
3. Prepare the family for the meeting by helping them formulate questions and understand the issues.
4. Share the information from the family with the other members of the multidisciplinary team before the meeting.
5. Assure that all pertinent topics are addressed and provide support and encouragement for the family during the meeting.
6. Provide post-meeting support and clarification for family. (Erickson, 2013; White, 2011)

When this model is applied to situations involving end-of-life decisions or uncertainty about the older adult's outcomes, nurses also provide anticipatory grief support by encouraging families to think about what it would mean to "hope for the best and prepare for the worst" (White, Cua, Walk et al., 2012).

Nurses also take a strong role in supporting and facilitating decisions about care during chronic conditions and end-of-life care. In particular, nurses provide information about the best types of services (e.g. hospice programs, palliative care) or place of care (e.g. hospital admission for long-term care residents when medical problems arise). Box 9-3 summarises a nursing model for facilitating decisions about long-term care for people with dementia.

Promoting carer wellness

As discussed previously, decisions about medical treatments are usually stressful and complex, not only for the older adult but also for families and carers. Stress is magnified when carers are responsible for decisions—including decisions that shorten life expectancy—with little or no input from the older adult. For example, when an older person is cognitively impaired and the surrogate decision makers have not previously discussed the care alternatives, the carer's stress is compounded by feelings of guilt and uncertainty.

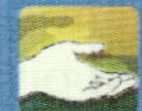

BOX 9-8
Model for facilitating decisions about the care of people with dementia

Step I: Assess the decision-making situation

- What is the decision-making ability of the person with dementia?
- What are the typical decision-making patterns in the family?
- Who influences the decision making, either directly or indirectly?
- How do family relationships help or hinder the decision-making process?
- Are there patterns of passive non-decisions as well as active decisions?
- What is each person's perception of the situation?
- How objective are the perceptions of the various decision makers?
- What does each person in the decision-making process have to gain or lose based on various decisions?

Step II: Obtain consensus about problems and needs

- Have each person involved with the care describe the problems and needs from their perspective.
- Provide additional assessment information about the needs of the person with dementia.
- Address the needs of the carers as well as the needs of the person with dementia.
- Summarise the identified needs of the older adult and the carers.

Step III: Discuss potential resources

- Ask carers to suggest potential solutions and resources.
- Identify resources for the carers' needs as well as for those of the person with dementia.
- Supplement the family's knowledge about resources and potential solutions.
- Discuss the positive and negative consequences of each option for the person with dementia and for the carers.
- As the family members discuss solutions, assess their attitudes about using various services and spending family resources to purchase services.
- Provide information about the long-range benefits that the carers might not perceive.
- Summarise important points on paper or a blackboard for all participants to review.

Step IV: Agree on a plan of action

- Obtain agreement about the most appropriate actions to take.
- Emphasise the fact that any plan of action will be given a trial period and should not be viewed as a permanent decision.
- Suggest a time frame and criteria for evaluating the plan of action.
- Identify one or two people who will evaluate the plan and make appropriate changes.

Step V: Involve the person with dementia

- Discuss the ability of the person with dementia to understand the decision.
- Identify the most realistic level of involvement for the person with dementia.
- Identify the best approach to take in involving the person with dementia.
- Identify the roles of carers and professionals in assisting the person with dementia to understand the decision.

Step VI: Summarise the plan and clarify roles

- Review and summarise the plan of action.
- Have the carers state their roles in very specific terms.
- Clarify the role of the nurse and other professionals.
- Assure carers that you will be available for further discussion and problem solving, or provide the name of someone who can assume this role.

Similarly, stress is magnified when family decision makers (e.g. siblings, spouses, in-laws) have differing perspectives or hold conflicting values about treatments. In all situations, nurses are the healthcare professionals who assume key support roles for carers, including teaching and advocacy. In addition to applying information already discussed (e.g. learning activities, communication strategies in Boxes 9-6 and 9-7), this chapter can be used to teach carers about healthcare decision making; it includes a list of helpful resources that carers can be encouraged to explore for additional information.

CHAPTER HIGHLIGHTS

Autonomy and rights

- Autonomy is the personal freedom to direct one's own life as long as it does not infringe on the rights of others.
- Adults are presumed to be competent and have the right to make health-related decisions unless they have been declared incompetent by a judge.
- Decision-making capacity describes one's ability to understand and process information, weigh alternatives, apply personal values, arrive at a decision, and communicate that decision to others.
- If an adult's decision-making capacity is questionable or compromised, his or her rights can be protected through legal documents, such as advance directives.

Living wills

- Living wills are legal documents (e.g. ADs, NFR orders) that make known to care providers and surrogate decision makers a person's wishes relative to medical treatments and care and lifestyle decisions.
- The legal terminology for surrogate or substitute decision makers within an AD varies, depending on the state or territory or country (Australia and New Zealand). Nurses play an important role in making sure these documents are available and their instructions are followed.
- Nurses must be familiar with the current laws that apply to living wills where they are practising.

Legal issues specific to long-term residential and community care settings

- Legislation applied to Australian and New Zealand long-term residential care facilities determines the standards of care, and assessments and documentation required. Nurses must comply with the legislation.
- All older adults receiving care are entitled to dignity, self-determination and the opportunity to communicate.
- Nurses must comply with the legal requirements when using restraint.
- Autonomy issues are frequently addressed by nurses in long-term care settings; balancing the rights of residents with institutional needs often poses a challenge.

Ethical issues commonly addressed when nursing older adults

- Values clarification is a tool that nurses can use as they address ethical issues in everyday care of older adults.
- Nurses are often involved in decisions about artificial hydration and nutrition.
- Assisting with care decisions during chronic illness is one of the most challenging aspects of nursing.

Cultural aspects of legal and ethical issues

- Language barriers are important to consider when discussing advance directives.
- Nurses should identify culturally influenced patterns of decision making when discussing advance directives and end-of-life care with older adults and their families.

Role of nurses regarding legal and ethical issues

- Advance care planning is a complex process for it involves ongoing communication about healthcare decisions that realistically reflect the person's values and preferences for treatments.
- Nurses have essential roles in working with older adults, their families, their healthcare proxies, and all healthcare professionals to implement advance directives.
- Nurses facilitate decision making about advance directives by providing information about advance directives and care options to older adults and to surrogate decision makers (Boxes 9-6 and 9-7).
- Nurses facilitate decisions about care of people with dementia by using the model in Box 9-8.

CRITICAL THINKING EXERCISES

1. You have been assigned to work with Mrs Murray, an 85-year-old widowed woman, who is in the hospital with heart failure. Her son and daughter tell you they would like to arrange for her to be discharged to a nursing home because they do not think she takes her medications correctly, and they are tired of her being admitted to the hospital every couple of months "to get her straightened out". The son and daughter live in another state and visit only when their mother is in the hospital. Mrs Murray has told you that she thinks her son and daughter would like to have her "put away in one of those homes" but she is adamantly opposed to leaving her home. She also has told you they think she is "senile" and she should stop driving her car, but she thinks she is quite capable of living alone, driving her car, and taking care of herself. Your observations are that she needs a lot of direction to take medications and participate in self-care activities, and she seems to be somewhat confused later in the day. What steps would you take to address her competency and decision-making abilities?
2. A Chinese woman, 78 years old, is being admitted to the hospital with hemiplegia after a stroke. There are no advance directives on her chart. What information would you want to know before you approached her about a living will and substitute decision maker? How would you explain these documents to her?
3. Mr Nikolaou is 78 years old and has been admitted for hip surgery after a fall-related fracture. He was diagnosed with Alzheimer's dementia 3 years ago and his family provides care for him in his home. His son has legal authority to make decisions for healthcare, but he will not make any decisions unless his three sisters agree to them. Mr Nikolaou does not have any other advance directives and the family says he never talked much about what medical care services he would want. He always told his family that they could make whatever decisions are best for him. The medical practitioner is considering the placement of a PEG tube because Mr Nikolaou's food and fluid intake are inadequate to meet his needs and one pressure area is beginning to develop on his buttocks. Mr Nikolaou's son and one daughter think that their father would have wanted to have every intervention possible in such a situation, and they think the PEG tube will improve his comfort and prevent the pressure ulcer. The other two daughters adamantly state that their father would never agree to such an invasive procedure and they aren't sure it will make him any more comfortable. They also worry about complications from having the tube. You are a member of the multidisciplinary team that is meeting with the family to help them come to an understanding about the use of a PEG tube in their father's situation. What points would you want to make during this family conference?

RESOURCES

For an extensive range of additional resources to enhance teaching and learning and to facilitate understanding of this chapter, please see the text's accompanying website located on thePoint at http://thepoint.lww.com.

Clinical tools

Advance Care Planning in NSW (Australia) (2015): http://advancecareplanning.org.au

Australian Government Department of Social Services, ageing and aged care (2012): *Decision-making tool: Supporting a restraint free environment in residential aged care*: www.dss.gov.au/our-responsibilities/ageing-and-aged-care/publications-articles/resources-learning-training/decision-making-tool-supporting-a-restraint-free-environment

Consumer's Tool Kit for Healthcare Advance Planning (despite being produced for the American context, this has some useful information): http://apps.americanbar.org/aging/publications/docs/consumer_tool_kit_bk.pdf

NSW Health (2013), Advance Planning for Quality Care at End of Life—Action Plan 2013–2018: www.health.nsw.gov.au/patients/acp/Pages/acp-plan-2013-2018.aspx

NSW Health (2014) (guidelines for end-of-life care and decision making): Advance end of life decisions, the law and clinical practice: www.health.nsw.gov.au/patients/acp/Pages/end-of-life-decisions-law-and-clinical-practice.aspx

NSW Health (2014) (compliance with this policy directive is mandatory): Using resuscitation plans in end of life decisions: www0.health.nsw.gov.au/policies/pd/2014/PD2014_030.html

Evidence-based practice

Hartford Institute for Geriatric Nursing: http://consultgerirn.org

Want to know more, search:

- Geriatric nursing protocol: Advance directives.
- Geriatric nursing protocol: Healthcare decision making.

Mitty, E. L. & Post, L. F. (2012). Healthcare decision making. In M. Boltz, E. Capezuti, T. Fulmer & D. Zwicker (Eds), *Evidence-based geriatric nursing protocols for best practice* (4th ed., pp. 562–578). New York: Springer.

Mitty, E. L. (2012). Advance directives. In M. Boltz, E. Capezuti, T. Fulmer & D. Zwicker (Eds), *Evidence-based geriatric nursing protocols for best practice* (4th ed., pp. 579–699). New York: Springer.

Joanna Briggs Institute (JBI): http://connect.jbiconnectplus.org

Evidence-based summaries:

- Chen, Z. (2013). Complementary therapies (aromatherapy and herbal medicine): Clinician information.
- Dao Le, L. K. (2014). Residential aged care: Physical restraint.
- D'Arcy, M. (2013). Informed consent: Clinician information.
- Fong, E. (2014). Physical restraint: Prone position.
- Jahan, N. (2013). Advance care planning/Advance directive.
- Jayasekara, R. (2014). Enteral delivery: Aged care.
- Read, S. (2013). Restraint (physical): Use.
- Sharma, L. (2014). Restraint standards: Clinical information.
- Slade, S. (2013). Admission: Residential aged care.

Recommended practices:

- JBI. (2013). Admission issues: Residential aged care.
- JBI. (2013). Restraint standards.
- McReynolds, T. (2013). Advance care planning.

Systematic review:

- Sze, T. W., Leng, C. Y. & Lin, S. K. (2012). The effectiveness of physical restraints in reducing falls among adults in acute care hospitals and nursing homes: A systematic review. *Joanna Briggs Institute Library of Systematic Reviews, 10*(5), 307–351.

Health education

Advance Care Planning Australia: www.advancecareplanning.org.au

Advance Care Planning Online Queensland: http://apps.health.qld.gov.au/acp/home.aspx

Age Concern New Zealand, Enduring Power of Attorney: www.ageconcern.org.nz

Aging With Dignity (*Five Wishes*): www.agingwithdignity.org/translated-five-wishes.php

American Association of Colleges of Nursing, End-of-Life Nursing Education Consortium Project (ELNEC): www.aacn.nche.edu

Australian Aged Care Quality Agency (AACQA), accreditation and education: www.aacqa.gov.au

Mental Health First Aid Australia, for cultural competence training: www.mhfa.com.au

TARS (The Aged Rights Service), Australia: www.tars.com.au

Training on respecting patient choices, Australia: www.advancecareplanning.org.au/training

REFERENCES

Abel, J., Pring, A., Rich, A. et al. (2012). The impact of advance care planning of place of death, a hospice retrospective study. *BMJ Supportive & Palliative Care, 3*, 168–173.

Aboriginal Mental Health First Aid Training and Research Program. (2008). Cultural considerations & communication techniques: Guidelines for providing mental health first aid to an Aboriginal or Torres Strait Islander person. Melbourne: Orygen Youth Health Research Centre, University of Melbourne and *beyondblue*. Accessed March 2015 via https://mhfa.com.au.

Advance Care Directives Working Party (NSW). (2004). Using advance care directives. Sydney: NSW Department of Health. Viewed March 2015 at www0.health.nsw.gov.au/policies/gl/2005/pdf/GL2005_056.pdf.

Advance Care Planning, Australia. (2015). A brief history of advance care planning. Accessed March 2015 at http://advancecareplanning.org.au/advance-care-planning/for-professionals/a-brief-history-of-advance-care-planning.

American Geriatrics Society. (2013). Feeding tubes in advanced dementia position statement. Viewed March 2015 via www.americangeriatrics.org.

Australian and New Zealand Society for Geriatric Medicine. (2007). *Under-nutrition and the older person*. Retrieved 3 January 2012 at www.anzsgm.org/documents/PosStatement6revisedsep07.pdf.

Australian and New Zealand Society for Geriatric Medicine. (2012). Position statement no. 2: Physical restraint use in older people. Revised September 2012. Available March 2015 via www.anzsgm.org/posstate.asp.

Australian Government Department of Health. (2014). Palliative care—Advance care planning. Accessed March 2015 at www.health.gov.au/internet/main/publishing.nsf/Content/acp.

Australian Government Department of Social Services. (2012). *Decision-making tool: Supporting a restraint free environment in residential aged care*. Canberra: Author. Accessible March 2015 via www.dss.gov.au.

Australian Government Department of Social Services. (2013). Rights and responsibilities—home care. At myagedcare portal, accessed March 2015 at www.myagedcare.gov.au/financial-and-legal/rights-and-responsibilities-home-care.

Australian Government Department of Social Services. (2014). Ageing and aged care. Accessed March 2015 at www.dss.gov.au/our-responsibilities/ageing-and-aged-care/aged-care-reform/overview.

Australian Government Department of Social Services. (2015). Charter of Residents' Rights and Responsibilities. Accessed March 2015 via www.dss.gov.au.

Aw, D., Hayhoe, B., Smajdor, A. et al. (2012). Advance care planning and the older patient. *Quarterly Journal of Medicine*, *105*, 225–230.

Beattie, E. (2009). Research participation of individuals with dementia. *Research in Gerontological Nursing*, *2*(2), 94–102.

Bischoff, K. E., Sudore, R., Miao, Y. et al. (2013). Advance care planning and the quality of end-of-life care in older adults. *Journal of the American Geriatrics Society*, *61*(2), 209–214.

Bradas, C. M., Sandhu, S. K., & Mion, L. C. (2012). Physical restraints and side rails in acute and critical care settings. In M. Boltz, E. Capezuti, T. Fulmer, & D. Zwicker (Eds), *Evidence-based practice protocols for best practice* (4th ed., pp. 229–245). New York: Springer.

Braun, U. K., Beyth, R. J., Ford, M. E. & McCullough, L. B. (2008). Voices of African American, Caucasian, and Hispanic surrogates on the burdens of end-of-life decision making. *Journal of General Internal Medicine*, *23*(3), 267–274.

Burkhardt, M. A. & Keegan, L. (2009). Holistic ethics. In B. M. Dossey & L. Keegan (Eds), *Holistic nursing: A handbook for practice* (5th ed., pp. 125–137). Boston, MA: Jones and Bartlett.

Carroll, D. W. (2010). Assessment of capacity for medical decision making. *Journal of Gerontological Nursing*, *36*(5), 47–52.

Chettin, M. (2012). Turning the lens inward: Cultural competence and providers' values in healthcare decision making. *Gerontologist*, *52*(6), 739–747.

Choice. (2013). Living wills. Accessed March 2015 at www.choice.com.au/reviews-and-tests/money/shopping-and-legal/legal/advance-care-directives.aspx.

Courtney, M., O'Reilly, M., Edwards, H. et al. (2010). Benchmarking clinical indicators of quality for Australian residential aged care facilities. *Australian Health Reviews*, *34*, 93–100.

Delegge, M. H. (2009). Tube feeding in patients with dementia: Where are we? *Nutrition in Clinical Practice: Official Publication of the American Society for Parenteral and Enteral Nutrition*, *24*(2), 214–216.

Ellison, S., Schetzer, L., Mullins, J. & Wong, K. (2004). *The legal needs of older people in NSW*. Sydney: Law and Justice Foundation of NSW.

Erickson, J. (2013). Bedside nurse involvement in end-of-life decision making. *Dimensions of Critical Care Nursing*, *32*(2), 65–68.

Fetherstonhaugh, D., Tarzia, L. & Nay, R. (2013). Being central to decision making means I am still here! The essence of decision making for people with dementia. *Journal of Aging Studies*, *27*, 143–150.

Gallagher-Lepak, S. & Kubsch, S. (2009). Transpersonal caring, a nursing practice guideline. *Holistic Nursing Practice*, *23*(3), 171–182.

Glass, A. P. & Nahapetyan, L. (2008). Discussions by elders and adult children about end-of-live preparation and preferences. *Preventing Chronic Disease Public Health Research, Practice, and Policy*, *5*(1), 1–8.

Goethals, S., de Casterle, B. D. & Gastmans, C. (2013). Nurses' decision making process in cases of physical restraint in acute elderly care: A qualitative study. *International Journal of Nursing Studies*, *50*, 603–612.

Green, M. J. & Levi, B. H. (2012). The era of "e": The use of new technologies in advance care planning. *Nursing Outlook*, *60*, 376–381.

Gulpers, M. J., Bleijlevens, M. H., Ambergen, T. et al. (2013). Reduction of belt restraint use: Long-term effects of EXBELT intervention. *Journal of the American Geriatrics Society*, *61*(1), 107–112.

Health & Disability Commissioner. (2009). *Your rights*. Accessed March 2015 via www.hdc.org.nz/.

Hands, J. (2006). *The family group conference as a means of decision-making in matters of adult guardianship*. Munich: GRIN Publishing GmbH.

Hospice and Palliative Nurses Association. (2011). HPNA position statement: Artificial nutrition and hydration in advanced illness. Available 18 June 2013 at www.hpna.org.

Joanna Briggs Institute (JBI). (2002). Physical restraint—Part 1: Use in acute and residential care facilities. *Best Practice: Evidence-Based Practice Information Sheets for Health Professionals*, *6*(3), 1–6.

Kuo, S., Rhodes, R. L., Mitchell, S. L., Mor, V. & Teno, J. M. (2009). Natural history of feeding-tube use in nursing home residents with advanced dementia. *Journal of American Medical Directors Association, 10*, 264–270.

Levinson, M., Mills, A., Hutchinson, A. M. et al. (2014). Comparison of not for resuscitation (NFR) forms across five Victorian health services. *Internal Medicine Journal, 44*(7), 671–675.

Malcomson, H. & Bisbee, S. (2009). Perspectives of healthy elders on advance care planning. *Journal of the American Academy of Nurse Practitioners, 21*(1), 18–23.

Mayo, A. M. & Wallhagen, M. I. (2009). Considerations of informed consent and decision-making competence in older adults with cognitive impairment. *Research in Gerontological Nursing, 2*(2), 103–110.

McMahan, R. D., Knight, S. J., Fried, T. R. et al. (2012). Advance care planning beyond advance directives: Perspectives from patients and surrogates. *Journal of Pain and Symptom Management, 46*(3), 355–365.

Medical Council of New Zealand. (2010). Best health outcomes for Pacific peoples: Practice implications. Accessed March 2015 at www.mcnz.org.nz/assets/News-and-Publications/Statements/Best-health-outcomes-for-Pacific-Peoples.pdf.

Mitty, E. L. (2012). Advance directives. In M. Boltz, E. Capezuti, T. Fulmer & D. Zwicker (Eds), *Evidence-based practice protocols for best practice* (4th ed., pp. 579–599). New York: Springer.

Mitty, E. L. & Post, L. F. (2012). Healthcare decision making. In M. Boltz, E. Capezuti, T. Fulmer & D. Zwicker (Eds), *Evidence-based practice protocols for best practice* (4th ed., pp. 562–578). New York: Springer.

Moorman, S. M. & Carr, D. (2008). Spouses' effectiveness as end-of-life healthcare surrogates: Accuracy, uncertainty, and errors of overtreatment or undertreatment. *Gerontologist, 48*(6), 811–819.

New Zealand Ministry of Health (NZMOH). (2011). Advance care planning: A guide for the New Zealand healthcare workforce. Accessed March 2015 at www.health.govt.nz/publication/advance-care-planning-guide-new-zealand-health-care-workforce.

New Zealand Ministry of Health (NZMOH). (2012). Māori health models. Accessible March 2015 at www.health.govt.nz/our-work/populations/maori-health/maori-health-models.

New Zealand Ministry of Health (NZMOH). (2014a). Certification of health care services. Accessed March 2015 at www.health.govt.nz/our-work/regulation-health-and-disability-system/certification-healthcare-services.

New Zealand Ministry of Health (NZMOH). (2014b). Health and Disability Services (Safety) Act 2001. Viewed March 2015 at www.health.govt.nz/our-work/regulation-health-and-disability-system/certification-health-care-services/health-and-disability-services-safety-act.

New Zealand Ministry of Social Development. (2011). Enduring Powers of Attorney: Protect your future. Accessed March 2015 at www.msd.govt.nz/what-we-can-do/seniorcitizens/your-rights/epa/index.html.

New Zealand National Health IT Board. (2015). Comprehensive clinical assessment for aged care (interRAI). Viewed March 2015 via www.ithealthboard.health.nz.

Okonkwo, O. C., Griffith, H. R., Copeland, J. N., Belue, K., Lanza, S., Zamrini, E. Y., . . . Marson D. C. (2008). Medical decision-making capacity in mild cognitive impairment, a 3-year longitudinal study. *Neurology, 71*, 1474–1480.

Pacquiao, D. F. (2011). Cultural competence in ethical decision-making. In M. M. Andrews & J. S. Boyle (Eds), *Transcultural concepts in nursing care* (6th ed.). Philadelphia, PA: Lippincott Williams & Wilkins.

Palecek, E. J., Teno, J. M., Casarett, D. J., Hanson, L. C., Rhodes, R. L. & Mitchell, S. L. (2010). Comfort feeding only: A proposal to bring clarity to decision-making regarding difficulty with eating for persons with advanced dementia. *Journal of the American Geriatrics Society, 58*, 580–584.

Parliamentary Counsel Office. (2010). Code of Health and Disability Services Consumers' Rights 1996. In Health and Disability Commissioner Act 1994. Accessed March 2015 via www.legislation.govt.nz.

Peereboom, K., & Coyle, N. (2012). Facilitating goals-of-care discussions for patients with life-limiting disease: Communication strategies for nurses. *Journal of Hospice and Palliative Nursing, 14*(4), 251–258.

Poppe, J., Burleigh, S. & Banerjee, S. (2013). Qualitative evaluation of advanced care planning in early dementia. *PLoS One, 8*(4), e6–e412.

Purnell, L. D. (2013). *Transcultural healthcare: A culturally competent approach* (4th ed.). Philadelphia, PA: F. A. Davis.

Retsas, A. P. (1998). Survey findings describing the use of physical restraints in nursing homes in Victoria, Australia. *International Journal of Nursing Studies, 35*(3), 184–191.

Sampson, E. L., Candy, B. & Jones, L. (2009). Enteral tube feeding for older people with advanced dementia. *Cochrane Database of Systematic Reviews, 2*. Art. no. CD007209.

Samsi, K. & Manthorpe, J. (2013). Everyday decision-making in dementia: Findings from a longitudinal interview study of people with dementia and family carers. *International Psychogeriatrics, 25*(6), 949–961.

Smebye, K. L., Kirkevold, M. & Engedal, K. (2012). How do persons with dementia participate in decision making related to health and daily care? A multi-case study. *BMC Health Services Research, 12*, 241. Available March 2015 at www.biomedcentral.com/1472-6963/12/241.

Standards New Zealand. (2009). *Health and disability services standards (restraint minimisation and safe practice)*. Standard no. NZS 8134.2:2008. Wellington: Author.

Suter, P. M., Rogers, J. & Strack, C. (2008). Artificial nutrition and hydration for the terminally ill, a reasoned approach. *Home Healthcare Nurse, 26*(1), 23–29.

Teno, J. M., Gozalo, P., Mitchell, S. L. et al. (2012). Feeding tubes and the prevention or healing of pressure ulcers. *Archives of Internal Medicine, 172*(9), 697–701.

Thomas, R., Wilson, D. M., Justice, C., Birch, S. & Sheps, S. (2008). A literature review of preferences for end-of-life care in developed countries by individuals with different cultural affiliations and ethnicity. *Journal of Hospice and Palliative Nursing, 10*(3), 142–160.

Waldrop, D. P. & Meeker, M. A. (2012). Communication and advanced care planning in palliative and end-of-life care. *Nursing Outlook, 60*, 365–369.

Wareham, P., McCallin, A. & Diesfeld, K. (2005). Advance directives: The New Zealand context. *Nursing Ethics, 12*(4), 349–359.

White, D. B. (2011). Rethinking interventions to improve surrogate decision making in intensive care units. *American Journal of Critical Care, 20*(3), 252–257.

White, D. B., Cua, S., Walk, R. et al. (2012). Nurse-led intervention to improve surrogate decision making for patients with advanced critical illness. *American Journal of Critical Care, 21*(6), 396–409.

Chapter 10

Elder abuse and neglect

By Carol Miller and Sharyn Hunter

LEARNING OBJECTIVES

After reading this chapter, you should be able to:

1. Define the various types of elder abuse.
2. Identify risk factors that contribute to elder abuse and neglect.
3. Describe nursing assessment aimed at identifying elder abuse and neglect, as well as risks for abuse and neglect.
4. Describe the nurse's opportunities for interventions for elder abuse in different practice settings.
5. Discuss the range of nursing and legal interventions directed towards preventing and alleviating elder abuse.

KEY POINTS

abandonment
domestic violence
elder mistreatment
emotional (psychological) abuse
financial or material exploitation
mandatory reporting
neglect
physical abuse
self-abuse
self-neglect
sexual abuse

Elder abuse and neglect is one of the most complex and serious functional consequences that affects vulnerable older adults—and one of the most challenging aspects when nursing older adults. Situations of elder abuse and neglect require an interdisciplinary approach, with nurses assuming essential roles in detection, assessment and interventions. This chapter presents the topic with emphasis on the key roles of nurses in addressing this complex issue.

OVERVIEW OF ELDER ABUSE AND NEGLECT

Certain members of any population are vulnerable to abuse and **neglect** by virtue of being physically or psychosocially impaired or subjugated. In developed countries today, vulnerable groups are protected and cared for through legislative mandates and social programs. In many countries, for example, children and people with developmental disabilities have been protected for many decades. In recent decades, additional groups have been recognised as needing protection: victims of partner and family violence, and abused or neglected older people. Although abuse or neglect of older adults is not new, elder abuse has received increased attention as a social problem, crime and health concern.

Definitions and characteristics of elder abuse

Definitions of elder abuse have changed over time in response to shifts in political climate, public sentiment, available funding, and increasing knowledge and professional interest. This section discusses the definitions and characteristics of elder abuse and the following section provides a historical perspective on elder abuse.

Both Australia and New Zealand define elder abuse as "... a single or repeated act, or lack of appropriate action, occurring within any relationship where there is an expectation of trust which causes harm or distress to an older person". It can be of various forms: physical, psychological, emotional, sexual, financial or simply reflect intentional or unintentional neglect (World Health Organization, 2002, p. 2). There are three basic categories of elder abuse:

- Domestic elder abuse
- Institutional elder abuse and
- **Self-neglect** or **self-abuse**. (National Center on Elder Abuse, 2015)

There are seven major types or forms of abuse and these are defined as:

- **Physical abuse**: use of physical force that may result in bodily injury, physical pain or impairment
- **Sexual abuse**: non-consensual sexual contact of any kind with an older adult
- **Emotional (psychological) abuse**: infliction of anguish, pain or distress through verbal or non-verbal acts
- **Neglect**: refusal or failure to fulfil any part of a person's obligations or duties to an older adult
- **Abandonment**: desertion of an elderly person by an individual who has assumed responsibility for providing care for the elder, or by a person with physical custody of the older adult
- **Self-neglect**: behaviour of an older adult that threatens his/her own health or safety
- **Financial or material exploitation**: the illegal or inappropriate use of an older adults funds, property or assets. (National Center on Elder Abuse, 2015)

The term **elder mistreatment** is also used to describe elder abuse. The Hartford Institute for Geriatric Nursing uses the term elder mistreatment to include self-neglect, carer/caregiver neglect, several types of abuse, and financial abuse/exploitation (Caceres & Fulmer, 2012).

Internationally, the concept of elder abuse has almost unlimited boundaries, as evidenced by the United Nations Second World Assembly on Aging (United Nations Economic and Social Council, 2002). This World Assembly viewed elder abuse as encompassing virtually anything that causes harm or distress to an older person and that occurs in a relationship with a trust expectation. This includes acts as wide ranging as direct forms of aggression, to denial of dignity to older people (United Nations Economic and Social Affairs, 2008).

Other examples of ever-expanding views include newspaper articles depicting older disaster victims as suffering from elder abuse, and legal services advertisements labelling compromised quality of care in long-term residential care facilities as elder abuse.

Efforts are currently underway to provide greater clarity to the meaning and dimensions of elder abuse. Conrad and associates (2011a; 2011b), for example, has applied sophisticated research methods, such as concept mapping, to financial exploitation. After national and local groups of elder abuse experts identified relevant statements for the construct, the statements were sorted, rated and depicted as conceptual maps. Then focus groups of practitioners and older adult service consumers reviewed these items, and elder abuse victims refined them before the items were subjected to tests of validity and reliability. The resulting older adult financial exploitation measure is intended to aid in the assessment of the problem by both clinicians and researchers.

Historical recognition of a social problem

In Australia, awareness of elder abuse as a social problem was not recognised until the late 1980s (Kurrle, 2004). Since the early 1990s various community responses have occurred to address the issue of elder abuse. Although the Australian Government is responsible for the aged care system, it is the state and territory governments that respond to elder abuse.

Each state and territory has developed its own approach to responding to elder abuse, which includes different funding strategies and elder abuse organisations (Australian Government Department of Health, 2015).

Both South Australia and Western Australia have an agency, Alliance for the Prevention of Elder Abuse (APEA), whose vision is to promote community awareness and response to elder abuse. Queensland has created an Elder Abuse Unit, while other states have a helpline. Victoria has published a guide for health and community services entitled *Elder abuse prevention and response guidelines for action 2012–2014* (State Government of Victoria, Department of Health, 2012). See Table 10-1 for the range of support services in Australian states and territories. Most organisations that provide services for older adults have developed protocols for the management of elder abuse. Many cases of elder abuse are assessed and managed by aged care assessment teams (ACATs).

In New Zealand by the late 1980s several reports had raised the social issue of elder abuse and neglect (Age Concern New Zealand [ACNZ], 2015). Seven intervention coordination Elder Abuse and Neglect Prevention Services (EANPs) were subsequently established to address this issue. Currently, 24 EANPs exist in New Zealand, most of which are partly funded by the Ministry of Social Development. The EANPs' objective is to ensure "the well-being, rights and safety of the older person and those who care for them" (ACNZ, 2007, p. 12). The Elder Abuse and Neglect Prevention Services across New Zealand provide information, advice or assistance about elder abuse and neglect. Specific services include:

- Training and education for professionals and carers
- Raising public awareness about the early identification and prevention of elder abuse and neglect
- Providing information, advice and advocacy
- Providing support and services about preventing abuse or neglect in the future

TABLE 10-1 Elder abuse prevention and advocacy information in Australia

State and territory	Service	Telephone numbers
ACT	Older Persons Abuse Prevention Referral and Information Line (APRIL)	02 6205 3535
NSW	NSW Elder Abuse Helpline	1800 628 221
NT	NT Police	131 444
QLD	Elder Abuse Prevention Unit	1300 651 192
SA	Aged Rights Advocacy Service	08 8232 5377 (Adelaide) or 1800 700 600 (rural)
TAS	Tasmanian Elder Abuse Helpline	1800 441 169
VIC	Seniors' Rights Victoria	1300 368 821
WA	Advocare Incorporated	1300 724 679 (Perth) 1800 655 566 (rural)

TABLE 10-2 Elder abuse prevention and advocacy information in New Zealand

Location	Organisation
Whangarei	Age Concern Whangarei
Auckland – Avondale	Age Concern Auckland
Auckland – Manurewa (Māori)	Te Oranga Kaumātua Kuia Disability Support Services
Auckland – Counties/Manukau	Age Concern Counties Manukau
Auckland – Manukau City (Pacific)	Toa Pacific
Auckland – North Shore	Age Concern North Shore
Hamilton City	Age Concern Hamilton
Tauranga	Age Concern Tauranga
New Plymouth	Tui Ora
Taupo	Age Concern Taupo
Gisborne	Age Concern Tairawhiti
Hastings	Age Concern Hastings
Palmerston North	Age Concern Manawatu
Levin	Age Concern Horowhenua
Kapiti (Paraparaumu)	Age Concern Kapiti Coast
Wanganui	Age Concern Wanganui
Masterton	Wairarapa Organisation For Older People
Wellington (including Lower Hutt & Porirua City)	Age Concern Wellington
Nelson	Age Concern Nelson
Buller	Buller REAP
Christchurch	Age Concern Canterbury
Timaru	Family Works, Presbyterian Support South Canterbury
Dunedin	Age Concern Otago
Invercargill	Age Concern Southland

- Assessing suspected elder abuse or neglect
- Managing intervention in cases of elder abuse or neglect
- Referring to other service providers, and coordinating and monitoring service plans.

(Family and Community Services, 2011)

Elder abuse prevention services and information for New Zealand are listed in Table 10-2. Elder abuse has become a global concern. First recognised in the U.S., Great Britain and Canada, elder abuse gained worldwide attention with the establishment of the International Network for the Prevention of Elder Abuse in 1997. Since the early 2000s, the United Nations World Assembly has focused on elder abuse as a major international concern (United Nations Economic and Social Affairs, 2008). As a global concern, elder abuse is typically seen as a violation of human rights or an act of oppression, with interventions often aimed at reforming national public policy to delineate and defend the rights of older people (Dow & Joosten, 2012).

Awareness of elder abuse has been increasing so that it is now recognised as a major social and health problem and a significant aspect of family violence. One indicator of increased global attention to elder abuse is the fact that World Elder Abuse Awareness Day has been commemorated since 2006 in countries worldwide on the 15th of June every year. This increasing attention can be attributed to such reasons as the following:

- The older adult population has been increasing rapidly, with the most vulnerable groups of older people (i.e. those who are 85 years of age and older) increasing at the fastest rate.
- Adult children increasingly are called upon to care for their elderly parents; however, some lack the capacity, skills, resources, availability or physical proximity to undertake this responsibility successfully.
- Researchers and clinicians are directing more attention to the problems that affect the most vulnerable older adults, leading to more information and publications.
- Educational efforts have made professionals and the public more aware of reporting laws and elder abuse services.
- Organisations have promoted professional networking and also advocated for public policy addressing elder abuse.

Nurses have been in the forefront of research, publications and practice innovations in elder abuse. Nursing journals have featured articles on elder abuse since the 1970s, and clinically oriented nursing texts on elder abuse have been co-authored by nurses since the 1980s. Since the mid

1980s, nursing has been represented in the field of elder abuse through the research of such scholars as Terry Fulmer, Linda Phillips and Elizabeth Podnieks. Nurses also have developed important clinical tools and protocols, particularly in the areas of screening and assessment. There is evidence of similar responses to elder abuse for nurses cross-culturally, suggesting a global humanitarian and nursing perspective to the problem (Erlingsson, Ono, Sasaki & Saveman, 2012; Sandmoe, Kirkevold & Ballantyne, 2011).

Prevalence and causes

Elder abuse is neither a rare nor an isolated phenomenon in Australia or New Zealand. Rather all indicators suggest that maltreatment of vulnerable older adults is widespread and occurs among all subgroups. Although estimates of elder abuse worldwide range from a low of 4% to a high of 47%, these estimates vary because of significant underreporting and differing definitions (Sooryanarayana, Choo & Hairi, 2013). Studies suggest that most maltreatment is repeated, is seldom reported to authorities, and represents more than one form of abuse.

Currently there is no national prevalence data available for Australia (Kurrle & Naughtin, 2008). Data has mostly been obtained from organisations that provide a service, or from state-based research. These sources do not provide a reliable estimate of prevalence. The NSW Elder Abuse Helpline has reported that 30% of all calls relate to financial abuse. A report about elder abuse in Western Australia also found that financial abuse was the most common form of abuse (Clare, Black Blundell & Clare, 2011). Reports suggest that the main abusers were adult children or other relatives. New Zealand elder abuse data reported by ACNZ (2015) is contained in Box 10-1.

Globally, 53 countries representing all six regions of the World Health Organization responded to a questionnaire and acknowledged elder abuse as a major local concern (Podnieks, Anetzberger, Wilson et al., 2010). Although elder abuse research is underway in both developed and developing countries, most countries report a need for more studies, particularly on prevalence. Some examples of studies on prevalence and types of elder abuse in countries are as follows:

- Ireland: 2.2%, with financial abuse most frequent (Naughton, Drennan, Lyons et al., 2012)
- United Kingdom: 2.6%, where neglect was most common (Biggs, Manthorpe, Tinker et al., 2009)
- Israel: 18.4%, where verbal abuse and financial exploitation dominated (Lowenstein et al., 2009)
- Older women in five European countries, that is, Finland, Austria, Belgium, Lithuania and Portugal: 18.1% (DeDonder, Lang, Luoma et al., 2011)
- Rural community in People's Republic of China: 36.2%, with carer neglect and physical mistreatment being the most commonly cited forms (Wu, Chen, Hu et al., 2012)
- Still other nations, such as Canada and India, are laying the foundation for improved elder abuse prevalence research (Podnieks, Rietschlin & Walsh, 2012; Shankardass, 2013).

Although the problem can affect any older person, the typical reported elder abuse victim is a socially isolated and physically or cognitively impaired woman of advanced age who lives alone or with the abuser and depends on the abuser for care. Studies have identified profiles of abused elders by type of abuse. For example, victims of self-neglect are likely to have the following characteristics: older age; chronic illness; functional limitations; solo living arrangements; social isolation; inadequate economic resources; and dementia, mental illness, substance abuse or hoarding behaviours (Day, Leahy-Warren & McCarthy, 2013; Ernst & Smith, 2011; Mosqueda & Dong, 2011). Finally, there may be some association between type of abuse and the sex of the perpetrator, with men being more likely to exploit or physically abuse elders, and women being more likely to physically neglect or psychologically abuse elders.

Studies of specific types of mistreatment indicate that elder abuse results from multiple, interrelated variables. Anetzberger (2013) summarised the risk factors associated with perpetrators, victims and perpetrator/victim environments (Box 10-2), emphasising that perpetrator risk factors were more powerful predictors of abuse occurrence than victim risk factors. Research on the risk factors of elder abuse points in the following directions:

- Risk factors vary by form of abuse.
- The aetiology of any form of abuse is a composite of several interrelated variables.
- The origins of elder abuse are found in both the victim and the perpetrator, as well as in the relationship between the two.
- The aetiology of elder abuse differs from that suggested for other abused populations in important ways (e.g. elder abuse is uniquely associated with ageism).

BOX 10-1
Elder abuse characteristics in New Zealand

- Psychological—up to 75%
- Material/financial—over 50%
- Physical—15% to 20%
- Neglect—10% to 15 %
- Self-neglect—10% to 15%
- Almost half of abused older adults are over the age of 80
- One-third of abused older adults live alone
- Three-quarters of alleged abusers are family members; and this often continues even when the older adult moves to residential care
- Almost half of alleged abusers are adult children
- Abusers are as likely to be female as male

Source: Age Concern New Zealand. (2015). Elder abuse and neglect prevention. Accessed March 2015 via www.ageconcern.org.nz.

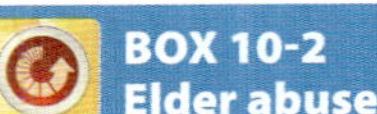

BOX 10-2
Elder abuse risk factors

Perpetrator risk factors
- Mental illness
- Alcoholism
- Hostility
- Financial dependency on the victim

Victim risk factors
- Dementia
- Problem behaviours
- Disability

Perpetrator/victim environment risk factors
- Shared living arrangements
- Social isolation or lack of social support

Cultural considerations

As a worldwide issue, elder abuse is being addressed in the context of the basic human right to be free from violence in the home. Cultural factors strongly influence how elder abuse is defined and perceived as well as broader aspects of elder abuse. For example, the value of *familism*, which emphasises needs of the family over those of the individual, can hinder the reporting of elder abuse as well as the use of support services (DeLiema, Gassoumis, Homeier et al., 2012). Even the definition of financial abuse can vary according to cultural expectations.

Cultural variation extends beyond race and ethnicity, of course. Although research in this area is minimal, some studies suggest that some groups may be more vulnerable to elder abuse, especially self-neglect, because of social isolation. In Australia and New Zealand, research about culture and elder abuse is limited (ACNZ, 2007; Black Blundell & Clare, 2012). One study conducted in Western Australia found that services for older adults who could not speak and/or read English were not adequate (Black Blundell & Clare, 2012). It found that older migrants were found to be at increased risk of isolation and therefore were more vulnerable to elder abuse because of difficulties communicating in English and the lack of informal support networks.

Further, there is little research about older adults who are vulnerable to self-neglect because of social isolation related to living in rural or remote areas. Similarly, older adults who experience stigma, such as lesbian, gay, bisexual and transgender (LGBT) elders, may place a high value on independence and avoid contact with senior service providers. For example, studies indicate that 65% of LGBT older adults reported victimisation due to sexual orientation, 8.3% reported they had been abused by a senior service provider because of homophobia, and 8.9% experienced blackmail or financial exploitation (National Center on Elder Abuse, 2013).

Although understanding cultural variations in the incidence and interpretations of elder abuse is important, nurses also should remember that individuals vary. Not all members of a cultural, religious or minority group behave according to reported trends.

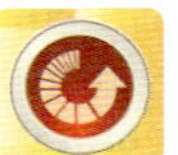

RISK FACTORS FOR ELDER ABUSE AND NEGLECT

Because risk for elder abuse and neglect is associated with a combination of characteristics and circumstances in the victim and perpetrator, identification of all risk factors is very complex. Most often, several risk factors must be present and these generally develop over a long period. Characteristics that tend to be common to most elder abuse situations are invisibility of the problem, vulnerability of the older person, and psychosocial and carer risk factors.

Invisibility and vulnerability

In contrast to most problems affecting older adults, one of the major risk factors for elder abuse is its invisibility. Despite the increasing attention given to elder abuse, the vast majority of cases are unreported, even in states with good reporting and intervention models. Factors that contribute to this invisibility and underreporting include the following:

- Older people generally have less contact with the community than do other segments of the population.
- Older people are reluctant to admit to being abused or neglected, because they fear reprisal or believe that alternative situations may be worse than the abusive one.
- Many myths and negative stereotypes associated with old age foster a strong denial of ageing and an even stronger denial of the social problems associated with vulnerable older people.

Vulnerability is associated with a combination of social, personal, situational and environmental factors. For example, elders may have significant psychosocial limitations resulting from conditions such as dementia, depression and mental illness. These conditions can increase their vulnerability to self-neglect or to abuse or exploitation by others; they also can affect the ability to seek help from others. Another factor that leads to vulnerability is the absence of close relatives or other support people who are able and willing to provide adequate and appropriate assistance.

WELLNESS OPPORTUNITY

By sensitively communicating care and concern, nurses encourage vulnerable older adults to talk about conditions that can be addressed to prevent abuse or neglect.

Cognitive and psychosocial factors

Impaired cognitive function is one of the most common characteristics of abused older adults. Considerable attention has been focused on dementia as a risk factor for self-neglect as well as psychological and physical abuse (Cooper et al., 2009). Impaired judgement, lack of insight, inability to make safe decisions and loss of contact with reality are specific impairments that can lead to abuse and neglect.

One study found that mistreatment was detected in 47.3% of a sample of 129 persons with dementia, with the following variables associated with increased occurrence of abuse: aggressive behaviours of the person with dementia, and carer's anxiety, depression, lower education and higher perceived burden (Wiglesworth, Mosqueda, Mulnard et al., 2010). In addition to dementia, depression and delirium are other conditions that can increase the risk for elder abuse and neglect. Characteristics of depression that contribute to its role in self-neglect include social isolation, a negative outlook, and lack of interest in self-care.

When the older adult denies the cognitive impairment or refuses help or evaluation, the risk for elder abuse increases. Older people who live alone and are aware of their impairments may be afraid of acknowledging them, because they fear they have an untreatable problem that will require a move to a long-term residential care facility. This fear may lead to social isolation, the overlooking of treatable or reversible causes of impairment, or a progressive but unnecessary decline in function.

Long-term mental illness also may predispose an older adult to abuse or neglect, especially in combination with other factors, such as dementia or the loss of a significant social support. Additional risk factors arise from social and environmental sources. The absence of a support system is one of the most common contributing factors to self-neglect, especially in people in their 80s, 90s or older who may have outlived most of the people whom once provided support and tangible services. This is especially problematic for people who have been lifelong recluses or who have no children or extended family.

Carer factors

Caregiving itself does not cause elder abuse; however, it can lead to abuse when those assuming the caregiving role are incapable of doing so because of life stress, pathological characteristics, personality characteristics, insufficient resources, or lack of understanding of the older adult's condition. Carers who perpetrate abuse often exhibit some of the same risk factors associated with abused elders, particularly if the carers themselves are older adults. Carer factors associated with elder abuse include poor health, cognitive impairment, social isolation, dependence and co-residence, and poor interpersonal relations with the dependent elder. It is not unusual to have a mutually neglectful or abusive situation when an older married couple has several of the psychosocial risk factors just identified and is, in addition, socially isolated. For example, a couple who both have dementia may unintentionally abuse each other and neglect themselves.

UNFOLDING CASE STUDY

Part A

Mrs Barnes is an 82-year-old widowed mother of four. She lives in a unit in a retirement village. The village has a bus service, which takes her to grocery stores and shopping malls and has a recreational centre. Mrs Barnes' eldest son died in an accident 12 years ago. Her daughter lives 65 kilometres away but visits once a week to do the grocery shopping and other errands. Two sons live within 4 kilometres of their mother's unit. Mrs Barnes lived in the home of one son and his wife until they argued 1 year ago. The other son lives alone in a small unit and visits his mother two or three times weekly and frequently takes her to lunch or dinner. Mrs Barnes has been hospitalised for major depression eight times since her eldest son's death. She also has been diagnosed as having hypertension, rheumatoid arthritis, and type 2 diabetes.

Mrs Barnes was referred to community nursing for follow-up after her last hospital stay because her medication regimen, which she had followed for 6 years, was changed while she was in the hospital. At the time of discharge Mrs Barnes was given a 30-day supply of medications set out in daily-dose medication containers for her. She was to take metformin 500 mg once a day; propranolol, 40 mg twice a day; paroxetine, 25 mg once a day; folic acid, 1 mg once a day; and methotrexate, 2.5 mg four tablets each Wednesday. Scheduled medication times were 8 a.m. and 8 p.m. The community nurse was to instruct Mrs Barnes in her medication regimen, including what medications she was to take, how she was to take them, what each medication was expected to do, and possible side effects. The nurse was also to assess Mrs Barnes' ability to follow instructions and her adherence to the medication regimen.

Because Mrs Barnes' vision was impaired from diabetes, she had difficulty managing her complex medication regimen. The visiting nurse arranged for unit-dose packaging for Mrs Barnes' prescriptions and visited twice a day for 2 days to observe Mrs Barnes' ability to take her medications accurately. On the third morning, the nurse telephoned Mrs Barnes at 8.15 a.m. and asked Mrs Barnes if she had any problems taking her pills. Mrs Barnes happily reported that she had taken all the pills, including the four methotrexate tablets, without any difficulty. The nurse then scheduled Mrs Barnes to be seen three times a week for ongoing assessment for several weeks.

Thinking points

- What are the factors that contribute to the risk of Mrs Barnes becoming abused or neglected?
- What are the factors that protect Mrs Barnes from becoming abused or neglected?
- As the visiting nurse, what concerns would you have about Mrs Barnes when you discharge her from your care, and how would you address these concerns?

ELDER ABUSE AND NEGLECT IN LONG-TERM RESIDENTIAL CARE FACILITIES

Elder abuse in long-term residential care was first brought to public attention during the early 1970s when reports about poor care in nursing homes were published. Although these reports led to improvements in overall care, neglect and physical abuse of older adults living in long-term residential care has been an ongoing concern.

However, evidence about elder abuse in long-term residential care continues to be limited.

New Zealand information suggests there is a higher proportion of neglect occurring in institutions as opposed to the community (ACNZ, 2007). In Australia since 2007, following changes to aged care legislation, **mandatory reporting** or compulsory reporting of elder abuse is required in long-term residential care. Guidelines are available that explain the reporting requirements (Australian Government Department of Social Services, 2015; Aged Rights Advocacy Service, 2015). A report must be made to the local police and the Aged Care Complaints Scheme (1800 550 552) of the incident involving suspected abuse within 24 hours of it being noted. Reportable abuse includes unlawful sexual contact and unreasonable use of force. A number of resources are available to help identify reportable elder abuse. Two examples are:

- Recognising, preventing and responding to abuse of older people living in the community: A resource for community care workers, available from the Benevolent Society via www.benevolent.org.au
- Compulsory reporting guidelines for approved providers of residential aged care, available from the Department of Social Security at http://guides.dss.gov.au/guide-aged-care-law/2/2/1#2.

There is no specific legislation in New Zealand in relation to long-term residential care and elder abuse. Age Concern New Zealand is the national coordinator of all the EANPs, and these organisations provide services to this context (ACNZ, 2015).

Research into elder abuse risk factors in long-term residential care facilities has identified many factors that stem from administrative problems within the institution, such as the lack of abuse prevention policies, insufficient staff screening, inadequate staff education and training, and staff shortages and turnover. Staff competencies for preventing elder abuse identified by direct care workers include understanding elder abuse risk factors, along with acquiring communication, relationship building and coping skills (DeHart, Webb & Cornman, 2009). Another contributing condition that is common in long-term residential care facilities is the challenge of dealing with resident-to-staff aggression. For example, a 2-week prevalence study of 1552 residents in large urban nursing homes found that 15.6% were aggressive towards staff during that period, with verbal abuse (12.4%) and physical aggression (7.6%) being the most common types (Lachs, Rosen, Teresi et al., 2013). Hirschel and Anetzberger (2012) reviewed the literature on risk factors for elder abuse in long-term residential care facilities and found that these can be divided into staffing characteristics (e.g. leading stressful lives and having negative attitudes toward residents), facility characteristics (e.g. inadequate supervision and harsh management practices), and resident characteristics, including social isolation and exhibiting difficult behaviours. Ultimately, effective strategies to address elder abuse in long-term residential care facilities must focus on all three areas of risk as well as their interrelationships.

Resident-to-resident aggression is a type of elder abuse that occurs in long-term residential care with a scope and incidence that has serious effects on safety and quality of life of many residents (Castle, 2012; Teresi, Ramirez, Ellis et al., 2013). Resident-to-resident aggression is defined as "negative and aggressive physical, sexual, or verbal interaction between long-term residential care residents that in a community setting would likely be construed as unwelcome and have high potential to cause physical or psychological distress in the recipient" (Pillemer, Chen, Van Haitsma et al., 2011, p. 25).

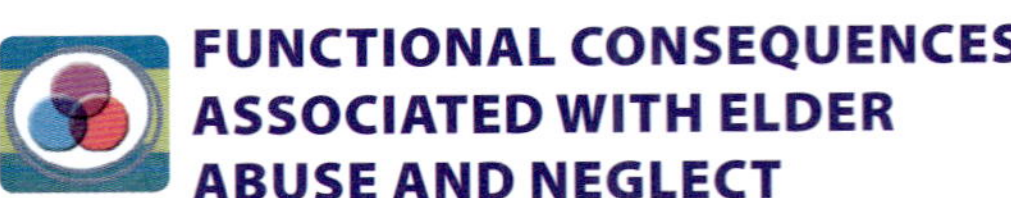

FUNCTIONAL CONSEQUENCES ASSOCIATED WITH ELDER ABUSE AND NEGLECT

Older people who have several risk factors are likely to become victims of elder abuse, as illustrated by the following case examples:

1. A middle-aged alcoholic man hit his aged father during an argument. In turn, both were beaten by their sons/grandsons, who wanted money for drugs. (*Physical abuse*)
2. An elderly woman never left home because she feared her memory lapses would prevent her from finding the way back. When she did venture out, she fell, and the ambulance was called. It was found she had no food in the house and was malnourished. (*Self-neglect*)
3. An unemployed couple kept their impaired grandparents confined to the house, refusing them visitors, abandoning them for days without adequate food, and denying them help for fear of losing access to their government pension. (*Psychological abuse and neglect*)
4. A son visited his mother in the nursing home and sexually assaulted her when staff members were not present. (*Sexual abuse*)
5. A depressed elderly woman refused to take a needed medication with the result that her legs became so swollen she could not leave her chair. (*Self-neglect*)
6. A woman in her 80s—who was weak, incontinent and had hypertension—was abandoned in an emergency department with a note reading, "Totally dependent! Handle with care." (*Abandonment*)

Specific actions that are defined in elder abuse laws include undue influence, unreasonable confinement, violation of rights, and denying privacy or visitors. Self-neglect and self-abuse are forms of elder abuse that differ from other types in that they have no perpetrator other than the older person himself or herself. In cases of self-neglect, the older person fails to meet essential needs, usually because of such factors as serious functional impairments or the desire to die (Day, McCarthy & Leahy-Warren, 2012). Studies indicate that prevalence of self-neglect is between 10% and 15% (Dong, Simon & Evans, 2012). Self-neglect develops gradually and is often associated with a lack of resources such as food, money and housing; at other times adequate resources are available but the older adult does not access appropriate resources. Many self-neglected older adults have underlying problems such as dementia, depression, psychosis or substance abuse disorders that affect their ability to seek assistance and accept help (Bond & Butler, 2013). Other times the person may refuse services because of a desire for privacy or fear of being forced to move or accept unwanted services.

Although elder abuse literature has not focused on situations that are mutually abusive or neglectful, nurses working in home settings have long encountered situations in which two people, often a married couple, abuse each other or are both neglected. These situations may be rooted in a long-term, mutually abusive relationship but usually evolve because of gradual declines in the functional abilities of both people. They also may be associated with the poor coping skills of a spouse or carer who is faced with increasing demands and little or no outside help. Many of these situations are now being recognised as partner violence (Roberto, McCann & Brossoie, 2013).

Since the late 1980s, partner or family violence in later life has been recognised as another aspect of elder abuse, with much of the focus on older women's experiences of intimate partner violence. Although this is a recognised and unique aspect of elder abuse, attention to and research about this topic remains limited. Some findings from a review of 32 studies by Weeks and LeBlanc (2011) are as follows:

- Abuse of women by their partners is a problem across all ages, races, religions and socioeconomic classes.
- Between 15% and 26.5% of women in midlife and older report intimate partner violence, with one study finding 3.5% of women aged 65 and older experiencing this in the past 5 years.
- Between 43% and 72% of abused older women do not report the abuse.
- Abuse of older women by their partners occurs in several contexts, including longstanding relationships, new relationships, or across several relationships, with the most common perpetuators being spouses (62%), current boyfriends (26%), and former spouses (12%).
- When intimate partner violence develops in later life, this may be associated with changes in health status or other ageing-related events (e.g. some men become more controlling after retirement).
- When abuse occurs throughout a long-term relationship it may shift from physical to emotional and financial abuse over time.
- Between 7.9% and 9% of women experiencing intimate partner violence reported that gun ownership and the presence of firearms greatly influenced the relationship dynamics.

Programs that address partner or family violence as an aspect of elder abuse are few and rare, especially in rural areas. Barriers to the use of available services include inaccessibility of programs, feelings of self-blame and shame, lack of information, reluctance of older victims to leave long-term relationships and lack of support from family and friends (Weeks & LeBlanc, 2011). Cultural expectations and norms also present barriers to reporting abuse and seeking help, particularly with regard to beliefs about traditional roles of women and the permanency of marriage. It is imperative that partner and family violence services suit the needs, beliefs, values and demographic and situational characteristics of individual older victims (Newman, Seff, Beaulaurier et al., 2013).

DIVERSITY NOTE

Rural culture can affect help-seeking behaviour in partner or family violence situations. Victims may stay in abusive relationships because they live in small, insulated communities with nearby family and strong social networks, especially if violence is an accepted part of life.

Although rape and other sexual violence perpetrated against older people received some attention during the late 1970s, the focus at that time was on sexual assault by strangers. During the 1990s, sexual assault by family members and paid carers became a widely recognised aspect of elder abuse. A landmark study of sexual abuse in care facilities found that the typical perpetrator was a man (78.4%) aged 56 (range 19 to 96) and almost as likely to be another resident (41%) as facility staff (43%). The victims were cognitively or physically impaired, with nearly half of the victims requiring assistance in all activities of daily living (ADLs). Sexual abuse most often was represented by molestation, which was four times more frequent than vaginal rapes, the second usual form (Ramsey-Klawsnik et al., 2008). Dementia increases the risk for sexual assault of older adults, in both long-term residential care and community settings (Connolly, Breckman, Callahan et al., 2012). Among the many barriers to the effective prevention of and response to elder sexual abuse—particularly for cognitively impaired victims—is the fact that many cases are not reported and very few are prosecuted (Payne, 2010).

CASE STUDY ONE

Part A

When Mr Popov's wife died, this frail man sought care in the home of a neighbour who offered both board and care in exchange for his monthly pension. In reality, the neighbour provided neither, but locked Mr Popov in the basement and gave him little food. If he complained about the treatment or refused to sign over the income or property, the carer hit or kicked him. After 4 years, the situation was discovered and reported to the local elder abuse organisation and the guardianship board.

Thinking points

- What type(s) of abuse does this case represent?
- What are some of the psychosocial consequences that Mr Popov is likely to have experienced in the past 4 years?
- What are some factors that contribute to this situation going on for 4 years?

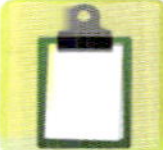

NURSING ASSESSMENT OF ABUSED OR NEGLECTED OLDER ADULTS

Elder abuse is not so much assessed as it is detected, so nurses often must assume the role of detective. Because elder abuse by its very nature is a hidden problem, assessment begins with a suspicion about its existence. Information may be purposefully withheld, and it is rarely volunteered, except in situations in which the older person or carer is desperate for help. Clues to elder abuse might first be noted when an older person is seen in an emergency department or admitted to a hospital. Most often, a home visit is an essential component of the assessment process, and gaining admission to the home is usually the first assessment challenge. Often the situation deteriorates so gradually that it is hard to determine the onset of abuse. In questionable situations, people who suspect that elder abuse is occurring may ignore the clues in hopes that the situation will resolve by itself.

WELLNESS OPPORTUNITY

Nurses pay particular attention to the older adult's relationships with others so that they can detect clues to elder abuse.

Unique aspects of elder abuse assessment

The assessment of elder abuse differs from usual nursing assessment in several respects. First, a major goal is to determine whether legal interventions are appropriate or necessary, in contrast to situations in which the primary focus is on specific health needs. In situations in which abuse is suspected, the immediate assessment focus is on the safety of the older person. This approach is similar to critical care nursing, in which basic life-sustaining needs are addressed immediately and other needs are considered later.

Second, realistic goals for elder abuse situations often are quite limited. Healthcare professionals sometimes have to accept basic safety as the only goal, especially when the elder and carer insist on choices that are not consistent with those recommended by healthcare workers. An assessment of risks to safety is essential, therefore, because choice of legal interventions is based partially on the degree of risk. Because the determination of safety often is based on medical and nursing information, the role of the nurse is especially important. In home settings in particular, the nurse may be the only healthcare professional who directly assesses the situation, and the nursing assessment may be the major determinant of recommendations for legal intervention.

Third, cases of elder abuse generally involve some element of resistance from the older person or carer(s). Only in rare situations do abused elders or their carers seek assistance from healthcare professionals. Although it might be impossible to establish a trusting relationship, the nurse must try, at the very least, to establish an accepting relationship. The initial assessment, therefore, is aimed at identifying ways of gaining access and at least passive acceptance.

Fourth, in contrast to most healthcare situations, the nurse may be viewed as a threat rather than a help. Thus, it may be difficult to gain access or to obtain adequate assessment information. When nurses are viewed as the "bad guy", they need to minimise the perceived threat even before the initial contact. Nurses can accomplish this by identifying someone who acknowledges that a problem exists and is willing to facilitate the assessment process. Any of the following people can be helpful in gaining access and acceptance:

- Neighbours or friends
- Relatives (especially family members who do not live in the problematic home setting)
- Staff from senior centres, offices on ageing, or healthcare or community agencies
- Doctors or any other health professionals
- Church-based people (e.g. clergy, parish nurses).

Fifth, when legal interventions are being considered, the legal rights of the person and the carers must be addressed. Nurses and other workers involved in elder abuse cases usually are uncomfortable making decisions that involve the rights of other adults. In institutional settings, legal and ethical decisions are guided by medical information and institutional policies, and the role of the doctor usually is the most important. In home settings, however, there are few clear guidelines and little or no doctor input.

Finally, the personal safety of the nurse is an assessment consideration in many elder abuse situations, especially when the nurse visits homes where the carer is a known or suspected perpetrator. In any situation that places a nurse at risk, an essential component of the assessment is ensuring that protections are in place for the nurse. For example, nurses can arrange their visits in conjunction with protective service workers visits or, if warranted, law enforcement officers. Some communities have law enforcement officers who are specially trained to deal with elder abuse situations. Whenever nurses visit older adults in places where the nurses' safety may be threatened, they need to be vigilant about potential risks and always be attentive to an escape route.

An elder abuse assessment instrument has been developed and this tool can be used by nurses to collect and organise all pertinent information. This tool is recommended as a *Try This: Best Practices in Nursing Care to Older Adults* resource by the Hartford Institute for Geriatric Nursing. Additional information and a cost-free video demonstrating the application of this tool in a clinical setting is available through collaboration of the Hartford Institute and the *American Journal of Nursing* at http://consultgerirn.org/resources, or at www.nursingcenter.com.

WELLNESS OPPORTUNITY

When making home visits, nurses pay particular attention to self-wellness by protecting themselves from risks.

Physical health

The nursing assessment of physical abuse and neglect focuses on the following: nutrition, hydration, bruises and injuries, degree of frailty, and presence of pathological conditions. The following sections discuss each of these aspects in relation to elder abuse and neglect.

Nutrition and hydration

Nutrition and hydration are important in determining not only the existence of physical neglect but also the seriousness and urgency of the situation. In community settings, nutrition and hydration status are crucial in determining if time allows for working with the elder in the home setting. The guidelines discussed in Chapter 18, particularly in Table 18-1 (Causes and consequences of nutrient deficiencies), can be applied to the detection of malnutrition and dehydration.

Skin turgor over the extremities is not necessarily a reliable indicator of hydration, especially for very old people or for people who have lost weight. Examination of the mucous membranes and an assessment of skin turgor over the sternum or abdomen provide more accurate clues to dehydration. The absence of thirst sensation is not necessarily an indicator of adequate hydration because older people may have a diminished thirst response. On the other hand, the presence of thirst sensation is a positive indicator of dehydration, a physiological disturbance, or an adverse medication effect. If a urine sample can be obtained, a measurement of specific gravity will provide information about hydration. When dipstick urinalysis is not available, a visual examination of urine concentration provides some clues about hydration.

When indicators of malnutrition or dehydration are identified, the next step is to determine whether the hydration or nutritional status can be improved adequately without removing the person from the setting. The role of the nurse can be especially important in assessing not only the nutrition and hydration status but also the measures required to alleviate these risks immediately. Sometimes, the provision of water and food is the most important intervention in neglect situations. In addition, this intervention is inexpensive and readily available and can be quite effective in establishing a relationship with a hungry or thirsty person.

Injuries, bruises and other physical harm

Assessment of indicators of physical harm is an important aspect of the detection of neglect or physical abuse. Any of the following conditions can be indicators of abuse or self-neglect: leg ulcers; pressure ulcers; dependent oedema; poor wound healing; burns from stoves, cigarettes or hot water; and bruises, swelling or injuries from falls, especially repeated falls. More than one of these indicators at the same time, or over a short period of time, should raise high levels of suspicion about neglect. The possibility of drug or alcohol abuse also should be considered when any of these indicators is identified, especially if the person is also depressed or socially isolated.

To detect physical abuse, the nurse should look for any indication of injury caused by people who live with or visit a vulnerable older adult. Examples are marks from cuts, bites, burns or punctures; bruises or injuries, especially on the face, head or trunk; bruises on both upper arms, as would result from being grabbed or shaken harshly; or bruises that reflect the shape of objects, like belts or hair-brushes. If evidence of injuries from falls is present, the nurse must consider the possibility that the person was shoved or otherwise caused to fall by someone else.

Nurses routinely assess the presence and characteristics of bruises, with particular attention to the onset of new bruises and the progression of bruises. Changes in colour have traditionally been considered indicators of the age of bruises, with the expectation that they progress from blue/black to green, then yellow, with red appearing at any time. A few studies have addressed progression of accidental bruises in relation to child abuse but there is little research on bruises in older adults. In 2002, Mosqueda and colleagues conducted a landmark study on the life cycle of bruises in older adults (Mosqueda, Burnright & Liao, 2005). Trained research assistants performed daily head-to-toe examinations of 101 older adults during the initial 14-day inspection period to identify the onset of new bruises. Seventy-three subjects had 108 bruises, which were documented and examined daily for up to 6 weeks. Researchers screened subjects to exclude any possibility of abuse and they considered variables such as medications, fall history, and medical conditions. The following findings from this study are pertinent to nursing assessment of bruises in older adults (Mosqueda et al., 2005):

- Accidental bruises occur in a predictable pattern in older adults, with nearly 90% appearing on extremities.
- No accidental bruises were observed on the neck, ears, genitalia, buttocks or soles of the feet.
- Bruise duration varied from 4 to 41 days, with 81% resolving by day 11.
- Red, yellow and purple are the most common discolourations during the early phase, but they can last throughout the life of the bruise.
- Yellow discolouration can begin within the first 24 hours after onset, tends to increase over time, and was the most common colour in bruises after 3 weeks.
- Subjects were more likely to know the cause when the bruises occurred on their trunks than when it was on their extremities.
- The most commonly reported cause was bumping into something.

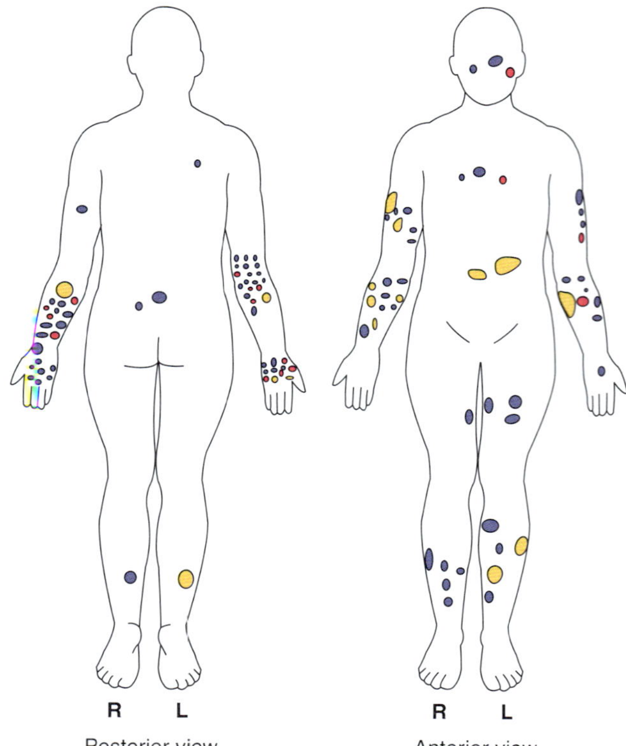

FIGURE 10-1 Most common sites of accidental bruises in older adults. (From Mosqueda, L., Burnright, K. & Liao, S. [2005]. The life cycle of bruises in older adults. *Journal of the American Geriatrics Society, 53*, 1339–1343. Used with permission from Wiley-Blackwell.)

- Subjects with compromised function and those on medications known to affect coagulation were more likely to have multiple bruises, with no differences in size, colour or location.

A second bruising study (Wiglesworth, Austin, Corona et al., 2009) investigated the characteristics of bruises sustained by physically abused older adults, as illustrated in Figure 10-1. A review of 839 injuries reported in nine studies, which included the study by Wiglesworth and colleagues, identified the following anatomical distribution of injuries related to elder physical abuse: upper extremity, 44%; head, neck, skull, brain, dental and maxillofacial area, 35%; lower extremity, 11%; and torso, 10% (Murphy, Waa, Jaffer et al., 2013).

In recent years there is increasing attention to evaluation and documentation of bruises and patterns of injuries as an indicator of physical abuse. In particular, researchers are trying to identify characteristics of injuries caused by a perpetrator, in contrast to those sustained accidentally. This is especially pertinent to identifying forensic markers of elder abuse that are needed to aid in the prosecution of perpetrators. Researchers are also investigating the causes of injuries sustained by abused older adults in relation to location of bruises, shown in the following relationships gleaned from the data analyses of 67 confirmed cases of those who reported physical elder abuse (Ziminski, Wiglesworth, Austin et al., 2013):

- Being choked—lumbar region, head and neck, and left anterior upper arm
- Being punched or hit—head and neck, right lateral upper arm
- Being grabbed—lateral or anterior arms, including left anterior upper and lower arm
- Being beaten—head and neck
- Being slammed against a wall—lumbar region.

Nurses also assess for indicators of abuse caused indirectly, as by a carer who gives the older adult excessive amounts of alcohol or drugs, especially psychoactive medications. Sometimes carers who abuse drugs or alcohol will give these substances to the people for whom they care, especially if the dependent person is not able or willing to refuse.

Another sign of abuse is excessive use of psychoactive medications solely for the carer's benefit so that the elder is more easily managed. Nurses are likely to observe any of the following indicators of overmedication in an elder: ataxia, somnolence, clouded mentation, slurred speech, staggering gait or extrapyramidal manifestations.

Aspects of physical neglect may include withholding therapeutic medications or interfering with medical care. For example, carers may decide not to purchase prescriptions or provide nursing care, medical equipment or comfort items because they do not want to spend the money, even though this care is necessary. If the older adult has not freely chosen to forego treatments, medications or assistance, then this may constitute physical neglect. If the carer is likely to inherit the money that is being saved, this may represent financial exploitation as well.

Degree of frailty

The degree of frailty of the older adult is another consideration in assessing actual or potential abuse or neglect. For example, an older adult who is slightly obese and fully ambulatory would not have the same degree of risk for fall-related injuries as one who weighs only 36 kilograms and ambulates unsteadily with a walker. Similarly, if the 75-year-old wife of an alcoholic man can easily escape to safety when he becomes violent, and she chooses to remain in the situation, she would not necessarily be considered a protective case. In contrast, if the woman is cognitively impaired, physically frail or unable to move quickly, and is the target of violence when her husband is inebriated, the situation could be defined as elder abuse.

Pathological conditions

In certain medical conditions, it is essential to assess the ability to follow medical regimens and the consequences of non-adherence. For example, consequences can be quite serious if an elder has diabetes or congestive heart failure and cannot take medications correctly. Nurses also assess whether the medical regimen can be modified to improve adherence and support the elder's ability to remain in an independent setting. For example, in an acute care setting, a therapeutic regimen might require the administration of some medications before meals and others after meals, and others three or four times a day at different times. Although this might be ideal for optimal effectiveness, elders or carers in a home setting may not be able to comply. A thorough nursing assessment can lead to interventions, such as education or simplification of the regimen, to achieve adequate adherence.

Activities of daily living

A major focus of assessment in elder abuse situations is to determine the necessity for legal interventions. Therefore, a nursing assessment of the person's potential for safe performance of activities of daily living (ADLs) is extremely important. This is particularly important when assessing self-neglect because impairments in instrumental ADLs are strongly associated with this type of abuse.

For community-living older adults, it is essential to assess the home environment and the elder's level of functioning in that environment. In addition, nurses often need to obtain information from carers. Home care workers provide valuable information, and they usually are more objective than family members. In some circumstances, it may be appropriate to involve occupational or physical therapists in the home assessment. When a difference of opinion exists, or when it is difficult to determine the safety of the situation, it may be helpful to have a team conference that includes all of the people who function in assessment or caregiving capacities and who have some degree of objectivity. In cases of suspected elder abuse, the assessment team may include many informal sources of help, such as family and neighbours, as well as formal sources of help, such as nurses and social workers.

Personal dress, hygiene and grooming are among the most visible and commonly appraised aspects of daily function. People often are viewed as neglected when they do not comply with socially defined standards of cleanliness, particularly when an unpleasant odour is noted. In elder abuse situations, nurses need to consider that poor hygiene and grooming are important reflections of many underlying problems, but they are not necessarily indicators of safety concerns. When families and healthcare or social service workers initially work with a neglected older person who is in need of much personal care, they often are tempted to begin by assisting the person with bathing and grooming. Although the workers may view this as a socially acceptable way to begin, the elder may perceive this as a threat to their pride and independence. Thus, nurses assess not only the impact of poor hygiene on the elder's health but also the consequences of imposing assistance when the elder is unwilling to accept help or acknowledge a hygiene problem. The nurse may determine that

TABLE 10-3 Risks to safety associated with functional limitations

Functional limitation	Risks to safety
Any mental or physical impairment, especially combined with social isolation and lack of a support system	Malnutrition and dehydration
Mobility limitations or seriously impaired vision, especially combined with poor judgement	Falls
Cognitive impairments in ambulatory people	Wandering, getting lost
Compromised mobility	Pressure sores
Cognitive impairment, especially poor judgement	Inability to get help
Poor judgement, especially when living in an unsafe neighbourhood	Basic safety and security

efforts to deal with personal hygiene would interfere with the short-term goal of establishing a relationship and the long-term goal of assisting with other aspects of daily function. Thus, nurses may need to begin by addressing nutrition, hydration and safety, while deferring attention to personal care issues associated with the most resistance.

Adequate nutrition, hydration and an ability to obtain help in an emergency are the basic human needs that are most often called into question in cases of elder abuse. Other basic needs may also be compromised, usually in relation to specific functional impairments and environmental circumstances. For instance, it is imperative to address bowel and bladder elimination for people who are confined to bed or a chair. For people with mobility limitations or serious vision impairments, safe ambulation and the ability to avoid falls are important considerations. Table 10-3 summarises some of the specific functional and environmental conditions that present risks to basic needs.

Cognitive and psychosocial function

Information in Chapters 13 (Cognitive and psychosocial assessment), 14 (Delirium and dementia), and 15 (Depression) is pertinent to assessing psychosocial function in relation to elder abuse. In addition, an important aspect of cognitive and psychosocial function for abuse situations is assessment of the elder's capacity for reasonable judgements about self-care. This is difficult because the determination of someone's ability to make appropriate judgements is based, at least in part, on subjective criteria and opinions.

People whose judgement is impaired to the point that they are at serious risk, especially if they do not acknowledge the risk, are usually considered to be incompetent or incapacitated. Thus, the crucial element of psychosocial assessment for elder abuse cases is a determination of risk (i.e. danger to the person) rather than a determination of whether other people would judge the decision as *good* or *appropriate*. When the competence of an older adult to make safe decisions regarding self-care is in doubt, nurses may be legally bound to make reports or consider other legal interventions. There are no federal guidelines for determining the mental capacity of abused or neglected older adults, and the legal criteria differ from state to state. Ethical and legal considerations related to elder abuse are discussed later in this chapter.

WELLNESS OPPORTUNITY

Nurses promote self-determination for older adults by respecting their rights to make decisions about their care, as long as their actions do not jeopardise safety for themselves or others.

Support resources

Support resources include those people, such as carers and friends, who influence a person's physical and psychosocial function. Some or all of the support people may directly cause the abusive situation or may actively or passively contribute to it. Therefore, nurses assess the support resources in terms of both helpful and detrimental effects. In addition, support resources not currently being used are identified as potential sources of help.

When the carers who perpetrate the abuse are also the support resources, nurses assess the potential for working with them to alleviate the negative consequences. Although it is not always easy to work with abusive carers, it may be even more difficult to eliminate their influence over an older adult. During the assessment, therefore, nurses identify any strengths of the carer and any willingness to change the situation voluntarily. If the carer is extremely stressed, then respite, along with individual or group support and counselling, may be effective interventions. In mutually abusive situations in which the designated carer also is abused or neglected, the nurse tries to identify any outside sources of support that have not been tapped. For example, in a mutually abusive situation involving a socially isolated married couple, the nurse might identify a relative or friend who is willing to assist with caregiving or decision-making responsibilities.

Because a carer's lack of knowledge can be an underlying factor in elder abuse, nurses assess the carer's understanding of the elder's needs. For example, carers may have good intentions when they use adult briefs for the control of incontinence and do not change them frequently, but they may not understand the potential for skin breakdown. Carers may administer excessive amounts of psychoactive medications because they do not understand the correct dosing schedule or the potential adverse effects. This is especially common when medications are ordered on an as-needed basis and the carer has not been given clear guidelines for determining when the medication is needed, or what the most effective dosage is. In these situations, nursing assessment of the carer's knowledge is especially important because educational interventions, role modelling, or the provision of additional services may alleviate the abuse.

In situations of neglect, there usually are very few support services to assess, and the task of the nurse is to identify potential sources of help and the barriers that interfere with the use of these resources. The assessment of barriers to the use of resources is discussed in Chapter 13 and is summarised in Box 13-8. It is especially important to identify these barriers because simple interventions, such as provision of information or assistance with transportation, may be effective in eliminating them. Cultural influences also must be assessed in relation to the use of support resources, as discussed in Chapter 2.

Environmental influences

As with other aspects of elder abuse, the primary purposes of assessing the environment are to identify the factors that create risks and to determine which of these factors can be alleviated through interventions. With regard to the immediate living conditions, the nurse assesses whether minimal standards of safety and cleanliness are being maintained. When nurses assess home environments that are terribly cluttered, they must make some determination of both the meaning and the consequences of the clutter. A massive collection of clutter from hoarding reflects an underlying disorder and may or may not be a risk factor that needs to be addressed. Consequences of hoarding range from socially unacceptable appearances to serious risks to health and safety. Therefore, the nurse must assess the person's ability to manoeuvre in the environment during daily activities, as well as the person's safety in emergency situations, such as a fire.

When nurses and other workers are initially exposed to massive amounts of clutter, their first inclination may be to think of a way to eliminate some of it. If this reaction is communicated to the resident of the cluttered home, however, it may become impossible to establish an accepting relationship, and the older adult may reject any further interventions. In assessing the home environment, therefore, nurses must be non-judgemental, except in circumstances in which the risks are so great that immediate action must be taken.

Nurses also assess the neighbourhood environment for its impact on the safety of the person. This is especially important when the older person lives in an area of high crime or extreme isolation and is vulnerable by virtue of impaired judgement, physical frailty, or a combination of physical and psychosocial impairments. People who are only moderately forgetful may be safe in an apartment or a suburban neighbourhood where neighbours watch out for them. In a high-crime neighbourhood, however, forgetting to lock the doors or to take other precautions may place the person at increased risk for physical harm, financial exploitation, or other serious abuses. Likewise, in a rural environment social isolation may increase the risks for vulnerable elderly people.

Finally, seasonal conditions can influence the degree of risk for self-neglect in people who have dementia and live in climates characterised by extreme heat or cold. For example, a person who does not pay utility bills may not be in any danger as long as the weather is mild, but when the temperature turns cold, that person would be at risk for hypothermia. The same is true for people who occasionally wander outside without dressing appropriately. As long as the neighbourhood is safe and the weather is mild, they may be relatively safe; however, they may be at increased risk during the cold months or very hot months, especially if they do not wear proper clothing. Nurses also assess any of the risk factors for hypothermia or heat-related illness.

Threats to life

The most immediate consideration in determining if legal interventions are necessary is the assessment of threats to life. Situations often are viewed as being of crisis proportions when they are first discovered, and the immediate reaction of the person who discovers the situation may be to remove a person from the environment. Many times, however, the person may not want to leave, or there may be no better setting in which the person can receive care immediately. In these situations, the nurse may be asked to assess the urgency and seriousness of the situation and to provide an opinion about whether legal interventions are justified. The nurse often is the person who can either convince the elder to accept help or convince the carers and social workers that the present situation is tolerable. For instance, when nurses determine that the situation is not life-threatening, they can reassure the person that they are trying to improve the situation and support the person remaining to be as safe and independent as possible. Examples of threats that nurses commonly assess in elder abuse situations include the following:

- History of physical violence on the part of the carer, especially when the elder is unable to escape or otherwise be protected
- Untreated wounds or infections
- Inability to administer insulin correctly
- Progressive gangrene or ulcerated conditions
- Inability to adhere to therapeutic regimens
- Consistent wandering in unsafe neighbourhoods or in very cold weather
- Misuse (usually unintentional) of certain medications, such as digoxin or insulin
- Excessive use of drugs or alcohol, either self- or carer-induced.

In situations in which the carer is the abuser, the nurse and other team members must assess whether or not the carer presents a threat to the life of the dependent older person.

When nurses do not have first-hand knowledge of the abused or neglected older person before being notified of a crisis situation, the first consideration is whether this is objectively a crisis or merely a crisis in the eyes of the person who just discovered the situation. Situations that appear the most appalling may actually represent a gradual deterioration over several months or years. Therefore, the initial assessment is aimed at determining any immediate threats to the life of the abused elder, such as malnutrition, dehydration, or an untreated medical condition. Finally, suicide potential must be assessed, especially in self-neglected elders who also are depressed and expressing feelings of hopelessness. Nurses can apply all of the principles of suicide assessment, discussed in Chapter 15, to abused and neglected elders.

Cultural aspects

Definitions and perceptions of elder abuse and neglect are influenced to a great extent by cultural norms. For example, Asian Indians may consider not visiting an older family member to be a form of psychological neglect, but Anglo Australians or New Zealanders may consider it to be a way of respecting privacy and autonomy. Very little evidence exists about aspects of elder abuse in different cultures. In Australia, an inquiry into Indigenous violence in remote communities found that abuse of older people existed and it was a recent development related to the loss of traditional values, especially the respect for elders (Australian Institute of Criminology, 2010).

In New Zealand it has been reported that the most common forms of elder abuse—psychological abuse, financial abuse or neglect—are the same for European, Māori and Pacific New Zealanders (ACNZ, 2007). Yet it was identified that the reason/s for this abuse or neglect varies and is dependent on the culture. It is recommended that when responding to elder abuse and neglect, Māori require a holistic approach involving *whānau*, traditional cultural values, and the four cornerstones of health to restore *manaakitanga* (Agewell, 2010). Therefore an understanding of culture is required so that a culturally appropriate management strategy can be implemented.

Cultural factors also have a strong influence on carer roles and responsibilities. Most families have culturally influenced expectations about which family members should provide care to dependent older adults and about whether it is acceptable to enlist the aid of paid carers. In some families, there may be conflicts about these expectations, particularly between older and younger generations. Sometimes, these conflicts may need to be identified and addressed before elder abuse or neglect can be resolved.

CULTURAL CONSIDERATIONS 10-1
Cultural considerations in assessing elder abuse and neglect

- What are the family and cultural expectations concerning family carers (e.g. is it acceptable to employ paid carers, or are family members expected to provide all the care)?
- Do family members differ in their perceptions about caregiving responsibilities?
- What are the family and cultural perspectives on autonomy and independence?
- Do family members differ in their perspectives on autonomy and independence?
- How are decisions made about care of the older adult (e.g. is it a patriarchal or matriarchal family)?
- Who are the acceptable sources of social support and personal assistance?
- Who are the acceptable sources of healthcare (e.g. herbalists, spiritual healers)?
- What are the acceptable healthcare practices (e.g. herbs, homeopathy, acupuncture, faith healing, folk remedies)?
- Are there language barriers that influence the care that is provided or that limit the number of care providers?
- How does skin colour affect assessment of bruises, pressure sores and other skin changes?

Nurses must identify cultural factors that influence the care that is provided—or not provided—to older adults. Cultural considerations 10-1 lists some of the assessment questions that should be considered in identifying cultural influences. When assessing family carer relationships, nurses should be sensitive to cultural variations in perspectives on family caregiving and respect differences, but they also must address abusive situations. In addition, cultural assessment information on the following topics should be considered: communication and cognitive and psychosocial assessment (see Chapter 13), nutrition (see Chapter 18), dementia (see Chapter 14), and depression (see Chapter 15).

In Australia a government-supported organisation Diversicare's project, Partners in Culturally Appropriate Care Program (PICAC), works to maintain links between older adults who live in long-term residential care or receive community services and their social, cultural and linguistic connections (available via http://diversicare.com.au). In New Zealand, Māori and Pacific people have a specific Elder Abuse and Neglect Prevention Service to address abuse issues within these cultural groups. See Box 10-3.

BOX 10-3
Dedicated Māori and Pacific People's elder abuse services

Dedicated Māori service Auckland region	Te Oranga Kaumatua Kuia Disability Support Services Trust 64 Mascot Ave, Mangere, Auckland 2022 Phone: 09 255 5470 Email: teorangakk@xtra.co.nz Website: www.teorangakk.org.nz
Dedicated Pacific People's service, Auckland region	TOA Pacific 214 Great South Rd, Otahuhu, Auckland 1062 Phone: 09 276 4596 Email: malia@toapacific.org.nz Website: www.toapacific.org

CASE STUDY TWO

Mrs Kirk is 80 years old and has been in a medical unit for 4 days. She was discharged at her request but "against medical advice" with no prescriptions for her medications or medical referral for home care. She has complex health conditions, including osteoarthritis, coronary artery disease, congestive heart failure, chronic obstructive pulmonary disease (COPD), depression, and type 2 diabetes (Insulin dependent). Although alert and oriented, Mrs Kirk has major deficits in her ability to perform daily living tasks. She also depends on a walker for ambulation and has a history of falling, including a fall that resulted in a hip fracture and her admission to a rehabilitation unit.

Mrs Kirk's support system is limited. Her son lives in another state but functions as power of attorney and provides some telephone reassurance. Her daughter is estranged from Mrs Kirk, and at their last meeting was verbally abusive to her. Mrs Kirk's older brother visits a few times weekly to help with meal preparation, grocery shopping, transportation, and medication pickups; however, his own health problems prevent him from providing more help.

Shortly after returning home, Mrs Kirk's precarious health status rapidly deteriorated. She became severely short of breath, requiring continuous oxygen. She began to hallucinate in the evening, believing that she alone had the responsibility of feeding all of the children in the neighbourhood. As her fears increased, so too did the calls to her brother. Eventually, she made several calls every night, overwhelming and exhausting him.

Thinking points

- What form(s) of elder abuse is (are) represented?
- What are signs or indicators of abuse that you as a nurse would be able to identify?
- What factors contribute to Mrs Kirk's current risks?
- How will you proceed in conducting a nursing assessment of Mrs Kirk?
- What barriers might you encounter in conducting the assessment? How will you overcome them?

NURSING ISSUES

Because elder abuse and neglect is so broad and complex, various nursing issues are applicable, depending on the situation. A nursing issue that would apply to many elder abuse situations where family members are carers is the family not coping. Related factors include changes in family roles, unrealistic expectations about caregiving, and changes in the health status of the older adult. If the nursing assessment identifies stressors related to family caregiving, the nursing issue of carer role strain might be applicable. Related carer factors include ineffective coping patterns, functional or cognitive impairments, and insufficient resources (e.g. respite, financial assets, assistance with care). Related factors involving the dependent older adult include increased dependence and the presence of difficult or unsafe behaviours (e.g. paranoia, wandering and incontinence).

The nursing issue of risk for injury might be used for older adults who are in self-neglecting situations, especially if the person lives alone and is physically and psychosocially impaired. The nursing issue of conflict about decision making might apply to abused or neglected older adults who live in an environment that places them at risk for harm because they are unable to make decisions about alternative environments. Related factors include fear, lack of information about alternatives, and impaired decision-making ability.

WELLNESS OPPORTUNITY

Nurses address body–mind–spirit interrelatedness by identifying nursing issues that address fear and other psychosocial consequences of abuse or neglect.

GOAL PLANNING FOR WELLNESS OUTCOMES

Nurses direct care for abused or neglected older adults towards addressing the complex needs of the elder as well as those of the family carers. Nursing goals that achieve wellness outcomes that are likely to pertain to the abused older adult includes abuse cessation, abuse protection, abuse recovery status, neglect cessation, risk control, self-care status, and social support. Goals related to abusive carers or family members include abusive behaviour self-restraint, improvement in carer emotional health and carer–older adult relationship, reduction in carer stressors, improvement in carer endurance potential, family coping and family social climate, and improvement in knowledge of health resources, role performance and stress levels.

WELLNESS OPPORTUNITY

Quality of life is a wellness outcome that is applicable to older adults and their carers when conditions contributing to abuse or neglect are alleviated.

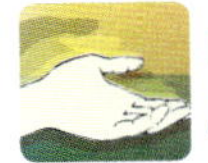

NURSING INTERVENTIONS TO ADDRESS ELDER ABUSE AND NEGLECT

From a healthcare perspective, abused elders can be described as the *intensive care patients* of the community because they require the highest level of skill from a variety of professionals. However, unlike intensive care patients in hospitals, the team members are not specialised healthcare professionals but rather are community-based workers and people who provide informal support. Nurses often assume the role of coordinator or team leader in implementing interventions that address the older adults, the carers, and the environment for these inherently complex and challenging situations.

Because of the extensive scope of elder abuse, there are numerous nursing interventions that could be applicable to both the abused or neglected elder and the carer. Some that would be appropriate in most situations are abuse protection support: crisis intervention, referral and risk identification for the elder; and support coping enhancement, referral and teaching for carers.

Interventions in elder abuse situations may involve legal actions when decision-making abilities of the older adult are impaired. Many situations involve carers who are not competent decision makers or are not acting in the best interest of the elder. Thus, many cases of elder abuse involve legal and ethical questions about the competency of the elder and the carers. Nurses often have a key role in advocating for the older adult and may feel unprepared or uncomfortable either making or participating in decisions that affect the rights of others. Similarly, nurses may feel torn between the right of the person to refuse treatment and the obligation to report abuse and neglect situations, as discussed later in this chapter.

Interventions for elder abuse are implemented in community settings, over a long period of time, by a team of formal and informal care providers. Nurses working in community settings have the most direct opportunities for both the prevention of and interventions for elder abuse. Home-delivered meals and nursing and medical strategies are interventions that are usually readily accepted and effective for addressing abused older adults in community settings. Nurses in institutional settings are likely to use interventions such as education and support of carers and facilitation of referrals to appropriate community agencies. Because the opportunities for intervention in institutional settings are quite different from those in community settings, each of these areas is discussed separately in the following sections.

Interventions in institutional settings

Nurses in acute and long-term residential care settings can intervene in cases of elder abuse when they interact with carers, who often seek advice from nurses about ways of providing care. For example, nurses can encourage carers to use a period of institutionalisation to re-evaluate the demands of the situation and to consider resources for support and assistance. Family may express ambivalence about managing the older adult's care at home, or they may be unsure or unrealistic about their own ability to provide appropriate care or to cope with the stress of the situation. In some cases, carers may be seeking approval for not providing care at home. In these situations, nurses can facilitate communication among all the decision makers, including the primary care provider, the older adult (if appropriate), and the various family members who are responsible for care. Sometimes, it is appropriate to suggest individual counselling or support groups, or make referrals for social services, particularly when carers are very stressed about care-related decisions.

When elder abuse occurs because of the carer's lack of information, nurses can be a role model and teach about appropriate caregiving measures. When carers need additional health education or support services, nurses can initiate a referral to a community agency for follow-up.

WELLNESS OPPORTUNITY

When vulnerable older adults are in an acute or a long-term residential care setting, nurses address the psychosocial needs of family carers by providing support and education; these are effective tools for preventing elder abuse.

Interventions in community settings

Families caring for people with dementia in home settings have identified professional advice about understanding and handling memory problems as important interventions for preventing elder abuse. Nurses in community settings have many opportunities for teaching carers about adequate care through role modelling and verbal and written instruction. For example, if carers have trouble managing complex medication regimens, nurses can use charts and organisers to facilitate adherence.

Nurses can also educate carers about basic care needs, such as nutrition, exercise and elimination. For example, nurses may suggest innovative ways of meeting the nutritional requirements of an elderly person who does not eat adequately. Home care nurses have the advantage of observing many creative and effective techniques used by carers that have never been described in any nursing texts. Thus, experienced home care nurses are continually expanding their repertoire of techniques for physical care and behavioural management, and these techniques can then be passed on to other family carers.

When elder abuse is rooted in carer stress, nurses can suggest services and help find ways of providing care so that the carer can use these resources for self-care. The following are examples of services aimed at reducing carer stress or dealing with carer problems:

- Alcoholics Anonymous for carers with alcoholism
- Individual counselling to learn coping skills
- Alzheimer's Association for support and education groups
- In-home or day care for respite.

Community care workers are the service providers who are most likely to care for abused elders in home settings, but they often are ill prepared to detect or address elder abuse. Nurses who provide home-based services, therefore, have a tremendous responsibility to help community care workers recognise and intervene in elder abuse situations. For example, nurses can teach about detecting clues to elder abuse, and they can address concerns about questionable conditions. If nurses cannot openly discuss the situation during home visits, they may have to arrange for a phone conversation with the community care workers.

In situations in which the older adult requires a significant degree of physical care or supervision, the services of a community care workers may be the most effective means of preventing elder abuse. Often, however, the retention of a community care workers in challenging situations depends largely on the degree of support and guidance provided by a professional nurse.

Nurses in other community settings, such as clinics or day-care centres, have opportunities to intervene in elder abuse. Nurses can prevent or alleviate elder abuse by facilitating referrals for appropriate community-based resources, such as adult day care or group or home-delivered meals. Even if nurses are not familiar with specific community services, they can discuss the advantages of various types of services and encourage older adults to contact these services. Compulsory reporting is also required in some community settings in Australia. If abuse is suspected of an older adult who receives home care through an Australian Government-funded aged care community service, then it must be reported to Aged Care Complaints Scheme on 1800 550 552.

WELLNESS OPPORTUNITY

Nurses help carers maintain self-wellness by identifying ways of alleviating stress associated with the demands of caregiving.

Referrals

Nurses often facilitate referrals for services that improve functioning for the older adult and decrease the burden of caregiving responsibilities. For instance, speech, physical and occupational therapies may be useful in improving the older person's ability to communicate, ambulate and perform ADLs. Referrals for community care services usually are made at the time of discharge from an institution; however, the older adult or family may have refused the services at that time.

Older adults who are not admitted to healthcare facilities may not know they qualify for aged care services, and a nurse making a home visit may be the first health professional to suggest these resources. Although older adults or their families may not know about or may have refused such services, nurses need to assess their willingness to accept help as conditions change.

Nurses also assess whether recent changes in the older adult qualify them for community care services. For example, a change in medications or a fall may qualify the person for community care. Another important role for nurses is suggesting types of medical equipment, disposable supplies, and assistive devices to improve function and safety for the elder and ease carer burden. For example, carers may respond positively to suggestions from the nurse about obtaining and using grab bars for preventing falls in the bathroom. Some durable medical equipment is covered by

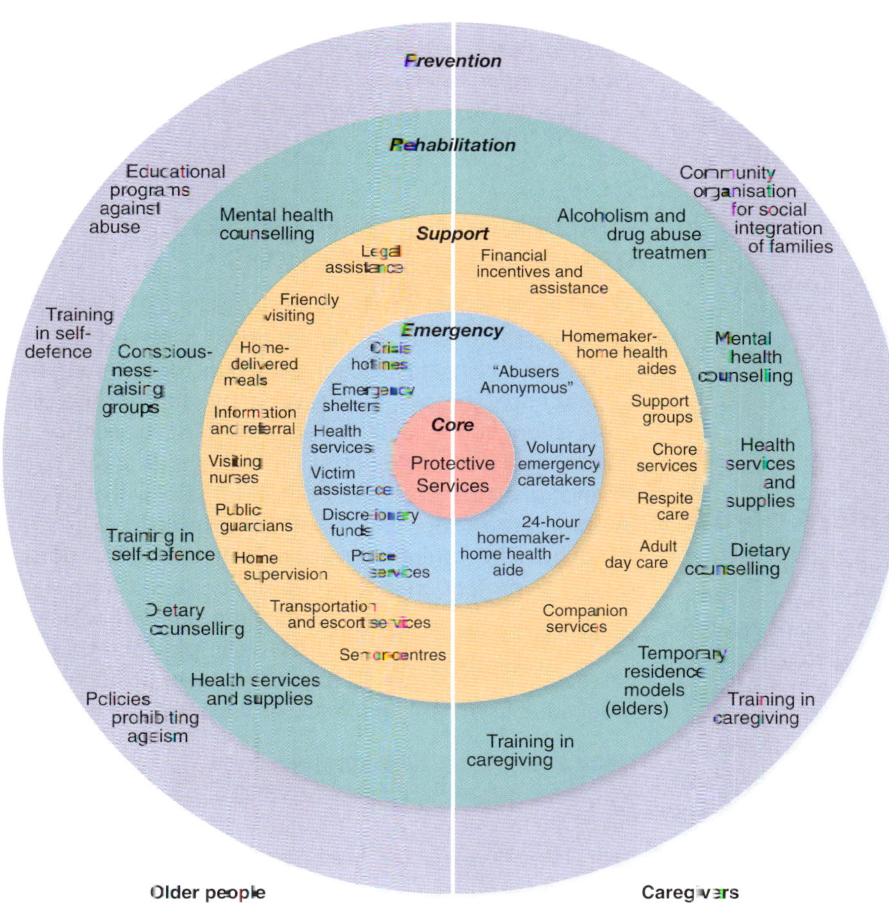

FIGURE 10-2 The types of services needed by abused older adults and their carers. (Used with permission from Anetzberger, G. J. [2010]. Report of the Elder Abuse Project: Recommendations for addressing the problem of elder abuse in Cuyahoga County. Cleveland, OH: Federation for Community Planning. Originally published in 1982.)

health insurance, and medical supply companies usually are quite helpful in advising people about specific equipment.

Prevention and treatment interventions

Abused elders and their carers or abusers typically need a wide range of interventions, which can be categorised according to basic function:

- Core, or essential, integrative services
- Emergency services, during crises or just before or after abuse or neglect occurs
- Support services for managing the problem and improving the situation
- Rehabilitative services to address problems of either the victim or the perpetrator
- Preventive services, including programs directed towards changing society in ways that diminish the likelihood of maltreatment or self-neglect.

Figure 10-2 identifies some of the specific types of services, arranged by function, which may be needed in elder abuse situations. Nurses are the healthcare professionals who are most accepted and qualified for implementing or arranging for many of the services for both the carers and abused or neglected older person(s).

Financial exploitation is an aspect of elder abuse that can be prevented through relatively simple and widely available measures to protect assets. For example, nurses can suggest that a trusted family member establishes a joint account with the older adult and keep track of all transactions. Out-of-town families can oversee financial transactions through online banking. Nurses can find information about programs directed towards the prevention of financial abuse and exploitation at the Internet sites listed in the resources section near the end of this chapter.

CASE STUDY THREE

Mr and Mrs Gradzki have been married for over 50 years and have six children, four of whom live in the area. Because of Mrs Gradzki's memory loss in recent years, Mr Gradzki has allowed home carers into the house to help her with eating and to perform personal care. The workers report that Mr Gradzki yells at his wife when she forgets things. On more than one occasion they witnessed him attempting to force feed her when she failed to eat an entire meal. After the couple has gone to their bedroom in the evening, the night carers have reported hearing screams, cursing and slapping sounds coming from behind the closed bedroom door. In the morning, Mrs Gradzki had bruises on her body and bumps on her head. When asked, Mr Gradzki denied hitting his wife. Mrs Gradzki cried when questioned, never providing an explanation for her injuries.

Mr Gradzki is reluctant to consider additional services, such as adult day care, citing cost as an issue. He had Mrs Gradzki change doctors several times in recent years because "they don't do anything to really help her". The children who live nearby have said that they do not want to get involved in their parents' situation. They describe years of their father physically and verbally abusing their mother and fear what might happen if any action is taken now.

Thinking points

- What interventions might be helpful in addressing the elder abuse evident in this situation?
- What is the role of the community nurse in introducing and implementing these interventions?
- What barriers might be encountered in acceptance of the interventions?
- As the community nurse in this situation, how will you help to overcome these barriers?

LEGAL INTERVENTIONS AND ETHICAL ISSUES

Most elder abuse situations require consideration of voluntary or involuntary legal interventions. Whenever feasible, problems should be remedied without the use of involuntary legal intervention. Because voluntary legal interventions require the consent of the older person, they cannot be initiated if the person is not mentally competent. Competent adults can revoke voluntary legal interventions at any time. Money management, power of attorney and various types of bank accounts, such as joint or direct deposit, are all interventions of this nature.

Other legal interventions that are useful for mentally competent older adults are discussed in Chapter 9. Some legal interventions, such as guardianship, are either voluntary or involuntary, but are most commonly used on an involuntary basis when the older person's safety or property is in jeopardy.

Because these legal interventions involve a much more extensive loss of personal freedom than voluntary ones, they should be used with extreme caution. A key consideration in the choice of legal interventions is determining the competency of the person to make decisions, as discussed in Chapters 9 and 13. Some measures, such as guardianship, may be easier to initiate than to discontinue.

Involuntary legal interventions are used when cognitive impairments—such as limited insight, judgement, memory or cognition—affect the ability of older people to function safely and meet their basic human needs. In general, involuntary legal intervention is indicated when assessment reveals all of the following conditions:

- Decisions must be made about the older person's health, living arrangements, money or property.
- The older person is not capable of making reasonable decisions.
- There is a risk to the older person's health, safety, money or property.
- The risk would be reduced or eliminated if someone else was empowered to make and implement decisions.

Legal interventions that address the abuser include **domestic violence** law and the criminal code.

WELLNESS OPPORTUNITY

Nurses support autonomy for older adults by identifying the least invasive legal interventions, while also ensuring the least amount of endangerment.

EVALUATING THE EFFECTIVENESS OF NURSING INTERVENTIONS

Nursing care of abused or neglected older adults is evaluated by the extent to which nursing goals are achieved. If a nursing goal is to alleviate the contributing factor of unnecessary dependence, the care is evaluated by whether the older adult is functioning at a higher level of independence. If a nursing goal is to address carer stress, the nursing care might be evaluated by the carer accepting help with the care, attending carer support groups, and expressing less stress about his or her caregiving responsibilities. When the nursing goal is to protect an incompetent older adult from harm, nursing care might be evaluated by the extent to which the least restrictive legal interventions are implemented. In such cases, nursing care is evaluated in terms of protecting the older adult from harm while also protecting his or her rights.

UNFOLDING CASE STUDY

Part B

Recall that Mrs Barnes is 82 years old and lives in a unit in a retirement village. After 2 months of receiving nursing visits, Mrs Barnes was discharged from the community agency because she was successfully managing her medications and other aspects of functioning adequately. Several months after she was discharged, the nurse in the medical practice noted a change in her mannerisms, accompanied by slurred speech and an unbalanced gait. Mrs Barnes had bruises on her arms, knees and forehead, but insisted that she had not fallen. After further investigation, the nurse found that her blood pressure was 210/104 mm Hg and that her blood glucose level was 16 mmol/L on the glucometer that the nurse kept in the clinic. A pill count revealed that Mrs Barnes had not taken her medications for 2½ days. After a consultation with her primary care provider, Mrs Barnes was admitted to the hospital. Tests revealed that she had suffered a stroke, resulting in left-sided weakness and short-term memory loss.

Mrs Barnes left the hospital against medical advice and returned to her unit, initially refusing visits from the community nurse. She insisted that her children come and administer her medications and prepare her meals because she was unable to do this for herself. Mrs Barnes reasoned that she had cared for her children when they were young, so they should come when she needed them. The children tried to assist Mrs Barnes for 4 days but were unable to meet both her demands and those of their jobs and families. Mrs Barnes reluctantly agreed to a visit from the community nurse who had visited her before. She expected that she would see the nurse once and that the nurse would "make my children do right".

Mrs Barnes' children were present for the initial assessment. Mrs Barnes was unable to stand or transfer to the commode without help. She could not use her chart and colour-coded boxes to take her pills. Mrs Barnes flatly refused to consider admission to an aged care facility for respite so she could regain her strength, and she would not consider living with her daughter or either son. The family told the nurse that they were exhausted and on the "verge of a breakdown" and could not continue to provide the care that Mrs Barnes needed. The nurse explained to Mrs Barnes that it was not safe for her to remain in her unit without assistance. She suggested that she hire an aide until other arrangements could be made, because her children were not obligated to lose their jobs or jeopardise their family relationships to care for her. Mrs Barnes accused her children of being greedy and caring only about themselves. She said that children have a duty to care for their parents and that she wasn't going to "have strangers doing the things that decent children should be doing". She directed her concluding remarks at the nurse, stating, "What's more, I don't need you to come back, either, because all you want to do is side with my children."

Thinking points

- What strategies would you use to establish a relationship with Mrs Barnes?
- What additional assessment information would you want to obtain, and how would you obtain it?
- What would your next steps be in working with Mrs Barnes?
- How would you work with the family?
- What other resources would you involve in planning and providing care for Mrs Barnes?

CHAPTER HIGHLIGHTS

Overview of elder abuse and neglect

- There are seven major forms of elder abuse: physical abuse, sexual abuse, emotional or psychological abuse, neglect, abandonment, financial or material exploitation, and self-neglect
- Awareness of elder abuse as a social problem began in the 1950s and 1960s and is now recognised as a major social and public health problem and a significant aspect of partner and family violence
- Studies of causes of elder abuse indicate that it differs from other forms of abuse and is complex
- Cultural differences in family and carer roles affect definitions of elder abuse

Risk factors for elder abuse and neglect

- Elder abuse is usually related to multiple risk factors that develop over a long period
- Invisibility and vulnerability are two risk factors that occur in most situations of abuse or neglect
- Common psychosocial risk factors: impaired cognition, long-term mental illness
- Carer factors: psychosocial impairments

Elder abuse and neglect in long-term residential care

- Elder abuse has been recognised as a problem in nursing homes since the 1970s, and studies indicate that it is widespread and underreported
- Mandatory reporting of suspected abuse is required in Australian long-term residential care facilities
- Age Concern New Zealand is responsible for the coordination of the 24 Elder Abuse and Neglect Prevention Services across New Zealand

Functional consequences associated with elder abuse and neglect

- Definitions: neglect, physical abuse, sexual abuse, emotional or psychological abuse, abandonment, self-neglect
- Partner and family violence, rape and sexual violence are unique aspects of elder abuse

Nursing assessment of abused or neglected older adults

- Unique aspects of elder abuse assessment: safety, limited goals, resistance, nurse viewed as threat, legal and ethical considerations, safety of nurse
- Physical health: nutrition, hydration, indicators of physical harm (Figure 10-1), degree of frailty, pathological conditions
- Activities of daily living: assess in relation to safety, basic needs, vulnerability (Table 10-3)
- Psychosocial function: impaired cognition, judgements about self-care
- Support resources: carers who also are perpetrators, lack of resources, barriers to using services
- Environmental influences: home, neighbourhood, seasonal factors
- Threats to life: degree of endangerment and ability to alleviate risks
- Cultural aspects: family and cultural expectations, perspectives on caregiving, barriers to assessment
- Cultural considerations 10-1

Nursing issues

- Compromised family coping
- Carer role strain (or risk of)
- Risk for injury
- Decisional conflict

Goal planning for wellness outcomes

- Quality of life
- Abuse cessation, protection, recovery status
- Neglect cessation
- Risk control
- Carer stressors, emotional health, endurance potential
- Family coping
- Social support

Nursing interventions to address elder abuse and neglect

- Role of the nurse in institutional settings (teaching carers, discharge planning, addressing carer stress, reporting elder abuse)

- Role of the nurse in community settings (teaching, supervising, providing direct care, working with community care workers, facilitating referrals, reporting elder abuse)
- Facilitating referrals (services for older adults and carers, medical equipment)
- Prevention and treatment interventions (types of core services, programs for preventing financial abuse; Figure 10-2)

Legal interventions and ethical issues

- Voluntary and involuntary interventions

Evaluating effectiveness of nursing interventions

- Higher level of functioning of older adult
- Alleviation of carer stress
- Use of least-restrictive legal interventions
- Protection of the older adult

CRITICAL THINKING EXERCISES

1. Identify factors in each of the following categories that currently contribute to elder abuse and neglect in the Australia or New Zealand:
   - Demographic statistics
   - Changes in families
   - Healthcare systems
   - Health status and other characteristics of older adults
   - Social awareness.
2. What is different about the nursing assessment of abused or neglected elders compared with the nursing assessment of other older adults?
3. What do you believe about family caregiving responsibilities? How would you deal with a family whose values about caregiving differ significantly from yours?
4. What are your beliefs about the degree of risk a frail elder should be allowed to take?
5. Under what circumstances would an elder be denied the right to remain in his or her own home?

RESOURCES

For an extensive range of additional resources to enhance teaching and learning and to facilitate understanding of this chapter, please see the text's accompanying website located on thePoint at http://thepoint.lww.com.

Clinical tools

Hartford Institute for Geriatric Nursing, ConsultGeriRN.org: http://consultgerirn.org/resources
Assessment tools *Try This®* series and *How to Try This* resources
General assessment series:
- *Try This*, issue 15: Elder mistreatment assessment. Fulmer, T. (2012). *Best Practices in Nursing Care to Older Adults*.
- *How to Try This* (article): Screening for mistreatment of older adults.
- *How to Try This* (video): *Elder mistreatment assessment*.

Evidence-based practice

Caceres, B. & Fulmer, T. (2012). Mistreatment detection. In M. Boltz, E. Capezuti, T. Fulmer & D. Zwicker (Eds), *Evidence-based geriatric nursing protocols for best practice* (4th ed., pp. 544–561). New York: Springer.

Joanna Briggs Institute: http://connect.jbiconnectplus.org
Evidence summaries:
- Battaglini, E. (2014). Elder abuse (community-dwelling elders): Mental health risk factors.
- Khanh, D. L. L. (2014). Elder abuse in residential aged care: Prevention.

National Guideline Clearinghouse: www.guideline.gov
Search for:
- Detection of elder mistreatment (2012). In *Evidence-based geriatric nursing protocols for best practice*.
- Elder abuse prevention (2004, revised 2010).
- Screening for intimate partner violence and abuse of elderly and vulnerable adults: U.S. Preventive Services Task Force recommendation statement (1996, revised 2013).

Health education

Advocare Incorporated, help with elder abuse: www.advocare.org.au
Age Concern New Zealand, elder abuse and neglect: www.ageconcern.org.nz
Aged Care Australia, article, Elder abuse: One report too many, by P. Sadler. (2009): www.agedcare.org.au/events-and-conferences/conferences/2009-acsa-national-conference/Paul%20Sadler.pdf/view
Aged Rights Advocacy Service (ARAS): www.sa.aged-rights.asn.au
Agewell New Zealand, elder abuse: www.agewell.org.nz
American Psychological Association, elder abuse and neglect: www.apa.org/pi/aging/resources/guides/elder-abuse.aspx
Diversicare, PICAC program: http://diversicare.com.au
Elder Abuse Prevention Unit: www.eapu.com.au/elder-abuse
myaged*care*, elder abuse concerns: www.myagedcare.gov.au
National Center on Elder Abuse (U.S.): www.ncea.aoa.gov
National Clearinghouse, abuse in later life: www.ncall.us
National Committee for the Prevention of Elder Abuse (U.S.): http://preventelderabuse.org

REFERENCES

Age Concern New Zealand (ACNZ). (2007). Elder abuse and neglect prevention: Challenges for the future. Viewed March 2015 at www.ageconcern.org.nz/files/EANP/Challenges%20for%20the%20Future,%20Stats%20report%20for%20Age%20Concern%202004-07.pdf.

Age Concern New Zealand (ACNZ). (2015). Elder abuse and neglect. Accessed March 2015 at www.ageconcern.org.nz/ACNZPublic/Services/EANP/ACNZ_Public/Elder_Abuse_and_Neglect.aspx?hkey.

Aged Rights Advocacy Service (ARAS). (2105). Residential care: Mandatory reporting. Accessed March 2015 at www.sa.agedrights.asn.au/residential_care/preventing_elder_abuse/elder_abuse_and_the_law/compulsory_reporting.

Agewell. (2010). Health topics: Elder abuse. Accessed March 2015 at www.agewell.org.nz/health_elder_abuse.html.

Anetzberger, G. J. (2010). Report of the Elder Abuse Project: Recommendations for addressing the problem of elder abuse in Cuyahoga County. Cleveland, OH: Federation for Community Planning.

Anetzberger, G. J. (2013). Elder abuse: Risk. In A. Jamieson & A. A. Moenssens (Eds), *Wiley encyclopedia of forensic science*. Chichester: John Wiley & Sons.

Australian Government Department of Health. (2015). Elder abuse. In myagedcare, portal accessed March 2015 at www.myagedcare.gov.au/financial-and-legal/elder-abuse-concerns.

Australian Government Department of Social Services. (2015). Alleged and suspected assaults. In Guide to aged care law, portal, accessed March 2015 at http://guides.dss.gov.au/guide-aged-care-law/2/2/1#2.

Australian Institute of Criminology. (2010). Appendix B. *Indigenous perpetrators of violence. Prevalence and risk factors for offending*. Research and public policy series no. 105. Canberra: Author. Accessed March 2015 at www.aic.gov.au/publications/current%20series/rpp/100-120/rpp105/10.aspx.

Biggs, S., Manthorpe, J., Tinker, A., Doyle, M. & Erens, B. (2009). Mistreatment of older people in the United Kingdom: Findings from the first national prevalence study. *Journal of Elder Abuse & Neglect, 21*(1), 1–14.

Black Blundell, B. & Clare, M. (2012). Elder abuse in culturally and linguistically diverse communities: Developing best practice. Perth: Advocare Incorporated. Accessed March 2015 via www.advocare.org.au.

Bond, M. C. & Butler, K. H. (2013). Elder abuse and neglect: Definitions, epidemiology, and approaches to emergency department screening. *Clinical Geriatric Medicine, 29*, 257–273.

Caceres, B. & Fulmer, T. (2012). Mistreatment detection. In M. Boltz, E. Capezuti, T. Fulmer, & D. Zwicker (Eds), *Evidence-based practice protocols for best practice* (4th ed., pp. 544–561). New York: Springer.

Castle, N. (2012). Resident-to-resident abuse in nursing homes as reported by nurses aides. *Journal of Elder Abuse & Neglect, 24*(4), 340–356.

Clare, M., Black Blundell, B. & Clare, J. (2011). Examination of the extent of elder abuse in Western Australia: A qualitative and quantitative investigation of existing agency policy, service responses and recorded data. Perth: Advocare Incorporated. Accessed March 2015 via www.advocare.org.au.

Connolly, M.-T., Breckman, R., Callahan, J. et al. (2012). The sexual revolution's last frontier: How silence about sex undermines health, well-being, and safety in old age. *Generations, 36*(3), 43–52.

Conrad, K. J., Iris, M., Ridings, J. W., Rosen, A., Fairman, K. & Anetzberger, G. J. (2011a). Conceptual model and map of psychological abuse of older adults. *Journal of Elder Abuse & Neglect, 23*(2), 147–168.

Conrad, K. J., Ridings, J. W., Iris, M., Fairman, K. P., Rosen, A. & Wilber, K. H. (2011b). Conceptual model and map of financial exploitation of older adults. *Journal of Elder Abuse & Neglect, 23*(4), 304–325.

Cooper, C., Selwood, A., Blanchard, M., Walker, Z., Blizzard, R. & Livingston, G. (2009). Abuse of people with dementia by family carers: Representative cross-sectional survey. *British Medical Journal, 338*, b155.

Day, M. R., Leahy-Warren, P. & McCarthy, G. (2013). Perceptions and views of self-neglect: A client-centered perspective. *Journal of Elder Abuse & Neglect, 25*(1), 76–94.

Day, M. R., McCarthy, G. & Leahy-Warren, P. (2012). Professional social workers' views on self-neglect: An exploratory study. *British Journal of Social Work, 42*(4), 725–743.

DeDonder, L., Lang, G., Luoma, M.-L. et al. (2011). Perpetrators of abuse against older women: A multi-national study in Europe. *Journal of Adult Protection, 13*(6), 302–314.

DeHart, D., Webb, J. & Cornman, C. (2009). Prevention of elder mistreatment in nursing homes: Competencies for direct-care staff. *Journal of Elder Abuse & Neglect, 21*(4), 360–378.

DeLiema, M., Gassoumis, Z., Homeier, D. et al. (2012). Determining prevalence and correlates of elder abuse using Promotores: Low income immigrant Latinos report high rates of abuse and neglect. *Journal of the American Geriatrics Society, 60*(7), 1333–1339.

Dong, X., Simon, M. & Evans, D. (2012). Elder self-neglect and hospitalization: Findings from the Chicago Health and Aging Project. *Journal of the American Geriatrics Society, 60*(2), 202–209.

Dow, B. & Joosten M. (2012). Understanding elder abuse: A social rights perspective. *International Psychogeriatrics, 24*(6), 853–855.

Erlingsson, C., Ono, M., Sasaki, F. & Saveman, B. I. (2012). An international collaborative study comparing Swedish and Japanese nurses' reactions to elder abuse. *Journal of Advanced Nursing, 68*(1), 56–68.

Ernst, J. S. & Smith, C. A. (2011). Adult protective services older adults confirmed for self-neglect: Characteristics and service use. *Journal of Elder Abuse & Neglect, 23*(4), 289–303.

Family and Community Services. (2011). Elder abuse and neglect prevention. Accessed March 2015 at www.familyservices.govt.nz/working-with-us/programmes-services/preventing-family-violence/elder-abuse-and-neglect-prevention-services.html.

Hirschel, A. & Anetzberger, G. J. (2012). Evaluating and enhancing federal responses to abuse and neglect in long-term care facilities. *Public Policy & Aging Report, 22*(1), 22–27.

Kurrle, S. (2004). Elder abuse. *Australian Family Physician, 33*(10), 807–812.

Kurrle, S. & Naughtin, G. (2008). An overview of elder abuse and neglect in Australia. *Journal of Elder Abuse and Neglect, 20*(2), 108–125.

Lachs, M. S., Rosen, T., Teresi, J. A., Eimicke, J. P., Ramirez, M., Silver, S. & Pillemer, K. (2013). Verbal and physical aggression directed at nursing home staff by residents. *Journal of General Internal Medicine, 28*(5), 660–667.

Lowenstein, A., Eisikovits, A., Band-Winterstein, T. et al. (2009). Is elder abuse and neglect a social phenomenon? Data from the first national prevalence survey in Israel. *Journal of Elder Abuse & Neglect, 21*(3), 253–277.

Mosqueda, L. & Dong, X. (2011). Elder abuse and self-neglect: "I don't care anything about going to the doctor, to be honest ...". *Journal of the American Medical Association, 306*(5), 532–540.

Mosqueda, L., Burnright, K. & Liao, S. (2005). The life cycle of bruises in older adults. *Journal of the American Geriatrics Society, 53*, 1339–1343.

Murphy, K., Waa, S., Jaffer, H. et al. (2013). A literature review of findings in physical elder abuse. *Canadian Association of Radiology Journal, 64*(1), 10–14.

National Center on Elder Abuse. (2013). Research brief, mistreatment of lesbian, gay, bisexual, and transgender (LGBT) elders. Accessible March 2015 via www.ncea.aoa.gov/Library/Review/Brief/Index.aspx.

National Center on Elder Abuse. (2015). What is elder abuse? Accessed March 2015 at www.ncea.aoa.gov/faq/index.aspx.

Naughton, C., Drennan, J., Lyons, I, Lafferty, A, Treacy, M., Phelan, A. & Delany, L. (2012). Elder abuse and neglect in Ireland: Results from a national prevalence survey. *Age & Ageing, 41*(1), 98–103.

Newman, F. I., Seff, L. R., Beaulaurier, R. L. & Palmer, R. C. (2013). Domestic abuse against elder women and perceived barriers to help-seeking. *Journal of Elder Abuse & Neglect, 25*(3), 205–229.

Payne, B. K. (2010). Understanding elder sexual abuse and the criminal justice system's response: Comparisons to elder physical abuse. *Justice Quarterly, 27*, 206–224.

Pillemer, K., Chen, E. K., Van Haitsma, K. S. et al. (2011). Resident-to-resident aggression in nursing homes: Results from a qualitative event reconstruction study. *Gerontologist, 52*(1), 24–33.

Podnieks, E., Anetzberger, G. J., Wilson, S. J., Teaster, P. B. & Wangmo, T. (2010). Worldview environmental scan on elder abuse. *Journal of Elder Abuse & Neglect, 22*(1–2), 164–179.

Podnieks, E., Rietschlin, J. & Walsh, C. A. (2012). Introduction. Elder abuse in Canada: Reports from a national roundtable discussion. *Journal of Elder Abuse & Neglect, 24*(2), 85–87.

Ramsey-Klawsnik, H., Teaster, P. B., Mendiondo, M. S., Marcum, J. L. & Abner, E. L. (2008). Sexual predators who target elders: Findings from the first national study of sexual abuse in care facilities. *Journal of Elder Abuse & Neglect, 20*, 353–376.

Roberto, K. A., McCann, B. R. & Brossoie, N. (2013). Intimate partner violence in late life: An analysis of national news reports. *Journal of Elder Abuse & Neglect, 25*(3), 230–241.

Sandmoe, A., Kirkevold, M. & Ballantyne, A. (2011). Challenges in handling elder abuse in community care: An exploratory study among nurses and care coordinators. *Journal of Clinical Nursing, 20*(23–24), 3351–3363.

Shankardass, M. K. (2013). Addressing elder abuse: Review of societal responses in India and selected Asian countries. *International Psychogeriatrics, 25*(8), 1229–1234.

Sooryanarayana, R., Choo, W. H. & Hairi, N. N. (2013). A review of prevalence and measurement of elder abuse in the community. *Trauma Violence & Abuse, 14*(4), 316–325.

State Government of Victoria, Department of Health (2012). Elder abuse prevention and response guidelines for action 2012–14. Accessed March 2015 at www.health.vic.gov.au/agedcare/policy/elder_abuse.htm#download.

Teresi, J. A., Ramirez, M., Ellis, J. et al. (2013). A staff intervention targeting resident-to-resident elder mistreatment in long-term care increased staff knowledge, recognition and reporting: Results from a cluster randomized trial. *International Journal of Nursing Studies, 50*(5), 644–656.

United Nations Economic and Social Affairs. (2008). Guide to the national implementation of the Madrid International Plan of Action on Aging. New York: United Nations Headquarters.

United Nations Economic and Social Council. (2002, February 25–March 1). Abuse of older persons: Recognizing and responding to abuse of older persons in a global context. Document of the Commission for Social Development presented at the Second World Assembly on Aging, New York.

Weeks, L. E. & LeBlanc, K. (2011). An ecological synthesis of research on older women's experiences of intimate partner violence. *Journal of Women & Aging, 23*, 283–304.

Wiglesworth, A., Austin, R., Corona, M. et al. (2009). Bruising as a marker of physical elder abuse. *Journal of the American Geriatrics Society, 57*(7), 1191–1196.

Wiglesworth, A., Mosqueda, L., Mulnard, R., Liao, S., Gibbs, L. & Fitzgerald, W. (2010). Screening for abuse and neglect of people with dementia. *Journal of the American Geriatrics Society, 58*, 493–500.

World Health Organization. (2002). The Toronto Declaration on the Global Prevention of Elder Abuse. Accessed March 2015 at www.who.int/ageing/projects/elder_abuse/alc_toronto_declaration_en.pdf.

Wu, L., Chen, H., Hu, Y. et al. (2012). Prevalence and associated factors of elder mistreatment in a rural community in People's Republic of China: A cross-sectional study. *PLoS One, 7*(3), e33857.

Ziminski, C. E., Wiglesworth, A., Austin, R. et al. (2013). Injury patterns and causal mechanisms of bruising in physical elder abuse. *Journal of Forensic Nursing, 9*(2), 84–91.

PART 3

PROMOTING WELLNESS IN PSYCHOSOCIAL FUNCTION

Chapter 11

Cognitive function

By Carol Miller and Sharyn Hunter

LEARNING OBJECTIVES

After reading this chapter, you should be able to:

1. Explain why an understanding of mild cognitive decline, dementia, delirium and depression (the "Ds") is essential for all nurses.
2. Describe age-related changes that affect cognitive abilities.
3. List risk factors that influence cognitive function in older adults
4. Discuss the functional consequences associated with cognition in older adults.
5. Identify nursing interventions to help older adults maintain or improve cognitive abilities.

KEY POINTS

"4 Ds"—mild cognitive impairment, dementia, delirium and depression
age-associated memory impairment
automatic and effortful processing theory
cognitive decline
cognitive reserve
contextual theories
continuum of processing
crystallised intelligence
developmental intelligence
empowering model
everyday problem solving
executive functions
fluid intelligence
memory
metamemory
mild cognitive impairment (MCI)
neuroplasticity
paradox of well-being
scaffolding theory of ageing and cognition
socioemotional selectivity
stage theories
wisdom

Cognition involves the processes of thinking, learning and remembering. The long-standing myths about cognitive ageing in society, which propose that cognitive impairment is normal with ageing, still exist. Even the adage that "you can't teach an old dog new tricks" underlies some of the most widely held and inaccurate perspectives on older adults' cognition. Research in recent decades supports a more optimistic view of cognitive ageing and recognises there are only minor cognitive changes that occur with normal ageing called **cognitive decline**. Research also continues to identify interventions that minimise ageing cognitive changes. One of the most significant ways in which nurses can promote wellness for older adults is by correcting myth-based views and encouraging older adults to engage in activities that foster cognitive fitness. However, it is also recognised that as people age, they are at increased risk of significant cognitive changes because of pathological conditions. Nurses commonly refer to impaired cognition as confusion, yet this term is ambiguous and does not adequately describe the cognitive changes. Today nurses in all settings frequently care for older adults who have cognitive impairment and it is essential that nurses understand the difference between normal ageing changes and the other types of cognitive impairment in older adults. This understanding will help nurses identify the type of cognitive impairment and provide appropriate care. Failure to do so can lead to increased morbidity and mortality.

TYPES OF COGNITIVE IMPAIRMENT IN OLDER ADULTS

There are currently four types of altered cognition that older adults might experience (Insel & Badger, 2002; Patel & Holland, 2012). They include *mild cognitive impairment, dementia, delirium* and *depression*. These can be referred to as the **"4 Ds"**. Each type has specific features, different treatment strategies and, importantly, they do not necessarily occur on their own. Combinations of the Ds can occur (e.g. a person living with dementia can develop delirium). The first D is the condition of mild cognitive impairment (MCI). MCI is different to the normal cognitive changes. Although this chapter focuses on normal cognitive ageing, MCI is also discussed so that the difference between the two is clarified. The other three Ds—dementia, delirium and depression—are caused by pathological changes. Chapter 14 discusses delirium and dementia, while Chapter 15 discusses depression in the older adult.

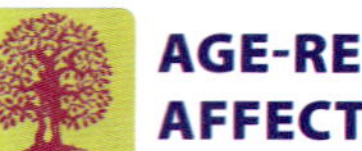

AGE-RELATED CHANGES THAT AFFECT COGNITION

Current theories about ageing and cognition differ significantly from those that were first proposed during the 1960s. Initial cross-sectional studies, which were based

Promoting cognitive wellness in older adults

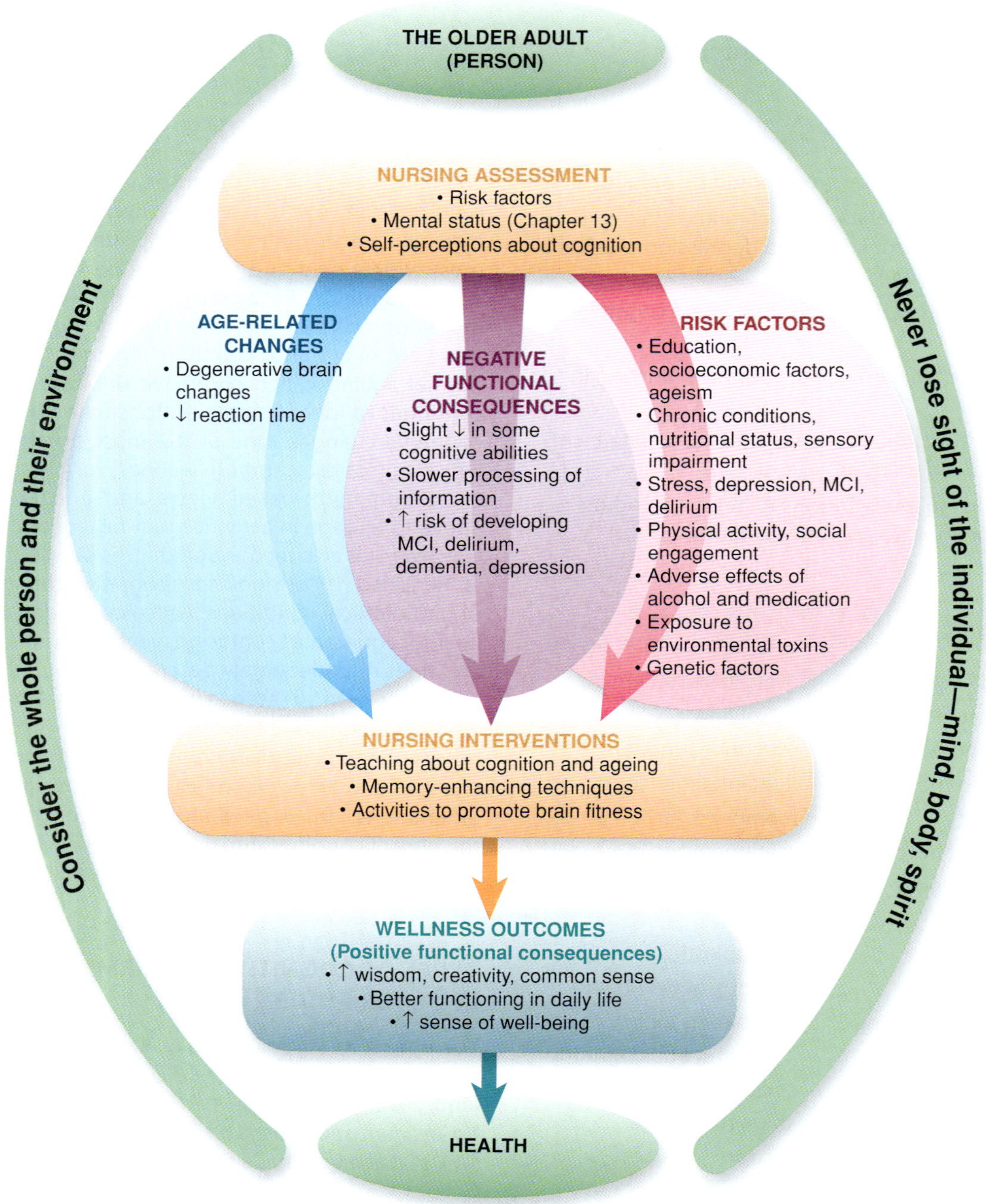

Consider the whole person and their environment

THE OLDER ADULT (PERSON)

NURSING ASSESSMENT
- Risk factors
- Mental status (Chapter 13)
- Self-perceptions about cognition

AGE-RELATED CHANGES
- Degenerative brain changes
- ↓ reaction time

NEGATIVE FUNCTIONAL CONSEQUENCES
- Slight ↓ in some cognitive abilities
- Slower processing of information
- ↑ risk of developing MCI, delirium, dementia, depression

RISK FACTORS
- Education, socioeconomic factors, ageism
- Chronic conditions, nutritional status, sensory impairment
- Stress, depression, MCI, delirium
- Physical activity, social engagement
- Adverse effects of alcohol and medication
- Exposure to environmental toxins
- Genetic factors

NURSING INTERVENTIONS
- Teaching about cognition and ageing
- Memory-enhancing techniques
- Activities to promote brain fitness

WELLNESS OUTCOMES (Positive functional consequences)
- ↑ wisdom, creativity, common sense
- Better functioning in daily life
- ↑ sense of well-being

HEALTH

Never lose sight of the individual—mind, body, spirit

on tests designed to predict school performance in children, led to the conclusion that a decline in cognitive abilities was a normal part of the ageing process. By the mid 1980s, results of longitudinal studies began showing that intellectual function remained the same or improved up to the age of 50 or 60 years, after which it gradually declined.

In recent decades researchers have focused on the interplay between cognitive abilities and such factors as emotions, environment, life experiences and socioeconomic conditions. Gerontologists are particularly interested in identifying interventions that improve cognitive abilities in older adults because studies indicate that the brain has the ability to change.

As with many other aspects of function in older adults, gerontologists are trying to distinguish between the cognitive changes that occur in healthy older adults and those that are associated with pathological processes such as dementia (discussed in Chapter 14). Age-related changes affecting cognition can be understood in terms of physical changes in the central nervous system and in theories about intelligence, **memory** and psychological development that attempt to explain the relationship between ageing and cognition.

Central nervous system

Knowledge about brain ageing is gleaned from many types of studies, including clinical, neuropsychological, neuropathological and neurochemical investigations. Initial studies of brain ageing relied on autopsy findings, but recent major advances in non-invasive neuroimaging techniques (e.g. functional magnetic resonance imaging) have significantly broadened the knowledge base. Recent studies continue to identify age-related changes in the brain, but they are inconclusive with regard to the impact of these changes on cognition. Current research findings are discussed here.

The brain is composed to two types of brain tissue, white and grey matter Grey matter contains the nerve cells while the white matter contains the nerve fibres and myelin. Loss of white matter is frequently noted on brain imaging tests in older adults, and these changes affect global functioning. However, studies indicate that these changes are due to small vessel disease associated with vascular risk factors rather than age-related changes alone (Inzitari et al., 2009).

Studies have also found decreased cerebral blood flow and cortical volume loss, particularly in the frontal lobes, but some studies suggest that the brains of older adults may be able to compensate for these changes (Sorond et al., 2008). Additional age-related changes in the brain and central nervous system that potentially affect cognitive abilities are reduced brain weight, diminished cerebral blood flow, enlarged ventricles and wider sulci, loss and shrinkage of neurons, reduced neurotransmitters or their binding sites, and accumulation of lipofuscin in nerve cell bodies. In addition to directly affecting cognitive skills, these age-related changes cause a slower reaction time and affect the speed of processing information.

> ### A student's perspective
>
> *The residents at the residential care facility continue to amaze me with their stories. There is so much one can learn just by listening, and the residents just want to share their stories and have our company more than anything—at least that is the impression I continually receive from them. They are all friendly, open people who are no different than the rest of us, but they have gained a large amount of knowledge over the years that many of us who are students probably have not acquired yet.*
>
> *Megan S.*

Gerontologists are emphasising that age-related degenerative changes in the neural structures do not totally determine cognitive abilities because cognitive potential can remain even when neural structures are compromised (Willis, Schaie & Martin, 2009). Researchers have proposed the **scaffolding theory of ageing and cognition** as a way of explaining the adaptive response of the brain to the declining neural structures and function. According to this theory, scaffolding is a normal process that involves the development and use of complementary and alternative neural circuits to achieve a cognitive goal (Goh & Park, 2009). This process protects cognitive abilities despite the presence of age-related changes (Park & Reuter-Lorenz, 2009).

The term **neuroplasticity** (also called *neural plasticity*) refers to the physiological ability of the brain and neural circuits to change and develop in response to environmental stimuli. The closely related concept of **cognitive reserve** refers to the capacity to continue to function at an adequate cognitive level despite the presence of age-related or pathological processes that affect the neural structures (Vance & Wright, 2009; Willis et al., 2009). Neuroplasticity is defined as positive when it promotes neuronal connections and increases cognitive reserve, and as negative when it inhibits the neuronal connections and decreases cognitive reserve (Vance & Wright, 2009).

Gerontologists are increasingly emphasising that cognitive development can occur at every stage of human development; however, older adults have more constraints and limits that need to be addressed (Willis et al., 2009). Studies based on the cognitive reserve model indicated that participation in creative activities (e.g. art, storytelling, dance classes) and leisure-time cognitive activities (e.g. reading, writing, group discussions, playing music) is associated with delayed onset of memory decline and improved cognition in older adults (Hall et al., 2009; McFadden & Basting, 2010).

Although research on brain ageing provides the biological base of information, psychological theories explain differences in cognitive abilities, as discussed in the following sections.

Fluid and crystallised intelligence

Cattell and Horn theory of fluid and crystallised intelligence, first proposed in the late 1960s, is one of the first theories that attempted to explain age-related changes in some cognitive abilities. **Fluid intelligence** depends primarily on central nervous system functioning as well as a person's inherent abilities, such as memory and pattern recognition. Fluid intelligence is associated with the cognitive skills of integration, inductive reasoning, abstract thinking, and flexible and adaptive thinking. This cognitive characteristic enables people to identify and draw conclusions about complex relationships. **Crystallised intelligence** refers to cognitive skills, such as vocabulary, information and verbal comprehension, which people acquire through culture, education, informal learning and other types of life experiences. This cognitive characteristic is strongly associated with **wisdom**, judgement and life experiences.

According to this theory, fluid and crystallised intelligence develop concurrently during infancy and childhood and are indistinguishable as the central nervous system is maturing. Age-related changes in neural structures cause a decline in fluid intelligence. Crystallised intelligence, however, continues to develop during adulthood because of accumulated experiences and learning. Crystallised intelligence, except for those processes that depend on the speed of response, does not decline with age, and it may even increase because of experiences that improve wisdom. Although fluid intelligence is thought to decline with increased age, a recent longitudinal study of 626 adults found that a strong sense of self-direction in work situations prevented declines in verbal memory and inductive reasoning, which are two aspects of fluid intelligence (Yu et al., 2009).

Memory

Memory is often conceptualised as a computer-like information-processing system in which information is first perceived, then stored, and finally retrieved when needed or wanted. *Primary memory* has a short duration and a very small capacity, and it serves as a holding tank for events of the immediate past few seconds rather than as a true memory storage system. Information in the primary memory can be either recalled for a brief time or transmitted to long-term storage. *Secondary memory* has longer duration and, therefore, is more important in terms of the retrieval, as well as the storage, of information.

Retrieval of information from storage is referred to as remote, tertiary or very long-term memory processing, and skills involved are classified as *recall memory* and *recognition memory*. Some theories associated with these concepts suggest that older people remember events of long ago better than recent events; however, studies indicate that both types of memory decline equally but older adults have a larger store of information about events of long ago (Botwinick, 1984). Studies have also found that older adults can remember the events that occurred but have more difficulty remembering the context in which they took place (Cansino, 2009).

More recently, gerontologists have viewed the information-processing model as too simplistic because it ignores the milieu in which the memory operates. Thus, newer **contextual theories** address variables that can affect memory. For example, slower speed of processing is an age-related change that can significantly affect memory and other cognitive skills. Other variables that can affect memory include motivation, expectations, experiences, education, personality, task demands, learning habits, intellectual skills, sociocultural background, physical and mental health, and style of processing information.

Recent studies found that memory and other cognitive skills of older adults are equal to or better than those of younger adults under some conditions (Labouvie-Vief, 2009a). For example, older adults have better memory recall and recognition than do younger adults when the information or emotional stimuli are positive in comparison to stimuli that are negative (Blanchard-Fields & Kalinauskas, 2009). Similarly, older adults are capable of using complex cognitive skills when the situation is highly interesting or has personal relevance (Hess et al., 2009).

Another theoretical approach emphasises encoding and analysing rather than storage and retrieval aspects of memory. According to this perspective, memory is a **continuum of processing**, ranging from shallow to deep levels; the deeper the level at which information is stored, the longer the memory will last. Any of the following variables can affect the depth of storage (Botwinick, 1984):

- Processing techniques, ranging from the shallowest levels used for sensory information to the deepest levels used for highly abstract information
- Elaboration, or quality, of processing conducted at any depth level
- Distinctiveness of the information, which depends partially on how well it is learned
- Depth and elaboration of retrieval processes.

Several studies based on this framework concluded that older adults have decreased memory function because of faulty processing mechanisms (Botwinick, 1984). A recent study suggested that the age-related reduction in memory accuracy is associated, at least in part, from poorer encoding (Pansky et al., 2009).

Another theoretical perspective that views memory as a continuum is the **automatic and effortful processing theory**, which was proposed by Hasher & Zacks (1979). At one end of the continuum is automatic processing, or those tasks that do not require attention or awareness and do not improve with practice. At the other end is effortful processing, or those tasks that demand high levels of attention and cognitive energy. With practice, effortful tasks require less attention and become more automatic. According to this theory, ageing does not affect automatic memory because these tasks require little or no cognitive energy. Effortful memory, however, declines with age because the limited cognitive resources that are available for memory functions begin to decline in early adulthood. Studies have confirmed declines in effortful processes (e.g. selective attention, mental imagery, verbal fluency, language production, and verbal and visuospatial working memory) and no declines in automatic cognitive functions (e.g. picture recognition and implicit and procedural memory) (Carstensen, Mikels & Mather, 2006).

Metamemory refers to self-knowledge and perceptions about memory, cognitive function, and development of memory. Metamemory is important in everyday activities because if people know what they can remember and how much effort they will need to remember certain things, they can plan efficient and effective strategies for remembering. Because older adults tend to perceive themselves as less competent than younger adults or less competent than they actually are in many cognitive tasks, gerontologists emphasise the importance of addressing ageist attitudes that contribute to negative self-stereotypes about cognitive abilities (Levy & Leifheit-Limson, 2009).

WELLNESS OPPORTUNITY

Nurses can influence attitudes by conveying positive beliefs about the ability of older adults to improve memory skills.

Adult psychological development

Theories about psychological development postulate that the thinking of older adults becomes increasingly complex and shows progressive reorganisation of intellectual skills (Labouvie-Vief & Blanchard-Fields, 1982). For example, a recent focus of these theories is on cognitive abilities associated with decision making and **everyday problem solving**. Conclusions from studies of decision-making skills are as follows (Mariske & Margrett, 2006):

- Affect and motivation are strong predictors of decision making in older adults.
- Older adults are more selective in the information they use for decision making (i.e. they base decisions on less information).
- Older adults require more time to make decisions that are equal in quality to those of younger adults, but they may choose to spend the same or less time.
- Increased task complexity is associated with more error and more inconsistencies for both older and younger adults.
- Task expertise and prior experience contribute to better decisions for both older and younger adults.

Nurses can apply conclusions from these studies when they involve older adults in decisions about self-care.

Stage theories of adult cognitive development were first developed during the 1970s as an extension of Piaget's theory of intellectual development in children and adolescents. One such theory postulated that children and adolescents focus on acquiring knowledge, and adults focus on applying knowledge in the following stages (Schaie, 1977–1978):

- *Achieving stage* (early adulthood): Adults apply acquired knowledge to demands and commitments, such as career and family; they use their intellectual abilities to establish their independence and develop goal-oriented behaviours.
- *Responsible stage* (late 30s to early 60s): Adults integrate long-range goals and attend to the needs of their family and society.
- *Executive stage* (a subset of the responsible stage): Applies to people who have high levels of social responsibilities.
- *Reintegration stage* (later adulthood): Intellectual tasks are to simplify life and select only those responsibilities that have meaning and purpose; older adults ask "Why should I know?" rather than "What should I know?"

More recently, Cohen (2005) developed an **empowering model** based on studies of more than 3000 older adults. This model describes the following four phases of mature ageing:

- *Midlife re-evaluation* (early 40s to late 50s): People confront their sense of mortality; plans and actions are shaped by a quest or crisis; brain changes spur developmental intelligence.
- *Liberation* (late 50s to early 70s): People feel a new sense of inner liberation; development in information-processing part of the brain increases desire for novelty; plans and actions are shaped by personal freedom; retirement allows time for new experiences.
- *Summing up* (late 60s through 80s): People are motivated to share wisdom; plans and actions are shaped by a desire to find meaning; brain development improves capacity for autobiographical expression; people may feel compelled to attend to unfinished business and unresolved conflicts.
- *Encore* (late 70s to the end of life): Plans and actions are shaped by the desire to restate and reaffirm major themes and to explore novel variations on those themes; brain changes promote positive emotions and morale; the desire to live well to the very end has a positive impact on others.

Gerontologists have also focused on the **paradox of well-being**, which describes the phenomenon of older adults suffering significant losses of health, cognition and social functioning but reporting high levels of well-being and positive emotions (Labouvie-Vief, 2009b). The **socioemotional selectivity** theory addresses this question in the context of motivation. According to this theory, older adults recognise that time is limited, so they are motivated to pursue emotional satisfaction. Thus, they shift their focus from the pursuit of knowledge and information gathering and concentrate on relationships that are closer and more intimate (Labouvie-Vief, 2009b).

Another current focus is on wisdom as an aspect of cognitive function, which is viewed as "a special type of expertise about the meaning of life and the pragmatics of how things work in a particular situation" (Zarit, 2009). A working definition of wisdom as an integral aspect of adult development includes the following (Knight & Laidlaw, 2009, p. 684):

- An accumulation of "knowing how" expertise over "knowing what"
- A greater ability to integrate and balance emotion and reason
- An awareness of the many contexts of life and how they change over the years
- An acceptance of uncertainty in life and an understanding of how to handle this
- An understanding of the relativism of individual values and an increased tolerance for individual differences.

A similar concept is **developmental intelligence**, defined as "the maturing of cognition, emotional intelligence, judgement, social skills, life experience, and consciousness and their integration and synergy" (Cohen, 2005, p. 35). Cohen's view of cognitive ageing, which is both optimistic and research based, emphasises that many older adults display the age-dependent quality of wisdom because they integrate all the components of developmental intelligence.

WELLNESS OPPORTUNITY

Nurses acknowledge the wisdom of older adults by asking such questions as, "Do you have some words of wisdom to share about that valuable experience?"

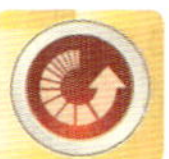

RISK FACTORS THAT AFFECT COGNITIVE WELLNESS

A multitude of internal and external conditions can affect cognitive function in people of all ages, but older adults are particularly vulnerable to these risk factors. Nurses need to pay particular attention to identifying the risk factors that are reversible and the ones that can be addressed through health promotion interventions.

Personal, social and attitudinal influences

Numerous personal, social and attitudinal factors affect cognitive abilities in people of any age, and researchers have tried to identify those that most significantly affect older adults. Quality and length of formal education is the factor most consistently associated with better cognitive performance and more cognitive reserve in older adults (Stine-Morrow & Chui, 2011). Other factors that affect cognitive function include occupation, social relations, socioeconomic status, hearing and vision problems, leisure and intellectual activities, and lifestyle factors (e.g. nutrition and physical activity).

Ageism and diminished expectations of older adults in modern societies can negatively affect cognitive function. Studies indicate that older adults internalise stereotypes about memory decline as an inevitable outcome of ageing and that these perceptions worsen their performance on tests of memory and other cognitive skills (Levy, Zonderman, Slade et al., 2011). Recent studies indicate that cognitive performance in older adults can be improved by providing positive stereotyping cues (Swift, Abrams & Marques, 2013).

WELLNESS OPPORTUNITY

Be aware of opportunities to dispel negative stereotypes about cognitive ageing when talking with older adults.

Health factors and health behaviours

Health conditions

Many chronic conditions affect cognitive abilities in older adults to such a degree that gerontologists are emphasising that researchers should view health conditions as the key explanatory variable in studies of cognitive ageing (MacDonald, DeCarlo & Dixon, 2011; Spiro & Brady, 2011). Pathological conditions that increase the risk for serious cognitive impairment due to dementia are discussed in Chapter 14, and this chapter discusses health factors associated with milder degrees of cognitive impairment. Some examples of chronic conditions associated with impaired cognitive function (with or without dementia) include stroke, diabetes and cardiovascular disorders. For example, longitudinal studies confirm that overall cardiovascular health before older adulthood is associated with better verbal memory, **executive functions** (problem-solving skills, inhibition and flexibility), and psychomotor speed during later adulthood (Reis, Loria, Launer et al., 2013).

A major focus of current research is on the effects of inflammatory conditions that affect the immune, neurological and cardiovascular systems, with emphasis on how these pathological processes can be a target for intervention (Barrientos, Frank, Watkins et al., 2012; Rosano, Marsland & Gianaros, 2012; Sartori, Vance, Slater et al., 2012). Specifically, one study concluded that a higher infectious burden (i.e. the cumulative effects of pathogens such as *Helicobacter pylori* and herpes simplex virus) was an independent risk factor for cognitive impairment (Katan, Moon, Paik et al., 2013). Studies also found that cognitive impairment is common after lacunar strokes, which are associated with cerebral small vessel disease (Kloppenborg, Nederkoorn, Grool et al., 2012; Makin, Turpin, Dennis et al., 2013).

Nutrition

Nutritional status is widely recognised as a health factor that can affect cognitive function regardless of a person's age. For example, low levels of beta-carotene and vitamins B, C and D are associated with poor cognitive function. Researchers have focused much attention on nutritional factors that affect cognition because these can often be addressed through relatively simple interventions. The following conclusions are based on recent studies:

- Lower haemoglobin levels (i.e. anaemia) are associated with cognitive decline in older adults (Shah, Schneider, Leurgans et al., 2012).
- Studies have found that low serum vitamin D levels were associated with poorer cognitive function and a higher risk for Alzheimer's disease (Annweiler, Rolland, Schott et al., 2012; Balion, Griffith, Strifler et al., 2012; Peterson, Mattek, Clemons et al., 2012; Slinin, Paudel, Taylor et al., 2012).
- Analysis of longitudinal data from the Framingham Heart Study of 549 community-dwelling older adults found that low levels of vitamin B are associated with cognitive decline (Morris, Selhub & Jacques, 2012).
- Analysis of data from blood tests of 104 subjects in the Oregon Brain Ageing Study found a positive correlation between high levels of vitamins B, C, D and E and better cognitive function; higher plasma transfat scores were associated with worse cognitive function (Bowman, Silbert, Howieson et al., 2012).
- Iron deficiency is associated with cognitive impairment, and its effect is independent of the presence of anaemia (Yavuz, Cankurtaran, Haznedaroglu et al., 2012).
- Dietary lutein and zeaxanthin can influence cognitive function in older adults (Johnson, 2012).

Senses

Sensory impairment is another aspect of health that affects cognitive processes because hearing or vision deficits limit the quantity and quality of information received from the environment. For example, studies have confirmed that hearing loss is independently associated with cognitive impairment and accelerated cognitive decline in community-dwelling older adults (Lin, Yaffe, Xia et al., 2013). Because sensory input significantly influences learning and other cognitive processes, nurses need to ensure optimal visual and hearing conditions when communicating with older adults (as discussed in Chapters 16 and 17).

Mental health

Researchers are also focusing on mental health factors that can affect cognitive function. A review of literature related to stress and cognition found consistent evidence that stress is negatively associated with cognitive function in older adults (Almeida, Piazza, Stawski et al., 2011). Studies indicate that chronic stress is associated with cognitive impairment by increasing levels of cortisol (Kremen, Lachman, Pruessner et al., 2012). Depression and even subclinical variations in depressive symptoms are strongly associated with impaired cognitive function (especially memory), as discussed in Chapter 15.

Lifestyle

Some studies focus on a combination of health-related factors, with emphasis on health behaviours that promote good cognitive function. Data from a 17-year study of 5100 men and women aged 42 to 63 years found an association between the number and the duration of unhealthy behaviours and lower scores on measures of cognitive function in later life (Sabia et al., 2012). Smoking is a health-related behaviour that is a risk for cognitive decline (Sabia, Elbaz, Dugravot et al., 2012). Many studies found that healthy lifestyle behaviours, such as physical activity and social engagement are associated with maintaining good cognitive function (e.g. Gow, Bastin, Munoz et al., 2012; Lovden, Xu & Wang, 2013; Miller, Siddarth, Gaines et al., 2012; Suzuki, Shimada, Makizako et al., 2012; Wang, Jin, Hendrie et al., 2013).

Medication effects

Prescription and over-the-counter medications can interfere with memory and other cognitive functions in a variety of ways. For example, anticholinergic ingredients, which are contained in numerous prescription and over-the-counter medications, significantly affect memory and other cognitive functions and are a common cause of changes in mental status in older adults (Pasina, Djade, Lucca et al., 2013). Because many medications have anticholinergic effects, researchers and clinicians have paid particular attention in recent years to the cumulative effects of these medications on acetylcholine, which is a neurotransmitter that directly affects cognitive function. Chapter 8 provides detailed information about anticholinergic and other types of medications that can interfere with cognitive function. Chapter 8, Table 8-9 contains information about specific medications and the modes of action that affect cognitive function.

Environmental factors

Researchers are also examining risk factors related to long-term exposure to environmental toxins. Studies indicate that exposure to second-hand smoke is associated with increased risk of cognitive decline (Orsitto, Turi, Venezia et al., 2012). Occupational and environmental exposure to lead can increase the risk for cognitive impairment, particularly through detrimental effects on neural processing speed (Grashow, Spiro, Taylor et al., 2013).

Neuropathology

MCI, delirium and depression increase the risk of an older adult developing dementia. Further discussion about these risks is provided later: MCI is described in this chapter; delirium in Chapter 14; and depression in Chapter 15.

WELLNESS OPPORTUNITY

From a holistic perspective, nurses help older adults identify risk factors such as nutrition and over-the-counter medications, which can be addressed through self-care actions.

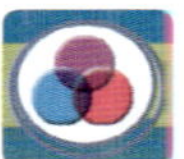

FUNCTIONAL CONSEQUENCES AFFECTING COGNITIVE FUNCTION

Healthy older adults will not experience any significant cognitive impairment that interferes with daily life, but they will notice minor deficits in some aspects of cognitive function and improvements in other aspects. Longitudinal studies have identified patterns of cognitive change that are likely to occur even in the absence of any pathological processes. These changes can be summarised as follows (Carlson et al., 2009; Caserta et al., 2009):

- Aspects of cognition that are involved with perceptual speed and numerical ability begin to decline during the third decade and continue to decline at a modest linear rate.
- Episodic memory (i.e. memory of personally experienced events) may begin to decline as early as the third or fourth decade.
- Decline of verbal ability and tasks of inductive reasoning occurs during the fifth or sixth decade.
- Changes that begin during earlier and middle adulthood are gradual and do not reach a level of significance until the seventh or eighth decade, at which point they may continue to decline.
- Executive functions (e.g. problem-solving skills, inhibition and flexibility) show considerable age-related declines.
- Word lexicon and general knowledge improve well into the sixth decade and remain stable during later adulthood.

It is important to keep in mind that these conclusions about patterns of change are based on well-designed studies, but gerontologists emphasise that there is a great deal of individual variation in cognitive changes, with some older adults showing no decline and a small percentage even showing improvement in cognitive abilities. Gerontologists also emphasise that studies focusing only on age-related cognitive changes do not address the strong interplay between cognition and other factors.

For example, researchers have found that social expertise and emotional processing and regulation remain stable and may even improve with increased age (Blanchard-Fields & Kalinauskas, 2009). Thus, cognitive function in older adults must be considered in relation to social, emotional and other factors.

This perspective is supported by recent studies which indicate that "healthy older brains are often as good as or better than younger brains in a wide variety of tasks" (Cohen, 2005, p. 4). Cohen cites the following evidence-based findings that support an optimistic view of cognitive ageing:

- New brain cells form throughout life.
- Experience and learning enable the brain to "resculpt" itself.
- Emotional circuitry of the brain matures and becomes more balanced during older adulthood.
- Functions of the left and right hemispheres of the brain become more integrated in older adults.

Another important consideration is that conclusions about cognitive ageing do not necessarily address cultural factors and, therefore, are limited by the factors cited in Cultural considerations 11-1.

An important implication of the findings discussed in this section and the section on risk factors is that numerous conditions affect cognitive function in older adults, and nurses can address many of these variables through educational interventions. In addition, nurses need to adapt their teaching methods to compensate for age-related changes in cognition that can affect learning. Box 11-1 summarises some research-based conclusions about cognitive ageing that are most relevant for identifying and implementing health education interventions for older adults.

WELLNESS OPPORTUNITY

Nurses promote wellness by encouraging older adults to identify ways in which their cognitive abilities have improved (e.g. wisdom based on experiences).

CULTURAL CONSIDERATIONS 11-1
Cultural factors and cognitive function

- It is important to recognise that the standards of intellectual performance have been developed for English-speaking people from a Western culture.
- It is important to recognise that cognitive abilities are highly influenced by health, education and socioeconomic status and that these factors and cultural factors are interrelated.
- Cultural and language factors may influence an older adult's perception and description of memory problems.

BOX 11-1
Functional consequences affecting cognition in older adults

Cognitive abilities in healthy older adults

- Skills that stay the same or improve: wisdom, creativity, common sense, coordination of facts and ideas and breadth of knowledge and experience
- Skills that decline slightly and gradually: abstraction, calculation, word fluency, verbal comprehension, spatial orientation, inductive reasoning and episodic memory
- Word finding may be more difficult (i.e. "tip-of-the-tongue" experiences), but total vocabulary increases
- Remote memory remains intact and holds a large store of information about the past
- Factors that interfere with cognitive function: anxiety, depression, diminished sensory input, poor health, negative beliefs, ageist attitudes, pathological processes (e.g. dementia)
- Factors that improve cognitive function: good nutrition, physical exercise, mental stimulation, challenging leisure activities, strong social networks, and activities that provide a sense of control and mastery.

Learning abilities

- Older adults are as capable of learning new things as younger people, but the speed with which they process information is slower.
- Older adults are more cautious in their responses and make more errors of omission.
- Potential barriers to learning in older adults include distractions, sensory deficits, lack of relevance, teacher–learner age differences and values that are incongruent with new knowledge.

PATHOLOGICAL CONDITIONS AFFECTING COGNITION: MILD COGNITIVE IMPAIRMENT

A number of pathological conditions affect the cognition of older adults. **Mild cognitive impairment (MCI)** is widely recognised as a heterogeneous syndrome characterised by cognitive function that is impaired beyond "normal ageing" but does not meet the criteria for mild dementia. Two subtypes of MCI are *amnesic MCI*, which involves memory loss, and *non-amnesic MCI*, which is the less common type. During the early 1960s, symptoms that are now categorised as MCI were referred to as *benign senescent forgetfulness*. During the 1980s and 1990s, labels of **age-associated memory impairment**, *mild neurocognitive decline*, or *cognitive impairment no dementia* were commonly applied to this constellation of symptoms. By the early 2000s, MCI was viewed as a precursor to Alzheimer's disease, but it is now considered a distinct syndrome with symptoms that can remain stable, resolve or progress (Patel & Holland, 2012). It is now known that MCI increases the risk for developing dementia, but it does not necessarily progress to dementia. Studies indicate that MCI improves significantly or reverts to baseline cognitive state in 15% to 40% of people (Patel & Holland, 2012). In contrast to those who revert or improve, people with MCI progress to Alzheimer's disease at the rate of 10% to 15% per year compared with a rate of 1% to 2% in control groups (Freitas, Simoes, Alves et al., 2013; Lopez, 2013).

Because MCI has only recently been defined as a distinct syndrome, diagnostic criteria are imprecise and current guidelines emphasise the need for a combination of clinical judgement, functional assessment and neuropsychological testing (Healey, 2012). Diagnosis of MCI depends on identifying declines in one or more of the cognitive domains (e.g. memory, attention, visuospatial abilities and executive functioning) without concurrent major effects on global cognition or daily functioning. Table 11-1 lists cognitive changes associated with normal ageing and MCI. In addition to cognitive characteristics, behavioural symptoms such as anxiety, depression and aggressiveness have been identified in 13% of people with MCI, as compared with 39% of those with Alzheimer's

TABLE 11-1 Distinguishing characteristics of normal cognitive ageing and mild cognitive impairment

Characteristic	Normal cognitive ageing	Mild cognitive impairment (MCI)	Mild dementia
Short-term memory changes	Preserved	Impaired in amnesic MCI, preserved in non-amnesic MCI	Noticeably impaired
Awareness of memory loss	Recognises and remembers details about memory limitations	Little or no recognition and memory of details about limitations	Limited or absent awareness
Mental status assessment	No significant changes from baseline	Mild or no significant impairment	Measurable declines from baseline
Social skills	No significant changes	Usually unchanged from normal	Impaired
Activities of daily living	Preserved	Preserved	Impaired
Instrumental activities of daily living	No significant changes from baseline	Limited changes, apparent in complex tasks (e.g. managing finances, and using appliances)	Impaired

Source: Patel, B. B. & Holland, N. W. (2012). Mild cognitive impairment: Hope for stability, plan for progression. *Cleveland Clinic Journal of Medicine, 79*(12), 857–864.

disease and 3% of controls (Van Der Mussele, Le Bastard, Vermeiren et al., 2013). Nurses can encourage older adults with noticeable cognitive deficits to obtain an appropriate evaluation, with emphasis on the importance of implementing interventions at a stage when progression to dementia could be delayed.

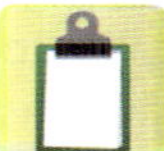

NURSING ASSESSMENT OF COGNITIVE FUNCTION

Formal assessment of intellectual performance involves administering psychometric tests, but nurses can informally assess memory and cognitive skills. In addition to assessing the intellectual performance of older adults, nurses can assess for risk factors that are likely to interfere with cognitive function. Because nursing assessment of cognition is an integral part of the psychosocial assessment, it is addressed comprehensively in a single chapter, Chapter 13. Nursing assessment of impaired cognitive function related to delirium and dementia is further addressed in Chapter 14, while depression is addressed in Chapter 15.

NURSING ISSUES

Healthy older adults experience some changes in cognitive function but, in the absence of pathological conditions and other risk factors, these changes do not significantly affect their overall functioning. The nursing issue of willingness for enhanced knowledge is appropriate for addressing normal cognitive ageing, because the focus is on health promotion interventions to maintain optimal cognitive functioning. Impaired memory may be appropriate for older adults with the amnesic type of MCI or memory limitations that affect daily functioning.

Issues related to cognitive impairment associated with dementia and acute confusional states such as delirium are discussed in Chapter 14, while depression is discussed in Chapter 15.

WELLNESS OPPORTUNITY

Nurses can use the wellness nursing issue of willingness for enhanced knowledge for older adults who are motivated to improve their cognitive skills.

GOAL PLANNING FOR WELLNESS OUTCOMES

When older adults have risks for cognitive impairment, goals are created to achieve wellness outcomes. These include improved cognition, increased concentration, improved information processing, increased knowledge about cognitive health, increased leisure participation, behaviour compensating for hearing impairment (e.g. the person will be wearing a hearing aid) and behaviour compensating for vision deficit.

A student's perspective

At the beginning of my placement, I didn't know what to expect. I didn't realise I would learn so much by just listening to the life story of someone who is 96 years old. I realised that many of these individuals have had quite an amazing life and have a lot of wisdom and knowledge to pass down.

Needless to say, my expectations changed dramatically! They went from just getting the placement over with, to me not wanting to leave. Many of the residents were still "with it" and could remember a lot about their childhood and past experiences. This is the information that I did my best to take in. How did they get to live to be 96 years old and be able to look back on their life and be proud of their accomplishments? That's the life I want to live!

Kim V.

WELLNESS OPPORTUNITY

Personal well-being is a wellness outcome that nurses can promote by supporting personal responsibility for actions that improve cognitive abilities.

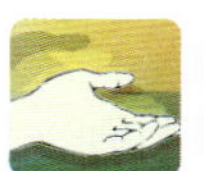

NURSING INTERVENTIONS TO PROMOTE COGNITIVE WELLNESS

Nurses have key roles in teaching older adults about the following evidence-based strategies for cognitive health and vitality (Gow, Bastin, Munoz et al., 2012; Guiney & Machado, 2013; Miller, Siddarth, Gaines et al., 2012; Stine-Morrow & Chui, 2011):

- Eat foods high in antioxidants (e.g. fruits and vegetable) and omega-3 fatty acids (e.g. fatty fish); limit salt, cholesterol and saturated fat.
- Maintain a healthy weight.
- Engage in regular physical activity, including aerobic activity, strengthening exercises, and flexibility and balance exercises.
- Engage in new learning experiences that are appealing and challenging.
- Practise body–mind activities such as tai chi and mindfulness-based meditation.
- Participate in leisure activities such as dancing, playing board games, playing a musical instrument, doing crossword puzzles and reading.
- Choose activities in which there is a sense of control and mastery, such as playing computer games or learning a new skill.
- Maintain strong and frequent social relationships with family and friends.

Many of the health promotion interventions that are discussed throughout this text provide specific examples of these types of activities. For example, interventions for cardiovascular wellness (see Chapter 20) are particularly relevant to promoting optimal cognitive function. Also, because vision and hearing impairments can interfere with cognitive abilities, any interventions directed towards improving sensory function (discussed in Chapters 16 and 17) may also be effective in improving cognitive function.

Nursing interventions related to cognitive wellness focus on: activity therapy; communication enhancement: hearing deficit; communication enhancement: visual deficit; exercise promotion; health education; learning facilitation; learning readiness enhancement; meditation facilitation; progressive muscle relaxation; role enhancement; self-awareness enhancement; self-responsibility enhancement; and individual teaching.

WELLNESS OPPORTUNITY

Nurses promote personal responsibility for wellness by helping older adults identify ways of incorporating "brain fitness" activities into their daily lives.

Health promotion: Teaching about memory and cognition

Teaching older adults about techniques to maintain or improve cognitive skills is within the realm of nursing responsibilities, as is teaching about maintaining and improving physical function. The concept of *metacognition* suggests that an understanding of one's own cognitive processes can influence performance. For example, someone who wants to remember a list of names needs both the intent to remember and knowledge about the techniques for remembering. Studies find that memory training can be effective in improving metamemory and other cognitive skills in older adults (Tullis & Benjamin, 2012).

In addition to addressing memory training techniques, it is important to address beliefs about cognition and ageing because these can significantly influence one's ability to learn. Thus, health education needs to include all of the following aspects:

- Correcting myths and misinformation
- Providing accurate information about age-related changes
- Communicating positive expectations
- Identifying goals for self-learning
- Providing information about techniques to enhance cognitive abilities
- Identifying the techniques that are most effective for the individual.

In community and long-term care settings, group sessions can effectively and efficiently address many psychosocial aspects of ageing, including cognitive function. The model developed by Turner Geriatric Services at the University of Michigan (Fogler & Stern, 2005) can be used to educate older adults about techniques for memory enhancement (see Box 11-2 on the following pages).

WELLNESS OPPORTUNITY

Nurses holistically address the learning needs of older adults by encouraging their participation in group programs, which have the additional benefit of offering social support.

Improving concentration and attention

When one's ability to attend to the environment and concentrate on visual and auditory cues is limited, the ability to learn and remember is also impaired. Thus, techniques such as relaxation, imagery and meditation, which enhance attention and concentration, may also improve memory and learning.

Likewise, any method that reduces environmental distractions may also improve one's cognitive abilities. Mindfulness (also called *mindfulness meditation*), which is the practice of focused awareness of the environment and one's reactions to it, is a self-care practice that can improve cognitive function and overall well-being. Many self-help books describe techniques for meditation, mindfulness and relaxation as ways of opening the mind to new learning. Nurses can teach the relaxation technique outlined in Chapter 24 to older adults for a variety of uses, including the enhancement of mental skills. Nurses can also promote personal responsibility for cognitive wellness by encouraging older adults to identify self-care practices that improve attention.

Encouraging participation in mentally stimulating activities

Because there is much evidence that participation in mentally stimulating activities is effective for promoting cognitive wellness, nurses can encourage older adults to participate in adult learning activities. In some settings, nurses can address health-related concerns of older adults through group health education programs, which have the additional benefit of providing social support. A process for implementing a nurse-led health education group is described in Chapter 12.

Nurses can also promote the use of computers by older adults for mental stimulation and practical benefits, such as increased communication with others and the acquisition of information that is relevant to their health and daily functioning. Nurses can encourage older adults to participate in educational opportunities in their local communities.

The University of the 3rd Age (U3A) is a worldwide organisation providing learning for personal enjoyment for those who have retired. There are many local U3A organisations across Australia and New Zealand that offer activities and courses for older adults. Although called a university, the courses do not have exams or confer degrees.

There is also a U3A Online organisation that provides resources and courses to those older adults who are unable

BOX 11-2
Memory training for older adults

Introduction

- Forgetting is a normal part of life for all people, but memory skills can be learned. The purposes of this program are to look at some reasons people forget things and to discuss ways of improving memory skills.
- When older adults are forgetful, they may blame it on old age, rather than seeing it as something that happens to everyone, regardless of age.
- Memory problems can be viewed as a challenge. Anyone can improve his or her memory, but as with any other skill, an effort must be made.

Stages of memory

- *Sensory memory* lasts only a few seconds. It involves the awareness of information obtained through vision, hearing, smell, taste and touch.
- *Short-term memory* is your working memory, or what is in your conscious thoughts. This, too, is very brief and contains small amounts of information. For example, this type of memory allows you to recall a telephone number as you dial it.
- *Long-term memory* is the memory bank, or what you depend on whenever you need to retrieve information. This memory bank is almost limitless and contains information you just learned, as well as information from long ago.

Memory changes and ageing

- Ageing is blamed for many memory problems, but very few changes occur solely because of ageing.
- In older adulthood, the processes of learning new information and recalling old information slow down a little. The overall ability to learn and remember, however, is not significantly affected in healthy older people.

Factors that interfere with memory

As people grow older, an increasing number of factors may interfere with their ability to remember, including the following:

- Not being attentive to the situation. This might be attributable, for example, to the fact that the situation is not relevant to you
- Being distracted by many things that interfere with your ability to concentrate. For example, this might be the result of worry or anxiety
- Feeling stressed
- Having a physical illness or being tired
- Having vision, hearing or other functional impairments that interfere with the ability to obtain information
- Feeling sad or depressed, or coping with loss or grief
- Not being intellectually stimulated (principle of "use it or lose it!")
- Not having cues to help you remember
- Not organising information for easy retention; not being organised in daily life
- Taking medications or alcohol that interfere with mental abilities
- Not being physically fit (e.g. as a result of poor nutrition or lack of exercise)

Ways of improving memory skills

- Write things down (e.g. use lists, calendars and notebooks).
- Use auditory cues (e.g. timers, alarm clocks) combined with written cues.
- Use environmental cues. For instance, you might remove something from its usual place, then return it to its normal location after it has served its purpose as a reminder.
- Assign specific places for specific items and keep the items in their proper place (e.g. keep keys on a hook near the door).
- Put reminders in appropriate places (e.g. place shoes that need to be repaired near the door).
- Use visual images. ("A picture is worth a thousand words.") Create a picture in your mind when you want to remember something; the more unusual the picture, the more likely it is that you will remember.
- Use active observation: pay attention to details of what is going on around you and be alert to the environment.
- Make associations, or mental connections. (For example, the phrase "spring ahead, fall back" can be recalled to ensure accuracy in changing clocks for seasonal time changes [from daylight savings time to standard time and vice versa].)
- Make associations between names and mental images (e.g. Carol and Christmas carol).
- Rehearse items you want to remember by repeating them aloud or writing the information on paper.
- Use self-instruction; say things aloud (e.g. "I'm putting my keys on the counter so I remember to turn off the stove before I leave.").
- Divide information into small parts that can be remembered easily. (For instance, to remember an address, divide it into groups.)
- Organise information into logical categories (e.g. shampoo and hair spray, toothpaste and mouthwash, and soap and deodorant).
- Use rhyming cues (e.g. "In 1492, Columbus sailed the ocean blue.").
- Use first-letter cues and make associations. (For example, to remember to buy carrots, apples, radishes, pickles, eggs and tea bags, remember the word CARPET.)
- Make word associations. (For instance, to remember the letters of your licence plate, make a word, such as camel, out of the letters CML.)
- Search the alphabet while focusing on what you are trying to remember. (For example, to remember that someone's name is Martin, start with names that begin with A and continue naming names through the alphabet until your memory is jogged for the correct one.)
- Make up a story to connect things you want to remember. (For instance, if you have to go to the cleaners and the post office, create a story about mailing a pair of pants.)

Conclusion

- Do not try to remember all of these techniques—you will need another method just to remember them all!

BOX 11-2
Memory training for older adults (*continued*)

- Select a few techniques that you like and use these whenever appropriate or needed.
- Minimise any distractions; pay attention to one thing at a time.
- Give yourself time to remember; forgetfulness is most likely to occur when you are in a hurry. Try to prepare in advance, when you have time to concentrate.
- Maintain some sense of organisation in your daily life, and devise systems to organise routine tasks such as taking medications.
- Carry a notepad or a calendar, and use written records so you do not have to rely entirely on mental cues.
- Relax and maintain a sense of humour. If you become anxious about your memory and are convinced you cannot remember, then you will create a self-fulfilling prophecy.

(Adapted with permission from Fogler, J. & Stern, L. [2005]. *Improving your memory: How to remember what you're starting to forget*. Baltimore: Johns Hopkins University Press.)

or not willing to physically attend a course. U3A Online can be found at http://u3aonline.org.au.

Road Scholar is a non-profit organisation that was founded in 1975 (called Elderhostel until 2009) to provide opportunities for lifelong learning by combining travel and education at a reasonable cost. In 2009, this program offered an extraordinary range of topics and formats in a wide range of affordable accommodations throughout more than 90 other countries. Nurses can encourage older adults to obtain additional information about this and other programs that are listed in the resources section at the end of this chapter.

WELLNESS OPPORTUNITY

Nurses promote personal responsibility by helping older adults identify activities that address their unique learning needs based on their life experiences and current interests.

Adapting health education materials

Much of the research on cognitive ageing has centred on factors that affect learning in older adulthood. Because many nursing interventions include health education, information about cognitive ageing can be used to adapt educational methods and materials to older adults. For example, nurses facilitate learning through the following adaptations: (1) allowing older adults enough time to process information; (2) providing small amounts of information over several sessions; 3) making referrals for home care nurses to follow up on teaching; (4) eliminating distractions in the learning environment; and (5) relating the information to past experiences and acquired wisdom (Cutilli, 2008). The suggestions presented in this text for communicating with older adults and compensating for hearing and vision deficit (see Chapters 13, 16 and 17) can be applied to health education. Nurses can apply the guidelines in Box 11-3 to educational interventions for older adults.

Adaptations of health education materials may also be necessary to ensure they are culturally appropriate. Many teaching materials are available in languages other than English. For instance, many sites listed in the resources section of Chapter 5 and other chapters provide health education materials in other languages.

Because there is growing emphasis on addressing needs of culturally diverse populations, nurses need to check the resources periodically and inquire about the availability of teaching materials for specific groups. Nurses can contact organisations, local hospitals, home care agencies and long-term residential care facilities, or check Internet sources, to inquire about health education materials available to address learning needs of culturally diverse populations in their service area. For example, organisations and state governments have developed advance directive forms and teaching tools that address the learning needs of specific cultural groups, as discussed in Chapter 9. Chapter 2 of this text further addresses the topic of culturally sensitive health education.

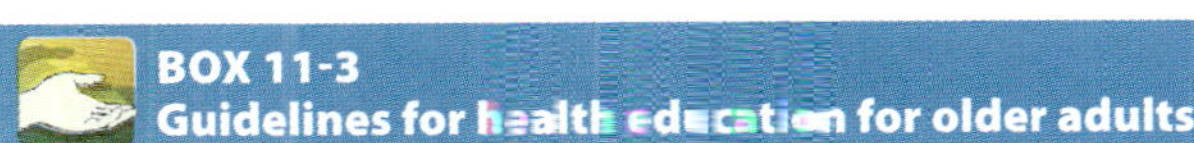

BOX 11-3
Guidelines for health education for older adults

Conditions that promote learning

- Supportive and rewarding contexts (e.g. praise and positive feedback) in contrast to those that are neutral, challenging or critical
- Environment that is pleasant, familiar, brightly lit, with little or no background noise and as few distractions as possible
- Personally relevant information that builds on prior experiences
- Information that is concrete rather than abstract
- Shorter, more frequent sessions

Presentation methods most conducive to learning

- Self-paced rate that allows time for assimilation
- Presentation of one idea at a time
- Emphasis on integration and application of knowledge and experience, rather than on acquisition of irrelevant information
- Visual aids for material that lends itself to thoughtful analysis
- Auditory aids, alone or with visual aids for information that is factual
- Advance organisers, such as outlines, overviews and written cues
- Reinforcement of the value of using organising aids

EVALUATING EFFECTIVENESS OF NURSING INTERVENTIONS

Effectiveness of nursing interventions is evaluated by the degree to which older adults are able to use their cognitive abilities to meet their daily needs. For example, older adults who forget to keep appointments might learn to use a calendar or other organisational aids to remember the appointments. In these situations, the effectiveness of interventions is measured by how well people remember to keep appointments. The effectiveness of nursing interventions also can be measured subjectively, based on the degree to which older adults express positive perceptions of their cognitive abilities and satisfaction with interventions, including self-care actions.

CASE STUDY

Mrs Cory is 71 years old and lives alone in her own home. She attends a local medical clinic for blood pressure checks, health screenings (e.g. cholesterol levels), and her annual flu shot. During her monthly visit for a blood pressure check, she confides that she is embarrassed about missing a dentist's appointment last week. She says she has been noticing increased difficulties with memory, and one of her friends has told her that she probably has Alzheimer's disease. She asks if there is a place where she can get a test for Alzheimer's disease.

Nursing assessment

Your nursing assessment indicates that Mrs Cory has missed a couple of healthcare appointments during the past year. She said she missed an eye appointment 6 months ago when she was very worried about her daughter, who was undergoing diagnostic tests for a lump in her breast. Last week, when she missed her dentist's appointment, she had been busy shopping for presents for her grandson's wedding. When you ask about additional problems with memory, Mrs Cory admits that she has more difficulty remembering people's names than she used to have. You do not identify any risk factors that might affect Mrs Cory's cognitive abilities (e.g. depression, medication effects, poor nutrition). Mrs Cory has never used calendars, and she says she remembers her doctor's appointments by keeping the appointment cards in her desk drawer along with her bills and her chequebook. She says that she checks her appointment cards every month, but she had not noticed the cards for the two appointments she missed.

Nursing issues

You use the nursing issue of health-seeking behaviours because Mrs Cory is interested in learning about memory training skills to assist her in remembering appointments. Mrs Cory has a poor understanding of age-related cognitive changes, and she indicates that she is interested in learning about ways to improve her memory.

Nursing care plan for Mrs Cory

Goals that support wellness outcomes	Nursing interventions	Nursing evaluation
Mrs Cory will express an interest in improving her memory skills.	• Use information in Box 11-1 to teach Mrs Cory about age-related changes that affect cognitive abilities.	• Mrs Cory agrees to participate in a discussion of memory training skills.
Mrs Cory will use memory training techniques to improve her functional level.	• Discuss the difference between dementia and age-associated memory impairment. • Emphasise that memory skills can be developed through memory training techniques. • Give Mrs Cory a copy of Box 11-2 and review the information. • Assist Mrs Cory in identifying one or two strategies for remembering appointments (e.g. begin using a calendar). • Assist Mrs Cory in identifying one or two strategies for remembering the names of people she meets (e.g. using visual images).	• Mrs Cory reports success in using a method for remembering appointments. • Mrs Cory reports success in using a method for remembering the names of people.

Thinking points

- What factors are likely to be contributing to Mrs Cory's forgetting about her appointments?
- What is the most effective way of using information in Boxes 11-1 and 11-2 to facilitate learning for Mrs Cory?
- What additional interventions would you suggest for Mrs Cory?

CHAPTER HIGHLIGHTS

Introduction

- Older adults are increasingly likely to experience changes in cognitive function
- Confusion is a term used by nurses to describe cognitive impairment
- Confusion is an ambiguous term and does not adequately describe the cognitive changes
- Nurses are required to understand the types of cognitive impairment of older adults to deliver optimal care
- Some cognitive changes are experienced by healthy older adults called cognitive decline.
- There are four types of altered cognition that may be experienced by the older adults: mild cognitive impairment, dementia, delirium and depression (the "4 Ds")
- The "4 Ds" are not associated with normal ageing changes in cognition

Age-related changes that affect cognition

- Central nervous system: degenerative changes in brain, slower reaction time
- Fluid intelligence (inductive reasoning, abstract thinking) declines, but crystallised intelligence (wisdom and judgement) improves
- Some, but not all, memory functions decline in healthy older adults
- Models of adult psychological development describe phases of mature ageing

Risk factors that affect cognitive wellness

- Personal and social influences: education, socioeconomic factors, ageism
- Physical health and functioning: chronic conditions, nutritional status, sensory impairment
- Mental health factors: stress, depression
- Health-related behaviours: physical activity, social engagement
- Adverse medication effects, especially from anticholinergics
- Neuropathological conditions: MCI, delirium, depression are risk factors for dementia
- Exposure to environmental toxins
- Genetic factors

Functional consequences affecting cognitive function

- Cognitive skills that decline with age: perceptual speed, numerical ability, episodic memory, verbal ability, inductive reasoning, executive functions
- Cognitive skills that improve with age: word lexicon, general knowledge
- Rapid or significant declines are due to pathological processes (e.g. strokes, dementia, delirium, MCI, depression)
- Cultural factors and cognitive function (Cultural considerations 11-1)
- Education, socioeconomic factors, ageism
- Increased risk of developing MCI, delirium, dementia, depression

Pathological conditions affecting cognition

- Delirium, dementia (Chapter 14) and depression (Chapter 15)
- MCI is not "normal ageing" but does not meet the criteria for mild dementia
- MCI may progress to Alzheimer's disease

Nursing assessment of cognitive function

- Refer to Chapter 13

Nursing issues

- Willingness for enhanced knowledge
- Health-seeking behaviours

Goal planning for wellness outcomes

- Cognition
- Concentration
- Health beliefs
- Health-seeking behaviour
- Information processing
- Knowledge about health promotion
- Leisure participation

Nursing interventions to promote cognitive wellness

- Evidence-based strategies for cognitive health: nutrition, mental exercise, physical exercise, challenging leisure activities, strong social networks, activities that foster a sense of control and mastery
- Teaching about memory and cognition for individuals and groups (Box 11-2)
- Improving concentration and attention (mindfulness, imagery, relaxation)
- Encouraging participation in mentally stimulating activities (computers, classes)
- Adapting health education materials (Box 11-3)

Evaluating effectiveness of nursing interventions

- The expression of satisfaction with improved cognitive abilities
- Ability to use cognitive skills in daily activities

CRITICAL THINKING EXERCISES

1. Identify the factors in your own life that interfere with cognitive function.
2. What memory aids do you use in your life? Are they effective? Would you like to develop additional memory aids?
3. You are a nurse working in a long-term residential care facility. Nearby is a retirement village that is owned by

the same organisation as the care facility. You have suggested to the director of the organisation that the residents of the facility and the retirement village would benefit from a series of short sessions discussing cognitive ageing changes. This suggestion is based on your observation that many of the older adults have asked you questions about memory problems, and some are concerned about Alzheimer's disease. Address each of the following issues:

- The director is a firm believer in the adage, "You can't teach an old dog new tricks." How would you convince the director that the classes you wish to offer are worthwhile?
- How would you structure the sessions (number and length of sessions, number of participants, and so forth)?
- Describe the content you would cover and the approach you would use for each topic. Include information about normal cognitive ageing, risk factors for impaired cognitive function and techniques for improving memory and other aspects of cognition.
- What audiovisual aids, including written materials, would you use?
- How would you adapt your teaching method and materials for the group?
- How would you evaluate the sessions?

RESOURCES

For an extensive range of additional resources to enhance teaching and learning and to facilitate understanding of this chapter, please see the text's accompanying website located on thePoint at http://thepoint.lww.com.

Clinical tools

Refer to Chapter 13: Cognitive and psychosocial assessment.

Evidence-based practice

Joanna Briggs Institute: http://connect.jbiconnectplus.org

- Caldwell, C., Fernandez, R., Traynor, V. & Perrin, C. (2014). Effects of spending time outdoors in daylight on the psychosocial well-being of older people and their family carers: A systematic review. *Joanna Briggs Institute Library of Systematic Reviews, 12*(9), 277–320.

Health education

AARP, Brain Games (free online): http://games.aarp.org/

American Society on Aging, MindAlert Lecture Monographs: http://asaging.org/mindalert-lecture-monographs

Better Health Channel, Healthy ageing, Stay mentally active: www.betterhealth.vic.gov.au/bhcv2/bhcarticles.nsf/pages/Healthy_ageing_stay_mentally_active?open

Brain Foundation, The Healthy Brain Program: http://brainfoundation.org.au/medical-info/healthy-brain

Road Scholar (formerly called Elderhostel): www.roadscholar.org

Healthy Brain Initiative, Centers for Disease Control and Prevention: www.cdc.gov/aging/pdf/TheHealthyBrainInitiative.pdf

Mind Your Mind, Alzheimer's Australia: http://mindyourmind.org.au

Neurological Foundation of New Zealand, Brain health: www.neurological.org.nz/brain-health

University of the Third Age: www.u3a.org.au

REFERENCES

Almeida, D. M., Piazza, J. R., Stawski, R. S., & Klein, L. C. (2011). The speedometer of life: Stress, health and aging. In K. W. Schaie & S. L. Willis. *Handbook of the psychology of aging* (7th ed., pp. 191–206). New York: Elsevier.

Annweiler, C., Rolland, Y., Schott, A. M. et al. (2012). Higher vitamin D dietary intake is associated with lower risk of Alzheimer's disease. *Journal of Gerontology: Medical Sciences, 67*(11), 1205–1211.

Balion, C., Griffith, L. E., Strifler, L. et al. (2012). Vitamin D, cognition, and dementia. *Neurology, 79*, 1397.

Barrientos, R. M., Frank, M. G., Watkins, L. R. et al. (2012). Aging-related changes in neuroimmune-endocrine function: Implications for hippocampal-dependent cognition. *Hormones and Behavior, 62*, 219–227.

Blanchard-Fields, F. & Kalinauskas, A. (2009). Theoretical perspectives on social context, cognition, and aging. In V. L. Bengston, M. Silverstein, N. M. Putney & D. Gans (Eds), *Handbook of theories of aging* (2nd ed., pp. 261–276). New York: Springer.

Bowman, G. L., Silbert, L. C., Howieson, D. et al. (2012). Nutrient biomarker patterns, cognitive function, and MRI measures of brain aging. *Neurology, 78*, 242.

Botwinick, J. (1984). *Aging and behavior* (3rd ed.). New York: Springer.

Cansino, S. (2009). Episodic memory decay along the adult lifespan: A review of behavioral and neurophysiological evidence. *International Journal of Psychophysiology, 71*, 64–69.

Carlson, M. C., Xue, Q-L., Zhou, J. & Fried, L. P. (2009). Executive decline and dysfunction precedes declines in memory: The Women's Health and Aging Study II. *Journals of Gerontology A: Biological Sciences, Medical Sciences, 64*(1), 110–117.

Carstensen, L. L., Mikels, J. A. & Mather, M. (2006). Aging and the intersection of cognition, motivation, and emotion. In J. E. Birren & K. W. Schaie (Eds), *Handbook of the psychology of aging* (6th ed., pp. 343–362). San Diego, CA: Academic Press.

Caserta, M. T., Bannon, Y., Fernandex, F., Giunta, B., Schoenbery, M. R. & Tan, J. (2009). Normal brain aging: Clinical immunological, neuropsychological, and neuroimaging features. *International Review of Neurobiology, 84*, 1–19.

Cohen, G. D. (2005). *The mature mind: The positive power of the aging brain.* New York: Basic Books.

Cutilli, C. C. (2008). Teaching the geriatric patient, making the most of "cognitive resources" and "gains". *Orthopaedic Nursing, 27*(3), 195–198.

Fogler, J. & Stern, L. (2005). *Improving your memory: How to remember what you're starting to forget* (3rd ed.). Baltimore: Johns Hopkins University Press.

Freitas, S., Simoes, M. R., Alves, L. et al. (2013). Montreal cognitive assessment. *Alzheimer's Disease & Associated Disorders, 27*, 38–43.

Goh, J. O. & Park, D. C. (2009). Neuroplasticity and cognitive aging: The scaffolding theory of aging and cognition. *Restorative Neurology and Neuroscience, 27*(5), 391–403.

Gow, A. J., Bastin, M. E., Munoz, M. et al. (2012). Neuroprotective lifestyles and the aging brain: Activity, atrophy, and white matter integrity. *Neurology, 79*(17), 1802–1808.

Grashow, R., Spiro, A., Taylor, K. M. et al. (2013). Cumulative lead exposure in community-dwelling adults and fine motor function. *Neurotoxicology, 35*, 154–161.

Guiney, H. & Machado, L. (2013). Benefits of regular aerobic exercise for executive functioning in healthy populations. *Psychonomic Bulletin & Review, 20*(1), 73–86.

Hall, C. B., Lipton, R. B., Sliwinski, M., Katz, M. J., Derby, C. A. & Verghese, J. (2009). Cognitive activities delay onset of memory decline in persons who develop dementia neurology. *American Academy of Neurology, 73*(5), 356–361.

Hasher, L. & Zacks, R. T. (1979). Autonomic and effortful processes in memory. *Journal of Experimental Psychology: General, 108*, 356–388.

Healey, W. E. (2012). Mild cognitive impairment and aging. *Topics in Geriatric Rehabilitation 28*(3), 157–162.

Hess, T. M., Leclerc, C. M., Swaim, E. & Weatherbee, S. R. (2009). Aging and everyday judgments: The impact of motivational and processing resource factors. *Psychological Aging, 24*(3), 735–740.

Insel, K. & Badger, T. A. (2002). Deciphering the 4 D's: cognitive decline, delirium, depression and dementia: A review. *Journal of Advanced Nursing, 38*(4), 360–368.

Inzitari, D., Pracucci, G., Poggesi, A., Carlucci, G., Barkhof, F. & Chabriat, H. (2009). Changes in white matter as determinant of global functional decline in older independent outpatients: Three-year follow-up of LADIS (leukoaraiosis and disability) Study cohort. *British Medical Journal, 339*, b2477 doi:10.1136/bmj.b2477.

Johnson, E. J. (2012). A possible role for lutein and zeaxanthin in cognitive function in the elderly. *American Journal of Clinical Nutrition, 96*(5), 1161S–1165S.

Katan, M., Moon, Y. P., Paik, M. C. et al. (2013). Infectious burden and cognitive function: The Northern Manhattan study. *Neurology, 80*(13), 1209–1215.

Kloppenborg, R. P., Nederkoorn, P. J., Grool, A. M. et al. (2012). Cerebral small-vessel disease and progression of brain atrophy. *Neurology, 79*(20), 2029–2036.

Knight, B. G. & Laidlaw, K. (2009). Translations theory: A wisdom-based model for psychological interventions to enhance well-being in later life. In V. L. Bengston, M. Silverstein, N. M. Putney & D. Gans (Eds), *Handbook of theories of aging* (2nd ed., pp. 693–705). New York: Springer.

Kremen, W. S., Lachman, M. E., Pruessner, J. C. et al. (2012). Mechanisms of age-related cognitive change and targets for intervention. *Journals of Gerontology: Medical Sciences, 67*(7), 760–765.

Labouvie-Vief, G. & Blanchard-Fields, F. (1982). Cognitive aging and psychological growth. *Ageing and Society, 2*, 183–209.

Labouvie-Vief, G. (2009a). Dynamic integration theory: Emotion, cognition, and equilibrium in later life. In V. L. Bengston, M. Silverstein, *Lancet Neurology, 11*(11), 1006–1012.

Labouvie-Vief, G. (2009b). Dynamic integration theory: Emotion, cognition, and equilibrium in later life. In V. L. Bengston, M. Silverstein, N. M. Putney & D. Gans (Eds), *Handbook of theories of aging* (2nd ed., pp. 277–293). New York: Springer.

Levy, B. R. & Leifheit-Limson, E. (2009). The stereotype-matching effect: Greater influence on functioning when age stereotypes correspond to outcomes. *Psychology and Aging, 24*(1), 230–233.

Levy, B. R., Zonderman, A. B., Slade, M. D. et al. (2011). Memory shaped by age stereotypes over time. *Journals of Gerontology: Psychological Sciences and Social Sciences, 67*(4), 432–436.

Lin, F. R., Yaffe, K., Xia, J. et al. (2013). Hearing loss and cognitive decline in older adults. *JAMA Internal Medicine, 173*(4), 293–299.

Lopez, O. L. (2013). Mild cognitive impairment. *Continuum, 19*(2), 411–424.

Lovden, M., Xu, W. & Wang, H. X. (2013). Lifestyle change and the prevention of cognitive decline and dementia: What is the evidence? *Current Opinions in Psychiatry, 26*(3), 239–243.

MacDonald, S., DeCarlo, C. A. & Dixon, R. A. (2011). Linking biological and cognitive aging. *Journals of Gerontology: Psychological Sciences and Social Sciences, 66B*(S1), i59–i70.

Makin, S., Turpin, S., Dennis, M. S. et al. (2013). Cognitive impairment after lacunar stroke: Systematic review and meta-analysis of incidence, prevalence and comparison with other stroke subtypes. *Journal of Neurology, Neurosurgery, and Psychiatry, 84*(8), 893–900.

Mariske, M. & Margrett, J. A. (2006). Everyday problem solving and decision making. In J. E. Birren & K. W. Schaie (Eds), *Handbook of the psychology of aging* (6th ed., pp. 315–342). San Diego, CA: Academic Press.

McFadden, S. H. & Basting, A. D. (2010). Healthy aging persons and their brains: Promoting resilience through creative engagement. *Clinics in Geriatric Medicine, 26*, 149–161.

Miller, K. J., Siddarth, P., Gaines, J. M. et al. (2012). The memory fitness program: Cognitive effects of a healthy aging intervention. *American Journal of Geriatric Psychiatry, 20*, 514–523.

Morris, M. S., Selhub, J. & Jacques, P. F. (2012). Vitamin B-12 and folate status in relation to decline in scores in the mini-mental state examination in the Framingham heart study. *Journal of the American Geriatrics Society, 60*(8), 1457–1464.

Orsitto, G., Turi, V., Venezia, A. et al. (2012). Relation of secondhand smoking to mild cognitive impairment in older inpatients. *Scientific World Journal*. Art. no. 726948. doi: 10.1100/2012/726948.

Pansky, A., Goldsmith, M., Koriat, A. & Pearlman-Avnion, S. (2009). Memory accuracy in old age: Cognitive, metacognitive, and neurocognitive determinants. *European Journal of Cognitive Psychology, 21*(2/3), 303–329.

Park, D. C. & Reuter-Lorenz, P. (2009). The adaptive brain: Aging and neurocognitive scaffolding. *Annual Review of Psychology, 60*, 173–196.

Pasina, L., Djade, C. D., Lucca, U. et al. (2013). Association of anticholinergic burden with cognitive and functional status in a cohort of hospitalized elderly. *Drugs & Aging, 30*(2), 103–112.

Patel, B. B. & Holland, N. W. (2012). Mild cognitive impairment: Hope for stability, plan for progression. *Cleveland Clinic Journal of Medicine, 79*(12), 857–864.

Peterson, A., Mattek, N., Clemons, A. et al. (2012). Serum vitamin D concentrations are associated with falling and cognitive function in older adults. *Journal of Nutrition, Health & Aging, 16*(10), 898–901.

Reis, J. P., Loria, C. M., Launer, L. J. et al. (2013). Cardiovascular health through young adulthood and cognitive functioning in midlife. *Annals of Neurology, 73*(2), 170–179.

Rosano, C., Marsland, A. L. & Gianaros, P. J. (2012). Maintaining brain health by monitoring inflammatory processes. *Aging and Disease, 3*(1), 16–33.

Sabia, S., Elbaz, A., Dugravot, A. et al. (2012). Impact of smoking on cognitive decline in early old age. *Archives of General Psychiatry, 69*(6), 627–635.

Sabia, S., Singh-Manoux, A., Hagger-Johnson, G. et al. (2012). Influence of individual and combined healthy behaviours on successful aging. *Canadian Medical Association Journal, 184*(18), 1985–1992.

Sartori, A. C., Vance, D. E., Slater, L. Z. et al. (2012). The impact of inflammation on cognitive function in older adults. *Journal of Neuroscience Nursing, 44*(4), 206–216.

Schaie, K. W. (1977–1978). Toward a stage theory of adult cognitive development. *Journal of Aging and Human Development, 8*, 129–138.

Shah, R. C., Schneider, J. A., Leurgans, S. et al. (2012). Association of lower hemoglobin level and neuropathology in community-dwelling older persons. *Journal of Alzheimer's Disease, 32*(3), 579–586.

Slinin, Y., Paudel, M., Taylor, B. C. et al. (2012). Association between serum 25(OH) vitamin D and the risk of cognitive decline in older women. *Journals of Gerontology: Biological Sciences and Medical Sciences, 67*(10), 1092–1098.

Sorond, F. A., Schnyer, D. M., Serrador, J. M., Milberg, W. P. & Lipstiz, L. A. (2008). Cerebral blood flow regulation during cognitive tasks: Effects of healthy aging. *Cortex, 44*, 179–184.

Spiro, A. & Brady, C. B. (2011). Integrating health into cognitive aging. *Journals of Gerontology: Psychological Sciences and Social Sciences, 66*(S1), i17–i25.

Stern, Y. (2012). Cognitive reserve in ageing and Alzheimer's disease. *Lancet Neurology, 11*(11), 1006–1012.

Stine-Morrow, E. & Chui, H. (2011). Cognitive resilience in adulthood. *Annual Review of Gerontology and Geriatrics, 32*, 93–114.

Suzuki, T., Shimada, H., Makizako, H. et al. (2012), Effects of multicomponent exercise on cognitive function in older adults with amnesic mild cognitive impairment. *BMC Neurology, 12*, 128. Accessed at www.biomedcentral.com/1471-2377/12/128.

Swift, H. J., Abrams, D. & Marques, S. (2013). Threat or boost: Social comparison affects older people's performance differently depending on task domain. *Journals of Gerontology: Psychological Sciences and Social Sciences, 68*(1), 23–30.

Tullis, J. G. & Benjamin, A. S. (2012). The effectiveness of updating metacognitive knowledge in the elderly. *Psychology and Aging, 27*(3), 683–690.

Van Der Mussele, Le Bastard, N., Vermeiren, Y. et al. (2013). Behavioral symptoms in mild cognitive impairment as compared with Alzheimer's disease and healthy older adults. *International Journal of Geriatric Psychiatry, 28*(3), 265–275.

Vance, D. E. & Wright, M. A. (2009). Positive and negative neuroplasticity, implications for age-related cognitive declines. *Journal of Gerontological Nursing, 35*(6), 11–18.

Wang, H., Jin, Y., Hendrie, H. C. et al. (2013). Late life leisure activities and risk of cognitive decline. *Journals of Gerontology: Medical Sciences, 68*(2), 205–213.

Willis, S. L., Schaie, K. W. & Martin, M. (2009). Cognitive plasticity. In V. L. Bengston, M. Silverstein, N. M. Putney & D. Gans (Eds), *Handbook of theories of aging* (2nd ed., pp. 295–322). New York: Springer.

Yavuz, B. B., Cankurtaran, M., Haznedaroglu, I. C. et al. (2012). Iron deficiency can cause cognitive impairment in geriatric patients. *Journal of Nutrition, Health & Aging, 16*(3), 220–224.

Yu, F., Ryan, L. H., Schaie, K. W., Willis, S. L. & Kolanowski, A. (2009). Factors associated with cognition in adults: The Seattle Longitudinal Study. *Research in Nursing and Health, 32*(5), 540–550.

Zarit, S. H. (2009). A good old age: Theories of mental health and aging. In V. L. Bengston, M. Silverstein, N. M. Putney & D. Gans (Eds), *Handbook of theories of aging* (2nd ed., pp. 675–691). New York: Springer.

Chapter 12
Psychosocial function

By Carol Miller and Sharyn Hunter

LEARNING OBJECTIVES

After reading this chapter, you should be able to:

1. Identify the life events that commonly occur in older adulthood.
2. Discuss theories related to stress and coping as they apply to older adults.
3. Identify the risk factors and cultural factors that influence psychosocial function in older adults.
4. Describe the functional consequences associated with psychosocial function in older adults.
5. Identify nursing interventions that promote psychosocial wellness in older adults.
6. Describe how to conduct a "healthy ageing class" for a small group of older adults.

KEY POINTS

anxiety
coping strategies
culture-bound syndromes
elderspeak
infantilisation
late-life anxiety disorder
learned helplessness
life events
life review
loneliness
reminiscence
resilience
self-esteem
spirituality
stress
stressors

Although the physiological changes and chronic illnesses associated with older adulthood may affect a person's functional abilities, the psychosocial changes are often the most challenging and demanding in terms of coping energy. Of course, many psychosocial challenges are strongly associated with compromised health and physical functioning, but some are attributable to changes in roles, relationships and living environments. Because many of the psychosocial changes are inevitable and somewhat predictable, older adults can prepare for and respond to psychosocial changes by developing and using effective **coping strategies**. Nurses can promote psychosocial wellness by supporting effective coping mechanisms and assisting in the development of new coping strategies.

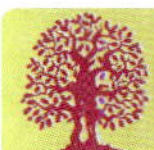

LIFE EVENTS: AGE-RELATED CHANGES AFFECTING PSYCHOSOCIAL FUNCTION

Life events are the major changes that occur at various times during the life cycle and significantly affect daily life. Certain events are commonly associated with different periods in one's life. For example, younger adults are likely to experience the following life events: establishing a career, moving away from the nuclear family, committing to a partner, creating a home, and beginning a family. The major life events of younger adulthood are familiar to us through either personal experiences or the shared experiences of friends. People usually view these events as positive gains and choose them purposefully. By contrast, life events of older adulthood might be unknown, unexpected, inevitable and, in fact, unwanted or even feared. Thus, older adults may experience a greater fear of losing control over their lives. In addition, life events during older adulthood are likely to involve losses of significant others and objects that have been part of life for many decades. Moreover, they tend to occur close together, with less time available for people to adjust to each event. Some life events evolve into chronic stresses. Dealing with ageist attitudes and behaviours of others is a life event that is specific to older adults.

Life events that are most likely to occur during older adulthood include retirement, relocation, chronic illness and functional impairments, decisions about driving a vehicle, widowhood, the death of friends and family and confronting ageist attitudes. Figure 12-1 illustrates some of the major life events that are likely to occur in older adulthood, as well as the related consequences. Although most of the consequences are negative, some consequences can be positive. For example, because of these life events, older adults may focus on achieving integrity and meaning in life and they may develop a greater acceptance of things that cannot be controlled. The illustration attempts to show the interrelatedness among the life events of older adulthood.

WELLNESS OPPORTUNITY

Nurses promote wellness by asking older adults to talk about the meaning of life events that they have experienced.

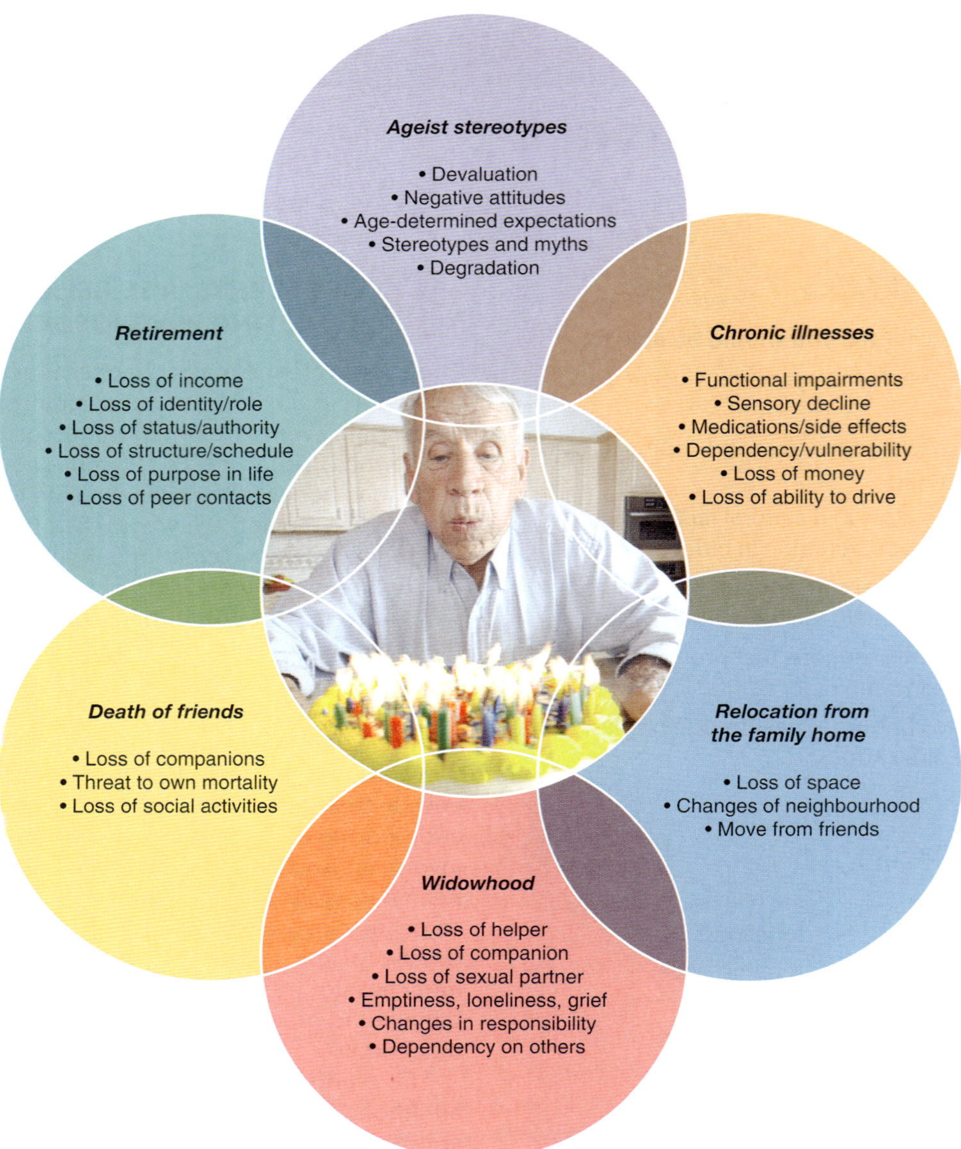

FIGURE 12-1 Psychosocial challenges of older adulthood.

Retirement

Retirement from employment is often viewed as a milestone that marks the passage into older adulthood. The age of 65 years is the traditional retirement age; however, there is a growing trend towards "bridge employment" involving a transition from full-time to part-time employment before retirement. Studies have found that bridge employment facilitates adjustment to retirement by helping older adults structure their time, offering opportunities for supplemental income and developing new routines and interests before full retirement (Mehrotra & Wagner, 2009).

Societal attitudes can influence one's adjustment to retirement, particularly in societies with a strong work ethic. In these societies, working people have a higher status than unemployed people and, among working people, status is based on the kind of job one holds and the salary one earns. Therefore, when people retire, they inevitably cope with a change in social status and the psychosocial challenge may be the greatest for people whose **self-esteem** (the extent to which one perceives oneself to be worthy or significant) and self-concept are based on job status. The following factors commonly influence the decision to retire: health, financial assets, job conditions, pension availability, family circumstances (e.g. care responsibilities), opportunities for continued employment and also the continued ability to perform job responsibilities. For married couples, both the worker and the spouse or partner must adjust to retirement. Sometimes the adjustment is more difficult for the partner who has not been employed.

DIVERSITY NOTE

Women, minority workers and people who live in rural areas are likely to have a sporadic work history and lower-paying jobs throughout their adult lives. They also may have lower retirement assets (Mehrotra & Wagner, 2009).

Relocation

Another common psychosocial adjustment for older adults is the decision to move from the family home because of such factors as loss of spouse, lack of available assistive services, a lack of a kinship network or carer/caregiver, chronic condition, and declining functional abilities and cognitive impairment or mental illness. Increased dependence on others because of health problems is a common reason for older adults to move to a facility where they can receive support services. Older adults whose adult children have moved to another place may relocate to be closer to them. Or older adults may choose to move to a desirable geographic location after they retire.

In addition to family and personal factors, many environmental conditions influence the decision to move. For example, older people in urban areas may find they are unsafe or socially isolated because the neighbourhood around them has changed and they are no longer surrounded by people with whom they can easily relate. In rural areas, geographic distance and lack of support services can have serious consequences for older adults who are functionally impaired, especially if they have few social supports. Problems also arise for older homeowners who find it more difficult to maintain their home and pay for utilities.

Relocation to long-term care is a significant life event for some older adults. Nurses caring for older adults in hospitals and in the community have important roles in assisting older adults and their families with relocation decisions and adjustments. It is not unusual for a decision to be made to discharge an older adult to long-term residential care from hospital after they have experienced an acute illness. This typically occurs when a narrow medical perspective rather than a broader psychosocial one is taken and the older adult does not have strong carer resources. Nurses are in key positions to address these decisions holistically, by exploring all options for care and ensuring psychosocial issues are considered alongside medical concerns. Nurses can ensure that older adults and their families are involved as much as possible in decisions and that these decisions support the psychosocial wellness of the older person. Nurses must be mindful that older adults' needs change and decisions will require review periodically.

WELLNESS OPPORTUNITY

Nurses promote psychosocial wellness by encouraging older adults to express their feelings about decisions related to long-term care plans and by helping them identify effective ways of coping, even when they are not happy about the decision.

Chronic illness and functional impairments

Another major life adjustment for many older adults is coping with chronic illnesses and functional limitations, particularly limitations that curtail their independence. Although the large majority of older adults experience one or more chronic conditions that affect their daily functioning, many have positive perceptions about their health. Seventy-four per cent of Australian people aged 65 to 74 years and 69% of Australian people aged over 74 years rate their health as excellent, very good or good (Australian Bureau of Statistics, 2013). Eighty-nine per cent of New Zealanders aged 65 to 74 years and 8?% of New Zealanders aged over 75 rated their health as excellent, very good or good (New Zealand Ministry of Health, 2013). However, most functional limitations necessitate only minor adjustments in daily living, but some, such as considerable cognitive, mobility or visual impairments, significantly increase a person's dependence on others. Other consequences of chronic illnesses include the following:

- Threats to self-esteem and altered self-concept
- Changes in lifestyle
- Unpredictability about one's ability to do what one wants to do
- Expenditures for assistance, medications and medical care
- Frequent trips to healthcare providers
- Adverse medication effects which sometimes cause further functional impairments
- Increased vulnerability to personal crimes and fear of crime.

Decisions about driving a vehicle

Decisions about driving a vehicle represent one of the most emotionally charged issues relating to functional impairment that older adults, their families and healthcare professionals face. Access to a car and the possession of a valid driver's licence not only provide transportation but also serve as significant indicators of autonomy. In fact, for many older adults, the ability to drive is synonymous with independence and the possession of a driver's licence, even one that goes unused, is a symbol of one's ability to shield oneself from dependence on others. Studies confirm that driving cessation is a stressful experience for many older adults, leading to depression, isolation, loss of identity, loss of self-esteem, feelings of diminished self-worth and diminished life satisfaction and quality of life (Kostyniuk, Molnar & Eby, 2009; Oxley & Charlton, 2009). Studies also indicate that driving status is a strong predictor of nursing home placement and of 3-year mortality risk (Edwards et al., 2009).

The loss of an independent means of transportation affects every aspect of an older person's life, from the acquisition of food and medicine to opportunities for social interaction. Because of this far-reaching impact, families and older persons may avoid dealing with driving-related issues.

Family members may be reluctant to suggest that an older relative give up driving for a number of reasons. For example, family members may not want to assume an authority role or they may lack acceptable alternatives for transportation. It is not surprising, then, that older adults and their families may avoid or resist the decision to stop driving. Neither is it surprising that when older adults give up or significantly curtail their driving, they face a difficult psychosocial challenge that may be viewed as a major life event.

Widowhood

The example of widowhood as a life event of older adulthood illustrates all of the characteristics discussed earlier. For most older couples, widowhood is inevitable and the chances are greater that women become widowed more than men. When widowhood occurs, there are additional consequences. Common additional consequences include the following:

- Loss of companionship and intimacy
- Loss of one's sexual partner
- Feelings of grief, loneliness and emptiness
- Increased responsibilities
- Increased dependence on others
- Loss of income and less efficient financial management
- Changes in relationships with children, married friends and other family members.

When a marriage or partnership has lasted for many decades, as is common in people who are in their 70s and 80s, the impact of the loss can be tremendous and the feelings of grief, loneliness and emptiness may be overwhelming. Despite the major impact of widowhood, however, some studies have found that spousal bereavement is associated with higher risk of mortality among middle-aged, but not older, adults (Aldwin, Hofer & McCammon, 2006). Another study found that older women experienced a negative impact on health and well-being soon after the loss of their spouse but that this was followed by a shift into a new and positive life phase of learning to live alone (Young & Cochrane, 2004).

Another characteristic of widowhood in older adulthood is that the chance of remarriage diminishes with advancing age. This is especially true for women because there are disproportionately fewer older men than older women due to greater longevity of women. In addition to the "shortage" of eligible men, other reasons that widows do not remarry are loyalty to their deceased husbands, family issues and a preference for their newly independent lives (Cattell, 2009). Even when widows or widowers do remarry, they need to adjust to entirely different roles with a new partner. If the married couple had clearly divided roles, as is common in the cohort of people who are old today, loss of the partner means an adjustment in important day-to-day tasks. For example, older couples often divide tasks so that only one of the two manages money, drives the vehicle, cleans the house, shops for groceries and does household repairs and maintenance. When the person responsible for a task no longer performs the role, the other person may be unable, unwilling or unprepared to assume this role.

WELLNESS OPPORTUNITY

When applicable, nurses encourage older adults to talk about their experience of widowhood by opening the conversation with a question such as, "How is your life different since your partner passed away?"

Death of friends and family

Like other life events of older adulthood, the loss of friends and family becomes inevitable with each year. Many people who are in their 90s have outlived most, if not all, of their friends and many of their relatives. Indeed, people who are in their 90s may not even know anyone who is older than they are. Moreover, as people are confronted with the death of others who are younger than or similar to them in age, they become increasingly aware of their own mortality. Older people may read obituaries and death notices in the newspaper as a daily activity. Although families may view this activity as a morbid preoccupation, it may, in fact, be an effective way for older people to learn what is happening to their friends. Because meaningful social relationships are an important predictor of well-being for older adults, loss of family and friends is likely to have a negative impact on psychosocial wellness. However, older adults who are able to adjust their expectations and do not feel a sense of social isolation may fare better than those who perceive themselves as socially isolated and disconnected (Cornwell & Waite, 2009).

Ageist attitudes

A life adjustment that, by its nature, is unique to older adulthood is the acceptance of being old. Because of the ageist attitudes common in modern industrialised societies, many older adults deny that they are old. Ageism can lead to prejudices, fear of ageing and feelings of devaluation and degradation (as discussed in Chapter 1). Studies indicate that positive or negative ageing stereotypes affect older adults' decisions and behaviours in beneficial or detrimental ways, respectively (Levy & Leifheit-Limson, 2009). Consequences of negative age-based stereotypes include impaired memory and decreased cognitive performance, declining will to live and diminished positive affect, negative effects on physical health (e.g. increased cardiovascular stress) and behavioural changes such as decreased walking speed and shaky handwriting (Kang & Chasteen, 2009). When negative ageist stereotypes are pervasive in a society, people with a good self-acceptance of being old may feel that it is socially unacceptable to admit that it is okay to be old.

Because of these societal attitudes, older adults may be confronted with age-determined expectations that dictate appropriate social behaviours. For example, public displays of affection are viewed as socially appropriate for teenagers and younger adults. However, when older adults hold hands or kiss in public, observers are likely to make comments like, "Isn't that cute; look at that old couple holding hands." Having sexual relationships outside of a marriage is another action that is generally overlooked when done by young adults, but that is likely to be criticised when done by older adults.

As an example of age-determined expectations, consider the following scene: a grey-haired man, who was clearly an older adult, was wearing headphones and listening to music on a portable radio. He was briskly moving along in a combination dance–walk tempo on a public footpath in an urban area. Observers remarked that the old man looked like he needed mental healthcare, whereas they ignored several teens nearby who were dancing and listening to music blaring from loudspeakers. The only apparent difference between the older adult and the teens was that the younger people were listening to louder music and demonstrating less control in their movements. The primary difference, however, was in the age-determined expectations in the eyes of the beholders!

WELLNESS OPPORTUNITY

Nurses can promote positive attitudes about ageing by talking about people who are examples of successful ageing.

THEORIES ABOUT STRESS AND COPING IN OLDER ADULTS

Theories about stress and coping attempt to answer such questions as, *How do life events affect older adults? Do coping patterns change in older adulthood?* and *How do stress and coping patterns affect health and functioning?* In keeping with the perspective of this text, these theories are discussed in relation to positive or negative functional consequences on psychosocial function. Additional psychological theories pertinent to older adults are discussed in Chapter 4.

Theories about stress

Hans Selye, who proposed the first major theory about stress in the mid-1950s, defined **stress** as the sum of all the effects of factors that act on the body (Selye, 1956). According to Selye's theory, **stressors** include normal activities and disease states; and all factors, whether pleasant or unpleasant, are equally important. Moreover, people respond to stressors in three stages: alarm, resistance and exhaustion. Limitations of this theory include the broad conceptualisation of stress, the lack of distinction between pleasant and unpleasant stressors and the failure to address the meaning of events for the person.

Holmes and Rahe (1967) proposed that stress was a mediator between a life event and adaptation to that event. They define life events as discrete and identifiable changes in life patterns that create stress and that can lead to negative health outcomes. According to this theory, stress causes physical and psychological harm that is in proportion to the intensity of the impact on and duration of a disruption in one's usual life pattern. Holmes and Rahe (1967) developed the Social Readjustment Rating Scale (SRRS) as a tool for measuring the duration and intensity of specific life events. The SRRS is a checklist of 43 life events, with relative weights assigned to each according to the usual amount of adaptive effort required by each event.

In addition to addressing the impact of major life events (e.g. acute stress), studies address the impact of chronic stressors, including those that evolve from a major life event. Scott and colleagues (2013) describe types of chronic stressors as (1) role strains from ongoing problems with work, family, relationships and caregiving, and (2) ambient stressors across life domains: health, finances, loneliness and neighbourhood. Daily hassles (i.e. relatively minor events arising from day-to-day living) are another source of stress that can negatively affect psychological well-being overall and cognitive function in particular (Stawski, Mogle & Sliwinski, 2013). Examples of hassles are misplacing or losing things and not having resources to meet demands (e.g. food, money, medications). When chronic stressors and daily hassles occur together—as is often the case—the negative effects are magnified, leading to declines in physical and cognitive functioning in older adults (Almeida, Piazza, Stawski et al., 2011). As summarised by Werner and colleagues (2012), "the level of stress experienced by individuals is dependent, in part, on all of the stressors they are currently experiencing and on their appraisal of any given situation" (p. 138).

A prominent current theme among gerontologists is expanding the "stress universe" to develop a more comprehensive approach to identifying many factors that affect the ways in which older adults experience and respond to stressors (George, 2011). In particular, researchers and clinicians focus attention on the connection between chronic stress and health. Currently, studies find that chronic stress increases the risk for all the following (Blume, Douglas & Evans, 2011; Gouin & Kiecolt-Glaser, 2011; Lyon, 2012):

- Onset of major illnesses (e.g. cancer, cardiovascular conditions)
- Exacerbation of chronic conditions (e.g. diabetes, multiple sclerosis, respiratory disease, inflammatory bowel disease)
- Symptoms (e.g. pain, fatigue, insomnia, headache, gastrointestinal distress)
- Delayed wound healing
- Depression.

Theories about coping

Theories about age-related differences in coping address the following types of internal mechanisms that people use to deal with stressful situations: seeking information; reframing the situation; maintaining a hopeful outlook; using stress-reduction techniques; channelling energy into physical activity; creating fantasies about various outcomes; finding reassurance and emotional support; identifying limited and realistic goals; identifying a positive purpose for the event; getting involved in other activities, such as work and family; and expressing oneself creatively, for example, through music, art or writing. These coping styles are categorised as *problem focused* (i.e. directed towards altering the source of stress) or *emotion focused* (i.e. directed towards regulating one's response). Studies indicate that older adults are more likely to use coping mechanisms that involve management of thoughts and feelings, whereas younger adults are likely to take direct approaches to modify the events or challenging situations in their lives (Brennan, Holland, Schutte et al., 2012; Mather, 2012). For example, a coping mechanism that promotes successful ageing is the ability of older adults to compensate for a diminished sense of control by adjusting their personal expectations (Hayward & Krause, 2013a).

In recent years, gerontologists have focused on both the meaning of the event to the individual and the coping resources available to the individual. Studies consistently identify strong social supports, especially religious supports, as a way of facilitating coping in older adults (George, 2011; Underwood, 2012). Social resources include instrumental support (e.g. meals, transportation, personal care), informational support (e.g. information about resources and services), and emotional support (e.g. communication that provides comfort, companionship, and other evidence that the person is loved, valued, esteemed and cared for).

Relevance for nurses

Nurses can use theories about stress and coping to identify interventions that help older adults maintain optimal functioning and quality of life when faced with the many challenges of ageing. A recent nursing study identified strategies used by older adults with chronic comorbid conditions to remain at home safely with optimal health and psychosocial well-being (Westra, Paitich, Ekstrom et al., 2013). The study identified two major themes related to coping with functional limitations: getting around at home and expanding life beyond self and home. Figure 12-2 provides an overview of strategies used by older adults for "getting on with living life". Many of the significant stresses, such as decreasing eyesight and hearing, can be addressed through nursing interventions to improve functional abilities, as discussed in all chapters of Part 4 in this text. Other significant stresses, such as losses of or changes in relationships, can be addressed through the psychosocial interventions discussed in the section on nursing interventions in this chapter.

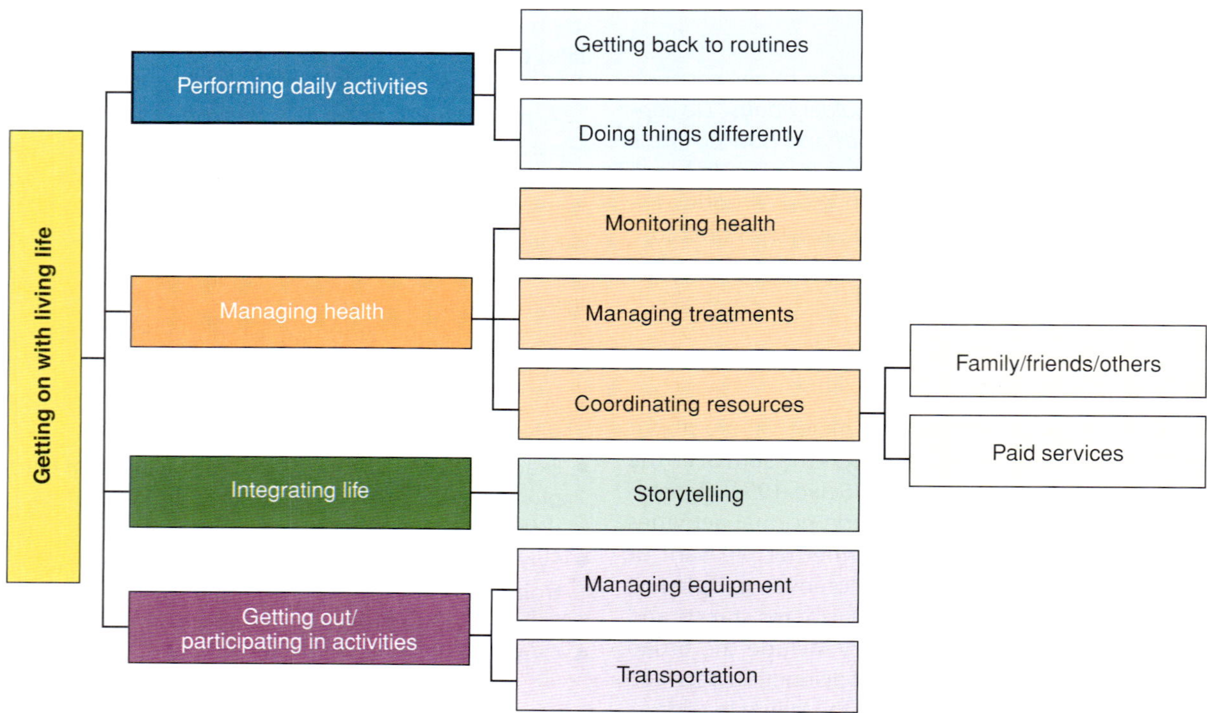

FIGURE 12-2 Strategies used by older adults to get on with living life. (Adapted with permission from Westra, B. L., Paitich, N., Ekstrom, D. et al. [2013]. Getting on with living life: Experiences of older adults after home care. *Home Healthcare Nurse, 31*[9], 493–501.)

FACTORS THAT INFLUENCE PSYCHOSOCIAL FUNCTION IN OLDER ADULTS

Psychosocial function is influenced by numerous factors, including personality, experiences, physical and emotional health, and socioeconomic and environmental conditions. Because many of the factors are beyond the usual scope of nursing, this section focuses on two aspects that are particularly pertinent to usual nursing care of older adults: religion and spirituality, and cultural considerations. Additional information about these topics is addressed in Chapter 13's section on assessing religion and spirituality, and Chapter 2, addressing diversity of older adults.

Religion and spirituality

Religion and spirituality are widely recognised as major coping resources that have a positive effect on many aspects of psychosocial function for older adults. Religion and spirituality are closely related but distinct concepts. Religion and religiosity, which have a strong social component, refer to an organised system of beliefs and behaviours that are shared by a group of people who are associated with a defined faith community. Examples of religious practices are rituals, prayers, meditation, worship services, attendance at church and adherence to certain dietary practices and styles of clothing. One of the intentions of religion is to nurture spiritual development; however, spirituality is broader and less structured and does not necessarily include membership in a formal religious group.

A student's perspective

When I interviewed one of the residents, I felt like I got a really good impression of the things he valued most and the exciting experiences in his life. I think the most significant part for me was when we talked about religion. When I asked him if he was religious, he answered very politely saying that his parents tried to raise him Catholic but that it was never really him. I then asked if he saw himself as spiritual and he said that he is very spiritual and that he definitely thinks there is something "more" after death.

Erika B.

Florence Nightingale viewed spirituality as intrinsic to human nature and emphasised that it was an individual's deepest and the most potent resource for healing. Definitions of spirituality generally include the following concepts: healing; wholeness; social justice; personal growth; interpersonal relationships; a sense of meaning and purpose to life; a transcendent relationship with a higher being; an association with reverence, mystery and inspiration; connectedness with nature, other people and the universe; and feelings of and behaviours arising from love, faith, hope, trust and forgiveness.

Current nursing references (for example, Burkhardt & Nagai-Jacobson, 2013, and Hendman, 2012) describe the following components of **spirituality**:

- Connectedness to self: joy, love, surrender, serenity, self-forgiveness, and meaning and purpose in life
- Connectedness with others: service, compassion, loving sexuality, forgiveness of others, shared genuine presence, meaningful interactions with significant others, and reciprocal giving and receiving
- Connectedness with a power greater than self: awe, prayer, ritual, reverence, meditation, reconciliation and mystical experiences
- Engagement in creative activities: art, music, nature, poetry, writing, singing and spiritual literature.

Gerontologists describe these "everyday spiritual experiences" as effective coping resources that enhance well-being for older adults (Whitehead & Bergeman, 2011). Gerontologists also emphasise the importance of religious beliefs and spirituality in helping older adults make sense of challenges inherent in ageing (Harris, Allen, Dunn et al., 2013; Manning, Leek, Radina, 2012).

WELLNESS OPPORTUNITY

Nurses promote wellness by asking older adults about relationships that provide meaning in their lives.

Cultural considerations

Cultural considerations are important for addressing many aspects of function, but they are especially important in relation to psychosocial function because a person's cultural background significantly influences the way a person defines and perceives all aspects of psychosocial function. In assessing psychosocial function in older adults, for example, it is essential to recognise that every society has standards of "normal" or "abnormal" behaviours and these standards provide guidelines for determining whether behaviours are healthy or unhealthy. However, many societies do not have the rigid distinctions between health and illness that are part of Western cultures, and concepts such as mental health have little meaning in many non-Western societies (Kavanagh, 2008). Cultural perceptions determine all of the following aspects of psychosocial function:

- Definition of mental health and mental illness
- Belief about the causes of mental health and illness
- Expression of symptoms or clinical manifestations of mental health and illness
- Criteria for labelling or diagnosing someone as mentally ill
- Decisions concerning appropriate healer(s)
- Choice of treatment(s) to cure mental illness
- Determination that mental health has been restored after an illness episode
- Relative degree of tolerance for abnormal behaviour by other members of society

CULTURAL CONSIDERATIONS 12-1
Cultural influences on psychosocial function

Cultural influences on beliefs about the cause of mental disorders

- In traditional Chinese culture, many diseases are attributed to an imbalance of yin and yang.
- Indigenous Australians, Pacific people and Māori view well-being from a holistic perspective. They may say they are unwell but not express specific symptoms. Mental health illness is often attributed to external forces or reasons (Vickery & Westerman, 2004; Māori Health, 2012; Medical Council of New Zealand, 2010).

Cultural influences on the manifestations of mental illness

- Cultural norms determine whether behaviours such as any of the following are viewed as either normal or abnormal: dreams, fainting, visions, trances, sorcery, delusions, hallucinations, intoxication, suicide, speaking in tongues, communicating with spirits, and the use of certain substances (e.g. alcohol, tobacco, peyote, marijuana and other drugs).
- Post-traumatic stress disorders are relatively common in immigrants and refugees.
- Filipino consider forgetfulness and anger to be mental health problems.
- Chinese and other groups are likely to express psychological distress through physical symptoms.
- Although psychotic disorders (i.e. loss of contact with reality) occur in every society and are characterised by similar primary symptoms (e.g. insomnia, delusions, hallucinations, flat affect and social or emotional withdrawal), the secondary features are highly influenced by cultural factors.
- In some groups, guilt and suicidal ideation do not accompany depression. For some peoples, suicide is an acceptable escape from problems.

Cultural influences on stress and coping

- Cultural factors often create barriers to the use of formal support services by ethnic elders, and these barriers may increase the feelings of burden experienced by carers.
- In Chinese families, cultural ideals promoting filial piety, family interdependence, veneration of elderly family members and acceptance of family caregiving roles may affect the way families experience and cope with stress related to their roles as carers.

Source: Andrews, M. M. & Boyle, J. S. (2011). *Transcultural concepts in nursing care.* Philadelphia, PA: Wolters Kluwer/Lippincott Williams & Wilkins.

Cultural considerations 12-1 identifies some of the cultural influences on psychosocial function and is particularly applicable to nursing care of older adults.

In some instances, people from diverse cultures may perceive or interpret physical symptoms and their related psychological or emotional components in a manner that is unfamiliar to professionals who do not share the same cultural background. This is likely to occur for **culture-bound syndromes**, which are specific manifestations that are unique to a particular cultural group (Ehrmin, 2012). In recent decades more than 200 culture-bound syndromes have been identified, and many of these are listed in official diagnostic manuals, which are periodically updated. Examples of culture-bound syndromes that nurses may encounter when caring for older adults include:

- *Dhat, Jiryan,* in people from India: dizziness, fatigue, weakness, loss of appetite, sexual dysfunction and feeling of guilt
- *Nervios,* in Latino people: irritability, tearfulness, sleep disturbances, difficulty concentrating, and feeling of vulnerability and emotional distress to stressful life experiences
- *Shenjing,* in Chinese people: depression, anxiety, dizziness, headaches, and sleep and gastrointestinal disturbances.

Professionals and folk or Indigenous healers with the same cultural background usually are knowledgeable about interventions for culture-bound syndromes. Older adults may be reluctant to discuss culture-bound syndromes or folk treatments with healthcare professionals, especially if the care provider has a different cultural background. The reasons for withholding such information are complex and may include fears that the nurse or other healthcare provider will disapprove, ridicule or fail to understand their folk or Indigenous healing system. Because of these factors, nurses may consider asking the person's permission to include folk or Indigenous healers in discussions about health-related issues. These healers frequently have considerable insight into the cultural and psychosocial aspects of human behaviour, and they may be remarkably successful in treating culture-bound syndromes and other disorders that have psychological and emotional components. Because herbal remedies that are sometimes used to treat culture-bound syndromes may interact with prescription or over-the-counter medications, nurses need to make every effort to elicit information about such remedies as part of an assessment (see Chapter 8).

CASE STUDY ONE

Mrs Malaquin is a 79-year-old native of the Philippines. She moved to Brisbane to be near her four children. She had lived in the same town in the Philippines for her entire adult life and had stayed there to care for her husband and her sister, who both required care for chronic conditions. Although she was a much-needed and highly esteemed member of her household in the Philippines, Mrs Malaquin, similar to many other immigrants, experienced role reversal when she lost her once-dominant position in the family and became financially dependent on her adult children after her relocation.

Similar to many older immigrants from the Philippines, Mrs Malaquin had a more active social network before her relocation. She, similar to many of her peers, spoke a dialect and did not speak Tagalog, the language spoken by many younger residents of the Philippines. After her relocation to Australia, her communication and interaction with others became restricted to her extended family because she did not feel confident using her limited English and could not find other speakers of her dialect. To buffer the disequilibrium she felt as a result of her migration, Mrs Malaquin sought comfort through prayer and regular attendance at the local Roman Catholic Church. She also began to regularly care for her two daughters' children.

You are the nurse at the local hospital who treated Mrs Malaquin in the emergency department after she fractured her wrist. During your assessment, you noted that Mrs Malaquin's injury would place a strain on the family because they would temporarily be without their child care provider.

Thinking points

- How would you involve the family members in the discharge plan for Mrs Malaquin so that her recovery could be ensured, she would not lose respect, and she would not feel responsible to assume her usual duties until her injury healed and she felt better?
- What problems would you anticipate with communicating with Mrs Malaquin in the emergency department? How would you handle these problems?
- What psychosocial repercussions did Mrs Malaquin's move to Australia have? Did she cope with these effectively? Would you have had any other suggestions for helping her to cope?
- How did Mrs Malaquin's culture influence her coping mechanisms?

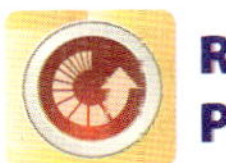

RISK FACTORS THAT AFFECT PSYCHOSOCIAL FUNCTION

Theories about stress and coping and research about causes of impaired mental health in older adults provide information about risks that can affect psychosocial function. The following factors contribute to high levels of stress and poor coping in older adults:

- Poor physical health
- Impaired functional abilities
- Weak social supports
- Lack of economic resources
- Immature developmental level
- Narrow range of coping skills
- Occurrence of unanticipated events
- Occurrence of several daily hassles at the same time
- Occurrence of several major life events in a short duration
- High social status and feelings of high self-efficacy in situations that cannot be changed or in which control cannot be exerted over the environment.

In addition, because the ability to determine the potential for change influences one's response to a stressful situation, people who cannot realistically appraise a situation may have more difficulty coping effectively. This is particularly pertinent with regard to health and functioning because ageist attitudes and stereotypes may contribute to the false belief that health changes and functional decline are inevitable consequences of ageing. Thus, nurses have important roles in teaching older adults about risk factors and potential interventions for health problems. For example, older adults who experience urinary incontinence or difficulties with sexual function may consider these changes to be inevitable consequences of age. On the basis of this appraisal, they are likely to use passive, emotion-focused coping mechanisms, trying simply to accept the situation. In addition, they are more likely to experience an unnecessary and unfortunate functional impairment and a diminished quality of life. By contrast, if the situation is appraised more accurately as a potentially treatable condition, more active and problem-focused coping mechanisms are likely to be used. Even when older adults accurately appraise health problems as changeable, they must identify healthcare professionals who understand the problem and who will attempt to find solutions. Thus, both older adults and healthcare professionals must accurately appraise the situation so they can initiate interventions and achieve wellness outcomes.

Older adults who normally have a sense of high self-efficacy may be particularly susceptible to disturbed self-esteem and feelings of powerlessness when they are in situations where they have little control over their environment. For example, studies have found that a sense of control over important aspects of one's life has positive effects on health and longevity, including improved general well-being and less depression (Angel, Angel & Hill, 2009; Jang, Chiriboga, Lee & Cho, 2009).

Learned helplessness is the experience of uncontrollable events that leads to expectations that future events will also be uncontrollable. Thus, actions that increase dependency or disempower older adults (e.g. providing assistance because this is more time-efficient rather than allowing the older person to function independently or with only a little assistance) are risk factors for diminished self-esteem and feelings of powerlessness. In addition, learned helplessness may contribute to depression, as discussed in Chapter 15.

WELLNESS OPPORTUNITY

Nurses promote wellness by allowing older adults to function as independently as possible and providing the supports they need, even if this is not as time-efficient as doing things for them.

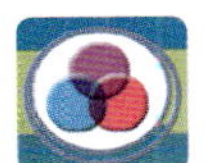

FUNCTIONAL CONSEQUENCES ASSOCIATED WITH PSYCHOSOCIAL FUNCTION IN OLDER ADULTS

Although negative functional consequences are commonly associated with psychosocial function in older adults, positive functional consequences also occur in older adults. This section reviews anxiety and loneliness as two negative functional consequences that nurses can address. In addition, cognitive impairment and depression are serious negative functional consequences that are discussed in Chapters 14 and 15, respectively. Resilience in later life, which is a topic that currently is receiving much attention in gerontological literature, is discussed in this section as a positive functional consequence.

Anxiety is a feeling of distress, subjectively experienced as fear or worry, and objectively expressed through autonomic and central nervous system responses. Prevalence of clinically significant anxiety symptoms in community-living older adults ranges from 15% to 52% (Yochim, Mueller, June et al., 2011). Mild and moderate anxiety can be beneficial because it motivates protective behaviours, but excessive anxiety is detrimental because it channels personal energy into defensive behaviours. Currently increasing attention is being paid to **late-life anxiety disorder**, a persistent condition of excessive anxiety characterised by uncontrollable worry that interferes with daily life and leads to serious physical and mental discomfort (Blay & Marinho, 2012). Serious consequences of anxiety disorders in older adults include sleep disturbances, diminished quality of life, and increased morbidity (Brenes, Miller, Williamson et al., 2012; Shrestha, Robertson & Stanley, 2011). Anxiety disorders are common in older adults and are often unrecognised and untreated (Lenze & Wetherell, 2011; Schuurmans & van Balkom, 2011). Information about nursing assessment of anxiety is discussed in Chapter 13. An important role for nurses is to facilitate referrals for professional interventions such as medications or cognitive behavioural therapy for older adults with anxiety disorders.

Older adults frequently experience feelings of loneliness, with studies consistently finding a 40% prevalence rate (Bekhet & Zauszniewski, 2012). **Loneliness** is defined as a feeling of emptiness or a lack of satisfying human relationships that is not alleviated by being around other people. Older adults are particularly vulnerable to experiencing loneliness because of the many losses associated with ageing, including loss of health, spouse, friends and social status (Smith, 2012; Stessman, Rottenberg, Shimshilashvili et al., 2013). In addition to widowhood, life events of older adulthood that increase the risk for loneliness include retirement, death of friends, relocation to new environments, and health-related problems (e.g. serious illness, significant vision or hearing impairment). Reviews of studies have disclosed that loneliness increases the risk for all the following: pain, anxiety, depression, cognitive decline, functional decline, impaired sleep, poor physical health and increased mortality (Park, Jang, Lee et al., 2013; Rote, Hill & Ellison, 2012; Smith, 2012).

Resilience

During the early 2000s, gerontologists began studying the concept of **resilience** in older adults, and currently this topic is of great interest in relation to psychosocial wellness. Resilient older adults can be described as "Despite various adversities they've faced throughout their lives, certain people inspire us by their gift of keeping positive and open as the years advance: still learning and contributing—still growing old and not just getting old" (Randall, 2013, p. 9).

A recent systematic review of 42 articles concluded that resilience in older adults is defined as the ability to bounce back and recover physical and psychological health in the face of adversity (van Kessel, 2013). Two key constructs identified in this review are (1) adversity, which is related to ongoing life experiences (e.g. ageing, poor health) rather than distinct events; and (2) ability, which included internal and external factors. Essential components of resilience include acceptance, meaningfulness, spirituality, caring for self, and social support and connectedness (van Kessel, 2013).

In addition to viewing resilience as a process of coping with adversity, resilience is discussed in the broader context of learning, growing and being positively transformed by adversity (Manning, 2013). As such, it is viewed as an outcome of increasing wisdom that is possible during later life. Examples of resilience of older adults in response to chronic illness include their ability to use coping mechanisms such as humour, acceptance, mindfulness, positive reframing, intellectual curiosity, and the realistic identification of the positive aspects in situations (Rybarczyk, Emery, Guequierre et al., 2012). Resilience also is closely linked to spirituality, a sense of hopefulness, and finding meaning in life and losses (Ramsey, 2012). These concepts are pertinent to caring for older adults because nurses have many opportunities to support resilience through the interventions for promoting psychosocial wellness discussed in this chapter.

NURSING ISSUES

The nursing issues of self-esteem disturbance, or the development of a negative perception of self-worth in response to the current situation (or risk of), are applicable in relation to some of the psychosocial adjustment issues of older adulthood. Related factors might be the internalisation of ageist attitudes, the loss of roles or financial security, the need for a change to a more dependent living arrangement and chronic illnesses that affect one's abilities and role identities.

If the nursing assessment identifies threats to the older person's sense of control, an appropriate nursing issue would be being powerless (or risk of). Common related factors for older adults are forced retirement, loss of the ability to drive a vehicle, lack of involvement in decision making, chronic conditions that cause progressive functional declines (e.g. dementia), and institutional constraints, such as lack of privacy and the need to follow schedules that do not meet the needs of the individual.

An issue of impaired social interaction may also apply. For example, this issue would be applicable when nurses make referrals for community resources to improve social supports for older adults.

Another nursing issue that might be applied to the psychosocial needs of older adults is ineffective coping. Other nursing issues that might be applicable with regard to specific aspects of psychosocial function include relocation stress syndrome (or risk for), anxiety, grieving, chronic sorrow and stress overload.

Nurses can use any of the following issues to address spiritual needs of older adults: spiritual distress (or risk for) or impaired religiosity (or risk for). In addition, nurses can use willingness for enhanced spiritual well-being when they are addressing older adults' sense of meaning and purpose.

WELLNESS OPPORTUNITY

Willingness for enhanced coping and for enhanced resilience are issues that focus on wellness that are applicable for many older adults who are experiencing psychosocial stress.

GOAL PLANNING FOR WELLNESS OUTCOMES

Goals that produce wellness outcomes related to psychosocial function focus on stress reduction, enhanced coping skills and improved quality of life. When planning wellness outcomes pertinent to low self-esteem due to a current situation (or risk for) or readiness for an enhanced self-concept, the following goals may be applicable: psychosocial adjustment to life change; adaptation to physical disability; improved body image and self-esteem; grief resolution; improved personal autonomy; reduced depression level; and improved quality of life.

Goals for older adults who experience being powerless include hope, improved personal autonomy and participation in healthcare decisions. Goals related to the nursing issue of social isolation include reduction in loneliness and improved social support, social involvement, leisure participation and personal well-being.

When nurses plan care for older adults with nursing issues of impaired adjustment, ineffective coping or readiness for enhanced coping, the following goals may apply: psychosocial adjustment to life change; acceptance of health status; adaptation to physical disability; and improved coping; decision making; knowledge about health resources; personal well-being; and reduced stress level.

WELLNESS OPPORTUNITY

Hope and quality of life may be applicable outcomes when nurses direct care towards improving psychosocial wellness.

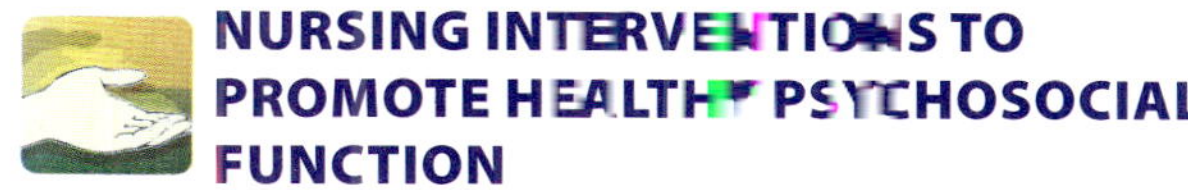

NURSING INTERVENTIONS TO PROMOTE HEALTHY PSYCHOSOCIAL FUNCTION

Nurses have many opportunities to promote healthy psychosocial function during the usual course of caring for older adults. For example, they can incorporate communication techniques and other interventions to enhance self-esteem, promote a sense of control and address spiritual needs. They also can use **life review** and **reminiscence** interventions, especially in home and long-term residential care settings. In addition to incorporating interventions in usual care, nurses promote psychosocial wellness by facilitating referrals for social supports. In some settings, nurses can implement group interventions such as healthy ageing classes, to help older adults cope effectively with the life events of older adulthood.

Nursing interventions which promote healthy psychosocial function would focus on: anxiety reduction; carer support; coping enhancement; decision-making support; emotional support; grief support; hope instillation; spiritual support; reminiscence therapy; resiliency promotion; role enhancement; self-esteem enhancement; socialisation enhancement; and facilitation of spiritual growth.

In addition to the interventions reviewed in this chapter, interventions that improve functional abilities promote psychosocial wellness because of the close relationship between physiological and psychosocial aspects of health and function. Thus, interventions to improve functional abilities, which are discussed throughout this text, also promote psychosocial wellness. In addition to having physical benefits, participation in physical activity is beneficial for many aspects of psychosocial function, such as alleviation of anxiety and depression.

A national longitudinal study of older adults concluded that physical activity interventions focused on improving mastery and fitness may have the greatest benefit in alleviating psychological distress (Cairney, Faulkner, Veldhuizen & Wade, 2009). Other studies indicate that tai chi, qigong and other meditative movement forms are especially beneficial for older adults (Rogers, Larkey & Keller, 2009).

Enhancing self-esteem

Self-esteem enhancement is an essential component of nursing care for older adults because self-esteem is an important coping resource and a factor that influences well-being. Self-esteem refers to the feelings one has about one's self. It is the emotional component of self-concept and is based on ones perceptions of other people's opinions about oneself. Good self-esteem is a characteristic that is associated with being happier, healthier, less anxious, more independent, more self-confident and more effective in meeting environmental demands than people with low self-esteem. Chapter 13 includes information on assessing self-esteem, whereas this chapter

(12) focuses on nursing interventions that enhance self-esteem, with emphasis on addressing factors that threaten it (e.g. dependence, devaluation, depersonalisation and powerlessness).

Many factors that are threats to self-esteem are associated with staff and environments of institutional settings and can be addressed through relatively simple nursing interventions. This is particularly important in environments such as long-term residential care settings where the care environment affects virtually every aspect of daily life for the residents. For instance, when older adults are admitted to institutional settings, nurses may be able to identify environmental or other factors that can quickly and easily be modified to promote a sense of control and minimise or eliminate a threat to self-esteem, as in the following examples:

- Ensuring easy access to their usual assistive devices (walkers, eyeglasses, hearing aids)
- Providing as much privacy as possible
- Asking about food preferences and ensuring as much choice as possible
- Asking open-ended questions, such as, "Is there anything that we can do to help you manage better while you're here?"
- Asking, "Is there anything you're worried about that I can help you with?"
- Ensuring that staff members address people by their preferred names
- Involving older adults as much as possible in decisions that affect them.

Threats to self-esteem also arise when carers promote unnecessary dependence for their own convenience. For example, using incontinence products and telling a bed-ridden person to wet the bed because it is easier to change the disposable pad or brief than to assist with toileting is a tremendous blow to the person's self-esteem. Thus, interventions that improve independent function, which are discussed throughout this text, are important for enhancing self-esteem.

Because self-esteem depends to some extent on the perceived appraisal of significant others, nurses can use communication interventions to increase the older adult's perception of self-worth. Nurses must be aware of their ageist attitudes and avoid reflecting these attitudes in verbal statements. For example, even a remark such as "You certainly look good for 85 years old", although said with good intentions, can reinforce ageist attitudes. Hidden messages in this statement may be that it is better to look younger and that, when you are old, you generally do not look good. Nurses can address ageism by avoiding even subtle messages that communicate negative attitudes. For instance, a statement, such as the following, might enhance an older person's self-esteem and challenge ageist attitudes: "At 85 years old, you must have a lot of wisdom. Can you share a bit of that wisdom with me?" Non-verbal communication may influence the person's perception of self-worth even more than verbal communication. For example, if a nurse walks past an older person sitting in a hallway without acknowledging his or her presence, this may be perceived as an indicator that the nurse does not value the older person. Even though the nurse may have been attending to responsibilities and had not intended to communicate a negative message, this action may adversely affect that older person's self-esteem. Thus, nurses must keep in mind that the perception of their actions is often more important than their intent and they must use verbal and non-verbal messages to communicate feelings of positive regard whenever possible.

For dependent older adults, the negative impact of disability and functional impairments on self-esteem is heightened by behaviours of others that convey attitudes of **infantilisation** (i.e. treating an adult in a way that is similar to the way infants are treated). For example, such remarks as "He acts just like a baby" or "Now, now, dear, let's be a good girl", convey infantilisation. Residents of nursing homes and assisted-living facilities view this kind of communication as being looked down upon by staff (Williams & Warren, 2009). The term **elderspeak**—also called "baby talk"—describes speech that is modified when addressed to older adults, usually by younger adults. Elderspeak is characterised by slowed speech, shortened sentences, elevated pitch and volume, simplistic vocabulary and grammar and inappropriately intimate terms of endearment (Williams et al., 2009). This type of communication is demeaning and patronising and it can have serious negative consequences. Researchers have found that elderspeak communication by nursing home staff caring for people with dementia was associated with increased resistance to care and with negative vocalisations (e.g. crying, screaming, yelling) (Herman & Williams, 2009; Williams et al., 2009). Moreover, it can reflect ageist attitudes or negative and inaccurate stereotypes. Thus, nurses need to monitor their communication with older adults to ensure that they avoid inappropriate terminology and elderspeak. Box 12-1 summarises nursing interventions for enhancing self-esteem in older adults.

WELLNESS OPPORTUNITY

Nurses can enhance self-esteem by pointing out an older adult's positive qualities during routine care activities.

Promoting a sense of control

Perceived control is a factor that significantly affects psychosocial wellness because higher levels of perceived mastery are associated with enhanced levels of well-being, alleviation of depression and increased participation in health promotion (Jang et al., 2009). Thus, nurses address psychosocial needs of older adults with interventions that promote a sense of control and that involve older adults in decisions. Nursing interventions to promote a sense of

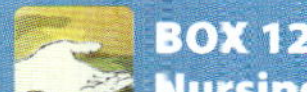

BOX 12-1
Nursing interventions to promote self-esteem

Communication techniques

- Acknowledge a person by using their preferred names and titles.
- When talking with older people, use the same tone of voice you use for your colleagues.
- Provide positive feedback for individual accomplishments, even in daily self-care tasks that require effort.
- Focus conversations on persons' strengths and positive attributes rather than on their limitations. (For example, for people who have physical impairments, focus on their non-physical attributes, such as personality characteristics or interpersonal relationships.)
- When negative functional consequences are attributed to old age, offer an alternative explanation and identify a contributing factor that is amenable to change. (For example, when older people attribute weakness 'simply' to being old, remind them they are recovering from hip surgery and should expect to improve with therapy.)
- Be cautious about communicating ageist attitudes, even inadvertently, in conversations.

Verbal communication to observe for and avoid

- Do not use names or phrases that reflect ageist attitudes (e.g. "little old lady", "dirty old man"), even in jest.
- Do not raise your voice except when necessary to facilitate communication with someone who has impaired hearing.
- Do not use terms that are associated with babies (e.g. *nappies*, *baby food*).
- Do not use *we* or *us* unless the term is accurate. (For example, do not say "Let's take our medicine now.")
- Do not use the term *senile*.

Non-verbal communication techniques and additional nursing actions

- When labelling clothing, put the person's name in an inconspicuous place.
- Use actions consciously to communicate positive regard (e.g. recognise the presence of someone as you walk past).

control for older adults include involving them as much as possible in organising their schedule and providing information about their plan of care.

Many studies have confirmed the importance of modifying the way people perceive and explain events, shifting attention to factors that can be changed or controlled. In the classic study by Rodin and Langer (1980), whenever a nursing home resident attributed a problem to being old, the staff provided another explanation and identified a causative factor that was amenable to change. For instance, when residents attributed feelings of fatigue to being old, they were reminded that they were awakened at 5:30 a.m. (Rodin & Langer, 1980). Nurses can listen for opportunities to challenge older adults' perceptions that promote a sense of hopelessness and rephrase the situation in a context that is empowering. For example, they can help older adults develop problem-focused coping mechanisms rather than passively and sometimes inaccurately, accepting the negative functional consequences of ageing.

Nursing interventions also address factors that can threaten perceived control, such as lack of privacy and loss of individuality, which commonly occur in institutional settings. Nurses can show respect for privacy by knocking on bedroom doors and asking permission before entering, by closing doors when privacy is desired, by asking permission before pulling bed curtains open and by being careful about moving personal belongings without permission from the older person. Encouraging the person to have personal belongings and to arrange these belongings in whatever fashion is desired also shows concern for individuality.

WELLNESS OPPORTUNITY

Nurses show concern for individuality by asking an older adult about a family photograph or greeting card that is in view.

Involving older adults in decision making

Older people are frequently left out of the decision-making process, even for those decisions that most profoundly affect their lives, such as moving to a long-term residential care facility. This lack of involvement occurs for a variety of reasons, related both to the older adult and to the decision makers. Some of the barriers within the older adult may be dementia, depression, long-term passivity regarding decisions, hearing impairments or other communication barriers. Some of the barriers within the decision makers that may thwart the decision-making process include stereotypes of older people as incompetent, perceptions that the older adult is not interested in or capable of making decisions and an unwillingness to deal with the older person's anticipated resistance to the desired outcome.

Many of the reasons for excluding older adults from the decision-making process are related to the attitudes of the family and of professional carers, so one nursing intervention is to challenge these attitudes. For example, in acute care settings, nurses can facilitate communication between older adults and their primary care provider to ensure that the older person is included in decisions about medical treatment and discharge plans. In long-term residential care settings, nurses have numerous opportunities to involve older adults in decisions about their daily care, medical interventions and discharge plans. In home settings, nurses can work with family members and older adults to ensure that the latter are involved in decisions about their care and that their rights are respected. In any setting, nurses may have to remind healthcare professionals, as well as family members and other carers, that although people may gain rights by virtue of being a certain age, they do not lose their rights just because they reach a certain age. For additional discussion of a nurse's role in decisions regarding long-term care for people with dementia, refer to Chapter 9.

Other aspects of decision making that can be addressed in nursing interventions are one's verbal interactions and choice of terminology. With regard to verbal communication, healthcare professionals often talk *about* older adults when in their presence rather than directing communication *to* them and focusing the conversation *on* them. This is especially common when family members or other carers are discussing situations with a nurse or other professional and the conversation takes place in the presence of the older person without directly involving him or her. In working with older adults, nurses need to pay particular attention to including older adults in conversations when the topic is directly related to them. When it is not appropriate to include the older adult in the conversation, the nurse can take steps to facilitate the conversation outside the presence of the older person. In these situations, the nurse can ask the older person's permission to discuss his or her situation with family member or carers and then report back to the older person, in language that the person can understand, about any discussions that take place or decisions that are made or pending.

With regard to terminology, the word "placement" is often used in reference to an older adult's admission to a nursing home. This term denotes passivity on the part of the older adult; it is closer to the terminology used when objects are placed on a shelf than to words normally used in reference to human beings. Nurses would communicate more positive feelings and a greater sense of control if they referred to an "admission" to a nursing home. The term admission suggests that certain criteria have been met and that an active decision has been made to determine whether the person meets these criteria. Even more important than using the correct terms, nurses must ensure that older adults are, in fact, actively involved in the decision-making process, rather than passively being "placed". Nurses can help older adults and their families with decisions about long-term residential care by helping them to assess their situation, by correcting misinformation, and by providing accurate information about the range of services and specific resources available (as described in Chapter 6).

Addressing role loss

Meaningful roles (e.g. spouse, carer, volunteer) are important determinants of feelings of worth, efficacy and self-esteem. Although role loss is a common occurrence in later adulthood, studies indicate that the development of new roles is an effective coping strategy for older adults (George, 2006). Participating in volunteer work is an excellent way of providing social interaction and a sense of purpose.

Volunteer work that extends work-related roles is particularly rewarding and psychologically uplifting because it provides new fulfilment, life meaning and life direction (Cook, 2013). Research reviews have identified the following positive health effects associated with volunteering: improved functioning, longer life expectancy, increased social interaction, reduced pain and depression, and increased life satisfaction and self-rated health (Jenkinson, Dickens, Jones et al., 2013; Li, Chen & Chen, 2013; Okun, Yeung & Brown, 2013).

Besides helping older adults develop new roles, nurses can focus on past and current achievements as an intervention for enhancing self-esteem, especially for older adults who must depend on others and have difficulty feeling a sense of accomplishment or even a sense of basic usefulness. Nurses implement this intervention, which may be especially helpful for older adults who have difficulty identifying meaningful roles, in a group setting or on an individual basis.

WELLNESS OPPORTUNITY

Nurses can ask older adults about their accomplishments in such areas as work and family, and give positive feedback about meaningful roles.

Encouraging life review and reminiscence

Life review and reminiscence are two closely related processes that are used to promote psychosocial health in older adults. Butler (2001) describes life review as a progressive return to consciousness of past experiences, particularly unresolved conflicts, for re-examination and reintegration. If the reintegration process is successful, the process gives new significance and meaning to life and prepares the person for death by alleviating fear and anxiety (Butler, 2001). Positive effects of life review include accepting one's mortality, righting of old wrongs, taking pride in accomplishments, gaining a sense of serenity and feeling that one has done one's best (Butler, 2001). Participants in a nursing study of life review in home settings reported that the intervention helped them integrate their lived experiences and was meaningful, pleasurable and healing (Binder et al., 2009).

Reminiscence is based on the same theoretical framework as life review; however, it can be done outside the life review process and it is more informal and less intense. Another difference is that life review addresses both pleasant and unpleasant issues of the past, whereas reminiscence focuses primarily on only pleasant and positive experiences. Reminiscence therapy as a nursing intervention is the recall of past events, feelings, images and memories that are associated with comfort, pleasure and pleasant experiences. As a group therapy, the reminiscence group is one of the most widely used interventions for older adults and it may be particularly effective for improving self-esteem, reducing social isolation and improving depression and cognitive functioning (Hsu & Wang, 2009; Huang, Li, Yang & Chen, 2009; Perese, Simon & Ryan, 2008).

A student's perspective

Performing a life review on anyone from a time other than your own is an interesting experience. I found it to be an amazing opportunity to sit down with Mrs B. and for her to open up to a 20-year-old girl that she had met only the week before. Within the first few minutes, she talked about her husband and I watched the tears roll down her face. This became the most significant part of our interview because I was able to understand how exposed she was allowing herself to be. It also made me realise how open older people can be when reminiscing about their lives and how important this topic is for them to share. It amazed me how just starting a conversation with an older person could bring so much emotion and joy at the exact same time. The interview with Mrs B. has affected my approach to older adults in clinical practice. I believe that a life review can be done on a daily basis while working with clients. This way, you can get to know each person on a personal level in order to provide individualised care. Each time you see a patient, you could continue the conversation and develop a relationship that benefits not only the client, but also yourself. I have learned that by showing interest in a person's life, you can allow them to discuss a significant part of who they have become, which is something they do not get to do on a daily basis.

Jillian B.

Fostering social supports

Nurses have many opportunities to foster the development of social networks for older adults and this is an appropriate intervention for addressing social isolation. In some situations, particularly in home and long-term residential care settings, nurses are an integral part of the older person's social network. Social isolation is likely to occur because of any of the following factors that commonly occur in older adulthood:

- Hearing impairments and other communication barriers
- Chronic illnesses that limit activity or energy
- A lack of social opportunities because of caregiving responsibilities
- Mobility limitations, including the inability to drive a vehicle
- Mental or psychosocial impairments that interfere with relationships
- Loss of spouse, friends or family through death, illness or physical distance.

Thus, nursing interventions that address these risk factors (e.g. improved mobility or sensory function) are also likely to have the positive consequence of improved social supports.

In long-term residential care settings, nurses can foster positive social interactions in group settings, such as dining and activity rooms. Sometimes, a very simple intervention, such as positioning chairs (including wheelchairs) so that people can interact with each other, can significantly influence social contacts, either positively or negatively. Wherever possible, nurses should arrange room assignments to encourage opportunities for positive social interactions. In addition, nurses can facilitate referrals for social and therapeutic activities in long-term residential care facilities.

In home settings, nurses can identify community resources, such as volunteer friendly-visitor and meal programs, to decrease social isolation. Support and education groups that primarily focus on coping with a chronic illness (e.g. stroke clubs or better breathing groups) also provide excellent opportunities for social contact and the development of friendships with people who are in similar situations. For people who are socially isolated because of their caregiving responsibility, carer support groups can enhance coping abilities and provide social support.

In any setting, nurses can encourage older adults to participate in structured group activities to enhance their well-being. A randomised control trial found that older adults who experienced loneliness showed significant health benefits from participation in weekly psychosocial groups for 3 months (Pitkala et al., 2011). In addition, one nursing study concluded that nurses have key roles in encouraging older women to make social connections because friendships are important in preventing loneliness, even when family members live nearby (Eshbaugh, 2009). Selected nursing interventions to promote psychosocial wellness are described in Box 12-2.

WELLNESS OPPORTUNITY

Nurses can talk with older adults about the benefits of support groups and provide a list of local resources that address the specific needs of older adults and their carers.

Addressing spiritual needs

Addressing spiritual needs of older adults is within the scope of nursing, as exemplified in the following interventions that are commonly included in nursing care:

- Intentionally communicating care and compassion
- Facilitating reminiscence
- Honouring a person's integrity
- Providing active and passive listening
- Making referrals for spiritual care
- Caring for someone who feels hopeless
- Arranging for participation in religious services
- Encouraging or facilitating participation in activities such as prayer and meditation.

Nursing interventions to address the spiritual needs of older adults need to be individualised and offered only if the person is receptive to the interventions. In addition, nurses need to be non-judgemental about religion and spirituality and avoid imposing their personal beliefs. Moreover, because cultural factors significantly influence a person's spirituality and religious beliefs, interventions must be culturally sensitive. Andrews and Hanson (2011) provide an excellent overview of specific cultural influences on religion and spirituality.

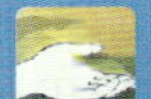

BOX 12-2
Nursing interventions to promote psychosocial wellness

Facilitating maximum independence

- Make sure that the person has access to all necessary assistive devices and personal accessories (e.g. wigs, canes, dentures, walkers and hearing aids).
- Allow enough time for the person to perform tasks at her or his own pace, and avoid unnecessary dependence that results from an overemphasis on time efficiency.
- Make sure that the environment has been adapted as much as possible to compensate for sensory losses and other functional impairments.

Promoting a sense of control

- Make a conscious effort to involve older adults in decisions regarding their care, both in small daily matters and in major healthcare concerns.
- Ask about likes and dislikes and try to address personal preferences.
- Whenever possible, allow people to choose between two alternatives, even if the options are in a very narrow range (e.g. "Would you prefer to wear the yellow jumper or the pink one today?").
- Ensure as much privacy, or perceived privacy, as possible.
- Knock on the door and ask for permission before entering a bedroom, even in institutional settings.
- Allow as much expression of individuality as possible in the personal environment (e.g. use personal furniture when possible and display family pictures in full view).
- Make sure that the call light is accessible for people who are confined.
- Do not talk about someone in his or her presence as if he or she does not exist.
- Avoid referring to nursing home *placement*. Refer instead to an *admission*, and include the person in the decision-making process.

Addressing role loss

- Identify new roles for people and acknowledge those past and present roles that are viewed positively.
- Encourage participation in reminiscence groups and other group therapies.
- Find opportunities to create meaningful roles, such as helper or assistant, by involving older adults in useful tasks, such as folding laundry.
- When older adults volunteer to assist others, acknowledge their contribution with a remark such as, "You certainly help us quite a bit when you take Mrs Smith to the dining room in her wheelchair."
- Acknowledge an older adult's non-physical assets and attributes, such as family relationships or a good sense of humour.
- Focus on positive relationships by acknowledging or asking about the receipt of flowers, greeting cards and other visible signs of concern expressed by others.
- Ask older adults about their responsibilities as parents, grandparents or roommates, and point out their positive contributions.
- Ask older adults about family photographs, initiate a discussion of positive relationships, and remind them that others care about them (e.g. encourage them to talk about their grandchildren and great-grandchildren).
- Ask older adults about accomplishments in such areas as work, family, hobbies and volunteer activities.
- Respond with such comments as "You must be proud of your children", or "You certainly have accomplished a lot."

Fostering social supports

- Use interventions to address hearing impairments and other communication barriers (see Chapter 16).
- Encourage participation in group activities.
- For people in wheelchairs, especially those who cannot move independently, position the chair in a way that promotes social interaction.
- For nursing home residents, plan table and room arrangements in a way that fosters social relationships.

In addition to addressing spiritual needs as a routine part of psychosocial nursing care, nurses often address spiritual needs during times of spiritual distress. For example, older adults are likely to express spiritual needs when they are coping with the loss of a significant relationship or dealing with news about a serious or terminal illness. Older adults who are carers for others, especially a spouse, are likely to express spiritual needs in relation to decisions about the care of the other person. For example, they may experience feelings of guilt about not being able to meet the needs of a dependent loved one or feelings of "playing God" with regard to decisions about cognitively impaired loved ones. In these circumstances, the provision of support, information and reassurance from a nurse who has dealt with these decisions in professional experiences may be an effective counselling intervention. At times, information from the primary care provider may be helpful in alleviating spiritual distress associated with end-of-life decisions or decisions about long-term care. In these cases, the nurse may be able to facilitate communication between the primary care provider and the family to alleviate the spiritual distress. Some nursing interventions that address spiritual needs of older adults are listed in Box 12-3.

Health promotion: Teaching about managing stress in daily life

Nurses have important roles in teaching older adults, as well as carers, about managing stress in daily life as an intervention for promoting psychosocial wellness. Although stress management is often overlooked, it is an essential aspect of health promotion for people of all ages. Nurses can encourage and demonstrate the use of simple relaxation techniques, such as deep breathing, during the usual course of caring for older adults and talking with carers. Nurses also can encourage participation in individual and group activities that are effective for reducing stress, such as yoga, meditation and tai chi. Box 12-4, Tips on managing stress in daily life, can be given to older adults and carers as a teaching tool.

BOX 12-3
Nursing interventions to address spiritual needs

Therapeutic communication interventions

- Use verbal and non-verbal communication to establish trust and convey empathic caring.
- Use active supportive listening.
- Convey non-judgemental attitudes.
- Communicate respect for individuality.
- Provide a supportive presence.
- Be open to expressions of feelings such as fear, anger, loneliness and powerlessness.
- Honour a person's integrity.
- Support the person in his or her feeling of being loved by others and by a higher power (e.g. God, Allah, Jehovah).
- Encourage verbalising feelings about the meaning of illness.
- Provide positive feedback about faith, courage, sense of humour, and other such feelings and experiences.
- Encourage discussion of events and relationships that provide spiritual support.

Actions to foster religious and spiritual activities

- Facilitate referrals for visits from religious care providers and sources of spiritual care (clergy, rabbis, church members, spiritual directors).
- Facilitate participation in religious services or activities (e.g. tapes, readings, videos, observations of "holy days").
- Assist with obtaining requested religious items (books, music, statues).
- Provide quiet and private time for individual spiritual or religious activities (e.g. prayer, reflection, meditation or guided imagery).
- Provide necessary support for religious rituals (e.g. lighting candles, receiving communion, praying the rosary).
- Encourage participation in relaxing and enjoyable activities (art, music, nature).

Interventions for specific circumstances

- Provide support and care during times of suffering.
- Assist in the process of dying.
- Assist a person who is fearful of the future.
- Provide care for the person who feels hopeless.
- Facilitate reconciliation among family members.
- Encourage participation in support groups.

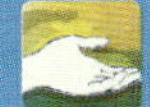

BOX 12-4
Tips on managing stress in daily life

Recognise the different types of stressors

- Events are stressful according to the degree to which they have an emotional impact and are perceived as desirable and controllable.
- Even events that are desirable, such as holidays and births and weddings of grandchildren, can be stressful.
- When stress cannot be alleviated, it is important to manage your perception of, and emotional responses to, the situation.
- Use problem-focused strategies to cope with situations that can be changed.

Coping strategies for situations that cannot be changed

- Develop an attitude of acceptance, reframe your perspective, and focus on what you can learn from this.
- Acknowledge and express feelings, even those that are unpleasant, such as grief, anger and sadness.
- Talk with someone and accept their caring and understanding: communicate to them that you do not expect to change the situation but appreciate an opportunity to express feelings.
- Foster supports for social, emotional and spiritual enrichment (e.g. friends, family, pets, hobbies, groups).
- Identify and use healthy ways of releasing tension and expressing emotions (e.g. physical activity, actions that lead to a sense of accomplishment).
- Engage in distracting activities, especially those that are pleasurable, health enhancing, and spiritually enriching.
- Use relaxation methods such as meditation, yoga, progressive relaxation.
- Express feelings and develop insights through such activities as journaling and self-talk.
- Seek guidance from counsellors or healthcare professionals.

Problem-focused coping strategies

- Time pressures: evaluate demands, determine priorities and plan a schedule for the most important things; include time for activities that relieve stress.
- Set realistic limits and become comfortable telling others what the limits are.
- Seek advice and reliable information from friends, family or professionals who can assist with developing a problem-solving plan.
- Adapt the environment so it is most conducive to your current needs.

Strategies to avoid

- Smoking
- Excessive eating or drinking (including alcohol or caffeine)
- Inappropriate use of medications or recreational drugs
- Inaccurately or inappropriately directing anger or emotions towards others
- Actions that are harmful to people, animals or the environment

Adapted with permission from Miller, C. A. (2013). Wellness activity tool for stress management. In C. A. Miller (Ed.), *Fast facts for health promotion in nursing: Promoting wellness in a nutshell* (pp. 61–63). New York: Springer.

Promoting wellness through healthy ageing classes

When older adults need assistance in coping with specific functional consequences or when they need education to clarify myths and misunderstandings about age-related changes, individual counselling may be the best intervention. When older adults need counselling about psychosocial adjustments, however, educational groups may be more effective. Nurses are often involved with establishing and leading support and educational groups for carers. Common themes that nurses can address in groups include use of resources, coping with losses, and promoting optimal functioning. An example of a nurse-led group intervention that allows for sharing of experiences among peers is the healthy ageing class, developed by Carol A. Miller. This intervention has been used successfully in the U.S. over the last two decades in a variety of settings with older adults who have different functional levels.

In Australia and New Zealand healthy ageing is desired by all stakeholders as both countries are experiencing unprecedented growth in their population of older adults. Healthy ageing supports the health and well-being of older people thus improving quality of life of the older adults and reducing the resources required to support this increased population. Healthy ageing classes conducted by nurses are an effective intervention to support healthy ageing. This model is based on the belief that older adults who are beginning to recognise age-related physical and psychosocial changes or who are already dealing with such changes can benefit from sharing their experiences with their peers. Nurses can use this model to enhance the coping skills of older adults who are adjusting to any of the challenges of older adulthood.

Healthy ageing model: Characteristics

Goals

Goals for older adults who participate in healthy ageing classes are as follows:

- Recognise the impact of common age-related physical and psychosocial changes.
- Support and encourage any of the effective coping mechanisms already being used.
- Develop new skills that could be effective for coping with current stressors.
- Obtain information that will facilitate problem-focused coping mechanisms for stressful situations that are amenable to change.
- Provide an opportunity for the sharing of similar experiences with peers.

Setting

Nurses in any setting can initiate healthy ageing classes, but long-term residential care institutions are perhaps the most conducive setting for the following reasons:

- Nurses have many opportunities to establish and lead groups.
- Residents of long-term residential care facilities:
  - Provide a captive audience from which to select group members
  - Usually are not acutely ill and they are dealing with psychosocial adjustments that are readily identified, and
  - Have in common at least one major life event, which is either a temporary or permanent move to a more dependent setting.

Community settings are also conducive to successful healthy ageing classes, but nurses may have to be more creative in gathering the group members. Nurses who provide health services or education programs for senior centres or assisted-living facilities might be able to establish ongoing healthy ageing classes as part of their responsibilities. In these settings, a healthy ageing class may be an efficient, as well as effective, way of providing health education using a format that has the additional advantage of enhancing coping mechanisms.

In acute care settings, nurses usually do not plan and implement group therapies, but in rehabilitative settings, nurses may have the opportunity to initiate healthy ageing classes.

Membership criteria

The primary criteria for group membership are that the person be willing to acknowledge age-related changes and be capable of acquiring insight into his or her adjustment to these changes. Group members may be coping with similar psychosocial stresses, but this is not necessarily a criterion for participation. For example, a healthy ageing class can comprise older adults who all have some degree of depression or who are coping with a particular stressful event, such as widowhood. An ideal group would include members who are coping with various life events commonly associated with older adulthood and who are motivated to learn effective coping styles.

The group works best if the membership is stable and closed, but this is not always possible. A disadvantage of an open group is that it is very difficult to develop cohesiveness. If the membership is open and changing, the leader must be more directive and the group as a whole will not be able to establish ongoing priorities for discussion topics. In addition, with changing membership, the leader has to focus more attention on the exchange of information about group members at the beginning of each session.

Size of group and length, duration and frequency of sessions

Although group size can range from 5 to 12 members, the ideal is about 8 members. Groups can be either ongoing or time-limited. When the membership is changing, such as in acute or rehabilitative settings, sessions can be an ongoing mode of therapy. In long-term residential care or community settings, it is best to schedule group meetings for a predetermined length of time, such as 8 to 10 weeks, and allow for changes in membership at the end of each period. One-hour sessions are held at weekly intervals, at a consistent time and place. In community settings, it can be helpful to convene the groups in conjunction with a meal program because participants will already have social relationships. As in institutional settings, a community centre offers an audience from which to select group members. Other potential community-based sites include assisted-living facilities and group settings, such as adult care homes (also called board-and-care homes).

Criteria for and responsibilities of group leaders

One nurse can lead group sessions, but it is often helpful to have a co-leader who has had social service training. An older adult who has made a positive psychosocial adjustment and who can serve as a role model also can be a good co-leader. The nurse must be able to clarify myths and misunderstandings about age-related changes and be skilled in group dynamics. As with the reminiscence group, the healthy ageing class is not an inter se psychotherapy session; therefore, the group leader is not required to be specially trained in mental health. To lead a healthy ageing class, however, a good understanding of both the physiological and the psychosocial aspects of ageing is essential.

The primary responsibilities of the group leaders are to facilitate the discussion of psychosocial adjustments of older adulthood and to provide feedback and clarification to the members. As with other groups, the leader must ensure that all members have an opportunity to participate and that the members attend to the identified topic. The leaders must also ensure that the group reaches some conclusions before the end of each session so that members leave with a feeling of accomplishment relating to at least one psychosocial challenge of older adulthood.

Format

As in all educational groups, the leader begins with an explanation of the purpose of the group and an introduction of the leaders and members. The leader also reviews the details of the sessions, such as their length, the duration of the group, the role of the leader and the expectations of the members. After addressing questions and introductory material, the leader introduces the concepts of life events and adjustments to the challenges of older adulthood. The leader can use a statement similar to the following:

> *Throughout life, certain events are likely to occur that affect us emotionally. These events may involve our health, our personal relationships, the place where we live, our job or career responsibilities, and opportunities or other events that require an adjustment on our part. These are called major life events and they often occur at certain points of life. To begin our discussion today, let's look at some of the major life events that are likely to occur in younger adulthood, around the age of 20 to 30 years.*

The group then identifies various life events, such as finding a job, moving from the family home, finding a partner and starting a family. The leader then asks members to identify life adjustments that are likely to occur between 30 and 50 years of age.

After the members have identified these life events, the leader emphasises that one purpose of the healthy ageing class is to identify effective ways of addressing the challenges inherent in the life events of older adulthood. The term "challenges" is used to communicate an active mode of addressing issues. The leader may want to discuss the phrase "challenges of being old" and allow the group members to comment on what they see as challenges in their lives. As the members identify the life events of older adulthood, the leader writes the events on a board or paper so that all the members can see the list. The leader can then ask about life events that the members think they are likely to experience in the next few years. As events are identified, the members are also asked to identify the consequences of the events that require an adjustment. Examples of these life events and consequences have been discussed earlier in this chapter and are summarised in Figure 12-1. If group members do not identify all of the life events, the leader may ask about a certain event, such as coping with one's own or a spouse's retirement. This discussion should continue until all the events and consequences in Figure 12-1 have been identified.

If the group is ongoing and has a stable membership, the leader may devote the majority of the first meeting to this discussion. The leader should emphasise that the rest of the meetings will be devoted to discussions of the identified issues and that the first meeting will set the stage for future sessions. If the group is open and has a changing membership, the leader may need to be more directing during this first phase to limit the time spent on this topic. With changing membership, this initial identification of issues would be limited to the first 20 to 30 minutes. The group can then discuss coping mechanisms for one specific issue during the latter half of the meeting.

After the issues are identified, the leader summarises the discussion, referring to the list of challenges written for the members to see. The members then share ideas about coping strategies that they have found to be helpful in adjusting to these changes. After the members have identified general coping mechanisms, the leader can suggest that the group choose one specific life event of older adulthood and discuss coping mechanisms that are helpful for addressing this challenge. Examples of coping strategies that might be discussed in relation to specific life events are summarised in Table 12-1. As these coping strategies are identified, they should be written on a board and members should be encouraged to relate their personal experiences.

As the cohesiveness and trust level among members increase, particularly in closed groups, the sharing of experiences may become very open and revealing. The task of the leader, then, is to keep the discussion focused on appropriate

TABLE 12-1 Coping strategies for the psychosocial challenges of older adulthood

Psychosocial adjustment	Coping strategy
Ageist stereotypes	Develop a firm self-identity, challenge the myths, question any behaviours that are based on age-determined expectations
Retirement	Develop new skills, use time for hobbies and personal pursuits, become involved with meaningful volunteer activities
Reduced income	Take advantage of discounts for seniors
Declining physical health	Maintain good health practices (nutrition, exercise, rest)
Functional limitations	Adapt the environment to ensure safety and optimal functional status, take advantage of assistive devices and equipment, accept help when necessary
Changes in cognitive skills	Take advantage of educational opportunities, enrol in classes, keep mentally stimulated, join a discussion group, use the library, avoid dwelling on the things you cannot do and focus on your abilities, take advantage of increased potential for wisdom and creativity
Death of spouse, friends and family members	Allow yourself to grieve appropriately, take advantage of opportunities for group or individual counselling and support, establish new relationships, renew old friendships, cherish the happy memories of the past, realise new freedoms
Relocation from family home	Look into the broad range of options for housing, appreciate the relief from the responsibilities of home ownership, take advantage of new services and opportunities for socialisation
Other challenges to mental health	Maintain a sense of humour, use stress-reduction techniques, learn assertiveness skills, participate in support groups

coping mechanisms. In cohesive groups with highly functional members, the leader might have an opportunity to discuss the difference between emotion-focused and problem-focused mechanisms. The depth of the discussion will depend on the degree of group cohesiveness and trust, the functional level of the members and the comfort level and willingness of the leader to deal with the identified issues.

During the last 10 minutes of each session, the leader should attempt to bring the discussion to some closure on at least one issue. This may be accomplished by summarising the issues and coping mechanisms that were identified. In open groups, the leader would end by encouraging those members who do not return to the group to look at coping mechanisms for their own specific issues, either by themselves or with a friend or confidant(e). For ongoing groups, the leader would end the session by facilitating agreement about the issues that will be discussed during the next session. The leader can also encourage members to think about the identified issues in the interim.

EVALUATING THE EFFECTIVENESS OF NURSING INTERVENTIONS

Nurses evaluate the effectiveness of interventions for older adults with self-concept disturbance by determining the extent to which older adults express positive views of themselves. Another measure of effective nursing care is that older adults no longer verbalise ageist attitudes. Nursing care of older adults who express a sense of being powerless is evaluated by the extent to which they become involved in decisions that affect them and the degree to which they express feelings of control over their lives. Nurses evaluate care for older adults with ineffective individual coping by observing behaviours that reflect the use of a variety of coping strategies (see Table 12-1). For example, an older adult might learn to use problem-focused coping strategies for a situation that he or she previously viewed as hopeless and unchangeable.

CHAPTER HIGHLIGHTS

Life events: Age-related changes affecting psychosocial function

- Retirement
- Relocation
- Chronic illness and functional impairments
- Decisions about driving a vehicle
- Widowhood
- Death of family and friends
- Ageist attitudes

Theories about psychosocial function in older adults

- Sources of stress for older adults are major life events, daily hassles and chronic stressors.
- Older adults are more likely to use emotion-focused coping styles that involve management of thoughts and feelings.
- Social supports are an important resource for coping in older adults.
- Nurses facilitate effective coping in older adults through interventions that improve their functional abilities.

Factors that influence psychosocial function in older adults

- Religion and spirituality are increasingly important resources for older adults.
- Cultural factors influence definitions perceptions of all aspects of psychosocial functioning (Cultural considerations 12-1).

CASE STUDY TWO

Mr Demetriou is 36 years old and was recently admitted to a long-term residential care facility. His medical diagnoses are type 2 diabetes, glaucoma, retinopathy and dementia of Alzheimer type. Mr Demetriou lived with his wife until 6 months ago, when she died after a brief illness. After her death, he needed help with all his activities of daily living, and his daughter arranged home care assistance for 2 hours a day. About 1 month ago, he started getting up and wandering outside at night. Once, he wandered off at 3:00 a.m., and the police had to take him home. After this episode, he was afraid to be alone, and he agreed to go to a long-term residential care facility.

During the first week in the long-term residential care facility, Mr Demetriou was cooperative with the staff and sociable with the other residents. He was resistant to the morning schedule of getting up at 6:00 a.m. and eating breakfast in the dining room at 7:30 a.m., but he passively complied when the staff firmly directed him. His daughter visited him daily and accompanied him to social and recreational activities with other residents. Mr Demetriou has been in the long-term residential care facility for 10 days, and he is becoming very resistant to staff efforts to get him dressed for breakfast. When he attends group activities, he is disruptive, yelling about being a hostage in a monastery. Mr Demetriou tells other residents that he was tricked into coming to this place and that the only reason he has to stay is because his daughter has taken over his house and is living there with her family. He frequently paces up and down the corridors and says he has to find his daughter to take him home because his wife is sick and she needs him to take care of her. You walk with him in the hallway, and he says, "I don't know why they keep me locked up here. I can't do anything like I used to do at home. It's like a monastery where you have to get up in the middle of the night and they make you get cleaned up and eat breakfast when it's still dark outside."

Nursing assessment

Your nursing assessment shows that Mr Demetriou needs supervision in all activities of daily living because of poor vision and memory impairment. He needs some assistance with personal care, but he can dress himself if staff set his clothes out for him. When Mr Demetriou was admitted to the facility, he was assigned to the "early wakers" group, which means that the night shift is responsible for waking him and getting him ready for breakfast by 7:30 a.m. The night-shift nursing assistants help him with showering, shaving and dressing.

During the admission interview, Mr Demetriou's daughter, Jane, said that his typical morning routine at home was to get up around 8:30 a.m. and get dressed independently, using the clothes that were set out for him by the community centre aide. He ate breakfast around 9:30 a.m. and then spent the day "working on his papers". Jane, who lives out of town, would call her father four times a week. When Jane talked with him on the phone, he always told her how busy he was working on his papers. Although Jane was paying all his bills from a joint bank account, Mr Demetriou would spend hours and hours with bill stubs, old bank statements and an inactive cheque account, thinking he was paying his bills.

Jane was staying at her father's house for the 2 weeks before his admission and for 1 week after admission to the nursing facility. She plans to return to town for a couple of days every other month and will visit her father at those times. The only nearby relative is a sister-in-law who comes to visit Mr Demetriou every 2 weeks.

Nursing issues

You use the nursing issue of powerlessness related to relocation to a facility and lack of control over activities of daily living. You select this issue, rather than impaired adjustment or ineffective individual coping, because Mr Demetriou focuses on a theme of loss of control. Your assessment identifies several factors that contribute to his powerlessness, and you address these factors in your nursing care plan.

Nursing care plan for Mr Demetriou

Goals for wellness outcomes	Nursing interventions	Nursing evaluation
Mr Demetriou will feel he has greater control over his morning schedule.	• Take Mr Demetriou off the "early wakers" list and allow him to sleep until 8 a.m. • Allow Mr Demetriou to wear his pyjamas and robe to breakfast and to shower, bathe and dress after breakfast.	• Mr Demetriou will no longer verbalise the feeling of being locked up in a monastery or a prison.
Mr Demetriou will function as independently as possible.	• The staff will set out Mr Demetriou's clothing and allow him to dress himself. • The staff will give Mr Demetriou positive feedback for dressing himself.	• Mr Demetriou dresses himself with minimal supervision. • Mr Demetriou performs his personal care activities at a pace that is comfortable for him.
Mr Demetriou will engage in a familiar activity that gives him a meaningful role.	• Ask Jane to send a set of bill stubs, old bank statements, and the inactive chequebook so that Mr Demetriou can do his "work". • Encourage Mr Demetriou to "work with his papers" in the activity room, where he can interact with other residents. • Give Mr Demetriou positive feedback when he interacts with other residents. • Compliment Mr Demetriou about doing his paperwork.	• Mr Demetriou resumes his former routine of working with his papers and will interact with other residents.

Risk factors that affect psychosocial wellness

- Physical, functional and psychosocial health significantly affect coping skills.
- The ability to appraise a situation accurately affects psychosocial function.
- Learned helplessness results when uncontrollable events reinforce the idea that future events will also be uncontrollable.

Functional consequences associated with psychosocial function

- Negative functional consequences include anxiety, loneliness, depression and cognitive impairment.
- Older adults also experience emotional well-being (e.g. joy, happiness, satisfaction, purpose in life and sense of mastery).
- Gerontologists are currently investigating the concept of resilience in older adults, which is defined as the ability to bounce back and recover physical and psychological health in the face of adversity.

Nursing assessment of psychosocial function

- Refer to Chapter 13.

Nursing issues

- Self-esteem disturbance
- Situational low self-esteem (or risk for)
- Being powerless
- Impaired adjustment
- Social isolation
- Willingness for enhanced coping
- Willingness for enhanced self-concept

Goal planning for wellness outcomes

- Psychosocial adjustment to a life change
- Adaptation to physical disability
- Improved personal autonomy
- Improved self-esteem
- Improved quality of life

Nursing interventions for psychosocial wellness

- Enhancing self-esteem: improving functioning, using verbal and non-verbal communication, avoiding elder-speak
- Promoting a sense of control: providing information, rephrasing events, addressing threats such as lack of privacy and loss of individuality
- Involving older adults in decision making: challenging attitudes, facilitating communication, using verbal and non-verbal communication techniques
- Addressing role loss: identifying meaningful roles
- Encouraging life review and reminiscence
- Fostering social supports
- Addressing spiritual needs: communicating caring and compassion, instilling hope, referring for spiritual care, encouraging participation in religious activities
- Teaching about managing stress in daily life
- Leading healthy ageing classes

Evaluating effectiveness of nursing interventions

- Positive self-perceptions
- Involvement in decisions
- Effective coping strategies

CRITICAL THINKING EXERCISES

1. Take a sheet of paper and draw two vertical lines to make three equal columns. Think of someone you know in your personal life or professional practice who is 80 years old or older. In the left column, list three or more life events that this person has experienced in later adulthood. In the centre column, describe the impact of the life event on the person's daily life. In the right column, list the coping mechanisms the person has used to deal with the life event. You can guess at the information, as needed, to complete the information in the centre and right columns.
2. Think of a recent life event in your own life and answer the following questions: How close in time was the life event to other stressful events in your life? What impact did the life event have and what were the manifestations of stress in your life (e.g. in your work, your health, your personal life, your relationships with other people)? What coping mechanisms did you use? Were the coping mechanisms effective? What coping mechanisms would you like to develop to prepare yourself for older adulthood?
3. You are asked to lead a 1-hour discussion titled "Mental Health and Ageing" for a group of 10 people at a senior citizen centre. Describe your approach to this topic. What would be your goals for the class? How would you involve the participants? What visual aids would you use?

RESOURCES

For an extensive range of additional resources to enhance teaching and learning and to facilitate understanding of this chapter, please see the text's accompanying website located on thePoint at http://thepoint.lww.com.

Clinical tools

Hartford Institute for Geriatric Nursing, ConsultGeriRN.org: http://consultgerirn.org/resources

Assessment tools *Try This*® series and *How to Try This* resources

General assessment series:

- *Try This*, issue 14: The Modified Caregiver Strain Index (CSI). Onega, L. L. (2013). *Best Practices in Nursing Care to Older Adults.*
- *How to Try This* (article): Helping those who help others: The Modified Caregiver Strain Index. Onega, L. L. *American Journal of Nursing, 108*(9), 62–69.

- *How to Try This* (video): *The Modified Caregiver Strain Index.*
- *Try This*, Issue 19: Horowitz's Impact of Event Scale: An assessment of post traumatic stress in older adults. Christianson, S. & Marren, J. (2013). *Best Practices in Nursing Care to Older Adults.*
- *How to Try This* (article): The Impact of Event Scale—Revised: A quick measure of a patient's response to trauma. Hyer, K. & Brown, L. (2008). *American Journal of Nursing, 108*(11), 60–68.
- *How to Try This* (video): *Horowitz Impact of Event Scale.*

Evidence-based practice

Joanna Briggs Institute: http://connect.jbiconnectplus.org

- Caldwell, C., Fernandez, R., Traynor, V. & Perrin, C. (2014). Effects of spending time outdoors in daylight on the psychosocial well-being of older people and their family carers: A systematic review. *Joanna Briggs Institute Library of Systematic Reviews, 12*(9), 277–320.
- Rathnayake, T. (2014). Healthcare staff and resident's family: Constructive relationships (evidence-based summary).

Health education

Age Concern New Zealand: www.ageconcern.org.nz

Search for:

- Wellbeing, health and happiness, recipes for life
- Accredited Visiting Service: Would you like more company?

COTA Australia: www.cotaaustralia.org.au

myaged*care*: www.myagedcare.gov.au

National Seniors Australia: www.nationalseniors.com.au

REFERENCES

Aldwin, D. F., Hofer, S. M. & McCammon, R. J. (2006). Modeling the effects of time: Integrating demographic and developmental perspectives. In R. H. Binstock & L. K. George (Eds), *Handbook of aging and the social sciences* (6th ed., pp. 20–38). Boston: Academic Press.

Almeida, D. M., Piazza, J. R., Stawski, R. S. et al. (2011). The speedometer of life: Stress, health and aging. In K. W. Schaie & S. L. Willis (Eds), *Handbook of the psychology of aging* (7th ed., pp. 191–206). New York: Elsevier.

Andrews, M. M. & Boyle, J. S. (2011). *Transcultural concepts in nursing care* (6th ed.). Philadelphia, PA: Wolters Kluwer/ Lippincott Williams & Wilkins.

Andrews, M. M. & Hanson, P. A. (2011). Religion, culture and nursing. In M. M. Andrews & J. S. Boyle (Eds), *Transcultural concepts in nursing care* (6th ed.). Philadelphia, PA: Lippincott Williams & Wilkins.

Angel, R. J., Angel, J. L. & Hill, T. D. (2009). Subjective control and health among Mexican-origin elders in Mexico and the United States: Structural considerations in comparative research. *Journal of Gerontology: Social Sciences, 64B*, 390–401.

Australian Bureau of Statistics (ABS). (2013). General health: Self-assessed health status. In *Profiles of health, Australia, 2011–13*. Cat. no. 4338. Canberra: ABS.

Australian Institute of Health and Welfare (AIHW). (2011). *Australian hospital statistics 2009–10*. Health services series no. 40. Cat. no. HSE 107. Canberra: AIHW.

Bekhet, A. K. & Zauszniewski, J. A. (2012). Mental health of elders in retirement communities: Is loneliness a key factor? *Archives of Psychiatric Nursing, 26*(3), 214–224.

Binder, B. K., Mastel-Smith, B., Hersch, G., Symes, L., Malecha, A. & McFarlane, J. (2009). Community-dwelling, older women's perspectives on Therapeutic Life Review: A qualitative analysis. *Issues in Mental Health Nursing, 30*, 288–294.

Blay, S. L. & Marinho, V. (2012). Anxiety disorders in old age. *Current Opinion in Psychiatry, 25*(6), 462–467.

Blume, J., Douglas, S. D. & Evans, D. L. (2011). Immune suppression and immune activation in depression. *Brain, Behavior and Immunology, 25*(2), 221–229.

Brenes, G. A., Miller, M. E., Williamson, J. D. et al. (2012). A randomized controlled trial of telephone-delivered cognitive-behavioral therapy for late-life anxiety disorders. *American Journal of Geriatric Psychiatry, 20*(8), 707–716.

Brennan, P. L., Holland, J. M., Schutte, K. K. et al. (2012). Coping trajectories in later life: A 20-year predictive study. *Aging & Mental Health, 16*(3), 305–316.

Burkhardt, M. A. & Nagai-Jacobson, M. G. (2013). Spirituality and health. In B. M. Dossey & L. Keegan (Eds), *Holistic nursing: A handbook for practice* (6th ed., Chapter 32). Boston, MA: Jones & Bartlett.

Butler, R. N. (2001). Life review. In M. D. Mezey (Ed.), *The encyclopedia of elder care* (pp. 401–402). New York: Springer.

Cairney, J., Faulkner, G., Veldhuizen, S. & Wade, T. J. (2009). Changes over time in physical activity and psychological distress among older adults. *Canadian Journal of Psychiatry, 54*, 160–169.

Cattell, M. G. (2009). Global perspectives on widowhood and aging. In J. Sokolovsky (Ed.), *The cultural context of aging: Worldwide perspectives* (3rd ed., Chapter 11, pp. 155–172). Santa Barbara, CA: Greenwood Press.

Cornwell, E. Y. & Waite, L. J. (2009). Social disconnectedness, perceived isolation and health among older adults. *Journal of Health & Social Behavior, 50*, 31–48.

Cook, S. L. (2013). Redirection: An extension of career during retirement. *Gerontologist*. doi:10.1093/geront/gnt105.

Edwards, J. D., Perkins, M., Ross, L. A. & Reynolds, S. L. (2009). Driving status and three-year mortality among community-dwelling older adults. *Journal of Gerontology: Medical Sciences, 64A*, 300–305.

Ehrmin, J. T. (2012). Transcultural perspectives in mental health nursing. In M. M. Andrews & J. S. Boyle (Eds), *Transcultural concepts in nursing care* (6th ed., pp. 243–276). Philadelphia, PA: Lippincott Williams & Wilkins.

Eshbaugh, E. M. (2009). The role of friends in predicting loneliness among older women living alone. *Journal of Gerontological Nursing, 35*(5), 13–16.

Folkman, S. & Lazarus, R. S. (1980). An analysis of coping in a middleaged community sample. *Journal of Health and Social Behavior, 21*, 219–239.

George, L. K. (2011). Social factors, depression, and aging. In R. H. Binstock & L. K. George (Eds), *Handbook of aging and the social sciences* (7th ed., pp. 149–162). New York: Elsevier.

Gouin, J.-P. & Kiecolt-Glaser, J. K. (2011). The impact of psychological stress on wound healing: Methods and mechanisms. *Immunology and Allergy Clinics of North America, 31*(1), 81–93.

Harris, G. M., Allen, R. S., Dunn, L. et al. (2013). "Trouble won't last always": Religious coping and meaning in the stress process. *Qualitative Health Research, 23*(6), 773–781.

Hayward, R. D. & Krause, N. (2013a). Trajectories of late-life change in God-mediated control. *Journals of Gerontology: Psychological and Social Sciences, 68*(1), 49–58.

Herdman, T. H. (Ed.). (2012). *NANDA International nursing diagnoses: Definitions and classification 2012–2014*. Oxford: Wiley-Blackwell.

Herman, R. E. & Williams, K. N. (2009). Elderspeak's influence on resistiveness to care: Focus on behavioral events. *American Journal of Alzheimer's Disease and Other Dementias, 24*, 417–423.

Holmes, T. H. & Rahe, R. H. (1967). The social readjustment rating scale. *Journal of Psychosomatic Research, 11*, 213–218.

Hsu, Y.-C. & Wang, J.-J. (2009). Physical, affective and behavioral effects of group reminiscence on depressed institutionalized elders in Taiwan. *Nursing Research, 58*, 294–299.

Huang, S.-L., Li, C.-M., Yang, C.-Y. & Chen, J.-J. (2009). Application of reminiscence treatment on older people with dementia: A case study in Pintung, Taiwan. *Journal of Nursing Research, 17*, 112–118.

Jang, Y., Chiriboga, D. A., Lee, J. & Cho, S. (2009). Determinants of a sense of mastery in Korean American elders: A longitudinal assessment. *Aging & Mental Health, 13*, 99–105.

Jenkinson, C. E., Dickens, A. P., Jones, K. et al. (2013). Is volunteering a public health intervention? A systematic review and meta-analysis of the health and survival of volunteers. *BioMed Central, 13*, 773. Available at www.biomedcentral.com/1471-2458/13/773.

Kang, S. K. & Chasteen, A. L. (2009). The development and validation of the age-based rejection sensitivity questionnaire. *Gerontologist, 49*, 303–316.

Kavanagh, K. H. (2008). Transcultural perspectives in mental health nursing. In M. M. Andrews & J. S. Boyle (Eds), *Transcultural concepts in nursing care* (5th ed., pp. 226–259). Philadelphia, PA: Lippincott Williams & Wilkins.

Kostyniuk, L. P., Molnar, L. J. & Eby, D. W. (2009). Safe mobility of older drivers: Concerns expressed by adult children. *Topics in Geriatric Rehabilitation, 25*, 24–32.

Lenze, E. J. & Wetherell, L. (2011). A lifespan view of anxiety disorders. *Dialogues in Clinical Neuroscience, 13*(4), 381–399.

Lyon, B. L. (2012). Stress, coping, and health. In V. H. Rice (Ed.), *Handbook of stress, coping, and health* (2nd ed., pp. 2–20). Thousand Oaks, CA: Sage.

Levy, B. R. & Leifheit-Limson, E. (2009). The stereotype-matching effect: Greater influence on functioning when age stereotypes correspond to outcomes. *Psychology and Aging, 24*, 230–233.

Li, Y.-P., Chen, Y.-M. & Chen, C.-H. (2013). Volunteer transitions and physical and psychological health among older adults in Taiwan. *Journals of Gerontology: Psychological Sciences and Social Sciences, 68*(6), 997–1003.

Manning, L. K., Leek, J. A. & Radina, M. E. (2012). Making sense of extreme longevity: Explorations into spiritual lives of centenarians. *Journal of Religion, Spirituality & Aging, 24*(4), 345–359.

Māori Health. (2012). Māori health models. Accessed February 2015 at www.health.govt.nz/our-work/populations/maori-health/maori-health-models.

Mather, M. (2012). The emotion paradox in the aging brain. *Annals of the New York Academy of Sciences, 1251*(1), 33–49.

Medical Council of New Zealand. (2010). Best health outcomes for Pacific peoples: Practice implications. Accessed March 2015 at www.mcnz.org.nz.

Mehrotra, C. M. & Wagner, L. S. (2009). Work, retirement and leisure. In C. M. Mehrotra & L. S. Wagner. *Aging and diversity* (2nd ed., pp. 253–315). London: Taylor & Francis.

Miller, C. A. (2013). Wellness activity tool for stress management. In C. A. Miller (Ed.), *Fast facts for health promotion in nursing: Promoting wellness in a nutshell* (pp. 61–62). New York: Springer.

New Zealand Ministry of Health. (2013). New Zealand Health Survey: Annual update of key findings 2012/13. Accessed March 2015 at www.health.govt.nz/publication/new-zealand-health-survey-annual-update-key-findings-2012-13.

Okun, M. A., Yeung, E. W. & Brown, S. (2013). Volunteering by older adults and risk of mortality: A meta-analysis. *Psychology and Aging, 28*(2), 564–577.

Oxley, J. & Charlton, J. (2009). Attitudes to and mobility impacts of driving cessation: Differences between current and former drivers. *Topics in Geriatric Rehabilitation, 25*, 43–54.

Park, N. S., Jang, Y., Lee, B. S. et al. (2013). The mediating role of loneliness in the relation between social engagement and depressive symptoms among older Korean Americans: Do men and women differ? *Journals of Gerontology: Psychological Sciences and Social Sciences, 68*(2), 193–201.

Perese, E. F., Simon, M. R. & Ryan, E. (2008). Promoting positive student clinical experiences with older adults through use of group reminiscence therapy. *Journal of Gerontological Nursing, 34*(12), 45–51.

Pitkala, K. H., Routasalo, P., Kautiainen, H. et al. (2011). Effects of socially stimulating group intervention on lonely, older people's cognition: A randomized, controlled trial. *American Journal of Geriatric Psychiatry, 19*(7), 654–663.

Ramsey, J. L. (2012). Spirituality and aging. *Annual Review of Gerontology and Geriatrics, 32*, 131–151.

Randall, W. L. (2013). The importance of being ironic: Narrative openness and personal resilience in later life. *Gerontologist, 53*(1), 9–16.

Rodin, J. & Langer, E. (1980). Aging labels: The decline of control and the fall of self-esteem. *Journal of Social Issues, 36*(2), 12–29.

Rogers, C. E., Larkey, L. K. & Keller, C. (2009). A review of clinical trials of tai chi and qigong in older adults. *Western Journal of Nursing Research, 31*, 245–279.

Rote, S., Hill, T. D. & Ellison, C. G. (2012). Religious attendance and loneliness in later life. *Gerontologist, 53*(1), 39–50.

Rybarczyk, B., Emery, E. E., Guequierre, L. L. et al. (2012). The role of resilience in chronic illness and disability in older adults. *Annual Review of Gerontology and Geriatrics, 32*, 173–188.

Schuurmans, J. & van Balkom, A. (2011). Late-life anxiety disorders: A review. *Current Psychiatric Reports, 13*(4), 267–273.

Scott, S. B., Whitehead, B. R., Bergeman, C. S. et al. (2013). Combinations of stressors in midlife: Examining role and domain stressors using regression trees and random forests. *Journals of Gerontology: Psychological Sciences and Social Sciences, 68*(3), 464–475.

Selye, H. (1956). *The stress of life*. New York: McGraw-Hill.

Shrestha, S., Robertson, S. & Stanley, M. A. (2011). Innovations in research for treatment of late-life anxiety. *Aging & Mental Health, 15*(7), 811–821.

Smith, J. M. (2012). Loneliness in older adults: An embodied experience. *Journal of Gerontological Nursing, 38*(8), 45–53.

Stawski, R. S., Mogle, J. A. & Sliwinski, M. J. (2013). Daily stressors and self-reported changes in memory in old age: The mediating effects of daily negative affect and cognitive interference. *Aging & Mental Health, 17*(2), 168–172.

Stessman, J., Rottenberg, Y., Shimshilashvili, I. et al. (2013). Loneliness, health, and longevity. *Journals of Gerontology: Biological Sciences and Medical Sciences, 69*(6), 744–750.

Underwood, P. W. (2012). Social support. In V. H. Rice (Ed.), *Handbook of stress, coping, and health* (2nd ed., pp. 355–380). Thousand Oaks, CA: Sage.

Van Kessel, G. (2013). The ability of older people to overcome adversity: A review of the resilience concept. *Geriatric Nursing, 34*, 122–127.

Vickery, D. & Westerman, T. (2004). "That's just the way he is": Some implications of Aboriginal mental health beliefs. *Australian e-Journal for the Advancement of Mental Health* (AeJAMH), 3(3).

Werner, J. S., Frost, M. H., Macnee, C. L. et al. (2012). Major and minor life stressors, measures, and health outcomes. In V. H. Rice (Ed.), *Handbook of stress, coping, and health* (2nd ed., pp. 126–154). Thousand Oaks, CA: Sage.

Westra, B. L., Paitich, N., Ekstrom, D., et al. (2013). Getting on with living life: Experiences of older adults after home care. *Home Healthcare Nurse, 31*(9), 493–501.

Whitehead, B. R. & Bergeman, C. S. (2011). Coping with daily stress: Differential role of spiritual experience on daily positive and negative affect. *Journals of Gerontology: Psychological Sciences and Social Sciences, 67*(4), 456–459.

Williams, K. N., Herman, R., Gajewski, B. & Wilson, K. (2009). Elderspeak communication: Impact on dementia care. *American Journal of Alzheimer's Disease and Other Dementias, 24*, 11–20.

Williams, K. N. & Warren, C. A. B. (2009). Communication in assisted living. *Journal of Aging Studies, 23*, 24–36.

Yochim, B. P., Mueller, A. E., June, A. et al. (2011). Psychometric properties of the Geriatric Anxiety Scale: Comparison to the Beck Anxiety Inventory and Geriatric Anxiety Inventory. *Clinical Gerontologist, 34*, 21–33.

Young, H. M. & Cochrane, B. E. (2004). Healthy aging for older women. *Nursing Clinics of North America, 39*, 131–143.

Chapter 13

Cognitive and psychosocial assessment

By Carol Miller and Sharyn Hunter

LEARNING OBJECTIVES

After reading this chapter, you should be able to:

1. Describe the purpose, scope of and procedure for a psychosocial assessment of older adults.
2. Describe communication techniques that are helpful for conducting a psychosocial assessment.
3. Describe how to assess each of the following specific components of mental status: physical appearance, motor function, social skills, response to an interview, orientation, alertness, memory, and speech and language characteristics.
4. Explain how to perform a nursing assessment of skills involved with decision making and executive function in older adults.
5. Describe how to assess each of the following components of affective function: mood, anxiety, self-esteem, depression, happiness and well-being.
6. Discuss distinguishing characteristics of delusions, hallucinations and illusions as they relate to the underlying conditions common in older adults.
7. Explain how to perform a nursing assessment of the following aspects of social supports: social network, barriers to services, and economic resources.
8. Explain how to perform a nursing assessment of the spiritual needs of older adults, including factors that cause spiritual distress as well as those that promote spiritual wellness.

KEY POINTS

abstract thinking
affect
akathisia
anxiety
circumstantiality
cognitive assessment tools
confabulation
decision making
delusions
executive dysfunction
generalised anxiety disorder (GAD)
hallucinations
illusions
insight
memory
mental status assessment
Mini-Cog
orientation
social supports

Cognitive and psychosocial assessments are complex and challenging but are also an essential aspect of nursing care for older adults. Although cognitive and psychosocial impairments are often attributed to factors relating to normal ageing or to untreatable conditions, careful assessment can identify the underlying cause(s) of cognitive changes, many of which can then be reversed or addressed through interventions.

Nurses can use assessment skills to improve the quality of life for older adults by ensuring that cognitive and psychosocial issues are identified and addressed. This chapter provides information about the assessment component of the nursing process related to cognitive and psychosocial function (Chapters 11 and 12). In addition, it supplements the assessment information in other chapters of this text, particularly the chapters on elder abuse (Chapter 10), dementia and delirium (Chapter 14), and depression (Chapter 15).

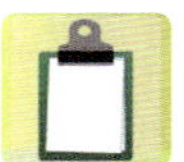

OVERVIEW OF COGNITIVE AND PSYCHOSOCIAL ASSESSMENT OF OLDER ADULTS

In contrast to physical and functional assessment procedures (which are viewed as routine measures to identify the causes of symptoms), cognitive and psychosocial assessment procedures are commonly perceived as formal psychological tests that analyse personality traits or identify the need for mental health treatment. Consequently, healthcare professionals may overlook the cognitive and psychosocial component of an assessment, or relegate it to the realm of mental health. However, an assessment of cognitive and psychosocial function is an essential component of holistic nursing care, which addresses the body–mind–spirit needs of older adults.

The first sections of this chapter cover the purposes and procedures of cognitive and psychosocial assessment, and the scope of psychosocial assessment that are applicable to nursing care of all older adults. The second major section reviews unique aspects of communicating with older adults and applies the concepts to cognitive and psychosocial assessment. The third section covers the assessment of the domains of cognitive and psychosocial assessment. Affective function, contact with reality, and **social supports** and other domains of psychosocial function are addressed in following separate sections. Nurses can use the assessment boxes as a guide to observations and communication techniques pertinent to each aspect of psychosocial assessment.

Purposes of the cognitive and psychosocial assessment process

From a wellness perspective, the purposes of psychosocial assessment include the following:

- Detecting asymptomatic or unacknowledged health problems at an early stage
- Identifying signs or symptoms of psychosocial dysfunction (e.g. anxiety, depression, memory problems, change in mental status)
- Identifying stressors and other risk factors (particularly those that are amenable to interventions) that affect cognitive, emotional or social function
- Obtaining information about the person's usual personality and coping mechanisms
- Assessing cognitive abilities
- Identifying social supports and other coping resources that could be supported or strengthened
- Identifying the older adult's personal goals for psychosocial wellness.

Nurses use this information to plan interventions that are based on realistic goals and expectations aimed at improving quality of life for older people.

When the nursing assessment identifies mental changes in an older adult, a multidisciplinary approach is important for further assessment and implementation of effective interventions. A common mistake is to label the changes as "normal for the person's age". Attributing changes to the ageing process is not only unfair to the older adult but can be detrimental, particularly if a treatable underlying condition is overlooked or appropriate interventions to improve functional abilities are neglected.

As should be clear from the discussion of cognitive function in Chapter 11 that age-related cognitive changes are rarely brought to the attention of healthcare professionals by the older person or carers/caregivers. For example, an older adult would be unlikely to make the following complaint: "I know I can learn new information, but I don't seem to be able to comprehend information as quickly as I used to." When mental changes are noted by other people or brought to the attention of healthcare professionals, it is more likely that they arise from pathological processes than from age-related processes. Therefore, whenever changes in psychosocial function are identified, healthcare professionals must make every effort to identify the underlying cause and not attribute the changes to age.

Scope of the psychosocial assessment

An important part of a psychosocial assessment is identifying the unique meaning of life events, with particular attention on identifying any effects on health. Initial questions can focus on events that occurred many years ago, such as "What kind of work did you do?" may prompt a discussion of feelings about retirement. Because changes in living arrangements can precipitate feelings of loss, a non-threatening question such as "What were the circumstances of your moving here?" might lead to further discussion of the meaning of the living arrangement for that person. People who have experienced the loss of a pet may be reluctant to acknowledge the depth of their feelings and they need to know that they will not be judged. Because pets may be particularly significant for older adults it is appropriate to include at least one question about pets in the psychosocial assessment of older adults.

Questions to assess the meaning of medical conditions and functional limitations are an essential component of the psychosocial assessment because coping with health changes is a common and challenging task for many older adults. Nurses also try to identify the person's concerns about the functional consequences that are likely to be associated with illness and disability. For example, older adults with diabetes may be less interested in knowing how the pancreas functions than in learning to cope with the attendant visual impairment or their fear of increasing dependence on others. Therefore, rather than focusing the assessment on medical diagnoses, ask a broader question such as "If you had to rate your health on a scale of 0% to 100%, what rating would you give it today?" After the person responds to this question, ask follow-up questions, such as "What would have to be changed for you to feel 100% healthy?" or "What rating would you have given yourself a year ago?" Answers to these questions can assist in establishing realistic and person-centred goals for interventions.

During a psychosocial assessment, nurses might hear information that is contrary to their own values or cultural expectations, such as the following examples:

- Expressions of racial prejudice, including use of derogatory labels
- Attitudes of extreme passivity about decisions involving the person's care
- Situations in which older adults are abused or exploited by friends, family or others
- Attitudes that are judgemental about women or other groups or not in accordance with the nurse's beliefs.

When dealing with these types of situations, it helps to be aware of one's own feelings and to address them accordingly.

Although it is essential to communicate a non-judgemental attitude during interactions with older adults, it also is important to acknowledge their feelings. For instance, if the person describes an episode of extreme exploitation and expresses feelings of anger about the situation, the nurse can show empathy and understanding with a statement such as "That sounds like a terrible situation to have been in." Nurses also need to consider that some of the information they obtain may involve legal or ethical issues that require further action. For example, information about recent or ongoing abuse or exploitation may necessitate a referral for further investigation as discussed in Chapter 10.

Procedure for the cognitive and psychosocial assessment

Nurses obtain cognitive and psychosocial assessment information by interviewing older adults and their carers and by observing older adults in their environments. Opportunities for performing these assessments vary in different healthcare settings, and nurses obtain much of the assessment information informally during the course of their usual care.

In acute care settings, nurses perform an assessment at the time of admission to establish a baseline for planning nursing care. Although the initial nursing assessment focuses on the person's immediate needs, nurses should not overlook the cognitive and psychosocial assessment, because it often provides clues to the causes of existing medical problems and insight into all the person's ongoing care needs.

As soon as the person's condition is medically stable, the nurse should begin addressing the older adult's cognitive and psychosocial issues as an important component of person-centred care and discharge planning. In long-term residential care settings, cognitive and psychosocial assessment information is obtained as an ongoing part of care and is commonly addressed in team conferences. When nurses provide care in home and community settings, they can obtain and record valuable assessment information by observing the interactions between older adults and their carers and environments.

In addition to interviewing and observing older adults, nurses obtain cognitive and psychosocial assessment information from other sources. For example, when the older person's cognitive function is compromised, it is essential to obtain information from family members and others who can provide a reliable history of the mental changes. In long-term residential care settings, the healthcare workers who spend the most time with the resident are an important source of information.

The tools for an effective cognitive and psychosocial assessment are a trusting relationship, a listening ear, an intuitive mind, a sensitive heart, and good communication skills. Although nurses routinely provide care involving physically intimate activities such as bathing, they may be less confident about discussing cognitive and psychosocial issues, particularly when the assessment involves concerns that would not normally be discussed with strangers. Older adults may feel threatened by cognitive and psychosocial assessment questions, particularly if they are trying to cover up cognitive deficits. Both the nurse and the older adult may initially feel uncomfortable during this assessment. Because increased awareness of one's own attitudes is an important first step in becoming comfortable with performing a psychosocial assessment, nurses can use a self-assessment guide (Box 13-1) to examine their own attitudes about older adults and identify areas of discomfort.

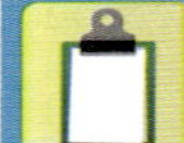

BOX 13-1
Self-assessment of attitudes about psychosocial aspects of ageing

What is my level of comfort in discussing psychosocial issues with older adults?

- How comfortable am I discussing emotional, cultural, spiritual and psychosocial subjects?
- Are there certain topics with which I am uncomfortable (e.g. death, suicide, alcoholism, sexuality, spirituality, terminal illness, abusive relationships)?
- Does the person's age influence my degree of comfort (e.g. Am I more comfortable discussing issues with someone who is in their 60s than with someone who is in their 90s?)
- Does the person's gender influence my degree of comfort?
- To what groups of older adults do I find it easy or difficult to relate?
- How do I feel about older adults who are single, divorced, widowed, separated or living together in a same-sex or heterosexual but unmarried relationship?

When I was growing up ...

- How were older adults in my family treated?
- What did I observe about the treatment of older adults in society?
- How were people with mental or emotional disorders viewed?
- What language was used to describe ageing, old age, and older adults with disturbed mental function?
- What words did my family use, and what was the connotative meaning of the words used, to describe older adults? Was it positive, negative or mixed?

What experiences have I had with older adults ...

- From different racial, ethnic, religious and socioeconomic backgrounds?
- With functional impairments or mental, psychological or emotional disorders?

The nurse may begin a cognitive and psychosocial assessment by explaining the purpose of the questions with a statement such as:

- "I'd like to get to know you better so we can make the best plans for follow-up after you leave the hospital."
- "I'd like to ask you some questions about your interests so we can plan for your care while you're here at the nursing facility."
- "I'd like to ask some questions about how you manage from day to day so we can identify any community services that might be helpful to you."

Nurses can ask initially about events of the remote past, such as where the person was born and grew up, as a nonthreatening way of leading into further questions. Incorporating some personal information in conversations can facilitate the establishment of a trusting relationship. For example, offering a little information about your own pets or family, for instance, might encourage an older adult to share feelings that they might not mention otherwise and may help to establish a framework of mutual interest. Sharing information about ethnic background also can be an effective and non-threatening way of obtaining information about possible cultural influences.

Formal cognitive and psychosocial assessment tools can be introduced when the older adult is more comfortable discussing issues. Because questions about memory can be very threatening, the topic might be introduced as follows: "I notice you have a hard time remembering dates. Have you noticed any other problems with your memory? Is it okay with you if I ask some questions about your memory?"

If no evidence of cognitive impairment is evident, but other people have expressed concern about the person's memory, a statement such as the following might be used: "Your daughter is concerned that you don't remember to keep appointments. Have you noticed any problems with your memory? Is it okay with you if I ask some questions about your memory?"

A student's perspective

My experience interviewing Mr M. was an amazing one. I learned a lot about older adults and also about my interview technique. I think several of my techniques helped Mr M. feel more comfortable and at ease. I told him if he felt uncomfortable answering any questions, he should feel free to pass and that did not happen once.

I started asking him easy questions about his job and things like that. Then I moved into more personal questions related to his childhood and whether he thought it had been easy or difficult. I thought he might not remember a lot of that time in his life, but he told me many stories from when he was younger. He also had a lot of pride in the work that he did as a middle-aged adult when he was foreman in a factory.

Another technique I used was to allow him to wander away from the "path" of the question that I had asked him, because I didn't want him to feel conformed to answer the specific question. By using this technique, I learned much more about him than the scope of my original question, and it also gave him time to tell me things at his own pace. I could also tell what information he valued as important and what he found more private.

Erin H.

DIVERSITY NOTE

Older adults from some Asian cultures may not approve of keeping dogs, cats and other domestic animals indoors because they are considered unclean carriers of fleas, ticks, rabies and other disease-causing organisms.

COMMUNICATION SKILLS FOR COGNITIVE AND PSYCHOSOCIAL ASSESSMENT

Analogous to the use of a stethoscope and other tools for assessing physiological function, nurses use skilful communication techniques as an essential tool for cognitive and psychosocial assessment. Good communication techniques are particularly important during these assessments because of the sensitivity of the topics and the importance of establishing a trusting relationship. When caring for older adults, however, nurses encounter many communication barriers that make it more difficult to discuss personal information, such as feelings and life events. Thus, to perform an effective cognitive and psychosocial assessment, nurses need to identify and address the barriers that commonly affect communication with older adults (as discussed in the following sections). In addition, techniques for communicating with people who have dementia are discussed in Chapter 14.

Identifying communication barriers

Non-verbal communication techniques are particularly important when discussing sensitive issues, but visual impairments can interfere with the older adult's ability to perceive non-verbal messages. Similarly, hearing impairment can be a source of uneasiness for both the nurse and the older adult if they need to speak loudly about sensitive topics or emotional issues.

External and internal distractions can interfere with the ability to focus on the conversation, particularly for older adults who are cognitively impaired. These barriers can occur in any of the following circumstances:

- Too much information being requested at one time (e.g. responding to questions about social background, cognitive abilities, and emotional function during a single interview)
- Too many people trying to communicate at one time (e.g. family members, carers or more than one professional)
- Environmental noise, particularly for people who use hearing aids, which usually magnify background noises
- Physical discomfort (e.g. pain, thirst, hunger, fatigue, bladder fullness or uncomfortable temperatures).

Communication barriers can also arise from pathological disorders and adverse medication effects. For example, neurological conditions (e.g. aphasia from strokes) often affect language and verbal skills, and cognitive impairments can interfere with a person's ability to listen, remember and respond to questions.

Similarly, people who are actively delusional or hallucinatory or who are not fully in touch with reality for any reason may have difficulty attending to the conversation. Adverse medication effects that can interfere with communication include mental changes and physical effects (e.g. dry mouth and tardive dyskinesia) as discussed in Chapter 8.

Sometimes nurses inadvertently use communication methods that are perceived as insensitive, uncaring, offensive or condescending, as in the following examples:

- Giving false reassurances (e.g. "Everything's going to be okay") when the person is facing overwhelming circumstances

- Offering trite responses (e.g. "Why cry over spilled milk?") when the person is seriously depressed
- Changing the subject to avoid sensitive issues
- Jumping to conclusions
- Giving unwanted advice
- Minimising the person's feelings.

These communication methods may interfere with the ability to develop the sense of trust that is necessary for discussing psychosocial issues.

Other verbal barriers include rapid or inarticulate speech and obstructive mannerisms, such as covering one's mouth or turning one's head away while talking. In institutional settings, much verbal communication takes place while nurses are walking down the hall, pushing a wheelchair, assisting with personal care, or performing other activities. During these activities, nurses can listen and engage in social conversation, but these are not the best times for asking personal questions or giving important information. Not only are the activities a distraction, but also they interfere with the face-to-face positioning that may be essential for effective communication (e.g. with people who are hearing impaired).

Cultural differences can create communication barriers that are difficult, and sometimes impossible, to overcome. For example, it is difficult to establish a trusting relationship when either the older adult or the nurse holds stereotypes or prejudices about the other person. Overseas-born culturally and linguistically diverse (CALD) people who have a condition that drains their energy or affects their cognitive function may revert to their native language, even if they spoke English well. In these situations, family members may be able to facilitate communication, or it may be appropriate to use interpreters, as discussed in Chapter 2. However, the nurse should consider the impact of the older adult's relationship with the interpreter upon his or her willingness to discuss psychosocial issues openly.

Enhancing communication with older adults

Because the initial *tone* of conversations influences further communication, nurses can use a simple introduction, which can establish rapport if it is done effectively. A verbal introduction is particularly important for older adults who have difficulty reading name tags or remembering names and for those who need assistance, because it is easier to ask for help when they can address someone by name. A more personal approach is to introduce yourself, explain your role, and to then ask the person his or her preferred name, and use the wristband to confirm information.

Touch is widely recognised as an important communication tool and is an intervention for many nursing issues that are applicable to older adults, including the feeling of hopelessness, being stressed because of relocation, and hearing and visionary deficits. Although older adults are generally quite receptive to touch, particularly by a nurse whose responsibilities naturally entail much physical contact, cultural and gender factors can influence perceptions of touch. Thus, before touching a person, nurses need to identify personal boundaries and assess the person's receptivity to being touched. Nurses can do this by asking permission to touch.

Hand massage and other modes of touch can be effective tools for promoting comfort and facilitating communication. Nursing studies identify intentional touch as an important holistic nursing intervention that transforms the relationship between nurses and older adults (Connor & Howett, 2009). In home and community settings, nurses can purposefully use a handshake to facilitate communication, particularly during an initial interaction with older adults. As not all people are receptive to this form of non-verbal communication, a response should not be forced. In addition, a handshake or similar form of touch can provide assessment information about skin temperature, the presence or absence of tremors, and other characteristics of one upper extremity. It also can provide clues about the person's social skills and awareness of others.

Attentive listening is an important communication skill, and it can be particularly effective as a psychosocial assessment tool and to communicate respect and caring. Usually, the best communication occurs when the nurse is verbally quiet and non-verbally responsive. Asking open-ended questions and non-verbally responding to indicate an interest in what the person is saying are usually effective in obtaining important information.

A student's perspective

The life-review interview with Mrs R. enlightened me for one very simple reason: she loves the life she lived. She has no regrets about her life and said she would change nothing. She is a very positive person, and hearing her outlook at life really got me thinking about the way I want to continue to live my life. It was inspiring to hear her views, and it takes away some of my fears of growing older.

The most significant point in the life-review interview is actually the same as the most difficult part. We were discussing family, and I wasn't sure if I should ask about her late husband because I didn't know how to bring him up. I finally found a way to ask about him and immediately her eyes filled with tears. She began to describe him and the things they used to do together. It was sad; yet hearing about how much she loved him was touching. She continued to cry as she said he was the best person she ever knew. Without even thinking, I grabbed her hand. As she squeezed my hand, I saw her become more at ease. With just that little action, I feel like I made her feel better. I had no idea that holding someone's hand could have such a powerful effect.

Molly D.

Non-verbal responses such as sustained eye contact—if culturally appropriate—and short verbal responses such as "And then what happened?" will encourage the person to elaborate on the information considered most important.

Nurses have many opportunities to identify psychosocial issues by listening for pertinent concerns and asking appropriate questions to obtain further information. For example, consider the response of Mrs P., who gave the following response to a question about where she lives:

> *I moved to Sunnybrook Retirement Village after my last stroke. I couldn't stay in my own home, because the bedrooms were on the second floor. The doctor told me I had to live where I could get help, and my daughter didn't want me with her. Now that I've fallen and broken my wrist, I'm not sure what the doctor will tell me. My daughter doesn't want to be bothered with me.*

This response gives clues to several potential issues, which the nurse can explore with any of the following questions:

- "What do you miss most since you moved?"
- "You mentioned that your daughter didn't want you living with her. Is that something you had hoped you could do?"
- "Do you worry that the doctor will suggest that you go to a nursing home?"
- "Do you see your daughter as often as you'd like?"

Answers to these questions might uncover psychosocial concerns that need to be addressed as a part of discharge planning.

When communicating about psychosocial issues, it is important to periodically clarify the messages. One clarification technique is to repeat part of a prior answer when asking further questions. For example, saying to Mrs P., "You mentioned that your daughter doesn't want you living with her ..." gives feedback about what the nurse heard and leads into further questions about underlying feelings.

Feedback can also be helpful when discrepancies between verbal and non-verbal communication are observed. A statement such as, "You look awfully sad. Are you sure it doesn't bother you?" might lead to an acknowledgement of feelings such as anger, rejection and loneliness.

When communicating with older adults, nurses might hear information that is contrary to their own values or cultural expectations, such as the following examples:

- Expressions of racial prejudice, including use of derogatory labels
- Attitudes of extreme passivity about decisions involving the person's care
- Situations in which older adults are abused or exploited by friends, family or others
- Attitudes about women or other groups that are judgemental or not in accordance with the nurse's beliefs.

When dealing with these kinds of experiences, it is helpful to be aware of one's own feelings and to address them accordingly. For example, during the psychosocial assessment, nurses must communicate a non-judgemental attitude, but afterwards they can share their feelings with colleagues.

In some situations, however, it is appropriate for nurses to acknowledge their feelings or opinions during the assessment. For instance, if the person describes an episode of extreme exploitation and expresses feelings of anger about the situation, the nurse can show empathy and understanding with a statement such as, "That sounds like a terrible situation to have been in."

Nurses also need to consider that some of the information they obtain during a psychosocial assessment may involve legal or ethical issues and that, even though this information is beyond the original intent of the assessment, nurses may be required to take further action. For example, information about recent or ongoing abuse or exploitation may necessitate a referral for further investigation, as discussed in Chapter 10.

A student's perspective

My communication with patients is something that I am always aware of. I have continued to learn something new each week. Silence during a conversation is something that is always uncomfortable for me. When talking with my client last week, I was trying to get a better sense of his level of family support. I began by asking him if he had any children. He indicated that he had two daughters, but they lived interstate. Normally I would have had a follow-up question for this response, but I decided to give the client some time to see if he would expand on his original response. It was an awkward few minutes—okay, it was probably just a few seconds that seemed like minutes—but he did open up tremendously. He went on to explain to me that he felt like they have abandoned him since their mother passed away. He began to tear up as he went on to explain that he has grandchildren he has only seen in pictures in Christmas cards. I was able to talk with him about his feelings about these issues and offer him some encouragement. Had I chosen to guide the conversation I would have most likely never had this opportunity. I continue to enjoy confronting uncomfortable communication situations so that I can overcome them and foster better therapeutic communication between myself and patients.

Amanda A.

Creating an environment that supports good communication

Face-to-face positioning facilitates verbal as well as non-verbal communication and is particularly important when visual or hearing impairments interfere with communication. Moreover, people usually feel more comfortable talking with others when they are at the same level of eye contact. Therefore, when conversing with someone in a bed or wheelchair, the nurse should sit in a chair. If possible, remove any physical barrier that interferes with direct face-to-face contact. For example, putting side rails down when talking with someone confined to bed or moving a walker that is in the line of vision can improve face-to-face communication. Before moving walkers or side rails, however, ask the older person's permission to do so; this demonstrates respect for the wishes of the individual. Nurses also need to ensure that these are left in the correct position before leaving.

Each person has his or her own "comfort zone" for communication, which is the physical space required for the person to feel at ease when communicating with others. This space varies according to the type of interactions and has been conceptualised as follows:

- Intimate distance is 0 cm to 45 cm
- Personal distance is 45 cm to 130 cm or 1.3 m
- Social distance is 1.3 m to 3.6 m.

The provision of nursing care often requires that interactions take place in the intimate or personal zones, even though the relationship would normally dictate that interactions take place in the social distance zone. Thus, nurses need to be aware of the influence of personal space on the comfort level of the older person and consider this during communication interactions. Because cultural factors strongly influence the perception of appropriate distance zones and many other aspects of non-verbal communication (e.g. touch, eye contact), it is essential to be sensitive to cultural differences that may affect communication. Cultural considerations 13-1 identifies some cultural influences on expressions of non-verbal communication.

During conversations with older adults, particularly when discussing psychosocial issues, nurses must provide as much privacy as possible. This may be difficult in institutional settings, particularly when older adults share rooms with others. Even in these situations, however, closing the door and pulling the bed curtain will increase the perception of privacy. In addition, nurses can take advantage of times when the roommate is out of the room, or it may be appropriate for the nurse to ask the roommate to allow private use of the room.

Eliminating distracting noises is also essential for establishing an environment that supports good communication. In institutional settings, closing a door to bedrooms not only increases privacy but also eliminates noises from the hallway. Before closing a door or bed curtains, however, the nurse should ask permission from the older person. Asking permission shows respect for the person's territory and may be particularly important when talking with people who become anxious when they are in closed spaces. If a radio or television is on, the nurse can ask permission to turn it off.

All the environmental modifications related to improving hearing and vision (discussed in Chapters 16 and 17, respectively) may be appropriate interventions for enhancing communication during a psychosocial assessment. One particularly easy and important consideration is the avoidance of

CULTURAL CONSIDERATIONS 13-1
Cultural influences on communication

Greetings

- Cultural groups that prefer to be greeted formally (e.g. Mr, Mrs, Ms) include Bosnians, Chinese, Filipino, Greeks, Italians, Japanese, Koreans, Russians, Turks.

Perception of personal space

- Cultural groups that are likely to have a closer range for personal distance include Arabs, Hispanics, Greeks, Japanese, Iranians, East Indian, Latin Americans and Middle Easterners.
- British, Canadians, Irish and Europeans are likely to require the most personal space.
- Men usually like to have a larger personal space than women.

Touch

- Cultural groups that are likely to be most comfortable with physical touch are Jews, French, Spanish, Italians, Indonesian, Māori, Pacific people and Indigenous Australians.
- Cultural groups that are likely to be uncomfortable with touch are British, Chinese, Germans, Hindus.
- Asians may believe that it is disrespectful to touch a person's head, because it is thought to be the source of their strength.
- Vietnamese view the human head as the seat of life and highly personal; they may feel anxious if touched on their head or shoulders; if any orifice of the head is invaded, they may fear these procedures could provide an escape for the essence of life.

Touch between men and women

- Cultural groups that do not allow physical touch between men and women outside the home include Bosnians, Middle Easterners, Somalis.
- In many Middle Eastern cultures, male healthcare providers may be prohibited from touching or examining part or all of the female body.
- In some Asian cultures, touching between persons of the same sex (but not between those of the opposite sex) is common and acceptable.

Eye contact

- People from some Asian, Hindi, Hmong, Indochinese and Middle Eastern cultures may consider direct eye contact impolite, immodest or aggressive, and they may avert their eyes when talking with healthcare professionals or, if female, when talking with men.
- Cultural groups that are likely to maintain steady eye contact during conversations include Arabs, Europeans, Greeks and Turks.
- Some cultural groups (e.g. Bosnians) maintain eye contact between women but not between men and women.

Facial expression

- Italians, Jews, Indigenous Australians and Māori smile readily and use many facial expressions along with words and gestures to communicate pain, happiness or displeasure.
- Irish, English and northern Europeans generally do not use facial expressions or other non-verbal expressions.

Source: Andrews, M. M. & Boyle, J. S. (2011). *Transcultural concepts in nursing care* (6th ed.). Philadelphia: Lippincott Williams & Wilkins; Purnell, L. D. (2009). *Guide to culturally competent health care* (2nd ed.). Philadelphia: F. A. Davis.

background glare. In hospital or long-term residential care settings, people often stand in front of a window when talking to an older adult/resident in a bed near the window. When the sun is shining or lights are reflected in the window, the background glare may interfere with the older adult's ability to see the person in front of the window. In these situations, simply closing the window curtains or sitting on the other side of the bed may significantly improve communication. In home settings, lack of lighting is a more common problem than glare. Asking the person's permission to turn on lights can be a very effective and easy way of improving communication.

After finishing the conversation, the nurse must remember to ask whether the person wants the environment returned to the way it was before. Turning on radios and televisions, replacing walkers and side rails, and leaving bed curtains and doors the way they were found shows respect for the person's preferences. Box 13-2 summarises verbal and non-verbal strategies to enhance communication with older adults and includes some strategies that are specific to communication during a psychosocial assessment.

A student's perspective

When I conducted a functional assessment, I found some communication techniques were therapeutic, whereas others were not.

One barrier that I encountered was the difficulty of understanding my client, because he did not have any teeth, and therefore, it was difficult for him to pronounce his words. Also, there was limited privacy, and the client seemed to be distracted by other people in the room. Another barrier was that I found myself looking down at the paper as opposed to maintaining consistent eye contact.

To combat these barriers, it would be important to provide more privacy and to minimise distractions. Also, because the client was difficult to understand, it would be important to ask for clarification about anything that was unclear. In addition, it is important to remember that a lack of eye contact is non-therapeutic.

*In order to improve on communication techniques, it is important to realise any barriers, identify ways to combat them, and think about what to do differently in the next situation. A helpful way to combat barriers is to remember the communication model of SOLER: **S**it facing the client, **O**bserve an open posture, **L**ean towards the client, **E**stablish and maintain intermittent eye contact, and **R**elax.*

Brittany D.

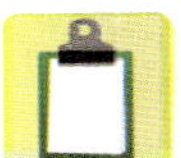

COGNITIVE AND PSYCHOSOCIAL ASSESSMENT

The **mental status assessment** is an organised approach to collecting data about a person's cognitive and psychosocial function. The mental status assessment collects information about the person's state of mind by observing and assessing a number of elements, including physical appearance, alertness and attention, motor function and praxis, social skills, response to interview, **orientation**, memory, speech and language characteristics, higher language skills, and executive function. Other aspects of psychosocial function, affective function, contact with reality and social supports, are discussed in separate sections.

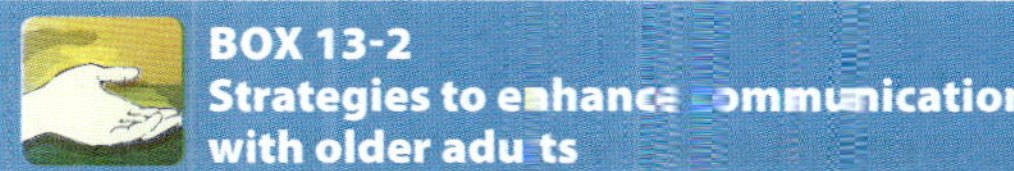

BOX 13-2
Strategies to enhance communication with older adults

General strategies

- Arrange for face-to-face positioning whenever possible.
- Ensure as much privacy as possible.
- Provide good lighting, and avoid background glare.
- Eliminate as much background noise as possible.
- Compensate as much as possible for vision or hearing impairments (e.g. make sure the person is using eyeglasses and hearing aid if appropriate).
- Begin contact with an exchange of names and, if appropriate, a handshake.
- Use culturally appropriate titles of respect, such as Mr, Mrs, Ms, Dr, Reverend, Elder, Bishop and so forth.
- Before calling a person by his or her first name, obtain permission or wait until you have been invited to use this familiar form of address. In some cultures, it is considered inappropriate or disrespectful for anyone but family or close friends to use first names.
- Be sure to pronounce names correctly. When in doubt, ask the older adult to say his or her name. Names that are difficult to pronounce may be written phonetically on the chart for later reference.
- Be aware of subtle linguistic messages that may convey bias or inequality.
- Avoid slang expressions such as "Pop", "Grandma", "dear", "chief" or similar terms, unless the older adult suggests that you do so.
- Never use slang, pejorative or derogatory terms to refer to ethnic, racial, religious or any other group (e.g. gays or lesbians).
- Use touch purposefully—provided that the person is open to this—to reinforce verbal messages and as a primary method of non-verbal communication.
- In all interactions, be aware of cultural differences that influence the perception and interpretation of verbal and non-verbal communication.

Strategies specific to a psychosocial assessment

- Explain the purpose of the psychosocial assessment in relation to a nursing goal; then, begin with questions about remote, non-threatening topics.
- Use open-ended questions and learn to use silence effectively and comfortably.
- Periodically clarify the messages.
- Maintain good eye contact, use attentive listening, and encourage the person to elaborate on information.
- Remain non-judgemental in your responses, but show appropriate empathy.
- Ask formal mental status questions, or the most threatening questions, towards the end of the interview.
- Gain the person's permission before asking formal assessment questions regarding memory and other cognitive abilities.

Mental status assessments are performed by various healthcare professionals, with each discipline specialising in various components. For example, psychiatrists are skilled in assessing affective and cognitive components, whereas social workers are skilled in assessing family relationship components. In relation to older adults, nurses assess the aspects of mental function that most directly influences the day-to-day activities of older adults; that is, cognition.

Cognitive assessment tools for older adults focus on measuring orientation, memory, higher language skills, executive function and praxis. There are a number of cognitive assessment tools that are used to screen for impaired cognition in the older adult.

The Mini-Mental State Examination (MMSE) has been widely used since the 1970s as a screening tool for cognitive impairment, but it takes at least 10 minutes to administer, and the formal tool must be purchased for use in any setting. Another concern about the MMSE is that it does not detect early stages of cognitive impairment, and scores are significantly influenced by such factors as education and culture (Pinto & Peters, 2009).

In recent years, healthcare professionals have recognised the need for an evidence-based screening tool that is widely available and easy to administer. The **Mini-Cog**, which consists of a three-item recall test and a simple clock-drawing test, is now widely used as a reliable and valid screening tool for cognitive impairment (Doerflinger, 2007). Another tool, the Abbreviated Mental Test Score (ATMS) is also useful to quickly screen cognition to establish if there are issues with memory and orientation. The ATMS contains 10 questions, and a score of less than 7 or 8 suggests cognitive impairment and that further assessment is required (see Figure 13-1).

Other tools have also been developed to address the lack of cultural sensitivity. The Rowland Universal Dementia Assessment Scale (RUDAS) and the Kimberley Indigenous Cognitive Assessment tool (KICA) are both validated cognitive screening tools for different cultures. The RUDAS has been developed to minimise the effects of culture and language on the assessment of cognition, while the KICA has been developed specifically for older Indigenous Australians living in rural and remote areas. Table 13-1 includes commonly used assessments to screen for cognitive impairment. The resources section at the end of this chapter includes materials that demonstrate the use of screening tools for assessing cognition. In addition, Chapters 14 and 15 address the assessment of other specific aspects of cognitive function related to pathological conditions. Screening tools are useful for identifying altered cognitive function, but they do not provide a broad or in-depth perspective on psychosocial function, as is presented in this chapter.

Physical appearance

Physical appearance is readily observed and reveals many aspects of psychosocial function. Clothing, grooming, cosmetics and hygiene provide many clues to psychological function, but they are only clues, and questions must be asked before any conclusions are drawn. For example, the

Question	Score 0 or 1
1. How old are you?	
2. What is the time (nearest hour)?	
3. Address for recall at the end of test – this should be repeated by the patient, e.g. 42 West Terrace	
4. What year is it?	
5. What is the name of this place?	
6. Can the patient recognise two relevant persons (e.g. nurse/doctor)	
7. What was the date of your birth?	
8. When was the second World War?	
9. Who is the present prime minister?	
10. Count down from 20 to 1 (no errors, no cues)	
TOTAL CORRECT	

FIGURE 13-1 Abbreviated Mental Test Score (ATMS). (Hodkinson, H. M. [1972]. Evaluation of a mental test score of mental impairment in the elderly. *Age Ageing, 1*, 233–238.)

TABLE 13-1 Tools commonly used to screen for cognitive impairment

Tool	Features
Abbreviated Mental Test (AMT)	Includes 10 items that assess memory and orientation
Folstein Mini-Mental State Examination (MMSE)	Assesses orientation, memory, attention, abilities to name, follow verbal and written commands, write a sentence spontaneously, and copy a complex polygon. Maximum of 30 points
Mini-Cog with Clock Drawing Test	Assesses cognitive function, memory, language comprehension, visual-motor skills, and executive function
Montreal Cognitive Assessment (MoCA)	Includes 30 items assessing short-term memory recall, visuospatial abilities, three-dimensional cube copy, and executive functions
Rowland Universal Dementia Assessment Scale (RUDAS)	Assesses memory, visuospatial orientation, praxis, visuo-construction drawing, judgement
Kimberley Indigenous Cognitive Assessment tool (KICA)	Has been developed for older Indigenous Australians living in rural and remote areas. Includes 18 questions
General Practitioner Assessment of Cognition (GPCOG)	Includes 5 items that assess short-term memory, orientation, visuo-spatial functioning, executive function
Psychogeriatric Assessment Scale (PAS)	Administered in long-term residential care in Australia
Modified Mini-Mental State (3Ms) Test	Developed in Australia; used instead of the MMSE

Source: Dementia Collaborative Research Centre (Australia). (2014). Assessment tools. Available at www.dementia-assessment.com.au/cognitive.

presence of body odour, poor hygiene and tattered clothing may be associated with any of the following conditions: depression, incontinence, impaired cognitive abilities, limited financial resources, overwhelming caregiving responsibilities, impaired vision or sense of smell, or lack of access to or inability to use bathing facilities

Observations about how clothing fits provide clues to weight changes (e.g. if clothing is too tight or loose, particularly in the waist). A history of weight loss may provide clues to depression, cognitive impairment, medical status or other barriers to adequate nutrition.

Observations about grooming practices, such as a woman's hair being dyed, can suggest any of the following questions about psychosocial function: Is this a reflection of positive or negative self-esteem? Does she want to appear younger than her age because she believes that old age is not as socially acceptable as youth? Does she want to deny her age because she associates old age with negative images? Similarly, an older woman's preference for wearing high-heeled shoes may be an indicator of self-image and of a desire to appear youthful. This is an important assessment issue because of the potential risk for falls and fractures.

Alertness and attention

Besides orientation, level of alertness is the mental status indicator that healthcare providers most frequently assess and document. Level of alertness is measured along a continuum, which includes stupor, drowsiness, somnolence, intermittent alertness/drowsiness and hyper alertness. An important aspect of assessing the person's level of alertness is the identification of any factors that can either increase or decrease alertness, with particular attention to those factors that can be addressed. For example, excessive daytime drowsiness can be associated with any of the following factors: medical problems, electrolyte imbalances, adverse medication effects (e.g. narcotics, anticholinergics, psychoactive medications), depression, dementia, excessive alcohol intake, or lack of sleep at night because of a variety of reasons (e.g. carer responsibilities).

In addition to assessing level of alertness, nurses also assess attention, which includes the ability to focus on a task and filter out distractions. Nurses can assess this mental status indicator by noting the older adult's ability to follow directions or respond appropriately to questions. When assessing responses, however, nurses need also to consider that information-processing skills may be affected not only by attention but also by other conditions such as cognitive or sensory impairments or pain.

Motor function and praxis

Assessment of motor function, which includes posture, movement and body language, can provide clues to broader aspects of psychosocial function. For example, stooped posture may be a clue to depression, whereas erect posture may indicate positive self-esteem. A shuffling, staggering or uncoordinated gait could indicate neurological deficits secondary to a disease process or adverse effects from alcohol or medications. Gait disturbances, as well as other abnormal movements, are possible signs of tardive dyskinesia or extrapyramidal symptoms. Evidence of tardive dyskinesia raises the question of past or present use of psychotropic medications (discussed in Chapter 8) and may give clues to mental health history.

Body language also provides clues to affective illnesses. Slouching and head hanging are common manifestations of withdrawal and depression. Poor eye contact, particularly looking at the floor, may be indicative of depression or the inability to answer questions, but nurses assess this in relation to cultural factors that influence the type and amount of eye contact considered to be appropriate.

Depression is usually associated with slowed psychomotor function, but excessive activity can be a clue to agitated depression. Agitation can be symptomatic of cognitive, affective, or other mental health disturbances; it may also be an adverse medication effect or an indicator of a physiological disturbance (e.g. dehydration, electrolyte imbalance) or a pathological condition (e.g. pneumonia, urinary tract infection), particularly in older adults with dementia.

Similarly, praxis performance is a part of the mental status assessment, because the ability to purposefully carry out simple motor skills is highly influenced by cognitive skills. Praxis performance requires basic motor ability, the cognitive knowledge of movement, and the ability to apply this knowledge into the motor function of moving. For example, observations of how someone navigates and avoids obstacles in the environment provide clues to the person's judgement and awareness of the environment. Nurses can assess psychomotor behaviours by asking the person to perform a simple activity of daily living (e.g. combing hair) and observing the person's ability to comprehend and perform the request.

Social skills

Assessment of social skills provides information about many aspects of psychosocial function. For example, friendly and cooperative people with good conversational skills may use social skills to hide their cognitive deficits, particularly if they are motivated to do so. By contrast, people with long-standing patterns of hostility, social isolation, poor social skills and a lack of ambition may be less motivated to perform well. In addition, people sometimes use the following social skills to cover up cognitive deficits: humour, evasiveness, leading the conversation, and making up answers to questions. Some older adults with dementia maintain very good social skills, even in the later stages of dementia when other skills have long since declined. Nurses also need to be aware of cultural factors that influence social skills and consider the cultural context of the relationship between the interviewer and the interviewee.

Response to the interview

The older adult's initial response to the interview, as well as changes that occur during the interview, can provide important assessment information. For example, an older adult may initially be very receptive to the questions but may become defensive or sarcastic when he or she is uncomfortable with the line of questioning. In addition, nurses need to assess the amount of time and effort expended in answering questions. This is particularly important when trying to differentiate between dementia and depression because cognitively impaired people may exert great effort in responding to questions, but depressed people may lack energy or motivation to respond. Two people may score the same on a formal mental status questionnaire, but one may miss the questions because of dementia and the other may miss them because of depression. When nurses suspect lack of motivation, they might clarify this by asking, "Is it that you don't know the answers, or that you just don't feel like answering the questions?"

Nurses are likely to encounter attitudes of hostility, resistance and defensiveness during the interview for a variety of reasons. A person who is depressed may be apathetic and may not want to expend the energy to answer the questions. A cognitively impaired person may be angry, hostile or defensive, particularly if he or she is trying to hide or deny cognitive deficits or does not understand the rationale for the questions. A person who has always been reclusive or suspicious may be unwilling to answer questions or may feel very defensive. Assessing the person's underlying attitude is as important as assessing the accuracy of responses to questions.

Assessing for **confabulation**, which is the process of making up information, is difficult when the nurse does not know the correct information. For example, questions about the person's place of birth or childhood experiences are not effective for assessing cognitive function unless the accuracy of the answers can be confirmed. **Circumstantiality**—another cover-up technique—involves the use of excessive details and roundabout answers in responding to questions.

Finally, nurses assess all information in relation to the person's usual personality traits. For example, highly sociable people might always use humour, whereas talkative people might naturally use circumstantiality. The use of humour and circumstantiality by people who are normally quiet and serious might indicate a great effort to cover up cognitive deficits. On the other hand, people who are normally quiet and withdrawn may be perceived falsely as being depressed. Finding out about the usual personality of an individual is difficult; however, nurses can ask a question such as, "Would you describe what you were like when you were 40 years old?" Family members and carers who have known the person for a long time are good sources of information about lifelong personality characteristics. Box 13-3 summarises guidelines for assessing physical appearance, motor function, social skills and responses to the interview in relation to the person's psychosocial function.

Orientation

Orientation to person, place and time is the indicator of mental status that is most frequently assessed and documented. Often, however, orientation is viewed as the primary indicator of cognitive function, rather than as one small piece of a larger picture. For example, the following questions are the gold standard for assessing orientation: "What is your name?"

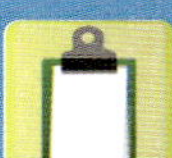

BOX 13-3
Guidelines for assessing physical appearance, motor function, social skills and response to the interview

Observations regarding physical appearance and motor function

- What is the person's apparent age in relation to his or her chronological age?
- How do the following factors reflect psychological function: hygiene, grooming, clothing, cosmetics?
- Does the person's physical appearance provide clues to dementia or depression or to other impairments of psychosocial function?
- What do the person's gait, posture and body language indicate about his or her psychological function?
- Is there any evidence of tardive dyskinesia or other adverse medication effects?
- How does the person manoeuvre in the environment, and what does this reflect regarding judgement, vision and other skills?

Observations regarding social skills and response to the interview

- What are the person's lifelong patterns of social skills, and how do these influence the assessment process?
- How do the person's social skills influence the interviewer's interpretation of other aspects of psychosocial function?
- Is the person motivated to answer questions?
- What is the person's attitude about the interview?
- If the person does not answer the questions, or gives incorrect answers, is it because of inability, cultural factors, or lack of motivation?
- Does the person use any of the following in an attempt to hide possible cognitive deficits: humour, sarcasm, avoidance, evasiveness, confabulation, circumstantiality, or leading the conversation?
- Does the person manifest any of the following characteristics: anger, hostility, resistance, defensiveness or suspiciousness?
- Do the person's underlying attitudes reflect his or her usual personality, or are they manifestations of cognitive or affective disturbances?

"Where are you?" and "What time is it?" Based on the accuracy of each answer, the person is then labelled as "oriented times one", "oriented times two", or "oriented times three". The superficial use of orientation questions and the subsequent labelling of the person as oriented times one, two or three, ignores important considerations, such as:

- Are any environmental clues available to the person to orient them to the time or place?
- Has the person been at the institution long enough to have learned its name?
- If the person cannot state the exact name of the facility, can they describe the type of facility it is or its general location?
- Do sociocultural factors influence the person's response to these questions?
- Can the person name familiar people, such as a spouse or children, even if they cannot state their own name?
- If the person cannot give specific names of other people, can they describe the correct role of the other person?
- If the person cannot state the exact time, can they give the general time of day?
- Does the person have medical problems that interfere with cognition?
- Is the person taking medications that can influence mental function?

A good assessment extends beyond the three classic questions and describes levels of orientation that are meaningful for the person in a particular setting. For example, the following description is far more useful than simply noting that the person is "oriented times one":

> *Mrs Smith could state her name but did not remember the name of this hospital. She could not give her daughter's name but was able to introduce her daughter to me without stating her name. She thought that the month was December because of the decorations in her room. She could not state the time because she did not have her watch with her, but she thought that it was afternoon because lunch had recently been served.*

If the nurse had used only the standard questions of "What is your name?" "Where are you?" and "What time is it?" Mrs Smith would be judged to be "oriented times one". Most healthcare providers, after reading the results of that assessment, would have assumed that Mrs Smith had serious cognitive impairment particularly if she were 85 years of age or older. Mrs Smith's actual responses, however, reflected various cognitive skills involved in organising information, making associations and using judgement. The more detailed description shows that Mrs Smith is probably quite a logical person who has not yet learned the name of the hospital and who might have some temporary memory impairment because of anxiety, medications or acute medical problems.

Memory

Formal **memory** testing assesses the person's memory of remote events, recent past events and immediate memory, which is further divided into retention, recall and recognition. Nurses can assess memory during regular conversations because all verbal communication depends to some degree on memory function. Nurses pay particular attention to assessing memory in relation to activities that are important in daily life, such as remembering to pay bills, take medications and shop for groceries. This assessment is made in relation to the expectations and demands of the person's usual environment. For example, if the person lives alone and manages finances independently the ability to pay bills is quite important. By contrast, if the person lives with a daughter and her family, remembering the birth dates of grandchildren may be an important memory task.

Assessment of memory is particularly challenging because memory complaints are common among older adults, but they are not necessarily based on actual deficits in memory function. For example, people who are depressed may perceive their memory skills as disproportionately impaired and may even exaggerate their deficits. In contrast to this situation, older adults with dementia may have little or no awareness of their memory deficits, or they may deny memory problems as a self-protective response. The question, "Do you ever have trouble remembering things?" may elicit a positive response, but the response is likely to tell you more about the person's perception of memory than about his or her actual memory function. Although this question may be quite useful in identifying any concerns that the older adult might have, it is not very useful in assessing memory function.

In addition to assessing memory directly, the nurse assesses the person's use of memory aids by posing a question such as, "Is there anything you do to help you remember appointments or other things?" Assessment of the extent to which the person depends on memory aids is useful in setting goals and planning for improved memory function. For example, if the person's memory function is barely adequate and is based heavily on memory aids, then the potential for further improvement is minimal. By contrast, if the person has some memory deficits but does not use any memory aids, then the potential for improvement increases. Observations about the use of memory aids also may provide clues to unacknowledged memory deficits. For example, if the person denies problems with memory, but repeatedly refers to written notes during an interview, then he or she may be compensating for an impaired memory. In this situation, the person is quite willing to use memory aids but is unwilling to acknowledge the need for such aids. Box 13-4 summarises guidelines for nursing assessment of orientation, alertness and memory and includes examples of appropriate questions for assessing the different types of memory.

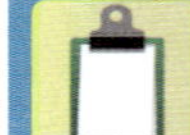

BOX 13-4
Guidelines for assessing orientation, alertness and memory

Interview questions to assess orientation

Note: Examples of direct questions are identified by quotation marks to distinguish them from the questions that are answered indirectly through observations.

- *Person:* "What is your name?" "What is your wife's name?" If names can't be given, can the person describe roles?
- *Place:* "What is your address?" "What is the name of this place?" "What kind of place is this?" "What is the name of this city?" "What is the name of this state?"
- *Time:* "What time is it?" "What day of the week is today?" "What month and date is it today?" "What season is it?"

Observations to assess alertness

- What is the person's level of alertness on the following continuum: hyper alert, alert, drowsy, somnolent, stuporous?
- Does the person's level of alertness fluctuate? If so, is there any pattern to the fluctuations?
- Are there physiological factors that might influence the person's level of alertness, such as medical conditions or effects of chemicals or medications?
- Are there psychosocial factors that might influence the person's level of alertness, such as anxiety, depression, night time caregiving responsibilities, or any other factor that might disrupt night time sleep?

Interview questions to assess memory

- *Remote events:* "Where were you born?" "Where did you go to high school?" "What was your first job?" "When were you married?"
- *Recent past events:* "Do you live with anyone?" "Do you have any grandchildren?" "What are the names of your grandchildren?" "When was the last time you went to the doctor?"
- *Immediate memory, retention:* State three unrelated words and ask the person to repeat the information, both immediately and again after 5 minutes.
- *Immediate memory, general grasp and recall:* Ask the person to read a short story and then to summarise the information presented in the story.
- *Immediate memory, recognition:* Ask a multiple-choice question and then ask the person to choose the correct answer.

Speech and language characteristics

Speech and language characteristics provide important information about many aspects of psychosocial function, such as the ability to organise and communicate thoughts. In addition, a good assessment of language skills helps the nurse to identify words and language patterns that are most appropriate for use with an older person. Because speech and language skills are highly dependent on cultural, educational and socioeconomic factors, it is important to consider these influences, particularly when assessing overseas-born older adults.

During any verbal interaction, nurses can assess all of the following speech and language characteristics: pace, tone, volume, articulation, ability to organise and communicate thoughts, and any abnormal speech or language characteristics. The following examples describe some common speech variations and associated conditions:

- *Rapid pace:* anxiety, agitation or mental illness
- *Slow-paced or excessively brief verbal communication:* depression, cognitive impairment or simple cautiousness
- *Tone of voice:* indirectly expressed feelings such as anger, hostility and resentment
- *Hypophonia* (i.e. an abnormally low volume of speech): depression, physical illness, low self-esteem, or long-standing speech habits
- *Abnormally loud volume:* impaired hearing or long-term experience communicating with someone who is hearing impaired
- *Poor articulation or slurred speech:* hearing impairment, ill-fitting dentures, lack of teeth or dentures, nervous system disorder, effects of alcohol or medications
- *Phonemic errors* (i.e. incorrect pronunciation): hearing impairment, cognitive deficits, educational and cultural influences

- *Semantic errors* (i.e. misinterpretation of the meaning of words): hearing impairment, cognitive deficits
- *Neologisms* (i.e. self-created and meaningless words): dementia, psychotic disorder (e.g. schizophrenia), repetition of a word that was not heard accurately
- *Incoherent speech:* dementia, aphasia, psychiatric disorders, alcohol or medication effects
- *Perseveration* (i.e. a repetitive or stuttering pattern of verbal or written communication) and *agnosia* (i.e. difficulty finding the correct words or the inability to name an object accurately, particularly if it is unfamiliar): dementia.

Aphasia is a communication disorder that is associated with neurological conditions such as stroke or vascular dementia. Expressive aphasia occurs when comprehension abilities are not affected but word retrieval or word-finding abilities are impaired. Receptive aphasia occurs when verbal and comprehension abilities are impaired but some language skills are retained. Global aphasia, which is a combination of receptive and expressive aphasia, results from more extensive neurological damage and is manifested by inconsistent and poorly controlled language skills. Therefore nurses need to be cognisant with the impact upon speech and language of an older adult's medical diagnosis and medical treatment regime.

Calculation and higher language skills

Reading, writing, spelling and arithmetic are *calculation* and higher language skills that are assessed as indicators of cognition. As with assessments of other indicators, the person's education, occupation and other influencing factors must be considered. Nurses can informally assess these skills in relation to how the person performs important daily activities. For example, for an older adult who lives alone, an assessment of the ability to pay utility bills and use money to purchase groceries is more valuable than a measurement of mathematical skills using a psychometric test. Likewise, a person's ability to read the daily newspaper or the markings on a thermostat may be a more valid gauge of functional ability than a score on a formal reading test.

Nurses can use written health education materials to assess reading and comprehension skills informally, and this method serves a practical purpose. For example, when collecting a urine sample, the nurse can give the person a list of instructions and ask him or her to read the instructions aloud. An observation of how well the person comprehends the instructions provides an assessment of reading skills that are important in daily life. Another opportunity for assessing reading comprehension may arise if the nurse observes that an older adult has a newspaper nearby. A non-threatening question such as, "What's new in the paper today?" can provide information about the person's interests in outside events and his or her ability to comprehend and remember written information.

Nurses can assess writing and other higher language skills by observing older adults during interactions that pertain to their care. For example, nurses can observe the way an older adult signs his or her name on documents such as permission forms. Nurses can also observe the older adult during the performance of more complex tasks such as compiling a written medication list or a list of questions to discuss with the primary care provider. Difficulty with writing skills is a common sign of early stages of dementia.

With traditional psychometric testing, calculation is measured with the "7s" test: the person is asked to subtract 7 from 100 and to continue subtracting 7s. Because this test is highly influenced by level of education, it is not necessarily the most appropriate test for older adults. It may be better to ask the older person to add 3 plus 3 and to continue adding 3s. Older adults who are depressed may not answer correctly because they do not want to expend the energy to calculate serial sevens. Older adults who have dementia may be able to perform well on this task if they try hard and if they previously had highly developed mathematical skills. Box 13-5 summarises the considerations that are important in assessing speech characteristics and calculation and higher language skills.

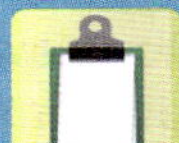

BOX 13-5
Guidelines for assessing speech characteristics and calculation and higher language skills

Observations to assess speech characteristics

- Is the pace of speech normal, slow or fast?
- Is the tone of voice suggestive of underlying feelings, such as anger, hostility or resentment?
- Is the volume abnormally soft or loud?
- Do the sentences flow coherently and smoothly?
- Is there evidence of any problem with integrating speech sounds into words (e.g. neologisms or phonemic or semantic errors)?
- Do any of the following factors affect the person's speech: dry mouth, poorly fitting dentures, absence of teeth or dentures, alcohol or medication effects, or neurological or other pathological processes?
- Does the person exhibit any of the following: agnosia; perseveration; or expressive, receptive or global aphasia?

Observations to assess calculation and higher language skills

- What is the person's ability to comprehend written materials encountered in the course of routine activities, such as the daily newspaper or instructions for medications?
- What is the quality of the person's handwriting (e.g. his or her signature)?
- Is the person able to perform mathematical computations necessary for daily activities?

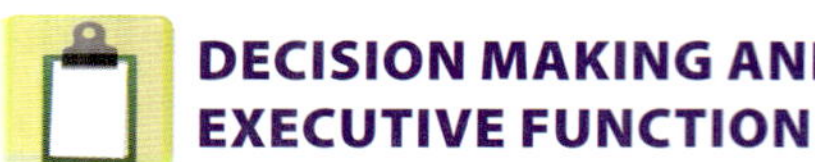

DECISION MAKING AND EXECUTIVE FUNCTION

The assessment of executive functioning is important to determine the ability of the older adults to participate in **decision making**. Decision making is one of the most important and complex of all cognitive abilities. It is also an important aspect of psychosocial function because all legally competent older adults, including those with dementia, have the right to be involved in decisions about their care.

Determination of competency is a complex issue, with many implications not only for older adults and their families and carers, but also for healthcare professionals (as discussed in Chapter 9). As an integral part of psychosocial nursing care, nurses assess cognitive skills—including **insight**, learning, memory, reasoning, judgement, problem solving and **abstract thinking**—that are involved with decision making.

An assessment tool that focuses specifically on decision making has not yet been developed; therefore nurses need to assess this aspect of psychosocial function by observing the abilities of older adults to solve problems during the course of daily activities and by asking pertinent assessment questions.

Abstract thinking is difficult to assess because it is strongly influenced by other factors such as education, personality and affective state. People who are very anxious or depressed may lack the attention or motivation required to respond to the questions typically used for the assessment of abstract thinking patterns. Similarity questions such as, "How are apples and oranges alike?" or "How are a table and chair alike?" are used to assess the person's ability to think abstractly.

During an interview, opportunities for assessing abstract thinking may arise, and the nurse listens for clues to the person's level of abstract versus concrete thinking. The following example illustrates one older adult's concrete thinking pattern:

Nurse: How did you feel about having to move from your home to live with your daughter and her family here?
Mr L.: I don't know; how would you feel?
Nurse: I'm not sure how I'd feel; that's never happened to me. I'm not in your shoes.
Mr L.: Well, here, put them on (stated emphatically while taking off his shoes to give to the nurse).

Nurses assess problem-solving abilities through observations about how older adults meet their needs in a particular situation. For instance, nurses can observe the ways older adults use call lights to meet their needs when confined to a bed or the ways in which they deal with complex decisions related to discharge planning.

Similarly, a very important problem-solving task for an older adult who lives alone may be meeting basic safety needs. Therefore, questions such as, "What would you do if you fell at home and could not get up?" or "What would you do if you woke up and smelled smoke?" might be an appropriate way of assessing judgement related to safety.

For an older adult who lives in a nursing home, a very important but complex problem-solving task may involve dealing with a disruptive roommate. In this situation, the answer to a question such as, "What would you do if your roommate started taking your belongings?" might provide the most pertinent information for assessing problem-solving skills.

Insight is the ability to understand the significance of the present situation. This skill is an important component of the problem-solving process, because it establishes a basis for planning care. Insight is influenced by psychosocial factors such as feelings, personality and coping mechanisms. *Denial* is a defence mechanism that is often used to protect oneself from unpleasant realities; the stronger the denial is, the more limited the insight is. It is important to assess for denial because, if the person refuses to acknowledge that he or she has a condition, it will be very difficult to plan interventions. The nursing assessment of insight concentrates on those areas of function that are pertinent to the care plan. For example, in assessing the insight of an older adult who has been brought to the hospital with malnutrition and uncontrolled hypertension, the nurse may ask such questions as the following:

- Why did your daughter bring you to the hospital?
- How do you manage with supermarket shopping and getting your meals?
- Do you take any medications?
- What are the medications for?
- What kinds of things does your daughter do for you?
- What kind of help do you think you might need when you leave the hospital?

Answers will facilitate care planning because they help the nurse assess the person's understanding of the present situation.

When the person has little or no understanding of his or her health situation, the nurse tries to identify the factors that interfere with insight. Insight may be absent or limited because of depression and feelings of hopelessness, lack of information about the medication regimen, denial of a reality that is too threatening, inability to remember information, or fear of losing independence.

An essential component of discharge planning is identifying both the level of insight and the factors that interfere with insight. In addition, the nurse attempts to identify factors that may improve the person's insight. If insight is lacking because of denial that stems from exaggerated fears, then alleviating the fears may facilitate insight.

Assessing executive function abilities in conjunction with determining an older person's capacity to safely and reliably plan and carry out activities related to daily living is important. Essential elements of executive function are abstract thinking and planning, initiating, sequencing, monitoring and stopping complex behaviour (Kennedy & Smyth, 2008). Cognitive abilities that are associated with executive function include insight, judgement, reasoning, attention, concept formation, cognitive flexibility, problem solving, abstraction and self-evaluation.

Executive dysfunction (also called executive function deficits) begins during the earliest stages of dementia and can be present even before memory problems are evident, particularly when the pathological processes affect the frontal lobes. The indicators of executive function deficits include diminished mental flexibility, limited ability to think abstractly, difficulty with problem solving, decline in ability to conceptualise, diminished ability to adapt to new situations, and difficulty shifting thought processes from one idea to another. People with executive cognitive dysfunction may perform well on the MMSE or other similar assessment tools but still not be able to perform essential daily activities safely and independently. Kennedy and Smyth (2008) have described and demonstrated the use of easy-to-use and evidence-based screening tools for executive dysfunction in article and video form (see the resources section towards the end of this chapter for information on accessing these online tools).

Because it is important to assess executive skills in relation to a previous level of function, it may be necessary to ask family members or the person being assessed if they have noticed changes in these abilities in recent years. When families or healthcare providers have serious questions about the decision-making abilities of an older person, or when a major decision must be made and there is disagreement about it, a more comprehensive assessment using neuropsychological tests may be warranted. For example, if a cognitively impaired older person expresses a strong desire to live alone but family members question the person's ability to function safely, a comprehensive geriatric assessment with emphasis on decision making and executive function skills will provide useful information.

AFFECTIVE FUNCTION

A person's **affect** refers to his or her mood, emotions and expressions of emotions. Happiness and sadness are feelings commonly associated with affective states, but all of the following have been identified as *primary affects* (also called *discrete emotions*): joy, awe, hope, fear, pain, rage, pride, guilt, shame, anger, regret, relief, hatred, surprise, interest, boredom, elation, confusion, jealousy, depression, suspicion, frustration, anxiety, bewilderment, amorousness and lack of feelings.

The components of affective state that are reviewed in this section are general mood, anxiety, self-esteem, depression and happiness. These five aspects were selected for the following reasons:

- An assessment of general mood assists the nurse in determining appropriate goals based on the person's usual affective state.
- Anxiety is a common factor in older adults that can often be alleviated or minimised through nursing interventions.
- Self-esteem is a major determinant of feelings, particularly depression and happiness.
- Self-esteem is particularly important because older adults can face many conditions that threaten their self-esteem.

Research into depression and happiness provides sound evidence for nursing practice.

Nursing interventions are directed towards all of these affective components to improve the quality of life of older adults.

Guidelines for assessing affective function

Affective function is assessed both quantitatively and qualitatively in relation to expectations about acceptable expressions of emotions. For example, people are expected to show some expression of sadness when talking about sad events. However, when the person's expression of feelings is not consistent with the external event, the affect is considered inappropriate. Affect is also assessed in relation to the personal meaning and the nearness in time of an event. People are expected to show greater feelings of sadness in response to tragic news than in response to neutral events. Likewise, people are expected to show a deeper affective response soon after experiencing a sad event than they would years after the event occurred.

The *depth and duration of affect*, which are important considerations in differentiating between dementia and depression in older adults, are also assessed. The affect of depressed people is generally sad and negativistic and is not influenced by external circumstances. By contrast, the affect of people who have dementia fluctuates more and changes in response to distractions. Emotional lability (i.e. emotional instability or fluctuation) is a characteristic of vascular dementia that is common in people who have had strokes

Non-verbal behaviours, such as those indicating anxiety, sadness and happiness, provide important information about a person's affective state that the person may not offer verbally. For example, despite a person's denial of feeling sad, he or she may exhibit the following non-verbal cues: crying, slouching over, looking at the ground, and having a mournful facial expression. The nurse uses this information as the basis for a leading comment such as, "You look like you're feeling sad."

Expressions of emotions are strongly determined by cultural norms and personality characteristics. In most Western societies, crying is more acceptable for women and children than for men and older boys, and showing anger and rage is more acceptable for men than for women.

Cultural expectations also influence the way a person expresses feelings in certain circumstances. For example, a person may be expected to cry and loudly proclaim mournful feelings at a funeral but may be prohibited from expressing any feelings in front of strangers or in a public place such as a hospital. Because some emotions such as anger or depression are viewed as less acceptable than others, such as happiness, people learn to deny and hide feelings that may be judged as unacceptable. Older adults, particularly, may have learned that certain feelings should not be expressed directly or verbally. It is particularly important to observe for any indirect or non-verbal clues of anger, depression and other less socially acceptable feelings.

In assessing the affective state of older adults, it is important to identify the terminology that is most acceptable. Many people will not admit to feeling anxious or depressed because they associate these terms with a serious mental illness or with a socially unacceptable state. Therefore, the nurse begins the assessment of affective state by focusing on feelings that are viewed positively or neutrally. If the person initiates the topic of feeling anxious or depressed, the nurse responds to those feelings and pursues a related line of questioning. However, in most circumstances it is best to begin with open-ended questions. A simple question such as, "How are you feeling today?" when asked with sincerity, is a familiar and comfortable way of eliciting information.

Mood

Mood is closely associated with emotions but differs in that it is more pervasive, less intense, and longer lasting. People are usually quite comfortable describing their mood as either bad or good and are more likely to offer information about their mood than their emotions. During a mental status examination, a question such as, "How would you describe your usual mood?" may be perceived as less threatening than the question, "How do you feel most of the time?" Non-verbal behaviours provide many clues about a person's mood and may be more accurate than verbal responses as an indicator of affective state. Joy, anger, anxiety, sadness, happiness and depression are examples of moods that are expressed in non-verbal behaviours in everyday life by most people.

Anxiety

Anxiety is defined as a feeling of distress, subjectively experienced as fear or worry and objectively expressed through autonomic and central nervous system responses. Moderate anxiety is beneficial because it motivates protective behaviours, but extreme anxiety is detrimental because it channels personal energy into defensive behaviours. Therefore, it is important to assess the degree of anxiety and the extent to which the anxiety is beneficial or detrimental.

In recent years, increasing attention has been given to **generalised anxiety disorder (GAD)**, which has a significant negative impact on health, functioning and quality of life for many older adults. GAD is characterised by persistent, excessive and uncontrollable worry accompanied by physiological symptoms such as fatigue, irritability, restlessness, sleep disturbances, difficulty concentrating and pervasive cognitive dysfunction (Allgulander, 2009). Despite the strong correlation between physical symptoms and emotional distress, older adults may not recognise the connection, and GAD is often unrecognised by healthcare providers (Calleo et al., 2009) (see Figure 13-2).

In assessing anxiety, nurses must identify the terminology that is most acceptable to the older adult. Words like "worries" and "concerns" are readily understood and usually elicit responses about sources of anxiety. Older adults also often use the phrases "nerve trouble" or "trouble with my nerves" in reference to anxiety states. Asking appropriate questions may elicit a response filled with information about their sources of anxiety.

Nurses observe for non-verbal manifestations of anxiety to supplement the information obtained from verbal communication. In any adult, anxiety may be manifested in the following non-verbal ways: pacing, shakiness, restlessness, irritability, fidgeting, diaphoresis, tachycardia, hyperventilation, dry mouth, voice changes, smoking habits, urinary frequency, increased muscle tension, poor eye contact, poor attention span, inability to sit still, changes in eating patterns, rapid or disconnected speech, or repetitive motions of facial muscles or any extremities. Although any of these indicators may be observed in older adults, the presence of mobility limitations or pathological conditions can interfere with some of them. For example, older adults who are confined to bed cannot pace but may experience subtle changes in eating or sleeping patterns because of anxiety. Older adults may be reluctant to report that they are worried or anxious; instead, they may focus on physiological symptoms (e.g. pain, fatigue, anorexia, insomnia or stomach distress).

Because anxiety is always a response to real or perceived threats, the nurse tries to identify sources of anxiety, even though they may not be readily apparent. Potential sources of anxiety (i.e. real or perceived threats) include health, assets, values, environment, self-concept, role function, needs fulfilment, goal achievement, personal relationships and sense of security.

Older adults do not always recognise the source of their anxiety because it may arise from unconscious conflicts, unacknowledged fears, maturational crises or developmental challenges. Even when people recognise the source of anxiety, they may be reluctant to discuss it, or they may refer to the threat only indirectly. For example, an older adult may have the perception that other people have the power to "put them away" in a nursing home simply because of slight memory impairment. If the person knows other older adults who have been admitted unwillingly to a nursing home, this fear may be exacerbated.

Further anxiety may arise from the person's fear of discussing the subject because of the perception that

Please answer the items according to how you've felt in the last week.

Check the column under Agree if you mostly agree that the item describes you;
check the column under Disagree if you mostly disagree that the item describes you.

	Agree	Disagree
* I worry a lot of the time.		
I find it difficult to make a decision.		
I often feel jumpy.		
I find it hard to relax.		
I often cannot enjoy things because of my worries.		
* Little things bother me a lot.		
I often feel like I have butterflies in my stomach.		
* I think of myself as a worrier.		
I can't help worrying about even trivial things.		
* I often feel nervous.		
* My own thoughts often make me anxious.		
I get an upset stomach due to my worrying.		
I think of myself as a nervous person.		
I always anticipate the worst will happen.		
I often feel shaky inside.		
I think that my worries interfere with my life.		
My worries often overwhelm me.		
I sometimes feel a great knot in my stomach.		
I miss out on things because I worry too much.		
I often feel upset.		

A score of 9 or more checks in the AGREE column indicates the need for further evaluation.

Items preceded by * are the ones most strongly associated with anxiety in older adults.

FIGURE 13-2 The Geriatric Anxiety Inventory. (Adapted with permission of UniQuest Pty Limited and the creators, Prof. Nancy Pachana and Prof. Gerard Byrne. Original GAI reference: Pachana, N. A., Byrne, G. J., Siddle, H., Koloski, N., Harley, E. & Arnold, E. [2007]. Development and validation of the Geriatric Anxiety Inventory. *International Psychogeriatrics*, 19, 103–114. © The University of Queensland 2010. Copyright in the Geriatric Anxiety Inventory is the property of The University of Queensland. All content is protected by Australian copyright law and, by virtue of international treaties, equivalent copyright laws in other countries. The Geriatric Anxiety Inventory may not be reproduced or copied without the prior written permission of UniQuest Pty Limited.)

initiating the topic might precipitate actions leading to nursing home admission. Rather than directly talking about the fears, the person may provide vague clues, for instance: "I felt so sorry for Maggie when her son put her in the nursing home."

Nurses must phrase questions aimed at identifying sources of anxiety in the least threatening way possible. When older adults express concerns about other older people, it may be appropriate to ask questions aimed at determining whether they have the same worries about themselves. For example, in response to the statement, "I felt so sorry for Maggie", the nurse might ask, "Do you ever worry that you'll have to go to a nursing home?" Nurses use open-ended questions that allow for a wide range of answers to identify sources of anxiety that might not otherwise be revealed. For example, nurses in institutional settings can ask, "What is your biggest worry about going home?" or "Do you have any worries about how you'll manage at home after you leave here?" In home settings, the nurse might ask an even broader question such as, "Do you have any concerns about the future?" or "What kinds of things do you worry about?" Answers to these questions are usually filled with clues to sources of anxiety and can lead to many additional questions.

Anxiety can be caused or exacerbated by physiological conditions that arise from disease processes or the adverse effects of bioactive substances, as in the following examples:

- Herbs, caffeine, nicotine and medications (both prescription and over-the-counter) can cause physiological anxiety reactions.
- Anxiety may be associated with withdrawal from nicotine or alcohol.
- Pathological processes that diminish cerebral oxygen, such as pulmonary or cardiovascular diseases, can cause anxiety reactions.
- Endocrine disorders, such as hyperthyroidism, may be manifested primarily by anxiety or other psychosocial symptoms.
- People with dementia may show signs of excessive anxiety when they are experiencing pain or physical discomfort, particularly if their verbal communication skills are impaired.
- Pacing is a commonly observed manifestation of anxiety in ambulatory older adults who have dementia.

Therefore, information about medical conditions and the older adult's use of herbs, caffeine and medications is an essential component of the anxiety assessment.

Medications that affect the central or autonomic nervous systems may precipitate or exacerbate anxiety. **Akathisia** is a frequently reported extrapyramidal effect of some neuroleptics that may subjectively or objectively be interpreted as anxiety. Akathisia is defined as an inner sense of restlessness that is worsened by inactivity and is manifested by motor restlessness. It is more common in women and older adults, and it can occur any time during the course of treatment with psychotropic medications. Therefore, if an older adult who is taking neuroleptics complains of certain feelings, such as "shaking on the inside", the possibility of adverse medication effects must be considered as a cause.

In addition to identifying sources and manifestations of anxiety, it is important to identify appropriate methods for reducing anxiety. Even if the sources of anxiety are not identified or cannot be changed, the experience of anxiety can be addressed through self-care interventions that improve coping. To this end, the nurse asks questions about usual coping methods. Questions such as "What do you do when you have trouble with your nerves?" or "What do you find helpful when your nerves are bad?" can pave the way for a discussion about coping with anxiety. If the person cannot identify effective coping mechanisms, the nurse offers suggestions in a non-judgemental way and assesses the person's response to them. For example, nurses can ask any of the following questions:

- "Does it help to talk to someone about your worries?"
- "Have you ever tried any relaxation methods when you are nervous?"
- "Do you find that taking a walk helps you when your nerves are bad?"

Evidence-based practice 13-1 summarises guidelines on detection and assessment of late-life anxiety, published by the University of Iowa College of Nursing.

Self-esteem

Self-esteem cannot be measured numerically, but nurses can observe for verbal and non-verbal indicators. For example, a statement such as, "You're wasting your time on me; you have more important things to do" is a clue to poor self-esteem. Non-verbal indicators of self-esteem include the way people dress, care for themselves, and present themselves to others.

Although interpreting behaviours in relation to self-esteem must be done with caution, the following behaviours

EVIDENCE-BASED PRACTICE 13-1
Detection and assessment of late-life anxiety

Statement of the problem

- Anxiety—defined as apprehensive expectation and excessive worry—ranges from normal reactions to everyday stress, to disabling levels, which are categorised as anxiety disorders.
- More than half of community-dwelling older adults report anxiety symptoms.
- Accurate assessment, referral and treatment are necessary because anxiety is associated with functional disability, reduced quality of life, lower life satisfactions, impaired physical and social function, and feelings of worthlessness.
- The following factors can interfere with recognition of anxiety in older adults: (1) stigma associated with mental illness, (2) older adults may focus on somatic symptoms and complaints, (3) manifestations may be considered normal consequences of ageing, (4) underreporting and denial of problems are common among older adults; (5) inability to determine the degree to which worry is associated with realistic concerns.
- Factors consistently associated with increased risk of late-life anxiety include physical illness, psychosocial stress, depression, cognitive impairment, and personal characteristics (i.e. female gender, advanced age, lower socioeconomic status, external locus of control, family history of anxiety disorder, alcohol or drug use).

Recommendations for nursing assessment

- Nurses should assess for anxiety in any older adult who expresses worry or fear and who is at risk due to physical illness, recent psychosocial stress, depression, cognitive impairment, or somatic complaints that are not associated with an identifiable underlying cause.
- Nurses can use such screening tools as the Geriatric Anxiety Inventory, Short Anxiety Screening Test, Hospital Anxiety and Depression Scale, or the Rating Anxiety in Dementia Scale.

Adapted from Smith, M., Ingram, T. & Brighton, V. (2009). Evidence-based practice guideline: Detection and assessment of late-life anxiety. University of Iowa Gerontological Nursing Interventions Research Center. Available at National Guideline Clearinghouse, www.guideline.gov.

may be associated with low self-esteem: rigidity, procrastination, unnecessary apologies, lack of confidence, expectations of failure, exaggeration of deficits, disappointment in self, self-destructive behaviours, constant approval seeking, overemphasis on weaknesses, inability to accept compliments, minimising personal capabilities, disregarding one's own opinions, inability to form close relationships, inability to accept help from others, and inability to say "no" when appropriate. It may be acceptable to ask some questions, however, particularly about the person's perception of positive qualities.

In addition to observing for indicators of self-esteem, nurses can ask questions that give insight into the older adult's self-perceptions. For example, a question such as, "What is the quality in yourself that other people admire the most?" is non-threatening. Moreover, this kind of question helps identify strengths that can be supported, and it provides clues to self-esteem. Nursing assessment is also directed towards identifying actual and potential threats to self-esteem so they can be addressed through interventions, as discussed in Chapter 12.

Because self-esteem is influenced by the person's perception of the opinions held by significant others, it is important to identify who the significant others are for a particular person (e.g. peers; spouse or partner; authority figures; and people in the work, church and social environments).

Culture often defines who adopts the role of the significant other. Some Chinese older adults, for example, expect their oldest son to look after their affairs and make key decisions about their health and well-being. Widows in some Middle Eastern and African cultures expect one of their husband's brothers to take care of them—an arrangement that fosters social and economic security for women who have lost a spouse. Being cared for by a family member (rather than by strangers) enhances self-esteem for older adults from all cultural backgrounds and increases the likelihood that their needs will be met as they age.

Depression

Depression is discussed as a general component of a psychosocial assessment in this chapter, and it is covered more comprehensively as an aspect of impaired psychosocial function in Chapter 15. Nurses can apply information in this chapter when assessing all older adults and use the information in Chapter 15 as a guide to assessing and caring for older adults who are depressed.

Nurses assess for depression by identifying verbal and non-verbal cues. Asking direct questions such as "Are you depressed?" is usually not effective in eliciting information because people may associate the word "depressed" with states of overwhelming grief. Older adults may be more comfortable responding to questions about whether they feel "sad", "blue" or "down in the dumps". Therefore, unless the older adult uses the term "depressed" to describe his or her feelings, other terminology is more likely to elicit an accurate response. As with other aspects of the mental status assessment, it is best to start with such open-ended questions as, "How are you feeling right now?" or "How have you been feeling this week?"

One of the purposes of an assessment of depression is to identify the person's usual patterns of coping with losses. For this reason, nurses encourage older adults to express their feelings about significant changes in their lives. For instance, when an older adult talks about a change that might be experienced as a loss, nurses can ask non-threatening questions that might lead to a discussion of their feelings, such as: "What's it like to live alone after 50 years of being married?" "How is life different since your friend moved away?" "Are there people you miss seeing since you retired?" "Are there any activities you miss doing since you no longer drive?"

If the questions do not elicit information about feelings, the nurse can comment on specific feelings that the person is likely to be experiencing. For example, a remark such as, "It seems like it would be pretty sad and lonely being here all by yourself after 55 years of marriage" allows the person to agree, disagree or offer an alternative to the suggested feelings. Be aware that, for older adults from some Asian and other cultures, expressing one's emotions overtly or discussing them with a stranger may be considered inappropriate.

Happiness and well-being

Happiness in relation to ageing is often equated with morale, wellness, contentment, well-being, life satisfaction, successful ageing, quality of life and "the good life". A recent literature review identified the following dimensions of well-being that can be addressed by healthcare professionals in relation to ageing (Kiefer, 2008):

- Staying active
- Interacting with peers
- Feeling financially secure
- Having a sense of personal autonomy
- Setting personal goals and challenges
- Having positive social interactions
- Developing effective coping strategies
- Participating in exercise and sports activities
- Actively contributing to society through paid or volunteer work.

Although nurses cannot address all these dimensions in a psychosocial assessment, they can include a few questions about happiness and well-being so that wellness can be promoted through nursing interventions. Psychologists sometimes use the following question to assess happiness: "Taking all things together how would you say things are today: would you say you're very happy, pretty happy, or not too happy these days?"

Nurses can ask a similar question such as, "If you had to rate your present level of happiness on a scale of 0% to 100%, what rating would you give it?" Nurses can use the

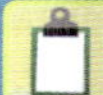

BOX 13-6
Guidelines for assessing affective function

General affective function

- Are the quantity and quality of emotions appropriate for the objective reality?
- What is the depth and duration of emotions regarding a particular event?
- What are the non-verbal cues to the person's affective state?
- How do sociocultural or environmental factors influence the person's expression of emotions?
- What terminology is acceptable to this person, particularly with regard to feelings such as anger, anxiety and depression?
- Does the person have any pets, or has he or she lost any pets?

Observations and questions to assess mood

- What is the person's usual affective state?
- What are the non-verbal indicators of the person's mood?

Observations and questions to assess anxiety

- What are the non-verbal indicators of anxiety?
- What real or perceived threats are present that might be sources of anxiety for the person?
- Might any of the following factors be contributing to the person's anxiety: caffeine, pathological conditions, medications, herbs, or interventions by folk or Indigenous healers that act on the central or autonomic nervous systems?
- What methods of coping has the person tried, and what have been the effects of these interventions?
- "What kinds of things do you worry about?"
- "Do you have any worries you'd be willing to discuss with me?"
- "Do you ever have trouble with your nerves?"

Observations and questions to assess self-esteem

- What verbal and non-verbal clues to self-esteem can be detected?
- What are the factors that influence self-esteem for this person?
- Does the environment present any real or potential threat to self-esteem?
- How are my actions as a nurse influencing the self-esteem of the older adults to whom I relate?
- Are carer attitudes, such as infantilisation, elderspeak or the promotion of unnecessary dependence, affecting the person's self-esteem?

Observations and questions to assess depression

- What are the verbal and non-verbal clues to depression?
- "Do you ever feel blue or down in the dumps?"
- "How has your life changed since your husband died?"
- "What do you miss the most since you moved from your family home?"

Observations and questions to assess happiness and life satisfaction

- How is the person's happiness and life satisfaction influenced by the following: functional abilities, personal relationships and socioeconomic resources?
- "On a scale of 0% to 100%, how happy would you say you are right now?"
- "If you could change one thing to increase your happiness rating, what would it be?"

person's response as a base for additional questions such as, "What would have to change to increase the rating by 10%?" "What kinds of things interfere with your happiness?" "If you could change one thing to be happier, what would it be?"

Older adults will usually respond to these questions in a realistic manner, and their answers will provide information for establishing appropriate goals. Box 13-6 summarises the considerations involved in assessing affective function in older adults.

CONTACT WITH REALITY

Although a certain amount of fantasy is acceptable in everyday patterns of thinking, people are expected to remain in contact with the world around them and respond appropriately to the same realities that others perceive. People lose contact with reality for numerous reasons, including dementia, delirium, psychotic disorders, and a transient denial of a threatening reality. Many of these underlying conditions are treatable; however, when older adults lose contact with reality, they are likely to be labelled as "senile". Because of stereotypes about older people, as well as the broad array of potential causes for loss of contact with reality, the assessment of an older person's contact with reality is particularly challenging.

Loss of contact with reality includes a wide range of behaviours ranging from simple and harmless misperceptions of reality to unyielding **delusions** or disturbing **hallucinations**. For example, people who are in the early stages of dementia may actively conceal or refuse to acknowledge memory deficits, and those in later stages of dementia may experience delusions that lead to behaviours that are inappropriate, or even dangerous. For instance, if someone believes that his belongings have been stolen, he may report the theft to the police or insist on going out to look for the robber. Three types of loss of contact with reality are delusions, hallucinations and **illusions**, which are defined as follows:

- *Delusions:* Fixed false beliefs that have little or no basis in reality and cannot be corrected by appealing to reason.
- *Hallucinations:* Sensory experiences that have no basis in an external stimulus. Visual and auditory hallucinations are most common, but tactile, olfactory and gustatory hallucinations also occur.
- *Illusions:* Misperceptions of an external stimulus. They may be mistaken for hallucinations, but differ in having some basis in reality, whereas hallucinations do not.

Just as a fever is one manifestation of a physical illness, loss of contact with reality is one manifestation of a mental health imbalance. For example, common manifestations of

TABLE 13-2 Distinguishing features of delusions, hallucinations and illusions

Underlying cause	Accompanying manifestations	Characteristics
Delirium	Diminished attention, a clouded state of consciousness, and other typical manifestations of delirium; metabolic disturbance, adverse medication effect, or other underlying cause.	*Delusions:* poorly organised, persecutory. *Hallucinations:* vivid, visual, colourful, threatening; accusatory auditory hallucinations induced by alcohol withdrawal. *Illusions:* brief, poorly organised.
Dementia	Cognitive impairment (particularly memory deficits); alert level of consciousness. Agitation, anxiety or wandering may be associated with loss of contact with reality. Neurological manifestations may accompany hallucinations, particularly when the underlying cause is vascular dementia.	*Delusions:* not fixed, loosely organised, readily changed or forgotten. Themes may include theft, fears, misidentification of places or people, and spousal infidelity. *Illusions:* occur more commonly than hallucinations; may be partially attributable to environmental factors. *Hallucinations:* more often visual than auditory; may be partially attributable to environmental factors.
Depression	Typical depressive symptoms, including anorexia, lack of energy, sleep disturbances and weight loss.	*Delusions:* Themes may include death, guilt, money, illnesses, self-reproach, gloomy foreboding, diminished self-esteem, and feelings of worthlessness. There may be some basis in reality, but perceptions are exaggerated. *Hallucinations:* typically auditory and derogatory.
Paranoid disorder	Absence of cognitive deficits or affective disorders; long-term social isolation or suspicious personality may be well hidden for years.	*Delusions:* fixed and well organised; may subside temporarily in different environments. Themes usually involve plots, noises, threats, obscenities or sexual assaults. *Hallucinations:* If present, these are related to the delusional themes.

loss of contact with reality in people with dementia include delusions, hallucinations, misidentification and also false accusations.

Certain characteristics of delusions, hallucinations and illusions are associated with specific conditions such as delirium, dementia and depression. In addition, loss of contact with reality typically occurs in combination with other manifestations of an underlying condition. Thus, an astute nursing assessment of contact with reality can provide essential information for identifying any underlying causes. Table 13-2 shows distinguishing features of delusions, hallucinations and illusions, and the following sections address these in relation to associated conditions that are most common in older adults.

Delusions

Delusions are a psychological mechanism that helps people preserve their egos, maintain control over threatening situations, and organise information that is difficult to process. Paranoia—defined as an extreme degree of suspiciousness—is one of the most common types of delusions in older adults. The following are typical paranoid complaints or behaviours of older adults:

- The accusation that others are stealing their money or belongings
- The perception that they are being cheated, observed, attacked, persecuted or sexually harassed
- The accusation that others are coming in and taking things, or messing up their belongings
- The belief that they have been injured by medical interventions such as pills or radiation.

Although the terms *paranoic* and *delusions* are sometimes used interchangeably in geriatric practice and references, this is inaccurate because there are many types of delusions.

In older adults, delusions can arise from pathological conditions such as delirium, dementia, depression and paranoid disorder. Delusions associated with each of these disorders are characterised in unique ways and occur in combination with other manifestations of the underlying condition, as discussed in the following sections. Additional information about psychotic symptoms of delirium and dementia is discussed in Chapter 14.

Delusions associated with pathological conditions

Delusions arising from delirium are only one manifestation of a complex pathological process that is further characterised by physiological disturbances, diminished attention, a clouded state of consciousness, and possibly hallucinations (described in Chapter 14) that subside once the delirium resolves. In addition to being associated with delirium, delusions may be caused by pathological conditions such as strokes or dementia. Delusions can also be an adverse medication effect, as in the common occurrence of delusional jealousy associated with dopamine agonists for treatment of Parkinson's disease (Perugi, Poletti, Logi et al., 2013). They also can be caused by abuse of or withdrawal from alcohol or drugs. Some of the physiological disorders

TABLE 13-3 Physiological disorders causing delusions or hallucinations

Type of disorder	Specific examples
Metabolic disorders	Uraemia, dehydration, electrolyte imbalance
Endocrine disorders	Hypoglycaemia, thyroid disorders
Neurological disorders	Stroke, cerebral trauma, cortical ischaemia
Deficiency states	Vitamin deficiencies (B_{12}, folate, niacin, thiamine)
Infections	Septicaemia, pneumonia, urinary tract infections, subacute bacterial endocarditis
Adverse medication effects	Anticholinergics, anticonvulsants, antidepressants, anti-parkinsonism agents, benzodiazepines, corticosteroids, digoxin toxicity, narcotics
Drug or alcohol	Alcohol, barbiturates, abuse or withdrawal

that are likely to cause delusions or hallucinations in older adults are listed in Table 13-3.

Delusions associated with dementia

Delusions are a neuropsychiatric symptom of dementia, with a prevalence rate ranging from 16% to 70% in various studies (Cohen-Mansfield & Golander, 2011). Common delusional themes in people with dementia are theft, abandonment, suspiciousness, spousal infidelity, misidentification of familiar places or people, and loved ones who have died are still alive. Delusions in people with dementia can lead to problematic behaviours, which often are repetitive or even obsessive, as in the following examples:

- Accusing someone of being intent on harming the person
- Perceiving a family member as a stranger
- Believing that a family carer is intent on leaving (i.e. abandoning) the person
- Accusing others of stealing things
- Demanding that a family member leave the home that is shared by the person with dementia
- Refusing to let a carer or family member provide care because the person with dementia does not trust that person
- Insisting that a spouse or family member is not the person he or she claims to be
- Requesting to go home, even when the person is already at home
- Believing that one's spouse is having an affair
- Looking for a spouse or parent who has been deceased for many years, then grieving when informed the person is dead
- Refusing to sleep in the same bed or room with spouse
- Believing that strangers are living in the house
- Insisting on leaving because "I need to go and take care of the babies".

Studies suggest that certain delusional themes are associated with pathological changes in specific brain regions, for example, delusions of theft, abandonment, infidelity and suspiciousness being associated with frontal and temporal regions (Nakatsuka, Meguro, Tsuboi et al., 2013; Nomura, Kazui, Wada et al., 2012; Sultzer, Leskin, Melrose et al., 2014). Other studies have found associations between types of delusion and stages of dementia, with persecutory delusions occurring earlier and misidentification delusions occurring during later stages (Ismail, Nguyen, Fischer et al., 2011; Reeves, Gould, Powell et al., 2012).

People with dementia will readily talk about delusions, whereas those who do not have dementia typically withhold or are secretive about information. The challenge in assessing these delusions, however, is to identify the possible reality of the situation. It is imperative to recognise that not all accusations are unfounded just because people have serious cognitive impairments. Before labelling ideas as delusional, assess for any basis in reality because even the most bizarre-sounding assertions may be totally or partially true.

Another consideration is that communication techniques differ for people with psychosis or dementia. For example, the usual psychiatric nursing approach for delusions associated with psychosis is to talk with the person about the delusional thoughts as a problem in his or her life. In contrast, for people with dementia, it is more appropriate to avoid arguing and provide distractions. In addition, it is essential to address underlying feelings of fear, anxiety and insecurity by providing reassurance. For example, it is usually effective to focus on the present with a reassuring statement such as, "I am staying here with you to make sure everything is okay, so let's have a little snack right now."

Delusions associated with depression

Persecutory and other delusions can be a manifestation of a major depression, but they are often overlooked or attributed to other factors, particularly in older adults living in community or long-term residential care settings. For example, when dementia and depression coexist, the delusions may be attributed to the dementia rather than considered as possible indicators of a treatable affective disorder.

Similarly, when a person with a paranoid personality becomes depressed, the delusions may be falsely attributed to the personality, particularly if the delusions are persecutory in nature. When delusions arise from depression, other manifestations of depression are usually identified in a thorough depression assessment, as discussed in Chapter 15.

Delusional themes may provide clues to an affective disorder, particularly if the focus is on a recent loss. Therefore, carefully listening to the content of the delusions is essential to an accurate assessment. In depressed older adults, the delusional themes often revolve around an exaggerated emphasis on guilt, money, illnesses, self-reproach, gloomy foreboding, diminished self-esteem, or feelings of worthlessness. Although some basis may exist in reality, the feelings of being persecuted and deserving of punishment are grossly exaggerated. The following are some examples of delusions arising from depression:

- Mrs N. believes that she is responsible for her husband's death; therefore, she believes she does not deserve help for her own illness.
- Ms K. has an unshakable belief that she has undiagnosed cancer and begins to plan for her funeral, even though numerous doctors have not found any disease process.
- Mr M., who recently had surgery for prostate cancer, is convinced his house is going to explode from a gas leak and repeatedly calls the gas company to come check it.

Delusions associated with paranoid disorder

Paranoid disorder—also called *paranoid ideation*—refers to a delusional disorder that is not associated with schizophrenia and is characterised by the tendency to view individuals or agencies with suspicion or as having harmful intentions. Factors associated with an increased risk for developing a late-life paranoid disorder include depression, social isolation, pathological conditions, sensory impairment, and sense of loss of control over the environment.

Common themes of paranoid delusions include spies, noises, threats, obscenities, lethal gases, bodily harm, stolen belongings, sexual infidelity or molestation, poisoned food or water, and having people enter living quarters by mysterious means at night. The delusions may occur more often when the person is socially isolated or in a particular environment, such as the home. If the person takes action based on the delusions, such as moving to another apartment or living with a family member, the delusions may subside temporarily.

Many people who have a paranoid disorder function well in the community, with the exception of one or two functional areas that are influenced by the delusions. Sometimes, a delusional state that was previously well-hidden may surface when the person is admitted to a long-term residential care facility, and the staff may think that the problem is new. In other situations, nurses will identify a paranoid disorder on making a home visit or interviewing an older person who has been admitted to the hospital. If the person also suffers from dementia, the delusions may be interpreted mistakenly as evidence of advancing dementia. When this occurs, a recommendation for long-term residential care may be made when other recommendations might be more appropriate.

Identifying a paranoid disorder in the psychosocial assessment is important so that the symptoms can be alleviated with appropriate interventions. When left unattended or written off as eccentricities, these disorders may progress to a point at which they seriously disrupt functional abilities. Therefore, when delusions and cognitive impairments coexist, it is essential to determine whether the delusions existed before the dementia and to what extent, if any, they interfered with daily activities.

If the delusions are part of a long-term pattern that has not interfered with the person's ability to function in daily life, the person may be able to remain in the community with support services and treatment directed towards the cognitive impairment. When the delusions interfere with daily activities, however, medical intervention (e.g. psychotropic medications) may be effective in eliminating the delusions or minimising their effects so that the person can maintain an independent level of function. When interventions are directed towards both the delusions and the cognitive impairment, the older person may be able to remain independent.

Hallucinations

In older adults, hallucinations are associated with dementia, depression, social isolation, sensory impairment and other physiological disturbances, including adverse medication effects. Visual hallucinations are common in people with Parkinson's disease and dementia with Lewy bodies and are related not only to the disease but also to the medications (e.g. levodopa) used for treatment (Sawada, Oeda, Yamamoto et al., 2013; Svetel, Smiljkovic, Pekmezovic et al., 2012). As with delusions, it is important to identify the underlying cause of hallucinations, because the selection of appropriate interventions depends on an accurate assessment.

Some older adults are aware of—and can describe—their hallucinatory experiences, particularly when hallucinations are caused by the adverse effects of medications (e.g. anticholinergics) or Parkinson's disease. However, in many situations, identification of hallucinations is based on astute observations of behaviours such as:

- Reaching out for objects that are not there
- Stepping over objects on the ground that are not visible to others
- Conversing with people who are not there
- Reporting sounds that have no environmental source (e.g. knocking, ringing).

An appropriate assessment technique is to elicit information from family and carers with a statement such as "Sometimes people see or hear things that others don't perceive. Do you notice any evidence of that happening to your father?" Because hallucinations are abnormal sensory experiences, it is essential to assess for environmental influences and to make sure that sensory deficits are compensated for as much as possible. This is especially important for people with dementia because they may have difficulty processing information. For example, an older adult who has dementia and is visually impaired may look at a chair and misperceive it as someone sitting. Similarly, auditory hallucinations are more common in people who have impaired hearing. In these situations, appropriate nursing interventions are implemented to compensate as much as possible for hearing and vision impairments and to facilitate referrals for hearing and vision evaluations.

Hallucinations associated with pathological conditions

Hallucinations are associated with a number of pathological conditions and a discussion about each follows.

Hallucinations are a common manifestation of delirium and are assessed within the larger context of this complex condition. Hallucinations associated with delirium are characterised as brief, vivid, visual, colourful, threatening and poorly organised. Occasionally, hallucinations are the earliest sign of delirium, and they may be overlooked or attributed to another condition (e.g. dementia). Visual hallucinations also are symptoms of ophthalmic conditions such as cataract, glaucoma or age-related macular degeneration (Hughes, 2013; Nguyen, Osterweil & Hoffman, 2013). Hallucinations arising from drug or alcohol withdrawal may occur during the first days of admission to an acute care setting or in any circumstance in which the person suddenly does not have access to their usual drugs or alcohol. Auditory hallucinations associated with alcohol withdrawal are typically accusatory and threatening, and they are sometimes organised into a complete paranoid system. The detection of alcohol-induced delirium is particularly important in acute care settings because people who are dependent on alcohol are more likely to acknowledge the problem and agree to appropriate interventions when they are in a crisis. Case study one illustrates such a situation.

CASE STUDY ONE

Mr Koch is 73 years old and has been caring for his wife, who has Alzheimer's disease, for several years. He is a very proud man who has difficulty accepting help.

One morning, Mr Koch begins vomiting coffee-ground emesis and is admitted to an acute care setting with the diagnosis of gastrointestinal bleeding. On admission, Mr Koch is very pleasant and expresses concern about his wife's care. The next morning, Mr Koch complains angrily to the nurses about the bars on the windows and is belligerent about the fact that he has been put in jail. He develops additional manifestations of delirium and is treated for alcohol withdrawal.

When the delirium has subsided, the nurse initiates a conversation about the care of his wife and asks him how he copes with the responsibility. Mr Koch admits that he has difficulty coping with his and his wife's declining health and his increasing loneliness and responsibilities. He has always been a social drinker, but he has gradually increased his consumption of alcohol to three six-packs of beer a day. As part of the discharge plan, Mr Koch agrees to talk with a sponsor from Alcoholics Anonymous.

Hallucinations are associated with dementia. Hallucinations and illusions may occur at any time in the course of a dementing illness and are also likely to occur during a transient ischaemic attack—a condition associated with vascular dementia. Visual hallucinations are a key diagnostic indicator of Parkinson's disease and dementia with Lewy bodies (Bertram & Williams, 2012; Hamilton, Landy, Salmon et al., 2012). When illusions occur, they are often related to environmental conditions that can be modified. For example, poor lighting or reflections from glass or mirrors can cause visual illusions, and background noise can contribute to auditory illusions, particularly for people with hearing aids. Psychiatric literature usually addresses illusions only with regard to misperceptions of visual or auditory stimuli, whereas an illusion, by definition, is a misinterpretation of any external stimulus. Nurses who care for people with dementia can cite numerous examples of behaviours that fit this broader definition of an illusion, such as the following:

- Mistaking the identities of carers, family members or other familiar people
- Perceiving an object as something other than what it really is
- Taking an object under the mistaken belief it belongs to them.

Table 13-3 summarises physiological disorders, including some adverse medication effects, which are most likely to cause hallucinations.

Hallucinations are associated with depression. Severely depressed older adults are more likely to experience delusions rather than hallucinations, but visual and auditory hallucinations of deceased loved ones commonly occur during periods of bereavement. Hallucinations associated with depression are likely to be auditory and derogatory, or they may involve visual perceptions of dead people. The following examples are typical of hallucinations arising from depression:

- Ms Cunningham reports that, at night, she hears the people in the next apartment saying she has cancer.
- Mr Terry reports hearing younger men say that he is sexually impotent and that he was not a good provider to his wife (who died within the past year).
- Ms Foshinger looks down from her second-floor window and sees a man, dressed in black, lying injured on the sidewalk.

Hallucinations are associated with paranoid disorder. If hallucinations are a symptom of paranoid disorder, they are likely to be closely related to the theme of the delusions. The following examples are characteristic of hallucinations arising from paranoid states:

- Mr Flicker says he hears people in the next apartment talking about him. These are the same people whom he believes will come in and steal things when he leaves the apartment.
- Ms Jennings reports seeing men observing her when she undresses or takes a bath. Moreover, when she goes to the supermarket, the man at the checkout always offers her money in exchange for sexual favours.

Special considerations for assessing contact with reality in older adults

Assessment of contact with reality presents a challenge for nurses for a variety of reasons:

- People often try to conceal delusions and hallucinations.
- When delusions and hallucinations arise from social isolation, the opportunities for assessment are extremely limited.
- To determine whether a reported experience is delusional, the nurse needs information about the reality, which is difficult to obtain if a reliable and objective observer is not available.
- Even after delusions or hallucinations are identified as such, the underlying factors may be difficult to identify.
- Older adults can often have more than one underlying condition, such as a delirium superimposed on a dementia.

Delusions are usually more readily acknowledged than hallucinations, and the most effective tools for assessing delusions are asking leading questions and listening attentively. Many older adults will confide their delusions to a nurse whom they perceive as interested, sympathetic and non-judgemental, particularly if a trusting relationship has been established.

Difficulty arises, however, when nurses hear information that may be interpreted as delusional but, in fact, is based wholly or partially in reality. For example, financial exploitation, violation of rights, and other aspects of elder abuse are not uncommon, particularly in older adults who are cognitively impaired or who live with family members who are psychosocially impaired. When older adults who have cognitive impairments or a lifelong suspicious personality describe abusive or exploitative situations, the assessment challenge is to determine what is real, what is distorted, and what is not based at all in reality.

Nurses also consider the potential effects of environmental and interpersonal factors in contributing to delusions, illusions or hallucinations. For example, the reflection of fluorescent lights on a highly polished floor can produce the illusion of water on the floor, and an older adult might walk around the reflection.

Stressful interpersonal relationships may contribute to the development of paranoid ideations, particularly in the context of past or present exploitation or abuse. Another important assessment consideration is whether a lack of assistive devices, such as eyeglasses and hearing aids, is contributing to altered perceptions. For example, if someone usually depends on eyeglasses, contact lenses or a hearing aid for adequate visual or auditory function, the absence of these items may contribute to the development of illusions or hallucinations.

During the assessment, nurses consider cultural factors that are likely to influence perceptions of reality and manifestations of mental illness, as discussed in Chapter 12. Religious background is a common cultural factor that can influence the content of delusions or hallucinations. For example, delusions and hallucinations in Irish Catholics are likely to focus on Jesus, a saint or the Virgin Mary. Similarly, Muslims with African, Asian or Middle Eastern cultural heritage may focus on the Prophet Mohammed. Box 13-7 summarises guidelines for assessing an individual's contact with reality.

BOX 13-7
Guidelines for assessing contact with reality

General principles

- In assessing any loss of contact with reality, the effects of alcohol, medications and physiological disturbances must always be considered as potential causative influences.
- People who are not cognitively impaired are usually more reluctant to talk about delusions and hallucinations than people who have dementia.
- When people talk about things that might be delusional, it is important to determine, through information provided by a reliable and objective observer, whether their perceptions have any basis in reality.
- When delusions are initially identified, it is important to determine whether they are of recent onset or have been long standing but only recently discovered.
- When delusions are identified in someone who has dementia, it is particularly important to consider the influence of treatable causative factors, such as depression or physiological disturbances.
- People who have dementia are likely to have illusions rather than hallucinations.
- People who are socially isolated are usually quite successful in concealing hallucinations.
- In assessing hallucinations and illusions, it is particularly important to consider the influence of the environment.

Interview questions to assess delusions, hallucinations and illusions

- "Do you have any thoughts you can't seem to get rid of?"
- "People sometimes have thoughts they're afraid to talk about because they believe others will think they're 'crazy'. Do you ever have thoughts like that?"
- "Do you sometimes hear voices when you're alone?"
- "Do you sometimes think you see things that other people don't see?"

Non-verbal clues to hallucinations

- Extreme withdrawal and isolation
- Contentment with social isolation, particularly if the person previously had many social contacts
- Gestures and other actions that normally occur in response to perceived stimuli

SOCIAL SUPPORTS

Social supports, which are categorised as *informal* and *formal*, refer to the services provided to address functional and psychosocial needs. Although even the most independent people receive social supports (e.g. emotional support from family and friends), social supports are usually discussed in relation to meeting the needs of people who depend on others in some way for assistance. While friends, family, clergy, neighbours or co-workers provide informal social support, workers who are paid by the older person or their family or by health and social service agencies or institutions provide formal social support.

Social supports significantly influence psychosocial function in older adults because they affect one's ability to cope with stressful life experiences by buffering them against harmful effects and improving one's physical and emotional well-being. Because the importance of social supports increases in relation to the degree of impairment of the older adult, it is essential to assess the social supports for any older adults who have conditions that affect their functional abilities.

The nursing assessment of social supports identifies not only the resources that are needed, available or being used to support the highest level of functioning, but also the barriers to the use of appropriate resources. The specific aspects of social supports that nurses assess include social networks, economic resources, and religion and spirituality. Box 13-8 summarises important questions and considerations involved in assessing social supports.

BOX 13-8
Guidelines for assessing social supports

Interview questions to assess social supports

- "On whom do you rely for help?"
- "Is there anyone who helps you with grocery shopping? Getting to doctor appointments? Getting prescriptions filled? Managing your money and paying bills?"
- "Is there anyone you can talk to when you have worries or difficulties?"
- "Is there anything you would like help with that you don't have help with now?"
- "Is there anyone in the family who could help with grocery shopping?"
- "Have you ever received information about transportation services (for meals, or other services)?"

Potential barriers to the use of formal supports

- Unwillingness to acknowledge, or lack of insight to recognise, the need for services
- Expectation that family members will provide the needed care
- Unwillingness to admit that family members cannot or will not provide the needed care
- Lack of financial resources to purchase services or unwillingness to spend money for services
- Perceived correlation between formal services and "welfare"
- Lack of transportation to access services
- Mistrust of service providers or an unwillingness to allow outsiders into the home
- Bad experiences with service providers or hearsay about the bad experiences of others
- Fear that the home situation will be judged as socially unacceptable, or embarrassment because it is socially unacceptable
- Fear that having outsiders in the house will lead to admission to a nursing home
- Lack of time, energy or problem-solving ability to obtain information about and select the appropriate services
- Fear that the service will be provided by someone about whom the care recipient holds prejudices
- Language and cultural barriers

Interview questions to assess financial resources

- "Do you have any money worries?"
- "Do you have any concerns about paying for services that you might need?"
- "Would you like to talk to someone about any financial concerns?"
- "Do you think you can afford the kind of help that your doctor recommended?"
- "Have you received any advice about financial planning for nursing home care?"

Interview questions to assess religious affiliation

- "Do you belong to any church, synagogue or mosque?"
- "Are you aware of any programs available at your church, synagogue or mosque that might be helpful to you?"

Social network

Nursing assessment of the social network addresses the social supports that are important for day-to-day functioning as well as those that affect the person's quality of life. The nurse can initiate the assessment by asking a broad question such as, "Whom do you rely on for help?" The nurse can then ask more specific questions about how the person accomplishes tasks that are most important for day-to-day function. For example, in discussing a follow-up appointment for medical care, the nurse may ask, "How do you get to your doctor appointments?"

Because a relationship with a confidant(e) is a significant predictor of quality of life for older adults, at least one question relating to this factor should be posed, such as, "Is there anyone you can talk to about your worries?" The answer to this question may also be important if the nurse or healthcare team is assisting the older adult with a decision about long-term care, because the older adult may want the confidant(e) to be involved in the decision-making process. In addition, the response to this question may provide important information about whether the older person has recently experienced a loss, or change in the availability, of a confidant(e).

After identifying any existing social networks, the nurse identifies the resources that might be helpful in addressing unmet needs. Such questions as, "Do you have any grandchildren or neighbours who could help with your garden?" are aimed at identifying informal supports that are available but are not currently being used. A question such as, "Are you aware there are services available to help you?" is aimed at identifying the person's awareness of formal supports that may not be in use.

Barriers to obtaining social supports

In addition to assessing the number and types of social supports available, nurses try to identify the barriers that interfere with the use of social supports. Many older adults who are eligible for service programs do not use these resources because they view them as costly, impersonal, overly structured, and hard to arrange.

Because older adults prefer to receive help from family and friends, negative attitudes about the use of formal social supports may be a source of resistance to their use. Without adequate informal supports, or when conflicts exist between older adults and their informal supports, an increase in dependence can trigger less effective coping mechanisms. An example is provided in Case study two.

CASE STUDY TWO

Mr and Mrs Sikorski always expected their children to care for them, but the children moved to other cities and visit several times a year. Mr and Mrs Sikorski refuse to accept any of the formal services that are available because of their cost, and also because they expect their children to provide the services out of filial responsibility. Furthermore, Mrs Sikorski cared for her parents when they were old, so she expects her daughter to do the same for her.

Mr and Mrs Sikorski frequently call their daughter and son-in-law to complain about their inability to get groceries and go to doctors' appointments. Rather than making use of transportation or other services available from the community, they neglect themselves. During the children's visit over the Christmas holiday, they find that their parents have not been eating adequately and are not taking their prescribed medications. When they mention these observations to their parents, Mr and Mrs Sikorski tell their children, "If you loved us, you'd be taking care of us, and this wouldn't be happening."

In addition to some older people's preference for obtaining services from families rather than outside agencies, there are many other barriers to the use of formal services. Fears about outsiders coming into the home rank high among the barriers to the provision of in-home services. Financial barriers also often exist, either because of an inability or an unwillingness to pay for services.

Additional barriers include unwillingness to accept help, lack of knowledge about types of services available, and not knowing where to go for specific services. The identification of these barriers is essential because counselling and educational interventions (e.g. providing information about services that are available) can address many of these issues.

Assessing barriers to support services can be challenging. Identification of these barriers is best accomplished by carefully listening to older people and their carers and by asking non-threatening questions. Attitudinal barriers, such as prejudices, may be identified through statements made by the carer about prior experiences of themselves or friends.

Economic resources

Financial issues are generally within the purview of social workers, and nurses usually prefer to avoid discussing money with older adults or their families. In planning for formal services for older adults, some assessment of financial assets is necessary, and the nurse is often the healthcare professional who obtains this information, particularly in home or other community settings. If no long-term residential care or community-based services are needed, the nurse can forego the financial assessment.

It is not always necessary to ask details about monthly income or the exact amount of savings and assets. Providing appropriate information about the available services and costs might reveal some anxieties and issues that can be discussed and resolved to the satisfaction of the older person and their significant other/s.

RELIGION AND SPIRITUALITY

As discussed in Chapter 12, religion and spirituality become more important in older adulthood, and these resources should be identified as a part of a comprehensive psychosocial assessment. A person's *religious affiliation* is assessed as a component of his or her social supports, whereas *spirituality* is assessed as a separate component of the psychosocial assessment. It is important that nurses recognise spirituality is an integral component of all humans, but not all people identify with a religious affiliation.

Identification of religious affiliation is a simple but important part of the psychosocial assessment, because available religion-based programs for older adults may be perceived as more acceptable than those provided by a public or non-religious agency. For example, an older Jewish person might be willing to go to the Jewish community centre for a senior meal program, and an older Roman Catholic adult might be willing to accept mental health services from Catholic social services, but these people might refuse to avail themselves of the same kinds of services when they are offered by another organisation.

Often, religion-based services are viewed by the older adult as services that they deserve as a reward for years of attendance at or service to a place of worship. Although most religion-based programs serve older adults regardless of their religious affiliations, the programs are often perceived as more appropriate if the person is of the same faith.

In addition to being perceived as more appropriate, some religion-based services are not available elsewhere, and they are often provided by trained volunteers free of charge. Examples of programs or services that may be available to members of a particular religious affiliation include transportation, respite care, peer counselling, chore assistance, friendly visiting, and telephone reassurance. Older adults can also take advantage of any religious program that is available for people of all ages.

Their identification of a specific place of worship is also important because attendance at religious services may be a significant factor in the older adult's social life. For many older adults, particularly those with limited mobility or those who have full-time caregiving responsibilities, attendance at religious services is their only opportunity for social interaction and personal support. Most people who are unable to attend religious services can arrange for home visits; indeed, these visits may be the only source of outside contact and emotional support that is acceptable to a home-bound older adult. Moreover, for people who are socially isolated, a visitor from their place of worship may be the only person monitoring the home situation. In these situations, health professionals who are concerned about home-bound older adults may be able to monitor their status through these visitors, as in Case study three.

CASE STUDY THREE

Mr Phillips was admitted to the hospital after a syncopal episode that resulted in a minor car accident. On admission, Mr Phillips was slightly unkempt and showed some memory deficits, but his self-care abilities improved during his 2-day hospitalisation. The nurse suggested Mr Phillips considers getting home-delivered meals and using other community resources, but he refused these services. The nurse was concerned because Mr Phillips lived alone and had no outside contacts other than Ms Croft, a lay minister who had visited weekly for 2 years. The nurse asked for and received permission from Mr Phillips to contact Ms Croft to inform her of available community services. Ms Croft was grateful for the information and said that she would contact the appropriate agencies if Mr Phillips' condition declined or if he agreed to accept help.

In this situation, information about the patient's religious affiliation enabled the nurse to implement an effective discharge plan that otherwise might not have been possible.

Although nurses do not always include spiritual needs as a routine part of the assessment, there are many times when a nursing assessment of the spiritual needs of older adults is warranted. When an older person provides clues about spiritual distress or discomfort, the nurse must be willing to respond to the older person rather than simply ignore the clues (as discussed in Chapter 12).

When a nurse is addressing quality-of-life issues, it is important to include questions about spirituality. For example, when planning long-term care, it is particularly important to assess and address spiritual needs. The assessment of spiritual needs focuses on a discussion of sources of strength and meaning in the older person's life, and is not intended to evaluate whether a person is more or less spiritual. As with all aspects of care, nurses need to be particularly aware of cultural influences on religious practices and expressions of spirituality, and be cautious about generalisations with regard to any cultural group.

Nurses may not be comfortable discussing spirituality, but they can increase their comfort level by recognising their own feelings and acknowledging that spirituality is a universal human need. Nurses might avoid discussion of spiritual needs because they believe that they are not skilled in meeting these needs. However, if nurses view the assessment of spiritual needs as an essential part of holistic care, they may become comfortable with addressing the spiritual needs of the older adults to whom they provide care. Nurses address the nursing aspects of those problems and refer the person to the appropriate resource for interventions that address the non-nursing aspects. In addition, nurses can suggest referrals to appropriate religious practitioners and support groups. Box 13-9 presents guidelines

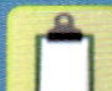

BOX 13-9
Guidelines for assessing spiritual needs

Guidelines for nursing assessment

- Be aware of your own feelings about spirituality, so that you can recognise and respond to the spiritual needs of others.
- Recognise that spiritual needs are a universal human phenomenon. Although not all people experience spiritual distress, all people have spiritual needs and the potential for spiritual growth.
- Recognise that it is within the realm of holistic nursing care to identify and plan interventions for spiritual growth as well as for spiritual distress.
- Convey a non-judgemental, open-minded attitude when you are eliciting information about a person's spirituality and religious beliefs.

Questions to assess spiritual health

- "What in your life is meaningful and important?"
- "What do you hope to accomplish in your life?"
- "What do you do that gives you pleasure and satisfaction?"
- "Who are the people you can turn to when you need someone to listen to you or to help you?"
- "Do you believe in a higher being?" (examples: God, Goddess Divinity) "How do you describe this being?"
- "Do you participate in any activities (rituals) that foster a connection with a higher being?" (examples: prayer or other religious activities)
- "What activities are helpful in bringing you inner peace and relieving stress?" (examples: meditation, walking in the woods)
- "What are your beliefs about death?"
- "Do you see a connection between your body, your mind, your emotions and your soul?"
- "Is there anything you need or would like to have to support your beliefs and your spiritual needs?" (example: Bible, sacred or revered object)
- "Would you like to arrange a visit from a spiritual leader?"
- "Are there any health practices that you would like to consider, even though our society may not consider them to be conventional?" (examples: therapeutic touch, guided imagery)

Observations/questions to assess spiritual distress

- During the psychosocial interview, listen for clues to spiritual distress, such as the following: suicidal ideation; anger towards God; inability to forgive others; feelings of hopelessness, uselessness, or abandonment; questions about the meaning of life, losses or suffering.
- "Are there any conflicts between your beliefs or values and actions that you feel you should be taking?" (example: feeling entitled to some time to oneself, which may be in conflict with the demands of caregiving for a spouse)
- "Are there any conflicts between what you believe in and what society or healthcare professionals are encouraging or suggesting you do?" (example: questioning the wisdom of using a feeding tube for a spouse who is chronically and severely impaired and unable to participate in the decision)
- "Do you have any special religious considerations that are not being addressed?" (examples: dietary practices, observance of religious holidays)
- *For people in institutional settings:* "Is there anything here that interferes with your spiritual needs?" (examples: noisy environment, lack of privacy)

for assessing spiritual needs. Assessment of spiritual needs includes not only the factors that cause spiritual distress but also the factors that are essential to spiritual growth, even in the absence of spiritual distress.

CHAPTER HIGHLIGHTS

Overview of cognitive and psychosocial assessment of older adults

- Cognitive and psychosocial assessment is a complex process that involves the use of good communication skills, appropriate interview questions, purposeful observations, and relevant assessment tools.
- Nurses can assess their own attitudes to increase their comfort level in performing a cognitive and psychosocial assessment of older adults (Box 13-1).

Communication skills for cognitive and psychosocial assessment

- Barriers to communication include visual and hearing impairments, internal and external distractions, pathological disorders, adverse medication effects, poor communication methods and cultural differences.
- Establishing rapport, using touch, listening, asking questions and giving feedback can enhance communication during psychosocial assessment.
- Nurses create an environment for effective communication by speaking face-to-face at eye level, respecting the person's comfort zone, ensuring privacy, eliminating distractions, and facilitating optimal vision and hearing functioning.

Cognitive and psychosocial assessment

- A mental status assessment includes both cognitive and psychosocial assessments. It involves the assessment of the following: physical appearance, alertness and attention, motor function and praxis, social skills, response to the interview, orientation, memory, speech characteristics, higher language skills and executive function. Assessment of executive function is particularly important for determining the ability of the older adult to participate in decision making. Insight, learning, memory, reasoning, judgement, problem solving and abstract thinking are some of the cognitive skills that are involved with decision making.
- Other domains of psychosocial assessment—affective function, contact with reality and social supports—are discussed below.
- A number of assessment tools can be used to screen for cognitive impairment (Table 13-1).

Decision making and executive function

- Assessment of cognitive skills such as executive function is particularly important for determining the ability of the older adult to participate in decision making.
- Insight, learning, memory, reasoning, judgement, problem solving and abstract thinking are some of the cognitive skills that are involved with decision making.

Affective function

- An assessment of affective function includes consideration of mood, anxiety, self-esteem, depression, and happiness and well-being.

Contact with reality

- Nurses assess contact with reality within the context of behavioural indicators to identify potential underlying causes of any loss of contact with reality.
- Three types of loss of contact with reality are delusions, hallucinations and illusions.

Social supports

- Psychosocial assessment identifies social supports and economic resources as well as any barriers to obtaining services.

Religion and spirituality

- A holistic nursing assessment addresses religious affiliation and spirituality.

CRITICAL THINKING EXERCISES

1. Complete the psychosocial self-assessment in Box 13-1.
2. Think of several different situations in the past few weeks in which you worked with older adults and answer the following questions:
   - What aspects of the person's psychosocial function did you observe?
   - What questions did you ask that would give you information about their psychosocial function?
   - What information did you obtain about their social supports?
3. Name at least three things you would observe or determine in order to assess each of the following when you are working with older adults: physical appearance, social skills, orientation, alertness and attention, memory, speech characteristics, higher language skills, decision-making skills, anxiety, self-esteem, depression, and contact with reality.
4. What questions would you ask an older adult to identify social supports and barriers to the use of services?
5. What approach would you use to assess an older adult's spiritual health and identify spiritual distress?

RESOURCES

For an extensive range of additional resources to enhance teaching and learning and to facilitate understanding of this chapter, please see the text's accompanying website located on thePoint at http://thepoint.lww.com.

Clinical tools

Alzheimer's Australia

- Rowland Universal Dementia Assessment Scale (RUDAS): www.fightdementia.org.au/understanding-dementia/rowland-universal-dementia-assessment-scale.aspx

Australian Indigenous Health*InfoNet*

- Kimberley Indigenous Cognitive Assessment tool (KICA) and instruction booklet: www.healthinfonet.ecu.edu.au/key-resources/promotion-resources?lid=1221

Dementia Collaborative Research Centre (Australia) lists recommended assessment tools: www.dementia-assessment.com.au/cognitive

General practitioner assessment of COGnition (GPCog): www.gpcog.com.au

Hartford Institute for Geriatric Nursing, ConsultGeriRN.org: http://consultgerirn.org/resources

Assessment tools *Try This*® series and *How to Try This* resources

General assessment series:

- *Try This,* issue 3: Mental status assessment of older adults: The Mini-Cog. Doerflinger, D. M. C. (2013). *Best Practices in Nursing Care to Older Adults.*
- *How to Try This* (article): The Mini-Cog. Doerflinger, D. M. C. (2007). *American Journal of Nursing, 107*(12), 62–71.
- *How to Try This* (video): *The Mini-Cog.*
- *Try This,* issue 3.2: Mental status assessment in older adults: Montreal Cognitive Assessment (MoCA). Version 7.1 (original version). Doerflinger, D. M. C. (2012). *Best Practices in Nursing Care to Older Adults.*
- *Try This,* issue 28: Preparedness for Caregiving Scale. Zwicker, D. (2010). *Best Practices in Nursing Care to Older Adults.*

Dementia series:

- *Try This,* issue D3: Brief evaluation of executive dysfunction: An essential refinement in the assessment of cognitive impairment. Kennedy, G. (2012). *Best Practices in Nursing Care to Older Adults with Dementia.*
- *How to Try This* (article): Screening older adults for executive dysfunction. Kennedy, G. J. & Smyth, C. A. (2008). *American Journal of Nursing, 108*(12), 62–71.
- *How to Try This* (video): *Brief evaluation of executive dysfunction: An essential refinement in the assessment of cognitive impairment.*

Evidence-based practice

National Guideline Clearinghouse: www.guideline.gov/index.aspx

- Milisen, K., Braes, T. & Foreman, M. D. (2012). Assessing cognitive function. In M. Boltz, E. Capezuti, T. Fulmer & D. Zwicker (Eds), *Evidence-based geriatric nursing protocols for best practice* (4th ed., pp. 122–134). New York: Springer.

Joanna Briggs Institute: http://connect.jbiconnectplus.org

Evidence-based summaries:

- Hong, C. (2014). Residential aged care: Suicide risk assessment.
- Le, L. K. D. (2014). White coat hypertension: Older people.

REFERENCES

Allgulander, C. (2009). Generalized anxiety disorder: Between now and DSM-V. *Psychiatric Clinics of North America, 32*, 611–628.

Andrews, M. M. & Boyle, J. S. (2011). *Transcultural concepts in nursing care* (6th ed.). Philadelphia, PA: Lippincott Williams & Wilkins.

Bertram, K. & Williams, D. R. (2012). Visual hallucinations in the differential diagnosis of parkinsonism. *Journal of Neurology, Neurosurgery & Psychiatry, 83*, 448–452.

Calleo, J., Stanley, M. A., Greisinger, A., Wehmanen, O., Johnson, M., Novy, D., . . . Kunik, M. (2009). Generalized anxiety disorder in older medical patients: Diagnostic recognition, mental health management and service utilization. *Journal of Clinical Psychology in Medical Settings, 16*, 175–185.

Cohen-Mansfield, J. & Golander, H. (2011). The measurement of psychosis in dementia: A comparison of assessment tools. *Alzheimer Disease and Associated Disorders, 25*, 101–108.

Connor, A. & Howett, M. (2009). A conceptual model of intentional comfort touch. *Journal of Holistic Nursing, 27*, 127–135.

Dementia Collaborative Research Centre (Australia). (2014). Assessment tools. Available via www.dementia-assessment.com.au/cognitive.

Doerflinger, D. M. C. (2007). *How to Try This* (article and video): The Mini-Cog. *American Journal of Nursing, 107*(12), 62–71.

Hamilton, J. M., Landy, K. M., Salmon, D. P. et al. (2012). Early visuospatial deficits predict the occurrence of visual hallucinations in autopsy-confirmed dementia with Lewy Bodies. *American Journal of Geriatric Psychiatry, 20*(9), 773–781.

Hodkinson, H. M. (1972). Evaluation of a mental test score of mental impairment in the elderly. *Age Ageing, 1*, 233–238.

Hughes, D. F. (2013). Charles Bonnet syndrome: A literature review into diagnostic criteria, treatment and implications for nursing practice. *Journal of Psychiatric and Mental Health Nursing, 20*(2), 169–175.

Ismail, A., Nguyen, M., Fischer, C. E. et al. (2011). Neurobiology of delusions in Alzheimer's disease. *Current Psychiatry Reports, 13*(3), 211–218.

Kennedy, G. J. & Smyth, C. A. (2008). Screening older adults for executive dysfunction. *American Journal of Nursing, 108*(12), 62–71.

Kiefer, R. A. (2008). An integrative review of the concept of well-being. *Holistic Nursing Practice, 22*, 244–252.

Nakatsuka, M., Meguro, K., Tsuboi, H. et al. (2013). Content of delusional thoughts in Alzheimer's disease and assessment of content-specific brain dysfunctions with BEHAVE-AD-FW and SPECT. *International Geropsychiatry, 25*(6), 939–948.

Nguyen, N. D., Osterweil, D. & Hoffman, J. (2013). Charles bonnet syndrome: Treating nonpsychiatric hallucinations. *Consults in Pharmacology, 28*(3), 184–188.

Nomura, K., Kazui, H., Wada, T. et al. (2012). Classification of delusions in Alzheimer's disease and their neural correlates. *Psychogeriatrics, 12*(3), 200–210.

Pachana, N. A., Byrne, G. J., Siddle, H., Koloski, N., Harley, E. & Arnold, E. (2007). Development and validation of the Geriatric Anxiety Inventory. *International Psychogeriatrics, 19*, 103–114.

Perugi, G., Poletti, M., Logi, C. et al. (2013). Diagnosis, assessment, and management of delusional jealousy in Parkinson's disease with and without dementia. *Neurological Science, 34*(9), 1537–1541.

Pinto, E. & Peters, R. (2009). Literature review of the Clock Drawing Test as a tool for cognitive screening. *Dementia and Geriatric Cognitive Disorders, 27*, 201–213.

Purnell, L. D. (2009). *Guide to culturally competent health care* (2nd ed.). Philadelphia, PA: F. A. Davis Co.

Reeves, S. J., Gould, R. L., Powell, J. F. et al. (2012). Origins of delusions in Alzheimer's disease. *Neuroscience & Biobehavioral Reviews, 36*(10), 2274–2287.

Sawada, H., Oeda, T., Yamamoto, K. et al. (2013). Trigger medications and patient-related risk factors for Parkinson disease psychosis requiring anti-psychotic drugs: A retrospective cohort study. *BMC Neurology, 13*, 145.

Smith, M., Ingram, T. & Brighton, V. (2009). Evidence-based guideline: Detection and assessment of late-life anxiety. *Journal of Gerontological Nursing, 35*(7), 9–15.

Sultzer, D. L., Leskin, L. P., Melrose, R. J. et al. (2014). Neurobiology of delusions, memory, and insight in Alzheimer disease. *American Journal of Geriatric Psychiatry, 22*(11), 1346–1355.

Svetel, M., Smilijkovic, T., Pekmezovic, T. et al. (2012). Hallucinations in Parkinson's disease: Cross-sectional study. *Acta Neurologica Belgica, 112*(1), 33–37.

Chapter 14

Impaired cognition: Delirium and dementia

By Carol Miller and Sharyn Hunter

LEARNING OBJECTIVES

After reading this chapter, you should be able to:

1. Describe person-centred care and explain why it is important to use this model of care for older adults with cognitive impairment.
2. Describe delirium, the predisposing and precipitating factors, and discuss nursing assessments and interventions related to delirium.
3. Explain the appropriate use of terminology that describes impaired cognitive function in older adults.
4. Describe characteristics of Alzheimer's disease, vascular dementia, frontotemporal dementia, and dementia with Lewy bodies.
5. List the factors that affect the risk for development of dementia.
6. Discuss the functional consequences of impaired cognitive function.
7. Describe guidelines for initial and ongoing assessment of cognitively impaired older adults.
8. Identify non-pharmacological interventions for addressing dementia-related behaviours, including environmental modifications and interaction and communication techniques.
9. Discuss medications for slowing the progression of dementia and for managing dementia-related behaviours.

KEY POINTS

Alzheimer's disease
behavioural and psychological symptoms of dementia (BPSD)
beta-amyloid
carer burden
Confusion Assessment Method (CAM)
delirium
dementia
excess disability
frontotemporal dementia
Lewy body dementia
mild cognitive impairment (MCI)
National Health Priority—dementia
person-centred care (PCC)
sundowning
vascular dementia

As people age, they are increasingly likely to experience pathological conditions that have a major impact on cognitive function.

Dementia and delirium are two main types of cognitive impairment that older adults may experience. This chapter discusses these two cognitive impairments, while the next chapter focuses on the other D, depression. Irrespective of the type of cognitive impairment, nurses must meet the challenge of preserving as much of the person's dignity and quality of life while they are receiving nursing care.

PERSON-CENTRED CARE

Increasingly healthcare delivery is moving away from task-focused, institution-driven care practices towards a holistic model of care, which focuses on the person receiving care, otherwise called **person-centred care (PCC)**.

This model of care was initially developed by Thomas Kitwood (1997) when he integrated his philosophy of personhood and the concept of person-centred approaches described by Dr Carl Rogers to develop person-centred care for people with dementia.

Kitwood was the first to recognise and promote that the person with dementia, despite their loss of cognitive abilities, is still a person. "Personhood is a standing or status that is bestowed upon one human being, by others, in the context of relationship and social being" (Kitwood, 1997, p. 8). Kitwood believed that when healthcarers/caregivers focus on the disease of dementia, the human being is disregarded. His work shifted the way people viewed the person with dementia from an object to a person with value and worth. Kitwood's work has been embraced internationally by healthcare practitioners, and person-centred care is no longer specific to people with dementia.

Person-centred care is particularly important for older adults because cognitive impairment and increasing frailty and disability puts them at an increased risk "… of disenfranchisement, loss of autonomy and loss of being recognised as a person or human" (McCormack, 2003, p. 204). Person-centred care begins by identifying the personhood of the person receiving care. This is achieved by recognising and engaging with them in their world. There are four elements of person-centred care that contribute to being recognised as a person or personhood. They are:

1. *Being in relation:* The person has relationships
2. *Being with self:* The person has a sense of being a person

3. *Being in a social world:* People are social beings
4. *Being in place:* Personhood is expressed in context. (McCormack, 2004, p. 33)

When nursing an older adult, particularly if they are cognitively impaired, delivering person-centred care will improve the older adult's quality of life and well-being. PCC enables nurses to meet the challenge of preserving their dignity.

DELIRIUM

Although **delirium** has been documented in patients for centuries, only in recent years have researchers and practitioners addressed delirium as an acute serious, preventable, treatable, commonly occurring but often unrecognised neuropsychiatric syndrome that disproportionately affects older adults (Fong, Tulebaev & Inouye, 2009). Delirium can develop over hours or days; fluctuate over the course of the day; and can persist for months. Changes in cognition involve problems with attention and consciousness as well as several or many additional changes, including altered sleep–wake patterns. Many diverse factors have been implicated in the development of delirium. However, delirium in older adults commonly occurs with an acute medical illness or medical complications. Because delirium has a variable presentation it can be often missed and underdiagnosed. At present the diagnosis of delirium is clinically based and depends on the presence or absence of certain features. Management strategies for delirium are focused on prevention and symptom management.

Prevalence, risk factors and functional consequences of delirium

Delirium results from an interaction between predisposing factors, which increase the person's vulnerability, and precipitating factors, which account for the immediate threat. The most commonly identified predisposing factors include advanced age, dementia, depression, functional dependency and number of medications. Common precipitating factors include surgery, infections, serious illness and physical restraints. The risk for developing delirium is highest for people with several predisposing factors in combination with one or more precipitating factors. Research found that several preoperative variables were significantly associated with an increased risk of delirium in older adults undergoing surgery, including older age, hypoalbuminaemia, impaired functional status, pre-existing dementia and pre-existing comorbidities (Robinson et al., 2009). Reviews of studies cite the following rates for delirium:

- 22% in community-living people with dementia
- 15% to 70% in long-term residential care residents
- 11% to 33% on admission to a hospital setting, with an additional 5% to 35% developing delirium after admission
- 80% or more in intensive care settings. (Cole, McCusker, Voyer et al., 2013; de Lange, Verhaak, van der Meer, 2013; Gofrey, Smith, Green et al., 2013; Popp, 2013)

Functional consequences include longer hospital stays, increased mortality, increased dependency, short- and long-term functional impairment, and higher rates of permanent residency in long-term care facilities (Fong, Jones, Marcantonio et al., 2012; Tullmann, Fletcher, Foreman, 2012). A study of outcomes during 1 month following hospitalisation found that those older adults who had dementia and were diagnosed as having delirium had a 25% short-term mortality rate, increased length of stay, poorer function at discharge, and greater functional decline at 1 month follow-up (Fick, Steis, Waller et al., 2013). Consistent evidence from longitudinal studies suggests that delirium strongly predicts development of dementia in the long term and acceleration of cognitive decline in people who already have dementia (Davis, Terrera, Keage et al., 2012; Macluluch, Anand, Davis et al., 2013).

Nursing assessment of delirium

Frequent assessment is imperative for effective detection of delirium because manifestations of delirium are wide ranging and can fluctuate quickly. Although nurses have essential roles in assessing delirium, studies indicate they have difficulty identifying manifestations of delirium, particularly in the hypoactive form and in people with dementia (Gordon, Melillo, Nannini et al., 2013; Solberg, Plummer, May et al., 2013; Steis & Fick, 2012). Delirium occurs commonly in hospitalised older adults and, because it is often unrecognised, routine cognitive screening is recommended as a standard part of care (Wand, Thoo, Ting et al., 2013). The **Confusion Assessment Method (CAM)**, which was developed in 1990, is the most widely used screening tool in acute and long-term residential care (Tullmann, Fletcher & Foreman, 2012). According to this method (Inouye, van Dyck, Alessi et al., 1990), delirium is diagnosed based on a four-point algorithm and by confirming the presence of features in points one and two, and either point three or point four, of the following:

1. Acute onset or fluctuating course: change in mental status from baseline or onset of abnormal behaviours that tend to come and go or increase and decrease in severity
2. Inattention: easy distractibility, difficulty focusing, diminished ability to keep track of conversations
3. Disorganised thinking: incoherent, disorganised, rambling, or illogical thinking or conversation
4. Altered level of consciousness: alert (normal), vigilant, lethargic, stupor, or coma.

An important consideration when using the CAM and assessing the feature of inattention is that a lack of response or the response of "don't know" may indicate inattention (i.e. feature 2) (Huang, Inouye, Jones et al.,

2012). Another consideration is that some people with delirium are aware of their cognitive deficits and can self-report. One study of 55 hospitalised adults with diagnosed delirium found that 31% recognised their delirium and this was associated with disorientation and acuity of onset (Ryan, O'Regan & Caoimh, 2013). Another assessment consideration is that, in addition to mental status changes, delirium subtypes are categorised according to motor and behavioural manifestations. Further information about the CAM is located in the resources section towards the end of this chapter.

Figure 14-1 illustrates a protocol for assessing and managing delirium in older adults, which was developed by the Hospital Elder Life Program (Sandhaus, Harrell & Valenti, 2006). A number of other algorithms have been developed by healthcare organisations in an attempt to increase the recognition and management of delirium in older adults. Nurses must be aware of institutional delirium protocols and ensure these are followed.

Three subtypes of delirium are characterised as follows:

- *Hyperactive:* restlessness, agitation, combativeness, anger, wandering, laughing, swearing, emotional lability and fast or loud speech
- *Hypoactive:* lethargy, staring, slowed movement, paucity of speech and unresponsiveness
- *Mixed:* fluctuations between hyperactive and hypoactive.

The hypoactive type may occur more commonly in older adults; however, it is not as easily recognised and manifestations may be dismissed as clinically unimportant (Blazer & van Nieuwenhuizen, 2012).

Nursing issue and outcomes

Acute confusional state is a term used to describe this nursing issue rather than using the medical term, delirium. Defining characteristics of an acute confusional state in older adults include fluctuation in cognition, consciousness or psychomotor activity; hallucinations or misperceptions; increased restlessness or agitation; and lack of motivation to initiate or follow through with purposeful or goal-directed behaviour.

Outcomes that address this issue and may be applicable are: reduction in anxiety level, improved cognition and cognitive orientation, concentration, distorted-thought self-control, information processing, memory, mood, neurological status and psychomotor energy. In addition, the outcomes may be applicable to address causative factors: electrolyte and acid/base balance, hydration, infection severity, nutritional status, control of risks for delirium, and sensory function status.

WELLNESS OPPORTUNITY

The wellness outcome of increased comfort level will holistically address the needs of older adults with delirium.

Nursing interventions for delirium

The complexity of delirium requires a multidisciplinary approach to management, with nurses having a key role in the prevention, early detection, ongoing assessment and management. Current emphasis is on implementing multifaceted programs in hospitals for prevention and early detection and treatment of delirium because outcomes are worse among those with more severe and persistent delirium. Reviews of studies suggest that multicomponent models of care, such as the Hospital Elder Life Program, are effective in preventing 33% to 40% of the incidence of delirium in hospitals (Godfrey, Smith, Green et al., 2013; Zauber, Murphy, Rizzuto et al., 2013). Current guidelines recommend the use of non-pharmacological interventions along with the avoidance of medications, such as benzodiazepines, that are associated with higher risk for delirium (Barr & Pandharipande, 2013; Davidson, Harvey, Bemis-Dougherty et al., 2013; Yevchak, Steis, Diehl et al., 2012). Pharmacological measures should be considered to control distressing symptoms or when safety is compromised (Australian and New Zealand Society for Geriatric Medicine, 2012). Small doses of antipsychotics have been found to be effective and appropriate in the short term. Initiating early and aggressive mobilisation is an evidence-based intervention that is effective for reducing delirium in intensive care patients; however, this intervention is only one component of a multifactorial care plan (Balas, Buckingham, Braley et al., 2013; Barr, Fraser, Puntillo et al., 2013; Desai, Chau, George, 2013).

Essential components of a multifactorial approach to delirium are staff education; comprehensive geriatric assessment; treatment of all contributing factors (e.g. pain, medical conditions, sleep deprivation, adverse medication effects, fluid and electrolyte imbalances, vision or hearing impairments); orientation interventions; environmental modifications; physical and occupational therapies; nutritional interventions; measures for preventing complications (e.g. falls, injuries, sleep problems, pressure ulcers, aspiration); encouraging the presence of family and other support people; and comprehensive discharge planning. Examples of interventions that are pertinent to nursing care plans are as follows:

- Provision of aids to orientation (e.g. clock, watch, calendar) and aids to improve sensory function (e.g. eyeglasses, hearing aids)
- Frequent verbal orientation and reminders about daily events
- Environmental modification (e.g. noise reduction, familiar objects)
- Psychological support (e.g. cognitive and social stimulation)
- Identification of adverse medication effects and discussion of medication regimen with prescribing practitioners
- Promotion of physiological stability (e.g. low-dose oxygenation, maintenance of fluid and electrolyte balance)

CARING FOR YOUR PATIENT WITH DELIRIUM

Features of delirium

- Acute onset of confusion with a fluctuating course
- Inattention: highly distractible, with difficulty focusing
- Disorganised thinking, altered level of consciousness, or both

Rule out physiological causes

NEURO EVENT

- Check level of consciousness
- History of recent head injury (subdural haematoma)
- Neurological check, noting motor deficit, pupil changes
- Diagnostic testing as ordered
- Lab studies (vitamin B_{12}, folate, blood chemistries, thyroid-stimulating hormone)

MEDICATION

- Check recent medication changes. Check drug levels. Avoid these medications: benzodiazepines, anti-cholinergics (diphenhydramine, oxybutynin, metoclopramide), steroids, histamine$_2$ blockers (famotidine, ranitidine HCl), drugs with high toxicity (digoxin, phenytoin sodium), psychotropics

INFECTION

- Consider urinary tract infection or pneumonia
- Check temperature and vital signs
- Lab work
- Chest x-ray
- Urinalysis (culture and sensitivity)
- Blood culture
- Sputum culture

DEHYDRATION

- Monitor intake and output
- Check serum glucose
- Give I.V. fluid as needed
- Review lab work
- Ensure adequate nutrition and hydration
- Check for electrolyte imbalance

HYPOXIA

- Pulse oximetry
- Respiratory rate
- Sputum
- Arterial blood gases
- Chest x-ray

Address physical needs

SAFETY

- Glasses
- Hearing device
- Orientation or reorientation
- Gentle reassurance
- Family at bedside
- Early mobilisation
- Fall-prevention protocol
- Consult physical therapy, occupational therapy

PAIN

- Provide comfort, supportive measures
- Give medication as ordered and assess pain control
- Avoid pethidine and propoxyphene-paracetamol, which may cause seizures, delirium in elderly
- Use paracetamol around the clock as first-line analgesic
- Add a laxative to any opioid regimen

ELIMINATION

- Frequent toileting
- Bowel regimen
- Remove urinary drainage catheter as soon as possible
- Treat constipation

SLEEP

- Use comfort measures, back rub
- Allow for long intervals of uninterrupted sleep
- Avoid sedative-hypnotic medications

NUTRITION

- Assist or feed
- Give supplements as required
- Consult speech pathologist for swallow evaluation, nutritionist
- Skin assessment

SOURCE: Adapted from a delirium algorithm developed at Moses Taylor Hospital.

FIGURE 14-1 Protocol for assessing and managing delirium in older adults published by the Hospital Elder Life Program. (Reprinted with permission from Sandhaus, S., Harrell, F. & Valenti, D. [2006]. Healthier aging: Here's help to prevent delirium in the hospital. *Nursing, 2006, 36*[7], 60–62.)

- Adequate pain management (refer to Chapter 28)
- Promotion of normal sleep–wake pattern (refer to Chapter 24)
- Maintenance of optimal bowel and bladder function (refer to Chapters 18 and 19)
- Physical activity (e.g. ambulation, physical therapy, occupational therapy)
- Provision of cognitively stimulating activities
- Encouragement of family and support people to be with the person.

Figure 14-1 illustrates a flowchart for nursing care of older adults with delirium (Sandhaus et al., 2006). Evidence-based resources that were originally developed by the noted delirium expert Dr Sharon K. Inouye and colleagues at the Yale University School of Medicine are available online for health professionals, families and the older adult for the recognition, assessment and treatment for delirium via www.hospitalelderlifeprogram.org. These resources also include the Hospital Elder Life Program (HELP), which provides optimal care for older persons while in hospital to prevent and manage delirium. Nursing interventions that are applicable for the nursing issue of acute confusion include anxiety reduction, behaviour management, cognitive stimulation, delirium management, energy management, environmental management, fluid/electrolyte management, hallucination management, mobility support, medication management, mood management, nutrition management, pain management, reality orientation and surveillance to ensure safety.

WELLNESS OPPORTUNITY

Nursing interventions to address holistically the needs of older adults during acute confusional states include use of a calming technique, emotional support, music therapy, presence and touch.

OVERVIEW OF DEMENTIA

Dementia is one of the most multifaceted topics discussed in this text, with evidence-based information rapidly emerging from many clinical, scientific, social and ethical perspectives. This overview section provides background information that is relevant to current understanding of dementia, and the remainder of this chapter applies the information to clinical practice.

Two considerations need to be addressed in relation to evidence-based information about dementia. First, it is important to recognise that recent developments in neuroimaging techniques have led to major improvements in the diagnosis of dementia, but these diagnostic methods are not widely available outside of research centres. Similarly, although many clinical trials of interventions for dementia are in progress, these are available only in research studies. Second, when reading results of studies of non-prescription products for the prevention of cognitive decline, it is crucial to pay close attention to the study design before drawing conclusions about the effectiveness of the product. For example, some studies indicate that resveratrol, vitamin E and *Ginkgo biloba* may prevent cognitive decline in some people, but more studies are needed before these products can be recommended. Because media attention often highlights so-called breakthroughs in the diagnosis of or treatments for dementia, nurses have important roles in teaching older adults and their carers about diagnosis and management of declines in cognitive function. In addition to keeping current on research and focusing on the clinical application of evidence-based recommendations, nurses can teach older adults about obtaining information from reliable sources, as discussed in the section on nursing interventions.

Terminology to describe dementia

An understanding of impaired cognitive function is complicated by the many terms used interchangeably—and sometimes inaccurately—to describe dementia. Recent research has greatly improved the ability of clinicians to diagnose and treat different types of dementia, but it has also brought about a confusing proliferation of dementia-related terminology. Perhaps more than any other terms used in reference to older adults, those associated with cognitive impairment are the most misused, misunderstood and emotionally charged. The following are some of the terms commonly used in reference to cognitive impairment in older adults: confusion, dementia, senility, Alzheimer's disease, small strokes, memory problems and organic brain syndrome. Different terms are more or less acceptable to different people and the selection of a term is often based on emotional preferences or lack of accurate information. Because cognitive impairment is an emotionally charged subject, it is imperative to use the most appropriate term based on an understanding of the underlying causes for the impairment and an assessment of what term is most acceptable to the older adult and his or her care partners.

Medical references to dementia can be traced back to 1906, when a German physician Alois Alzheimer described neuritic plaques in the autopsied brain of a woman who was 55 years old at the time of her death and had experienced cognitive and behaviour changes for about 5 years before her death. By building on earlier studies indicating that hardening of the arteries caused cognitive impairment in *older* adults, Alzheimer concluded that neuritic plaques caused cognitive impairment in *younger* adults. By 1910, Alzheimer's disease (i.e. presenile dementia) was considered a distinct disease differentiated from senile dementia by younger age at onset. This viewpoint was not challenged until the 1960s when autopsy studies indicated that many of the brain changes attributed to irreversible pathological conditions were actually manifestations of treatable conditions. Landmark studies by Tomlinson, Blessed and Roth (1968, 1970) led to the conclusion that the neuropathological changes of Alzheimer's disease represent a single disease process, regardless of the age at onset. In 1974, another landmark study by Hachinski, Lassen and Marshall found that cerebral atherosclerosis was both a major cause of cognitive impairments and the most common medical *mis*diagnosis. Moreover, these scientists denounced the use of the phrase "hardening of the arteries" and introduced the term "multi-infarct dementia" to describe dementias of cerebrovascular origin. Based on recent research, the term vascular dementia is more appropriate than either of these terms, as discussed in the section on types of dementia.

In clinical settings, dementia is the medical term that includes a group of brain disorders characterised by a gradual decline in cognitive abilities (e.g. memory, understanding, judgement, decision making, communication) and changes in personality and behaviour. Because Alzheimer's disease is a type of dementia that occurs most commonly and has the longest history of recognition, *Alzheimer's disease* and *dementia* are sometimes used interchangeably, although this is not always accurate. Because the term "dementia" is closely associated with the uncomplimentary use of the term "demented", a phrase such as "a person living with dementia" is more appropriate when referring to the medical syndrome of impaired cognitive function. Several leading gerontologists recently suggested that clinicians use the term "aging-associated cognitive challenges" to emphasise that this condition is something that can serve as a source of growth for older adults (George, Qualls, Camp et al., 2012).

An additional point must be emphasised with regard to the term *dementia*. Dementia is not a single disease but a group of diseases, and each type is associated with a different cause and unique combination of manifestations. Additional considerations that complicate the use of terms related to impaired cognitive function are as follows:

- Two or more types of dementia can develop at the same time or sequentially.
- Commonly available diagnostic techniques cannot always determine the type of dementia.
- Terms may be used inaccurately even by healthcare professionals.
- Because the ability to differentiate between types of dementia is still in early stages, many of the studies on Alzheimer's disease have included subjects with other types of dementia.

In this chapter, the term *dementia* is used except when the information is pertinent to a particular type. The text refers to Alzheimer's disease when a source has used that term; however, it is important to recognise that many of the citations on Alzheimer's disease refer to dementia in the broader sense.

Types of dementia

Even with current advances in technology, the diagnosis of dementia is as much of an art as a science, and pathological brain changes can be clearly identified only on autopsy. The current approach to diagnosing dementia can be likened to the approach taken to diagnosing an infection. An infection is a generic diagnosis indicating the presence of a constellation of signs and symptoms (e.g. malaise, elevated temperature), but it does not indicate the causative factor.

As additional information is collected, the specific type of infection is identified (e.g. pneumonia, urinary tract infection, bacterial, viral), and sometimes, more than one infection is discovered. Until the specific causative agent is identified, generic measures are taken (e.g. antipyretics, broad-spectrum antibiotics).

After the specific causative agent is identified (e.g. through culture and sensitivity tests), the infection is treated with very specific antimicrobial agents. At all stages, comfort measures are used.

Analogously, dementia is a generic diagnosis indicating a constellation of signs and symptoms (e.g. memory impairment, personality changes), but there are no clear indicators during early stages of most types of dementia. As the condition progresses and further information develops, one or more causative factors is likely to be identified. However, there is no diagnostic equivalent of a "culture and sensitivity" test for dementia, so it is difficult to distinguish between the different types of dementia. Thus, diagnosis of specific types of dementia is based on clinical observations, history of risk factors, and information from brain imaging and other available diagnostic data.

Based on current scientific literature, the four most commonly recognised types of dementia are **Alzheimer's disease, vascular dementia, Lewy body dementia** and **frontotemporal dementia**. It is important to realise that research is evolving, and there are significant overlaps in manifestations of the different types of dementia. Another complicating factor is that two (or more) types of dementia can—and often do—coexist in the same person and, as the pathological processes progress, it becomes more difficult to distinguish one type of dementia from another.

Autopsy studies of older people who have died with dementia find that various pathologies account for most cases of dementia. Multiple neuropathologies are particularly common among those over the age of 80 years (Flicker, 2010; Jellinger & Attems, 2010) and this type of dementia is referred to as *mixed dementia*. This chapter presents information that is clinically important in relation to each of the four most common types of dementia; however, information about functional consequences, assessment and interventions applies to all types. Table 14-1

TABLE 14-1 Distinguishing features of common types of dementia

Type	Onset and course	Typical manifestations
Alzheimer's disease	Insidious onset; diagnosis often made retrospectively; slowly progressive over 5 to 10 years, with accelerated decline associated with concomitant conditions (e.g. heart failure, delirium)	Early cognitive changes, usually but not always involving memory loss. Gradual loss of other cognitive abilities (e.g. decision making, language) and communication skills. Gradual onset of behaviour and personality changes (e.g. depression, irritability, agitation, indifference)
Vascular dementia	Abrupt onset due to cumulative effects of small strokes or sudden onset if related to major stroke. History of vascular risks (e.g. stroke, hypertension). Irregular course or improvement is possible depending on causative factors	Manifestations consistent with area of brain that is affected: aphasia, memory impairment, apathy, depression, emotional lability and sensory-motor deficits (e.g. hemiparesis, gait disturbances, hemisensory loss, urinary incontinence)
Lewy body dementia	Insidious onset with a progressive decline in cognitive, behavioural and motor symptoms; manifestations similar to Parkinson's disease	Significant cognitive impairment; fluctuating levels of cognition; parkinsonism; hallucinations; sleep disturbances; loss of postural stability; highly sensitive to neuroleptic medications
Frontotemporal degeneration	Gradual onset between the ages of 50 and 70; family history common; progressive decline in functioning	Early and progressive changes in behaviour, motor abilities, or speech-language skills. Memory impairments occur later during the course of the disease
	Gradual onset typically before the age of 65 years; family history common; progressive decline in functioning	Early and progressive changes in behaviour, motor abilities and/or speech-language skills. Memory impairments occur later during the course of the disease

describes the distinguishing features of the four most common types of dementia.

DIVERSITY NOTE

It has been reported that the prevalence of dementia among Indigenous people in a rural and remote region of Australia is four to five times higher than other Australians (Smith et al., 2008). However, the prevalence of dementia in older Māori is not significantly different to non-Māori (New Zealand Ministry of Health, 2011).

Alzheimer's disease

Alzheimer's disease accounts for 60% to 80% of the cases of dementia (Alzheimer's Association, 2013) and, as already discussed, is the type of dementia with the strongest research base. Hallmark pathological characteristics of Alzheimer's disease are as follows:

- Amyloid plaques in the spaces between the neurons: abnormal deposits of a protein fragment called **beta-amyloid**, which is formed from the breakdown of a larger protein called amyloid precursor protein
- Neurofibrillary tangles inside the neurons: abnormal clusters of a protein called tau
- Loss of synaptic connections between neurons
- Cell death causing brain atrophy.

All of the above lead to a marked reduction in brain weight, as illustrated in Figure 14-2.

The gradual progression of brain atrophy is correlated with stages of Alzheimer's, from preclinical to severe, as illustrated in Figure 14-3.

In 2011, the National Institute on Aging and the Alzheimer's Association published the first major update on diagnostic guidelines for Alzheimer's since 1984. These guidelines, which are similar to those published by the International Working Group on Alzheimer's Disease, define Alzheimer's disease as a neurological condition that begins with a preclinical stage and progresses to the clinical diagnosis

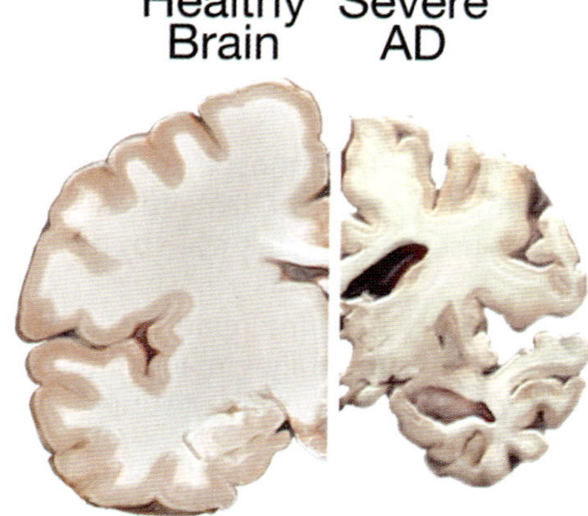

FIGURE 14-2 Pathological brain changes cause significant atrophy. (Courtesy of the National Institute on Aging/National Institutes of Health.)

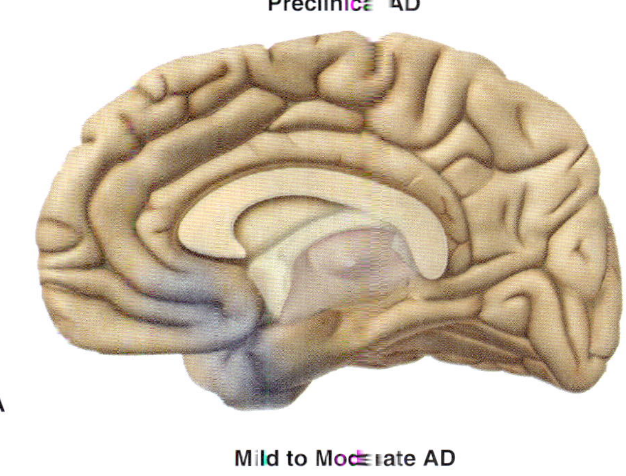

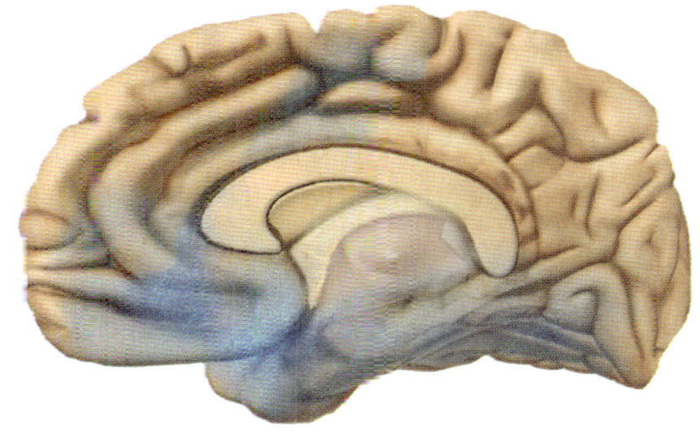

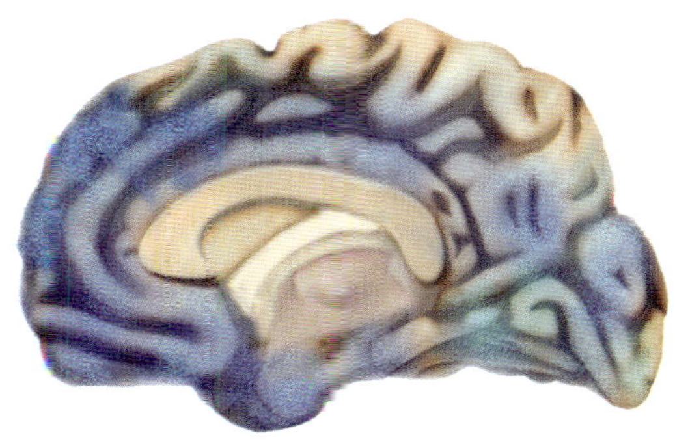

FIGURE 14-3 (**A**) During preclinical Alzheimer's disease, subtle degenerative changes begin to occur, and the person develops mild cognitive impairment. (**B**) In mild to moderate stages of Alzheimer's disease, pathological changes affect the areas of the brain that control memory, language and reasoning. (**C**) In the severe stage of Alzheimer's disease pathological changes cause significant atrophy in many areas. (Courtesy of the National Institute on Aging/National Institutes of Health.)

of dementia. Box 14-1 presents evidence-based information from these guidelines and additional pertinent research information about additional aspects of Alzheimer's disease.

Vascular dementia

Vascular dementia refers to cognitive impairment, ranging from mild to severe, which is caused by the death of nerve cells in the regions nourished by the diseased vessels. Estimated prevalence is between 11% and 18% for vascular dementia alone and between 22% and 34% for a combination of vascular dementia and Alzheimer's disease (Kling, Trojanowski, Wolk et al., 2013). Underlying pathological processes include clinical stroke (e.g. haemorrhage or occlusion of blood vessels) or subclinical vascular brain injury (e.g. lacunar strokes of the small arteries). Although vascular dementia has been viewed as a distinct type of dementia, reviews of recent studies indicate that cerebrovascular damage most often occurs concurrently with the neuropathological changes of other dementias (Gorelick & Nyenhuis, 2013; Kling, Trojanowski, Wolk et al., 2013). As with all types of dementia, manifestations range from mild to severe and fluctuations are associated with progression of the disease and the onset of concurrent conditions. Factors that are strongly associated with increased risk for vascular dementia include stroke, hypertension, hypercholesterolaemia, obesity, diabetes and atrial fibrillation. Table 14-1 provides information about the onset, course and typical manifestations of vascular dementia.

Lewy body dementia

Lewy body dementia is part of a group of disorders called *Lewy body diseases*, which also includes Parkinson's disease and Parkinson's disease with dementia. Lewy body dementia and Parkinson's disease with dementia account for between 15% and 20% of dementia diagnoses (Gealogo, 2013). The hallmark pathological characteristic of Lewy body disease is the presence of abnormal proteins (i.e. Lewy bodies) in the brain that eventually damage the neurons and affect all the following cognitive abilities, motor function, sensory function, sleep patterns and autonomic function. Clinically it is difficult to differentiate between Lewy body dementia and Alzheimer's disease because they have overlapping features and often occur together. Features that are more characteristic of dementia with Lewy bodies (compared with Alzheimer's disease) include more pronounced cognitive fluctuations, spontaneous parkinsonism and visual hallucinations as an early and recurrent manifestation (Hanagasi, Bilgic & Emre, 2013; Huang & Halliday, 2013). Table 14-1 lists distinguishing features of Lewy body dementia.

People with Lewy body dementia are highly sensitive to medications with anticholinergic properties and they can develop extreme, idiosyncratic or fatal reactions to even low doses of certain medications such as phenothiazines and newer antipsychotics (Kaur, Harvey, DeCarli et al., 2012). For example, sedatives or antipsychotics may cause hallucinations, agitation or extreme somnolence. Thus, anticholinergic medications, including over-the-counter products, should be avoided, and if they are used, doses should be minimal, and the older adult should be observed carefully for adverse effects. Another clinically important characteristic is that people with Lewy body dementia may decompensate rapidly and significantly when they have a medical condition (e.g. minor infection) or when their

BOX 14-1
Dementia (D) and Alzheimer's disease (AD) in the Australia and New Zealand: Facts, figures and overview

Australia marked dementia as a **National Health Priority** in 2012 and, as a result, collaboration between Australian governments and health sector organisations is facilitated to improve the delivery of dementia care.

In 2013 the New Zealand Ministry of Health published the *New Zealand framework for dementia care*, which guides the District Health Boards and the health and social support sectors with the development of their dementia care pathways.

Prevalence of D

- In 2014, 332,000 Australians have been diagnosed with D
- In 2011, 48,000 New Zealanders had D
- Figures are expected to increase by 2050: in Australia to approx. 1 million; New Zealand to approx. 150,000
- In Australia three in ten people over the age of 85 have D
- In Australia each week, 1700 new cases of D equates to approx. one person diagnosed every 6 minutes

Consequences of D

- D is the third leading cause of death (the second leading cause in women) in Australia
- D is the third cause of significant health loss in older adults aged 75 years and over in New Zealand

Stages of AD as proposed by 2011 Criteria of the National Institute on Aging and the Alzheimer's Association

- Preclinical AD: Pathological changes begin 20 years or more before the onset of symptoms; this stage cannot be diagnosed in usual clinical settings, but is being used for research purposes
- **Mild cognitive impairment (MCI)** due to AD: Measurable changes in cognitive abilities that are noticeable to the person affected and to people who have frequent contact with the person; cognitive changes do not significantly affect the person's everyday activities
- Dementia due to AD: Memory, thinking and behavioural symptoms that impair the person's ability to function in daily life

Symptoms of AD

- Memory loss that disrupts daily life
- Challenges in planning or solving problems
- Difficulty completing familiar tasks at home, at work, or at leisure
- Confusion with time and place
- Trouble understanding visual images and spatial relationships
- Changes in language or writing skills
- Misplacing things and losing the ability to retrace steps
- Impaired judgement
- Withdrawal from work or social activities
- Changes in mood and personality

Factors that increase the risk for AD

- Family history: increased risk in people who have first-degree relative with AD (i.e. parent or sibling)
- Inheriting the ApoE-E4 gene from one or both parents
- Diagnosis of MCI in combination with memory impairment, delirium
- Risks for cardiovascular disease: smoking, obesity, diabetes, hypertension, hypercholesterolaemia
- Traumatic brain injury

Factors that decrease the risk for AD

- Physical activity
- Diet that is low in saturated fats and rich in vegetables and vegetable-based oils
- Higher levels of education, which help build a "cognitive reserve"
- Engaging in social and cognitive activities

Source: Alzheimer's Australia (2014); Alzheimer's New Zealand (2012); Alzheimer's Association (2013).

environment is changed. Also, cognitive fluctuations commonly occur over minutes, hours or days. It is important to be alert to the possibility that people with Lewy body dementia may be misdiagnosed as having Alzheimer's disease or they may have both types of dementia.

Frontotemporal dementia

Frontotemporal degeneration (also called frontotemporal disorders and formerly called frontotemporal dementia) describes a type of dementia caused by neurodegenerative conditions involving the frontal or temporal lobes or both, which collectively are referred to as frontotemporal degeneration. Pick's disease was first identified as a type of frontotemporal dementia in 1892 and, in recent years, frontotemporal degeneration is recognised as a major cause of young-onset dementia. Symptoms of frontotemporal degeneration typically begin during the sixth decade of life but may begin as early as the third decade (Warren, Rohrer & Rossor, 2013).

Manifestations of frontotemporal degeneration vary widely according to the order in which the frontal or temporal lobes of the brain are affected. Types of frontotemporal degeneration as classified by symptoms are as follows:

- Progressive behavioural and personality decline: apathy, disinhibition, emotional lability, changes in behaviour and personality, and diminished concentration, attention, reasoning, judgement
- Progressive language decline: loss of abilities related to speaking, writing and language comprehension
- Progressive motor decline: falls, gait changes, movement disorders, muscle rigidity, difficulty with tasks involving fine motor skills.

Diagnosis of frontotemporal degeneration is difficult because manifestations vary widely and overlap with those of other types of dementia. People with frontotemporal degeneration are often misdiagnosed as having a psychiatric illness because of their younger age, better performance on usual cognitive tests, and lack of insight. Because of its early onset and prominent and difficult-to-manage behavioural manifestations, frontotemporal degeneration is associated with significant stress and financial burden for spouses and other care partners (Massimo, Evans, Benner, 2013).

A consideration related to management is that usual medications for dementia (i.e. cholinesterase inhibitors or memantine) are not effective for frontotemporal degeneration. However, there is some evidence that trazodone at a dose of 100 mg three times a day may be helpful for managing symptoms (Chow & Alobaidy, 2013). In addition, because usual non-pharmacological management strategies for dementia, such as redirecting the person, have limited effectiveness, nurses need to be creative in developing individualised care plans. For example, nurses can facilitate and coordinate an interdisciplinary team approach, including all the following: speech-language therapists to address speech, language and swallowing problems; physical and occupational therapists to address progressive motor decline; and social workers and mental health professionals to address behavioural and emotional components.

FACTORS ASSOCIATED WITH DEMENTIA

From a wellness perspective, it is important to recognise not only the factors that increase the risk for dementia but also those that protect against cognitive impairment. Researchers and policy makers are increasingly emphasising the importance of addressing modifiable risk factors as an intervention for preventing dementia. In December 2013, 109 scientists from 36 countries issued a statement calling for international attention to making prevention of dementia a major health issue. Some highlights of the statement, which was published in the *Journal of Alzheimer's Disease* (Smith & Yaffe, 2014), are as follows:

- The same public health approach that has been effective for about half of the reduction in deaths from heart disease and stroke should be applied to dementia.
- About half of Alzheimer's disease cases worldwide might be attributable to known risk factors. Taking immediate action on known risk factors could perhaps prevent up to one-fifth of predicted new cases by 2025.
- There is already sufficient evidence to justify trials related to all the following: exercise, diabetes management, depression treatment, blood pressure control, B vitamins, omega-3 fatty acids, cognitive training and social activities.
- Public health policies should "tell people that adopting a healthy lifestyle may help ward off dementia as it does for other diseases".

A consistent conclusion of studies related to risks for dementia is that behaviours and interventions that are effective for preventing cardiovascular disease and promoting overall health (e.g. physical activity and healthy dietary practices) are also associated with improved cognitive function (Alzheimer's Association, 2013; Barnett, Hachinski & Blackwell, 2013; Justin, Turek, Hakim, 2013; Mangialasche, Kivipelto, Solomon et al., 2012; Prince et al., 2014).

WELLNESS OPPORTUNITY

Nurses can teach all adults that engaging in social, mental and physical activity is a risk-free way of promoting cognitive wellness and may also prevent dementia.

As discussed in Chapter 11, there is increasing research interest in understanding of the role *cognitive reserve* has in the maintenance of cognitive function despite brain pathology. Nurses have suggested that interventions to enhance cognitive reserve in people with early stage dementia may also be interventions to prevent delirium (Fick et al., 2009). Specific preventive strategies suggested by Fick and colleagues (2009) include physical activity, social interaction, challenging mental activities, and avoidance of inappropriate medications.

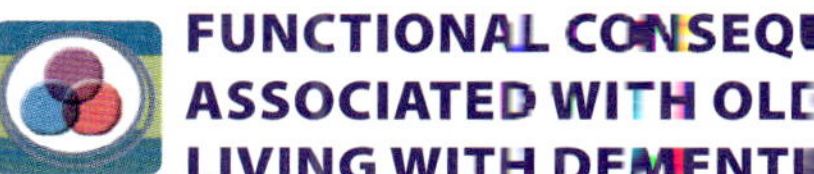

FUNCTIONAL CONSEQUENCES ASSOCIATED WITH OLDER ADULTS LIVING WITH DEMENTIA

Functional consequences related to Alzheimer's disease have been studied since the 1950s, but research on the unique manifestations of different dementias is in very early stages. Many functional consequences are common to all of the dementias and, as the disease progresses, manifestations of all types of dementia become more similar. However, it is important to recognise that during all stages and in all types of dementia, functional consequences vary tremendously among individuals because of unique personality characteristics, coexisting conditions (e.g. depression, functional impairments), and other influences.

It also is imperative to acknowledge that the *personhood* of each individual who has dementia is always present and needs to be addressed in every interaction. Acknowledging personhood in people living with dementia involves recognising the needs, wants, emotions, personality, relationships, life story and need for connectedness of the individual (Palmer, 2013). Although dementia has long been associated with a "loss of self", a recent study stated that "personhood can be understood as increasingly concealed rather than lost" (Smebye & Kirkevold, 2013, p. 29). This perspective highlights the responsibility of nurses and all who provide care to acknowledge and discover the underlying personhood of each person who has dementia. In this and the following sections of this chapter, the experiences of people living with dementia are described in boxes to illustrate the unique ways in which dementia affects individuals and their care partners. In addition to the functional consequences that directly affect the person living with dementia, carers and families of people living with dementia also experience significant consequences.

Stages of dementia

In the mid 1980s an American psychiatrist named Reisberg proposed a seven-stage model for describing the functional consequences of Alzheimer's disease (Reisberg, 1986). Reisberg's staging schema, which has been updated and refined, is referred to as the Global Deterioration Scale/ Functional Assessment Staging, or GDS/FAST. This staging system is widely used and has been found to be valid and reliable for staging Alzheimer's disease in diverse settings (Sabbagh et al., 2009). Table 14-2 summarises the functional consequences associated with each of the seven stages of the GDS/FAST. According to this framework, the diagnosis of Alzheimer's disease is made retrospectively because it is based on a progression of manifestations.

Gerontologists, clinicians, people living with dementia, and families and carers are intensely interested in identifying factors that influence not only the course of the disease but the person's survival time. One review of 48 studies that evaluated dementia prognosis and survival found that increased age, male gender, decreased functional status and medical comorbidities were associated with a higher mortality rate in people living with dementia (Lee & Chodosh, 2009).

Because dementia is strongly associated with shortened life expectancy, it is widely recognised as a terminal illness, with death being the ultimate functional consequence. Thus, in recent years, there has been increasing recognition of the need to provide hospice and palliative care services during late-stage dementia.

Self-awareness of people living with dementia

One of the myths associated with dementia is that people living with dementia deny their symptoms or have no awareness of their deficits. Unfortunately, this fallacy has led to serious misunderstandings on the part of some healthcare professionals, as exemplified by statements such as, "If they can ask if they have Alzheimer's disease, then they don't have it."

In recent years, this perception of a high prevalence of so-called denial in people living with dementia has diminished, and gerontologists are researching insight and self-awareness through all stages of dementia.

Lack of awareness of cognitive deficit, called *anosognosia*, is now recognised as a core diagnostic feature of frontotemporal dementia; it also occurs with Alzheimer's dementia when the frontal cortex is affected (Salmon et al., 2008; Shibata et al., 2008). However, increasing evidence shows that even when people living with dementia have anosognosia, they maintain self-awareness of their needs and feelings, called *retained awareness*, from early stages to later stages (Bossen, Specht & McKenzie, 2009).

TABLE 14-2 Global Deterioration Scale/Functional Assessment Staging (GDS/FAST) of Alzheimer's disease

Stage	Effects on functioning
1: Normal adult	No deficits or complaints
2: Age-associated	Deficits consistent with normal ageing (i.e. memory impairment no objective findings, difficulty with word finding, forgets location of objects)
3: Mild cognitive	Some deficits in performing complex tasks, impairment particularly in demanding social and employment settings; diminished organisational skills; deficits noted by others for the first time
4: Mild dementia	Diminished ability to perform complex tasks (e.g. meal planning, financial management); decreased knowledge of current and recent events; flattened affect and withdrawal from challenging situations
5: Moderate dementia	Obvious cognitive deficits; unable to manage complex daily tasks without some supervision or assistance; difficulty remembering names of familiar people
6: Moderately severe	Increasingly obvious cognitive deficits (e.g. dementia disorientation, significant short-term memory impairment); personality and emotional changes (e.g. anxiety, delusions) Loss of abilities in the following order: (a) Difficulty putting clothing on properly without assistance (b) Unable to bathe independently (c) Unable to handle all aspects of toileting (e.g. does not wipe properly) (d) Occasional or frequent urinary incontinence (e) Occasional or frequent faecal incontinence
7: Severe dementia	Progressive loss of all verbal and psychomotor abilities: (a) Verbal abilities limited to six or fewer different words (b) Verbal abilities limited to a single intelligible word (c) Unable to walk without assistance (d) Unable to sit without assistance (e) Unable to smile (f) Unable to hold up head independently

Source: Reisberg, B. (1986). Dementia: A systematic approach to identifying reversible causes. *Geriatrics, 41*(4), 30–46.

Although studies are just beginning to shed light on this multidimensional topic, research indicates that many people with dementia are aware of their deficits and that some level of awareness is retained as the dementia progresses (Clare, Nelis, Martyr et al., 2012; Clare, Whitaker, Roberts, 2013; Mardh, Karlsson & Marcusson, 2013). Studies also indicate that a higher level of awareness is associated with greater levels of anxiety and depression (Horning, Melrose, Sultzer, 2014; van Vliet, de Vugt, Kohler et al., 2012;

Verhulsdonk, Quack, Gof: et al., 2013). Even in later stages, the personhood of people living with dementia is increasingly changed and hidden but it is not lost (Edvardsson, Winbad & Sandman, 2008).

Programs emphasising the provision of person-centred care through all stages of dementia are based on these research findings. Studies of the feelings and experiences of individuals living with dementia provide important insight into the awareness they retain, as described in boxes throughout this chapter, with direct quotes from people living with dementia. Box 14-2 summarises statements of people living with dementia about how they are perceived by others.

BOX 14-2
Lived experiences: How people with dementia feel about others' perceptions

- It would be nice if a lot of people had more understanding and appreciate what you have got. I was in town, and this other lady started laughing because of the way I was trying to struggle to talk and that started to make me feel uncomfortable; I thought if only she understood then perhaps she wouldn't stand there and laugh.
- If you say to someone, "Can you wait a couple of minutes; I've got dementia and I want to explain", they look at you and think there is nothing wrong with you; you should be able to talk. Then again, you get some who say, "HOW ARE YOU?" and you think, "Grr ... I'm not that bad."
- It's as though, that's it, you are dribbling and nodding, and that's the picture of Alzheimer's. But we are all sitting here and talking perfectly normally. We have got Alzheimer's of some form; we are not nodding and dribbling.
- The stigma is far more than cancer, far more ... and people still do not talk about dementia; they still try to avoid it.
- I'm trying to guard that I don't get looked down on. I don't want the feeling of being back in first grade or whatever ... of going in the other direction, of decreasing instead of improving, and I have inward anger.
- Everybody I have met has been absolutely amazed that (a) I can still talk and still think, and (b) that I have a diagnosis of dementia. They do not understand it.
- How another person reacts to you can make you very unhappy.
- No one really understands how hard it is to live life like this, so people tend to trivialise how you feel, patronise you, and make out that they feel the same way.
- Written off as being devoid of feelings and needs ... It was clear to me that my dementia negated the things that I said. It was very painful.
- It has been proven by thousands of early stage people with dementia to be capable and intelligent beings just moving a little slower.
- My family members' relationships with me changed as soon as they found out that I was "no longer competent". The things that I say seem to be a lot more subject to question than they used to be. It's as if I can't possibly know anything anymore. At least that's the way I feel.
- Nobody thought to consider my background; nobody wanted to know about that. 'Oh no, that doesn't matter, let's just look at you now.' I think the difficulty is that you need a snapshot of how you were to compare it to how you are. They have no interest in that.

Source: Alzheimer's Society (2008); Alzheimer Society (2010a); Alzheimer's Society (2010b); Beard & Fox (2008); Beard, Knauss & Moyer (2009); Clare, Rowlands & Quin (2008).

Personal experiences of dementia

During the early stages, only the individual living with dementia and the people who live, work or have close contact with the person notice the initial changes, such as impaired judgement and short-term memory. When the changes are noticed, numerous explanations may be applicable, and the deficits may be attributed to such factors as depression or the occurrence of a major life event (e.g. retirement, widowhood).

People in the early stages of dementia may withdraw from complex tasks as a way of protecting themselves from the effects of diminishing cognitive abilities. For example, employed people may retire without acknowledging cognitive impairments as the reason. People who do not have to perform complex intellectual or psychomotor tasks may be able to conceal or compensate for the cognitive losses until the deficits seriously interfere with *activities of daily living* (ADLs). As the disease progresses, however, the person living with dementia is less able to cover up the changes, and people with less intimate contact will begin to question the underlying cause of the deficits.

Many first-person accounts of the lived experiences of people living with dementia have been published since the 1990s. Although most of these memoirs describe dementia as an overwhelming challenge to be struggled with, defeated by, or succumbed to, some personal narratives reflect positive themes such as resilience, a strong sense of self, and striving for normalcy. Thus, it is important that healthcare practitioners recognise that the extent to which dementia is viewed as problematic does vary. A study by Hulko (2009) suggested that people who are "more privileged" are more likely to view dementia negatively, and those who are more "marginalised" will dismiss the significance of dementia and resist being viewed as the sum of their symptoms (Hulko, 2009). Box 14-3 describes the experiences and feelings of people living with dementia about the earliest changes and their diagnoses.

Common emotions and behaviours of people living with dementia include loss, fear, shame, anger, sadness, anxiety, frustration, loneliness, depression, uncertainty, sense of uselessness, self-blame, diminished affect and withdrawal from challenging activities. A major focus of emotional responses, particularly during the early stages, is on readjusting one's self-concept, trying to maintain a sense of normalcy, and developing cognitive, social and behavioural strategies to improve confidence (Cotter, 2009). Even during the later stages of dementia, when cognitive abilities are severely impaired, emotional responses are directed towards preserving a sense of self. Dominant

BOX 14-3
Lived experiences: Feelings about earliest dementia changes

- I knew my brain wasn't what it used to be because I've always remembered that I gave birth to my girls and one time I thought, "I can't remember what their birthday is."
- To sing a song that I have sung 100 times before to music I have heard 100 times before and I'm standing there thinking, "What the hell am I doing here and what am I going to sing?" This started to happen more and more, and when you are out on the stage on your own and you don't know what you are doing, it is a terrifying prospect.
- If I was getting dressed in the morning, I would put my clothes on, and I would guarantee you there was at least a pair of trousers, a shirt, or a hat and coat—and it had all gone on upside down, back to front.
- I was struggling at work. I became disorganised and was losing control of the class, which is something I had never done.
- I'm still the same person I've always been. It's just that now I'm *me* with Alzheimer's. I am still loving and caring, and I still have feelings, and I would like to think that I haven't changed in myself.
- Although I was expecting it by then, the words were still devastating to hear.
- I feel like I still have enough intelligence to be a person and not just someone you pat on the head as you go by … It's devastating, and it takes away your sense of self. I feel like I'm still a person and my wants and desires should at least be considered before decisions are made.
- I felt I had a shock. I just thought it can't be. I said it's for other people.
- The angst and anger that I went through during the diagnostic process, I could have actually gone and thumped people.
- It was as if the thunderclouds had been taken away because they had given an answer to me why I was treating my family so like a louse that I was.
- I was relieved really that what I was trying to convince people had been verified.
- I think the word Alzheimer's puts like a fear in you, like cancer does.
- I still have a memory so that's the good part. I forget that I have got dementia.
- It is a really frightening thing when no one can tell you how fast you will deteriorate. It is hard to get across how that feels, but it gnaws at you continually, and each day you wonder what faculty will be lost next.
- It is quite strange because dementia seems to hit people in very different ways. There are little threads of commonality in it, but everyone is affected in a slightly different way.
- I think I have a very different view about how long I'll be around, or when life will come to an end, or when I'll be incompetent than I did before the diagnosis. No question.
- I certainly think that it's important to let family be aware of one's problems. Not to the extent of complaining and complaining, but this is what it is, and I have to deal with that. I wouldn't deny it ever.

Source: Alzheimer's Society (2008); Alzheimer's Society (2010a); Alzheimer's Society (2010b); Beard & Fox (2008); Beard, Knauss & Moyer (2009); Clare, Rowlands & Quin (2008).

emotions during later stages of dementia include feelings of loss, anger, frustration, uncertainty and lack of control or self-determination (Clare, Rowlands & Quin, 2008). It is imperative to recognise that emotional responses of people living with dementia may be blunted or altered, but they are never absent. As dementia progresses, the person is likely to express emotions non-verbally and behaviourally. Thus, two important responsibilities of carers are to encourage and interpret non-verbal communication, which becomes the primary mode of communication during later stages of dementia.

WELLNESS OPPORTUNITY

Nurses holistically address psychosocial needs by recognising that individuals vary significantly in their emotional responses, but people living with dementia never lose the ability to respond to others.

Behavioural and psychological symptoms of dementia (BPSD)

Significant behavioural disturbances, called **behavioural and psychological symptoms of dementia (BPSD)** (also called *neuropsychiatric symptoms*), occur at some point during the course of dementia in nearly all people living with dementia (Burke, Hall, Tariot et al., 2013; Selbaek, Engedal & Bergh, 2013). Some examples of BPSD are as follows:

- Agitation: abnormal level of verbal, vocal or motor activity (e.g. aggression, screaming)
- Psychiatric symptoms: delusions, hallucinations
- Personality changes, disinhibition
- Mood disturbances: apathy, depression, euphoria, emotional lability
- Aberrant motor movements: pacing, rummaging, wandering
- Changes in sleep, eating, appetite
- Hypersexual behaviour: inappropriate statements, sexually aggressive actions, masturbation in public places.

When BPSD or increased confusion or restlessness occur only or primarily in the early evening, this is called **sundowning**. Factors associated with sundowning include fatigue, overstimulation, fear of darkness and altered circadian rhythm.

Aggression and agitation are types of BPSD that are strongly associated with serious functional consequences, including distress and reduced quality of life for the person living with dementia and for those who are care partners, and increased risk for being admitted to a hospital or long-term care setting (Ballard & Corbett, 2013; Toot, Devine, Akporobaro et al., 2013). Conditions associated with physical and verbal aggressive behaviour include depression, psychosis, poor physical health, severe cognitive impairment, and lack of environmental stimuli. Conditions associated with agitation include pain, overstimulation, social isolation, disruption of usual routines, and unmet physical needs related to sleep, thirst, hunger, fatigue or elimination (Morgan, Sail, Snow et al., 2013).

Although BPSD occurs in almost all people living with dementia, these symptoms vary widely and none of these behaviours occurs in all people living with dementia. Also, manifestations of BPSD change during the course of the illness in each person and many resolve as dementia progresses. It is not unusual for one or more manifestation of BPSD to resolve at the same time that new ones develop. Because of the wide variability in these symptoms, many people, including healthcare professionals, hold stereotypes or misunderstandings about BPSD. Remarks such as, "I know he doesn't have Alzheimer's disease because he doesn't hallucinate", or "I know she doesn't have Alzheimer's disease because she's not violent", reflect a false belief that certain difficult behaviours are an inevitable consequence of dementia. Similarly, a question such as "Can you tell if my mother will be the 'nice kind' or the 'mean kind' as her Alzheimer's gets worse?" indicates the need for accurate information about BPSD. Another consideration is that spouses and other family members may have difficulty distinguishing between long-term personality patterns and behaviours arising from dementia. This is especially challenging when the person living with dementia has a history of dysfunctional behaviours (e.g. alcohol abuse, anger management) or unhealthy relationships.

A serious consequence of these misunderstandings is that the symptoms are misinterpreted and causative factors are not addressed. Responsibilities of nurses include dispelling myths and misunderstandings and helping carers identify triggers. In addition, it is important to avoid terminology that perpetuates misunderstandings, such as the commonly used term "refuses to …". Table 14-3 summarises some common misperceptions and related facts about dementia-associated behaviours.

A major nursing responsibility is to look for contributing causes and implement strategies to prevent BPSD or minimise the effects of these behaviours. Common contributing causes include pain, fatigue, physical discomfort, environmental conditions, changes in routine, overstimulation or lack of stimulation. It also is imperative to recognise that behavioural manifestations in people living with dementia can be caused, at least in part, by delirium superimposed on dementia, as discussed in the section on delirium. Strategies for addressing behavioural symptoms are discussed in the section on nursing interventions.

Another nursing responsibility, which is consistent with a person-centred approach to care, is to identify the feelings and experiences that the person living with dementia is attempting to communicate through his or her behaviour. Results of a study by Dupuis and colleagues (2012) suggest that professionals replace the concept of challenging behaviour with the term *responsive behaviour* in people living with dementia. This approach emphasises that behaviours are meaningful and "moves us away from judging behaviours to understanding meaning in actions and responses. It means moving away from a focus on dysfunction, deficit and decline, to recognising, valuing and believing in the continued abilities of persons living with dementia to express their experiences and act in purposeful, meaningful and even intentional ways" (Dupuis, Wiersma & Loiselle, 2012, p. 170).

TABLE 14-3 Misperceptions and realities about dementia-associated behaviours

Misperceptions of behaviours	Realities
"He refuses to …"	He has no idea about what is offered; needs to do something else before agreeing to the activity; wants to feel he has a choice; may not have ability to carry out the activity.
"She fights me when I …"	She may be experiencing pain or discomfort, which is exacerbated by activity; she may not understand the activity.
"He denies any problem."	The person may not have insight, awareness or ability to understand.
"There's no reason for him to act that way."	There usually is a triggering event or an unmet need and the behaviour is a way to cope, adapt, respond or express a need.
Manipulative, deliberate actions to get attention.	The person probably does not have enough insight or intent to be manipulative; may be the only way the person is able to express needs.
Nothing to do to prevent the behaviour.	Care partners can be proactive in identifying and addressing triggers.
Interventions that were effective in the past will be effective now	If usual interventions no longer work, be flexible, creative and try something else; use a "trial and error" approach by trying variations of interventions that worked.

Adapted from Miller, C. A. (2012). *Fast facts for dementia care: What nurses need to know in a nutshell*. Used with permission from Springer Publishing Company.

A student's perspective

There is a woman at my nursing home who has severe dementia, to the point where she often is not very kind to the nurses, physios, OTs and other staff. For most of our clinical rotation, I only heard reports of her being angry and sometimes insulting. This can be comical at times, and we all know not to take it personally because we know her attitude is a result of her disease. Understanding the chance I was taking, I went to talk to her during breakfast because she was just staring off into space. Kneeling at her eye level and placing my hand on her shoulder, I began by asking how her morning was. She complained about the cold weather and about how aggressive the OTs were in dressing her. I let her vent, I made some positive remarks, and I complimented her on how beautiful she looked that day.

As I rose to my feet to leave her a few minutes later, she reached for my arm and said, "You're such a sweetheart; you're so kind." My first internal reaction was to be blown away! I had never heard of this woman delivering compliments! But throughout the rest of the day, I couldn't keep the smile off my face. This encounter helped me realise that this woman's beautiful personality is still with her and will always be a part of her. Yes, right now it's being masked most of the time by her dementia, but she still has feelings of kindness and a desire for happiness that fight past her disease every once in a while. I'm just glad I got to be part of that moment and discover that she's still there and needs to be treated like it always. One day she'll have the opportunity and power to express her thanks for those who showed her love and patience.

Shannon H.

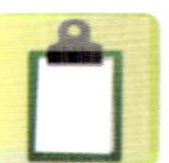

NURSING ASSESSMENT OF DEMENTIA IN OLDER ADULTS

Dementia is a complex syndrome that usually involves a long course of manifestations and intermittent fluctuations. Thus, assessment is an ongoing process that focuses on identifying contributing and treatable conditions and negative consequences that develop during the course of dementia. It also is important to identify and address conditions that interfere with the assessment of dementia.

Factors that influence the assessment of dementia

Attitudes, myths and lack of information are risk factors that interfere with an appropriate assessment of, and interventions for, dementia. In recent years, tremendous progress has been made in understanding and identifying causes of impaired cognitive function; however, many older adults and their families and carers still view serious cognitive impairments as an expected and normal concomitant of ageing. When this happens, treatable conditions are likely to be overlooked, and older adults are denied the appropriate interventions to treat or manage their conditions. Even in the absence of curative treatments, many interventions are effective in delaying the progression of the condition, managing symptoms, and assisting with long-term planning.

WELLNESS OPPORTUNITY

Nurses have many opportunities to teach older adults and their carers about the importance of evaluating any significant cognitive impairment.

Cultural factors that influence perceptions about ageing and illness can significantly affect both the evaluation and treatment of dementia. For example, some cultural groups accept cognitive impairment as "normal ageing", whereas others view dementia-related behaviours as shameful. Gerontologists are just beginning to study various aspects of cultural influences on perception of mental changes and acceptance of interventions.

Initial assessment

With the exception of delirium and post-stroke dementia, impaired cognitive function is a slowly progressive process that requires careful assessment to correctly identify underlying causes. Often, the changes occur slowly over a period of years, and an assessment is delayed until the changes significantly interfere with normal functioning. The assessment process usually takes place over weeks or months and involves the compilation of information about both medical and psychosocial functioning.

Because progressive cognitive impairment is a very complex phenomenon, the assessment process generally is multidisciplinary, requiring input from primary care providers, psychiatrists, nurses, social workers and rehabilitation therapists.

Members of the assessment team must work with the family and other carers to obtain information and determine the appropriate level of involvement of the cognitively impaired person with regard to discussing assessment results and planning care. The major nursing focus is to determine the person's level of function, to identify the factors that affect the person's level of function, and to identify the person's response to his or her illness.

Frequently, the nurse serves as the team leader and is responsible for coordinating information and facilitating communication among team members and with the older adult and his or her family or other carers. Nurses can use Box 14-4 as a guide for assessing progressive cognitive impairments in older adults.

Key assessment tools used to assess cognition and cognitive impairment that apply to dementia are discussed comprehensively in Chapter 13 on cognitive and psychological assessment.

Ongoing assessment of consequences

Because dementia is a progressive condition that commonly coexists with other conditions, all people living with dementia require ongoing assessment of all of the following:

- Changes in cognitive and psychosocial function related to the dementia (e.g. a decline in cognitive abilities, the onset of anxiety or depression)
- Changes in cognitive status related to concurrent conditions (e.g. delirium due to a medical condition or adverse medication effects)
- Changes in functional abilities
- Causes of behavioural changes related to treatable conditions (e.g. anxiety, physical discomfort, environmental factors).

A major goal of ongoing assessment is to identify factors that interfere with the person's level of functioning or

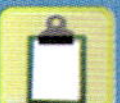

BOX 14-4
Assessing progressive cognitive impairment in older adults

General principles

- Assessment of impaired cognitive function usually takes place during several visits, and it might include a home assessment.
- The person with impaired cognitive function may not be a reliable reporter, but his or her perceptions should be an integral part of the assessment and the accuracy of information should be validated.
- Healthcare professionals must respect the person's rights and ask permission before obtaining information from others, including family members.
- Do not assume that the family has drawn accurate conclusions about events of the past (e.g. family members may state that the person retired and then showed cognitive deficits when, in reality, the person retired because of an inability to cope with job demands).

Focus of the assessment

- The primary purpose of the assessment is to identify the causes of the cognitive impairment.
- An assessment of a person with impaired cognitive function is multidisciplinary and includes the following components: complete medical history and physical examination, including a review of all medications; a functional assessment; a comprehensive psychosocial and formal mental status assessment; and an assessment of environmental and carer influences, with particular emphasis on those factors that affect safety and functional abilities.
- The assessment includes an interview with carers, family members and other people who can describe the progression of the manifestations of impairment.
- Information about lifelong patterns of personality, coping and performance characteristics is considered in relation to the person's current functional level.
- It may be necessary to ask probing questions to help family members recognise clues to cognitive deficits retrospectively.

Considerations in assessing risk factors contributing to impaired cognitive function

- Never assume that all cognitive impairments and behavioural manifestations stem from a dementing illness.
- Because risk factors can either cause the initial cognitive impairments or develop later, causing additional impairments, they must be reassessed periodically.
- The following categories of risk factors must be assessed, both initially and on an ongoing basis: depression, physiological alterations, functional impairments, adverse medication effects, and environmental and psychosocial influences.
- Early in the assessment, ensure that vision and hearing impairments are compensated for as much as possible and that the environment does not interfere with the person's performance (e.g. as possible, make sure the person is using eyeglasses and a hearing aid if needed, and make sure the lighting is optimal).
- A priority is to identify and treat those factors that are reversible before deciding on a long-term management plan.

quality of life, so that interventions can be initiated to alleviate these contributing factors. Even though dementia is a progressive condition that gradually affects all levels of functioning, some of the changes that occur are caused by concurrent conditions rather than by the dementia itself. Thus, ongoing assessment to identify all factors that affect level of functioning is essential. Another goal of ongoing assessment is to identify the person's strengths and limitations in order to plan individualised interventions to improve the person's functioning and quality of life.

Because of the progressive and fluctuating nature of impaired cognitive function, the person's strengths and limitations will change periodically, so care plans must be updated frequently. One way of assessing strengths and weaknesses is to inquire about the ways in which dementia has affected daily living and how the person has coped with, or adjusted to, these changes. Box 14-5 summarises some statements of people living with dementia about ways of coping and daily living.

Nurses can use Table 14-2 as a guide to assessing the progression of dementia from early to later stages. The following guides in this text are pertinent for ongoing assessment of the many aspects of functional consequences associated with the progression of dementia: functioning and safety (Chapter 7), psychosocial function and depression (Chapters 12 and 15), hearing and vision (Chapters 16 and 17), urinary function (Chapter 19), fall risks (Chapter 22), and sleep and rest (Chapter 24).

Nurses also can use the assessment tools in the chapters on medications (Chapter 8) and pain (Chapter 28) to address those aspects of care that are particularly important for people living with dementia. In addition, the assessment tools available from the Hartford Institute for Geriatric Nursing listed in the clinical tools section towards the end of this and other chapters are applicable to assessing aspects of functioning and care for people living with dementia.

WELLNESS OPPORTUNITY

Nurses promote wellness by identifying factors that support optimal functioning rather than focusing only on those that are problematic.

NURSING ISSUES

A nursing issue commonly experienced by people living with dementia is chronic confusion or impaired cognition. Additional nursing issues that are applicable to functional consequences associated with psychosocial responses to dementia include fear, anxiety, hopelessness, social isolation, self-esteem disturbance, and ineffective individual coping. During the later stages, when dementia affects the person's functional abilities, applicable nursing issues include wandering, imbalanced nutrition, urinary incontinence, self-care

BOX 14-5
Lived experiences: Coping and daily living with dementia

About ways of coping

- I think it is alright to allow yourself a bit of time to focus on the pain and fear. That is only human; but it is important to move away from the sad focus and not let it consume you.
- I try to be more patient with myself and forgive myself.
- Staying busy doing what I love to do really keeps me going and gets me through. I'm in two support groups; I have weekly mandolin lesions; I do a weekly men's meditation class with daily homework; I'm reading about consciousness and healing that supports my living in the now and taking care of my spirit.
- I try to do something that I can still do—not as well as before—but something that I can still do.
- It's very important to laugh and enjoy a joke or pleasantries with people.
- We have this problem and we can't change that, but we can improve our lives by not letting it just bring us unhappiness 24 hours a day.
- Usually I just slow down, and reset my expectations. Expecting that you can be who you used to be is just a recipe for pain and sadness.
- I need to have the knowledge that I'm doing what I can. Because oftentimes it's so subtle, and I curse it every now and then and that helps.
- I ask people not to expect me to remember to do things.
- Ahh! I have a great lack of ease with not remembering things. Oh God, it drives me crazy … but we have to accept what we cannot change.
- Going to church; I sing … makes me happy.

About day-to-day living

- Tomorrow I'll have little memory of today, and this makes living today like pushing the rock up the hill knowing it will roll back.
- Inertia is a serious problem with me, and sometimes I seem glued to my chair. Likely it's just that it's so much effort to get myself organised to do things, that I'm mentally exhausted before I even start.
- I streamline everything and get rid of everything I don't use very often. Keeping the house clutter-free helps to minimise the time necessary to find misplaced items.
- I try to find ways to compensate. For example, I now use a GPS to help me from getting lost when I drive.
- My brother-in-law removed all my cabinet doors in my kitchen so I can see all my food in my pantry when I walk into my kitchen.
- I think it would be better if I did not drive; and actually mentally, it is much better that I make that decision than somebody makes that decision for me. Psychologically, it is very good that I am actually in a position where they said, "Okay, you can drive", and just left it at that, and I turned around and said, "Well, thanks very much, but I am actually not going to drive."

Source: Alzheimer's Society (2008); Alzheimer's Society (2010b); Beard & Fox (2008); Beard, Knauss & Moyer (2009); Clare, Rowlands & Quin (2008).

deficit, impaired verbal communication, risk for falls, risk of injury, disturbed sensory perception, and disturbed sleep pattern. If cognitive deficits interfere with the person's ability to take medications accurately, the issue of ineffective medication management will apply.

Nursing issues also address the needs of carers because much of the care of people living with dementia focuses on helping the family and other carers address the day-to-day needs and issues of the person living with dementia. Nursing issues that might be used to address carer needs include family coping and carer role strain (or risk for carer role strain). During the later stages of dementia, the nursing issue of anticipatory grieving may be appropriate, particularly for spousal carers.

WELLNESS OPPORTUNITY

Willingness for enhanced coping is a wellness nursing issue that nurses can apply for people living with dementia as well as their carers.

GOAL PLANNING FOR WELLNESS OUTCOMES

During all stages of dementia, nursing care is directed towards promoting the highest level of functioning, while also supporting the highest quality of life. Nursing goals created that produce wellness outcomes for older adults living with dementia can include: decreased anxiety level, improved cognition, cognitive orientation, comfort level, communication, coping, memory, mood, nutritional status, quality of life, self-care status, sleep, social interaction skills, and increased leisure participation.

When friends, family members or paid carers care for the person living with dementia, nurses plan outcomes to promote carer wellness. In the early stages of dementia, the carer's foremost need might be for information about the disease and about resources that address the changing needs of the person living with dementia and the carer's own needs.

As the dementia progresses, carers are likely to need emotional support and practical assistance. Some goals that may be applicable to carers include decreased anxiety level, improved cognition, cognitive orientation, comfort level, communication, coping, memory, mood, nutritional status, quality of life, self-care status, sleep, social interaction skills, and increased leisure participation.

WELLNESS OPPORTUNITY

Hope is an outcome that would be applicable when nurses plan for wellness to address the body–mind–spirit needs of both people living with dementia and their carers.

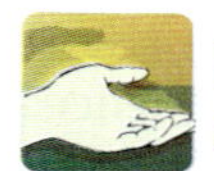

NURSING INTERVENTIONS TO ADDRESS DEMENTIA

Information about interventions to address dementia is evolving at a rapid pace, and research by nurses and other healthcare professionals is shedding light on appropriate interventions for treating the disease and managing the functional consequences. Many interventions are applicable to all people living with dementia and are individualised according to specific manifestations (e.g. reassurance for anxiety and confusion, redirection for unsafe or inappropriate behaviours). Similarly, health promotion interventions (e.g. exercise and nutrition) are applicable for primary and secondary prevention in all people living with dementia. Because a major focus of research is on identifying interventions specifically to address BPSD, information about interventions for dementia-related behaviours is presented in this section. In addition, because carers are an essential component of interventions at all stages of dementia, additional information about addressing the needs of carers is also discussed.

Another consideration for nurses about interventions for dementia is that they have key roles in planning and implementing interventions. Effective care for people living with dementia requires consistent and significant input from many healthcare professionals and other care partners. It is imperative to address nursing interventions in the context of comprehensive, multidisciplinary and person-centred approach to the complex issues related to dementia. Because a comprehensive discussion of interventions for dementia is beyond the scope of this chapter, the topic is addressed by reviewing theoretical frameworks, applying general principles in different clinical settings, and giving an overview of nursing interventions that are applicable in all settings.

Many practical references are also available on the management of dementia. Table 14-4 lists examples of nursing studies of non-pharmacological interventions for dementia-related behaviours. In addition to professional nursing references, numerous books have been written by highly qualified and experienced carers that are excellent references for any nurse caring for people living with dementia. The Alzheimer's Australia and Alzheimer's New Zealand

TABLE 14-4 Research on non-pharmacological interventions for people living with dementia

Intervention	Results	References
*Reviews of studies** related to exercise programs for people living with dementia	Regular exercise interventions can improve mood, behaviour and functioning in people living with dementia; some, but not all, studies show that participation in regular exercise is associated with improved cognitive function in people living with dementia	Amoyal and Fallon (2012); Forbes, Thiessen, Blake et al. (2013); Kirk-Sanchez and McGough (2014)
*Cochrane review** of studies of reality orientation as a form of cognitive stimulation	Consistent evidence shows that reality orientation is a beneficial form of cognitive stimulation for people living with mild to moderate dementia	Woods, Aguirre, Spector et al. (2012)
*Research reviews** on cognitive stimulation for mild cognitive impairment	Reviews of studies indicate that people with mild cognitive impairment and dementia can benefit from cognitive rehabilitation strategies such as memory aids and visual imagery	Cotelli, Manenti, Zanetti et al. (2012); Hopper, Bourgeois, Pimentel et al. (2013); Simon, Yokomizo, Bottino (2012)
*Meta-analysis review** of 23 studies on non-pharmacological interventions for behavioural manifestations of dementia in community-living people with dementia	Support and educational sessions (in-person and by telephone) for carers using multiple components over 3 to 6 months are effective for addressing behaviours such as agitation, aggression, depression, and repetitive behaviours	Brodaty and Arasaratnam (2012)
Learning therapy: cognitive intervention using reading and arithmetic tasks carried out for 15 to 20 minutes, 5 days weekly	Improved and sustained cognitive function after 6 months, compared with control group	Kawashima (2013)
Watermemories Swimming Club: 45-minute classes twice weekly for 12 weeks for people living with dementia	Positive effects on quality of life, social interactions, and functional abilities (no control group)	Neville, Clifton, Henwood et al. (2013)
Leisure activities 3 times per week for 12 weeks, 110 nursing home residents, with outcome measures at baseline and 3, 6 and 9 months	Residents in mah-jongg group (for cognitive stimulation) showed slower rate of global decline compared with control group	Cheng, Chow, Song et al. (2014)
Qualitative study of music-based interventions for residents of a care home	Music is important during all stages of dementia for reducing behavioural and psychological symptoms and promoting interpersonal connectedness	McDermott, Orrell and Ridder (2014)

*Italics differentiate research reviews from individual studies.

provide health education materials and additional reliable information about interventions for people living with dementia and their carers.

DIVERSITY NOTE

A comprehensive resource where information about provision of culturally appropriate dementia care can be found at the Centre for Cultural Diversity in Ageing website, www.culturaldiversity.com.au/resources/practice-guides/dementia-care.

This text addresses nursing interventions by reviewing theoretical frameworks, applying general principles in different clinical settings, and giving an overview of nursing interventions that are applicable in all settings.

Nursing that may be applicable to caring for people living with dementia include active listening, activity therapy, anxiety reduction, behaviour management, calming technique, dementia management, wandering management, emotional support, environmental management, exercise promotion, fall prevention, humour, memory training, mood management, music therapy, presence, reality orientation, reminiscence therapy, self-care assistance, spiritual support *and* touch. When addressing carer needs, interventions would focus on: carer support, consultation, coping enhancement, counselling, decision-making support, humour, referral, respite care, simple relaxation therapy, spiritual growth facilitation and teaching.

WELLNESS OPPORTUNITY

Hope instillation is an outcome that nurses address when they help people living with dementia and their carers to identify a positive meaning for their situation.

Non-pharmacological interventions for promoting wellness for people living with dementia

Interventions must be highly individualised and frequently modified for those living with dementia. An intervention that works for one person may not work for others, and interventions that are effective one day will not necessarily be effective the next day. A dominant theme of research and practice is the implementation of person-centred interventions that are based on a comprehensive and ongoing assessment of the person's unique and changing needs. Caring for people living with dementia is a creative and challenging process.

One way in which nurses promote wellness for people living with dementia is by addressing concerns that improve quality of life. The consequences of dementia significantly affect all aspects of a person's life—most often in undesirable ways—but achieving quality of life is still possible. A review of studies identified the following key domains of quality of life for people living with dementia: health, independence, self-determination, social interaction, financial security, psychological well-being, security and privacy, religion and spirituality, and being of use or giving meaning to life (Alzheimer's Society, 2010b).

BOX 14-6
Lived experiences: Needs and quality of life

About needs

- Just explain it a bit more, like when he said, "I will refer you to the memory clinic", you know, another two or three sentences. I just want to put you in the picture as to what will go on there, what it's for, what the set up is.
- To be taken seriously.
- As you have been diagnosed, there should be a follow-up with information on what you have got, how do you cope with it, what to look for, what's gonna happen.

About quality of life

- Quality of life is living with your family—your circle of friends and family.
- Friendship is good. Very important to have friends.
- Oh, there's nothing better than peace and quiet to be happy and comfortable, but if you ain't got peace, you're upset, and when you've got peace and quiet, you don't have anything in the mind.
- To feel safe. I've lived here for about 2 years and feel secure and safe. No accidents. This is important.
- I want to keep my own environment . . . because I am familiarised with it.
- It's not just the environment in the house, it's when you go out . . . in the bank, environment in the shops you go into, or restaurants is another environment, which you have got to overcome.
- I think your physical health is very important because even though I've got problems in myself, with my brain through my vascular dementia, I feel that if you have got your physical fitness then it still gives you that form of independence that you can still do things. Like I can still go to the bathroom and shave, where if you haven't got good health and you start having problems as well, it must be horrendous.

Source: Alzheimer's Society (2008); Alzheimer's Society (2010b).

An essential intervention for promoting wellness is to pay careful attention to the verbal and non-verbal ways in which the person living with dementia communicates his or her needs and feelings. Box 14-6 provides statements of people living with dementia about their needs and quality of life.

Another way of promoting wellness for people living with dementia is through interventions that support the person's strengths and individuality during all stages of dementia by providing person-centred care, as described in the following sections. Nurses also promote wellness through interventions that support optimal levels of functioning. For example, at least some of the functional decline associated with dementia can be categorised as **excess disability**, which is defined as limitations that are beyond what is to be expected. Environmental factors that do not support optimal functioning of people living with dementia are another source of excess disability (Slaughter & Hayduk, 2012). Another major focus of current research is on non-pharmacological interventions to improve functioning and quality of life for people living with dementia and their care partners, as described in Table 14-4. Nurses can facilitate referrals for these interventions, which are particularly important during early and moderate stages of dementia. These interventions address aspects of functioning and quality of life, but they are not necessarily applicable to addressing dementia-related behaviours, which are discussed in a separate section.

Improving safety and function through environmental modifications

Environmental modifications are important interventions for people living with dementia because environmental factors profoundly affect their safety, functioning and quality of life. During the 1960s, gerontologists initially emphasised the importance of cognitive stimulation and suggested that reality orientation programs be widely implemented, particularly in nursing homes and other residential care settings.

Reality orientation involves the repeated use of verbal and non-verbal indicators of time, place and person in the context of the individual, group and environment. Reality orientation interventions include frequent verbal reminders about the time of day from all staff and "reality orientation boards" that display information in large print about the day, date and weather. Improving the person's self-esteem and sense of control, and reducing confusion, anxiety and disorientation are the goals. Reality orientation may be effective for some people living with dementia, particularly when combined with other strategies, but this intervention must be tailored to individual needs rather than universally applied.

Currently, gerontologists emphasise the important role of the total physical and psychosocial environment as an intervention not only for safety and independent functioning but also for quality of life of people living with dementia (Kiser & Zasler, 2009). In addition, environmental interventions are essential for preventing and addressing problematic behaviours such as wandering. A review of studies related to the therapeutic effects of music emphasises that music improves cognition, communication and quality of life in many ways for people living with dementia (Foster, 2009). Examples of environmental factors that significantly affect the safety, functioning, behaviours and well-being of people living with dementia are:

- Noise
- Music
- Floor surfaces
- Colours and colour contrast
- Lighting (e.g. glare, shadows, brightness)
- Design and placement of exits and bathrooms
- Living things (e.g. plants, birds, fish, pets)
- Furniture (seating, placement, heights of tables and chairs)
- Safety devices (e.g. rails, grab bars)
- Provisions for privacy and social interaction
- Items that improve comfort and hominess (e.g. decorative items, textured items, meaningful personal belongings)
- Absence of potentially harmful items (e.g. clutter, obstacles, sharp knives, cleaning solutions and other potentially toxic products.

Box 14-7 summarises environmental interventions and techniques to address safety and independence in ADLs.

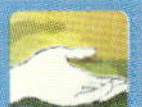

BOX 14-7
Environmental adaptations and techniques for improving safety and functioning in people living with dementia

General environmental modifications

- Modify the environment to compensate as much as possible for sensory deficits and other functional impairments. (Refer to interventions in Chapters 16 through 19 and 22).
- Use clocks, calendars, daily newspapers, and simple written cues for orientation (e.g. day, date, names, place and events).
- Use simple pictures, written cues and colour codes for identifying items and places (e.g. toilet, bedroom).
- Use simple written cues to clarify directions for operating radios, televisions, appliances and thermostats (e.g. on, off, directional arrows).
- Place pictures of familiar people in highly visible places, but use non-glossy pictures and non-glare glass in picture frames.
- Turn lights on as soon as or before it gets dark.
- Use night lights, or leave dim lights on during the night.
- Provide adequate environmental stimuli while avoiding overstimulation.

Techniques to ensure safety

- Make sure the person carries some form of identification, along with the phone number of someone to call.
- Adapt the environment for safety (e.g. use alarm devices on doors to prevent wandering).
- Keep the environment uncluttered.
- Keep medications, cleaning solutions, and any poisonous chemicals in inaccessible places.

Techniques to facilitate independent performance of ADLs

- Keep all activities as simple and routine as possible.
- Establish routines that allow for maximum independence and the least amount of frustration.
- While keeping the routines as consistent as possible, recognise that they will have to be changed as the person's level of function changes.
- Lay out one set of clothing in the order in which the items are to be donned.
- If the person needs assistance with hygiene, use matter-of-fact statements such as "It's time for your bath."
- Arrange personal care items such as grooming and hygiene aids, in a visible and uncluttered place, in the order in which the items are to be used.
- Leave a toothbrush on the bathroom sink with toothpaste already on it.
- Establish an individualised toileting plan that allows for the person's maximum independence but minimal risk for incontinence episodes.
- Offer finger foods and nutritious snacks if the person will not sit at the table to eat a meal.

Interacting and communicating with older adults living with dementia

Verbal and non-verbal communication techniques are widely recognised as essential interventions for people living with dementia throughout the entire course of the disease. Nurses need to pay particular attention to the effects on communication of touch, facial expressions, tone of voice and body language. Box 14-8 summarises techniques for facilitating communication with people living with dementia. These techniques are general guidelines, and it is important to adapt communication to the particular needs of each person living with dementia. An assessment and intervention tool for addressing communication needs of people living with dementia, including a cost-free video demonstrating the application of this tool, is available from the Hartford Foundation for Geriatric Nursing at http://consultgerirn.org/resources, or at www.nursingcenter.com.

Interactions with older adults living with dementia should also focus on maintaining their personhood. Nurses do this by delivering care that is person-centred. Nurses begin this process by undertaking a nursing history and performing cognitive and psychosocial assessments. Nurses would also endeavour to address the four elements of PCC. For instance, nurses would explore the element:

1. *Being in relation* by asking such questions as, "Who are the important people in this person's life?" and "Who provides emotional support to this person?"
2. *Being with self* by asking the questions, "What is this person's preferred name?" and "What are their abilities, their likes, dislikes and their routines?"
3. *Being in a social world* by asking the questions, "What occupation did this person perform?" and "What is their life story?" and
4. *Being in place* by asking the questions, "Will the care environment impact on this person", and "How will it impact upon them?"

Gathering this information will ensure that the older adult's personhood is preserved. This information provides the basis for all interactions.

Other interactions have also been identified that support the older adult's personhood and maintains their dignity and well-being (Kitwood, 1997). These are listed and described in Box 14-9. Negative interactions that lead to deterioration in the older adult living with dementia are listed in Box 14-10, and these should be avoided. An excellent educational resource for undergraduate healthcare students about person-centred care and personhood is available from the weblink http://nursing.flinders.edu.au/comeintomyworld. A comprehensive description of Kitwood's positive and negative interactions is contained in this resource. This resource is scenario based and enables students to explore the concepts of person-centred care and personhood, and Kitwood's interactions with people who are living with dementia in different care situations.

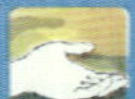

BOX 14-8
Facilitating communication with people who have dementia

Verbal communication

- Adapt your level of communication to the abilities of the person living with dementia.
- Use very simple sentences.
- Present only one idea at a time.
- Allow enough time for processing.
- Avoid infantilisation (e.g. do not use baby talk or use a demeaning or condescending tone of voice).
- Assist with word finding (e.g. supply missing words, repeat the person's sentence with the correct word).
- Avoid shaming the person (e.g. do not emphasise deficits).
- Paraphrase what the person says, and ask for clarification about the meaning.
- If the person does not understand a statement, repeat the statement using the same words, or simplify the wording.
- Do not argue with the person, unless it is a matter of safety.
- Avoid complex or sarcastic humour.
- Use positive statements (i.e. avoid using statements containing the word "don't" or other negative commands).
- Involve the person with decisions to the best of his or her ability by offering simple and concrete choices (e.g. "Do you want chicken or steak?" rather than "What do you want to eat?").
- Do not ask questions that you know the person cannot answer correctly.
- Do not test the person's memory unnecessarily.
- Listen to the feelings the person is trying to express and respond to the feelings, rather than the statement.
- When discussing activities of daily living (ADLs), avoid statements, such as "You need a bath now", which may be interpreted as judgemental.

Non-verbal communication

- Attract and maintain the person's attention (e.g. through eye contact, pleasant facial expressions).
- Use a relaxed and smiling approach.
- Reinforce verbal communication with appropriate non-verbal communication (e.g. demonstrate what you are asking the person to do).
- Use simple pictures rather than written cues.
- Use appropriate touch for communication (e.g. to gain the person's attention or reinforce feelings of concern), unless the person responds negatively to touch.
- Be aware of your own non-verbal communication.
- Keep in mind that your non-verbal cues will probably communicate more than your spoken words and will not necessarily be interpreted correctly.
- Closely observe all non-verbal cues exhibited by the person, particularly those that express feelings.
- Assume that all non-verbal expressions of the person living with dementia are attempts to communicate needs or feelings.

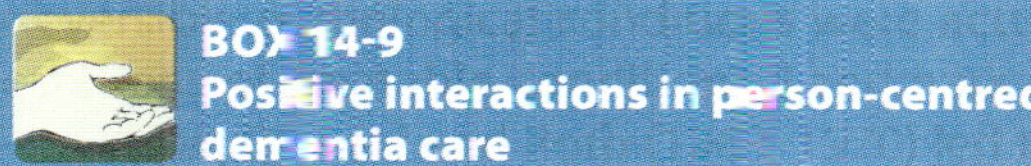

BOX 14-9
Positive interactions in person-centred dementia care

Social interaction

Recognition	Individual known as a unique person by name; involves verbal communication and eye contact
Negotiation	Individual consulted about preferences, choices, needs
Collaboration	Carer aligns himself or herself with care recipient to engage in a task
Play	Encouraging expressions of spontaneity and of self
Stimulation	Engaging in interactions using senses
Celebration	Celebrating anything the individual finds enjoyable
Relaxation	Providing close personal comfort (e.g. holding hands)

Psychotherapeutic interactions

Validation	Acknowledging person's emotions and feelings and responding to them; empathy
Holding	Providing a space where the individual feels comfortable in self-revelation
Facilitation	Enabling a person to use their remaining abilities, not emphasising errors

Roles in which people living with dementia can take a lead

Creation	Individual spontaneously offers something to the interaction; affirmation of this
Giving	Individual offers him/herself in a positive emotional or helpful way

Source: Kitwood, T. (1997). *Dementia reconsidered: The person comes first.* Buckingham: Open University Press; Epp, T. D. (2003). Person-centred dementia care: A vision to be refined. *Canadian Alzheimer Disease Review, April*, 14–18.

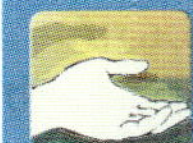

BOX 14-10
Negative interactions in person-centred dementia care

- Accusation
- Banishment
- Disempowerment
- Disparagement
- Disruption
- Ignoring
- Imposition
- Infantilisation
- Intimidation
- Invalidation
- Labelling
- Mockery
- Objectification
- Outpacing
- Stigmatisation
- Treachery
- Withholding

Source: Kitwood, T. (1997). *Dementia reconsidered: The person comes first.* Buckingham: Open University Press.

WELLNESS OPPORTUNITY

Nurses promote emotional wellness by encouraging older adults living with dementia to talk about happy memories of earlier years and by affirming the pleasant feelings the person experiences when recalling these events.

Interventions for dementia-related behaviours

Healthcare professionals increasingly recognise that dementia-related behaviours (see previous discussion about BPSD) reflect an attempt to communicate needs the person may not consciously recognise and cannot express verbally. Nurses must direct their interventions towards the underlying needs of the person living with dementia, referred to as their "unmet needs".

Hall and Buckwalter (1987) proposed a theoretical framework for addressing dementia-related behaviours called the Progressively Lowered Stress Threshold (PLST) model. Briefly stated, this model posits that dysfunctional behaviours indicate a progressive lowering of the stress threshold, which in turn, interferes with the person's functioning and ability to interact with the environment. Common stressors associated with dysfunctional episodes are fatigue; change of environment, routine or carer; misleading stimuli or inappropriate stimulus levels; internal or external demands that exceed functional capacity; physical stressors (e.g. pain, illness, depression); and affective response to loss.

The goal of nursing care, then, is to maximise the person's function by relieving stressors that cause excess disability. The choice of interventions is based on an ongoing assessment of anxiety "as a barometer to determine how much activity and stimuli the anxious person can tolerate at any point during their illness. As anxious behaviours occur, activities and environmental stimuli are modified and simplified until the anxiety disappears" (Hall & Buckwalter, 1987, p. 403). This approach (summarised in Box 14-11) is highly individualised; from a nursing perspective, it is analogous to adjusting insulin doses for people with diabetes according to serum glucose levels. Box 14-12 contains more information related to managing difficult behaviours in institutional settings without the use of antipsychotic medications.

There are a number of resources that are available to assist nurses in understanding and providing support to carers regarding dementia related behaviours. In both Australia and New Zealand the Alzheimer's organisations have many printed and video resources (see the resources at the end of the chapter). In Australia there is a telephone service, Dementia Behaviour Management Advisory Service (DBMAS), available nationally for families and care workers who are concerned about the behaviours of people living with dementia. The service provides advice, assessment, intervention, education and support 24 hours a day, seven days a week, and it can be contacted on 1800 699 799.

Two Australian practice guidelines are available about BPSD. One released in 2012, Behaviour management—A

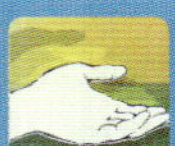

BOX 14-11
Nursing interventions for people living with dementia based on the Progressively Lowered Stress Threshold Model (PLST)

- Maximise safety by modifying the environment to compensate for cognitive losses.
- Control any factors that increase stress, such as fatigue; physical stressors; competing or overwhelming stimuli; changes in routine, carer or environment; and activities or demands that exceed the person's functional ability.
- Plan and maintain a consistent routine.
- Implement regular rest periods to compensate for fatigue and loss of reserve energy.
- Provide unconditional positive regard.
- Remain non-judgemental about the appropriateness of all behaviours except those that present threats to safety.
- Recognise individual expressions of fatigue, anxiety and increasing stress, and intervene to reduce stressors as soon as possible.
- Modify reality orientation and other therapeutic interventions to incorporate only that information needed for safe function.
- Use reassuring forms of therapy, such as music and reminiscence.

Source: Hall, G. R. & Buckwalter, K. C. (1987). Progressively lowered stress threshold: A conceptual model for care of adults with Alzheimer's disease. *Archives of Psychiatric Nursing, 1,* 399–406.

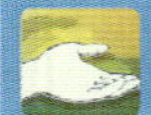

BOX 14-12
Non-drug management of difficult behaviours and BPSD in persons living with dementia

Step 1: Assess and treat contributing factors

FOCUS on one behaviour at a time
- Note how often, how bad, how long and document specific details
- **Ask:** What is really going on? What is causing the problem behaviour? What is making it worse?

IDENTIFY what leads to or triggers problems (unmet needs)
- **Physical:** pain, infection, hunger/thirst, other needs?
- **Psychological:** loneliness, boredom, nothing to do?
- **Environment:** too much/too little going on; lost?
- **Psychiatric:** depression, anxiety, psychosis?

REDUCE, ELIMINATE things that lead to or trigger the problems
- Treat medical/physical problems
- Offer pain medications for comfort or to help cooperation
- Address emotional needs: reassure, encourage, engage
- Offer enjoyable activities to do alone, 1:1, small group
- Remove or disguise misleading objects
- Redirect away from people or areas that lead to problems
- Try another approach; try again later
- Find out what works for others; get someone to help

DOCUMENT outcomes
- If the behaviour is reduced or manageable, go to Step 3
- If the behaviour persists, go to Step 2

Step 2: Select and apply interventions

CONSIDER retained abilities, preferences, resources
- Cognitive level
- Physical functional level
- Long-standing personality, life history, interests
- Preferred personal routines, daily schedules
- Personal/family/facility resources

DEVELOP a person-centred plan
- Adjust carer approaches
- Adapt/change the environment
- Select/use best evidence-based interventions tailored to the person's unique needs/interests/abilities

ADJUST your approach to the person
- **Personal approach:** cue, prompt, remind, distract; focus on person's wishes, interests, concerns; use/avoid touch as indicated. Do not try to reason, teach new routines, or ask to "try harder".
- **Daily routines:** simplify tasks and put them in a regular order; offer limited choices; use long-standing patterns and preferences to guide routines and activities
- **Communication style:** simple words and phrases; speak in short sentences; speak clearly; wait for answers; make eye contact; monitor tone of voice and body language
- **Unconditional positive regard:** do not confront, challenge or explain misbeliefs (hallucinations, delusions, illusions); accept belief as real to the person; reassure, comfort and distract

ADAPT or CHANGE the environment
- **Eliminate things that lead to confusion:** clutter, TV, radio, noise, people talking; reflections in mirrors/dark windows; misunderstood pictures or decor
- **Reduce things that cause stress:** caffeine; extra people; holiday decorations; public TV
- **Adjust stimulation:** if overstimulated, reduce noise, activity and confusion; if under-stimulated (bored), increase activity and involvement
- **Help with functioning:** signs, cues, using pictures to help way-finding; increase lighting to reduce misinterpretation
- **Involve in meaningful activities:** personalised program of 1:1 and small group or large group as needed
- **Change the setting:** secure outdoor areas; decorative objects; objects to touch and hold; homelike features; smaller, divided recreational and dining areas; natural and bright light; spa-like bathing facilities; signs to help way-finding

SELECT and USE evidence-based interventions
- Work with the team to fit the intervention to the person
- Check care plan for additional information
- Contact supervisor with problems/issues

Step 3: MONITOR outcomes and adjust course as needed
- Track behaviour problems using rating scale(s)
- Assure adequate "dose" (intensity, duration, frequency) of interventions
- Adapt/add interventions as needed to get the best possible outcomes
- Make sure all people working with the person understand and cooperate with the treatment plan and are trained as needed

Reprinted with permission from Carnahan, R., Smith M. & Reist, J. et al. (2012). Improving antipsychotic appropriateness in dementia patients. POGOe—Portal of Geriatrics Online Education. Available March 2015 at www.pogoe.org/productid/21209 and via www.healthcare.uiowa.edu/igec/iaadapt.

guide to good practice: Managing behavioural and psychological symptoms of dementia (BPSD), provides evidence-based guidance for clinicians and both formal and informal carers. Access to this document is obtained through the Dementia Collaborative Research Centres at www.dementiaresearch.org.au.

The other title, *Assessment and management of people with behavioural and psychological symptoms of dementia (BPSD): A handbook for NSW Health clinicians*, was published in 2013 by the New South Wales' Ministry of Health and the Royal Australian and New Zealand College of Psychiatrists to provide a practice guide for clinicians working for NSW Health. The document can be accessed via www.ranzcp.org.

Pharmacological interventions promoting wellness in people living with dementia

Medications are becoming increasingly important in treating dementia because recent studies and guidelines support and encourage certain medications to slow the progress of the disease. However, despite intense and ongoing research related to the development of drugs for the modification of the disease, there is still no drug available (Anand, Gill & Mahdi, 2014). Nurses have important roles in teaching carers about medications for dementia. Nurses are also frequently involved with decisions about medications for managing dementia-related symptoms.

Medications for reducing symptoms of dementia

In 1993, tacrine was approved as the first medication for the treatment of Alzheimer's disease. By the turn of the century, three cholinesterase inhibitors were approved for use. Now three medications—donepezil (Aricept), rivastigmine (Exelon) and galantamine (Reminyl)—are the standards for mild to moderate Alzheimer's disease because they have fewer adverse effects. Reviews of studies consistently find that these medications exert modest positive effects in improving the symptoms of some kinds of dementia. They can improve cognitive ability, motivation and reduce apathy, and may have some effects on other behavioural changes. They have also been shown to delay the progression of functional decline and cognitive and behavioural symptoms (e.g. Prvulovic, Hampel & Pantel, 2010; Seltzer, 2010).

In 2003, memantine (Ebixa) became the first medication approved for treatment of moderate to severe Alzheimer's disease. The physiological action of this medication, which differs from that of cholinesterase inhibitors, blocks the neural toxicity associated with excess release of glutamate. Studies consistently show that memantine reduces symptoms and slows the rate of decline in the older adults in moderate to later stages of Alzheimer's disease (Thomas & Grossberg, 2009).

The usual pharmacological approach is to begin a cholinesterase inhibitor before or during the moderate stage of dementia, and to add memantine during the moderate or later stages. These drugs are usually started at a low dose, which is increased gradually if it is well tolerated. The most common adverse effects of cholinesterase inhibitors are nausea, vomiting, diarrhoea, weight loss and loss of appetite. The adverse effects of memantine include dizziness, headache, constipation and increased confusion.

Medications for managing dementia-related symptoms

Decisions about the use of psychotropic medications for dementia-related disruptive behaviour are complex for several reasons. First, because dementia-related behaviours are often precipitated by modifiable factors, including medical conditions environmental influences and adverse medication effects (e.g. anticholinergic medications), initial interventions should always address any contributing factors. For example, if behaviours are due to the adverse effects of medications, initial interventions focus on eliminating or reducing the dose. Second, there is always a risk that medications will further interfere with function and perhaps even cause serious harm, such as further reduction in cognitive function or increased risk for falls. A third consideration is whether the behaviours justify the risks associated with medications. Bothersome or socially inappropriate behaviours may best be ignored or tolerated than treated with medications. However, if the behaviour is unsafe, uncomfortable or interferes with the function of the person living with dementia or the rights or safety of others, then pharmaceutical intervention may be appropriate, but only if other interventions are not successful. In any situation, healthcare professionals should view behaviour-modifying medications as one component of a comprehensive management plan that addresses the complex nature of dementia-related behaviours.

Although antipsychotics have been used for the management of dementia-related behaviours for many decades, there is increasing concerns about serious adverse effects and lack of effectiveness in people living with dementia. Concerns about safety of so-called first-generation antipsychotics (e.g. haloperidol) led to increased use of newer antipsychotics (called atypical antipsychotics), including olanzapine (Zyprexa), quetiapine (Seroquel) and risperidone (Risperdal). Current systematic reviews of studies conducted since 2000 indicate that all types of antipsychotics are associated with safety risks, including increased risk of death (e.g. Gareri, De Fazio, Manfredi et al., 2014; Langballe, Engdahl, Nordeng et al., 2014; Seitz, Gill, Herrmann et al., 2013). Because no medication is both safe and consistently more effective than pharmacological interventions for BPSD, there is much support for non-pharmacological approaches. Box 14-13 contains information to assist nurses with decisions about behaviour-modifying medications for people living with dementia.

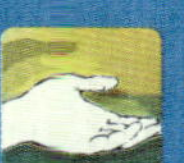

BOX 14-13
Guidelines for decisions about behaviour-modifying medications for people living with dementia

Considerations regarding behaviour-modifying medications

- Identify contributing factors (e.g. environmental conditions; psychosocial factors such as anxiety or depression; or physiological factors such as pain, discomfort or medical disorders). If any of these factors are implicated, interventions should be directed at the causative factor.
- Explore whether the behaviours are caused by adverse medication effects? In this case, the appropriate intervention might be to reduce the dose of or discontinue a medication, rather than begin a new medication.
- Use medications only after non-pharmacological measures have been implemented.
- Determine whether the behaviours truly justify the use of medications, or are the carers requesting medications for their own comfort and convenience?

Considerations regarding the choice and dose of medications

- Be sure the specific goals of and expectations for the medication interventions are clear to all carers.
- If the person is depressed, explain that antidepressants may be effective in treating the depression and that some functional improvement may occur, as the depression is alleviated.
- Don't assume that, just because medications are necessary and appropriate during one stage of dementia, they will be necessary and appropriate on an ongoing basis.
- Re-evaluate medication regimens as the dementia progresses or as other conditions, such as medical disorders, affect the person's functional level.
- Select a particular medication based on current manifestations as well as prior experiences with medications because people living with dementia exhibit a wide range of responses to various medications.
- Remember that some people living with dementia, particularly those with dementia with Lewy bodies, are highly sensitive to even minute doses of psychotropic medications.
- Keep in mind that any behaviour-modifying medication is likely to interfere with cognitive function and that the type of behaviour-modifying medication should be appropriate for the type of behavioural manifestations (e.g. antipsychotics for delusions and hallucination, antianxiety agents for anxiety).
- When introducing an initial dose of medication, give one-half to one-third the normal adult dose.
- Increase dosage gradually until therapeutic effects are achieved; all the while, observe the person for adverse effects.
- Consider the half-life of a medication when determining the frequency of doses. Avoid medications with long half-lives (e.g. diazepam).

WELLNESS OPPORTUNITY

Nurses holistically address behavioural symptoms by trying to identify non-pharmacological interventions that improve quality of life for the person with dementia and his or her carers.

Considerations for non-Alzheimer's dementia

As already mentioned, more information is available for Alzheimer's disease than for other types of dementia. However, information specific to other types of dementia is increasingly becoming available, particularly for Lewy body dementia, as in the following considerations that pertain to nursing care:

- Use anticholinergic medications (e.g. antipsychotics and benzodiazepines) with caution, and only in very low doses.
- Assess for physiological disorders at the first sign of changes in behaviour, because people with Lewy body dementia decompensate more when they have a medical condition.
- Assess for signs of autonomic nervous system dysfunction affecting swallowing, digestion, blood pressure, temperature regulation, and bowel and bladder control.
- Consider referrals for occupational and physical therapy because movement and balance disorders occur early in the disease.

A consideration related to vascular dementia is that management of cardiovascular risk factors (e.g. lipids, blood pressure, lifestyle interventions) is an integral part of the treatment plan.

General principles of nursing interventions in different settings

Irrespective of the setting, all older people who have a diagnosis of dementia will receive care that is person centred and individualised.

Long-term residential care settings

In recent years, there has been increasing implementation of multifaceted models of care for people living with dementia in long-term residential care settings. Many of these facilities have specially designed areas of care for people living with dementia called dementia-specific units (DSUs). Essential features of these units for cognitively impaired residents include environmental modifications, family involvement, individualised care plans, dementia-specific activity programs, and specially trained and selected staff. Many long-term residential care facilities incorporate these features into all care units and address the individualised needs of the residents, as discussed in Chapter 6. These facilities typically address the needs of people who are in moderate to severe stages of dementia, although some residents are in the early stages. Box 14-14 summarises statements of people with moderate to severe dementia in a long-term residential care home about their experiences.

Acute care settings

Older adults are rarely hospitalised for an initial evaluation of dementia, but they are frequently admitted to acute

BOX 14-14
Lived experiences: People with moderate to severe dementia in long-term residential care homes

I still am somebody

- I can remember all those things, and they come back. And I know I can't do them now but if I think about them, I'm sort of living them again, so that's really nice.
- Well, I ebb and flow a bit because I'm older and I've had heart trouble for years, so I think, really, I do ever so well. I've got no complaints at all.
- I used to do a lot. I may get back to it and particularly if we get a nice spring sort of thing, it might be better for me.
- I'm thankful for what I can do, you know what I mean? I won't give in.

Nothing's right now

- Don't lose me, will you? Please don't lose me.
- Things you like to remember, you can't remember, and things that you can remember easily drift away in front of you.
- I don't know what's the matter with me and why people don't talk to me much. I feel to be an outsider.
- I don't know whether I'm stuck here for the rest of my life or what's happening really.
- I'm frightened, please help me to know.
- Nobody wants me. I mean, that's the case, nobody does. If I was wanted by anybody, I could be quite useful. But nobody knows that I want a job.

I'm all right; I'll manage

- I wouldn't say it was as good as home at a place like this. You're just one of a number—group—who are pretty well in a similar position, but you do your best and give as much help. I've been sorting books out all morning.
- It's not as nice as I'd like it to be, but I have to be satisfied with small things these days.
- I haven't got to do any shopping, I haven't got to cook any meals, and that's a lot, isn't it? You've gotta get used to it, haven't you?
- I never thought I'd come to a place like this, but I'm quite happy.
- I've got a pal; she helps me out.

It drives me mad

- I'd rather be doing something, yes, although there's not a lot I can do … I'm capable of doing.
- I get bored here. They go to sleep and I feel like throwing something at them, because they … nobody talking or nobody goes walking. You've gotta do something, haven't you, to help you go through? Because it wasn't the things I've been used to. They just sit there; it drives me mad.
- I want to be free … or die. I don't mind dying, but I don't want to be coddled here.

Source: Clare, Rowlands, Bruce, Surr & Downs (2008); Clare, Rowlands & Quin (2008).

care settings for evaluation and treatment of medical problems that are superimposed on the dementia. Consequently, nurses in hospital settings usually deal not only with the acute illness but also with the dementia-related behaviours, which are exacerbated by the medical problem, the hospital environment, the unfamiliar carers, and the change in routines. Thus, nurses in acute care settings face a tremendous challenge in caring for people living with dementia.

One of the most important initial interventions is to involve at least one of the older adult's usual carers in planning and implementing the care for the cognitively impaired person. Although the person living with dementia is likely to exhibit different behaviours in the hospital than at home, nurses must begin by identifying any interventions that were effective in the home environment. During the admission process, nurses may save a lot of time and frustration by interviewing the carers about specific methods that help or hinder care. For example, if nurses know that the person eats only sandwiches or needs assistance with a specific toileting routine, they can incorporate appropriate intervention in their care plans. Because many people living with dementia have lost the ability to express their needs verbally, nurses need to obtain information from family carers who understand how the person expresses their needs.

In addition to obtaining information from a usual carer, nurses may consider involving the carer in the person's care or asking him or her to provide a familiar presence during the hospitalisation. Despite a need for respite from caregiving responsibilities, family and other carers may be willing to provide assistance and guidance. This may be particularly helpful during the first few days of hospitalisation as the older person can be very unsettled in an unfamiliar environment with strange people. Nurses can find assessment and intervention tools for addressing the needs of hospitalised people living with dementia, including videos demonstrating the application of these tools, at http://consultgerirn.org/resources or at www.nursingcenter.com.

Community settings

In community settings, the role of nurses is to work with family members or paid carers to provide appropriate interventions that focus on improving functioning for the person living with dementia, alleviating the burden for the carers and improving quality of life for all. An intervention that might be most effective, as well as efficient, is to encourage carers' participation in educational or support groups, which often are led or co-led by nurses. The number of groups addressing the needs of carers is increasing rapidly, and information about these groups is available from Alzheimer's associations or local hospitals. Nurses also can encourage carers to purchase one of the many carer guides that are available in bookstores or through the Internet and other resources.

In addition to educating carers about specific management problems, nurses in community settings must be ready to discuss resources for medical care, home services, and other community-based aged care services for older adults living with dementia and their carers. As the number and range of services increase, it is becoming more and more difficult to keep up to date on the resources in one's own community. Although nurses cannot be expected to know all the details about all available community services, they should know generally about the services available.

Another major focus of community-based programs is health promotion for people with early stage dementia. Findings from research reviews and focus groups indicate the need for support programs, health promotion programs, and activities to help the person manage the disease and to "normalise" life (e.g. exercise programs, fall prevention, cognitive stimulation) (Burgener et al., 2009).

One nursing study of people who had early stage dementia and who participated in a 12-week health promotion course showed significant improvements in measures of cognition and depression (Buettner & Fitzsimmons, 2009). There also is increasing evidence that cognitive training and memory rehabilitation programs can effectively improve functioning and quality of life during early stage dementia (Nomura et al., 2009; Yu et al., 2009). Nurses have important roles in referring people living with dementia to support groups and other community-based resources. Box 14-15 summarises statements of people living with dementia about their lived experiences related to needing help from others and being part of a support group.

Assessing carer burden

Carer burden differs from caregiving in that it involves the carer's response to the numerous stressors associated with caregiving (Etters, Goodall & Harrison, 2008). Carer burden is associated with poor outcomes for both the carer and person living with dementia and an early placement in long-term residential care.

Irrespective of the setting, to provide appropriate interventions that focus on minimising carer burden—and thereby improving the quality of life of both the person living with dementia and the carer—nurses have a responsibility to detect and prevent carer burden. Interventions appropriate to reducing carer burden depend on several factors such as the type of relationship (spouse versus other), the progression of the disease, gender, culture and personal characteristics (Etters, Goodall & Harrison, 2008).

A number of tools commonly used by nurses to assess carer burden are the Zarit Burden Interview (ZBI), the Caregiver Strain Index (CSI), and the Screen for Caregiver Burden (SCB). The completion of one of these tools, as well as the collection of other clinical information about the carer and the person living with dementia, can assist with the detection of carers who are at risk. Regular screening for carer burden is also recommended to assist with early detection (see Chapter 27).

BOX 14-15
Lived experiences: Interventions, experiences and feelings

About needing help from others

- When the day comes that I have got to start asking for help and if that independence is taken away, then I would like to think that I could still be consulted and still have some say in my independence.
- It is very beneficial, when I am unable to verbalise what I want, for my wife to display multiple options and allow me to choose one.
- If all else fails, I rely on my partner and my family to come up with solutions I cannot solve.
- I think it would be nice if people gave you the courtesy of time to finish what you are trying to say.
- You can't do what you want. You have to ask. So you have to adjust your schedule to someone else's. I guess the best word for it is that it is somewhat humiliating to be in that position when you're used to running your own life.
- I had somebody helping me cook for a while and that really bothered me. It makes me feel "less than myself".
- Before I'd take a walk around the block rather than blow my stack. By the time I got back, my feet hurt so much that I quit worrying about what I was mad about. Now my husband will go with me, and that doesn't do it.

About being part of a support group

- Since it is difficult to maintain my old social networks, I reach out to others online through e-mail groups and chat rooms for people living with dementia. These can be real life-savers some days.
- It is that bit of extra that you know these people are having the same problems and *really* understand.
- I commiserate with my friends going through the same things.
- When I've gotten real down, it seems as though my failure in things I do is exaggerated many times. I feel as though my power has been lost to do anything about it. I feel hopeless and helpless. Thank God for my chat group sticking with me to crawl out.
- I participate in the group in hopes that people living with dementia will begin to be treated with more respect and dignity and to help others recognise how much coping we must do to accomplish even simple things throughout a normal day.
- I have always been a person who has wanted to make a difference in the world, and through the group, I feel I have been able to change a small part of the way some people think about early-stage dementia.
- Let's work together to change paradigms about what persons living with dementia can and can't do. Don't limit us—help us push the envelopes of our new abilities.
- The benefits to me personally are so important, as I can still feel that I am a valuable contributing member of society, even though I'm "cognitively disabled".
- Today I have met people who are in very much the same boat as I am with things they can and can't do, so for me it's a relief to find that there are others in the same boat.

Source: Alzheimer's Society (2010b); Beard & Fox (2008); Beard, Knauss & Moyer (2009); Clare, Rowlands & Quin (2008).

EVALUATING THE EFFECTIVENESS OF NURSING INTERVENTIONS

Nurses can evaluate the care of people living with dementia according to the extent to which they receive necessary supports and maintain their dignity and quality of life. Because a decline in function is an inherent part of dementia, nursing care is evaluated on an ongoing basis as the person's condition changes and in relation to appropriate and changing goals. Nurses evaluate the degree to which quality of life is maintained by obtaining feedback about life satisfaction, which people in the early and middle stages of dementia usually can express verbally or non-verbally. For example, nurses can evaluate the extent to which the person enjoys or participates in meaningful activities and interactions. As dementia progresses, it becomes more difficult to obtain this kind of information, and nurses rely more on feedback from carers and their own judgement. During the later stages of dementia, measures of quality of life focus more on comfort and basic physical needs. Throughout the dementia course, care can be evaluated by the extent to which the person is free from pain, fear and anxiety.

Another evaluation consideration is the extent to which the needs of carers are met. One evaluation criterion is whether carers express satisfaction with their own quality of life, despite the demands of the situation. Other criteria may be a carer's attendance at support groups and his or her use of resources to assist with or guide care.

CASE STUDY

Mrs Padmakumar is 85 years old and lives with her 86-year-old husband in a unit in a retirement village. Mrs Padmakumar was born in India and migrated to Australia when she was aged 32 years. She has never been employed outside the home and her life has always centred on her husband and children. Two years ago, Mrs Padmakumar was diagnosed with Alzheimer's disease but she was able to participate in her usual activities until the past year. Now she is neglecting her personal care and is unsafe during meal preparation.

When she wakes up several times nightly to go to the bathroom, she sometimes goes to the front door rather than returning to the bedroom. Mr Padmakumar worries that she will leave in the middle of the night. This disrupts his sleep because he maintains a state of constant vigilance. Mr Padmakumar has called the Aged Care Assessment Team (Australia) or Needs Assessment and Service Coordination (New Zealand).

Nursing assessment

During your initial assessment, you find that Mrs Padmakumar is pleasant and receptive but has little insight into her need for help. She acknowledges that her doctor told her she has "a memory problem" but reports that this problem doesn't affect her daily life, except that her husband has to remind her about things like turning the stove off after cooking meals. She acknowledges being lonely and says she misses being able to read books and talk to people. Mrs Padmakumar takes donepezil and vitamin E and is otherwise physically healthy.

With regard to ADLs, Mrs Padmakumar has not taken a bath or shower in several months, and she gets very angry if Mr Padmakumar suggests that she take one. She gets confused about her clothing and sometimes wears her underwear over her regular clothes or wears a skirt and slacks at the same time. She insists on doing the meal preparation, but she is not safe while using the stove and gets confused about ingredients in recipes (e.g. she has used salt instead of sugar). Mrs Padmakumar has always done the laundry and housekeeping but in the past months, she "made a lot of mistakes", such as using powdered milk for laundry detergent.

Mr Padmakumar reports feeling very stressed about the full-time responsibilities of caring for his wife. This stress has escalated in the past month because he no longer feels he can leave her alone. Mrs Padmakumar "shadows" him and feels very insecure if he is out of her sight for more than a few minutes. Mr Padmakumar took her everywhere with him for the past year but in the last few months, this has become increasingly difficult. For example, when they are grocery shopping, Mrs Padmakumar gets very impatient and pushes the trolley into other people. Then, while they are waiting in the checkout line, she insists on taking one of each of the nearby magazines, and she creates a scene if Mr Padmakumar doesn't buy them for her.

Mr Padmakumar confides that he expected to be able to care for his wife at home "until the end", but now he has doubts about his ability to keep her at home. He perceives her as "senile" and feels he should be able to meet her needs. There are no nearby family members who can help with her care, but his son and daughter have offered to help pay for some services. Mr Padmakumar is aware of Alzheimer's support groups, but he has not attended any because he cannot leave his wife alone. When asked about his health, Mr Padmakumar says, "I see the doctor for my arthritis and heart problems, but I get along okay, except that I'm supposed to have cataract surgery, and I don't know how I'll manage to get that done."

Nursing issues

Your nursing issue for Mrs Padmakumar is altered thought processes related to the effects of dementia. You use the nursing issue of carer role strain for Mr Padmakumar because you recognise the need to address Mr Padmakumar's problems. Your immediate goal is to arrange for supportive services and assistance with Mrs Padmakumar's care because this will improve the quality of life for both Mr and Mrs Padmakumar, and it will alleviate some of the carer stress for Mr Padmakumar. A long-term goal is to arrange for respite services, so Mr Padmakumar can undergo cataract surgery. You also recognise the need for educational and support services for Mr Padmakumar.

Nursing care plan for Mr and Mrs Padmakumar

Goals for wellness outcomes	Nursing interventions	Nursing evaluation
Mrs Padmakumar will function at her highest level of independence.	• Work with Mr Padmakumar to identify ways to improve Mrs Padmakumar's ability to function safely and independently in performing activities of daily living (ADLs). (For instance, Mr Padmakumar can involve Mrs Padmakumar in selecting an outfit to wear and can set out the clothing in the order in which it should be donned.) • Arrange for a community carer to work with Mrs Padmakumar and assist her with complex tasks such as laundry, housekeeping and meal preparation. • Teach the community carer to assume an "assistant" and "friend" role by providing only subtle supervision and minimal direct help with activities such as laundry.	• Mrs Padmakumar performs ADLs and instrumental activities of daily living (IADLs) with minimal assistance.
Mrs Padmakumar's quality of life will be maintained.	• Work with Mr Padmakumar and the community carer to identify activities that are interesting, satisfying and intellectually stimulating (e.g. "word find" games). • Explore the possibility of Mrs Padmakumar's attending an older person day care program for group activities. • Support Mrs Padmakumar in carrying out familiar roles and meaningful activities.	• Mrs Padmakumar continues to engage in activities that are satisfying.
Mr Padmakumar will use sources of support to alleviate carer-related stress.	• Arrange the community carer's schedule to enable Mr Padmakumar to attend carer support groups and educational programs. • Help Mr Padmakumar in identifying one activity per week that he could do to promote his own well-being (e.g. going to lunch with a friend). • Provide community carer assistance for 4-hour periods to allow Mr Padmakumar time for grocery shopping and pursuing his own interests. • Provide Mr Padmakumar with information about carer support networks available through Alzheimer's associations and suggest he join a support network.	• Mr Padmakumar verbalises feelings of being able to cope effectively with caregiver responsibilities. • Mr Padmakumar participates in one activity per week focused on his own needs and interests.

Thinking points

- Use the GDS/FAST in Table 14-2 to assess Mrs Padmakumar's stage of dementia.
- What would you identify as Mr Padmakumar's needs as a carer?
- What health education information would you plan for Mr Padmakumar?
- What approaches and resources would you suggest for Mr Padmakumar and community care workers for communicating with Mrs Padmakumar?
- What challenges would you anticipate having to address as you provide ongoing supervision of the community carer and continue to work with Mr and Mrs Padmakumar?

CHAPTER HIGHLIGHTS

Person-centred care

- Increasingly healthcare delivery is moving away from task-focused, institution-driven care practices towards a holistic model of care, which focuses on the person receiving care or person-centred care (PCC)
- When nursing an older adult, particularly when they have a cognitive impairment, delivering PCC will improve their quality of life and preserve their dignity and personhood

Delirium

- Characteristics: acute onset; fluctuating course; disturbances in thought, memory, attention, behaviour, perception, orientation and consciousness
- Hyperactive delirium is easily recognised, and hypoactive deliriums is common but unrecognised in older adults
- Risk factors include advanced age, pain, dementia, surgery, medications, physiological disturbances and pathological conditions

- Functional consequences include decline in functioning, increased mortality, and permanent residency in long-term residential care facilities
- Nursing assessment: the Confusion Assessment Method (CAM)
- Nursing issue: acute confusional state
- Nursing outcomes: improved cognition, concentration, information processing, memory
- Nursing interventions: addressing risk factors (Figure 14-1)

Overview of dementia

- Terminology (senility, hardening of the arteries, organic brain syndrome) reflects complexity of causes and types of dementia
- Dementia is a syndrome of impaired cognition caused by brain dysfunction
- Theories to explain dementia are still evolving
- Diagnosis of specific types of dementia is based on clinical observations, history and available diagnostic data

Types of dementia

- There are four main types of dementia that have been identified (Table 14-1):
  - Alzheimer's disease (Figures 14-2 & 14-3)
  - Vascular dementia
  - Lewy body dementia
  - Frontotemporal dementia

Risk factors associated with dementia

- Factors that increase the risk for dementia include genetic factors, lifestyle factors and health status
- Factors under investigation for protecting against dementia include physical exercise, omega-3 fatty acids, and engaging in socially and cognitively stimulating and meaningful activities Box 14-1

Functional consequences associated with dementia

- Stages of progression (Table 14-2)
- Self-awareness, common emotions and behaviours (Boxes 14-2 & 14-3)
- Behavioural and psychological symptoms of dementia

Nursing assessment of dementia

- Initial assessment: multidisciplinary, focus on level of function, response to illness (Box 14-4)
- Ongoing assessment of consequences (Box 14-5; Table 14-2, assessment guides in other chapters and clinical tools section)

Nursing issues

- Wellness nursing issue for person living with dementia and carers: willingness for enhanced coping
- Person living with dementia: chronic confusion or impaired cognition, anxiety, impaired memory, risk for injury, self-care deficit, disturbed sleep pattern, imbalanced nutrition, wandering, urinary incontinence
- Carers: family coping and carer role strain (or risk for), anticipatory grieving

Goal planning for wellness outcomes

- Person living with dementia: decreased anxiety level, and improved orientation, comfort level, communication, memory, mood, nutritional status, self-care status and sleep
- Cares: carer emotional or physical health, carer stressors, caregiving endurance potential
- For both the person living with dementia and his or her carers: coping, quality of life

Nursing interventions to address dementia

- Nursing studies of non-pharmacological interventions for dementia-related behaviours (Table 14-4)
- Addressing quality of life (Box 14-5)
- Improving safety and functioning through environmental modifications (Box 14-7)
- Interacting and communicating with older adults who have dementia (Box 14-8, Box 14-9, Box 14-10, clinical tools)
- Dementia related behaviours—PLST model and BPSD (Boxes 14-11 & 14-12)
- Teaching about medications for slowing the progression of dementia
- Teaching about medications for managing dementia-related symptoms (Box 14-13)
- General principles in long-term residential care settings, acute care (clinical tools from Hartford Institute for Geriatric Nursing), and community settings (Boxes 14-14 & 14-15)

Evaluating the effectiveness of nursing interventions

- Maintenance of dignity and quality of life for the person living with dementia
- Extent to which needs of carers are met

CRITICAL THINKING EXERCISES

1. Define each of the following terms, and describe the relevance of each term according to our current understanding of impaired cognitive function: senility, organic brain syndrome, hardening of the arteries, delirium, dementia, and Alzheimer's disease.
2. Describe the distinguishing features of each of the following types of dementia: Alzheimer's disease, vascular dementia, Lewy body dementia, and frontotemporal dementia.
3. You are working in a medical clinic as practice nurse. How would you respond to the following questions posed by a 74-year-old woman: "I've been having memory problems lately, but I know it's not Alzheimer's,

because I haven't done anything really stupid. What do you think I should do? My friend says ginkgo helps her a lot, and I was thinking of trying that. Do you know how much of it I should take?"

4. You are planning an in-service program to deliver to long-term care staff about medications used in the treatment of dementia and the management of dementia-related behaviours. What information would be able to you present?

RESOURCES

For an extensive range of additional resources to enhance teaching and learning and to facilitate understanding of this chapter, please see the text's accompanying website located on thePoint at http://thepoint.lww.com.

Clinical tools

Delirium: Hospital Elder Life Program (HELP) for Prevention of Delirium: www.hospitalelderlifeprogram.org

Hartford Institute for Geriatric Nursing, ConsultGeriRN.org: http://consultgerirn.org/resources

Assessment tools *Try This*® series and *How to Try This* resources

General assessment series:

- *Try This*, issue D9: Decision making in older adults with dementia. Mitty, C. (2012). *Best Practices in Nursing Care to Older Adults.*
- *Try This*, issue D10: Working with families of hospitalized older adults with dementia. Hall, G. & Maslow, K. (2007). *Best Practices in Nursing Care to Older Adults.*
- *How to Try This* (article): Working with families of hospitalized older adults with dementia. Bradway C. & Hirschman, K. (2008). *American Journal of Nursing, 108*(10), 52–60. (Look for May 2015 update.)
- *How to Try This* (video): *Working with families of hospitalized older adults with dementia.*
- *Try This*, issue D11.1 (2007): Eating and feeding issues in older adults with dementia, Part I: Assessment. Amella, E. (2007). *Best Practices in Nursing Care to Older Adults.*
- *How to Try This* (article): The Edinburgh Feeding Evaluation in Dementia Scale: Determining how much help people with dementia need at mealtime. Stockdell, R. & Amella, E. (2008). *American Journal of Nursing, 108*(8), 46–54. (Look for May 2015 update.)
- *How to Try This* (video): *Eating and feeding issues in older adults with dementia.*
- *Try This*, issue D11.2: Eating and feeding issues in older adults with dementia, Part II: Interventions. Amella, E. (2007). *Best Practices in Nursing Care to Older Adults.*
- *Try This*, issue D12: Home Safety Inventory for Older Adults with Dementia. Lach, H. (2012). *Best Practices in Nursing Care to Older Adults.*
- *Try This*, issue D13: Use of the Functional Activities Questionnaire in Older Adults with Dementia. Lach, H. (2012). *Best Practices in Nursing Care to Older Adults.*
- *Try This*, issue D14: The AD8: The Washington University Dementia Screening Test: Eight-item Interview to Differentiate Aging and Dementia. Galvin, J. (2013). *Best Practices in Nursing Care to Older Adults.*

Evidence-based practice

Fletcher, K. (2012). Dementia. In Boltz, M., Capezuti, E., Fulmer, T. & Zwicker, D. (Eds), *Evidence-based geriatric nursing protocols for best practice* (4th ed. pp. 163–185). New York: Springer.

Tullmann, D., Mion, L., Fletcher, K. & Foreman, M. (2012). Delirium. In Boltz, M., Capezuti, E., Fulmer, T. & Zwicker D. (Eds), *Evidence-based geriatric nursing protocols for best practice* (4th ed. pp. 186–199). New York: Springer.

Joanna Briggs Institute: http://connect.jbiconnectplus.org

Evidence summaries:

Behaviour

- Challenging behaviour (acute care): Older person. Jayasekara, R. (2013).
- Challenging behaviour: Assessment tools. Seraji, H. (2013).
- Challenging behaviour (older person): Non-pharmacological management. Slade, S. (2013).
- Challenging behaviour in older adults with dementia (nursing home): Assessment and non-pharmacological management. Khanh, D. L. L. (2014).
- Physical activity (older adults): Behavior. Chen, Z. (2014).

Delirium

- Delirium: Management. Seraji, H. (2013).
- Delirium: Occupational therapy. Seraji, H. (2013).
- Delirium: Screening and assessment. Seraji, H. (2014).
- Postoperative delirium (geriatrics): Clinician information. Slade, S. (2014).

Dementia

- Advanced dementia: Clinical care with eating and drinking. Kunde, L. (2014).
- Behavioral and psychological symptoms of dementia: Non-pharmacological management. Battaglini, E. (2014).
- Challenging behaviour in older adults with dementia (nursing home): Assessment and non-pharmacological management. Khanh, D. L. L. (2014).
- Preserving cognitive function (older people without dementia): Exercise and physical activity. Campbell, J. (2014).
- Dementia: Cognitive leisure activities. Rathnayake, T. (2014).
- Dementia: Communication skills for staff. Slade, S. (2013).
- Dementia: Family support following diagnosis. Battaglini, E. (2014)
- Dementia: Informed consent. Slade, S. (2014).
- Dementia with Lewy bodies: Management. Clark, L. (2014).
- Dementia: Massage and touch. Battaglini, E. (2014).
- Dementia: Montessori-based interventions. Seraji, H. (2013).

- Dementia: Music therapy. Battaglini, E. (2014).
- Dementia: Pharmacological interventions. Seraji, H. (2013).
- Delirium: Prevention. Seraji, H. (2013).
- Dementia: Psychosocial interventions. Slade, S. (2014).
- Dementia: Reminiscence therapy. Vijay, A. (2014).
- Dementia: Occupational therapy intervention. Battaglini, E. (2014).
- Dementia: Oral hygiene care. Tolu, F. G. (2014).
- Dementia: Wandering. Battaglini, E. (2014).

Recommended practices:

- Dementia: Communication difficulties (2013).
- *Dementia*: Consent issues (2013).
- Dementia: Family support following diagnosis (2013).
- Occupational therapy interventions for persons with dementia. Guthrie, S. (2013).
- Postoperative delirium (geriatrics): Surgical strategies (2013).
- Wandering management (2013).

Systematic reviews:

- Petriwskyj, A., Parker, D., Robinson, A., Gibson, A., Andrews, S. & Banks, S. (2013). Family involvement in decision making for people with dementia in residential aged care: A systematic review of quantitative and qualitative evidence. *Joanna Briggs Institute Library of Systematic Reviews, 11*(7), 131–282.
- Thomas, E., Smith, J., Forrester, A., Heider, G., Jadotte, Y. & Holly, C. (2014). The effectiveness of non-pharmacological multi-component interventions for the prevention of delirium in non-intensive care unit older adult hospitalized patients: A systematic review. *Joanna Briggs Institute Library of Systematic Reviews, 12*(4), 180–232.
- Fox, B., Hodgkinson, B. & Parker, D. (2014). The effects of physical exercise on functional performance, quality of life, cognitive impairment and physical activity levels for older adults aged 65 years and older with a diagnosis of dementia: A systematic review. *Joanna Briggs Institute Library of Systematic Reviews, 12*(9), 158–276.

National Guideline Clearinghouse: www.guideline.gov

Search for:

- Delirium
- Dementia
- Caregivers

Health education

Alzheimer's Association (US): www.alz.org/index.asp

Alzheimer's Australia: www.fightdementia.org.au

Alzheimer's Disease Education and Referral (ADEAR) Center: http://alzheimers.org

Alzheimer's New Zealand: www.alzheimers.org.nz

Dementia Advocacy and Support Network (DASN) International: http://dasninternational.org

Health Direct Australia, Seniors' health: www.healthdirect.gov.au/alzheimers-disease

MyDr—Alzheimer's disease and dementia: www.mydr.com.au/topics/alzheimers-disease-and-dementia

National Institute on Aging (NIA): www.nia.nih.gov/alzheimers

Neurological Foundation of New Zealand: www.neurological.org.nz/disorders/alzheimers

REFERENCES

Alzheimer's Association. (2013). 2013 Alzheimer's disease facts and figures. *Alzheimer's & Dementia, 9*, 208–245.

Alzheimer's Australia. (2014). *Summary of dementia statistics in Australia*. Accessed March 2015 at https://fightdementia.org.au/about-dementia-and-memory-loss/statistics.

Alzheimer's New Zealand. (2012). Updated *Dementia economic impact report, 2011, New Zealand*. Report prepared by Deloitte Access Economics for Alzheimer's New Zealand, Wellington. Accessed March 2015 at www.alzheimers.org.nz/files/reports/Updated_Dementia_Economic_Impact_Report_2012_New_Zealand.pdf.

Alzheimer's Society. (2008). *Dementia: Out of the shadows*. London: Alzheimer's Society.

Alzheimer's Society. (2010a). *My name is not dementia: People with dementia discuss quality of life*. London: Alzheimer's Society.

Alzheimer's Society. (2010b). *My name is not dementia: Literature review*. London: Alzheimers Society.

Amoyal, N. & Fallon, E. (2012). Physical exercise and cognitive training clinical interventions used in slowing degeneration associated with mild cognitive impairment. *Topics in Geriatric Rehabilitation, 28*(3), 208–216.

Anand, R., Gill, K. D. & Mahdi, A. A. (2014). Therapeutics of Alzheimer's disease: Past, present and future. *Neuropharmacology, 76*(Part A), 27–50.

Australian and New Zealand Society for Geriatric Medicine. (2012). Delirium in older people: Position statement 13. Accessed March 2015 via www.anzsgm.org/posstate.asp.

Balas, M., Buckingham, R., Braley, T. et al. (2013). Extending the ABCDE Bundle to the post-intensive care unit setting. *Journal of Gerontological Nursing, 29*(8), 39–50.

Ballard, C. & Corbett, A. (2013). Agitation and aggression in people with Alzheimer's disease. *Current Opinions in Psychiatry, 26*(3), 252–259.

Barnett, J. H., Hachinski, V. & Blackwell, A. D. (2013). Cognitive health begins at conception: Addressing dementia as a lifelong and preventable condition. *BioMed Central Medicine, 11*, 246. Accessed January 2014 via www.biomedcentral.com.

Barr, J., Fraser, G. L., Puntillo, K. et al. (2013). Clinical practice guidelines for the management of pain, agitation and delirium in adult patients in the intensive care unit. *Critical Care Medicine, 41*(1), 263–306.

Barr, J. & Pandharipande, P. P. (2013). The pain, agitation, and delirium care bundle: Synergistic benefits of implementing the 2013 pain, agitation, and delirium guidelines in an integrated and interdisciplinary fashion. *Critical Care Medicine, 41*, S99–S115.

Beard, R. L. & Fox, P. J. (2008). Resisting social disenfranchisement: Negotiating collective identities and everyday life with memory loss. *Social Science & Medicine, 66*, 1509–1520.

Beard, R. L., Knauss, J. & Moyer, D. (2009). Managing disability and enjoying life: How we reframe dementia through personal narratives. *Journal of Aging Studies, 23*, 227–235.

Blazer, D. G. & van Nieuwenhuizen, A. O. (2012). Evidence for the diagnostic criteria of delirium: An update. *Current Opinion in Psychiatry, 25*, 239–243.

Bossen, A. L., Specht, J. K. P. & McKenzie, S. E. (2009). Needs of people with early-stage Alzheimer's disease. *Journal of Gerontological Nursing, 35*(3f), 8–14.

Brodaty, H. & Arasaratnam, C. (2012). Meta-analysis of nonpharmacological interventions for neuropsychiatric symptoms of dementia. *American Journal of Psychiatry, 169*(9), 946–953.

Buettner, L. L. & Fitzsimmons, S. (2009). Promoting health in early-stage dementia: Evaluation of a 12-week course. *Journal of Gerontological Nursing, 35*(3), 39–49.

Burgener, S. C., Buettner, L. L., Beattie, E. & Rose, K. M. (2009). Effectiveness of community-based, nonpharmacological interventions for early-stage dementia, conclusions and recommendations. *Journal of Gerontological Nursing, 35*(3), 48–58.

Burke, A., Hall, G. & Tariot, P. N. (2013). The clinical problem of neuropsychiatric signs and symptoms in dementia. *Continuum, 19*(2 Dementia), 382–396.

Carnahan, R., Smith M. & Reist, J. et al. (2012). Improving antipsychotic appropriateness in dementia patients. POGOe—Portal of Geriatrics Online Education. Available March 2015 at www.pogoe.org/productid/21209.

Cheng, S. T., Chow, P. K., Song, Y. Q. et al. (2014). Can leisure activities slow dementia progression in nursing home residents? A cluster-randomized controlled trial. *International Psychogeriatrics, 26*(4), 637–643.

Chow, T. & Alobaidy, A. (2013). Incorporating new diagnostic schemas, genetics, and proteinopathy into evaluation of frontotemporal degeneration. *Continuum, 19*(2), 438–456.

Clare, L., Nelis, S. M., Martyr, A. et al. (2012). Longitudinal trajectories of awareness in early-stage dementia. *Alzheimer's Disease and Associated Disorders, 26*(2), 140–147.

Clare, L., Rowlands, J., Bruce, E., Surr, C. & Downs, M. (2008). The experience of living with dementia in residential care: An interpretative phenomenological analysis. *Gerontologist, 48*(6), 711–720.

Clare, L., Rowlands, J. M. & Quin, R. (2008). Collective strength: The impact of developing a shared social identity in early-stage dementia. *Dementia, 7*(1), 9–30.

Clare, L., Whitaker, C. J., Roberts, S. M. et al. (2013). Memory awareness profiles differentiate mild cognitive impairment from early-stage dementia: Evidence from assessments of performance monitoring and evaluative judgment. *Dementia and Geriatric Cognitive Disorders, 35*(5–6), 266–279.

Cole, M. G., McCusker, J., Voyer, P. et al. (2013). Symptoms of delirium predict incident delirium in older long-term care residents. *International Psychogeriatrics, 25*(6), 887–894.

Cotelli, M., Manenti, R., Zanetti, O. et al. (2012). Non-pharmacological intervention for memory decline. *Frontiers in Human Neuroscience, 6*, article 46. Accessed 15 January 2014 via www.frontiersin.org.

Cotter, V. T. (2009). Hope in early-stage dementia: A concept analysis. *Holistic Nursing Practice, 23*(5), 297–301.

Davidson, J. E., Harvey, M. A., Bemis-Dougherty, A. et al. (2013). Implementation of the pain, agitation, and delirium clinical practice guidelines and promoting patient mobility to prevent post-intensive care syndrome. *Critical Care Medicine, 41*(9), S136–S145.

Davis, D. H. J., Terrera, G. M., Keage, H. et al. (2012). Delirium is a strong risk factor for dementia in the oldest-old: A population-based cohort study. *Brain: Journal of Neurology, 135*, 2809–2816.

de Lange, E., Verhaak, P. F. & van der Meer, K. (2013). Prevalence, presentation and prognosis of delirium in older people in the population, at home and in long term care: A review. *International Journal of Geriatric Psychiatry, 28*(2), 127–134.

Desai, S., Chau, T. & George, L. (2013). Intensive care unit delirium. *Critical Care Nursing Quarterly, 36*(4), 370–389.

Dupuis, S. L., Wiersma, E. & Loiselle, L. (2012). Pathologizing behavior: Meanings of behaviors in dementia care. *Journal of Aging Studies, 26*, 162–173.

Edvardsson, D., Winblad, B. & Sandman, P. O. (2008). Person-centered care of people with severe Alzheimer's disease: Current status and ways forward. *Lancet Neurology, 7*, 362–367.

Epp, T. D. (2003). Person-centred dementia care: A vision to be refined. *Canadian Alzheimer Disease Review, April*, 14–18.

Etters, E., Goodall, D. & Harrison, B. E. (2008). Caregiver burden among dementia patient caregivers: A review of the literature. *Journal of the American Academy of Nurse Practitioners, 20*(8), 423–428.

Fick, D. M., Kolanowski, A., Beattie, E. & McCrow, J. (2009). Delirium in early-stage Alzheimer's disease. *Journal of Gerontological Nursing, 35*(3), 30–38.

Fick, D. M., Steis, M. R., Waller, J. L. et al. (2013). Delirium superimposed on dementia is associated with prolonged length of stay and poor outcomes in hospitalized older adults. *Journal of Hospital Medicine, 8*(9), 500–505.

Flicker, L. (2010). Cardiovascular risk factors, cerebrovascular disease burden, and healthy brain aging. *The Clinics in Geriatric Medicine, 26*, 17–27.

Fong, T. G., Jones, R. N., Marcantonio, E. R. et al. (2012). Adverse outcomes after hospitalization and delirium in persons with Alzheimer disease. *Annals of Internal Medicine, 156*(12), 848–856.

Fong, T. G., Tulebaev, S. R. & Inouye, S. K. (2009). Delirium in elderly adults: Diagnosis, prevention and treatment. *Nature Reviews Neurology, 5*, 210–220. doi:10.1038/nrneurol.2009.24.

Forbes, D., Thiessen, E. J., Blake, C. M. et al. (2013). Exercise programs for people with dementia. *Cochrane Database Systematic Reviews*. Art. ID CD006489. doi:10.1002/14651858.CD006489.pub3.

Foster, B. (2009). Music for life's journey: The capacity of music in dementia care. *Alzheimer's Care Today, 10*(1), 42–49

Gareri, P., De Fazio, P., Manfredi, V. G. et al. (2014). Use and safety of antipsychotics in behavioral disorders in elderly people with dementia. *Journal of Clinical Psychopharmacology, 34*(1), 109–123.

Gealogo, G. A. (2013). Dementia with Lewy bodies: A comprehensive review for nurses. *Journal of Neuroscience Nursing, 45*(6), 347–358.

George, D. R., Qualls, S. H., Camp, C. J. et al. (2012). Renovating Alzheimer's: "Constructive" reflections on the new clinical and research diagnostic guidelines. *Gerontologist, 53*(3), 378–387.

Godfrey, M., Smith, J., Green, J. et al. (2013). Developing and implementing an integrated delirium prevention system of care: A theory driven participatory research study. *BMC Health Services Research, 13*, 341. Accessed 15 January 2014 via www.biomedcentral.com.

Gordon, S. J., Melillo, K. D., Nannini, A. et al. (2013). Bedside coaching to improve nurses' recognition of delirium. *Journal of Neuroscience Nursing, 45*(5), 288–293.

Gorelick, P. B. & Nyenhuis, D. (2013). Understanding and treating vascular cognitive impairment. *Continuum, 19*(2), 425–437.

Hachinski, V. C., Lassen, N. A. & Marshall, J. (1974). Multi-infarct dementia: A cause of mental deterioration in elderly. *Lancet, 2*, 207–209.

Hall, G. R. & Buckwalter, K. C. (1987). Progressively lowered threshold: A conceptual model for care of adults with Alzheimer's disease. *Archives of Psychiatric Nursing, 1*, 399–406.

Hanagasi, H. A., Bilgic, B. & Emre, M. (2013). Neuroimaging, biomarkers, and management of dementia with Lewy bodies. *Frontiers in Neurology, 4*, article 151. Accessed 15 January 2014 via www.frontiersin.org.

Hopper, T., Bourgeois, M., Pimentel, J. et al. (2013). An evidence-based systematic review on cognitive interventions for individuals with dementia. *American Journal of Speech Language Pathology, 22*(1), 126–145.

Horning, S. M., Melrose, R. & Sultzer, D. (2014). Insight in Alzheimer's disease and its relation to psychiatric and behavioral disturbances. *International Journal of Geriatric Psychiatry, 29*(1), 77–84.

Huang, L.-W., Inouye, S. K., Jones, R. N. et al. (2012). Identifying indicators of key diagnostic features of delirium. *Journal of the American Geriatrics Society, 60*(6), 1044–1050.

Huang, Y. & Halliday, G. (2013). Can we clinically diagnose dementia with Lewy bodies yet? *Translational Neurodegeneration, 2*, 4. Accessed 15 January 2014 at www.translationalneurodegeneration.com/content/2/1/4.

Hulko, W. (2009). From "not a big deal" to "hellish": Experiences of older people with dementia. *Journal of Aging Studies, 23*, 131–144.

Inouye, S. K., van Dyck, C. H., Alessi, C. A., Balkin, S., Siegal, A. P. & Horwitz, R. I. (1990). Clarifying confusion: The confusion assessment method. A new method for detection of delirium. *Annals of Internal Medicine, 113*(12), 941–948.

Jellinger, K. A. & Attems, J. (2010). Prevalence of dementia disorders in the oldest-old: An autopsy study. *Acta Neuropathologica, 119*(4), 421–433.

Justin, B. N., Turek, M. & Hakim, A. M. (2013). Heart disease as a risk factor for dementia. *Clinical Epidemiology, 26*(5), 135–145.

Kaur, B., Harvey, D. J., DeCarli, C. S. et al. (2012). Extrapyramidal signs by dementia severity in Alzheimer disease and dementia with Lewy bodies. *Alzheimer's Disease and Associated Disorders, 27*(3), 226–232.

Kawashima, R. (2013). Mental exercises for cognitive function: Clinical evidence. *Journal of Preventive Medicine & Public Health, 46*, S22–S27.

Kirk-Sanchez, N. & McGough, E. L. (2014). Physical exercise and cognitive performance in the elderly: Current perspectives. *Clinical Interventions in Aging, 9*, 51–62.

Kiser, L. & Zasler, N. (2009). Residential design for real life rehabilitation. *NeuroRehabilitation, 25*, 219–227.

Kitwood, T. (1997). *Dementia reconsidered: The person comes first*. Buckingham: Open University Press.

Kling, M. A., Trojanowski, J. Q., Wolk, D. A. et al. (2013). Vascular disease and dementias: Paradigm shifts to drive research in new directions. *Alzheimer's and Dementia, 9*(1), 76–92.

Langballe, E. M., Engdahl, B., Nordeng, H. et al. (2014). Short- and long-term mortality risk associated with the use of antipsychotics among 26,940 dementia outpatients: A population-based study. *American Journal of Geriatric Psychiatry, 22*(4), 321–331.

Lee, M. & Chodosh, J. (2009). Dementia and life expectancy: What do we know? *Journal of the American Medical Directors Association, 10*(7), 466–471

Macluluch, A. M., Anand, A., Davis, D. H. et al. (2013). New horizons in the pathogenesis, assessment and management of delirium. *Age and Ageing, 42*, 667–674.

Mangialasche, F., Kivipelto, M., Solomon, A. et al. (2012). Dementia prevention: Current epidemiological evidence and future perspective. *Alzheimer's Research & Therapy, 4*, 6. Accessed 15 January 2014 via http://alzres.com/content/4/1/6.

Mardh, S., Karlsson, T., Marcusson, J. (2013). Aspects of awareness in patients with Alzheimer's disease. *International Psychogeriatrics, 25*(7), 1167–1179.

Massimo, L., Evans, L. K. & Benner, P. (2013). Caring for loved ones with frontotemporal degeneration: The lived experiences of spouses. *Geriatric Nursing, 34*, 302–306.

McCormack, B. (2003). A conceptual framework for person-centred practice with older people. *International Journal of Nursing of Nursing Practice, 9*, 202–208.

McCormack, B. (2004). Person-centredness in gerontological nursing: An overview of the literature. *International Journal of Older People, 13*, 3a, 31–38.

McDermott, O., Orrell, M. & Ridder, H. M. (2014). The importance of music for people with dementia: The perspectives of people with dementia, family carers, staff and music therapists. *Aging and Mental Health, 18*(6), 706–716.

Miller, C. A. (2012). *Fast facts for dementia care: What nurses need to know in a nutshell.* New York, NY: Springer.

Morgan, R. O., Sail, K. R., Snow, A. L. et al. (2013). Modeling causes of aggressive behavior in patients with dementia. *Gerontologist, 53*(5), 738–747.

Neville, C., Clifton, K., Henwood, T. et al. (2013). Watermemories: A swimming club for adults with dementia. *Journal of Gerontological Nursing, 39*(2), 21–25.

New South Wales' Ministry of Health & Royal Australian and New Zealand College of Psychiatrists. (2013). *Assessment and management of people with behavioural and psychological symptoms of dementia (BPSD): A handbook for NSW Health clinicians.* Sydney: NSW Ministry of Health.

New Zealand Ministry of Health (NZMOH). (2011). *Tatau Kura Tangata: Health of older Māori chart book 2011.* Wellington: Author. Accessed March 2015 at www.health.govt.nz/publication/tatau-kura-tangata-health-older-maori-chart-book-2011.

Nomura, M., Makimoto, K., Kato, M., Shiba, T., Matsuura, C., Shigenobu, K., . . . Ikeda, M. (2009). Empowering older people with early dementia and family caregivers: A participatory action research study. *International Journal of Nursing Studies, 46*(4), 431–441.

Palmer, J. L. (2013). Preserving personhood of individuals with advanced dementia: Lessons from family caregivers. *Geriatric Nursing, 34,* 224–229.

Popp, J. (2013). Delirium and cognitive decline: More than a coincidence. *Current Opinion in Neurology, 26*(6), 634–639.

Prince, M., Albanese, E., Guerchet, M., Prima, M. (2014). *World Alzheimer's Report 2104: Dementia and risk reduction*. London: Alzheimer's Disease International.

Prvulovic, D., Hampel, H. & Pantel, J. (2010). Galatamine for Alzheimer's disease. *Expert Opinion on Drug Metabolism and Toxicology, 6*(3), 345–354.

Reisberg, B. (1986). Dementia: A systematic approach to identifying reversible causes. *Geriatrics, 41*(4), 30–46.

Robinson, T. N., Raeburn, C. D., Tran, Z. V.; Angles, E. M.; Brenner, L. A. & Moss, M. (2009). Postoperative delirium in the elderly: Risk factors and outcomes. *Annals of Surgery, 249*(1), 173–178.

Ryan, D. J., O'Regan, N. A., Caoimh R. O. et al. (2012). Delirium in an adult acute hospital population: Predictors, prevalence and detection. *British Medical Journal Open Access, 3*, e001772.

Sabbagh, M. N., Cooper, K., DeLange, J., Stoehr, J. D., Thind, K., Lahti, T., . . . Beach, T. G. (2009). Functional, global and cognitive decline correlates to accumulation of Alzheimer's pathology in MCI and AD. *Current Alzheimer's Research, 7*(4), 280–286.

Salmon, E., Perani, D., Collette, F., Feyers, D., Kalbe, E., Holthoff, V., . . . Herholz, K. (2008). A comparison of unawareness in frontotemporal dementia and Alzheimer's disease. *Journal of Neurology, Neurosurgery, and Psychiatry, 79*(2), 176–179.

Sandhaus, S., Harrell, F. & Valenti, D. (2006). Healthier aging: Here's help to prevent delirium in the hospital. *Nursing, 36*(7), 60–62.

Seitz, D. P., Gill, S. S., Herrmann, N. et al. (2013). Pharmacological treatments for neuropsychiatric symptoms of dementia in long-term care: A systematic review. *International Psychogeriatrics, 25*(2), 185–203.

Selbaek, G., Engedal, K. & Bergh, S. (2013). The prevalence and course of neuropsychiatric symptoms in nursing home patients with dementia: A systematic review. *Journal of the American Medical Association, 14*, 161–169.

Seltzer, B. (2010). Galantamine-ER for the treatment of mild-to-moderate Alzheimer's disease. *Clinical Intervention in Aging, 5*, 1–6.

Shibata, K., Narumoto, J., Kitabayashi, Y., Ushijima, Y. & Fukui, K. (2008). Correlation between anosognosia and regional cerebral blood flow in Alzheimer's disease. *Neuroscience Letters, 435*(1), 7–10.

Simon, S. S., Yokomizo, J. E. & Bottino, C. (2012). Cognitive intervention in amnesic mild cognitive impairment: A systematic review. *Neuroscience and Biobehavioral Reviews, 36*, 1163–1178.

Slaughter, S. E. & Hayduk, L. A. (2012). Contributions of environment, comorbidity, and stage of dementia to the onset of walking and eating disability in long-term care residents. *Journal of the American Geriatrics Society, 60*(9), 1624–1631.

Smebye, K. L. & Kirkevold, M. (2013). The influence of relationships on personhood in dementia care: A qualitative, hermeneutic study. *BioMed Central Nursing, 12*(1), 29.

Smith, A. D. & Yaffe, K. (2014). Dementia (including Alzheimer's disease) can be prevented: Statement supported by international experts. *Journal of Alzheimer's Disease, 38*, 699–703.

Smith, K., Flicker, L., Lautenschlager, N. T., Almeida, O. P., Atkinson, D., Dwyer, D. & LoGiudice, D. (2008). High prevalence of dementia and cognitive impairment in Indigenous Australians. *Neurology, 71*(19), 1470–1473.

Solberg, L. M., Plummer, C. E., May, K. N. et al. (2013). A quality improvement program to increase nurses' detection of delirium in an acute medical unit. *Geriatric Nursing, 34*, 75–79.

Steis, M. R. & Fick, D. M. (2012). Delirium superimposed on dementia: Accuracy of nurse documentation. *Journal of Gerontological Nursing, 38*(1), 32–42.

Thomas, S. J. & Grossberg, G. T. (2009). Memantine: A review of studies into its safety and efficacy in treating Alzheimer's disease and other dementias. *Clinical Interventions in Aging, 4*, 367–377.

Tomlinson, B. E., Blessed, G. & Roth, M. (1968). Observations on the brains of non-demented old people. *Journal of Neurological Science, 7*, 331–356.

Tomlinson, B. E., Blessed, G. & Roth, M. (1970). Observation on the brains of demented old people. *Journal of Neurological Science, 11*, 205–242.

Toot, S., Devine, M., Akporobaro, A. et al. (2013). Causes of hospital admission for people with dementia: A systematic review. *Journal of the American Medical Directors Association, 14*(7), 463–470.

Tullmann, D. F., Fletcher, K. & Foreman, M. D. (2012). Delirium. In M. Boltz, E. Capezuti, T. Fulmer & D. Zwicker (Eds), *Evidence-based practice protocols for best practice* (4th ed., pp. 186–199). New York, NY: Springer.

van Vliet, D., De Vugt, M. E., Kohler, S. et al. (2012). Awareness and its association with affective symptoms in young-onset and late-onset Alzheimer disease. *Alzheimer's Disease and Associated Disorders, 27*(3), 265–271.

Verhulsdonk, S., Quack, R., Groh, B. et al. (2013). Anosognosia and depression in patients with Alzheimer's dementia. *Archives of Gerontology and Geriatrics, 57*(3), 282–287.

Wand, A., Thoo W., Ting, V. et al. (2013). Identification and rates of delirium in elderly medical inpatients from diverse language groups. *Geriatric Nursing, 34*, 355–360.

Warren, J. D., Rohrer, J. D. & Rossor, M. N. (2013). Frontotemporal dementia. *British Medical Journal Open Access, 347*.

Woods, B., Aguirre, E., Spector, A. E. et al. (2012). Cognitive stimulation to improve cognitive functioning in people with dementia. *Cochrane Database of Systematic Reviews*. Art. ID CD005562. doi:10.1002/14651858.pub2.

Yevchak, A., Steis, M., Diehl, T. et al. (2012). Managing delirium in the acute care setting: A pilot focus group study. *International Journal of Older People Nursing, 7*(2), 152–162.

Yu, F., Rose, K. M., Burgener, S. C., Cunningham, C., Buettner, L. L., Beattie, E., . . . McKenzie, S. E. (2009). Cognitive training for earlystage Alzheimer's disease and dementia. *Journal of Gerontological Nursing, 35*(3), 23–28.

Zauber, T. S., Murphy, K., Rizzuto, L. et al. (2013). Quality improvement and cost savings with multicomponent delirium interventions: Replication of the Hospital Elder Life Program in a community hospital. *Psychosomatics*, March 11, p. ii. S0033–3182(13)00011-X. doi:10.116/j.psym.2013.01.010.

Chapter 15

Impaired cognition: Depression

By Carol Miller and Sharyn Hunter

LEARNING OBJECTIVES

After reading this chapter, you should be able to:

1. Describe theories that explain late-life depression.
2. Examine risk factors that cause or contribute to depression in older adults.
3. Discuss the functional consequences of late-life depression.
4. Describe the following aspects of nursing assessment: unique manifestations of late-life depression, depression in cognitively impaired older adults, cultural factors related to depression and use of screening tools.
5. Identify interventions for addressing risk factors, improving psychosocial function and teaching about antidepressants, psychosocial therapies and complementary and alternative modalities.
6. Discuss nursing responsibilities related to assessing and preventing suicide in older adults.

KEY POINTS

Alzheimer's disease
antidepressants
bright-light therapy
cognitive triad theory
Cornell Scale for Depression in Dementia (CSDD)
depression
electroconvulsive therapy (ECT)
Geriatric Depression Scale—Short Form (GDS-SF)
late-life depression
learned helplessness theory
post-stroke depression
psychomotor agitation
psychomotor retardation
psychosocial therapies
selective serotonin reuptake inhibitors (SSRIs)
serotonin and noradrenaline reuptake inhibitors (SNRIs)
St John's wort
suicide
vascular depression

Despite the common occurrence of **depression** in older adults, it is often undetected and untreated. The term depression is difficult to define because it is considered a mood, a complaint, a syndrome and a disease. However, gerontological references commonly use the term *depressive symptoms* to describe a constellation of symptoms that profoundly affect the cognition and quality of life of older adults. Gerontologists have developed theories to explain depression in older adults, which is often called late-life depression, and healthcare practitioners have developed assessment tools to identify depression in older adults. Nurses have important roles in addressing depression because there is a range of nursing interventions that can have a significant positive impact on the quality of life of older adults.

Although psychiatric references describe many types of depression, which are also called mood disorders, the two types most commonly discussed in relation to older adults are major depression (also called major depressive disorder) or sub-threshold (also called minor, subclinical, or non-major) depression. Diagnostic criterion for major depression includes depressed mood and/or loss of interest or pleasure along with at least five of the following signs and symptoms: weight loss; appetite change; sleep disturbances; observable, psychomotor agitation or retardation (i.e. slowness); fatigue or loss of energy; feeling worthless or excessively guilty; cognitive impairment; and recurrent thoughts of death or suicide (Snowden & Almeida, 2013). A defining characteristic of major depression is that it noticeably interferes with usual functioning and is associated with significantly diminished quality of life. Minor depression is characterised by these same signs and symptoms, but they are not as severe and their effects on functioning and quality of life are not as serious. Rather than defining types of depression in distinct categories, it should be viewed as a continuum of symptoms that should not be overlooked (Lee, Hasche, Choi et al., 2013).

Late-life depression refers to the onset of depression after age 65. Although manifestations differ only slightly in older adults, causative factors are more complex and it often occurs concomitantly with other conditions. In addition, late-life depression is associated with more serious consequences and is often unrecognised and undertreated. Much of the current research focuses on the relationships between late-life depression and chronic conditions that are common in older adults such as pain, stroke, dementia and cardiovascular disease. Estimates of prevalence of late-life depression in community settings range from 10% to 25% depending on the definition and subgroup studied (Almeida, 2012; Forlani, Morri, Ferrari et al., 2014).

THEORIES ABOUT LATE-LIFE DEPRESSION

Late-life depression is a multifaceted condition, which is caused by complex relationships and numerous other factors that commonly occur in older adults. Although no single theory can explain why older adults are likely to become depressed, some of the more common psychosocial, cognitive and biological theories explain causative factors from various perspectives. A major focus of recent research is the relationship between dementia and depression, and studies are just beginning to address questions about the very common co-occurrence of these two conditions.

Psychosocial theories

Psychosocial theories focus on the impact of loss as well as the buffering effects of social supports and the social network in protecting against depression. Blazer (2002) reviewed the psychosocial theories related to late-life

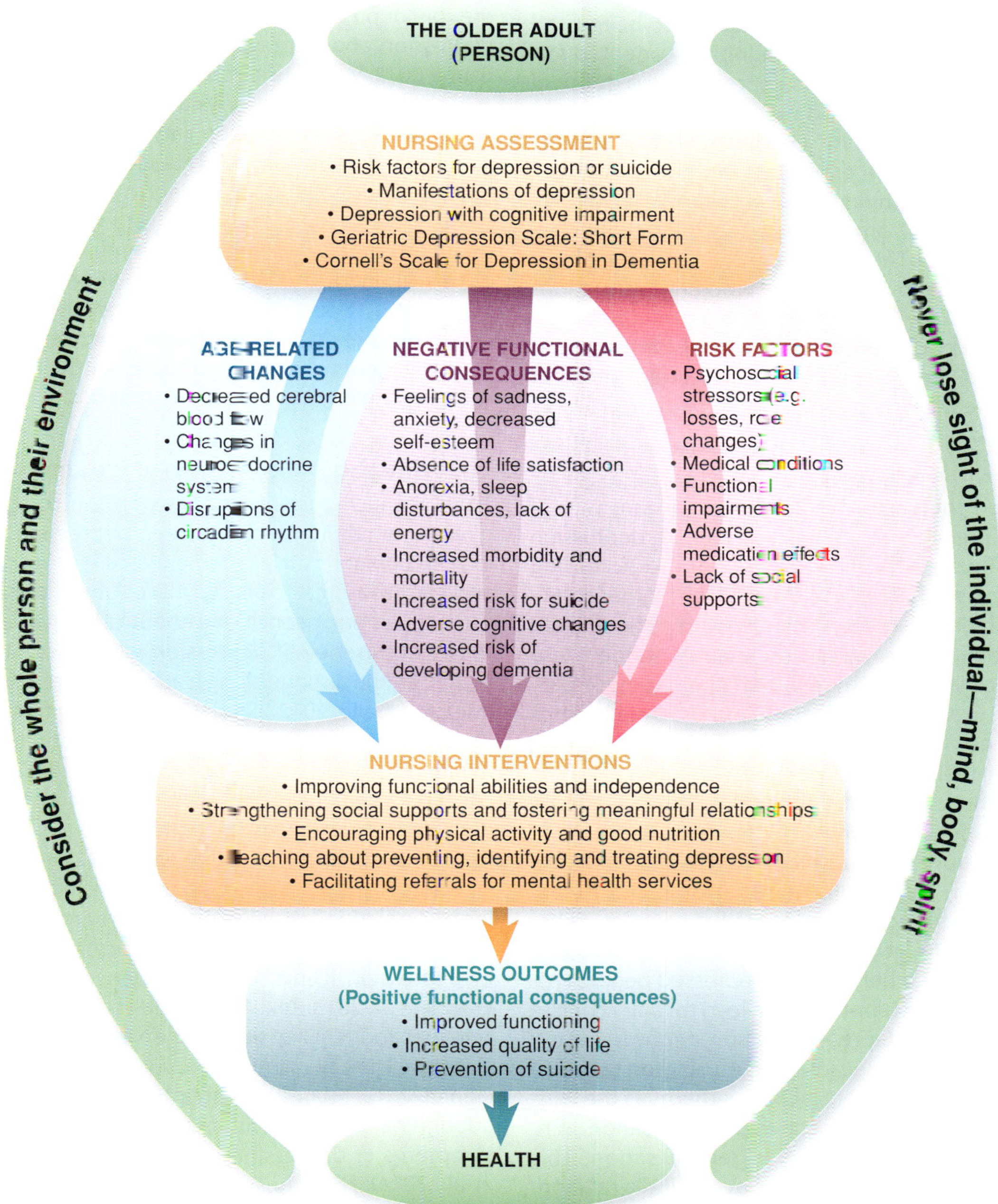

depression and identified the following potential contributing factors:

- Ageism, loss of social roles and lower socioeconomic status
- Early experiences, including impoverishment and childhood trauma
- Recent social stressors, including stressful life events
- Inadequate social network (e.g. no spouse/partner, few friends, small family network)
- Diminished social interaction
- Poor social integration (e.g. unstable environment, lack of strong religious affiliation)
- A combination of the preceding factors.

The **learned helplessness theory** has also been used to explain late-life depression. A cognitively oriented formulation of this theory describes depression as a deficit in the following four areas: cognitive, motivational, self-esteem and affective-somatic (Seligman, 1981). Depression occurs when people expect bad things to happen, believe they can do nothing to prevent them and perceive that the events result from internal, stable and global factors (Seligman, 1981). This theory would explain the occurrence of depression in older adults who are in situations over which they have little control. The learned helplessness theory supports the use of nursing interventions directed towards improving self-efficacy and a sense of control over one's environment.

Cognitive triad theory

Beck proposed the **cognitive triad theory** as a way of explaining depression in general, and late-life depression in particular (Beck, Rush, Shaw & Emery, 1979). According to this theory, people appraise themselves by the "cognitive triad" of their self-image, their environment or experiences, and their future. Depressed people judge these three realms as lacking some features that are necessary for happiness. Examples of negative appraisals are feelings of worthlessness, interpretations of neutral events as bad, and unrealistic feelings of hopelessness.

Beck postulates that depression is caused not by adverse events but by distorted perceptions, which impair one's ability to appraise oneself and the event in a constructive manner. The second element of Beck's theory involves schemas, or consistent cognitive patterns. Schemas are assumptions, or unarticulated rules, that influence thoughts, feelings and behaviours. Depressed people typically hold negative assumptions that lead to faulty conclusions. For instance, a depressed person might believe "I must not be important because the nurse didn't stop to see me." The third component of Beck's theory is the existence of certain logical errors such as personalisation, minimisation, magnification and over-generalisation. This theory is supported by studies that have found a relationship between late-life depression and cognitive distortions or negative cognitions (Blazer, 2002).

Biological and genetic theories

Biological theories about late-life depression investigate the relationships among ageing, depression, and changes in the brain, nervous system and neuroendocrine system. These theories focus on the changes in the neuroendocrine system that are associated with depression, such as alterations in cortisol levels and increased activity in the hypothalamic–pituitary–adrenal axis. A current focus of neurobiological research is the potential role of inflammatory mechanisms as causative factors for depression (Catena-Dell'Osso et al., 2013). Studies are also addressing neurobiological mechanisms that are associated with increased risk for suicide (Pandey, 2013). These theories led to a better understanding of the role of physical activity as an effective intervention for depression and depression-like behaviours (Eyre, Papps & Baune, 2013; Matta Mello Portugal et al., 2013).

Other biological theories address anatomical changes (e.g. lesions in white or deep gray matter), neurophysiological brain changes (e.g. decreased cerebral blood flow), and disruption of the circadian rhythms (e.g. sleep patterns). For example, longitudinal studies indicate that the age-related atrophy of brain volume contributes to the development of late-life depression (Ribeiz, Duran, Oliveira et al., 2013). Researchers have also focused on the interrelationship between biological and genetic variables, for example, genetic variations that affect the release of neurotransmitters under stressful conditions.

Theories about depression and dementia

There is much current emphasis on the complex and bidirectional relationships between depression and pathological conditions such as dementia, cerebrovascular disease and cardiovascular disease. Although studies related to these topics are inconclusive about causative relationships the co-occurrence of depression with medical conditions is cited as "the distinguishing feature of depression in late life" (Mezuk & Gallo, 2013). Studies consistently find that the co-occurrence of depression with chronic conditions in older adults is associated with more serious negative functional consequences, including all the following: greater pain, diminished functioning, lower quality of life, and increased risk for suicide (Byma, Given & Given, 2012).

Since the early 2000s, gerontologists have recognised a high correlation between depression and dementia, with cognitive deficits being both a predictor and consequence of depression (Diniz, Butters, Albert et al., 2013; Vilalta-Franch et al., 2013; Zeki Al Hazzouri et al., 2014). Studies indicate that about half of the people with **Alzheimer's disease** also have clinically significant depression (Bewernick & Schlaepfer, 2013; Knapskog, Barca, Engedal, 2013). In addition about 20% of people with mild cognitive impairment have symptoms of depression (Polyakova, Sonnabend, Sander et al., 2014). Hypotheses about the relationship between depression and cognitive changes that are currently being investigated are as follows: (1) depression is a precursor of early manifestation of dementia; (2) depression occurs early in the course of dementia as a psychological reaction to eroding cognitive abilities; (3) depression and cognitive decline are associated with a common pathway of neurological changes; and (4) depression causes neurological and neuroendocrine changes that accelerate the rate of cognitive decline (Clazaran, Trincado, Bermejo-Pareja, 2013; Richard, Reitz, Honig et al., 2013; van den Kommer, Comijs, Aartsen et al., 2013). Distinguishing features of depression in people with dementia include increased manifestations related to motivation (e.g., apathy and less overt mood complaints (Marano, Rosenberg & Lyketsos, 2013).

Another area of intense investigation is the common co-occurrence of depression and cerebrovascular disease caused by strokes or cumulative effects of ischaemic episodes. **Post-stroke depression** is the most common neuropsychiatric consequence of a stroke, with prevalence rates ranging from 9% to 34% during the first 6 months and up to 70% of all stroke survivors over the longer term (da Rocha e Silva et al., 2013; Flaster, Sharma & Rao, 2013; Taylor-Piliae, Hepworth & Coull, 2013). Poststroke depression is most likely to occur in people with greater functional and cognitive impairment and is associated with increased mortality and poor recovery (DeRyck, Brouns, Fransen et al., 2013; Hornsten, Lovheim & Gustafson, 2013).

Vascular depression occurs in the context of cerebrovascular disease without evidence or history of major stroke. Although research about vascular depression is in an early stage, studies indicate that the brain changes associated with cerebrovascular disease are strongly linked to the occurrence and worsening of depression in older adults (Taylor, Aizenstein & Alexopoulos, 2013; Volk & Steffens, 2013). Vascular depression is characterised by apathy, functional impairment, psychomotor retardation and cognitive impairments, including poor insight and executive dysfunction.

The relationship between depression and cardiovascular disease is another current focus of intense investigation by cardiologists and gerontologists. During the past two decades, researchers have identified all the following links: (1) depression is an independent risk factor for cardiac disease; (2) depression is often chronic and recurrent in people with cardiovascular disease; and (3) depression is an independent risk factor for adverse cardiovascular outcomes, including poor recovery and increased mortality (Huffman, Celano, Beach et al., 2013). Because depression occurs so frequently in people with cardiovascular disease, it is recommended that routine screening for depression occurs in all people with coronary heart disease (Whooley & Wong, 2013).

WELLNESS OPPORTUNITY

From a holistic nursing perspective, it is important to recognise there are many types of depression and, in older adults particularly, depression is complex and likely to occur concomitantly with dementia and other conditions.

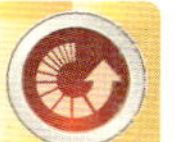

RISK FACTORS FOR DEPRESSION IN OLDER ADULTS

Risk factors that are likely to cause or contribute to depression in older adults include demographic factors and psychosocial influences, medical conditions and functional impairments, and the effects of medications and alcohol. Although these factors can increase the risk for depression in people of any age, older adults are more likely than younger people to have one or more of these variables. The following sections discuss each category of risk in relation to older adults. Additional risk factors for depression include cognitive impairments and dementia, as discussed in other sections of this chapter.

Demographic factors and psychosocial influences

Demographic factors and psychosocial influences that are associated with depression in older adults include:

- Female sex
- Personal or family history of depression
- Bereavement, loss of significant relationships
- Loneliness
- Chronic stress
- Recent social stressors
- Stressful social environment
- Loss of meaningful social interaction
- Lack of social supports
- Loss of significant roles
- Current or previous experiences of abuse or neglect
- Being a carer/caregiver (including assuming primary care of a grandchild).

Although losses and stress can be risk factors for depression, social supports (e.g. having at least one close relationship) and effective coping mechanisms can protect older adults from depression. Thus, the stressors alone are not the primary risk factor for depression; rather, it is the combination of stressors and the absence of social supports that increases the risk for depression. In addition to causing the onset of depression, psychosocial factors can affect the duration of depression.

Medical conditions and functional impairments

Medical conditions that are considered causative factors for depression are listed in Box 15-1. Some of these conditions are related to electrolyte imbalances or nutritional deficiencies, which can be easily identified and treated. For example, recent studies show that low levels of serum 25(OH)D (vitamin D) are associated with increased depression in older adults; supplemental vitamin D is associated with reduced depressive symptoms in women (Shipowick, Moores & Corbett, 2009).

The relationships between medical conditions, functional impairments and depression are complex and interactive, with depression contributing to medical illness and disability, and medical illness and disability contributing to

BOX 15-1
Medical conditions that can cause depression

Central nervous system disorders
Parkinson's disease
Dementia
Strokes
Haemorrhage or haematoma
Tumours
Neurosyphilis
Normal-pressure hydrocephalus

Nutritional deficiencies
Folate or vitamin B_{12} deficiency
Pernicious anaemia
Iron deficiency
Vitamin D deficiency

Cardiovascular disturbances
Myocardial infarction
Congestive heart failure
Coronary artery bypass surgery

Miscellaneous
Rheumatoid arthritis
Cancer, particularly of the pancreas or intestinal tract
Tuberculosis
Hip fracture
Alcohol/drug abuse

Metabolic and endocrine disorders
Diabetes
Hypothyroidism/hyperthyroidism
Hypoglycaemia/hyperglycaemia
Parathyroid disorders
Adrenal diseases
Hepatic or renal disease

Fluid and electrolyte disturbances
Hypercalcaemia
Hypokalaemia
Hyponatraemia

Infections
AIDS
Meningitis
Viral pneumonia
Hepatitis
Urinary tract infections

Chronic conditions
Chronic obstructive pulmonary disease
Chronic kidney disease

depression. Some examples of interrelationships between depression and medical conditions or functional impairments include the following:

- Depression in medically ill older adults is associated with increased mortality, longer hospitalisations and extended recovery time.
- Medical illnesses can threaten survival, independence, self-concept, role functions, economic resources and sense of well-being.
- Disability leads to depression because it causes social isolation, low self-esteem, restricted social activity, strained interpersonal relationships and loss of perceived control.
- Depression in medically ill older adults can lead to other health problems such as hip fractures and increased susceptibility to infection.
- Chronic pain is a common cause of depression, and it is sometimes a symptom of depression.
- Depression worsens pain, and pain worsens depression.
- Functional impairment is associated with depression as both a contributing factor and a consequence.
- Depression is a common cause of nutritional deficits in older adults and nutritional deficiencies can be a risk factor for depression.

Gerontologists emphasise that depression is a treatable component of medical conditions that has a significant negative effect on health-related quality of life for older adults (Gallegos-Carrillo et al., 2009). One study found that depression was more burdensome than physical symptoms in people with Parkinson's disease (Jones, Pohar & Patten, 2009). Studies that address depression in people with diabetes, cardiovascular disease, chronic obstructive pulmonary disease and chronic kidney disease consistently emphasise that depression occurs commonly with these conditions, is an independent risk for poorer outcomes and should be identified and treated (de Voogd et al., 2009; Hedayati et al., 2009; Lin et al., 2009; Omachi et al., 2009; Subramaniam et al., 2009). Studies also found that improvement in depression can lead to improved functioning and have a meaningful effect on the ability to live at home (Li & Conwell, 2009).

Another risk factor is that depression often goes unrecognised as a concomitant condition in older adults with medical conditions. For example, depression in long-term care residents is often overlooked as a treatable condition (Thakur & Blazer, 2008). Although this is not a risk factor for causing depression, it is a risk factor for the progression of depression, subsequent functional decline and increased morbidity and mortality.

Effects of medications and alcohol

People of any age may experience depression as an adverse medication effect, but older adults are at higher risk because they take more medications. Medications may be risk factors for depression in the following ways:

- Adverse medication effects can cause a depressive syndrome that improves or disappears when the medication is stopped.
- Adverse medication effects can induce a depression that does not remit when the medications are stopped.
- Adverse medication effects can simulate a depressive syndrome by causing lethargy, insomnia and irritability.
- The withdrawal of certain medications, such as psychostimulants, can cause a depressive syndrome.

BOX 15-2
Examples of medications that can cause depression

Analgesics
Indomethacin
Narcotics

Antihypertensives and cardiovascular agents
Beta blockers
Clonidine
Digoxin
Hydralazine
Methyldopa

Anti-parkinsonism agents
Levodopa

Central nervous system agents
Alcohol
Barbiturates
Benzodiazepines
Fluphenazine
Haloperidol

Histamine blockers
Cimetidine

Steroids
Corticosteroids
Oestrogen

Anti-cancer (chemotherapeutic) agents

Depression as an adverse effect of medications is usually related to the use of medications, such as those listed in Box 15-2, which are prescribed for chronic conditions. However, depression can also be an adverse effect of alcohol or drugs that are abused (e.g. benzodiazepines). Moreover, although people of any age might experience adverse effects from alcohol, older people are more sensitive to these adverse effects because of age-related changes. Alcohol and depression have a synergistic relationship: alcohol causes depression and depression leads to alcohol abuse, which in turn exacerbates the depression.

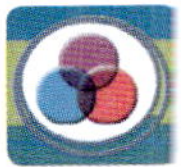

FUNCTIONAL CONSEQUENCES ASSOCIATED WITH DEPRESSION IN OLDER ADULTS

Depression has serious functional consequences for people of any age, but for frail and seriously depressed older adults, the effects can be life-threatening. Functional consequences range from a negative impact on well-being and quality of life to the most serious consequence, which is **suicide**. These negative functional consequences are associated not only with major depression but also with minor and subclinical depression in older adults; these consequences often progress if treatment is not initiated (Lyness et al., 2009). This section discusses the wide range of functional consequences that are associated with depression. Suicide is addressed as a separate topic at the end of this chapter because nurses need to address it not only as the most serious consequence of depression but also as an entity in itself.

Physical health and functioning

A decline in physical functioning is one of the most consistently identified functional consequences of depression in older adults, particularly in those who are also cognitively impaired (Hybels, Pieper & Blazer, 2009; Steffens, 2009). Additional functional consequences that affect health and functioning are a high number of physical complaints, perception of worse health and inability to carry out important life functions such as managing money or medications (Licht-Strunk et al., 2009b). Many studies in a variety of settings found that depression is an independent risk for excess morbidity and mortality (Barca et al., 2009; Schoevers et al., 2009; Wolinsky et al., 2009). It is important to recognise that some of these consequences, such as the inability to manage money or medications, may be a central factor in preventing the person from living independently. Box 15-3 lists ways in which depression affects physical health and functioning.

Appetite disturbances, particularly anorexia, are among the most common physical complaints of depressed older adults. Sometimes, the depressed person does not complain

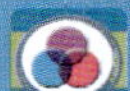

BOX 15-3
Functional consequences of late-life depression

Impact on physical function

- Loss of appetite
- Weight loss
- Digestive system complaints, particularly dysphagia, flatulence, constipation, stomach distress or early satiety
- Insomnia, hypersomnia, frequent awakening, early-morning awakening and other sleep disturbances
- Fatigue, loss of energy
- Pain, discomfort, dyspnoea, general malaise
- Slowed or increased psychomotor activities
- Loss of libido or other problems with sexual function

Impact on cognitive and psychosocial function

- Affect: sad, low, "blue", worried, unhappy, 'down in the dumps'
- Absence of feelings; feeling numb or empty
- Diminished life satisfaction
- Low self-esteem
- Loss of interest or pleasure
- Passivity, lack of motivation to do things
- Inattention to personal appearance
- Feelings of guilt, hopelessness, self-blame, unworthiness, uselessness, helplessness
- Anxiety, worry, irritability
- Slowed thinking, poor memory, inability to concentrate, poor attention span, inability to make decisions, exaggeration of any mental deficits
- Rumination about past and present problems and failures

of anorexia and may even deny the problem, but a carer or family member may note that the person is not interested in food and is losing weight. Other gastrointestinal complaints that may be functional consequences of depression include flatulence, constipation, early satiety and attention to bowels. Any of these disturbances may be attributed to or caused by other factors such as medical conditions or adverse medication effects; however, depression must be considered as a possible underlying factor. Chronic fatigue and diminished energy are additional functional consequences of late-life depression that are likely to be attributed to or caused by other conditions.

Like weight loss and diminished appetite, sleep changes commonly occur in older adults, and they may or may not be caused by depression. Waking up more frequently during the night and early morning awakening are two changes in sleep patterns that are characteristic of depression. Current research is exploring the bidirectional relationship between sleep changes and depression, with studies pointing towards insomnia being a risk factor for and a functional consequence of depression (Baglioni, Berger & Rieman, 2013; Krystal, Edinger & Wohlgemuth, 2012).

Older adults are similar to other depressed people of any age and experience psychomotor agitation or retardation. **Psychomotor retardation** is manifested as slowed body movements and slowed verbal responses, sometimes to the point of muteness. A monotonous or whispering tone of voice might also be an indicator of psychomotor retardation. Affected people often complain of feeling extremely fatigued and having little or no energy. In contrast to people with psychomotor retardation, people with **psychomotor agitation** present an atypical picture of depression. These people manifest high levels of activity such as pacing and hand wringing. They may be unable to sit still and may have verbal outbursts, such as shouting. Another activity associated with psychomotor agitation is compulsive behaviour such as frequent toileting or hand washing.

In addition to direct functional consequences on health and functioning, late-life depression is associated with increased risk for developing medical conditions, including cancer, coronary disease and type 2 diabetes (Park & Unutzer, 2013). Moreover, a review of studies concluded there is strong evidence that depression increases morbidity and mortality (i.e. poor recovery, more complications and higher death rate) in people with all the following medical conditions: cancer, dementia, diabetes, osteoporosis, chronic pain, cardiovascular disease, and cerebrovascular disease (Park & Unutzer, 2013).

Cognitive and psychosocial function and quality of life

Cognitive impairments can occur because of depression and, in older adults, these deficits are likely to be viewed as a primary problem rather than as a consequence of another problem. Depressed older adults may, in fact, exaggerate cognitive deficits and make statements about global deficits, such as, "I can't remember anything at all." In particular, they may emphasise memory deficits and attribute these to normal ageing or be concerned they are developing dementia when the underlying problem is actually a depression-related difficulty in concentrating. See Box 15-3 for a list of the functional consequences of depression that affect cognitive and psychosocial function.

Depression is usually characterised by a depressed mood or sad affect, but older adults may not perceive or acknowledge these mood disturbances in themselves. Rather than acknowledging that they are depressed, older adults are more likely to talk about being "blue" or "down in the dumps". Depressed older people may feel like crying but may not be able to cry or identify the underlying reason for their sadness. Another psychosocial consequence of depression is the absence of life satisfaction, even when the person has reasons to feel satisfied.

Anxiety, irritability, diminished self-esteem and negative feelings about self are some of the more generalised affective consequences of depression. Studies indicate that the co-occurrence of anxiety and depression is associated with increased cognitive impairment (Beaudreau & O'Hara, 2009). The absence of feelings, or a feeling of emptiness, can also be a functional consequence of depression. A loss of interest in social activities may be the depression-related psychosocial change that is most obvious to others. Similarly, other people are likely to observe that the depressed older person has little or no concern about personal appearance. In addition, the depressed person may be overly or unrealistically worried about illnesses, financial affairs and family issues.

Depression has a major negative impact on quality of life. For example, depressed older adults report unsatisfactory social functioning, lower levels of life satisfaction and poor perceptions of physical and mental health. In addition, many of the symptoms of depression (e.g. worry, fatigue, sad affect, sleep disturbances, loss of interest) directly interfere with well-being and quality of life. Moreover, depressed older adults often feel a sense of hopelessness. One study of community-living older adults found that feelings of sadness, irritability, worries about the future and lack of positive affect were significant characteristics of older adults with subclinical depression (Adams & Moon, 2009).

WELLNESS OPPORTUNITY

Because people who are depressed tend to have very low self-esteem, nurses can point out concrete examples of positive qualities that they see in the person.

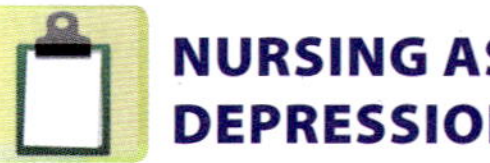

NURSING ASSESSMENT OF DEPRESSION IN OLDER ADULTS

Whereas Chapter 13 addressed all aspects of psychosocial assessment, this section focuses on the following specific

TABLE 15-1 Comparison of depression in younger and older adults

Depressed younger adults	Depressed older adults
More likely to report emotional symptoms	Report more cognitive and physical symptoms
Sense of hopelessness, uselessness and helplessness	Apathy; exaggeration of personal helplessness
Negative feelings towards self	Sense of emptiness, loss of interest, withdrawal from social activities
Insomnia	Hypersomnia; early morning awakening
Eating disorders	Anorexia, weight loss
More verbal expressions of suicidal ideation than successful attempts; more passive means of suicide	Less talk about suicide, but more successful attempts and more violent means of suicide

aspects of late-life depression: identifying the unique manifestations of depression in older adults, identifying depression in people with dementia and using screening tools to identify late-life depression. Assessing the suicide risk in older adults is discussed in the section on suicide. The assessment information in Chapter 13, particularly Box 13-7, can be used with the information in the following sections as a guide for assessing depression in older adults.

WELLNESS OPPORTUNITY

Nurses can ask a depressed older adult, "Can you think of one thing that we can do to improve your quality of life today?"

Identifying the unique manifestations of depression

Assessment of late-life depression is complicated by a wide array of possible manifestations, as reviewed in the functional consequences section. Moreover, manifestations of depression in older adults may differ from those in younger adults. One study found that older adults are less likely to show affective symptoms and are more likely to have cognitive changes, physical complaints and a loss of interest than younger adults (Fiske, Wetherell & Gatz, 2009). Although it is difficult to generalise about manifestations of depression according to age categories, some conclusions about the differences in younger and older adults are summarised in Table 15-1.

In assessing depression in any cognitively impaired older adult, it is often difficult to distinguish between manifestations of depression and dementia. Table 15-2, which identifies specific features that are most likely to be associated with either dementia or depression, can be used as a guide for nursing assessment to differentiate between these two conditions. It is important to keep in mind that older adults frequently have both depression and dementia, so manifestations will not always be clearly distinguishable.

Cultural factors can influence one's perception of depression, and nurses must consider these, particularly during their assessments. Nurses can use the information in Cultural considerations 15-1 to identify some of the cultural variations in expressions of depression. In addition, nurses need to be aware of and sensitive to the fact that many cultural groups attach a strong stigma to depression and other forms of mental illness. Thus, they need to use

TABLE 15-2 Distinguishing features of dementia and depression

Parameter	Dementia	Depression
Onset of symptoms	Gradual onset, recognised only by hindsight	Abrupt onset, possibly involving a triggering event
Presentation of symptoms	Unawareness of symptoms, or attribution to non-pathological causes	Exaggeration of memory problems and other cognitive deficits
Memory and attention	Impaired memory, particularly for recent events; poor attention; strong attempts to perform well	Memory and attention deficits attributable to lack of motivation and inability to concentrate
Emotions	Labile affect that changes in response to suggestions; possible apathy owing to cognitive impairments	Consistent feelings of sadness and being "down in the dumps"; unresponsive to suggestions
Response to questions	Evasive, angry, sarcastic; use of humour, confabulation or social skills to cover up deficits	Slowed, apathetic, frequent response of "I don't know", with no effort expended
Personal appearance	Inappropriate dress and actions owing to impaired perceptions and thought processes	Little or no concern about appearance because of lack of motivation or diminished self-esteem
Physical complaints	Vague fatigue and weakness; complaints are inconsistent and easily forgotten	Anorexia, weight loss, constipation, insomnia, decreased energy
Neurological features	Aphasia, agnosia, agraphia, apraxia, perseveration	Complaints of dysphagia without any physical basis
Contact with reality	Denial of reality; illusions more predominant than hallucinations; if present, delusions are aimed at explaining deficits	Exaggerated sense of gloom; possible auditory hallucinations or self-derogatory delusions

CULTURAL CONSIDERATIONS 15-1
Cultural variations in expressions of depression

Cultural group	Common expressions of depression
Bosnians	Express emotional distress in somatic symptoms such as gastrointestinal or respiratory complaints
British	Associate depression with genetic predisposition, traumatic childhood or poor relationship with mother
Chinese	Shameful to discuss; may be called "neurasthenia" (i.e. symptoms produced by social stressors)
Filipinos	Shameful to discuss; may refer to *Lungknot* (i.e. sadness)
Greeks	Emotional distress is likely to present with somatic complaints such as dizziness and paraesthesias
Hindus	Psychological distress is expressed through physical symptoms such as headaches, burning sensation in feet or forehead and tingling pain in lower extremities
Indigenous Australians*	Mental illness is considered shameful. It is not uncommon for these people to see spirits or hear voices of deceased loved ones. However, in the absence of other mental health symptoms, these are not sufficient for diagnosing a mental illness.
Japanese	Because of shame and stigma, emotional distress may be expressed through physical symptoms and may become severe before help is sought
Koreans	Emotions are expressed as physical complaints, including headaches, insomnia, anorexia, lack of energy
Māori**	Mental and behavioural states can be quite different. For example, *whakamā* is a mental and behavioural state that occurs when there is a sense of disadvantage or loss of standing. It presents as slowness and a lack of responsiveness and this state is not to be confused with depression.
South Asians	References to *Dil uddas hona*, associated with spiritual unhappiness
People from countries with a recent history of war, violence or political upheaval	May be associated with post-traumatic stress disorder; feelings of helplessness; memories of war-related brutalities; may be at increased risk for suicide

Sources: Andrews, M. M. & Boyle, J. S. (2011). *Transcultural concepts in nursing care* (6th ed.). Philadelphia, PA: Lippincott Williams & Wilkins; Lawrence et al. (2006) Concepts and causation of depression: A cross-cultural study of the beliefs of older adults. *The Gerontologist, 46,* 23–32; Lipson, J. G. & Dibble, S. L. (2005) *Culture and clinical care.* San Francisco: UCSF Nursing Press; and Purnell, L. D. (2014). *Guide to culturally competent health care* (3rd ed.). Philadelphia: F.A. Davis Co.; *Aboriginal Mental Health First Aid Training and Research Program. (2008). Cultural considerations & communication techniques: Guidelines for providing mental health first aid to an Aboriginal or Torres Strait Islander person. Available March 2015 via https://mhfa.com.au; **bpac[nz] better medicine. (2010). Recognising and managing mental health disorders in Māori. *Best Practice Journal, 28,* 8–17.

appropriate communication techniques when assessing for depression and discussing interventions with older adults and their carers.

WELLNESS OPPORTUNITY

Nurses respect individual preferences by listening carefully to identify acceptable terminology in older adults who do not want to acknowledge being "depressed".

Using screening tools

Concerns about depression being unrecognised and undertreated in older people have stimulated the development of very brief screening tools that healthcare professionals can use in a variety of settings.

The **Geriatric Depression Scale—Short Form (GDS-SF** or GDS-15) is a 15-question screening tool that is widely used across healthcare settings for older adults and can be administered in 5 to 7 minutes. Studies have found that the GDS-SF is reliable, effective and easily used to detect depression in older adults, including those with cognitive impairment (Greenberg, 2012; Harvath & McKenzie, 2012). Another advantage is that the tool and scoring form can be downloaded for free in English and more than 30 other languages from www.stanford.edu/~yesavage/GDS.html. The Hartford Institute for Geriatric Nursing recommends the GDS-SF (Figure 15-1) as an evidence-based screening tool for late-life depression (Greenberg, 2012).

Another tool, the **Cornell Scale for Depression in Dementia (CSDD)**, has been designed to assess signs and symptoms of major depression in adults with dementia. The CSDD uses an interview approach to obtain information about the person's psychosocial function, involvement in activities and physical signs from the person and from others. This tool can be used when the older adult is unable to comprehend the questions used in the GDS-SF. In Australia the CSDD is a part of the Aged Care Funding Instrument and it is used in the Australian long-term residential care sector to screen all new admissions for depression. In the resources section under clinical tools at the end of this chapter there are weblinks where more information about the GDS-SF and the CSDD can be obtained.

Depression screening for older adults in residential settings is recommended. The Patient Health Questionnaire (PHQ-2) is a two-item screening tool that is recommended for community-based settings because of its brevity, sensitivity and ease of use (Watson et al., 2009). The two screening questions recommended by the USPSTF and the PHQ-2

Geriatric Depression Scale (Short Form)		
1. Are you basically satisfied with your life?	Yes	No
2. Have you dropped many of your activities and interests?	Yes	No
3. Do you feel that your life is empty?	Yes	No
4. Do you often get bored?	Yes	No
5. Are you in good spirits most of the time?	Yes	No
6. Are you afraid that something bad is going to happen to you?	Yes	No
7. Do you feel happy most of the time?	Yes	No
8. Do you often feel helpless?	Yes	No
9. Do you prefer to stay at home rather than go out and do new things?	Yes	No
10. Do you feel you have more problems with memory than most?	Yes	No
11. Do you think it is wonderful to be alive now?	Yes	No
12. Do you feel pretty worthless the way you are now?	Yes	No
13. Do you feel full of energy?	Yes	No
14. Do you feel that your situation is hopeless?	Yes	No
15. Do you think that most people are better off than you are?	Yes	No
Score ___/15 One point for "No" to questions 1, 5, 7, 11, 13	Normal	3 ± 2
One point for "Yes" to other questions	Mildly depressed	7 ± 3
	Very depressed	12 ± 2

FIGURE 15-1 Geriatric Depression Scale (Short Form). (From Yesavage, J. A. et al. [1983]. Development and validation of a geriatric depression screening scale: A preliminary report. *Journal of Psychiatric Research, 17*, 37–49. Available at www.stanford.edu/~yesavage/gds.html.)

are: (1) During the past 2 weeks (or month), have you felt down, depressed or hopeless? and (2) During the past 2 weeks (or month), have you felt little interest or pleasure in doing things? A positive response to either of these two questions warrants further assessment with a formal depression scale. This type of screening has been included in the Australian best practice assessment for older people in long-term residential care, the NATFRAME (see Chapter 7). The tool, the Preliminary Depression Assessment, screens for depression in newly admitted residents.

NURSING ISSUES

The following nursing issues may be applicable to an older person who is diagnosed with depression: ineffective coping, hopelessness, chronic low self-esteem, social isolation, being powerless, carer role strain and risk for imbalanced nutrition. Related factors commonly found in older adults are relocation, ageist attitudes, financial concerns, social isolation, caregiving responsibilities, multiple social stressors, loss of significant roles or relationships, functional impairments (including cognitive deficits) and increased dependence (e.g. owing to the loss of the ability to drive). Risk for compromised resilience may also be an applicable issue.

WELLNESS OPPORTUNITY

Nurses can use the wellness issue of willingness for enhanced coping for older adults who are interested in improving their coping skills to address depressive symptoms that are not severe.

GOAL PLANNING FOR WELLNESS OUTCOMES

When caring for older adults who are depressed, nurses identify goals that support wellness outcomes as an essential part of the planning process. Goals applicable to depressed older adults include improving coping, hope, increased self-esteem, social support and social involvement, improved role performance, and carer emotional health. Specific interventions to achieve wellness outcomes related to depression and suicide are discussed in the following sections.

WELLNESS OPPORTUNITY

Quality of life is a wellness outcome that is achieved by addressing the functional and psychosocial consequences of depression.

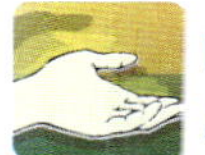

NURSING INTERVENTIONS TO ADDRESS DEPRESSION

Although all nurses are responsible for addressing depression in older adults, those who work in community-based and residential care settings have the most ongoing opportunities to identify manifestations of depression and to request further evaluation and treatment. In recent years, general practitioners have been the healthcare professionals evaluating and managing depression, and referrals to psychiatrists and other mental health professionals for depression have become less common. This trend is due to the emphasis on cost-effectiveness and the availability of safer and more effective antidepressant medications. Nursing protocols for depression in older people emphasise the important responsibility of nurses in reducing the negative consequences of depression through early recognition, intervention and referral of people with depression (Harvath & McKenzie, 2012).

Interventions for older adults who are depressed focus on the following: carer support, coping enhancement, counselling, crisis intervention, emotional support, exercise promotion, grief work facilitation, hope instillation, mood management, music therapy, role enhancement, self-esteem enhancement, suicide prevention and individual teaching. The next sections review the role of the nurse in planning and implementing interventions for late-life depression.

Alleviating risk factors

Nurses promote wellness for depressed older adults by addressing the many risk factors that are well within the realm of nursing, such as functional impairments, adverse medication effects and excess alcohol use. Many nursing interventions that improve the level of functioning are also effective for alleviating or preventing depression. For example, dementia, sensory impairments, urinary incontinence and mobility impairments are examples of conditions that can contribute to depression and will respond to nursing interventions (refer to Chapters 14, 16, 17, 19 and 22).

WELLNESS OPPORTUNITY

Nurses promote wellness by challenging ageist stereotypes that falsely attribute functional impairments to inevitable consequences of ageing.

If adverse medication effects are a risk factor for depression, nurses can educate the person about this potential relationship and identify problem-solving strategies to address the adverse effects. One such strategy, particularly for older adults who are unaccustomed to raising questions about their medications, is to teach them about communicating with the prescribing medical practitioner (as discussed in Chapter 8). For example, if the older person understands that there is a wide array of antihypertensive medications and that not all of them will cause depression, the person can use this information in discussing the problem with his or her medical practitioner. Nurses can also reassure the older adult that it is acceptable to initiate this kind of problem-solving discussion with medical practitioners. When the nurse, rather than the person, is the one who communicates with the medical practitioner, the nurse can raise appropriate questions about depression as an adverse medication effect. This problem-solving approach is particularly important when the medical practitioner is considering adding an antidepressant medication to a regimen that includes a depression-inducing medication.

In these situations, the solution may be to change medications rather than to add another medication and increase the risk for adverse effects.

If excess alcohol use is a risk factor for depression, individual and group interventions can be effective, particularly when the alcohol abuse is a reaction to recent losses. Alcoholics Anonymous (AA) is the most widely used group program for alcoholics of any age, and in some areas, age-homogeneous groups have been established, including some for older adults. Nurses can encourage older adults to initiate contact with AA, or they might directly facilitate the referral if the person agrees to this. Individual and family counselling may also be effective, and nurses can suggest or facilitate referrals for these mental health services.

Improving psychosocial function

Nurses can use health promotion interventions, such as the ones discussed in Chapter 12, for addressing risk factors for and symptoms of depression. In any clinical setting, nurses can focus on interventions to promote autonomy, personal control, self-efficacy and decision making about daily care as an intervention for depression (Harvath & McKenzie, 2012).

Interventions to strengthen social supports and foster meaningful roles are particularly pertinent and relatively easy to implement. Nurses have many opportunities to encourage participation in group meals or social programs. Many local communities have some social programs for older adults, and many provide transportation. Many churches and religious organisations also have programs designed to meet the social needs of isolated older adults. Volunteer visitor or phone call programs, for example, are sometimes available to address the needs of people who have difficulty with getting out of the house. Other programs such as pet therapy or "Adopt-a-Grandparent" are available in some home, community-based and long-term residential care settings, and they can be helpful in alleviating loneliness and depression.

Comprehensive information about support services for older adults in New Zealand is located at Eldernet at www.eldernet.co.nz. Older Australian adults can find government support services for older adults at www.myagedcare.gov.au. Nurses can also encourage older adults to maintain social contacts through simple measures such as phone calls.

Involvement in volunteer activities can enhance self-esteem and provide meaningful roles for older adults who are mildly depressed. Nurses can suggest that older adults explore opportunities for volunteer activities through such organisations as Volunteering Australia and Volunteering New Zealand. See the following weblinks for information about these organisations: www.volunteeringaustralia.org and www.volunteeringnz.org.nz.

WELLNESS OPPORTUNITY

Nurses promote quality of life by encouraging an older adult to engage in activities that are pleasant and meaningful to that person.

Promoting health through physical activity and nutrition

The beneficial effects of exercise as an intervention for depression have been documented in research reviews

(Cooney, Dwan, Greig et al., 2013; Joutsenniemi et al., 2013). However, older adults might not view exercise as important, or they may be reluctant to participate in exercise programs because of chronic illnesses such as arthritis. If older adults understand the benefits of exercise for both their physical and mental health, and if an individually tailored program is developed for them, they may be more willing to become involved in exercise programs. In community and long-term care settings, nurses can facilitate the establishment of group exercise programs and encourage depressed older adults to participate in them. In addition to encouraging participation in exercise programs, nurses can encourage participation in many other forms of physical activity. Even in hospital settings, nurses can facilitate referrals to physical, occupational and recreational therapists as a psychosocial nursing intervention (Harvath & McKenzie, 2012).

Nutrition is an important consideration as an intervention for depression for three reasons. First, depression often negatively affects nutritional status, and this can cause additional negative consequences. Second, good nutrition has a positive effect on mental health and cognitive function. Third, constipation is both a consequence of depression and an adverse effect of some antidepressant medications, and nutritional interventions can be effective in alleviating it. During phases of serious depression, malnutrition can lead to medical problems, which may progress to the point of being life-threatening. When depression is severe enough to lead to malnutrition, the older person must be evaluated for in-patient psychiatric care. Interventions for less severely depressed older people are aimed at maintaining adequate hydration and nutrition and preventing or managing constipation (as discussed in Chapter 18).

WELLNESS OPPORTUNITY

Nurses address the body–mind–spirit interrelationship by incorporating interventions for optimal nutrition as an essential component of care for depressed older adults.

Providing education and counselling

Many types of individual and group **psychosocial therapies** are effective interventions for late-life depression. For example, when multiple stressors challenge the person's coping abilities and contribute to depression, individual or group therapy can be an important intervention for improving the person's psychosocial health and alleviating depression. Nurses can provide counselling and emotional support for all depressed older adults, and in some situations, they can provide specific psychosocial therapies. Some examples of holistic interventions that are within the scope of nursing include the following (Helming & Jackson, 2009):

- Helping older adults identify non-verbalised fears and provide reality-based information to help them evaluate the fear
- Assisting older adults to verbalise emotions by identifying and labelling them so they can communicate more effectively about their emotions and fear
- Providing counselling based on basic psychological theories and concepts
- Encouraging "storytelling" and helping older adults to acknowledge their strengths as well as weaknesses through the power of storytelling
- Facilitating referrals to appropriate mental health services.

Nurses need to be sufficiently familiar with psychosocial therapies that are commonly used for depressed older adults, so they can encourage or facilitate referrals for interventions. Evidence-based guidelines identify the following therapies as effective for depression in older adults (Blazer, 2002; Ekers, Richards & Gilbody, 2008; Laidlow et al., 2003):

- Behaviour therapy (e.g. problem solving, practising assertiveness, setting up a daily schedule)
- Cognitive therapy (e.g. conscious restructuring of negative thought processes)
- Interpersonal therapy (e.g. modification of relationships or expectations about relationships)
- Supportive therapy (e.g. evaluating the strengths and weaknesses and facilitating choices that improve coping abilities).

In addition to these types of "talking therapies", self-care interventions that address the body–mind connection can alleviate symptoms of depression. One study found that an 8-week mindfulness-based psycho-educational intervention was effective in reducing anxiety and depression in adults who had chronic heart failure (Sullivan, 2009).

In recent years, group therapies have been recognised as an effective and efficient intervention for depressed older adults. Group therapy is effective for depressed older adults because it imparts information, improves self-esteem, enhances social interaction, encourages attitudinal changes and facilitates personal development (Blazer, 2002). Support and self-help groups are two commonly used types of interventions to improve psychosocial function and alleviate depression in older adults who are coping with life events such as caregiving, widowhood or grief reactions; nurses can educate older adults about the availability of such groups. Other group models used as interventions for late-life depression include reminiscence, relaxation, art therapy, focused imagery, creative movement and cognitive-behavioural strategies. Although adult day-care programs are not primarily group therapy for depressed older adults, they are a commonly available resource for providing structured social and therapeutic activities. Similarly, many community-based senior programs provide opportunities for group meals, exercise and social interaction, and these can be effective therapies for alleviating mild to moderate depression in older adults. Information about these and other group programs for older adults can be obtained from local networks on ageing, and nurses can encourage older adults or their carers to seek out and take advantage of these programs.

Facilitating referrals for psychosocial therapies

Nurses have important roles in facilitating referrals for appropriate psychosocial therapies, particularly for older adults who are seriously depressed. In addition to facilitating referrals for mental health services, nurses often have opportunities to initiate discussion of psychosocial therapies during the course of their usual work with older adults. Interdisciplinary geropsychiatric and geriatric assessment offer assessment and treatment of late-life depression, and some community mental health centres have programs for depressed older adults. In Australia, when nurses are concerned about an older person's mental health, they can refer to a mental health team for older persons. A major consideration with regard to referrals for depression interventions is that there is compelling evidence to support the effectiveness of many psychosocial therapies as well as the use of antidepressant medications, either alone or in combination (Harvath & McKenzie, 2012; Trangle et al., 2012). Researchers also emphasise the need to persist with the treatment of depression and to try different treatments if the first or second approaches are not effective (Kok, Nolen & Heeren, 2009).

WELLNESS OPPORTUNITY

Nurses promote wellness when they convince an older person that depression is not a necessary consequence of ageing but is a condition that can respond to treatment.

Health promotion: Teaching about and managing antidepressant medications

Types of antidepressant medications

Nurses need to understand the types of **antidepressants** available in order to educate older adults about their medications. Biochemical theories of depression have guided the development of various antidepressant medications. For example, the observation that depression was a common adverse effect of drugs that deplete the brain of catecholamine led to the development of tricyclic and other cyclic antidepressants, which block the reuptake of chemical messengers at neuronal synapses in the brain. As scientists have discovered more information about brain function and neurotransmitters, pharmaceutical companies have made major advances in developing safe and effective antidepressants. Major types of antidepressants are monoamine oxidase inhibitors, cyclic antidepressants, selective serotonin reuptake inhibitors, serotonin and noradrenaline inhibitors and atypical antidepressants (i.e. those that do not fit any other category).

Monoamine oxidase inhibitors (MAOIs) were the first medications used as antidepressants. After their use became widespread in the 1960s, it was discovered that medications in this category can cause dangerous and even fatal adverse effects (e.g. hypertensive crisis) when they interact with numerous other medications and with certain types of food. Another disadvantage of using MAOIs is the common occurrence of confusion, restlessness, agitation and paranoid ideation in older adults who are cognitively impaired (Blazer, 2002). Because there are so many contraindications to the use of MAOIs in older adults, they are used with extreme caution and only when other therapies have been ineffective. Thus, older adults who are taking an MAOI are usually very closely supervised and evaluated by a psychiatrist or other primary care practitioner. Examples of MAOIs are phenelzine and tranylcypromine.

Cyclic antidepressants—used widely since the late 1950s—are considered particularly effective in alleviating the following depression-related symptoms: loss of libido, sleep and appetite disturbances, and loss of interest and pleasure in activities. Cyclic antidepressants are usually categorised as tricyclic antidepressants (which were the first ones developed) and second-generation agents (which have been widely used since the mid 1980s).

Cyclic antidepressants differ more in their potential for adverse effects than in their therapeutic effects. Because cyclic antidepressants affect several neurotransmitters, they are associated with a variety of anticholinergic and other detrimental effects. Two particular areas of concern in geriatric care are the potential for adverse cardiovascular and anticholinergic effects. The most likely cardiovascular effects are orthostatic hypotension and altered cardiac rate and rhythm. Serious anticholinergic effects include blurred vision, urinary retention and cognitive impairments.

Additional common side effects are sedation, constipation, dry mouth and weight gain. Because of these side effects, people with glaucoma, prostatic hyperplasia or cardiac conduction abnormalities should not take cyclic antidepressants. In addition, cyclic antidepressants should be avoided in people with dementia or Parkinson's disease because of the potential adverse effect of cognitive impairment. As a rule of thumb for older adults, cyclic agents with weaker anticholinergic effects should be prescribed over those with stronger anticholinergic effects.

During the late 1980s pharmaceutical companies developed two classes of antidepressants that were chemically unrelated to and more selective in their action than the cyclic antidepressants. **Selective serotonin reuptake inhibitors (SSRIs)** relieve symptoms of depression by blocking the reuptake of serotonin, so the level of this neurotransmitter is increased in the brain cells. **Serotonin and noradrenaline reuptake inhibitors (SNRIs)** increase the levels of both serotonin and noradrenaline by inhibiting the reuptake of these neurotransmitters in the brain cells. This type of antidepressant is also called dual reuptake inhibitors. The therapeutic effectiveness of SSRIs and SNRIs is similar to that of cyclic antidepressants, but they have minimal cholinergic, histaminic, dopaminergic and noradrenergic effects. SSRIs are currently considered the first-line medications for depression because they are effective for most people and their adverse effects are more tolerable and less dangerous (Blazer, 2002). For example, an important consideration for older adults is that SSRIs are less likely than cyclics to cause orthostatic hypotension and anticholinergic effects. This is particularly important for older adults who have cognitive impairments and for those who are at high risk for falls.

Although SSRIs are safer than other types of antidepressants, nurses need to be aware of important adverse effects and drug interactions. For example, because SSRIs are metabolised in the liver and some of them are highly bound to plasma protein, SSRIs may interact with other drugs that are metabolised in the liver or are highly protein-bound. Nurses also need to know that hyponatraemia is an adverse effect that occurs in up to 32% of older adults who take SSRIs (Bowen, 2009). In addition, nurses need to observe for potential interactions between SSRIs and nicotine, alcohol and other medications (including some over-the-counter products). For example, the risk for gastrointestinal bleeding is increased when SSRIs are used concurrently with non-steroidal anti-inflammatory drugs or low-dose aspirin. Also, serious adverse effects can occur when an SSRI is taken with another drug or dietary supplement that increases serotonin levels in the brain (e.g. pethidine, L-tryptophan, St John's wort). Drug interactions may occur even after an SSRI with a long half-life (e.g. fluoxetine) has been discontinued.

Common adverse effects of SSRIs include nausea, vomiting, diarrhoea, headache, nervousness, insomnia, tremor, dry mouth and sexual dysfunction. Withdrawal effects of SSRIs include nausea, tremor, anxiety, dizziness, palpitations and paraesthesia.

A meta-analysis of randomised controlled trials comparing 12 commonly prescribed antidepressants identified mirtazapine, escitalopram, venlafaxine and sertraline as the most efficacious medications, with escitalopram and sertraline having the most favourable results with regard to both efficacy and acceptability (Cipriani et al., 2009). Desvenlafaxine is a newer SNRI antidepressant (related to venlafaxine) that is both efficacious and well-tolerated but it has not been compared with other antidepressants in long-term trials (Perry, 2009; Soares, 2009; Thase et al., 2009).

Antidepressants that are commonly used for older adults are listed in Table 15-3 according to their classifications. Special considerations in the use of some of these antidepressants are as follows: venlafaxine may cause an increase in blood pressure; mirtazapine can be helpful for stimulating appetite, but it also can be sedating; bupropion has a stimulating effect, which can sometimes be therapeutic but is contraindicated in people with a seizure disorder; bupropion and mirtazapine have the lowest rate of sexual side effects. Also, it is important to monitor serum sodium levels initially and periodically for older adults who are taking SSRIs.

Nurses also need to be aware that the following antidepressants are contraindicated in older adults due to their adverse effects: amitriptyline, doxepin and fluoxetine daily dose (Prozac). Psychomotor stimulants (e.g. methylphenidate) have been used for decades for certain types of depression, but they are not commonly used for older adults.

TABLE 15-3 Antidepressants commonly used for older adults

Category	Examples
Selective serotonin reuptake inhibitors (SSRIs)	Citalopram Escitalopram Fluvoxamine Paroxetine Sertraline
Serotonin and noradrenaline reuptake inhibitors (SNRIs)	Desvenlafaxine Venlafaxine
Serotonin modulators	Trazodone
Dopamine reuptake inhibitors	Bupropion
Cyclic antidepressants	Imipramine Nortriptyline
Tetracyclic antidepressants	Mirtazapine

Nursing responsibilities regarding antidepressants

An important nursing responsibility regarding antidepressants is to educate older adults about the primary purpose of these medications, which is to alleviate depressive symptoms so that the person is able to respond to additional interventions such as psychosocial therapy. For older adults who have both depression and dementia, antidepressant medications may improve the affective symptoms so that overall abilities are improved and the person is able to function more effectively and independently.

Nursing responsibilities regarding antidepressant medication therapy include observing for both adverse and therapeutic effects and educating the older adult about the unique aspects of these medication therapies. Another important responsibility is educating older adults about the need for ongoing evaluation and treatment of depression, including the monitoring of antidepressant medication use. Older adults who have been diagnosed with major depressive disorder are at high risk of recurrence, and this risk is increased if antidepressant medications are not maintained for at least 6 months. Older adults often want to discontinue medications when their depressive symptoms resolve, and nurses need to teach them about the importance of ongoing antidepressant therapy and periodic re-evaluations after medications are discontinued. This is particularly important because a person's beliefs about the use of medications affect adherence; therefore, beliefs need to be explored before and during medication therapy. Box 15-4 summarises guidelines for the nursing responsibilities regarding antidepressant medications.

Health promotion: Teaching about complementary and alternative interventions

There has been increasing interest in the use of herbs and other natural remedies for depression. **St John's wort** (*Hypericum perforatum*) is widely used in Europe and is the most commonly used antidepressant in Germany. Since 1998, the National Institutes of Health Office of Alternative Medicine

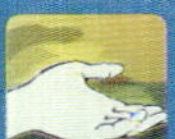

BOX 15-4
Health education about antidepressant medications

Information to be shared with the older adult

- Immediate improvement will not be evident, but a fair trial must be given to the medication as long as serious adverse effects are not noticed.
- The fair trial may take as long as 12 weeks, but some positive effects should be noticed within 2 to 4 weeks.
- If one type of antidepressant is not effective, another type may be effective.
- Antidepressants cannot be used on an "as needed" basis.
- Antidepressants should be viewed as part of a comprehensive approach to treating depression, and psychosocial therapies should be considered along with antidepressants.
- Antidepressants can interact with alcohol, nicotine and other medications, including over-the-counter medications, possibly altering the effects of the medication or increasing the potential for adverse effects.
- The prescribing medical practitioner should be asked about potential adverse effects and drug–drug or food–drug interactions.
- The prescribing medical practitioner should be consulted before discontinuing an antidepressant.
- If postural hypotension occurs, the effects can be minimised through such interventions as changing position slowly and maintaining adequate fluid intake.
- If monoamine oxidase inhibitors (MAOIs) are prescribed, certain medications must be avoided, and a low-tyramine diet must be followed (i.e. avoidance of beer, yoghurt, red wine, fermented cheese and pickled foods, as well as excessive amounts of caffeine and chocolate).

Principles regarding dosage and length of treatment

- Older adults should be started at half to a third the normal adult dose.
- Dosages can be increased gradually until maximal therapeutic levels are reached, while observing for adverse effects.
- Age-related changes may increase the time needed for medication to reach maximal effectiveness.
- A once-daily regimen usually is effective.
- Bedtime administration of an antidepressant may facilitate sleep as a result of the drug's hypnotic effects, but some antidepressants (e.g. fluoxetine) may be better taken in the morning because of side effects such as agitation.
- The length of treatment is usually 6 months for a first-time depression, 1 to 2 years for people with a history of a prior depressive episode and lifetime maintenance for people with a history of three or more depressive episodes.

has sponsored randomised, controlled, double-blinded studies in the U.S. to compare placebo, St John's wort and prescription antidepressants. A comprehensive review of recent studies concluded that St John's wort is an effective treatment for some types of depression (e.g. minor depression), but it also has adverse effects and interactions that nurses need to be aware of (Carpenter et al., 2008). Common side effects include fatigue, headache, restlessness, anorgasmia, polyuria, hypothyroidism, pruritus, photosensitivity, dry mouth and gastrointestinal effects. Drug interactions identified in studies include antidepressants, carbamazepine, digoxin, simvastatin, theophylline and warfarin. St John's wort is widely available and relatively inexpensive, but products are not standardised or regulated for quality (see Chapter 8 for further considerations regarding herbs).

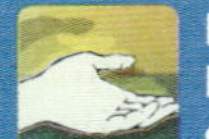

BOX 15-5
Interventions commonly used for preventing or alleviating depression

Health promotion interventions

- Participate in enjoyable exercise for a minimum of 30 minutes five times weekly.
- Seek individual or group counselling to address stressful situations.
- If symptoms of depression affect daily functioning or quality of life, seek evaluation and treatment from a medical practitioner.

Nutritional considerations

- Ensure adequate intake of (or use supplements of) the following nutrients: vitamins B, C and D; magnesium; selenium.

Complementary and alternative therapies

- St John's wort, 300 mg three times daily, may be effective in reducing the symptoms of mild to moderate depression; however, do not take this with an antidepressant, and be sure to talk with your medical practitioner about using it. Observe for interactions with other medications.
- Bright-light therapy for half an hour, daily
- Art, dance, music, drama, yoga, tai chi, qigong, massage, imagery, meditation, relaxation, stress management, spiritual healing

Bright-light therapy is an evidence-based treatment of some types of depression, including those with seasonal effective disorder (SAD), both as a stand-alone intervention and to enhance the effects of antidepressants (Howland, 2009). This type of therapy has been used as a method of resetting the circadian rhythm and treating the depression. Nurses can use Box 15-5 as a guide to teaching older adults about interventions that may be helpful for preventing or alleviating depression.

Health promotion: Teaching about electroconvulsive therapy

Electroconvulsive therapy (ECT), which involves the electrical induction of seizures, is a treatment that is highly effective for treating severe depressive episodes. Studies consistently find that ECT is the most rapid and effective treatment for major depression in older adults and, in fact has many potential advantages over antidepressants (McDonald & Vahabzadeh, 2013; Oudman, 2012; Weiner & Krystal, 2012). Evidence-based guidelines recommend consideration for ECT in any of the following circumstances (Trangle, Dieperink, Gabert et al., 2012):

- Geriatric depression
- When antidepressants are ineffective, not tolerated, or pose significant medical risk
- When any of the following conditions exist: catatonia, severe risk of suicide, depression with psychosis

- When the person's health is significantly compromised due to depression (e.g. not eating, functional impairment)
- Combination of depression and Parkinson's disease.

Prevalent negative attitudes about ECT are attributable, in part, to the alleged inhumane use of this procedure when it was first developed half a century ago. However, in recent years the technique for administering ECT has been refined, and the risks, discomfort and side effects are now quite minimal. Adverse effects include headache, nausea, disorientation, memory loss, impaired attention and decreased concentration. Adverse effects usually are transient; however, the adverse cognitive effects may be more extensive or even permanent, particularly after several courses of ECT. Studies are inconclusive with regard to increased vulnerability of older adults to adverse cognitive effects, but at least one study (Verwijk, Comijs, Kok et al., 2013) found improvements in cognitive function 6 months after ECT treatments in depressed people aged 55 or older. After an initial course of ECT, antidepressants and maintenance treatments of ECT are effective for maintaining positive results and preventing a relapse (Rapinesi, Kotzalidis, Serata et al., 2013; Weiner & Krystal, 2012).

With the exception of psychiatric settings, nurses will not be involved with the care of people who are undergoing ECT. However, nurses caring for depressed people in any setting need to be aware of evidence-based guidelines for the use of ECT and maintain an open mind about this therapy. In addition, nurses may be in a position to encourage older adults or their carers to seek advice about ECT from knowledgeable professionals.

EVALUATING THE EFFECTIVENESS OF NURSING INTERVENTIONS

Nurses evaluate their care of depressed older adults by documenting improved coping skills and diminished manifestations of depression. For example, the person may report diminished feelings of hopelessness and improved appetite and sleep. Another measure reflecting improved quality of life would be the older adult's interest and participation in meaningful activities. Effectiveness of nursing interventions may also be evaluated by whether the older adult has begun taking antidepressant medications and participating in individual or group therapies. Evidence-based guidelines 15-1 summarises guidelines for nursing assessment and interventions related to depression in older adults.

SUICIDE IN LATE LIFE

Although suicide is the most serious functional consequence of late-life depression, nurses and other healthcarers tend to overlook this risk. This tendency is partially attributable to the fact that old age is associated with passivity and non-violence,

EVIDENCE-BASED PRACTICE 15-1
Depression in older adults

Statement of the problem

- Depression is highly prevalent in older adults and is not a natural part of ageing.
- Depressive symptoms are associated with higher morbidity and mortality rates in older adults; specific consequences of depression include heightened pain and disability, delayed recovery from illness or surgery, worsening of medical conditions and suicide.
- Depressive symptoms are more common in older adults who have dementia or more severe or chronic disabling conditions.
- Nurses are at the front line in the early recognition of depression and the facilitation of mental health services.

Recommendations for nursing assessment

- Depression may range in severity from mild symptoms to more severe forms, both of which can persist over longer periods and have serious negative consequences for the older adult.
- Depression can occur for the first time in late life or it can be part of a long-standing affective disorder.
- Recognition of depression in older adults is hindered by the coexistence of medical illnesses, disability, cognitive dysfunction and psychosocial adversity in older adults.
- The nursing standard of practice for depression in older adults includes the following assessment parameters: identifying risk factors and high-risk groups, using GDS-SF or CSDD for screening, performing a focused depression assessment on all high-risk groups, obtaining and reviewing medical history and physical/neurological examination, assessing for medications and medical conditions that may contribute to depression, assessing cognitive function and level of functioning.
- Risks for late-life suicide include depressive symptoms, perceived health status, sleep quality, absence of a confidant, disruption of social support, family conflict, loneliness.

Recommendations for care

- For severe depression (e.g. GDS 11 or greater), refer for mental health evaluation and treatment with medication, psychosocial therapies, hospitalisation or ECT.
- For less severe depression (e.g. GDS score between 6 and 10), refer to mental health services for psychosocial therapies and determination whether antidepressant therapy is warranted.
- For all levels of depression develop an individualised plan integrating nursing interventions that address issues such as safety, nutrition, risk factors, health education, social support, pleasant reminiscence and relaxation therapies.

Recommendations for teaching older adults

Teach older adults and carers about the following:

- Depression is common, treatable and not the depressed person's fault.
- Adherence to the prescribed treatment regimen, including medications, is imperative to prevent recurrence.
- It is important to be aware of the therapeutic and adverse effects of the prescribed antidepressant

Source: Horvath, T. A. & McKenzie, G. (2012). Depression. In M. Boltz, E. Capezuti, T. Fulmer & D. Zwicker (Eds), *Evidence-based geriatric nursing protocols for best practice* (4th ed., pp. 135–162). New York: Springer.

whereas suicide is associated with aggressiveness and violence. The following statistics demonstrate that suicide is a serious issue for other aged groups as well as older adults:

- The suicide rate for older adults over 65 years in New Zealand in 2007 was 10%. The highest suicide rate of 23% was reported for the 35 to 44 years age group in the same year (World Health Organization [WHO], 2011).
- The suicide rate for older adults over 65 years in Australia in 2006 was almost 15%. The highest suicide rate of 22% was reported for the 35 to 44 years age group (WHO, 2011).
- The suicide rate in 2011 for Australian men aged 85 years and over was 32 suicides per 100,000 population. This rate is four times higher than women aged 85 years and over and twice that for men of all ages (Australian Institute of Health and Welfare, 2013).

DIVERSITY NOTE

Both Indigenous and Māori older adults have a lower suicide mortality rate than non-Indigenous Australians and non-Māori people.

Official data about suicide do not include information about suicidal events that are unreported for such reasons as family efforts to conceal evidence and difficulty determining the true cause of death in medically ill people. Nor do these rates reflect the unrecognised suicidal acts that older adults indirectly or subtly use to take their own lives such as refusing to eat, failing to take medically necessary medications and other means of self-neglect.

DIVERSITY NOTE

At all ages and by race and ethnicity, the suicide rates are higher for males than for females.

Assessing the risks for suicide

Nursing assessment of suicide risk is particularly important because many older people give clues, sometimes to many people, about potential suicide. These clues, however, may be subtle, and the person who hears them may not associate them with suicide risk, particularly in older adults. By identifying risk factors, nurses can initiate interventions to prevent suicide. This is particularly important because three-quarters of older people who commit suicide visit their primary care provider within 1 month before the act, but they are not likely to directly express suicidal ideation. Thus, healthcare providers need to assess for risks and identify those older adults who may be contemplating suicide. The following are some of the more commonly identified risks for suicide in older adults (Cukrowicz et al., 2009; Hicks & Woods, 2009; Liu & Chiu, 2009; Mitty & Flores, 2008):

- Depression, which may be masked by excessive focus on physical complaints
- Personal or family history of depression
- Past suicide attempts
- Loneliness, limited social support
- Family discord
- Feelings of abandonment
- Recent bereavement
- Presence of chronic or severe pain.

Because depression is the factor most consistently identified across studies as a risk factor for suicide, it is important to assess for suicidal ideation in any depressed older adult. In addition to these factors that alert the nurse to risk for suicide, the factors that are most strongly predictive of actual suicide are a history of previous attempts and current suicide ideation that includes a plan or evidence of preparation of a plan.

When risk factors or clues to potential suicide are identified, the nurse must further assess the actual risk for a suicide attempt. This assessment is multilevel, with each level of questions depending on the response to the previous level. Nurses begin the assessment with level 1 questions to determine the presence or absence of suicidal thoughts. Although healthcare professionals may be reluctant to initiate questions about suicide because they fear that this line of questioning may "put ideas in the person's head", this fear is unfounded. People who do not have suicidal thoughts usually respect the necessity of the questions but do not begin thinking about suicide just because the topic was broached. Even so, rather than beginning with a blunt question such as "Do you ever think about committing suicide?", the nurse can phrase the question in such a way that the person will give clues to his or her intent if it exists but will not be offended by the question if it does not (see Box 15-6 for examples).

Nurses need to recognise that older adults may express a loss of interest in living and may even state that they wish they were dead, but these verbalisations are not necessarily associated with suicidal thoughts. Many times these expressions arise from feelings of being overwhelmed with an illness or stressful situation, and they are not indicators of a desire to take one's own life. These expressions may also be related to dementia or an inability to express one's feelings accurately, which sometimes occurs after strokes. In these situations, nurses need to assess further for depression and identify stressful conditions that can be addressed through interventions.

If suicidal thoughts are suspected or identified at level 1, nurses ask level 2 questions, which are aimed at determining the presence or absence of thoughts about self-harm. If the answer to any of these questions is positive, nurses ask level 3 questions, which are very direct and specific because this information is crucial to assessing the immediate risk for suicide. If the person describes a detailed plan and has access to all the necessary implements, the potential for suicide is extremely high. By contrast, if the person has a plan that is vague or that cannot possibly be carried out, the immediate potential for suicide is lower. For example, if the plan involves a gun, but the person does not have a gun and cannot get out of the

BOX 15-6
Guidelines for assessing suicide risk

Risk factors for suicide in older adults

- Demographic factors: white race, male gender
- Depression, particularly when accompanied by insomnia, agitation and self-neglect
- Chronic illness with increasing dependence and helplessness; diagnosis of cancer or a terminal illness
- Poor social supports; social isolation, particularly recent isolation
- History of mental health illness, particularly major depression
- Onset of major depression within the past year
- Family history of suicide; personal or family history of suicide attempts
- Patterns of impulsive behaviour
- Alcohol abuse
- Poor communication skills

Verbal clues to suicide intent

- "Pretty soon you won't have to worry about me."
- "I would be better off dead."
- "I'll make sure I won't be a burden to others."
- Expressions of hopelessness
- Remarks about life being unbearable
- Reflections on the worthlessness of life

Non-verbal clues to suicide intent

- Making a will; giving belongings away; preparing for own funeral
- Serious self-neglect, particularly in people who have no cognitive impairments
- Frequent visits to medical practitioners
- Excessive use of medications or alcohol
- Accumulation of prescription medications
- Unusual preoccupation with self and withdrawal from others

Interview questions to assess the immediate risk of suicide

- "Do you think that life is not worth living?"
- "Do you think about escaping from your problems?"
- "Do you wish you were dead?"
- "Do you think about harming yourself?"
- "Do you think about ending your life?"
- "Do you have a plan?"
- "What would you do to take your life?"
- "Have you ever started to act on a plan to harm yourself?"
- "Under what circumstances would you act on that plan?"
- "What prevents you from acting on the plan?"

house, then the chance of a successful suicide is low. By contrast, if the person threatens to consume the bottle of barbiturates that is readily available in the medicine cabinet, then the chance of a successful suicide is quite high.

Nurses proceed to level 4 questions to assess the immediacy of the risk when the person has described a plan. When answers to levels 3 or 4 are positive, the nurse must plan immediate interventions to deal with the suicide risk. An essential nursing responsibility with regard to level 4 questions is to ask what prevents the person from carrying out the plan because this information provides a base for supporting important person-centred reasons for living.

Nursing issues and outcomes

If the nursing assessment identifies risk factors for suicide, an applicable issue would be risk for suicide. Related factors would include any risk factors and verbal and non-verbal clues to suicide. An example is an 85-year-old widower who says his life is no longer worthwhile and who makes frequent visits to his doctor for complaints of weight loss and sleep disturbance. Outcomes for older adults at risk for suicide include suicide self-restraint and safe personal behaviour.

Nursing interventions for preventing suicide

Nurses do not routinely encounter suicidal older adults, but they need to be prepared to implement immediate interventions whenever they identify a person at risk. The most important intervention is to seek mental health resources and activate referrals to the appropriate protective service agency rather than attempting to deal with potentially suicidal people without the help of specialised resources. One study found that the provision of care management services significantly reduced suicidal ideation in depressed older adults (Alexopoulos, 2009). All communities have some emergency mental health resources, and nurses can follow institutional policies regarding referrals for appropriate services. In any situation, nurses use appropriate communication techniques to address potentially suicidal older adults. Some guidelines for working with people who are potentially suicidal are listed in Box 15-7.

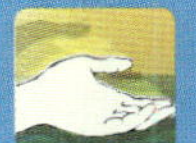

BOX 15-7
Nursing interventions for people who are potentially suicidal

Communicating with someone who is potentially suicidal

- Be direct and honest; do not be afraid to ask direct questions, such as "Are you thinking of hurting yourself?"
- Express feelings of concern and confidence.
- Acknowledge the person's feelings of helplessness and hopelessness.
- Encourage the person to talk about the precipitating event, if there is one.
- Emphasise that suicide is only one of several options; then explore other options.
- Emphasise positive relationships; talk about the negative impact of suicide on survivors.
- Maintain a non-judgemental attitude.
- Make a contract: ask the person to agree to do certain things for limited amounts of time and to call for help if he or she cannot keep the agreement.
- Discuss reasons that the person identifies for not carrying out a suicide plan and find ways to support and strengthen these.
- Discuss the problems openly with the family and carers.

Crisis intervention

- Focus on the immediate precipitating event.
- Reduce the immediate danger by removing the implements, interfering with the plan and providing constant supervision.
- Obtain psychiatric help; call a suicide hot line or activate emergency mental health services if necessary.

Evaluating the effectiveness of nursing interventions

Nursing care of older adults who are at high risk for self-harm are evaluated by the prevention of harm. Another measure is the degree to which the older adult develops coping skills to deal with the issues that underlie his or her suicidal thoughts. Nurses can also find out whether the older adult obtained suggested mental health services and determine the effectiveness of any referrals that were made.

CASE STUDY

Mrs Tong is 81 years old. Recently, she was diagnosed with vascular dementia. She lives with her husband, who has diabetes, macular degeneration and severe arthritis. Mrs Tong had managed all household and financial responsibilities until approximately 1 year ago, when she began having trouble with her memory. Mrs Tong was evaluated by her medical practitioner where you work as a practice nurse. She was advised to stop driving and to arrange for some help with complex tasks such as bill paying and grocery shopping. Two months after the initial evaluation, Mrs Tong returns for follow-up and informs you that she limits her driving to short, daytime trips in familiar areas. When asked about getting help with complex tasks, she states, "I just don't have any energy to make all those calls you suggested. Besides, I don't want anyone else looking at my finances or going to the shop for me."

Nursing assessment

A cognitive assessment indicates that Mrs Tong's level of cognitive impairment is unchanged since her initial evaluation. She has some deficits in calculation, short-term memory, abstract thinking, problem solving and language skills. Your psychosocial assessment reveals that Mrs Tong has a very sad affect and low self-esteem, and she expresses feelings of hopelessness and helplessness. She admits to being overwhelmed with feelings of responsibility for herself and her husband, and she says she feels "paralysed because there's no light at the end of the tunnel". She scored 11 on the GDS-15.

When you ask about her daily life, Mrs Tong says she spends most of her time at home because she does not have the energy to go out. She admits that she has difficulty falling asleep at night, and she wakes up at around 4 a.m. and is unable to return to sleep. She naps for a couple of hours in the morning and in the afternoon because "I feel tired all the time, and I can't go out and do things anyway." Her appetite is poor, and in the past 2 months, her weight declined from 64 kilograms to 58 kilograms (her height is 167 centimetres). She complains of constipation and "heartburn".

When you ask about meaningful activities, she tells you she no longer goes to her weekly bowling club because it meets in the evening, and she does not want to drive at night. She has also given up her church activities (Thursday discussion club and Sunday service) because she does not want to inconvenience anyone by having them drive her. She feels it is "demeaning to have to tell my friends that I need a ride". She used to enjoy reading, but she has not felt like going to the library, and she is not interested in any of the books she has at home.

Nursing issues

You use the nursing issue of ineffective individual coping, related to depression, and declining cognitive abilities. Evidence comes from Mrs Tong's sad affect, low self-esteem, loss of interest in activities, feelings of hopelessness and helplessness, inability to address her problems effectively and a GDS-15 score indicative of depression. Physical manifestations are her poor appetite, weight loss, sleep disturbances and complaints about constipation and heartburn.

Nursing care plan for Mrs Tong

Goals for wellness outcomes	Nursing interventions	Nursing evaluation
Mrs Tong will be able to identify her coping patterns.	• Ask Mrs Tong to describe her prior experiences in dealing with her husband's illness. • Help Mrs Tong to identify coping strategies that have been helpful in the past.	• Mrs Tong recognises and acknowledges the coping strategies that have been helpful in the past.
Mrs Tong will learn about depression and be encouraged to obtain further evaluation of her depression.	• Talk with Mrs Tong about her signs and symptoms of depression, emphasising the fact that depression is a treatable condition. • Discuss the relationship between depression and the inability to cope effectively with stressful situations. • Ask Mrs Tong if she is willing to see a psychiatrist, or talk to her general medical practitioner for further evaluation and treatment. • Explain that antidepressant medications can be very effective when combined with counselling.	• Mrs Tong follows through with an appointment with a psychiatrist or talks with her medical practitioner.

Goals for wellness outcomes	Nursing interventions	Nursing evaluation
Effective coping strategies for addressing Mrs Tong's declining abilities will be identified.	• Discuss with Mrs Tong several options for ongoing support and counselling to assist her in coping with her declining abilities (e.g. support group for people with memory loss; or individual counselling sessions with the social worker). • Emphasise the importance of developing short-term goals that can be addressed through problem solving (e.g. suggest that Mrs Tong begin to address her lack of meaningful activities by going to the library for reading material).	• Mrs Tong attends one support group on a trial basis and talks with you about the experience at her next appointment in 1 month. • Mrs Tong makes an appointment for counselling with the social worker. • Mrs Tong participates in one meaningful activity each week for the next month.

Thinking points

- What risk factors are likely to be contributing to Mrs Tong's depression?
- What further assessment information would you obtain?
- What questions on the GDS-15 (Figure 15-1) do you think would be indicative of depression for Mrs Tong?
- What additional interventions would you suggest for Mrs Tong?

CHAPTER HIGHLIGHTS

Depression in older adults

- Signs and symptoms of depression in older adults are on a continuum of severity from major depression to subthreshold depression.
- Depression is characterised by depressed mood and/or loss of interest, along with additional manifestations, including weight loss, appetite change, sleep disturbances, psychomotor agitation or retardation, fatigue, cognitive impairment, feeling worthless or excessively guilty, and recurrent thoughts of death or suicide.
- Late-life depression refers to the onset of depression after the age of 65 years.

Theories about late-life depression

- Psychosocial (impact of losses, learned helplessness)
- Cognitive triad (negative appraisals cause distorted perceptions and lead to faulty conclusions)
- Biological and genetic (changes in the nervous system, genetic variables)
- Depression and dementia (common neuropathological changes, vascular depression)

Risk factors for depression in older adults

- Demographic and psychosocial
- Pathological conditions and functional impairment (Box 15-1)
- Effects of alcohol and medications (Box 15-2)

Functional consequences associated with depression in older adults

- Reduced physical health and functioning
- Impaired cognitive and psychosocial function and reduced quality of life
- Increased risk of developing dementia

Nursing assessment of depression in older adults

- Unique manifestations in older versus younger adults (Table 15-1)
- Differentiating between the features of dementia and depression (Table 15-2)
- Cultural variations in expressions of depression (Cultural considerations 15-1)
- Screening tools: GDS-SF (Figure 15-1) and CSDD

Nursing issues

- Willingness for enhanced coping
- Ineffective coping
- Hopelessness
- Carer role strain
- Risk for imbalanced nutrition
- Risk for compromised resilience

Goal planning for wellness outcomes

- Coping
- Hope
- Carer emotional health
- Nutritional status
- Physical well-being

Nursing interventions to address depression

- Alleviating risk factors (addressing functional limitations, teaching about adverse effects of medications and excessive alcohol)
- Improving psychosocial function (e.g. social supports, meaningful activities)
- Promoting health through physical activity and nutrition
- Providing education and counselling (individual and group psychosocial interventions)

- Facilitating referrals for psychosocial therapies
- Teaching about antidepressant medications (Table 15-4)
- Teaching about ECT
- Teaching about alternative care practices (e.g. St John's wort, bright-light therapy)

Evaluating the effectiveness of nursing interventions

- Improved coping skills
- Fewer manifestations of depression
- Expressed feelings of improved quality of life
- Effective use of appropriate mental health services

Suicide in late life

- Suicide rates and mechanisms
- Nursing assessment of suicide risk (Box 15-6)
- Nursing issues and outcomes
- Nursing interventions for preventing suicide (Box 15-7)
- Evaluating effectiveness of interventions

CRITICAL THINKING EXERCISES

1. Think of an older adult in your personal life or professional practice who is or has been depressed. What are (were) the risk factors in that person's situation that might play (have played) a part in the depression?
2. Describe at least four cultural variations in the way depression might be expressed.
3. What assessment observations would you make and what questions would you ask to differentiate between dementia and depression in older adults?
4. Make up a case example of someone who is potentially suicidal and who would require all four levels of suicide assessment. Describe how you would phrase the questions for each of the levels.
5. Describe a teaching plan for an 84-year-old woman for whom paroxetine, 10 mg daily, has been prescribed.

RESOURCES

For an extensive range of additional resources to enhance teaching and learning and to facilitate understanding of this chapter, please see the text's accompanying website located on thePoint at http://thepoint.lww.com.

Clinical tools

Cornell Scale for Depression in Dementia Administration & Scoring Guidelines: www.umaryland.edu/media/umb/oaa/gerontology-programs/documents/The-Cornell-Scale-for-Depression-in-Dementia.pdf0.pdf

Hartford Institute for Geriatric Nursing, ConsultGeriRN.org: http://consultgerirn.org/resources

Assessment tools *Try This*® series and *How to Try This* resources

General assessment series:

- *Try This,* issue 4: The Geriatric Depression Scale (GDS). Greenberg, S. A. (2012). *Best Practices in Nursing Care to Older Adults.*
- *How to Try This* (article): The Geriatric Depression Scale: Short Form. Morrow, S. (1999). *American Journal of Nursing,* 99(1), 24.
- *How to Try This* (video): *GDS Short Form Assessment.*

Evidence-based practice

Agency for Healthcare Research and Quality: www.ahrq.gov/professionals/clinicians-providers/guidelines-recommendations/index.html

- Screening for depression in adults (2013): Summary of the evidence.

Harvath, T. A. & McKenzie, G. (2012). Depression in older adults. In M. Boltz, E. Capezuti, T. Fulmer & D. Zwicker (Eds), *Evidence-based geriatric nursing protocols for best practice* (4th ed., pp. 135–162). New York: Springer

Joanna Briggs Institute: http://connect.jbiconnectplus.org

- Depression (older men): Testosterone supplementation therapy. Kunde, L. (2014).

National Guideline Clearinghouse: www.guideline.gov

- AAFP guideline for the detection and management of post-myocardial infarction depression (revised 2014). American Academy of Family Physicians.

Search: Depression

- Depression in older adults (2012). In *Evidence-based geriatric nursing protocols for best practice.*
- Diagnosis and treatment of depression in adults: 2012 clinical practice guideline.
- Recommendations on screening for depression in adults (revised 2013).
- Screening for delirium, dementia and depression in older adults (revised 2010).

National Center for Biotechnology Information (NCBI) National Institute of Health

- Brown, E. L. & Tilter, M. G. (2009). Evidence based guideline detection of depression in older adults with dementia. *Journal of Gerontology Nursing, 35*(2), 11–15.

Health education

beyondblue, older people: www.beyondblue.org.au/resources

Geriatric Mental Health Foundation: www.gmhfonline.org

Health and Disability Commissioner, mental health and addictions, New Zealand: www.hdc.org.nz/about-us/mental-health-and-addictions

Mental Health First Aid Australia, cultural competence training: www.mhfa.com.au

National Institute of Mental Health, depression: www.nimh.nih.gov/health/topics/depression/index.shtml

New Zealand Mental Health Foundation: www.mentalhealth.org.nz

Transcultural Mental Health, Australia: www.dhi.health.nsw.gov.au

REFERENCES

Aboriginal Mental Health First Aid Training and Research Program. (2008). Cultural considerations &

communication techniques: Guidelines for providing mental health first aid to an Aboriginal or Torres Strait Islander person. Melbourne: Orygen Youth Health Research Centre, University of Melbourne and *beyondblue*. Accessed March 2015 via https://mhfa.com.au.

Adams, K. B. & Moon, H. (2009). Subthreshold depression: Characteristics and risk factors among vulnerable elders. *Aging & Mental Health, 13*(5), 682–692.

Alexopoulos, G. S. (2009). Reducing suicidal ideation and depression in older primary care patients: 24-month outcomes of the PROSPECT study. *American Journal of Psychiatry, 166*, 882–890.

Almeida, O. P. (2012). Approaches to decrease the prevalence of depression in later life. *Current Opinion in Psychiatry, 25*(6), 451–456.

Andrews, M. M. & Boyle, J. S. (2012). *Transcultural concepts in nursing care* (6th ed). Philadelphia, PA: Lippincott Williams & Wilkins.

Australian Institute of Health and Welfare (AIHW). (2013). *Australia's welfare 2013*. Series no. 11. Cat. no. AUS 174. Canberra: AIHW.

Baglioni, C., Berger, M. & Rieman, D. (2013). Bidirectional relationships between sleep, insomnia, and depression. In H. Lavretsky, M. Sajatovic, & C. F. Reynolds, III (Eds), *Late-life mood disorders* (pp. 347–360). Oxford: Oxford University Press.

Barca, M. L., Engedal, K., Laks, J. & Selbaek, G. (2009). A 12 months follow-up study of depression among nursing-home patients in Norway. *Journal of Affective Disorders, 120*, 141–148.

Beaudreau, S. A. & O'Hara, R. (2009). The association of anxiety and depressive symptoms with cognitive performance in community-dwelling older adults. *Psychology and Aging, 24*, 507–512.

Beck, A. T., Rush, A. J., Shaw, B. & Emery, G. (1979). *Cognitive therapy of depression*. New York: Guilford Press.

Bewernick, B. H. & Schlaepfer, T. E. (2013). Chronic depression as a model disease for cerebral aging. *Dialogues in Clinical Neuroscience, 15*(1), 77–82.

Blazer, D. G. (2002). *Depression in late life* (3rd ed.). New York: Springer.

Bowen, P. D. (2009). Use of selective serotonin reuptake inhibitors in the treatment of depression in older adults: Identifying and managing potential risk for hyponatremia. *Geriatric Nursing, 30*, 85–88.

bpac[nz] better medicine. (2010). Recognising and managing mental health disorders in Māori. *BPJ, 28*, 8–17. Accessed February 2015 at www.bpac.org.nz/magazine/2010/june/mentalhealth.asp.

Byma, E. A., Given, C. W. & Given, B. A. (2012). Associations among indicators of depression in Medicaid-eligible community-dwelling older adults. *Gerontologist, 53*(4), 608–617.

Carpenter, C., Crigger, N., Kugler, R. & Loya, A. (2008). *Hypericum* and nurses: A comprehensive literature review on the efficacy of St. John's wort in the treatment of depression. *Journal of Holistic Nursing, 26*, 200–207.

Catena-Dell'Osso, M., Rotella, F., Dell'Osso, A. et al. (2013). Inflammation, serotonin and major depression. *Current Drug Targets, 14*(5), 571–577.

Cipriani, A., Santilli, C., Furukawa, T. A., Signoretti, A., Nakagawa, A., McGuire, H., . . . Barbui, C. (2009). Escitalopram versus other antidepressive agents for depression. *Cochrane Database of Systematic Reviews, 2*, CD006532. doi:10.1002/14651858.CD006532.pub2.

Cooney, G. M., Dwan, K., Greig, C. A. et al. (2013). Exercise for depression. *Cochrane Database of Systematic Reviews, 19*(9), CD004366. doi:10.1002/14651858.CD004366.pub6.

Cukrowicz, K. C., Duberstein P. R., Vannoy S. D., Lynch T. R., McQuoid, D. R. & Steffens, D. C. (2009). Course of suicide ideation and predictors of change in depressed older adults. *Journal of Affective Disorders, 113*(1–2), 30–36. doi:10.1016/j.jad.2008.05.012.

Da Rocha e Silva, C. E., Alves Brasil, M. A., Matos do Nascimento, E. et al. (2013). Is poststroke depression a major depression? *Cerebrovascular Diseases, 35*(4), 385–391.

de Voogd, J. N., Wempe, J. B., Koeter, G. H., Postema, K., van Sonderen, E., Ranchor, A. V., . . Sanderman, R. (2009). Depressive symptoms as predictors of mortality in patients with COPD. *Chest, 135*(3), 619–625.

DeRyck, A., Brouns, R., Fransen, E. et al. (2013). A prospective study on the prevalence and risk factors of poststroke depression. *Cerebrovascular Diseases, 3*(1–13). doi:10.1159/000345557.

Diniz, B. S., Butters, M. A., Albert, S. M. et al. (2013). Late-lie depression and risk of vascular dementia and Alzheimer's disease: Systematic review and meta-analysis of community-based cohort studies. *British Journal of Psychiatry, 202*(5), 329–335.

Ekers, D., Richards, D. & Gilbody, S. (2008). A meta-analysis of randomized trials of behavioural treatment of depression. *Psychological Medicine, 38*, 611–623.

Eyre, H. A., Papps, E. & Baune, B. T. (2013). Treating depression and depression-like behavior with physical activity: An immune perspective. *Frontiers in Psychiatry, 4*(3). doi:10.3389/fpsycht.2013.00003.

Flaster, M., Sharma, A. & Rao, M. (2013). Poststroke depression: A review emphasizing the role of prophylactic treatment and synergy with treatment for motor recovery. *Topics in Stroke Rehabilitation, 20*(2), 139–150.

Fiske, A., Wetherell, J. L. & Gatz, M. (2009). Depression in older adults. *Annual Review of Clinical Psychology, 5*, 363–389.

Forlani, C., Morri, M., Ferrari, B. et al. (2014). Prevalence and gender differences in late-life depression: A population-based study. *American Journal of Geriatric Psychiatry, 22*(4), 370–380.

Gallegos-Carrillo, K., Garcia-Pena, C., Mudgal, J., Romero, X., Duran-Arenas, L. & Salmeron, J. (2009). *Journal of Psychosomatic Research, 66*, 127–135.

Greenberg, S. A. (2012). *How to Try This*: The Geriatric Depression Scale—Short Form. Available at www.consultgerirn.org.

Harvath, T. A. & McKenzie, G. (2012). Depression. In M. Boltz, E. Capezuti, T. Fulmer & D. Zwicker (Eds), *Evidence-based geriatric nursing protocols for best practice* (4th ed., pp. 135–162). New York: Springer.

Hedayati, S. S., Minhauddin, A. T., Toto, R. D., Morris, D. W. & Rush, A. J. (2009). Prevalence of major depressive episode in CKD. *American Journal of Kidney Disease, 54*, 399–402.

Helming, M. B. & Jackson, C. (2009). Relationships. In B. M. Dossey & L. Keegan (Eds), *Holistic nursing: A handbook for practice* (5th ed., pp. 367–391). Boston: Jones and Bartlett Publishers.

Hicks, L. E. & Woods, N. (2009). Depression and suicide risks in older adults: A case study. *Home Healthcare Nurse, 27*(8), 482–487.

Hornsten, C., Lovheim, H. J. & Gustafson, Y. (2013). The association between stroke, depression, and 5-year mortality among very old people. *Stroke, 44*(9), 2587–2589.

Howland, R. H. (2009). Somatic therapies for seasonal affective disorder. *Journal of Psychosocial Nursing and Mental Health Services, 47*, 17–20.

Huffman, J. C., Celano, C. M., Beach, S. R. et al. (2013). Depression and cardiac disease: Epidemiology, mechanisms, and diagnosis. *Cardiovascular Psychiatry and Neurology*, article ID 695925, 14p. doi:10.1155/2013/695925.

Hybels, C. F., Pieper, C. F. & Blazer, D. G. (2009). The complex relationship between depressive symptoms and functional limitations in community-dwelling older adults: The impact of sub-threshold depression. *Psychology and Medicine, 39*, 1677–1688.

Jones, C. A., Pohar, S. L. & Patten, S. B. (2009). Major depression and health-related quality of life in Parkinson's disease. *General Hospital Psychiatry, 31*, 334–340.

Joutsenniemi, K., Tuulio-Henriksson, A., Elovainio, M. et al. (2013). Depressive symptoms, major depressive episodes and cognitive test performance: What is the role of physical activity? *Nordic Psychiatry, 67*(4), 265–273.

Knapskog, A. B., Barca, M. L. & Engedal, K. (2013). Prevalence of depression among memory clinic patients as measured by the Cornell Scale of Depression in Dementia. *Aging & Mental Health, 18*(5), 579–587.

Kok, R. M., Nolen, W. A. & Heeren, T. J. (2009). Outcome of late-life depression after 3 years of sequential treatment. *Acta Psychiatrica Scandinavica, 119*, 274–281.

Krystal, A. D., Edinger, J. D. & Wohlgemuth, W. K. (2012). Sleep and circadian rhythm disorders. In D. G. Blazer & D. C. Steffens (Eds), *Essentials of geriatric psychiatry* (2nd ed., pp. 209–221). Washington, DC: American Psychiatric Publishing.

Laidlaw, K., Thompson, L. W., Dick-Siskin, L. et al. (2003). Cognitive behaviour therapy with older people. Chichester: John Wiley.

Lawrence, V., Murray, J., Banerjee, S., Turner, S., Sangha, K., Byng, R., . . . Macdonald, A. (2006). Concepts and causation of depression: A crosscultural study of the beliefs of older adults. *Gerontologist, 46*, 23–32.

Lee, M. J., Hasche, L. K., Choi, S. et al. (2013). Comparison of major depressive disorder and subthreshold depression among older adults in community long-term care. *Aging & Mental Health, 17*(4), 461–469.

Li, L. W. & Conwell, Y. (2009). Effects of changes in depressive symptoms and cognitive functioning on physical disability in home care elders. *Journal of Gerontology. Medical Sciences, 64A*, 230–236.

Licht-Strunk, E., van Marwijk, H., Hoekstra, T., Twisk, J., De Haan, M. & Beekman, A. (2009b). Outcome of depression in later life in primary care: Longitudinal cohort study with three years' follow-up. *British Medical Journal, 338*, a3079.

Lin, E., Heckbert, S., Rutter, C., Katon, W., Ciechanowski, P., Ludman, E., . . . Korff, M. (2009). Depression and increased mortality in diabetes: Unexpected causes of death. *Annals of Family Medicine, 7*(5), 414–421.

Lipson, J. G. & Dibble, S. L. (2005). *Culture and clinical care*. San Francisco: UCSF Nursing Press.

Liu, I. C. & Chiu, C. H. (2009). Case-control study of suicide attempts in the elderly. *International Psychogeriatrics, 21*, 896–902.

Lyness, J. M., Chapman, B. P., McGriff, J., Drayer, R. & Duberstein, P. (2009). One-year outcomes of minor and subsyndromal depression in older primary care patients. *International Psychogeriatrics, 21*, 60–68.

Marano, C. M., Rosenberg, P. B. & Lyketsos, C. G. (2013). Depression in dementia. In H. Lavretsky, M. Sajatovic & C. F. Reynolds, III (Eds), *Late-life mood disorders* (pp. 177–205). Oxford: Oxford University Press.

Matta Mello Portugal, E., Cevada, T., Sobral Monteiro, R. et al. (2013). Neuroscience of exercise: From neurobiology mechanisms to mental health. *Neuropsychology, 68*(1), 1–14.

McDonald, W. M. & Vahabzadeh, A., (2013). Electroconvulsive therapy and neuromodulation in the treatment of late-life mood disorders. In H. Lavretsky, M. Sajatovic & C. F. Reynolds, III (Eds), *Late-life mood disorders* (pp. 406–431). Oxford: Oxford University Press.

Mezuk, B. & Gallo, J. J. (2013). Depression and medical illness in late life. In H. Lavretsky, M. Sajatovic & C. F. Reynolds, III (Eds), *Latelife mood disorders* (pp. 270–294). Oxford: Oxford University Press.

Mittey, E. & Flores, S. (2008). Suicide in late life. *Geriatric Nursing, 29*, 160–165.

Olazaran, J., Trincado, R. & Bermejo-Pareja, F. (2013). Cumulative effect of depression on dementia risk. *International Journal of Alzheimer's Disease, 2013.* Article ID 457175. doi:10.1155/2013/457175.

Omachi, T. A., Katz, P. P., Yelin, E. H., Gregorch, S. E., Iribarren, C., Blanc, P. D. & Eisner, M. D. (2009). Depression and health-related quality of life in chronic obstructive pulmonary disease. *American Journal of Medicine, 122*(778), e9–e15.

Oudman, E. (2012). Is electroconvulsive therapy (ECT) effective and safe for treatment of depression in dementia? A short review. *Journal of ECT 28*(1), 34–38.

Pandey, G. N. (2013). Biologic basis of suicide and suicidal behavior. *Bipolar Disorders, 15*(5), 524–541.

Park, M. & Unutzer, J. (2013). Public health burden of late-life mood disorders. In H. Lavretsky, M. Sajatovic & C. F. Reynolds, III (Eds), *Late-life mood disorders* (pp. 42–60). Oxford: Oxford University Press.

Perry, R. (2009). Desvenlafaxine: A serotonin-norepinephrine reuptake inhibitor for the treatment of adults with major depressive disorder. *Clinical Therapeutics, 31*(PT), 1374–1404

Polyakova, M., Sonnabend, N., Sander, C. et al. (2014). Prevalence of minor depression in elderly persons with and without mild cognitive impairment: A systematic review. *Journal of Affective Disorders, 152–154*, 28–38.

Purnell, L. D. (2014). *Guide to culturally competent health care* (3rd ed.). Philadelphia: F.A. Davis Co.

Rapinesi, C., Kotzalidis, G. D., Serata, D. et al. (2013). Prevention of relapse with maintenance electroconvulsive therapy in elderly patients with major depressive episodes. *Journal of ECT, 29*(1), 61–64.

Ribeiz, S., Duran, F., Oliveira, M. et al. (2013). Structural brain changes as biomarkers and outcome predictors in patients with late-life depression: A cross-sectional and prospective study. *PLoS One, 8*(11), e80049.

Richard, E., Reitz, C., Honig, L. H. et al. (2013). Late-life depression, mild cognitive impairment, and dementia. *Journal of the American Medical Society Neurology, 70*(3), 364–382.

Schoevers, R. A., Geerlings, M. I., Deeg, D. J., Holwerda, T. J., Jonker, C. & Beekman, A. T. (2009). Depression and excess mortality: Evidence for a dose responsive relation in community living elderly. *International Journal of Geriatric Psychiatry, 24*(2), 169–176.

Seligman, M. E. P. (1981). A learned helplessness point of view. In L. P. Rehm (Ed.), *Behavior therapy for depression* (pp. 123–141). New York: Academic Press.

Shipowick, C. D., Moore, C. B. & Corbett, C. (2009). Vitamin D and depressive symptoms in women during the winter: A pilot study. *Applied Nursing Research, 22*, 221–225.

Snowden, J. & Almeida, O. P. (2013). The diagnosis and treatment and unipolar depression in late life. In H. Lavretsky, M. Sajatovic & C. F. Reynolds, III (Eds), *Late-life mood disorders* (pp. 79–103). Oxford: Oxford University Press.

Soares, C. N. (2009). Assessing the efficacy of desvenlafaxine for improving functioning and well-being outcome measures in patients with major depressive disorder: A pooled analysis of 9 double-blind, placebo-controlled, 8-week clinical trials. *Journal of Clinical Psychiatry, 70*(10), 1365–1371.

Steffens, D. C. (2009). A multiplicity of approaches to characterize geriatric depression and its outcomes. *Current Opinion in Psychiatry, 22*(6), 522–526.

Subramaniam, M., Sum, C. F., Pek, E., Stahl, D., Verma, S., Liow, P. H., Chong, S. A. (2009). Comorbid depression and increased health care utilization in individuals with diabetes. *General Hospital Psychiatry, 31*(3), 220–224.

Sullivan, M. J. (2009). The support, education, and research in chronic heart failure study (SEARCH): A mindfulness-based psychoeducational intervention improves depression and clinical symptoms in patients with chronic heart failure. *American Heart Journal, 157*(1), 84–90.

Taylor, W. D., Aizenstein, H. J. & Alexopoulos, G. S. (2013). The vascular depression hypothesis: Mechanisms linking vascular disease with depression. *Molecular Psychiatry, 18*(9), 963–974.

Taylor-Piliae, R. E., Hepworth, J. T. & Coull, B. M. (2013). Predictors of depressive symptoms among community-dwelling stroke survivors. *Journal of Cardiovascular Nursing, 28*(5), 460–467.

Thakur, M. & Blazer, D. G. (2008). Depression in long-term care. *Journal of the American Medical Directors Association, 9*(2), 82–87.

Thase, M. E., Kornstein, S. G., Germain, J. M., Jiang, Q., Guico-Pabia, C. & Ninan, P. T. (2009). An integrated analysis of the efficacy of desvenlafaxine compared with placebo in patients with major depressive disorder. *CNS Spectrums, 14*(3), 144–154.

Trangle, M., Dieperink, B., Gabert, T. et al. (2012). Health care guideline: Major depression in adults in primary care. Bloomington, MN: Institute for Clinical Systems Improvement. Available February 2015 via www.icsi.org.

Van den Kommer, T. N., Comijs, H. C., Aartsen, M. J. et al. (2013). Depression and cognition: How do they interrelate in old age? *American Journal of Geriatric Psychiatry, 21*(4), 398–410.

Verwijk, E., Comijs, H. C., Kok, R. M. et al. (2014). Short- and long-term neurocognitive functioning after electroconvulsive therapy in depressed elderly: A prospective naturalistic study. *International Psychogeriatrics, 26*(2), 315–324.

Vilalta-Franch, J., Lopez-Pousa, S., Llinas-Regla, J. et al. (2013). Depression subtypes and 5-year risk of dementia and Alzheimer disease in patients aged 70 years. *International Journal of Geriatric Psychiatry 28*(4), 341–350.

Volk, S. & Steffens, D. C. (2013). Post-stroke depression and vascular depression. In H. Lavretsky, M. Sajatovic & C. F. Reynolds, III (Eds), *Late-life mood disorders* (pp. 24–269). Oxford: Oxford University Press.

Watson, L. C., Zimmerman, S., Cohen, L. W. & Dominik, R. (2009). Practical depression screening in residential care assisted living: Five methods compared with gold standard diagnoses. *American Journal of Geriatric Psychiatry, 17*(7), 556–564.

Weiner, R. D. & Krystal, A. D. (2012). Electroconvulsive therapy. In D. G. Blazer & D. C. Steffens (Eds), *Essentials of geriatric psychiatry* (2nd ed., pp. 305–318). Washington, DC: American Psychiatric Publishing.

Whooley, M. A. & Wong, J. M. (2013). Depression and cardiovascular disorders. *Annual Review of Clinical Psychology, 9*, 327–354.

Wolinsky, F. D., Mahncke, H. W., Vander Weg, M. W., Martin, R., Unverzagt, F. W., . . . Tennstedt, S. L. (2009). The ACTIVE cognitive training interventions and the onset of recovery from suspected clinical depression. *Journal of Gerontology: Psychological Sciences, 64B*(5), 577–585.

World Health Organization (WHO). (2011). *Mental health atlas—2011 country profiles.* Australia and New Zealand. Available February 2015 via www.who.int/mental_health/evidence/atlas/profiles/en.

Yesavage, J. A., Brink, T. L., Rose, T. L., Lum, O., Huang, V., Adey, M. et al. (1983). Development and validation of a geriatric depression screening scale: A preliminary report. *Journal of Psychiatric Research, 17*, 37–49. Scale available February 2015 at www.stanford.edu/~yesavage/GDS.html.

Zeki Al Hazzouri, A., Vittinghoff, E., Byers, A. et al. (2014). Long- term cumulative depressive symptom burden and risk of cognitive decline and dementia among very old women. *Journals of Gerontology: Biological Sciences and Medical Sciences, 69*(5), 595–601.

PART 4

PROMOTING WELLNESS IN PHYSICAL FUNCTION

Chapter 16

Hearing

By Carol Miller and Sharyn Hunter

LEARNING OBJECTIVES

After reading this chapter, you should be able to:

1. Describe age-related changes that affect hearing.
2. Identify risk factors that affect hearing wellness.
3. Discuss the functional consequences that affect hearing wellness.
4. Conduct a nursing assessment of hearing, with emphasis on identifying opportunities for health promotion.
5. Identify nursing interventions to promote hearing wellness for older adults by addressing risk factors that interfere with hearing.

KEY POINTS

assistive listening device
cerumen
conductive hearing loss
hearing aid
mixed hearing loss
noise-induced hearing loss (NIHL)
otosclerosis
presbycusis
sensorineural hearing loss
tinnitus

Performance of many important daily activities—including communicating, protecting oneself from danger and enjoying music, voices and sounds—is highly dependent on good hearing. In older adults, age-related changes combine with risk factors to affect hearing wellness. Nurses promote wellness for older adults when they use health promotion interventions to improve hearing and communication. This chapter addresses the functional consequences associated with hearing in older adults and provides guides for nursing assessment and interventions.

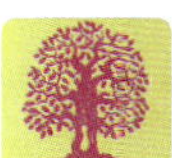

AGE-RELATED CHANGES THAT AFFECT HEARING

Auditory function depends on a sequence of processes, beginning in the three compartments of the ear and ending with the processing of information in the auditory cortex of the brain (see Table 16-1). Sounds are coded according to intensity and frequency. Intensity or amplitude reflects the loudness or softness of the sound and is measured in decibels (dB). Frequency, which is measured in cycles per second (cps) or hertz (Hz), determines whether the pitch is high or low. Sound intensity and frequency may be altered if certain risk factors come into play. Even in the absence of risk factors, normal age-related changes affect frequency, causing hearing problems for many older adults.

External ear

Hearing begins in the external or outer ear, which consists of the pinna and the external auditory canal (Figure 16-1). These cartilaginous structures localise sounds so the person can identify the sources. The pinna undergoes changes in size, shape, flexibility and hair growth with increasing age, but these changes do not affect the conduction of sound waves in healthy older adults. The auditory canal is covered by skin and lined with hair follicles and cerumen-producing glands. **Cerumen** or earwax is a natural substance that is genetically determined to be either dry (flaky and grey) or wet (moist and brown or tan). The function of cerumen is to cleanse, protect and lubricate the ear canal. Cerumen is naturally expelled, but it can build up in older adults because of age-related changes, such as an increased concentration of keratin, the growth of longer and thicker hair (especially in men) and the thinning and drying of the skin lining the canal. An age-related diminution in sweat gland activity further increases the potential for cerumen to accumulate by making the wax drier and more difficult to remove. A prolapsed or collapsed ear canal

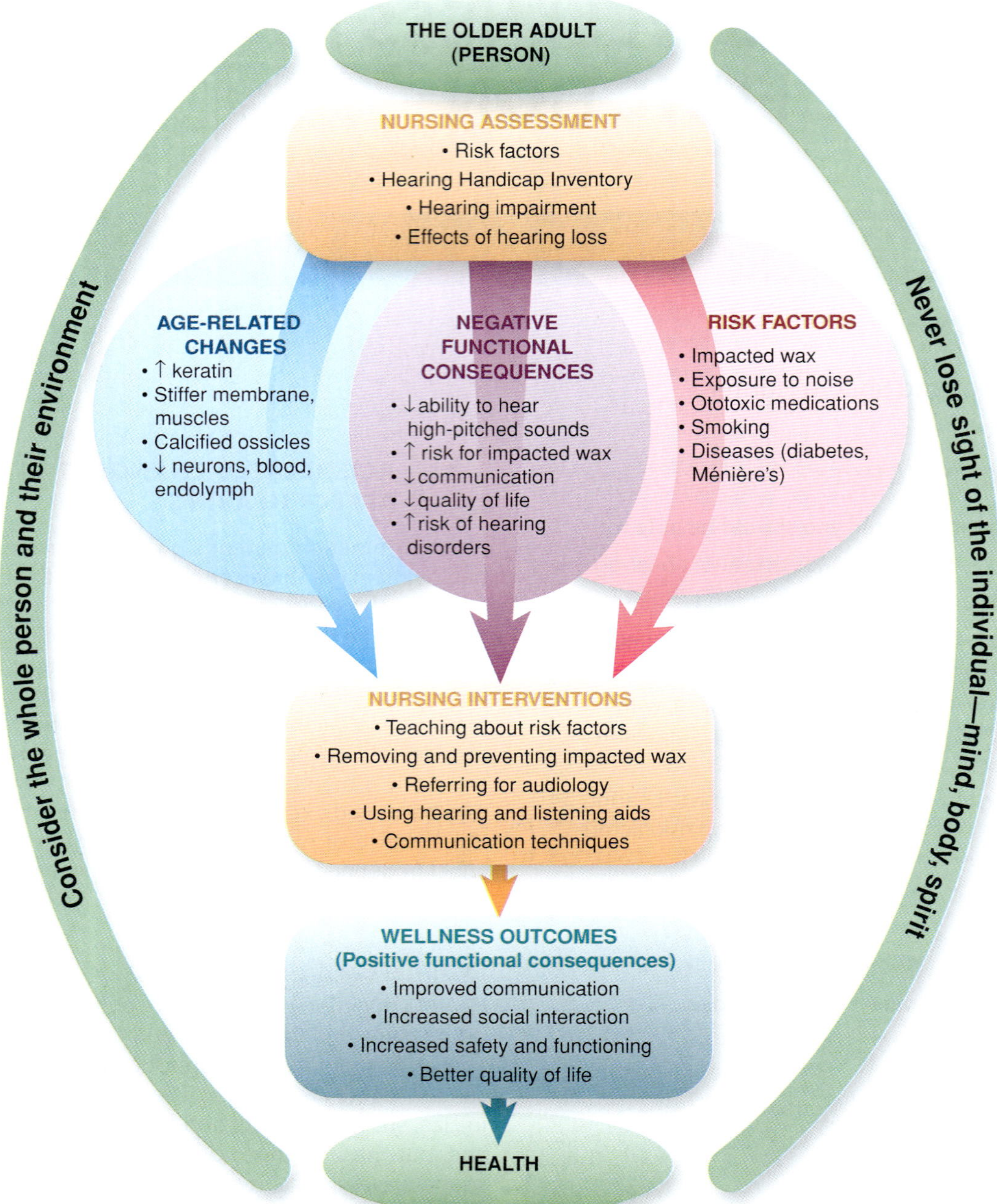

is another age-related condition that can occur and affect localisation and perception of high-frequency sounds.

DIVERSITY NOTE

Caucasians are likely to have wet cerumen, whereas Asians are likely to have dry cerumen.

Middle ear

The tympanic membrane is a transparent, pearl-grey, slightly cone-shaped layer of the flexible tissue separating the outer and middle ear. Its primary functions are to transmit sound energy and protect the middle and inner ear. With increased age, collagenous tissue replaces the elastic tissue, resulting in a thinner and stiffer eardrum. Sound vibrations pass through the tympanic membrane to the three auditory ossicles: the malleus, incus and stapes. These bones are connected to each other but move independently, acting as a lever to amplify sound. Their primary function is to transmit vibrations across the air-filled middle ear, through the oval window and into the fluid-filled inner ear. The transmission of sound is influenced by the

TABLE 16-1 Functional consequences of age-related changes affecting hearing

	Change	Consequence
External ear	• Longer, thicker hair • Thinner, drier skin • Increased keratin	Potential for impacted cerumen and subsequent impaired sound conduction
Middle ear	• Diminished resiliency of tympanic membrane • Calcified, hardened ossicles • Weakened and stiff muscles and ligaments	Impaired sound conduction
Inner ear and nervous system	• Diminished neurons, endolymph, hair cells and blood supply • Degeneration of spiral ganglion and arterial blood vessels • Decreased flexibility of basilar membrane • Degeneration of central processing systems	*Presbycusis:* diminished ability to hear high-pitched sounds, especially in the presence of background noise

frequency of each sound and is the most effective in the middle-frequency range of normal voices, and the least effective at the lowest and highest frequencies. Age-related calcification of the ossicular bones can interfere with the transfer of sound vibrations from the tympanic membrane to the oval window.

The middle ear muscles and ligaments contract in response to loud noises, stimulating the acoustic reflex. This protects the delicate inner ear and filters out auditory distractions originating from one's own voice and body movements. With increased age the middle ear muscles and ligaments become weaker and stiffer and have a detrimental effect on the acoustic reflex. In addition, these degenerative changes diminish the resiliency of the tympanic membrane.

Inner ear

In the inner ear, vibrations are transmitted to the cochlea, where they are converted to nerve impulses and coded for intensity and frequency. Nerve impulses stimulate fibres of the eighth cranial nerve and send the auditory message to the brain. This process transpires primarily in the sensory hair cells of the organ of Corti in the cochlea.

Age-related changes of the inner ear include loss of hair cells, a reduction of blood supply, the diminution of endolymph production, decreased basilar membrane

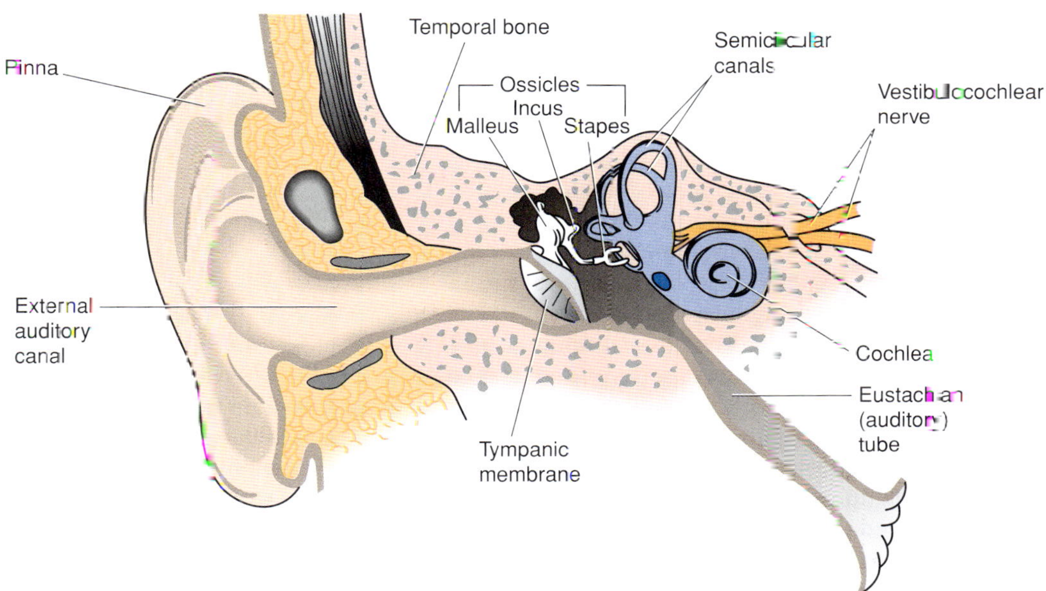

FIGURE 16-1 The ear. Age-related changes in structures of the ear can affect hearing in older adults.

flexibility, degeneration of spiral ganglion cells and loss of neurons in the cochlear nuclei. These inner ear changes result in the degenerative hearing impairment termed **presbycusis**. One classification system for presbycusis is based on the specific structural source of the impairment as follows:

- *Sensory presbycusis* is associated with degenerative changes of the hair cells and the organ of Corti and is characterised by a sharp hearing loss at high frequencies.
- *Neural presbycusis* is caused by degeneration of nerve fibres in the cochlea and spiral ganglion and is characterised by reduced speech discrimination.
- *Metabolic presbycusis* is caused by degenerative changes in the stria vascularis and a subsequent interruption in essential nutrient supply. Initially, these changes reduce the sensitivity to all sound frequencies; eventually, they interfere with speech discrimination.
- *Mechanical presbycusis* results from mechanical changes in the inner ear structures and is characterised by a hearing loss that initially involves lower frequencies and gradually spreads to higher frequencies and interferes with speech discrimination.

Although useful for explaining the physiological basis for various types of presbycusis, in reality, presbycusis usually involves several age-related processes.

Auditory nervous system

From the inner ear, the auditory nerve fibres pass through the internal auditory meatus and enter the brain. Functions of the auditory nerve pathway include localising sound direction, fine-tuning auditory stimuli and transferring information from the primary auditory cortex to the auditory association area. The auditory nervous system is affected by all of the following age-related changes: degenerative changes in the inner ear, narrowing of the auditory meatus from bone apposition; diminished blood supply; and central nervous system changes (e.g. diminished speed of information processing). Recent studies indicate that the age-related changes in central auditory function account for a significant component of hearing loss in older adults (Gates, Feeney & Mills, 2008).

Risk factors that affect hearing wellness

In addition to the age-related changes that affect hearing, factors associated with lifestyle, heredity, environment, medications, impacted wax and disease conditions can cause hearing loss. Reviews of studies identified the following risk factors for hearing impairment: male gender, increased age, genetic predisposition, exposure to noise, impacted cerumen, smoking, exposure to second-hand smoke, use of ototoxic medications, education level less than or equal to a high school qualification, and certain medical conditions (e.g. stroke, diabetes, hypertension, cardiovascular disease) (Adobamen & Ogisi, 2012; Fabry, Davila, Arheart et al., 2011; Kiely, Gopinath, Mitchell et al., 2012; Lin, Chien, Li et al., 2012; Mahboubi, Zardouz, Oliaei et al., 2013).

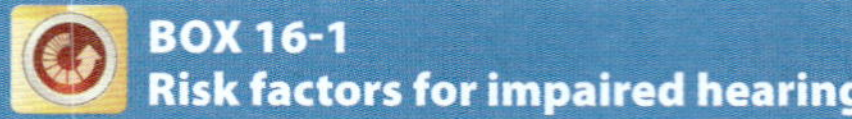

BOX 16-1
Risk factors for impaired hearing

Genetic predisposition
Increased age
Recreational or occupational exposure to noise
Cigarette smoking
Ototoxic medications
- Aminoglycosides
- Aspirin and other salicylates
- Cisplatin
- Erythromycin
- Ibuprofen
- Imipramine
- Indomethacin
- Loop diuretics
- Quinidine
- Quinine

Ototoxic environmental chemicals
- Carbon monoxide
- Fuels
- Lead
- Mercury
- Organophosphates
- Styrene
- Toluene

Much of the research on risk factors focuses on modifiable risk factors, such as noise, that can be addressed through health promotion interventions. Research is also focusing on the interrelationship between risk factors such as noise and ototoxic substances (e.g. medications or environmental toxins). For example, people who are genetically predisposed to hearing loss may be more susceptible to the damaging effects of noise exposure or ototoxic drugs. Because age-related changes increase the risk for hearing loss, it is especially important to identify modifiable risk factors in older adults so that those risks can be addressed. Most likely, some hearing loss attributed to age-related changes actually results from risk factors, such as exposure to noise or ototoxic substances. Box 16-1 summarises some factors that interfere with hearing wellness, either alone or in combinations.

Lifestyle and environmental factors

A commonly occurring risk factor for impaired hearing is prolonged or intermittent exposure to noise, which can be viewed as both a lifestyle choice and an environmental factor. In fact, environmental noise has been compared to second-hand smoke in that it is an unwanted airborne pollutant produced by others without consent and at times, places and volumes over which bystanders have no control (Tompkins, 2009). Studies indicate that although age-related changes account for a greater amount of hearing loss than occupational noise exposure, **noise-induced hearing loss (NIHL)** is still the most important preventable cause of hearing loss in the U.S. (Dobie, 2008). Occupations associated with an increased risk for NIHL include farmers, musicians, truck drivers, armed services members and aviation workers (Jansen et al., 2009; Helfer et al., 2010; Karimi et al., 2010; McCullagh & Robertson, 2009; Wagstaff, 2009). Use of headphones and earphones with personal music players is an example of a recreational activity that increases the risk of NIHL (Kim et al., 2009; Vogel et al., 2010).

Some older adults may have worked in occupational settings before safe noise level recommendations were enforced by the Safety Institute of Australia (SIA) or in New Zealand by the Institute of Safety Management (NZISM). For instance, older people who were once employed as weavers or textile workers are likely to have been exposed to detrimentally noisy environments during their work years. Because the effects of NIHL and age-related changes are cumulative, the hearing loss may not be noticed until later adulthood.

Exposure to toxic chemicals in the workplace or the environment is another risk factor for hearing loss that has been under investigation since the 1990s, with current research focusing on metals, solvents, asphyxiants and pesticides/herbicides. Cigarette smoking, as well as living in a household with a smoker, is another factor being investigated both as an independent risk and as a condition that potentiates the effects of noise to cause hearing loss.

Shooting, woodworking and other leisure-time activities can also contribute to NIHL, especially if people engaging in these activities do not use protective ear devices. Other activities that are likely to cause sensorineural damage unless protective mechanisms are used include listening to loud music; operating tractors, chain saws or leaf blowers; and riding motorcycles, aeroplanes, snowmobiles or motorboats. Figure 16-2 illustrates the noise levels of various activities. Sounds louder than 80 dB are considered potentially ototoxic.

DIVERSITY NOTE

Moderate to severe age-related hearing loss in women is strongly associated with a maternal family history of hearing loss and in men is significantly, but less strongly, associated with a paternal family history (McMahon et al., 2008).

Impacted cerumen

Impacted cerumen is common in older adults as a leading cause of hearing loss. Age-related changes, which make the cerumen dryer, harder and coarser, increase the risk of impaction. The use of hearing aids also increases the possibility of impacted wax which can damage or interfere with the function of the hearing aid. In addition to causing a hearing loss, impacted cerumen can cause pain, infection, tinnitus, dizziness or chronic coughing (due to stimulation of a branch of the vagus nerve) (McCarter, Courtney & Pollart, 2007; University of Texas School of Nursing, 2007). Cerumen accumulation is preventable and treatable and, most importantly, it is readily amenable to nursing interventions, as discussed later in this chapter. Studies indicate that up to 57% of older long-term care residents have impacted cerumen (Roland et al., 2008). Moreover, studies of hospitalised older adults indicate that 75% of those who had earwax removed had improved hearing (McCarter et al., 2007).

Ototoxic medications

Medications can cause or contribute to hearing impairments by damaging the cochlear and vestibular divisions of the auditory nerve. Despite the fact that quinine and salicylate ototoxicities were first observed more than a century ago, the ototoxic effects of medication have received little attention in clinical settings. Although age alone does not increase the risk for ototoxicity, older adults are more likely to be taking ototoxic medications, such as aspirin and frusemide.

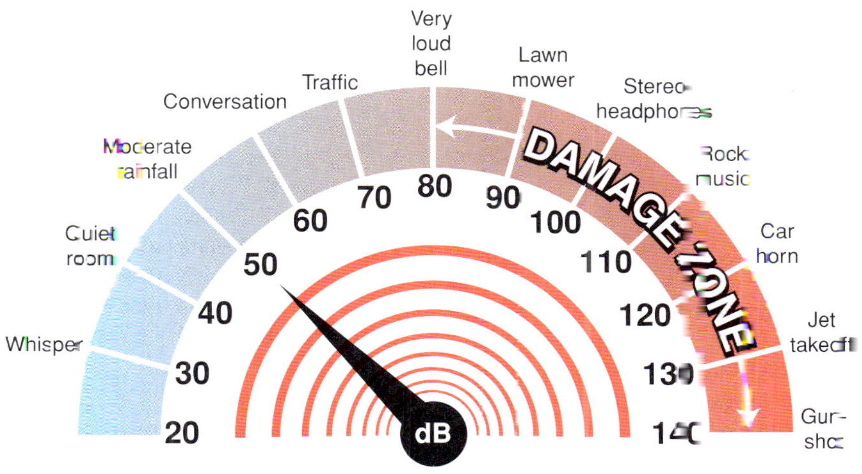

FIGURE 16-2 Noise levels associated with common activities are measured in decibels (dB). Sounds louder than 80 dB are potentially harmful to ears.

Other contributing factors that commonly occur in older adults and increase the risk for ototoxicity include renal failure, long-term use of ototoxic medications and potentiation between two ototoxic medications, such as furosemide and aminoglycoside antibiotics. Box 16-1 lists medications that are likely to be ototoxic. Ototoxicity is often dose related and hearing loss may be temporary if medications are discontinued or the dose is reduced. Although ototoxicity is potentially reversible, medications may be overlooked as a causative factor if the hearing loss is mistakenly ascribed to inevitable and irreversible degenerative changes.

Disease processes

Otosclerosis is a hereditary disease of the auditory ossicles that causes ankylosis of the footplate of the stapes to the oval window. Otosclerosis usually begins in youth or early adulthood, but the hearing loss may not be detected until middle or later adulthood, when age-related middle ear changes compound the disease-related changes. Otosclerosis primarily causes a conductive hearing loss, but some sensorineural loss also may occur. Initially, it is difficult to hear soft and low-pitched sounds. As the hearing loss worsens, the person is likely to experience dizziness, tinnitus or balance problems.

WELLNESS OPPORTUNITY

Modifiable and preventable risk factors for hearing loss include noise, medications and impacted cerumen.

UNFOLDING CASE STUDY

Part A

Mr Hilde is 60 years old and owns a small building business. He has been a carpenter for 38 years, but in the past 9 years, he has spent most of his time in the office, managing his business. He enjoys hunting and fishing on weekends. He has smoked two packs of cigarettes a day since he was 16 years old. His wife has been telling him she thinks he hears only what he wants to hear. Mr Hilde admits that he turns the television volume up louder than he used to but denies having any "real hearing problem".

Thinking points

- What age-related changes and risk factors could contribute to Mr Hilde's hearing loss?
- Describe the hearing loss that Mr Hilde is likely to be experiencing.
- What environmental conditions will contribute to Mr Hilde's hearing difficulty?

Ménière's disease and acoustic neuromas are auditory system diseases that commonly cause hearing impairment. Studies have found that diabetes is an independent risk factor for hearing impairment (Bainbridge, Hoffman & Cowie, 2008). Other conditions and systemic diseases that can cause or contribute to hearing impairment include syphilis, myxoedema, hypertension, meningitis, hypothyroidism, head trauma, high fevers, Paget's disease, radiation for head and neck cancers and viral infections (e.g. measles and mumps).

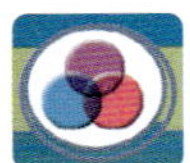

FUNCTIONAL CONSEQUENCES AFFECTING HEARING WELLNESS

Three-quarters of Australians aged 70 and over have hearing loss (Access Economics, 2006). Hearing impairment is most likely to occur in men, people of low socioeconomic status and people exposed to prolonged job-related or recreational noise. Poor health is also associated with a higher risk for impaired hearing, as is a family history of otosclerosis. Hearing loss in men in Australia aged 70 years and over contributes to a significant amount of disability in this age group (Access Economics, 2006). In New Zealand, 36.7% of women and 57.4% of men 65 and over have hearing impairment (New Zealand Ministry of Health, 2006).

DIVERSITY NOTE

Australian Hearing (www.hearing.com.au) has resources available in five different languages.

Hearing losses are categorised according to the site of the impairment. Abnormalities of the external and middle ear impair the sound conduction mechanism and are classified as **conductive hearing losses**. Abnormalities of the inner ear interfere with the sensory and neural structures and are classified as **sensorineural hearing losses**. Sensorineural hearing loss is often age related or noise induced. A hearing loss that involves both conductive and sensorineural impairments is called a **mixed hearing loss**.

Effects on communication

Accurate comprehension of speech depends on speech pace, sound frequencies, environmental noise and internal auditory function. Hearing acuity for high-frequency tones begins to decline in early adulthood; by the age of 30 years for men and 50 years for women, there is some decline in hearing sensitivity at all frequencies.

DIVERSITY NOTE

In addition to having an earlier age of onset for hearing loss, hearing levels decline more rapidly in men, so the cumulative effects are usually noticed by men in their 50s and women in their 60s. In both Australia and New Zealand there is a higher prevalence of older men than older women with hearing impairment.

Speech comprehension is most directly influenced by the frequency of *phonemes*, the smallest units of sound. Each phoneme in a word has a different frequency; generally, vowels have lower frequencies and consonants have higher frequencies. Although most word phonemes have lower-range frequencies, sibilant consonants (those that have a whistling quality, such as *ch, f, g, s, sh, t, th* and *z*) have higher-range frequencies. Because the earliest and most universal age-related changes affect one's ability to code higher-frequency sounds, words rich in sibilants will be most affected by age-related changes of the auditory system.

Presbycusis as mentioned earlier, is the sensorineural hearing loss associated with an age-related degeneration of the auditory structures. Presbycusis usually occurs in both ears, but the degree of impairment in each ear can vary. An early functional consequence of presbycusis is the loss of ability to hear high-pitched sounds and sibilant consonants. When high-pitched sounds are filtered out, words become distorted and jumbled and sentences become incoherent. For example, someone with presbycusis might interpret a sentence like "I think she should go to the store" as "I wish we could go to the show". This characteristic, known as *diminished speech discrimination*, is influenced by the speaker's rate of speech: rapid, slow or slurred speech patterns make it increasingly difficult for the older person to discern words. As the hearing loss progresses, explosive consonants, such as *b, d, k, p* and *t* also become distorted.

Background noise and environmental conditions, such as echoing or poor acoustics, compound the effects of sensorineural hearing loss and can interfere with the ability to recognise words, even in the absence of a significant hearing loss. Thus, older adults in a hospital or long-term residential care facility, for example, may be particularly sensitive to background noises to which the staff may have become accustomed. One nursing study identified the following sources of noise that were most bothersome to hospitalised older adults: voices, carts, foot traffic, overhead pages and alarms from monitoring devices (Dube et al., 2008). People with sensorineural hearing loss are sometimes hypersensitive to high-frequency sounds, causing a very narrow range in which sound is heard adequately and comfortably. A conductive hearing loss is characterised by a reduced intensity of sounds and difficulty hearing vowels and low-pitched tones. In contrast to presbycusis, all frequencies of sounds are heard equally once the sound threshold is reached and background noise does not interfere as much with speech comprehension. Often there is a history of otosclerosis, perforated eardrum or other ear disease. In older adults, impacted cerumen is also a common contributing factor. Depending on the causative factor conductive hearing loss occurs in one or both ears. See Table 16-1 for a summary of the functional consequences of age-related changes that affect hearing.

Effects of hearing loss on overall wellness

Adequate hearing is a primary component of communication that enables people to enjoy humour, appreciate music, obtain information, relate to others, and respond to threats. Thus, hearing deficits inevitably affect safety, functioning and quality of life in many ways. Reviews of studies have identified all the following effects of hearing loss on overall wellness and quality of life of older adults:

- Diminished physical and cognitive function
- Functional decline
- Perception of quality of life as excellent: only 39% of subjects with hearing loss, compared with 68% of those without
- A source of loneliness, isolation and diminished participation in social activities
- Increased self-perception of poor social skills, which can result in diminished self-esteem
- Increased prevalence of depression
- Decreased autonomy
- Increased dependence on others. (Ciorba, Bianchini, Pelucchi, et al., 2012; Hawkins, Bottone, Ozminkowski, et al., 2012; Li-Korotky, 2012; Mondelli & de Souza, 2012)

A study assessing the association between hearing impairment and activity limitation concluded that severely diminished hearing loss can make the difference between independent living and the need for formal support services or placement (Gopinath, Schneider, McMahon et al., 2012).

Although researchers have found a strong association between hearing loss and impaired cognitive function, many questions remain about the cause–effect relationship. For example, Lin (2011) analysed data from a nationally representative sample of older adults in the U.S. and found that hearing loss is independently associated with lower cognitive function scores, but it is unclear whether hearing loss is a modifiable risk factor or an early indicator of cognitive decline. Longitudinal data indicate that hearing loss is associated with both accelerated decline and an increased incidence of cognitive impairment in community-dwelling older adults (Lin, Yaffe, Xia et al., 2013). A study of long-term care residents found that those with a more severe hearing loss also had poorer cognitive function (Jupiter, 2012).

It is important to consider the effect of hearing loss on cognitive function because any reduction in sensory stimuli can interfere with information perception and processing. Hearing loss also may affect performance on mental status assessments because people who cannot discriminate words may be reluctant to respond to questions and may refrain from answering rather than risk feeling foolish. Poor performance on tests of cognitive abilities can mistakenly lead to a perception that the person has cognitive impairments or dementia when, in fact, the person has a hearing loss. In addition, when hearing loss interferes with one's ability to perceive reality accurately, it can lead to suspiciousness, paranoia, and loss of contact with reality. When only parts of a conversation are heard, a person is likely to believe that the conversation is about him or her, and persecutory delusions can develop.

DIVERSITY NOTE

Hearing loss may have a greater social impact on older men and a greater emotional impact on older women. Thus, men may withdraw from social interactions and women may continue to be active but worry about how well they can participate (Taylor & Jurma, 2003).

In addition to having a negative influence on the quality of life, hearing deficits can affect the safety and functioning of older adults. For example, people with hearing impairments are likely to be less responsive when warning signals are sounded for fires, ambulances and other emergencies. Besides creating actual safety hazards, the hearing deficit can lead to fear and anxiety about personal safety. Even mild hearing impairment in older adults is associated with functional decline and increased dependency in daily activities.

Negative societal attitudes about ageing and hearing loss can result in a doubly negative effect on the person who is old as well as hard of hearing. The older person may be reluctant to acknowledge a hearing deficit, choosing to limit opportunities for communication rather than face the stigma associated with hearing impairments. These attitudes and accompanying behaviours can cause other psychosocial consequences such as loneliness, social isolation and even a more rapid progression of the hearing loss. Geropsychologists who studied the relationship between age stereotypes and hearing loss found that negative perceptions of ageing—particularly those related to physical appearance—were associated with a greater decline in hearing over a 3-year period (Levy, Slade & Gill, 2006). Moreover, Levy and colleagues (2006) found that age stereotypes had a greater influence on hearing loss than other risk factors such as age, sex, depression or smoking history.

WELLNESS OPPORTUNITY

Nurses can initiate conversations that reflect positive and nonjudgemental attitudes about ageing and hearing loss.

UNFOLDING CASE STUDY

Part B

Mr Hilde is now 69 years old and has been retired for several years. He spends several days a week working in his shed and fishing seasonally. He also enjoys making small pieces of furniture and doing other woodworking. He continues to smoke but has cut down to one pack per day. Mr Hilde and his wife regularly visit the general practice where you work as the practice nurse. They make an appointment to talk with you because Mrs Hilde is concerned about her husband's hearing. Mr Hilde, who blames his problem on "old age", refuses to have an evaluation for a hearing aid because he does not think an aid would do any good and "besides, it would stick out like a sore thumb".

Thinking points

- What factors contribute to Mr Hilde's hearing loss?
- What environmental and other conditions might make the hearing loss worse?
- What myths or misunderstandings are likely to influence Mr Hilde's perception of his hearing problem and potential interventions for it?

PATHOLOGICAL CONDITION AFFECTING HEARING: TINNITUS

Tinnitus is the persistent sensation of ringing, roaring, blowing, buzzing or other types of noise that do not originate in the external environment. Tinnitus is a common pathological condition in older adults that is highly associated with hearing loss, ototoxic medications and Ménière's disease. It can be caused by impacted wax, especially if the wax is attached to the tympanic membrane. Caffeine, alcohol or nicotine can exacerbate tinnitus. People with tinnitus should be evaluated for associated pathological conditions or any of the contributing factors. Examples of contributing conditions that should be evaluated for medical treatment include hypertension, cerebrovascular disease and inflammatory or allergic conditions of the nose and adjacent structures (Shulman & Goldstein, 2009). Studies suggest that intensity of tinnitus is worsened by increased age and amount of exposure to noise and has a significant negative effect on psychological quality of life (Muluk & Oguztürk, 2008).

WELLNESS OPPORTUNITY

Nurses can teach people who have tinnitus about the exacerbating effects of conditions, including smoking cigarettes and drinking alcoholic or caffeinated beverages that can be addressed through self-care actions.

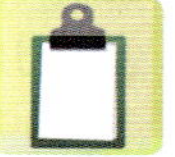

NURSING ASSESSMENT OF HEARING

Nursing assessment of hearing is aimed at identifying the following:

- Factors that interfere with hearing wellness
- Actual hearing deficit
- The impact of any hearing deficits on safety and quality of life
- Opportunities for improving hearing wellness
- Barriers to implementing interventions.

Each of the above factors is important in helping older adults and their carers/caregivers compensate for hearing deficits. Assessment is accomplished through interviewing, observing behavioural cues and administering hearing tests.

Interviewing about hearing changes

Interview questions are used to acquire information about (1) present and past risk factors, (2) the person's awareness and acknowledgement of a hearing impairment, (3) the psychosocial impact of any hearing deficit and (4) attitudes that might influence health promotion interventions (Box 16-2). The hearing assessment interview begins with questions about family history of hearing impairments and a personal history of prolonged exposure to loud noises. Identification of ototoxic medications as a risk factor can be included as part of the hearing assessment or as part of the medication history. Nurses can use questions to prompt the person to acknowledge a hearing problem, particularly if they discuss these factors in relation to increasing the risk for hearing loss.

If the older adult does not initiate a discussion of hearing problems, the nurse asks direct questions about the person's discernment of a hearing deficit. If the older adult denies having a hearing problem but shows behavioural cues indicative of a hearing deficit, the nurse elicits further information by asking leading questions such as "I notice you turn your left ear towards me. Is your hearing better in that ear?"

Nurses ask questions about changes in the older adult's social activities to identify psychosocial consequences of hearing impairment that can be addressed through interventions. If no hearing impairment is present, questions about lifestyle do not necessarily have to be included as part of the hearing assessment. When a person acknowledges the existence of a hearing impairment, however, the nurse then asks about any associated changes in social and occupational activities.

WELLNESS OPPORTUNITY

Nurses address the whole person by including questions about the impact of a hearing loss on his or her quality of life.

The nurse assesses the older person's attitudes towards hearing loss, hearing aids and assistive listening devices because these attitudes influence his or her acceptance of interventions. This is an important aspect of promoting hearing wellness because more than one-third of older adults could benefit from a hearing aid but 89.3% of those do not own one (Hidalgo et al., 2009).

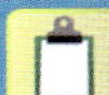

BOX 16-2
Guidelines for assessing hearing

Questions to identify risk factors for hearing loss

- Do you have a family history of hearing loss or deafness?
- Have you been exposed to loud noises in your job or leisure activities?
- Do you have a history of any of the following: diabetes, hypothyroidism, Ménière's disease, or Paget's disease?
- What medications do you take? (Refer to Box 16-1 to identify potentially ototoxic medications.)
- Have you ever had impacted wax in your ears?

Questions to assess awareness and presence of hearing deficit

- Do you have any trouble with your hearing?
- Have you noticed any change in your ability to understand conversations or hear words?
- Are you bothered by any noises in your ears, such as ringing or buzzing?

Questions to ask if hearing loss is acknowledged

- How long have you noticed a hearing loss?
- Do you notice differences in hearing in your left ear, versus your right ear?
- Has there been a progressive loss, or did the hearing problem begin suddenly?
- Describe your hearing difficulty.
- Are there any conditions such as noisy environments or particular voices or sounds that especially interfere with your hearing?
- Does your hearing loss interfere with your ability to communicate with others, either individually or in groups?
- Are there any activities that you would like to do but feel you cannot because of hearing problems?
- Have you ever had, or thought about having, an evaluation for a hearing aid?
- Have you ever tried using a hearing aid?

Questions to identify opportunities for education about disease prevention and health promotion

- Does the person engage in any activities that expose him or her to loud noises, such as woodworking or lawn mowing? If so, does he or she understand the importance of wearing ear protectors?
- If the person has a history of impacted wax, does he or she take preventive measures?
- Does the person smoke cigarettes or live in a household with a smoker? If so, does the person realise that this is a risk factor for hearing loss?
- What are the person's attitudes about hearing loss?
- Is hearing loss considered normal and untreatable?
- Is a hearing aid considered to be a stigma?
- If the person is resistant to an audiological evaluation, what are the barriers? (For example, are there financial or transportation limitations that interfere with obtaining a hearing aid?)
- Does the hearing loss contribute to a sense of isolation, depression, paranoia or low self esteem?
- What are the person's usual communication opportunities, and how does the hearing loss influence these usual patterns? (For instance, does the person live in an environment where it is important to be able to use the phone?)
- Does the person live in a noisy environment and find relief in the hearing impairment?
- If the person lives in an environment where group activities are a large part of daily activities, does the person want to participate in these activities?

ITEM	YES (4 pts)	SOMETIMES (2 pts)	NO (0 pts)
Does a hearing problem cause you to feel embarrassed when you meet new people?	____	____	____
Does a hearing problem cause you to feel frustrated when talking to members of your family?	____	____	____
Do you have difficulty hearing when someone speaks in a whisper?	____	____	____
Do you feel handicapped by a hearing problem?	____	____	____
Does a hearing problem cause you difficulty when visiting friends, relatives or neighbours?	____	____	____
Does a hearing problem cause you to attend religious services less often than you would like?	____	____	____
Does a hearing problem cause you to have arguments with family members?	____	____	____
Does a hearing problem cause you difficulty when listening to TV or radio?	____	____	____
Do you feel that any difficulty with your hearing limits or hampers your personal or social life?	____	____	____
Does a hearing problem cause you difficulty when in a restaurant with relatives or friends?	____	____	____

RAW SCORE______ (sum of the points assigned each of the items)

INTERPRETING THE RAW SCORE
0 to 8 = 13% probability of hearing impairment (no handicap/no referral)
10 to 24 = 50% probability of hearing impairment (mild-moderate handicap/refer)
26 to 40 = 84% probability of hearing impairment (severe handicap/refer)

FIGURE 16-3 The screening version of the Hearing Handicap Inventory for the Elderly (HHIE-S). (Reprinted with permission from Ventry, I. & Weinstein, B. [1983]. *Identification of elderly people with hearing problems* [pp. 37–42]. Rockville, MD: American Speech-Language-Hearing Association. Copyright, American Speech-Language-Hearing Association.)

When nurses identify attitudinal barriers, they can plan health education interventions to address myths or misunderstandings. For example, older adults may believe that hearing aids are too costly or of little use or they may be embarrassed to use a device that is visible to others. They also may not know how to go about arranging for an evaluation and may distrust advertisements about hearing aids. Resistance towards hearing aids can also arise from lack of money, transportation or motivation to communicate. Thus, the nurse focuses part of the assessment on barriers that are likely to interfere with interventions for hearing wellness.

The Hearing Handicap Inventory for the Elderly (HHIE-S) is a 10-item questionnaire that can be administered to older adults in approximately 5 minutes (Figure 16-3).

This tool was developed in the early 1980s for use with cognitively intact older adults in a variety of clinical and community settings. During the 25 years since its publication, it has been translated into nine languages and studies have found it is a valid tool for measuring clinical outcomes (Montano, 2007). The HHIE-S questionnaire can be administered to assess the presence and functional consequences of hearing loss. The Brief Hearing Loss Screener is a simple seven-question-assessment self-reporting tool recommended by the Hartford Institute for Geriatric Nursing.

WELLNESS OPPORTUNITY

Nurses promote self-care by asking an older adult to use the HHIE-S and then reviewing the results of this assessment to identify goals.

Observing behavioural cues

Behavioural cues related to hearing loss provide important information about the presence of a hearing impairment, the psychosocial consequences of any such impairment and the person's attitudes about assistive devices. If the older adult denies a hearing deficit that has been noticed by others, behavioural cues can be an important source of assessment information. Denial of a hearing deficit can be rooted in lack of awareness of the impairment because of gradual onset or, if the older person is socially isolated, can be caused by a paucity of opportunities for communication. Feelings of embarrassment or misconceptions that the hearing loss is an inevitable and untreatable consequence of ageing can also contribute to denial. Box 16-3 lists behavioural cues the nurse should observe as part of the hearing assessment.

Using hearing assessment tools

Nurses assess hearing by using an otoscope to examine the ear and a tuning fork to check hearing. The purpose of the otoscopic examination is to identify impacted wax and other factors that can interfere with hearing, whereas the purpose of the tuning fork test is to detect hearing impairments and to differentiate between conductive and sensorineural losses. Box 16-4 describes the procedure for performing a nursing assessment of hearing using the otoscope and tuning fork. A handheld audio scope is another assessment tool that is recommended in nursing guidelines; however, this tool is not as widely available as an otoscope or tuning fork. When a hearing deficit is identified, the nurse can recommend that further evaluation be

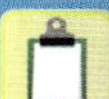

BOX 16-3
Guidelines for assessing behavioural cues related to hearing

Behavioural cues to a hearing deficit

- Inappropriate or no response to questions, especially in the absence of opportunities for lip reading
- Inability to follow verbal directions without cues
- Short attention span, easy distractibility
- Frequent requests for repetition or clarification of verbal communication
- Intense observation of the speaker
- Mouthing of words spoken by the speaker
- Turning of one ear towards the speaker
- Unusual physical proximity to the speaker
- Lack of response to loud environmental noises
- Speech that is too loud or inarticulate
- Abnormal voice characteristics, such as monotony
- Misperception that others are talking about him or her

Behavioural cues about psychosocial consequences

- Uncharacteristic avoidance of group settings
- Lack of interest in social activities, especially those requiring verbal communication or those that the person enjoyed in the past (e.g. bingo, card games)

Behavioural cues about assistive devices

- Not using a hearing aid that has been purchased
- Failure to obtain batteries for a hearing aid
- Expression of embarrassment about using assistive devices

BOX 16-4
Guidelines for otoscopic and tuning fork assessment

Using the otoscope to assess factors that could interfere with hearing

- Hold the otoscope upside down, resting your hand on the person's head to stabilise the instrument.
- Before inserting the speculum, pull the pinna upwards and backwards, while tilting the person's head slightly back and towards the opposite shoulder.
- If cerumen has accumulated to the point of interfering with the examination or occluding the canal, follow the cerumen removal procedure described in the section on nursing interventions.
- Normal otoscopic findings in older adults include the following:
  - Small amount of cerumen
  - Pinkish-white epithelial lining, no redness or lesions
  - Pearl-grey tympanic membrane, which is less translucent than in younger adults
  - Light reflex anteroinferiorly from the umbo
  - Visible landmarks

Using the tuning fork to detect hearing impairment

- Use a tuning fork with frequency of 512 to 1024 cps (Hz).
- Hold the tuning fork firmly at the stem.
- Strike the fork against the palm of your hand, or strike the fork with a rubber reflex hammer, to set it in motion.

Weber test

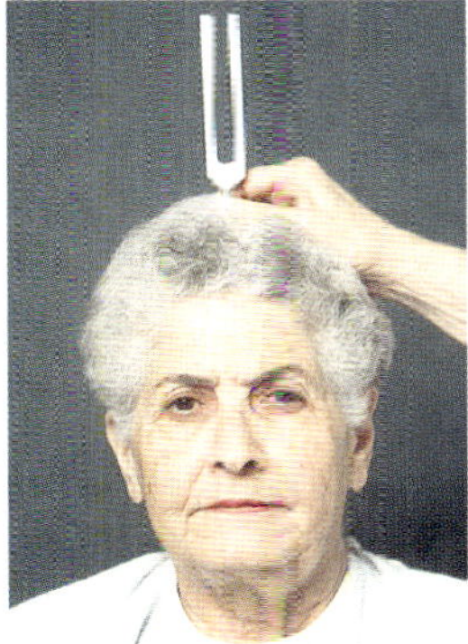

Reprinted with permission from Bickley, L. (2013). *Bates' guide to physical examination and history taking* (11th ed.). Philadelphia: Lippincott Williams & Wilkins.

- **Procedure:** Place the tip of a vibrating tuning fork at the centre of the person's forehead. Ask where they hear the sound and whether it is louder in one ear than in the other.
- **Normal finding:** The sound from the tuning fork is heard equally in both ears.
- **Abnormal finding:** The sound from the tuning fork is heard better in one ear, indicating a possible hearing loss.

Rinne test

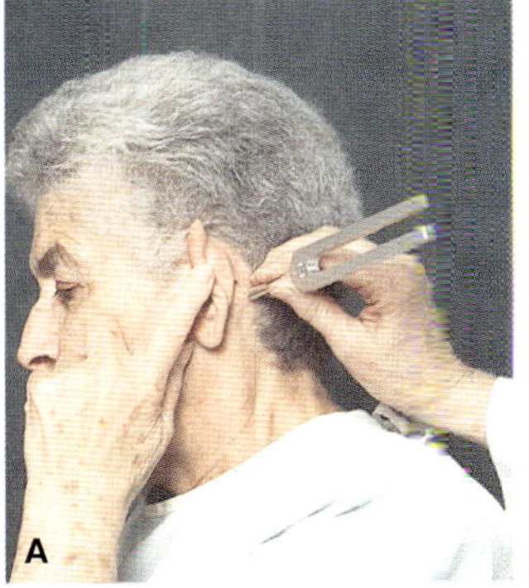

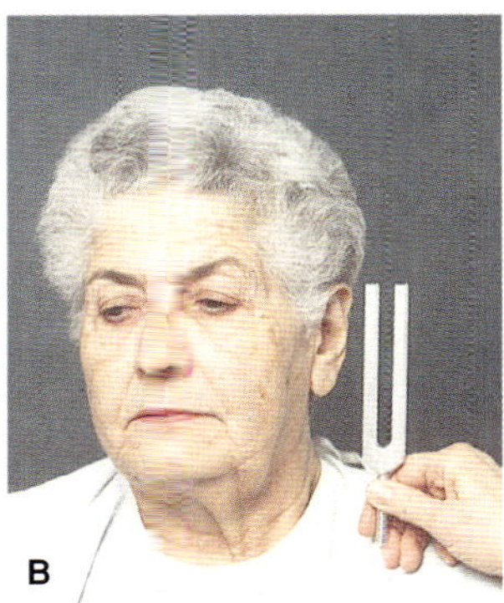

Reprinted with permission from Bickley, L. (2013). *Bates' guide to physical examination and history taking* (11th ed.). Philadelphia: Lippincott Williams & Wilkins.

- **Procedure:** Mask one ear, then place a vibrating tuning fork on the mastoid process of the opposite ear until the person indicates that the sound from the vibrations can no longer be heard. Then, quickly place the tuning fork in front of the ear canal with the top near the ear canal.
- **Normal finding:** The duration the tuning fork vibrations can be heard over the ear canal is approximately twice as long as the time it can be heard over the mastoid bone.
- **Abnormal finding:** The length of time the tuning fork vibrations are heard in front of the ear is shorter than twice as long as the time it can be heard when placed on the mastoid process. In such a case, the person should undergo further tests for impaired hearing.

conducted at a speech and hearing centre or by a specialised doctor, such as an otolaryngologist.

UNFOLDING CASE STUDY

Part C

Recall you are the practice nurse at the local medical centre. You have an appointment with Mr Hilde, who is 69 years old, and his wife. Mrs Hilde is worried about Mr Hilde's hearing.

Thinking points

- Which of the questions and considerations in Boxes 16-2 and 16-3 would you use in assessing Mr Hilde?
- Would you involve Mrs Hilde in any part of the assessment? If so, how would you involve her?
- What health promotion advice would you give Mr Hilde at this time?

NURSING ISSUES

On the basis of the nursing assessment, the nurse might identify an actual hearing deficit or risk factors for impaired hearing. An appropriate nursing issue for an older adult with a hearing impairment would be disturbed sensory perception: auditory. When nurses focus on promoting wellness, one issue that may be pertinent is the person's willingness for enhanced communication, where the exchange of information and ideas can be improved for the older adult.

If psychosocial consequences are identified, other pertinent nursing issues might include anxiety, impaired social interaction and ineffective coping. When the hearing impairment is severe and uncompensated to the point that the person does not function safely, then risk for injury might be an applicable nursing issue.

WELLNESS OPPORTUNITY

Nurses can use the wellness nursing issue of willingness for enhanced communication for older adults who are willing to explore possibilities for improving their hearing through health promotion interventions.

GOAL PLANNING FOR WELLNESS OUTCOMES

When older adults experience impaired hearing or when risk factors threaten hearing wellness, nurses create goals that achieve wellness outcomes as an essential part of the planning process. Goals for hearing deficit can include developing hearing compensation behaviour and improved sensory function—hearing. In addition, the following goals related to hearing are relevant: increasing personal safety behaviour for hearing to reduce the risk of hearing impairment, and reducing loneliness through improved communication ability, social interaction skills and social involvement. Specific interventions to achieve these goals are discussed in the following section.

WELLNESS OPPORTUNITY

Quality of life is a wellness outcome that is achieved through nursing interventions that improve communication for older adults with impaired hearing.

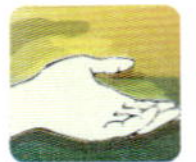

NURSING INTERVENTIONS FOR HEARING WELLNESS

Nursing interventions aim to promote hearing wellness through preventing hearing loss, assisting older adults to compensate for hearing deficits and using communication methods that facilitate optimal communication. Specific interventions to achieve these goals are discussed in detail in the following sections. Nursing interventions include communication enhancement for hearing deficit, ear care and environmental management: safety, health education, health screening, health system guidance and risk identification.

WELLNESS OPPORTUNITY

Nurses can emphasise that even though interventions to prevent hearing loss ideally begin early in life, it is never too late to begin protecting ears from noise.

Promoting hearing wellness for all older adults

For all older adults, nurses can challenge the perception that hearing loss is an inevitable consequence of growing older by teaching about interventions to protect hearing, with emphasis on NIHL. Many older adults engage in recreational or occupational activities that can cause NIHL and may not realise that age-related changes increase their susceptibility to development of hearing loss. Nurses can also teach about the importance of having a hearing screening done by self-assessment (e.g. using the HHIE-S) or by audiometry. Nurses can use Box 16-5 and resources listed at the end of this chapter to teach older adults about health promotion actions they can take to prevent or address hearing loss.

For older adults with modifiable risk factors, such as smoking and the use of ototoxic medication, nurses can focus their health education on alleviating the risks. For example, nurses can teach older adults and their carers about the potential ototoxicity of the medications listed in Box 16-1. This information is particularly important for older adults who have additional risk factors for impaired hearing. When effective medication alternatives are available or when the older adult is experiencing hearing difficulties, efforts should be made to avoid the use of these medications. As with other questions about medication, older adults and their carers should be advised to discuss their concerns about ototoxic medications with their GP.

Nurses can also teach about the interacting effects of two or more risk factors, such as smoking and age-related changes, or medication effects and a genetic predisposition to ototoxicity. People who already experience a mild

BOX 16-5
Health promotion teaching about hearing

Prevention of hearing loss

- Because exposure to loud noise is a major contributing factor to hearing loss, it is important to limit your exposure or use ear protectors that are appropriate to the task (e.g. when mowing the lawn, using equipment with gas or electric motors).
- Because smoking increases the risk of hearing loss, consider this as another reason to quit smoking.

Early detection and treatment of hearing loss

- Because some medications and medical conditions can cause hearing problems, ask your medical practitioner to thoroughly evaluate for these conditions.
- Have your ears checked for impacted wax and talk with your medical practitioner about preventing impacted wax if this has been a problem for you.
- Obtain evaluation at a speech and hearing centre for a hearing aid, assistive hearing device or aural rehabilitation services.
- Consider using an amplifying device (e.g. for phones, radios, doorbells) or sound substitution devices (e.g. flashing lights, closed-captioned television) as might be needed for safety and improved quality of life.
- Take advantage of available assistive listening devices in public places (e.g. churches, theatres, government buildings).

hearing impairment may be motivated to protect their hearing by avoiding hazardous noise and protecting their ears when they are exposed to noise. Similarly, if they are experiencing a hearing loss and recognise that nicotine can be ototoxic, they may be more motivated to stop smoking.

Whenever a nursing assessment identifies a hearing impairment, nursing interventions should focus on a referral for medical and audiology evaluations. Sometimes the nursing interventions also need to address barriers to obtaining a hearing aid, as discussed in the section on hearing aids. Nurses in community or residential settings for older adults may be able to find an audiologist who is willing to provide screening programs at little or no cost. As long as the sponsors of these programs do not have a vested interest in promoting a particular type of hearing aid, they may be effective resources for screening programs.

Preventing and alleviating impacted cerumen

Nurses can promote hearing wellness through interventions and health education aimed at alleviating or preventing hearing impairment caused by impacted wax.

It has been reported that up to 57% of long-term care residents in Australia have received ear syringing for impacted cerumen (Bird, 2008). See Evidence-based practice 16-1 for information on assessment, health promotion and removing impacted cerumen.

Compensating for hearing deficits

Interventions for hearing-impaired people should be considered only after a medical evaluation is performed to identify treatable causes of the hearing loss. An audiologist can then evaluate and more thoroughly determine the best approach for facilitating communication. People who have irreversible hearing deficits and who are interested in corrective measures can be encouraged to participate in an aural rehabilitation program. Individualised aural rehabilitation programs consist of counselling, together with any or all of the following services: amplification devices, auditory training, lip reading and speech skills. These programs are available at hearing centres, which are often affiliated with hospitals and medical centres. Internet resources, such as Australian Hearing and others, can provide information about local resources for the evaluation and treatment of hearing disorders. Nurses play a role in suggesting referrals for aural rehabilitation, discussing such programs with older adults and their carers, and facilitating or encouraging the use of recommended sound amplification devices.

Sound amplification is generally achieved by using hearing aids or assistive listening devices. Hearing aids are individually prescribed and require audiology services, whereas assistive listening devices are not individualised and are available without professional assistance or recommendation. These two types of sound amplification are discussed in the following sections.

Surgical implantation of an electronic device, such as a cochlear implant, may be indicated to compensate for damaged or non-functional parts of the inner ear. Adults who have lost all or most of their hearing later in life are candidates for this type of surgery, but extensive evaluation of the person is necessary to determine the appropriateness of the procedure. As this procedure becomes more common, nurses will be caring for more older adults who have had cochlear implants. One nursing implication is that the implanted devices are not compatible with magnetic resonance imaging (MRI), so nurses need to make sure that MRIs are not ordered for people with cochlear implants.

Sound amplification

Sound amplification is achieved by using hearing aids or assistive listening devices, often in combination. Hearing aids are individually prescribed and require audiology services, whereas assistive listening devices are not individualised and are available without professional assistance or recommendation.

Any device that amplifies or replaces sounds for individual communication or group communication is categorised as an **assistive listening device**, as in the following examples:

- A stethoscope is an assistive listening device commonly used by healthcare workers.
- Megaphones and microphones are used for group communication.
- Closed-captioned televisions substitute visual cues for auditory cues.

EVIDENCE-BASED PRACTICE 16-1
Impacted cerumen

Statement of the problem

- Cerumen is normally expelled from the ear canal by a self-cleaning mechanism, but excessive or impacted cerumen occurs in high-risk populations, which include older adults, people who are cognitively impaired and people who use hearing aids.
- Impacted cerumen, which affects between 19% and 65% of older adults aged 65+ years, is underdiagnosed and undertreated.
- Impacted cerumen can cause hearing loss (ranging from 5 dB to 40 dB); diminished cognitive function; and symptoms such as pain, itching, tinnitus, cough, dizziness and sensation of fullness.
- Cerumen impaction may interfere with hearing aid performance by reducing the intensity of sound, changing the resonance properties of the ears, or causing feedback and poor fitting.
- Cerumen impaction is the cause of damage to 60% to 70% of hearing aids that are sent for repair.
- There are strong data indicating that removal of impacted cerumen can improve hearing.
- Older adults are often unaware they have a cerumen impaction potentially impairing their hearing or that removal of the impaction may improve their hearing; they may even rate their hearing ability as good or fair.

Recommendations for nursing assessment

- Arrange for or perform an otoscopic examination whenever any of the following manifestations occur: hearing loss, ear pain, tinnitus, cough or vertigo.
- Arrange for or perform an otoscopic examination at intervals of 3–12 months for older adults who use hearing aids.

Recommendations for health promotion: Teaching older adults

Teach older adults and carers about the following measures:

- Use the following measures to reduce the risk of developing impacted cerumen: instil ceruminolytic agents prophylactically and have the ear canal irrigated by a healthcare professional.
- Do not insert cotton-tipped applicators or any other foreign object in ear canals.
- Make sure that hearing aids are properly cleaned and cared for.
- If you have an increased risk for cerumen impaction, have your ears cleaned and checked by a qualified healthcare practitioner every 6–12 months.

Recommendations for care

Ceruminolytic agents

- Ceruminolytics are wax-softening agents that disperse the cerumen and reduce the need for other interventions.
- Three types of ceruminolytics are water-based (e.g. water, saline, docusate sodium, hydrogen peroxide, sodium bicarbonate); oil-based (e.g. almond oil, mineral oil, olive oil); and non-water-, non-oil-based (e.g. Debrox, EarClear).
- Studies comparing two or more ceruminolytic agents indicate that any type of ceruminolytic is better than no treatment, but no particular agent is more effective than others.

Aural irrigation

- Irrigating the ear canal with a stream of water is effective in removing impacted cerumen.
- Instillation of ceruminolytic agents 15 minutes or for several days prior to the irrigation improves the success of the treatment.
- Irrigation can be done with an ear syringe or an electronic jet irrigator; oral/dental jet irrigators can be equipped with specially designed tips to prevent overinsertion and direct the water away from the tympanic membrane.
- Medical doctors often delegate the task of aural irrigation to nurses but only if there are no contraindications and the nurse has received training in this intervention.
- Ear irrigation should not be performed on people with a history of ear surgery or those who have any abnormality of the ear canal or a non-intact tympanic membrane; it should be used cautiously in older adults with diabetes.

Manual removal

- Manual removal is the use of an instrument (e.g. ear curettes or probes) by a skilled practitioner to remove the impacted cerumen.

Potentially harmful interventions

- Cotton-tipped swabs should not be used because they can cause further impaction and other complications.
- Home use of oral jet irrigators and cotton-tipped swabs are associated with increased risk of damage to the ear canal.
- Ear candling (also called *ear coning* or *thermo-auricular therapy*) is a commonly used alternative practice for cerumen removal. Research indicates that ear candling is not effective and is associated with considerable risks.

Source: Roland, P. S., Smith, T. L., Schwartz, S. R., Rosenfeld, R. M., Ballachanda, B., Earll, J. M., … Wetmore, S. (2008). Clinical practice guideline: Cerumen impaction. *Otolaryngology—Head and Neck Surgery, 139*, S1–S21.

- A personal listening system, which consists of a small, battery-powered amplifier and headphones, can be used easily in any setting.
- A small amplifying device can be attached to a telephone receiver.
- Some mobile phones are designed to accommodate people who use hearing aids or need amplification. Visual stimuli, such as flashing lights, can be used as a signal for a doorbell.
- Vibratory stimuli can be used as a substitute for an alarm clock.

The advantages of assistive listening devices over hearing aids include lower cost (usually) and the ability to share a device among several people. In addition, these devices are less intrusive than hearing aids and do not require as much manual dexterity. Assistive listening devices can be used alone or with hearing aids. Figure 16-4 shows several examples of devices that can be used to enhance communication with someone who is hard of hearing.

Nurses can teach older adults and their carers about using assistive listening devices as a substitute for or as an adjunct to hearing aids. For example, people may not realise

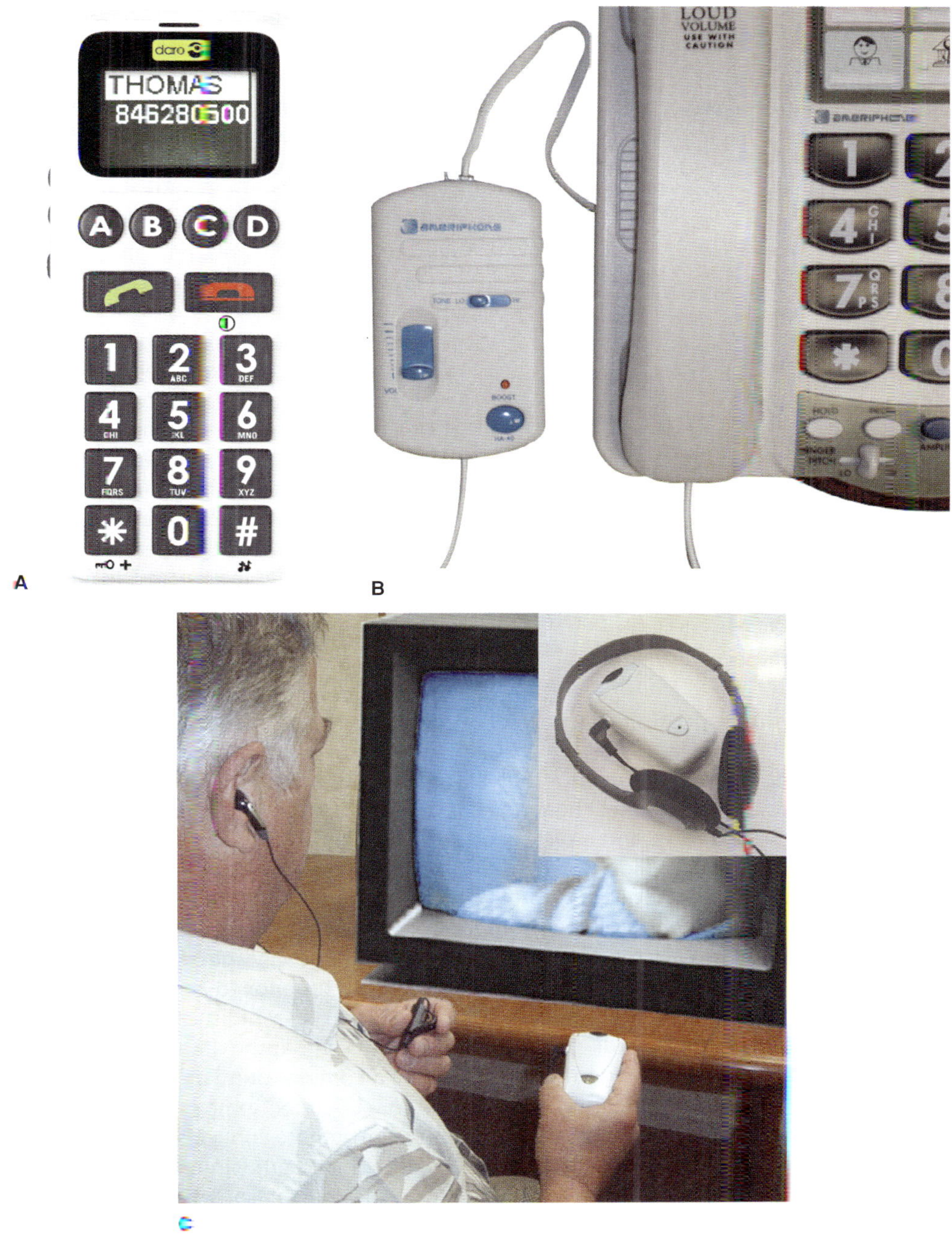

FIGURE 16-4 (**A**) Mobile phone with amplification, large keypad, two-way speakerphone, and vibrating ringer alert. (**B**) Easy-to-use in-line phone amplifier. (**C**) Personal sound amplifier with volume control, swivelling microphone, and lightweight ear-bud headphones. (Courtesy of ActiveForever.com.)

that since 1990, all televisions with screens 13″ or larger are required to include a closed-caption option, and this feature is available for many programs. Many public places, including churches, theatres and government buildings, provide portable assistive listening devices, and hearing-impaired people can ask about the availability of such a device.

Hearing aids

A **hearing aid** is a battery-operated device that consists of an amplifier, a microphone and a receiver. Hearing aids can be classified by size, location worn and technology. The largest are approximately the size of a deck of cards and are worn on the body, whereas the new, smaller types fit completely in the ear canal. These smaller types can be seen only with close inspection of the ear and have a nylon string attached for insertion and removal. Some preferred hearing aid locations include in-the-ear, in-the-canal and completely in-the-canal (Figure 16-5). Body-worn and behind-the-ear hearing aids have become much less popular in recent years because of the availability of smaller,

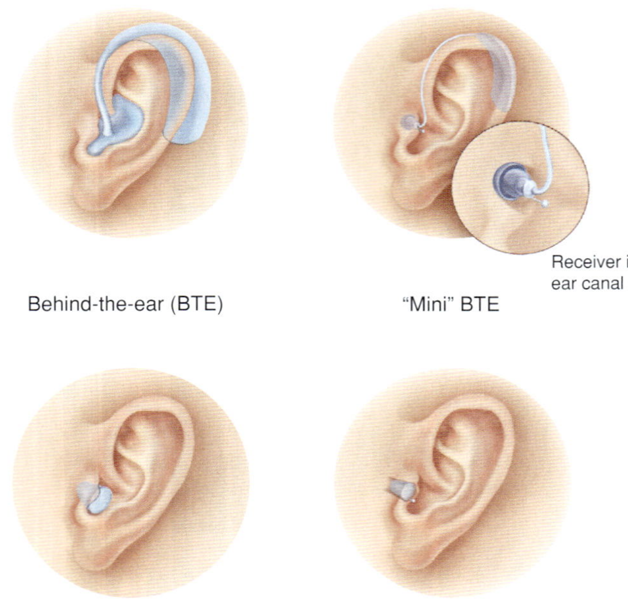

FIGURE 16-5 Examples of four types of hearing aids.

more powerful hearing aids made possible by newer technology.

Until recently, the amplifying power of a hearing aid was strongly associated with its size because most hearing aids used the same type of technology and severely impaired people needed larger, body-worn aids. However, new technology has made available a variety of types of hearing aids that can be programmed and adjusted for individual differences. Currently, the effectiveness of a hearing aid is associated more with the type of technology used than with its size. Hearing aids are classified by whether they are analogue or digital and according to the degree of individualised adjustments or programming possible. As discussed later, the cost of hearing aids increases as the programming becomes more adjustable and individualised.

Conventional, or traditional, hearing aids use analogue technology to amplify sound but they do not correct distortions. These aids are the simplest type and are adjusted by the manufacturer on the basis of an evaluation by an audiologist. Although the person wearing the aid can adjust its volume and the audiologist can make some minor adjustments, the aid becomes less effective as the person's hearing changes and may need to be replaced if the hearing loss progresses. Because analogue aids amplify all sounds equally, they tend to be unsatisfactory for people who have only a mild high-frequency hearing loss and may be more beneficial to people with impairments at multiple frequencies. This characteristic also makes analogue aids difficult to use in noisy environments, but older adults may find that they are satisfactory in quiet situations and one-on-one conversations.

Nurses may need to encourage the selective use of analogue aids in their appropriate environments. These aids are the least expensive type, costing hundreds rather than thousands of dollars. In Australia, cost is not as important a consideration as in New Zealand. Australia has a comprehensive community-based service, which is free for those aged 65 and over and who are eligible for a government pension (Australian Hearing, 2014). About 50% of the clients receiving services from Australian Hearing are 80 years and over.

However, cost is an important consideration for older Australians who are not eligible for a pension. If the older person has private health insurance, this will assist with costs. Out-of-pocket expenses depend on the type and level of private health insurance. The New Zealand Ministry of Health (2014) provides some funding towards the cost of hearing aids for older people in New Zealand, but not for the hearing assessment, fitting fee or the cost of repairs and batteries. The New Zealand Ministry of Health provides a booklet, Guide to getting hearing aids: Hearing aid subsidy scheme, available via www.health.govt.nz. A variation of the conventional hearing aid is the recently developed disposable hearing aid, which lasts for approximately 30 to 40 days. They were developed for people with a mild to moderate hearing loss and are about as effective as other analogue hearing aids. Because they are not customised, they may not fit as well and are more likely to be associated with discomfort or feedback problems. These aids are available in the U.S. but are not yet available in Australia or New Zealand.

Programmable analogue hearing aids are more advanced than conventional hearing aids because they are selectively programmed to meet the needs of a hearing-impaired person. A major advantage of these hearing aids is they are acoustically superior to conventional models and can be adjusted for different listening situations. Some programmable aids can automatically adjust their volume to the level of incoming sound by making soft sounds louder and loud sounds softer. Some programmable aids are equipped with a tiny remote control device, so that the user can conveniently make adjustments for different environments. Remote devices are sometimes built into a wristwatch. Disadvantages include the need to train the wearer, the cost of up to several thousand dollars and the need for frequent adjustments by the hearing healthcare professional.

Digital hearing aids use the most advanced technology and cost significantly more than the analogue hearing aid. The digital aids are the most flexible for individual needs because the audiologist uses a computer to program the aid to amplify specific frequencies for each person's hearing loss. The digital technology examines the incoming sounds and adapts the amplification without adding noise or distortion. In addition, some of these aids have directional microphones, enabling them to collect sounds from two directions and allowing the wearer to adjust the directionality. These aids can be programmed for different listening environments and the wearer can use a remote control device to adjust the aid for various listening situations. The only disadvantage of these aids is their high cost, which is at least several thousand dollars.

Despite the major improvements in hearing aids in the last decade, only approximately 20% of people who could benefit from a hearing aid actually use one. Nurses can address negative attitudes and have a positive effect on the use of hearing aids by helping older adults to explore the many options for amplification and by encouraging them to obtain accurate information from audiologists and reputable organisations listed in the resources section at the end of this chapter.

Nurses can encourage older adults and their families to obtain initial information about hearing aids from consumer and healthcare organisations, rather than primarily from a hearing aid dealer who sells only one kind of device. Many websites provide objective information about the various types of hearing aids and some of these are listed in the resources section at the end of the chapter.

If transportation limitations are problematic for an older person who is otherwise receptive to obtaining a hearing aid, nursing interventions can be aimed at identifying community resources to address this issue.

In addition to the high cost of hearing aids, common barriers to obtaining and using them are the high levels of manual dexterity, fine motor movement and good vision required to adjust the volume and other controls and to change batteries. Many of these barriers can be addressed by selecting the most appropriate hearing aid and by working closely with the audiologist to identify ways of simplifying the process.

Nurses who work with older adults in residential care settings can teach about the most effective use of hearing aids in different circumstances. For example, the older adult can be encouraged to use the aid for one-on-one conversations but to remove it in the dining area or other large social areas where there is much background noise. Nurses promote realistic expectations with regard to hearing aids by explaining that hearing aids do not restore normal hearing but do improve communication and the quality of life. Nurses also need to work with carers to provide additional support during the initial adjustment period.

Although it is impossible to know about all the available hearing aids, nurses need to keep up to date on various types and their implications for older adults. For example, it is important for nurses to know whether a person has an analogue or a digital hearing aid, because the person with an analogue aid may not be willing to use it in settings where background noise is problematic. It is also important for nurses to know whether the person has a remote control device for the hearing aid, so the nurse can assist with adjusting the settings and give special attention to keeping track of the device.

Nurses must be familiar enough with hearing aids to assist older adults and their carers with their use and care. Although nurses can expect that the initial hearing-aid use and care instructions will be given by the hearing aid provider, these instructions may have to be reviewed or revamped as dependency needs and carer roles change. Older adults who normally depend on family members for assistance with their hearing aid may not be able to use and care for it properly when they are in a hospital or nursing home. Likewise, nurses in home settings may have to teach carers about hearing aids if the older adult needs assistance that was not previously provided by that carer. This situation is likely to arise if the carer changes or if the older adult becomes more dependent because of increased functional impairment. Box 16-6 summarises the teaching points related to the use and care of hearing aids.

BOX 16-6
Use and care of hearing aids

Guidelines for insertion and use

- With the volume of the device turned off and the canal portion pointing into the ear, insert the hearing aid.
- Make sure the aid fits snugly in the ear canal.
- The M, T and O settings designate microphone, telephone and off, respectively.
- Turn the M-T-O switch to M.
- Turn the volume up slowly, beginning at a third to a half volume until a comfortable level is reached.
- If whistling (feedback) occurs, check the position of the device in the ear and the volume. The aid may not fit snugly enough, or the volume may be too high.
- Begin wearing the aid for short periods in a familiar and quiet environment and in one-on-one conversations.
- Gradually increase the duration the aid is worn, the variety of environments and the number of people included in conversations.
- Allow several months before expecting to feel totally comfortable with the hearing aid.
- Avoid noisy environments and eliminate background noise when possible (e.g. turn off televisions and radios; close doors to rooms).
- Use the appropriate setting (T) for telephone calls.
- Understand that hearing aids do not restore hearing to normal, but rather amplify sound, including all environmental noises.

Guidelines for care and maintenance

- Keep a fresh battery available (batteries can be expected to last for 70–85 hours), but do not purchase batteries more than 1 month in advance.
- Turn off the hearing aid before changing the battery.
- Remove the battery or turn off the aid when not in use.
- Clean the aid as per manufacturer's directions.
- Never use alcohol on the earmold because this will cause drying and cracking.
- Check the earmold for cracks or scratches.
- Avoid extreme heat, cold or moisture (e.g. do not leave the hearing aid near the stove; do not wear it while using a hair dryer and do not wear it outside in rainy or extremely cold weather unless it is protected well).
- Avoid exposure to chemicals, such as hairspray or permanent solutions.
- Avoid dropping the aid on a hard surface; when handling it, keep it over a soft or padded surface.

Auditory rehabilitation

Auditory rehabilitation (also called aural, hearing or audiological rehabilitation or rehab) refers to the services that improve communication for people who are hearing impaired. Auditory rehabilitation programs provide the following services: counselling, education, amplification aids, communication methods, and management of the environment. Studies indicate that, although auditory rehabilitation programs can improve cognitive and social function in older adults, the rates of utilisation and compliance are very low (Li-Korotky, 2012; Parham, Lin, Coelho et al., 2013). Nurses play an important role in discussing such programs with older adults and their carers and suggesting referrals for auditory rehabilitation. Speech and hearing centres are good sources of information about auditory rehabilitation programs. Information is also available through Internet resources located at the end of the chapter in the health education section.

WELLNESS OPPORTUNITY

Nurses promote self-care by providing educational brochures about the types and benefits of amplification devices and encouraging older adults to ask their GP about an audiology referral.

Surgical interventions

Cochlear implants have been used for several decades, but the criteria for this type of intervention have been narrow. In recent years there have been remarkable developments in inner- and middle-ear implants and bone-conduction hearing devices as interventions for hearing loss. These developments have been accompanied by expanded criteria for surgical interventions, which are increasingly being used for hearing-impaired older adults. A recent review of data from 12 years of cochlear implants in adults aged 60 years and older found that this intervention consistently improved speech understanding scores. Older adults who were younger at implantation and had higher preoperative speech scores derived the greatest benefit (Lin, Chien, Li et al., 2012). Based on current evidence, it is important to encourage older adults to explore options for surgical interventions when hearing loss is not adequately improved with other interventions.

When older adults have surgically implanted hearing devices, it is important to find out if an external component is attached to the body, inserted in the ear, or kept close to the body. When this is the case, nurses document information in the person's chart and also assist with keeping track of all components. Another nursing implication is that some implanted hearing devices are affected by or interfere with magnetic resonance imaging (MRI), so it is essential to obtain information about their compatibility if an MRI is being considered.

Communicating with hearing-impaired older adults

Good communication techniques are essential in assisting older adults to compensate for any hearing deficits. The primary functional consequence of presbycusis is a diminished acuity for high-frequency sounds, which is exacerbated by fast-paced speech and environmental noise. Therefore, most communication interventions are directed towards improving the clarity of words, slowing the rate of speech and eliminating environmental noise and distractions. Verbal techniques that enhance auditory communication should be augmented by non-verbal techniques, such as body language and written communication, as described in Box 16-7. Nurses can apply these techniques and use this box for teaching carers how to improve communication with hearing-impaired people. In recent years, increased attention has been directed towards planning or modifying environments to diminish background noise and to improve the ability of people to hear. Although some noise-control modifications such as curtains are relatively simple and can be applied to many settings, other measures, such as the selection of building materials, need to be implemented while environments are being designed.

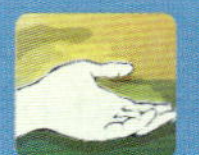

BOX 16-7
Techniques for communicating with hearing-impaired people

- Stand or sit directly in front of, and close to, the person.
- Talk toward the better ear, but make sure your lips can be seen.
- Make sure the person pays attention and looks at your face.
- Address the person by name, pause, and then begin talking.
- Speak distinctly, slowly, and directly to the person.
- Do not exaggerate lip movements because this will interfere with lip reading.
- Avoid chewing gum, covering your mouth, or turning your head away.
- If the person does not understand, repeat the message using different words.
- Avoid or eliminate any background noise.
- Do not raise the volume of your voice; rather, try to lower the tone while still speaking in a moderately loud voice.
- Keep all instructions simple and ask for feedback to assess what the person heard.
- Avoid questions that elicit simple yes or no answers.
- Keep sentences short.
- Use body language that is congruent with what you are trying to communicate.
- Demonstrate what you are saying.
- Use large-print written communication and pictures to supplement verbal communication.
- Make sure only one person talks at a time; arrange for one-on-one communication whenever possible.
- If eyeglasses normally are worn to improve vision, make sure they are clean.
- Provide adequate lighting so that the person can see your lips; avoid settings in which there is glare behind or around you.

UNFOLDING CASE STUDY

Part D

Mr Hilde is now 83 years old and has been a widower for 1 year. He has given up woodworking because he developed Parkinson's disease 11 years ago and cannot manage the necessary fine motor movements. He continues to fish seasonally, play poker monthly and smoke one pack of cigarettes per day. In addition to Parkinson's disease, he has hypertension and coronary artery disease. He still lives in his own home and attends a senior centre for meals and social activities three times a week. His hearing loss has progressed to the point that he has difficulty with phone conversations and has to turn the television up loud. He cannot hear the doorbell. At the senior centre, participants avoid conversations with him because he has difficulty hearing.

You are the practice nurse at the local medical centre where Mr Hilde visits regularly. At one visit, he tells you that his daughter is upset with him because he never answers his phone when she calls, and she cannot have a decent phone conversation with him. She lives in another state and worries about him. She has offered to pay for a hearing aid evaluation for him, but he has told her, "Those things stick out like a sore thumb and they don't do any good, anyway. I can hear anything I want to hear and there's a lot I don't care to hear, so why should you spend a lot of money for something that I won't use?" He asks your opinion about this and is wondering whether he should at least get a checkup to pacify his daughter. He expects he will be told that nothing can be done and that his daughter will have to be satisfied with the situation.

Thinking points

- Which information in Box 16-2 would be most pertinent to obtain at this time?
- What myths and misunderstandings influence Mr Hilde?
- What nursing issues would you apply to Mr Hilde?
- Which information in Box 16-5 would be pertinent to this situation?
- What health promotion teaching would you do to address Mr Hilde's resistance to having his hearing evaluated?
- What additional health promotion advice would you give?
- Because you usually see Mr Hilde weekly, you can develop a long-term teaching plan. How would you establish priorities for immediate and long-term goals?

EVALUATING THE EFFECTIVENESS OF NURSING INTERVENTIONS

Nurses observe the compensatory behaviours of hearing-impaired older adults to evaluate the effectiveness of interventions for the nursing issue of disturbed sensory perception: auditory. The following are indicators of successful interventions:

- Improved ability to communicate
- Effective use of hearing aids and amplification devices
- Increased participation in social activities
- Environmental modifications to eliminate background noise
- Appropriate participation in aural rehabilitation program.

Evaluation of effectiveness of interventions varies in different healthcare settings. For example, nurses in short-term settings provide health education as part of a discharge plan that includes information about resources for hearing evaluations. Evaluation of the effectiveness of this intervention is based on the person's positive response to the nurse's suggestions, but the nurse is not likely to know whether the person followed through with the referral and had beneficial outcomes. In home, community and long-term residential care settings, nurses address long-term goals by facilitating referrals for audiology services. In these settings, the evaluation of interventions is based on the person's use of additional resources to improve communication abilities.

UNFOLDING CASE STUDY

Part E

Mr Hilde is an 89-year-old widower who has had Parkinson's disease for 17 years. Presbycusis is listed as an additional diagnosis on his medical record. He is being admitted to long-term residential care because his condition has declined to the point that his daughter, Ms Davis, can no longer manage his care in her home, where he has lived for several years. He is medically stable but needs assistance in all activities of daily living.

Nursing assessment

During the admission interview, you notice that Mr Hilde has difficulty hearing your questions and he frequently asks his daughter to give the requested information. He shows no significant cognitive deficits, but he seems to have difficulty understanding verbal communication. When you ask about any hearing impairment, Ms Davis tells you that her father has used hearing aids for 5 years and has been re-evaluated periodically at a hearing centre. Two months ago, he obtained new hearing aids, but wears them only for one-on-one conversations with her. Because of Mr Hilde's tremors and difficulty with fine motor movements, Ms Davis cares for his hearing aids and assists with their insertion and removal.

Ms Davis has encouraged her father to wear his hearing aids during family gatherings, but he says the noise from small children is too annoying. Except for family gatherings, Mr Hilde has very few opportunities for social interaction, and he has become more and more withdrawn. He used to enjoy playing poker, but has not played for several years because all of his friends have died. Now he spends much of his time watching closed-captioned television programs. Ms Davis hopes that her father will respond to the opportunities for social interaction provided at the nursing home and that his quality of life will improve.

Nursing issues

In addition to nursing issues related to Mr Hilde's chronic illness and self-care deficits, you identify impaired social interaction related to the effects of hearing loss. You select this rather than disturbed sensory perception: auditory because Mr Hilde's hearing impairment has already been evaluated and sound amplification devices are available to him.

Nursing care plan for Mr Hilde

In your care plan, you address the psychosocial consequences of Mr Hilde's hearing impairment. Your nursing care is directed towards improving his social interaction through the use of available devices and through other communication techniques that will enhance his social interaction skills.

Goals for wellness outcomes	Nursing interventions	Nursing evaluation
Mr Hilde will develop effective communication techniques for resident–staff interactions	• During the initial interview, talk with Mr Hilde and Ms Davis about the importance of good verbal communication with staff; emphasise the need for the staff to get to know Mr Hilde so his needs can be addressed. • Ask Mr Hilde to wear his hearing aids during all one-on-one interactions with staff. • Use good communication techniques when talking with Mr Hilde (as in Box 16-7). • Make sure all staff members provide appropriate assistance with the insertion and removal of Mr Hilde's hearing aids. • Include hearing aid maintenance as part of the daily responsibilities of the nursing aide.	• Mr Hilde wears his hearing aids during all one-on-one conversations with staff. • Mr Hilde reports satisfactory verbal interactions with the staff. • Mr Hilde's hearing aids are maintained in good operating condition.
Mr Hilde will engage in social interaction with one other resident.	• During the initial care plan conference, identify several other residents who might converse with Mr Hilde. • Ask the staff to encourage one-on-one conversations between Mr Hilde and the selected resident (e.g. suggest that they watch closed-captioned television programs together). • Ask Mr Hilde to wear his hearing aids during one-on-one interactions with residents. • Provide assistance with inserting and removing hearing aids as needed. • Provide a quiet environment for one-on-one conversations with other residents.	• Mr Hilde wears his hearing aids at least once daily for a conversation with one other resident.
Mr Hilde will engage in small group activities with other residents.	• During the first monthly care review conference, ask the activities staff to invite Mr Hilde to a poker game with three other residents in the small-group room. • Make sure that environmental noise is controlled as much as possible.	• By the second month in this facility, Mr Hilde participates in weekly poker games with three other residents.

Thinking points

- What nursing responsibilities would you have with regard to addressing Mr Hilde's hearing impairment? How would you work with other staff to implement the care plan described in the concluding case example?
- What are some of the advantages and disadvantages of hearing aids in a long-term residential care setting? How would you address the disadvantages?
- How would you involve Ms Davis in the care plan to address Mr Hilde's hearing impairment?
- If Mr Hilde were in an acute care setting, how would you address his hearing problem?

CHAPTER HIGHLIGHTS

Age-related changes that affect hearing

- External ear: thicker hair, thinner skin, increased keratin
- Middle ear: less resilient tympanic membrane, calcified ossicles, stiffer muscles and ligaments
- Inner ear and auditory nervous system: fewer neurons and hair cells, diminished blood supply, degeneration of spiral ganglion and central processing systems

Risk factors that affect hearing wellness

- Lifestyle and environmental factors: smoking, background noise, exposure to noise or toxic chemicals
- Genetic predisposition to otosclerosis
- Impacted cerumen
- Ototoxic medications: aminoglycosides, aspirin, loop diuretics, quinine
- Disease processes: diabetes, Paget's disease, Ménière's disease

Functional consequences affecting hearing wellness

- Presbycusis: diminished ability to hear high-pitched sounds, especially in the presence of background noise
- Predisposition to impacted cerumen
- Psychosocial consequences: depression, social isolation, declines in cognitive function, diminished quality of life
- Increased risk of hearing disorders

Pathological condition affecting hearing

- Tinnitus: persistent sensation of noises that do not originate in the external environment

Nursing assessment of hearing

- Screening tool: the Hearing Handicap Inventory for the Elderly
- Past and present risk factors (e.g. use of ototoxic medications, noise exposure, family history of otosclerosis)
- Attitudes about hearing aids if impairment is present
- Impact of hearing impairment on communication and quality of life
- Behavioural cues to impaired hearing
- Otoscopic examination for impacted cerumen
- Tuning fork tests for hearing

Nursing issues

- Willingness for enhanced communication
- Disturbed sensory perception: auditory
- Additional issues that address the functional consequences of impaired hearing are: impaired communication, anxiety, impaired adjustment, impaired social interaction, ineffective individual coping and risk for injury

Goal planning for wellness outcomes

- Improved communication
- Increased social interactions
- Improved quality of life
- Increased safety and functioning

Nursing interventions for hearing wellness

- Teaching about interventions to address modifiable risk factors: smoking, exposure to noise, use of ototoxic medications
- Removing and preventing impacted cerumen
- Promoting referrals for audiology services
- Using assistive listening devices
- Teaching about the use and care of a hearing aid
- Communicating with hearing-impaired older adults
- Compensating for hearing deficit by using hearing devices and hearing aids

Evaluating effectiveness of nursing interventions

- Improved communication
- Use of appropriate amplification aids
- Appropriate environmental modifications
- Increased participation in social activities

CRITICAL THINKING EXERCISES

1. Describe presbycusis and explain the functional consequences of this condition as it affects the everyday life of an older adult.
2. What risk factors would you consider in an 83-year-old person who complains of recent problems with hearing?
3. What advice would you give to someone who asks you about a brochure she received from a hearing aid company that offers free hearing screenings describing a new high-powered hearing aid? The person has trouble hearing but has never had an evaluation.
4. Describe at least 10 ways in which you can adapt your communication for a hearing-impaired person.
5. Find at least one resource (*not* a hearing aid dealer) in your community that you could recommend to an older adult who needs a hearing evaluation.
6. Visit at least three Internet sites that provide educational materials about hearing impairment and choose the one you think would be best for obtaining health information brochures.

RESOURCES

For an extensive range of additional resources to enhance teaching and learning and to facilitate understanding of this chapter, please see the text's accompanying website located on thePoint at http://thepoint.lww.com.

Clinical tools

Hartford Institute for Geriatric Nursing http://consultgerirn.org/resources

General assessment series:

- *Try This*, issue 12: Hearing screening in older adults: A brief hearing loss screener. Demers, K. (2012). *Best Practices in Nursing Care to Older Adults.*

Evidence-based practice

Adams-Wendling, L. & Pimple, C. (2008). Evidence-based guideline: Nursing management of hearing impairment in nursing facility residents. *Journal of Gerontological Nursing, 34*(11), 9–17.

Cacchione, P. Z. (2012). Sensory changes. In M. Boltz, E. Capezuti, T. Fulmer & D. Zwicker (Eds), *Evidence-based geriatric nursing protocols for best practice* (4th ed. pp. 48–73). New York: Springer.

Australian Indigenous Health*InfoNet*, ear health: www.healthinfonet.ecu.edu.au/other-health-conditions/ear

Joanna Briggs Institute: http://connect.jbiconnectplus.org

Consumer information sheet:

- Schneller, L. E. (2010). Ear wax/drops.

Evidence summaries:

- Campbell, J. (2014). Dual sensory loss (older people): Mental health.
- Chu, V. (2014a). Ear irrigation.
- Chu, V. (2014b). Ear syringing.
- Chu, V. (2014c). Ear wax: Aural toilet.
- Chu, V. (2014d). Hearing aids.
- Dao Le, L. K. (2014). Hearing loss: Screening (people with dementia).

Recommended practices:

- Ear irrigation (electronic irrigator) (2013).
- Ear syringing (2013).
- Ear toilet (2014).
- Hearing aids: Care and maintenance (2013).
- Hearing aids: Insertion and troubleshooting (2013).

National Guideline Clearinghouse: www.guideline.gov/index.aspx

Search for: Hearing loss/impairment

- Evaluation and management of obstructing cerumen (2007).
- Hearing impairment in nursing facility residents (2007).
- Screening for hearing loss in older adults: U.S. Preventive Services Task Force recommendation statement (revised 2012).

Health education

Australian Hearing: www.hearing.com.au

Australian Indigenous Health*InfoNet*, ear health: www.healthinfonet.ecu.edu.au/other-health-conditions/ear

Better Hearing Australia: www.betterhearingaustralia.org.au

Deaf Aotearoa New Zealand: www.deaf.org.nz

Hearing Association New Zealand: www.hearing.org.nz

Hearing Loss Association of America (formerly Self Help for Hard of Hearing People): www.hearingloss.org

International Hearing Society: www.ihsinfo.org

National Foundation for the deaf: www.nfd.org.nz

National Institute on Deafness and Other Communication Disorders: www.nidcd.nih.gov

REFERENCES

Access Economics. (2006). Listen Hear! The Economic Impact and Cost of Hearing Loss in Australia. Report commissioned by the Cooperative Research Centre for Cochlear Implant and Hearing Aid Innovation and Victorian Deaf Society. Accessed February 2015 at www.audiology.asn.au/public/1/files/Publications/ListenHearFinal.pdf.

Adobamen, P. R. & Ogisi, F. O. (2012). Hearing loss due to wax impaction. *Nigerian Quarterly Journal of Hospital Medicine, 22*(2), 117–120.

Australian Hearing. (2014). Health professionals. Available February 2015 at www.hearing.com.au/category/healthprofessionals.

Bainbridge, K. E., Hoffman, H. J. & Cowie, C. C. (2008). Diabetes and hearing impairment in the United States: Audiometric evidence from the National Health and Nutrition Examination Survey, 1999–2004. *Annals of Internal Medicine, 149*(1), 1–10.

Bickley, L. (2013). *Bates' guide to physical examination and history taking* (11th ed.). Philadelphia: Lippincott Williams & Wilkins.

Bird, S. (2008). Ear syringing: Minimising the risks. *Australian Family Physician, 37*(4), 359–360.

Ciorba, A., Bianchini, C., Pelucchi, S. et al. (2012). The impact of hearing loss on quality of life of elderly adults. *Clinical Interventions in Aging, 7*, 159–163.

Dobie, R. A. (2008). The burden of age-related and occupational noise-induced hearing loss in the United States. *Ear and Hearing, 29*(4), 565–577.

Dube, J. A., Barth, M. M., Cmiel, C. A., Cutshall, S. M., Olson, S. M., Sulla, S. J., . . . Holland, D. E. (2008). Environmental noise sources and interventions to minimize them: A tale of 2 hospitals. *Journal of Nursing Care Quarterly, 23*(3), 216–224.

Fabry, D. A., Davila, E. P., Arheart, K. L. et al. (2011). Secondhand smoke exposure and the risk of hearing loss. *Tobacco Control, 20*(1), 82–85.

Gates, G. A., Feeney, M. P. & Mills, D. (2008). Cross-sectional age-changes of hearing in the elderly. *Ear and Hearing, 29*(6), 865–874.

Gopinath, B., Schneider, J., McMahon, C. M. et al. (2012). Severity of age-related hearing loss is associated with impaired activities of daily living. *Age & Ageing, 41*(2), 195–200.

Hawkins, K., Bottone, F. G., Ozminkowski, R. J. et al. (2012). The prevalence of hearing impairment and its burden on the quality of life among adults with Medicare Supplement insurance. *Quality of Life Research, 21*(7), 1135–1147.

Helfer, T. M., Canham-Chervak, M., Canada, S. & Michener, T. A. (2010). Epidemiology of hearing impairment and noise-induced hearing injury among U.S. military personnel, 2003–2005. *American Journal of Preventive Medicine, 38*(Suppl. 1), S71–S77.

Hidalgo, J. L.-T., Gras, C. B., Lapeira, J. T., Verdejo, M.-A. L., del Campo del Campo, J. M., Rabadán, F. E. (2009). Functional status of elderly people with hearing loss. *Archives of Gerontology and Geriatrics, 49*, 88–92.

Jansen, E. J., Hellerman, H. W., Dreschler, W. A. & deLaat, J. A. (2009). Noise induced hearing loss and other hearing complaints among musicians of symphony orchestras. *International Archives of Occupational and Environmental Health, 82*(2), 153–164.

Jupiter, T. (2012). Cognition and screening for hearing loss in nursing home residents. *Journal of the American Medical Directors Association, 13*(8), 744–747.

Karimi, A., Nasiri, S., Kazerooni, F. K. & Oliaei, M. (2010). Noise induced hearing loss risk assessment in truck drivers. *Noise and Health, 12*(46), 49–55.

Kiely, K. M., Gopinath, B., Mitchell, P. et al. (2012). Cognitive, health, and sociodemographic predictors of longitudinal decline in hearing acuity among older adults. *Journals of Gerontology: Medical Sciences, 67*(9), 997–1003.

Kim, M. G., Hong, S. M., Shim, H. J., Cha, C. I. & Yeo, S. G. (2009). Hearing threshold of Korean adolescents associated with the use of personal music players. *Yonsei Medical Journal, 50*(6), 771–776.

Kozak, A. T. & Grundfast, K. M. (2009). Hearing loss. *Otolaryngology Clinics of North America, 42*, 79–85.

Levy, B. R., Slade, M. D. & Gill, T. M. (2006). Hearing decline predicted by elders' stereotypes. *Journals of Gerontology: Series B, Psychological Sciences and Social Sciences, 61*, P82–P87.

Li-Korotky, H-S. (2012). Age-related hearing loss: Quality of care for quality of life. *Gerontologist, 52*(2), 265–271.

Lin, F. R. (2011). Hearing loss and cognition among older adults in the United States. *Journals of Gerontology: Medical Sciences, 66A*(10), 1113–1135.

Lin, F. R., Chien, W. W., Li, L. et al. (2012). Cochlear implantation in older adults. *Medicine, 91*(5), 229–241.

Lin, F. R., Yaffe, K., Xia, J. et al. (2013). Hearing loss and cognitive decline in older adults. *Journal of the American Medical Association Internal Medicine, 21*, 1–7.

Mahboubi, H., Zardouz, S., Oliaei, S. et al. (2013). Noise-induced hearing threshold shift among US adults and implications for noise-induced hearing loss: National Health and Nutrition Examination Surveys. *European Archives of Otorhinolaryngology, 270*(2), 461–470.

McCarter, D. F., Courtney, A. U. & Pollart, S. M. (2007). Cerumen impaction. *American Academy of Family Physicians, 75*, 1523–1528, 1530.

McCullagh, M. & Robertson, C. (2009). Too late smart: Farmers' adoption of self-protective behaviours in response to exposure to hazardous noise. *American Association of Occupational Health Nurses Journal, 57*(3), 99–105.

McMahon, C. M., Kifley, A., Rochtchina, E., Bewall, P. & Mitchell, P. (2008). The contribution of family history of hearing loss in an older population. *Ear and Hearing, 29*(4), 578–584.

Mondelli, M. F. & de Souza, P. J. (2012). Quality of life in elderly adults before and after hearing aid fitting. *Brazilian Journal of Otorhinolaryngology, 78*(3), 49–56.

Montano, J. (2007). An advocate for self-assessment: Barbara Weinstein. *ASHA Leader, 12*(14), 42–43.

Muluk, N. B. & Oguztürk, O. (2008). Occupational noise-inducted tinnitus: Does it affect workers' quality of life? *Journal of Otolaryngology: Head and Neck Surgery, 37*(1), 65–71.

New Zealand Ministry of Health. (2006). *Older people's health chart book 2006*. Wellington: Author. Available February 2015 at www.health.govt.nz/system/files/documents/publications/older-peoples-health-chart-book-2006-new.pdf.

New Zealand Ministry of Health. (2014). Guide to getting hearing aids: Hearing aid funding scheme. Accessed February 2015 at www.health.govt.nz/publication/guide-getting-hearing-aids-hearing-aid-funding-scheme.

Parham, K., Lin, F. R., Coelho, D. H. et al. (2013). Comprehensive management of presbycusis: Central and peripheral. *Otolaryngology—Head & Neck Surgery, 148*(4), 537–539.

Roland, P. S., Smith, T. L., Schwartz, S. R., Rosenfeld, R. M., Ballachanda, B., Earll, J. M. . . . Wetmore, S. (2008). Clinical practice guideline: Cerumen impaction. *Otolaryngology—Head and Neck Surgery, 139*, S1–S21.

Shulman, A. & Goldstein, B. (2009). Subjective idiopathic tinnitus and palliative care: A plan for diagnosis and treatment. *Otolaryngologlocal Clinics of North America, 42*, 15–37.

Taylor, K. S. & Jurma, W. E. (2003, 3 November). Gender-specific audiologic rehabilitation programs and self-perception of handicap in the elderly. *Audiology Online*. Viewed February 2015 at www.audiologyonline.com/articles/gender-specific-audiologic-rehabilitation-programs-1109 and www.audiologyonline.com/articles/article_detail.asp?article_id=509.

Tompkins, O. S. (2009). Secondhand noise and stress. *American Association of Occupational Health Nurses Journal, 57*(10), 436.

University of Texas School of Nursing. (2007). Evaluation and management of obstructing cerumen. National Guideline Clearinghouse. Available via www.guideline.gov.

Ventry, I. & Weinstein, B. (1983). *Identification of elderly people with hearing problems* (pp. 37–42). Rockville, MD: American Speech-Language-Hearing Association.

Vogel, I., Verschuure, H., van der Ploeg, C. P., Brug, J. & Raat, H. (2010). Estimating adolescent risk for hearing loss based on data from a large school-based survey. *American Journal of Public Health, 100*(6), 1095–1100.

Wagstaff, A. S. (2009). Hearing loss in civilian airline and helicopter pilots compared to air traffic control personnel. *Aviation, Space and Environmental Medicine, 80*(10), 857–861.

Chapter 17
Vision

By Carol Miller and Sharyn Hunter

LEARNING OBJECTIVES

After reading this chapter, you should be able to:

1. Describe age-related changes that affect vision.
2. Identify risk factors that can affect visual wellness.
3. Discuss the functional consequences that affect visual wellness.
4. Describe three pathological conditions that cause vision impairments in older adults.
5. Conduct a nursing assessment of vision, with emphasis on identifying opportunities for health promotion.
6. Identify nursing interventions to facilitate visual wellness in older adults by addressing risk factors that interfere with vision.

KEY POINTS

accommodation
acuity
age-related macular degeneration (AMD)
arcus senilis
blepharochalasis
cataracts
colour perception
critical flicker fusion
dark adaptation
depth perception
dry eye syndrome
ectropion
enophthalmos
entropion
glare
glaucoma
low-vision aids
ophthalmologists
optical technicians
optometrists
presbyopia
visual field
visual impairment

Important daily activities—including communicating, enjoying visual images and manoeuvring in the environment—are highly dependent on eyesight. Visual impairments can profoundly affect a person's safety, functioning and quality of life. Although age-related changes and risk factors affect visual wellness, nurses have an array of interventions to assist older adults in maintaining optimal visual function. This chapter addresses the functional consequences affecting vision in older adults and focuses on the role of nurses in assessing vision and helping older adults to achieve visual wellness.

AGE-RELATED CHANGES THAT AFFECT VISION

Visual function depends on a sequence of processes, beginning with the perception of an external stimulus and ending with the processing of neural impulses in the cerebral cortex. Age-related changes affect all of the structures involved in visual function. However, in the absence of disease processes, these gradual changes have only a subtle impact on the daily activities of the older person.

Eye appearance and tear ducts

During early stages, age-related changes in the appearance of the eye and eyelids do not interfere with visual function, but they may progress to the point of requiring interventions. For example, drooping of the upper eyelid initially is a cosmetic issue, but if it progresses to the point of interfering with vision, a minor surgical intervention might be appropriate. Table 17-1 summarises age-related changes in appearance and tear ducts and the associated effects on visual function.

DIVERSITY NOTE

Arcus senilis—a ring around the iris—is more common in men and dark-skinned people than in women or light-skinned people (Fernandez et al., 2007).

The eye

Age-related changes in the eye itself also affect visual wellness. Specific structures of the eye that change with age include the cornea, lens, iris and pupil, ciliary body, vitreous and retina (see Figure 17-1).

The *cornea* is a translucent covering over the eye that refracts light rays and provides 65% to 75% of the focusing power of the eye. As the eye ages the cornea becomes opaque and yellow, interfering with the passage of light—especially ultraviolet (UV) rays—to the retina. Other corneal changes, such as the accumulation of lipid deposits, can cause an increased scattering of light rays and have a blurring effect on vision. In addition, age-related changes in the curvature of the cornea influence the refractive ability.

The *lens* consists of concentric and avascular layers of clear, crystalline protein. The lens has no blood supply, so it depends on the aqueous humour for metabolic and support functions. *Aqueous humour* is a clear fluid that is produced in the anterior chamber of the eye and normally maintains eye pressure between 10 and 20 mm Hg. The transparent lens

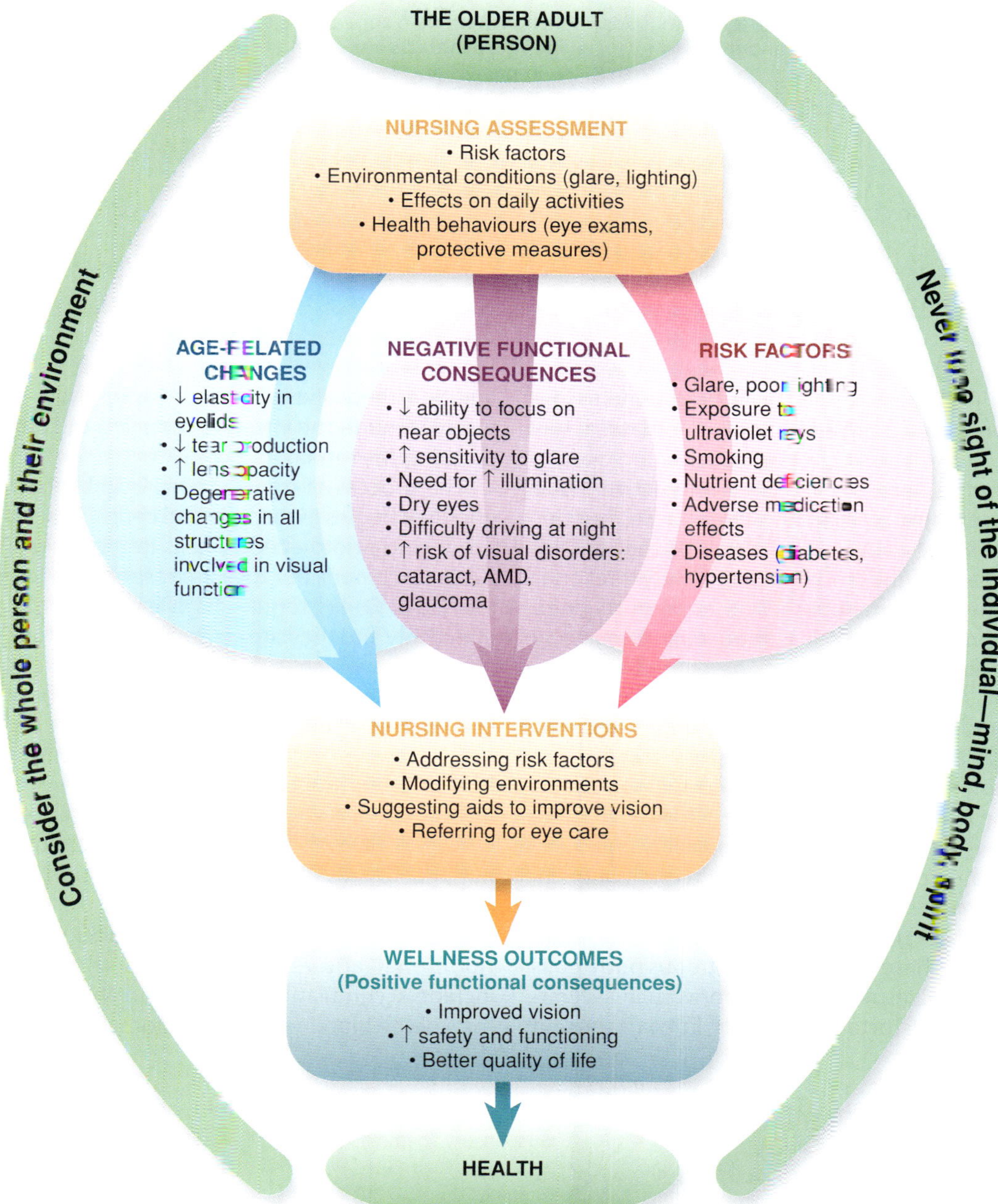

fibres are continually forming new layers without shedding the old layers. As new layers form peripherally, the old layers are compressed inwards towards the centre of the lens, where they eventually become absorbed into the nucleus. This process gradually increases the size and density of the lens, causing a tripling of its mass by the time the person reaches 70 years of age. Thus, the lens gradually becomes stiffer, denser and more opaque.

Because of these age-related changes, the lens moves forwards in the eye and is less responsive to the ciliary muscle. These changes also interfere with the transmission of light rays, diffusing the rays that pass through the lens and reducing the amount of light reaching the retina. These changes do not affect all wavelengths equally; rather, the most detrimental effect occurs with the shorter blue and violet wavelengths.

The *iris* is a pigmented sphincter muscle that dilates and contracts to control pupillary size and regulate the amount of light reaching the retina. With increasing age, the iris becomes sclerotic and rigid and the *pupil* becomes smaller.

TABLE 17-1 Effects of age-related changes in appearance and tear ducts

Age-related changes	Effect
Loss of orbital fat, decreased elasticity of eyelid muscles, accumulation of dark pigment around the eyes	**Enophthalmos** = appearance of sunken eyes **Blepharochalasis** = drooping of upper eyelid, which can eventually impair vision
Relaxation of lower eyelid	**Ectropion** = lower eyelid falls away from conjunctiva, causing decreased lubrication **Entropion** = lower eyelid becomes inverted and eyelashes irritate the cornea
Accumulation of lipids in outer part of the cornea	**Arcus senilis** (also called corneal arcus) = development of yellow or grey-white ring around the iris
Narrowing of tear duct opening, reduced production of tears	**Dry eye syndrome** = excessive tearing, watery eyes, irritation and inflammation

These changes interfere with the ability to respond to low levels of light and reduce the amount of light that reaches the retina.

The *ciliary body* is a mass of muscles, connective tissue and blood vessels surrounding the lens. These muscles regulate the passage of light rays through the lens by changing the shape of the lens. The ciliary body is responsible for **accommodation**, a process that controls one's ability to focus on near objects. In addition, the ciliary body produces aqueous fluid. Because of age-related changes, muscle cells are replaced with connective tissue and the ciliary body gradually becomes smaller, stiffer and less functional. With advanced age, diminished secretion of aqueous humour interferes with the nourishment and cleansing of the lens and cornea.

The *vitreous* is a clear, gelatinous mass that forms the inner substance of the eye and maintains its spherical shape. Age-related changes cause the gelatinous substance to shrink and a proportionate increase in the liquid portion. Because of these changes, the vitreous body pulls away from the retina, resulting in symptoms such as floaters, blurred vision, distorted images or light flashes. In addition, these changes can cause light to scatter more diffusely through the vitreous, reducing the amount of light reaching the retina.

The process of transforming visual stimuli into neural impulses begins in the rods and cones, which are pigment-producing photoreceptor cells in the *retina*. Rods do not perceive colours, but they are responsible for vision under low light. Cones require high levels of light to function effectively and they are responsible for **colour perception** and **acuity**, which is the ability to detect details and discern objects. Rods are distributed throughout the peripheral retina and cones are concentrated in the central and most sensitive part of the macula—the *fovea*. Although both the rods and cones diminish with increasing age, the impact of these changes is minimal because loss of cones occurs primarily in the periphery of the retina, with only a minimal loss in the fovea. Also, although the number of rods declines in the central retina, the remaining rods increase in size and maintain their ability to capture light. Additional age-related changes in retinal structures include accumulation of lipofuscin and thinning and sclerosis of the blood vessels and pigment epithelium.

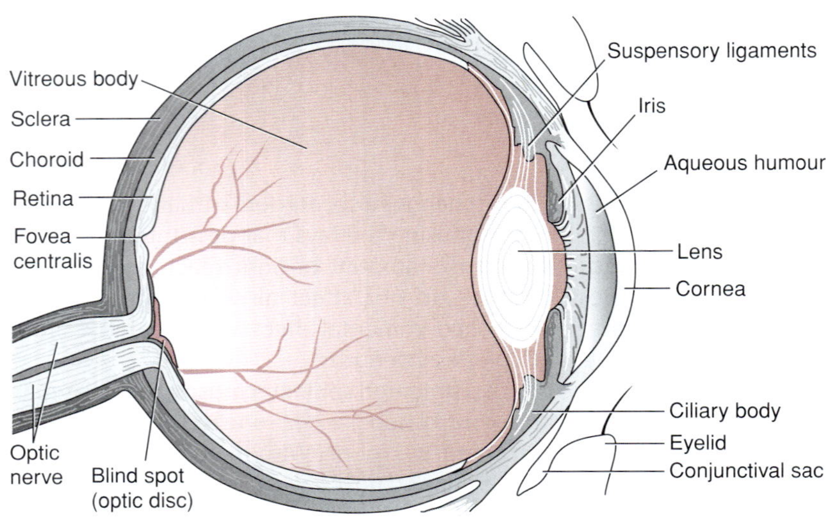

FIGURE 17-1 The eye. Age-related changes in structures of the eye can affect vision in older adults.

The retinal–neural pathway

Photoreceptor cells converge in the ganglion cells of the optic nerve. Neurosensory information is passed from the optic nerve, through the thalamus, to the visual cortex. Age-related changes affecting these neurons, as well as other central nervous system changes that affect cognitive function, can interfere with visual function in older adults.

EFFECTS OF AGE-RELATED CHANGES ON VISION

Best-corrected visual acuity begins to decrease in adults—regardless of race, sex, ethnicity or socioeconomic status—after age 50, even in the absence of any risk factors. Even an exceptional person who has 6/6 visual acuity at the age of 90 can experience subtle changes in overall vision and optical quality. However, despite the universal prevalence of age-related vision changes, most older adults can perform their usual activities by using low-vision aids and modifying their environment (e.g. Evidence-based practice 17-1). **Visual impairment**, defined as vision loss that cannot be corrected by eyeglasses or contact lenses alone, ranges from mild impairment to blindness. Mild visual impairments are caused by normal age-related changes, but they are significantly exacerbated by environmental conditions such as glare and poor lighting. Compensatory interventions for the effects of age-related vision changes are quite effective for promoting visual wellness. These mild visual impairments are illustrated in Figure 17-2 and discussed in the following sections; the consequences of more significant visual impairments are discussed later in the section on pathological conditions affecting vision.

Loss of accommodation

Presbyopia is the loss of accommodation, or the inability to focus clearly and quickly on objects at various distances.

EVIDENCE-BASED PRACTICE 17-1
Vision changes

Statement of the problem

- Older adults experience the following age-related changes and functional outcomes affecting vision:
  - Decreased dark adaptation, increasing the safety risk when environmental lighting changes
  - Pupils become smaller, diminishing the ability to adjust to glare and changes in lighting conditions
  - Decreased upward gaze, which decreases the field of vision
  - Smaller visual field, which increases the safety risk for driving and manoeuvring in the environment
  - Decreased sensitivity of the cornea, resulting in delayed recognition of injury
  - Decreased production of tears, leading to dryness and irritation.
- Presbyopia, which is due to normal age-related loss of elasticity of the lens, leads to a decrease in the eyes' ability to focus on near objects and adapt to light.
- In addition to the effects of age-related vision changes, there is a high prevalence of visual impairment among older adults resulting from the following conditions: cataracts, macular degeneration, glaucoma, diabetic retinopathy, hypertensive retinopathy, temporal arteritis and detached retina.
- Older adults account for 30% of all visually impaired people.
- Studies have found a prevalence rate of visual impairment of 40% to 50% of older adults in long-term care settings.

Recommendations for nursing assessment

Assess all the following parameters in relation to vision:

- Health history of any conditions that predispose older adults to visual impairment (e.g. diabetes, hypertension)
- Specific questions related to visual health (e.g. last eye examination, usual eyesight, changes in vision, use of eye drops, history of trauma or surgery, family history of eye problems)
- Medications that may exacerbate sensory problems (e.g. anticholinergics)
- External structures to identify eyelid lag or lens cloudiness
- Older adult's interest in receiving treatment for visual impairment.
- Use screening tests for distance and near vision, contrast sensitivity and visual fields.

Recommendations for health promotion: Teaching the older adult

Teach older adults and carers/caregivers about the following measures:

- Obtain an annual eye examination with either an optometrist or an ophthalmologist.
- Add colour contrast to fixtures in the home (e.g. light switches, taps) to create a safer and more functional environment.

Recommendations for care

- Be aware of the impact of vision change on safety and quality of life: increased risk of falls, difficulty or inability to read (including medication labels), difficulty driving, difficulty navigating environments (especially stairs or curbs), diminished ability to remain independent.
- Obtain a medical history and develop a care plan that ensures continuation of ongoing therapeutic regimens for people with chronic eye conditions (e.g. eye drops for glaucoma).
- Provide adequate non-glare lighting and identify the lighting that is best for each individual.
- Encourage the use of the person's eyeglasses and additional magnification if appropriate.
- Add colour contrast to fixtures and electronics in the room if appropriate.
- For older adults living with diabetes or hypertension, schedule an annual dilated-eye examination by an ophthalmologist.
- In long-term care settings initiate a mechanism to trigger a reminder about annual eye examinations for residents.
- When vision is worse than 20/125, refer older adults to a low-vision specialist to provide training in the use of visual assistive devices.

Source: Cacchione, P. Z. (2008). Sensory changes. In E. Capezuti, D. Zwicker, M. Mezey & T. Fulmer (Eds), *Evidence-based geriatric nursing protocols for best practice* (3rd ed., pp. 477–502). New York: Springer. A modified version is available online via http://consultgerirn.org

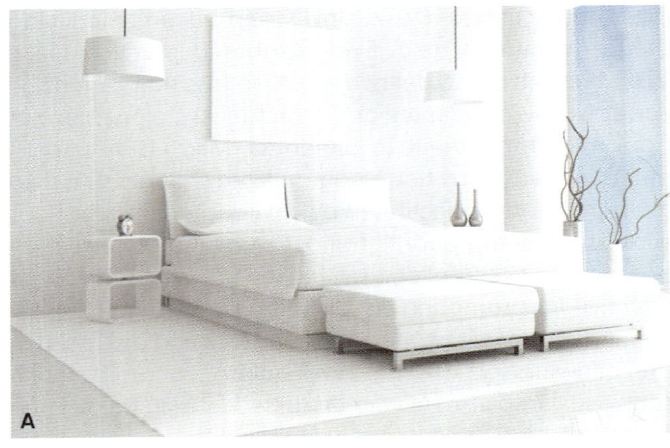

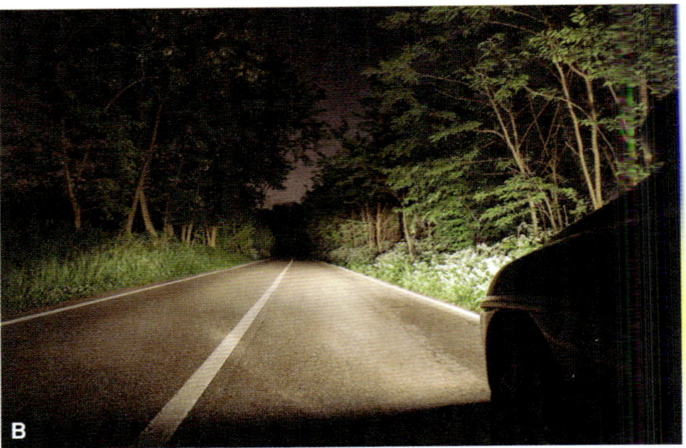

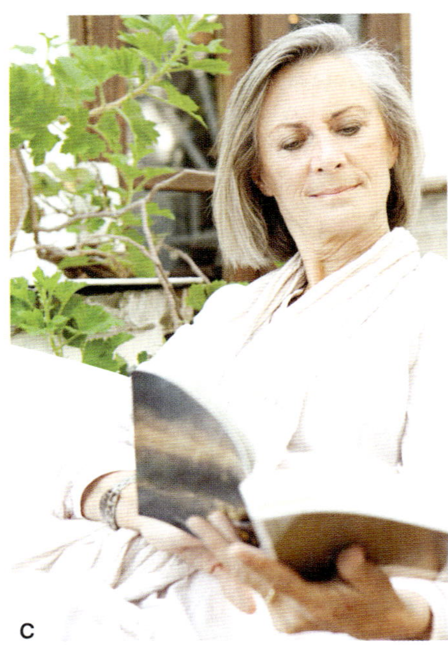

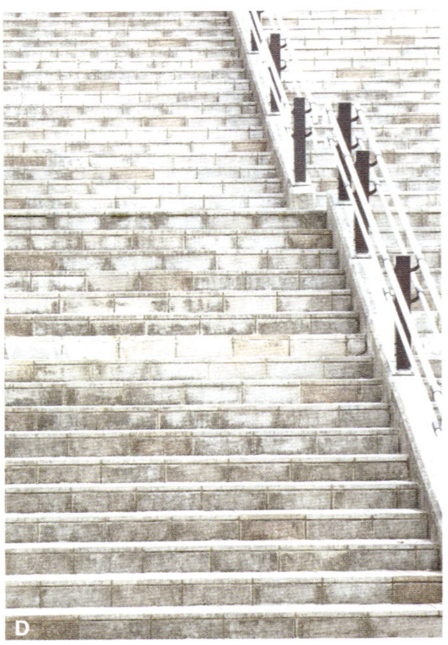

FIGURE 17-2 Mild visual impairments include (**A**) reduced contrast sensitivity, (**B**) increased sensitivity to glare and difficulty with night driving, (**C**) increased lighting requirements and decreased ability to focus close up, and (**D**) decreased ability to judge depth perception. (All images from shutterstock.com; copyrights: A [archideaphoto], B [ollyy], C [MJTH], and D [Sakarin Sawasdinaka].)

Presbyopia is an initial and universal age-related vision change, which begins in early adulthood and affects all humans to some degree by their mid 50s (Ferrer-Blasco, Gonzalez-Meijome & Montes-Mico, 2008). This vision change is caused by degenerative changes in the lens and the ciliary body. Functionally, accommodative changes gradually extend the near point of vision, which is the closest point at which a small object can be seen clearly. A typical example of the effects of presbyopia is the need to hold reading materials farther from the eye to focus clearly on the print.

Diminished acuity

Visual acuity is customarily assessed by using a Snellen chart and it is measured against a normal value of 6/6. The first number represents the distance in metres used for testing. This is usually one, three or six metres. The second number represents the size of the symbol read, where a bigger second number means a larger size of symbol. The bigger second number reflects poorer vision. Visual acuity is best around age 30, after which it gradually declines. Diminished acuity results from age-related ocular changes, including decreased pupillary size, scatter of light in the cornea and lens, opacification of the lens and vitreous, and loss of photoreceptor cells in the retina. These changes interfere with the passage of light to the retina, causing a threefold reduction in retinal illumination between the ages 20 and 60. Acuity is also influenced by conditions, such as size and movement of the object and the amount of light reflected off an object. Because poor illumination compounds the effects of age-related ocular changes with regard to visual acuity, most older people require more illumination to see objects clearly. In addition, because visual acuity is more impaired for moving objects than for stationary objects, it becomes more impaired with increasing speed of the object. These changes in visual acuity can particularly affect night driving competence.

Delayed dark and light adaptation

The ability to respond to dim light—**dark adaptation**—begins to decline around the age of 20 years and diminishes more markedly after age 60. This decline is associated with decreased retinal illumination and other age-related changes in the retina and retinal–neural pathways. As a result, the older adult requires more time to adapt to dim lighting when moving from a brighter to a darker environment. For instance, when entering a darkened movie theatre, an older person needs extra time to adapt to the changes in lighting before proceeding to a seat.

Age-related changes in the lens and pupil interfere with the response to bright lights because they reduce the amount of light reaching the retina. In practical terms, this means that an older person responds more slowly to lights, such as car or bus headlights, and requires more time to recover from exposure to glare and bright lights.

Increased glare sensitivity

Glare occurs when scattered light in the optic media reduces the clarity of visual images. Glare is experienced when light is reflected from shiny surfaces, when the light is excessively bright or inappropriately focused or when bright light originates from several sources at once. Glare is classified according to three types: veiling, dazzling and scotomatic. *Veiling glare* is caused by the scattering of light over the retinal surface and results in diminished contrast of the viewed object. Veiling glare occurs, for example, when bright fluorescent lights in a grocery store reflect on the clear plastic covering over food products in a white case. *Dazzling glare*, which is caused by bright visual displays, interferes with the ability to discern details. Glass-covered directories in brightly lit shopping centres produce a dazzling glare that interferes with a person's ability to read the words in the directory, particularly if there is poor contrast between the letters and the background. *Scotomatic glare* is a blinding glare caused by loss of retinal sensitivity and overstimulation of retinal pigments during exposure to bright lights. For example, sunshine can create scotomatic glare, especially at sunrise or sunset.

Beginning in the fifth decade, age-related changes increase a person's sensitivity to glare as well as the time required to recover from glare. Glare sensitivity is influenced primarily by opacification of the lens; however, it is affected also by age-related changes in the pupil and vitreous. Functionally, these changes can significantly affect the person's ability to read signs, see objects, drive at night and manoeuvre safely in bright environments. In many modern buildings and shopping centres, the bright lights, large windows and highly reflective floors generate glare that can lead to accidents and inaccurate perceptions.

Reduced visual field

A **visual field** is an oval-shaped area encompassing the total view that people perceive while looking at a fixed point straight ahead. The scope of the visual field narrows slightly between the ages of 40 and 50 years and then declines steadily. Functionally, the visual field is important when people engage in tasks that require a broad perception of the environment and moving objects. Walking in crowded places and driving a vehicle are examples of activities that depend on the visual field.

Diminished depth perception

Depth perception is the visual skill responsible for locating objects in three-dimensional space, judging differences in the depth of objects and observing relationships among objects in space. Functionally, depth perception enables people to use objects effectively and to manoeuvre safely in the environment. *Stereopsis* or the disparity between retinal images that is caused by the separation of the two eyes is the primary ocular characteristic that affects depth perception. Additional factors that influence depth perception include prior perceptual experiences of the observer; movement of the observer's head or body; and characteristics of the object, such as size, height, distance, texture, brightness and shading. Although depth perception declines with increasing age, studies indicate that despite age-related changes in stereopsis, older adults are able to discriminate depth differences in a manner that is similar to younger adults (Norman et al., 2008).

Altered colour vision

Pigments in the retinal cones absorb light in the red, blue or yellow ranges of the spectrum. As with many other visual functions, colour perception is influenced by the type and quantity of light waves reaching the retina. Consequently, any age-related changes that interfere with retinal illumination—including lens opacification, pupillary miosis, retinal or retinal–neural changes—can interfere with accurate colour perception. Opacification and yellowing of the lens interferes most directly with shorter wavelengths, causing an altered perception of blues, greens and violets. Low levels of illumination and other environmental factors also interfere with colour perception.

Functionally, altered colour perception is manifested as a relative darkening of blue objects and a yellowed perception of white light. Accurate colour perception is not essential in all daily activities, but it is important, for instance, in differentiating between medications that are similar in colour or tone, especially those in the blue–green and yellow–white ranges. In addition, altered colour perception can interfere with the detection of spoiled food.

TABLE 17-2 Age-related changes affecting vision

Changes	Consequences
• Corneal yellowing and increased opacity	• Diminished acuity
• Changes in the corneal curvature	• Slower response to changes in illumination
• Increase in lens size and density	• Increased sensitivity to glare
• Sclerosis and rigidity of the iris	• Narrowing of the visual field
• Decrease in pupillary size	• Diminished depth perception
• Atrophy of the ciliary muscle	• Altered colour perception
• Shrinkage of gelatinous substance in the vitreous	• Distorted perception of flashing lights
• Atrophy of photoreceptor cells	• Slower processing of visual information
• Thinning and sclerosis of retinal blood vessels	
• Degeneration of neurons in the visual cortex	
• Decreased tears	• Potential for dry eye syndrome

Diminished critical flicker fusion

Critical flicker fusion is the point at which an intermittent light source is perceived as a continuous, rather than flashing, light. The ability to perceive flashing lights accurately is a function of the retinal receptors and is influenced by extra ocular factors, such as the size, colour and luminance of the object. Age-related changes in the retina and retinal–neural pathway, as well as changes that decrease retinal illumination, interfere with critical flicker fusion. Low levels of illumination further exacerbate the effects of these changes. Functionally, diminished critical flicker fusion distorts the perception of a flashing light, making it appear to be a continuous light. Thus, diminished critical flicker fusion can interfere with the discernment of emergency vehicles and road construction lights, especially at night.

Slower visual information processing

Age-related changes of the retinal–neural pathway affect the accuracy and efficiency of visual information processing. Thus, older adults generally need more time to process visual information, but the effects are minimal or negligible when tasks are familiar. Table 17-2 summarises age-related vision changes and their effects on vision.

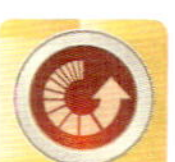

RISK FACTORS THAT AFFECT VISUAL WELLNESS

Lifestyle, nutritional and environmental factors—including both immediate and long-term conditions—exacerbate age-related vision changes and interfere with visual wellness. For example, long-term exposure to UV light (i.e. sunlight) is associated with the development of **cataracts** (age-related changes in the lens) and loss of photoreceptor cells, particularly the cones. Furthermore, older adults are more vulnerable to eye damage from sunlight because age-related changes alter the protective response to harmful UV light. Warmer environmental temperatures are associated with an earlier age of onset for presbyopia (i.e. loss of near vision). Dry eyes can be caused by environmental conditions such as wind, sunlight, low humidity and second-hand smoke. Other environmental influences on visual wellness include glare, dim lighting and poor colour contrast. Studies found that poor nutrition increases the risk for **age-related macular degeneration (AMD)** (Montgomery et al., 2010). Cigarette smoking is a lifestyle factor that increases the risk for cataracts and macular degeneration. One study found that smoking was associated with approximately four times higher odds of visual impairment (Jin & Wong, 2008).

WELLNESS OPPORTUNITY

Poor lighting and exposure to sunlight are risk factors that can readily be addressed through simple self-care practices.

Chronic conditions can adversely affect visual function in various ways. Vision impairments commonly occur in people with Alzheimer's or Parkinson's disease, even during the early stages. Dementia with Lewy bodies is commonly characterised by visual hallucinations and impairments of visuospatial skills (Hamilton et al., 2008). People with diabetes are at increased risk for developing cataracts, glaucoma and diabetic retinopathy. People with hypertension or hypercholesterolaemia are at higher risk for AMD. Malnutrition has been associated with cataract development, and vitamin A deficiency has been associated with dry eyes from reduced tear production.

Medications that are associated with adverse effects on vision include aspirin, haloperidol, non-steroidal anti-inflammatory agents, tricyclic antidepressants, digoxin, anticholinergics, phenothiazines, isoniazid, tamoxifen, amiodarone, sildenafil and oral or inhaled corticosteroids. Cataracts are common in people with glaucoma because of the anticholinesterase drugs used in glaucoma treatment.

Medications that can cause or contribute to dry eyes include oestrogen, diuretics, antihistamines, anticholinergics, phenothiazines, beta-blockers and anti-parkinsonism agents. Systemic anticoagulants can precipitate intraocular haemorrhage in people with pre-existing macular degeneration.

UNFOLDING CASE STUDY

Part A

Mrs Fuller is 50 years old and has used reading glasses for 15 years but has never needed glasses for anything other than reading and sewing. She recently noticed that she has trouble reading the glass-enclosed directory at the shopping centre. She works in an office building with an atrium that has skylights, and she has trouble reading the signs on the doors.

Thinking points

- What age-related factors contribute to the vision changes that Mrs Fuller notices?
- What environmental factors are likely to contribute to Mrs Fuller's difficulty when she is in the shopping centre or at work?
- When Mrs Fuller is in her home environment, what tasks might be more difficult because of age-related vision changes?

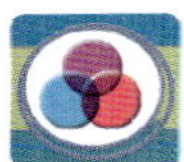

FUNCTIONAL CONSEQUENCES AFFECTING VISUAL WELLNESS

The most serious visual impairments that affect older adults are associated with pathological conditions such as cataracts, glaucoma or AMD, all of which are increasingly likely to occur with advanced age. Visual impairments are categorised as "functional" when acuity is <6/18–6/60, as "low vision" when it is between <6/60–3/60 and as "blindness" when it is <3/60 or worse.

In Australia and New Zealand, AMD is the primary cause of blindness in older adults (Australian Institute Health and Welfare [AIHW], 2013; Blind Foundation [BF], 2011). Cataract is the primary cause of visual impairment in older Australians (AIHW, 2013). The following sections describe the functional consequences that are associated with the types of visual impairments that are most likely to occur in older adults.

DIVERSITY NOTE

It is estimated that 35% of Indigenous Australian adults have not had an eye examination (AIHW, 2011). It has been reported that the lack of specialist eye services in remote and Indigenous communities may be a contributing factor to the low levels of eye examination. The 2008 National Indigenous Eye Health Survey (NIEHS) found blindness rates in Indigenous adults were six times higher than surveyed Australian adults (Australian Indigenous Health*InfoNet*, 2014). The prevalence of vision impairment and blindness in Māori adults aged 45–74 years is twice that of non-Māori adults (BF, 2011).

Effects on safety and function

Because visual impairments are associated with many aspects of safety and functioning, people who are visually impaired are likely to be more dependent in their activities of daily living. Age-related vision changes most directly influence the following activities:

- Getting outside
- Driving a vehicle
- Shopping for groceries
- Going up and down stairs
- Getting in and out of bed or a chair
- Manoeuvring safely in dark or unfamiliar environments
- Seeing markings on clocks, radios, thermostats, appliances and televisions
- Reading newspapers, directories, small-print signs and posters, and labels on food items and medication containers.

Most of these activities are affected not only by alterations in visual skills but also by environmental conditions, such as glare and lighting.

Visually impaired people enter care homes 3 years earlier, have twice the risk of falls and four times the risk of hip fractures than other residents (Eichenbaum 2012). Studies have found that people with impaired vision not only have an increased risk of falls but also experience greater fear of falling and activity limitation due to fear of falling (Ramulu, van Landingham, Massof et al., 2012; Tanabe, Yuki, Ozeki et al., 2012; Wang, Rousseau, Boisjoly et al., 2012).

Specific age-related vision changes that increase the risk for falls include diminished acuity, reduced visual field, diminished depth perception, reduced contrast sensitivity, and increased sensitivity to glare. In addition, delayed processing of visual information can interfere with the quick responses necessary for avoiding falls.

Effects on quality of life

Age-related vision changes develop gradually and often go unnoticed for many years. As the changes progress and interfere with usual activities, older adults may withdraw from activities rather than acknowledge a vision problem or adjust to the changes. Studies find that visual impairments are associated with anxiety, depression and lower levels of psychological well-being (Tabuchi, Yochimura, Kashiwagi et al., 2012; Mathew, Delbaere, Lord et al., 2011; Popescu, Boisjoly, Schmaltz et al., 2011).

Of course, a person's usual lifestyle influences the extent of any psychosocial impact related to vision changes. For example, if the preferred leisure activities require good visual skills, the older adult is likely to become bored and even depressed when vision changes interfere with endeavours such as reading or craftwork. Similarly, when artistic pursuits and entertainment events are important activities, diminished visual function can interfere with the person's quality of life. By contrast, the effect of vision impairment on lifestyle may be minimal for people who prefer music or other activities that are less dependent on visual skills.

One's living environment and support systems are other determinants of the psychosocial consequences of vision changes. Good visual skills are more important for people who live alone or who provide care for others than they are for people who live with, or have frequent contact with, others who have good vision. Also, psychosocial consequences will be minimised if visually impaired people can modify their living environment to compensate for the impairments. By contrast, people who live in institutional settings may experience relatively greater negative consequences because of their inability to alter environmental conditions.

Some older adults who notice declines in vision develop fears that negatively affect their quality of life. For example, people may mistakenly fear going blind if they think they have a serious and progressive disease when, in reality, they have a treatable condition. Fear of blindness may be based on myths, inaccurate information or the experiences of friends who have serious visual impairments. Negative or hopeless attitudes about vision changes can deter the older person from acknowledging the problem or seeking help. Fear of falling is another source of anxiety associated with impaired vision. Inaccurate depth perception can lead to frequent bumping into objects, and the older adult may feel insecure and unsafe, even in familiar environments. If the person has experienced falls or tripping, or knows someone who suffered a fracture as a result of falling, the fears may be magnified.

WELLNESS OPPORTUNITY

Nurses assess the impact of vision impairment on the whole person so they can address fears, anxieties and other responses that affect quality of life.

Effects on driving

Vision changes can significantly affect driving skills and exert a profound impact on older adults, their families and the society. Because driving is associated with considerable safety and independence concerns for drivers and their families—and because unsafe drivers place others at risk—there has been intense and increasing interest in the effects of vision changes on the driving skills of older adults. Visual dimensions that influence driving abilities are near vision, visual search, dynamic vision, contrast sensitivity, depth perception and visual processing speed. Consequences of visual impairment with regard to driving include the following:

- Slower dark and light adaptation creates problems when driving in and out of tunnels and when driving at night on streets with variable lighting
- Decreased peripheral vision interferes with the wide visual field that is important for avoiding collisions
- Decreased acuity interferes with the perception of moving objects, especially fast-moving vehicles
- Diminished accommodation and acuity create problems when the older adult tries to read dashboard indicators after focusing on the road
- Glare interferes with the perception of objects and is heightened by rainy, snowy or sunny conditions
- Bright sunlight shortly after sunrise or before sunset can significantly interfere with the perception of red and green traffic lights because of increased sensitivity to glare
- If the car has tinted windows, the diminished illumination further interferes with visual skills
- Decreased depth perception can cause the person to follow too closely thus increasing the risk of collision.

In recent years, gerontologists and clinicians are focusing their attention on identifying variables that affect driving in older adults and many studies address visual skills as an important factor. For example, Baldock, Berndt and Mathias (2008) found that drivers with deficits in contrast sensitivity are likely to approach points on a road at which a manoeuvre is required (e.g. an intersection) too quickly. Studies have also found an association between driving cessation and all the following visual function measures: cataracts, glaucoma, contrast sensitivity, baseline visual acuity and peripheral visual field deficits (Ackerman et al., 2008; Ramulu et al., 2009).

WELLNESS OPPORTUNITY

Nurses need to be aware of the far-reaching implications of the ability to drive not only on the safety of the individual and others but also on independence and the quality of life.

PATHOLOGICAL CONDITIONS AFFECTING VISION

Chronic conditions that interfere with visual wellness occur very commonly in older adults, so nurses have important roles in detecting and managing these conditions. Health promotion interventions are particularly important with conditions such as glaucoma because interventions can prevent vision impairment. However, this condition is often undiagnosed so the interventions are not implemented in a timely manner. Among older adults, the three most common pathological eye conditions are cataracts, AMD and glaucoma (Figure 17-3, Table 17-3).

DIVERSITY NOTE

Worldwide, women account for nearly two-thirds of people who are blind. Most of these women are older than 60 years and 90% of them live in poverty (Gilbert & Bassett, 2007).

Cataracts

Cataracts are a leading and reversible cause of visual impairment, affecting approximately 50% of people aged 80 years and older. Cataracts are caused by the progression of age-related changes in the lens that begins around age 40 and eventually can progress to total opacification. As cataracts develop, the normally transparent lens becomes

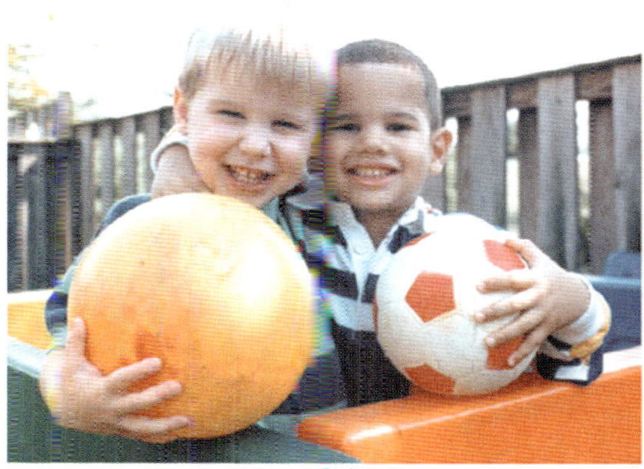

Normal vision

Cataracts

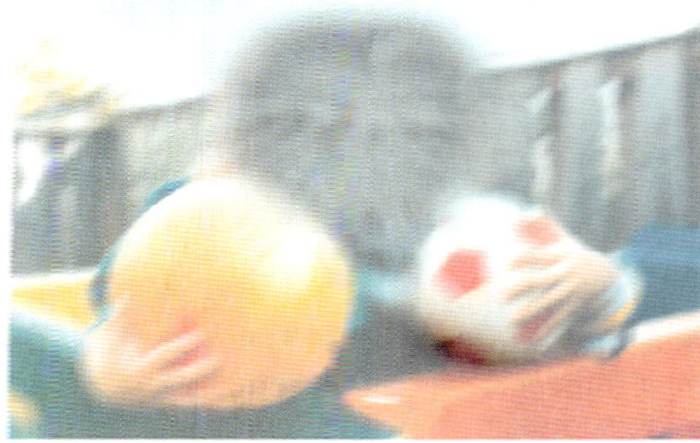

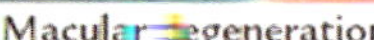

Macular degeneration

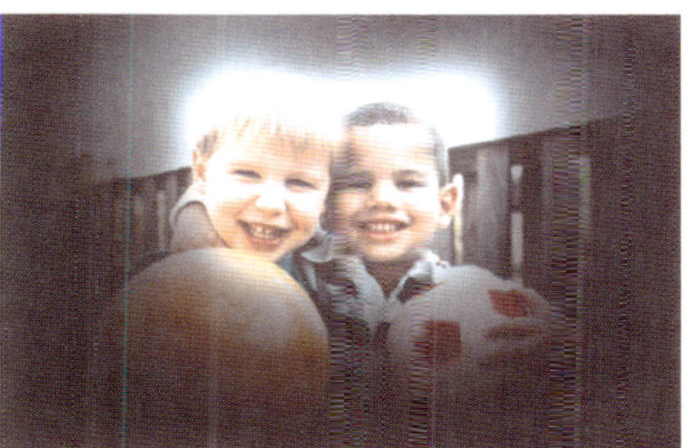

Glaucoma

FIGURE 17-3 Examples of normal vision, vision with cataracts, vision with age-related macular degeneration and vision with glaucoma. (Courtesy of the National Eye Institute, National Institutes of Health.)

TABLE 17-3 Common disease conditions affecting vision

Condition	Risk factors	Symptoms	Management
Cataract	Advanced age, exposure to sunlight, smoking, diabetes, malnutrition, trauma or radiation to the eye or head, medications (corticosteroids, phenothiazines, amiodarone, benzodiazepines, anticholinesterases)	Increased sensitivity to glare, decreased contrast sensitivity, blurred vision, distorted images, double vision, diminished colour perception, frequent eyeglass prescription changes	Surgical removal of lens followed by implantation of an intraocular lens
Age-related macular degeneration (AMD)	Advanced age, white ethnicity, family history of AMD, smoking, hypertension, hyperlipidaemia, medications (tamoxifen, phenothiazines, chloroquine)	Gradual progressive loss of central vision, distorted straight lines, blurred vision	Visual rehabilitation programs, argon laser therapy for wet type, experimental treatments under investigation for both types
Glaucoma	Advanced age, family history of glaucoma, diabetes, medications (anticholinergics, corticosteroids)	**Chronic:** Slow onset, diminished vision in dim light, increased sensitivity to glare, decreased contrast sensitivity, diminished peripheral vision **Acute:** sudden onset, intense pain, blurred vision, halo around lights, nausea and vomiting	**Chronic:** Medical therapy with miotics, adrenergic agonists, carbonic anhydrase inhibitors, beta-blockers, and prostaglandins (administered as eye drops) **Acute:** immediate treatment with medications to reduce pressure, followed by laser surgery

cloudy, transmission of light to the retina is diminished and vision is impaired. In addition to being caused by age-related changes, risk factors include systemic disease, medications and environmental factors, as summarised in Table 17-3. Also, cataracts are likely to occur more commonly after glaucoma surgery or other types of eye surgery. The most modifiable and preventable risk factors for cataracts are cigarette smoking and exposure to sunlight.

Cataracts usually occur in both eyes but they do not necessarily progress bilaterally at the same rate. Cataracts are classified according to their location: *cortical* cataracts occur in the cortex, *nuclear* cataracts occur in the nucleus and *posterior sub-capsular* cataracts occur on the back of the membrane that surrounds the lens. The location of cataracts significantly influences their impact, with nuclear cataracts interfering the most with vision.

In their early stages, cataracts do not necessarily affect visual acuity, but as they progress, they cause difficulty performing activities such as reading and night driving (see Figure 17-3). People with cataracts are likely to experience any of the following vision changes:

- Dimmed or blurred vision
- Distorted or double images
- Frequent changes in corrective lenses
- An increased sensitivity to glare
- A need for more light when reading
- The perception of a "film" over the eye
- A diminished ability to discern contrast
- The perception of halos around bright lights
- Distorted or diminished colour perception (e.g. blue appears dulled and red, yellow and orange appear brighter).

Cataracts cannot be treated with medication, but in the early stages, they are managed by the prescription of stronger eyeglasses or contact lenses. When visual acuity declines to the point that it affects the person's safety or the quality of life and provides a reasonable likelihood of improved vision, cataract surgery is usually recommended. When surgery is required for both eyes, the procedure is usually done on one eye at a time, with the second surgery being done after the first one heals completely. However, a recent study of immediate versus delayed sequential cataract surgery found that subjects who had cataract surgery on both eyes in one session experienced greater improvements and a more rapid visual rehabilitation (Nassiri et al., 2009). An optometrist can screen for cataracts and an ophthalmologist can diagnose cataracts and perform cataract surgery. This is the most commonly performed operation today.

Surgeons typically remove the affected lens through a process called *phacoemulsification*, in which they break up the clouded lens with ultrasound waves and then aspirate the tiny particles with a suction device. After the cataract is removed, the surgeon implants an intraocular lens. The surgical procedure is done with local anaesthesia, takes less than one hour and has a very low rate of complications. If the person needed corrective lenses before the surgery, the surgeon can insert an intraocular lens that mimics the natural focusing ability of the eye and results in improved vision, with little or no need for additional correction. One drawback of the intraocular lens is that some older people report continued difficulty with glare and halos.

Nurses have an important role in dispelling myths that might interfere with older adults obtaining surgical treatment for cataracts. For example, older adults might think that cataract surgery is riskier or more complicated than it actually is because they are familiar with experiences of friends or relatives who had cataract surgery many years ago. Nurses can emphasise that advances in surgical techniques for cataract surgery have significantly improved both the process and the outcomes of cataract surgery for older adults in recent years. In addition, nurses can emphasise that there are many benefits, especially when the vision impairment interferes with safety and the quality of life.

DIVERSITY NOTE

Indigenous Australians are less likely than other Australians to undergo cataract surgery (AIHW, 2011).

Although nurses need not be thoroughly familiar with the surgical techniques, they can emphasise that the cataract surgery today is much simpler and has an extremely high success rate in significantly improving safety, functioning and the quality of life. Moreover, nurses can encourage older adults to seek reliable information and periodic evaluations from eye care professionals, rather than simply tolerating a loss of vision because of cataracts.

WELLNESS OPPORTUNITY

Nurses promote responsible decision making by encouraging older adults and their carers to explore risks and benefits of cataract surgery.

Age-related macular degeneration

Age-related macular degeneration (AMD) is the leading cause of severe vision loss and blindness in people older than 55 years in the developed countries (Coleman, Chan, Ferris & Chew, 2008). AMD affects one-in-seven Australians over 50 years (Van Newkirk et al., 2000) and is the primary cause of 48% of the cases of blindness in Australians 65 years and over (AIHW, 2013), and in New Zealand for people over 50 years (BF, 2011). AMD is associated with the risk factors summarised in Table 17-3. Longitudinal studies found that AMD is significantly associated with serious function consequences, including higher rates of blindness, depression, hip fracture and residence in long-term care facilities (Wysong, Lee & Sloan, 2010). Prevention of AMD focuses on control of modifiable risk factors, such as smoking, and the use of a nutritional supplement that contains all of the following: vitamin C 500 mg, vitamin E 400 IU, beta-carotene 15 mg, zinc oxide 80 mg and cupric oxide 2 mg (Coleman et al., 2008).

DIVERSITY NOTE

AMD is more common in light-skinned individuals than in people of any other ethnic origin; in people 75 years and older, female gender may be a risk factor (Coleman et al., 2008).

Early in the disease, deposits of yellow by-products of retinal pigment called *drusen*, build up in the macula, which is the area in the middle of the retina where visual acuity is the best. As the disease progresses, it is classified either as *dry type*, which accounts for 80% to 90% of cases or *wet (exudative) type*. In the dry type, damage is caused by the death of the photoreceptors, which is seen on funduscopy as tiny areas of atrophy of the retinal pigment epithelium. The dry type of AMD usually progresses slowly and does not cause total blindness; however, if the wet type develops, visual loss can be rapid and severe. In the wet type, the damage is caused by the formation of new blood vessels in the choroid, a process called *choroidal neovascularisation*, followed by haemorrhage into the sub-retinal space.

In the early stage of AMD, the person will experience blurred vision and will have difficulty reading, especially in dim light. Similar to most other eye conditions, AMD occurs in both eyes, but it can appear initially in only one eye and its course may differ in each eye. As AMD progresses, it affects central vision and significantly interferes with such activities as reading, driving, watching television, recognising people and performing many self-care activities (see Figure 17-3). The primary treatment goal for older adults with either type of AMD is to reduce the risk of further vision loss.

Laser photocoagulation and photodynamic therapy are two interventions that are used for treating the choroidal neovascularisation that occurs in the wet type of AMD for people who meet the medical criteria for these two treatments. A disadvantage of these treatments is that many people do not experience significant long-term effects. Some progress is being made with regard to biological or pharmacological agents that halt the disease process, so nurses can encourage anyone with AMD to obtain information about clinical trials and new developments through such sources as Vision Australia, the Save Sight Society (New Zealand) and other organisations listed in the resources section at the end of the chapter. Nurses can serve in support roles for people with AMD by encouraging them to participate in vision rehabilitation programs so they can learn the most effective ways of compensating for declining vision. People with AMD are usually taught to test their eyes daily by using the Amsler grid (Figure 17-4) so they will be aware

A

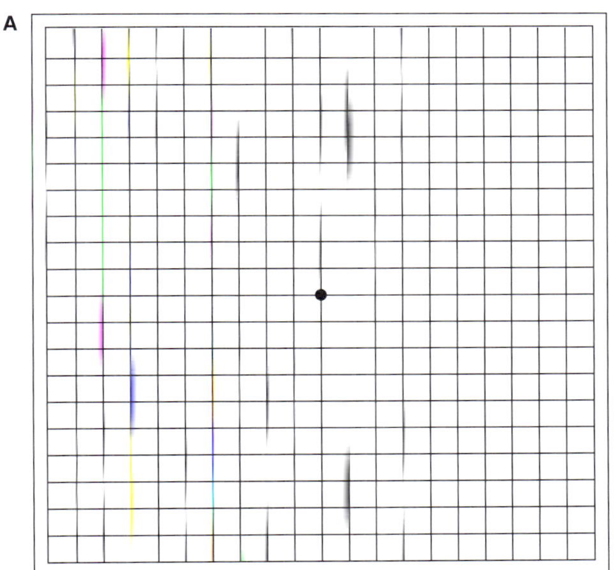

B

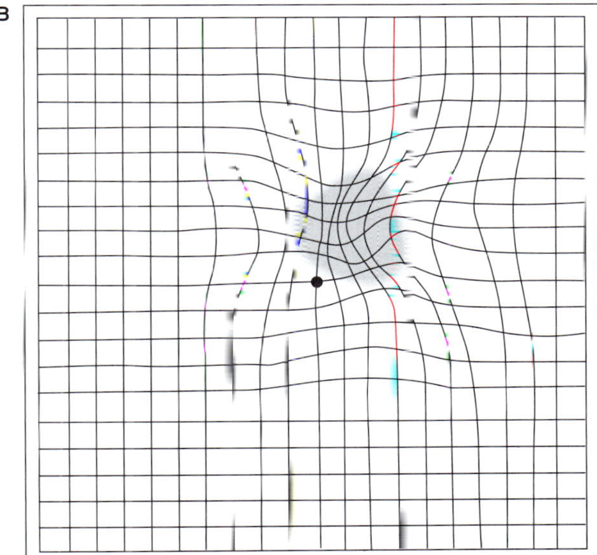

Instructions for Use

1. Tape this page at eye level where light is consistent and without glare.
2. Put on your reading glasses and cover one eye.
3. Fix your gaze on the centre black dot.
4. Keeping your gaze fixed, try to see if any lines are distorted or missing.
5. Mark the defect on the chart.
6. TEST EACH EYE SEPARATELY.
7. If the distortion is new or has worsened, arrange to see your ophthalmologist at once.
8. **Always** keep the Amsler grid the **same distance** from your eyes each time you test.

FIGURE 17-4 Amsler grid. (**A**) People with age-related macular degeneration (AMD) use the Amsler grid to perform a simple daily test for sudden changes in their condition. (**B**) This is what the Amsler grid might look like to someone with AMD. (Part A: Reprinted with permission from American Macular Degeneration Foundation, 888-MACULAR, www.macular.org.)

of sudden changes. In long-term residential care settings and for older adults with memory problems, nurses may have to provide daily reminders or assistance with performing this task. Nurses also need to encourage people with AMD to receive ongoing evaluation by eye care practitioners to detect treatable aspects of this disease.

Glaucoma

The term **glaucoma** refers to a group of eye diseases in which the ganglion cells of the optic nerve are damaged by an abnormal build-up of aqueous humour in the eye. If the fluid cannot flow out of the anterior chamber of the eye through the channel between the iris and the cornea, it accumulates and pushes the optic nerve into a cupped or concave shape. The resulting damage to the optic nerve causes a loss of peripheral vision. If left untreated, the damage can progress to blindness.

DIVERSITY NOTE

Glaucoma and age-related macular degeneration are still uncommon causes of vision loss in Aboriginal and Torres Strait Islander people (AIHW, 2011).

Chronic (open-angle) glaucoma, which accounts for most cases of glaucoma, occurs when the drainage canals become clogged. This condition has an insidious onset and affects vision when the optic nerve becomes damaged. Early signs include increased intraocular pressure, poor vision in dim lighting and increased sensitivity to glare. If the condition progresses, manifestations include headaches, "tired eyes", impaired peripheral vision, a fixed and dilated pupil, the perception of halos around lights and frequent changes in the prescription for corrective lenses. Chronic glaucoma usually occurs in both eyes, but it can begin in only one eye and does not necessarily progress at the same rate in both eyes. Because chronic glaucoma progresses slowly and causes little or no visual impairment in the early stage, annual assessments of intraocular pressure are necessary to detect the condition before visual impairments occur. Chronic glaucoma is most commonly managed with medications, but surgical treatment options include laser surgery and other types of eye surgery. Medication management commonly includes one or more of the following types of eye drops: miotics, prostaglandins, beta-blockers, adrenergic agonists and carbonic anhydrase inhibitors.

Normal-tension glaucoma is another type of glaucoma that occurs in older adults. With this type of glaucoma, the intraocular pressure is within the normal range, but the optic nerve is damaged and the visual field is narrowed (see Figure 17-3). This condition is often managed with the same medications and surgical approaches that are used for chronic glaucoma.

Acute (closed-angle) glaucoma is caused by a sudden complete blockage of the flow of aqueous humour. This condition has an abrupt onset in one or both eyes and should be considered a medical emergency. People with acute glaucoma present with increased intraocular pressure, severe eye pain, clouded or blurred vision, dilation of the pupil, and nausea and vomiting. This condition can be precipitated by medications that cause pupil dilation, such as anticholinergics. Immediate treatment with medications is usually effective for acute attacks, but surgical intervention is often needed.

Health education for older adults with glaucoma focuses on the importance of adhering to ongoing medication routines and regularly being evaluated by their eye care practitioner. If older adults with glaucoma are admitted for institutional care, nurses need to ensure that prescribed eye drops are administered as ordered. In home care situations nurses may need to develop a plan for administering eye drops on a daily or more frequent basis. If an older adult has memory problems, establishing a routine for administering eye drops can be quite challenging. Many times, complicated eye drop regimens can be simplified by working with the eye care practitioner to decrease the number of eye drops that are necessary or to prescribe a longer-acting medication that can be administered less frequently.

WELLNESS OPPORTUNITY

Nurses promote self-care by teaching people with glaucoma to be aware of prescription and over-the-counter medications that can exacerbate glaucoma.

UNFOLDING CASE STUDY

Part B

Mrs Fuller is now 72 years old and has been retired for several years. You are the practice nurse at her local medical centre. Mrs Fuller's medical history indicates that she has smoked a packet of cigarettes a day for 40 years, and has been taking medications for hypertension and osteoarthritis for 5 years. When you meet Mrs Fuller at her regular appointment, she mentions that during a recent medical check-up her doctor said she thought she had early cataracts. The doctor told her it was too early to do anything about them. She has never had an eye examination, other than what her regular doctor does periodically. When asked about her symptoms, Mrs Fuller tells you that she sometimes feels like there is a film over her eyes and she has trouble seeing when she is outside on sunny days. Mrs Fuller says that she never liked wearing sunglasses and hopes she will not have to start wearing them now. She has recently purchased stronger reading glasses, and these help a little with reading and sewing.

Thinking points

- What factors likely contributed to the development of Mrs Fuller's cataracts?
- When Mrs Fuller is driving during the day, what difficulties might she notice because of vision changes? Because of environmental conditions?
- When Mrs Fuller is driving at night, what difficulties might she notice because of vision changes? Because of environmental conditions?
- When Mrs Fuller is in her home, what changes in visual abilities might she notice because of cataracts?

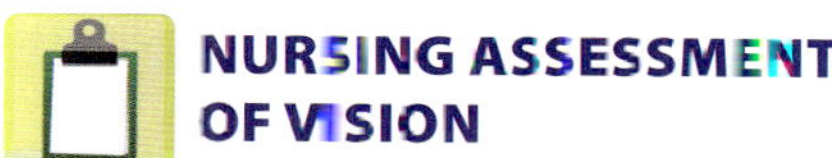

NURSING ASSESSMENT OF VISION

Nursing assessment of vision is aimed at identifying the following:

- Factors that interfere with visual wellness
- Vision problems
- The impact of vision changes on safety, independence or the quality of life
- Opportunities for promoting visual wellness
- Barriers to implementing interventions.

Nursing assessment of visual function is not a substitute for an examination by an eye care specialist. Where the purpose of an examination by an eye care specialist is to detect and initiate appropriate treatment of vision problems, the goal of the nursing assessment is to assist the older adult in minimising the negative consequences of vision changes. Nursing assessment also aims at identifying modifiable risk factors that can be addressed through health promotion. Nurses assess visual abilities by interviewing the older adult (or carers of dependent older adults), by observing the older adult's ability to perform activities of daily living and by testing the older adult's visual skills.

Interviewing about vision changes

Nurses use interview questions to elicit the following information: past and present risk factors for vision impairment, the person's awareness of any vision changes, the impact of these changes on daily activities and the quality of life, and the person's attitudes about interventions (Box 17-1). The interview begins with direct questions about the person's awareness of any changes in vision. If the person acknowledges a visual impairment, nurses elicit additional details about the onset and progression of vision changes. Nurses also ask about symptoms that cause discomfort or that indicate the possible presence of disease processes.

Nurses then ask about the impact of vision changes on the person's usual or desired activities. If the person has acknowledged vision changes, nurses can ask specific questions about how these changes have influenced usual activities. If the person is not aware of vision changes, nurses inquire about any difficulties performing complex activities, such as driving, shopping and meal preparation. Questions about leisure interests are incorporated into the interview to obtain information about the psychosocial consequences of vision impairments. Although the older adult may not associate lifestyle changes with vision impairments, questions about changes in hobbies and leisure activities can help nurses identify the need for interventions to improve visual wellness. Because poor vision increases the risk for falls, especially tripping-related falls, nurses ask about a history of tripping, falling and near-falling.

WELLNESS OPPORTUNITY

Nurses assess the impact of vision changes on the person's relationships with other people as one aspect of the quality of life.

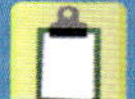

BOX 17-1
Guidelines for assessing vision

Questions to assess awareness and presence of vision impairment

- Have you noticed any changes in your vision during the past few years?
- Do you experience any uncomfortable symptoms, such as dry eyes?
- Do you have difficulty managing any of your usual activities because you have trouble seeing? (Consider asking about the following: sewing, reading, driving, grooming, hobbies, preparing meals, watching television, managing money, writing letters, using the telephone, using dials on appliances, shopping for groceries, and going up and down stairs.)
- Have you ever tripped or fallen because you had trouble seeing?
- Have you stopped doing any activities because of vision problems? (For example, have you stopped driving at night because of difficulty seeing?)
- Are there things you would do if you could see better?

Questions to ask if vision loss is acknowledged

- When did you first notice a loss of vision or a change in your ability to see?
- Have the changes been gradual, or did you notice sudden changes at any particular time?
- How would you describe the changes in your ability to see?
- Have you noticed pain, blurred vision, burning or itching, halos around lights, intolerance to bright light, a difference between day and night vision, or spots or flashing lights in front of your eyes?
- What kind of medical evaluation and care, if any, have you had for this problem?

Questions to identify opportunities for education about disease prevention and health promotion

- When was the last time you had your eyes checked?
- Where do you go for eye care?
- Have you ever had your eyes checked for cataracts, glaucoma and other eye conditions?
- What do you think about going for regular check-ups for glaucoma and other eye problems?

Questions to identify risk factors for vision loss

- When you spend time outdoors in the sun, do you use sunglasses or a hat to protect your eyes from bright light?
- Do you smoke cigarettes?
- Do you have a history of diabetes or hypertension?
- Do you have a family history of glaucoma or macular degeneration?
- What medications do you take? (Refer to Table 17-3 to identify medications that may increase the risk for vision loss.)

Identifying opportunities for health promotion

Nurses identify opportunities for health promotion by asking about the person's usual eye care practices and about factors that can interfere with visual wellness. Information about the source, frequency and dates of the person's eye examinations is particularly useful for planning health promotion interventions that address the early detection of eye disease. Nurses also listen for indicators of myths or misunderstandings that should be addressed through health education. If the person has cataracts, glaucoma or another chronic condition affecting their vision, nurses ask questions to ascertain the person's self-care practices and attitude towards eye examinations and disease management. If no visual impairment is reported, nurses assess attitudes about early detection of treatable conditions.

Last, identification of modifiable risk factors provides an opportunity for health education. For example, it is especially important to ask about cigarette smoking if the person has cataracts, AMD or a family history of AMD. If the older person is likely to spend time outdoors in sunny climates, nurses ask about exposure to sunlight. Placing this question towards the end of the interview sets the stage for health education about protective measures, such as the use of sunglasses.

WELLNESS OPPORTUNITY

Nurses pave the way for teaching about self-care by assessing attitudes about preventive and protective activities, such as obtaining eye examinations and wearing sunglasses.

Observing cues to visual function

Reliable information about a person's visual function can be obtained simply by being observant. For example, nurses can observe for any abnormalities of the eyelids, such as serious eyelid lag, that might interfere with visual wellness. Nurses can detect other, more subtle, indications that visual function is impaired by observing the person's appearance and ability to perform daily activities. Finally, community-based nurses may have opportunities to observe older adults in their usual environments to assess their functioning and conditions that can affect visual abilities. When assessments cannot be performed in the person's usual environment, nurses can ask the older person and carers for information about the person's abilities in the home setting.

Nurses consider their observations in relation to the person's usual patterns of activities and personal care. For example, observation of spots and soiled marks on clothing would be interpreted differently for someone known to be meticulous about his or her appearance than for someone who had never showed much concern about this. When assessing older people in a clinical setting or their usual environment, the nurse should note any circumstances that might influence their visual performance, either positively or negatively. An example of a positive influence might be the presence of good lighting and colour contrast. Some negative influences, such as glare from fluorescent lights reflecting on highly polished floors, are more likely to exist in an institutional setting than a home setting. Assessment of the person's visual performance also must take into account the influences of factors such as illness, medication effects, psychological stress, unfamiliar environments (in clinical setting) and unavailability of corrective lenses (if not being used). These influences are of particular concern because they are likely to have a negative impact on the older person's performance of daily activities. Suggestions for observing behavioural and environmental cues related to visual function are listed in Box 17-2.

BOX 17-2
Guidelines for assessing behavioural and environmental cues related to visual performance

Behavioural cues

- Is clothing spotted, soiled or mismatched, in contrast to a former pattern of neatness and sense of style?
- Is make-up applied in heavy quantities, in contrast to the usual manner of application?
- Does the person rely heavily on non-visual cues in performing usual activities, especially manoeuvring in the environment (e.g. using the hands to find objects or to probe for obstacles?

Environmental cues

- What kind of lighting is used for various tasks? If the lighting is not adequate, can adjustments be made to improve the person's visual abilities?
- Does the person try to economise at home by using dim lights or no lights at all? If so, does this interfere with visual abilities or safe functioning?
- Where does the person usually sit in relation to light sources Does glare from a window interfere with vision? Do shadow from lamps interfere with vision? Do overhead lights cause glare? Are light bulbs of sufficient wattage?
- What are the sources of light on stairways and hallways?
- Is there sufficient colour contrast in the following areas: walls and floors; stairs and landings; furniture; eating utensils and place settings; cooking utensils and counter tops; markings and background on appliance dials?
- Are nightlights used in hallways and bathrooms?

Using standard vision tests

Nurses can assess vision by using both formal and informal tests. Before testing, however, nurses should eliminate sources of glare, make sure the testing materials have good colour contrast and place a light source above the person's head to provide good lighting while avoiding shadows. If the person normally wears corrective lenses, make sure that they are clean and in place. Test each eye separately, using an appropriate eye cover; avoid using a hand as a cover. Recognise that the accuracy of some tests is influenced by the nurse's own vision. The nursing assessment of vision is not a substitute for a complete eye examination, but its purpose is to provide information that is useful for planning care and identifying the need for further evaluation.

Vision assessment tools that nurses can use in clinical settings include the Snellen chart, pinhole assessment, the Cardiff Acuity Test and the Amsler grid (as described in detail by Kalinowski, 2008). Nurses use these tests with interviews and observations, as described earlier. Box 17-3 summarises guidelines for using the Snellen chart and the Confrontation Test, which nurses can use to assess distance acuity and peripheral vision.

Nurses can informally test near acuity by asking the person to read a newspaper or other printed material of various type sizes. Another method is to ask the person to read a line or two of a form that needs to be signed and then observe the person's ability to find the signature line. Nurses can create additional opportunities for assessing

BOX 17-3 Guidelines for using vision screening tests

Using the Snellen chart to assess distance acuity

- Position the chart 6 metres away from the person, at eye level.
- If space does not permit a 6-metre distance, the distance between the person and the chart should be either 4.5 or 3.0 metres, with final measurement adjusted for distance. Alternatively, a scaled-down Snellen card can be used, if available.
- If the person usually wears corrective lenses, test the corrected vision.
- Ask the person to start reciting the letters in the line that can be read most easily; then ask him or her to read as many letters as possible in the lines directly below that line.
- Document the findings for each eye by noting the figure at the end of the last line on which at least half of the letters were read correctly.
- The upper figure denotes the distance of the person from the chart, whereas the lower figure denotes the distance from the chart at which a person with normal vision would be able to read the line. (That is, a vision measurement of 20/50 indicates that the person being tested can see things at a distance of 6 metres that a person with normal vision would be able to see at a distance of 15 metres.)
- Normal Snellen chart test results for older adults are as follows:
  - A corrected vision of 20/20 is considered to be normal.
  - If a distance of 3 metres is used, the corrected vision should be 10/10.
  - The average corrected vision for older adults ranges from 20/20 to 20/50.

Performing the confrontation test to assess peripheral vision

- Sit directly across from the older person, about half a metre away.
- Cover your left eye and have the examinee cover his or her right eye.
- Instruct the examinee to focus on your right eye while you focus on the examinee's left eye.
- Fully extend your right arm midway between you and the examinee.
- While holding a pencil, slowly move your right hand, with the fingers wiggling, from the outer periphery towards the centre, testing visual fields from top to bottom.
- While maintaining continuous eye contact, ask the examinee to report the point at which the pencil is visualised.
- Repeat these steps, covering your right eye and the examinee's left eye and using your left arm.
- Normal confrontation test results for older adults: the pencil in your hand should be seen simultaneously by both you and the older person in all quadrants.

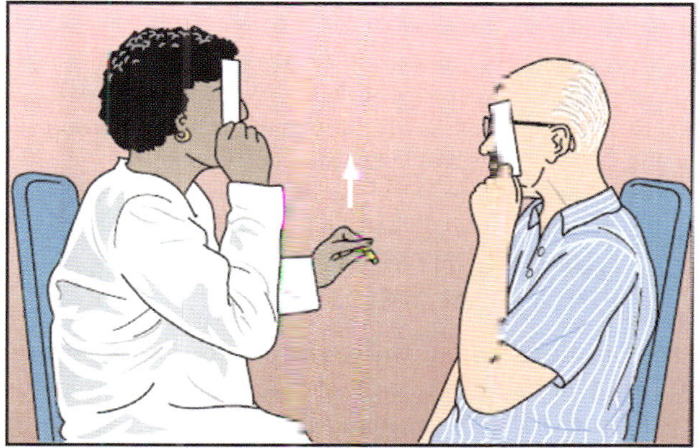

FIGURE A. Performing the confrontation test.

acuity by providing written educational materials and asking the person to read a specific part, such as a phone number. Nurses can informally assess distance acuity by asking the person to look out a window or down a hallway and to describe certain details, such as the words on a sign.

UNFOLDING CASE STUDY

Part C

Recall you are the practice nurse at the local medical centre. Several months have passed since you spoke to Mrs Fuller about her "early cataracts". Today, she again tells you she feels there is a "film" over her eyes, and she has trouble seeing when she is outside on sunny days. No further assessment of her eyes has occurred since your previous discussion.

Thinking points

- Which questions from Box 17-1 would you ask Mrs Fuller at this time?
- What sort of information might you be able to glean from behavioural or environmental cues about Mrs Fuller's ability to see? (See Box 17-2.)
- Would assessing Mrs Fuller's vision by using vision screening tests be appropriate? (See Box 17-3.) If so, which tests would you perform?
- What health promotion education would you give Mrs Fuller at this time?

NURSING ISSUES

On the basis of the nursing assessment, the nurse might identify actual vision impairment or risk factors for impaired vision. An appropriate nursing issue for an older adult with impaired vision would be disturbed visual sensory perception. Related factors that commonly affect older adults include age-related vision changes (e.g. presbyopia), sensory organ alterations (e.g. glaucoma) and environmental factors (e.g. glare, dim lighting or poor colour contrast). The care plan at the end of this chapter is based on a nursing issue of disturbed visual sensory perception related to age-related changes, sensory organ alterations and environmental factors. Other nursing issues might be addressed if the visual impairment interferes with the older adult's safety, quality of life or performance of activities of daily living. Possible issues to address these functional consequences include anxiety, ineffective coping, self-care deficit, risk for injury, impaired social interaction, readiness for enhanced coping and readiness for enhanced self-care.

WELLNESS OPPORTUNITY

The wellness nursing issue of willingness for enhanced knowledge to improve vision would be applicable for older adults who are willing to explore interventions that improve their vision.

GOAL PLANNING FOR WELLNESS OUTCOMES

When older adults experience vision impairments or have risk factors that affect visual functioning, nurses develop goals that achieve wellness outcomes as an essential part of the planning process. Goals that most directly relate to interventions to improve vision for older adults are developing vision compensation behaviour and improving visual sensory function. In addition, other goals related to vision are improved coping: adaptation to physical disability; improved self-care: activities of daily living; reduced stress level; increased knowledge: personal safety and fall prevention behaviour; and reduction in risk for visual impairment. Specific interventions to achieve these goals are discussed in the following section.

WELLNESS OPPORTUNITY

Quality of life is a wellness outcome that is achieved through nursing interventions that improve visual function.

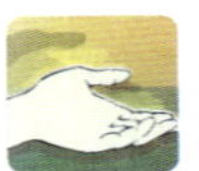

NURSING INTERVENTIONS FOR VISUAL WELLNESS

Nurses promote visual wellness through interventions directed towards preventing vision loss, promoting comfort measures for dry eyes and implementing or teaching about methods to foster optimal visual function. Interventions to achieve these goals are discussed in detail in the following sections. The following pertinent nursing interventions include: communication enhancement: visual deficit; coping enhancement, eye care; and environmental management: safety, health education, health screening, health system guidance, risk identification and fall prevention.

Health promotion for visual wellness

Health promotion interventions focus on maintaining vision at an optimal level by compensating for any visual deficits and identifying any treatable conditions at an early stage. Nurses can teach older adults about preserving optimal visual function by reducing or eliminating risk factors that can cause visual impairments. For example, the use of broad-brimmed hats and close-fitting sunglasses with UV-B–absorbing lenses have the long-range effect of protecting the eyes from harmful rays and the immediate benefit of screening out sun glare that can interfere with visual function. In addition, nurses can teach about preventing eye disease through nutritional interventions. Studies confirm that consumption of foods high in lutein—a carotenoid found in corn, egg yolk and leafy green vegetables—can improve vision and protect against cataracts and AMD (Najm & Lie, 2008). Health promotion teaching also emphasises the importance of annual eye examinations and timely evaluation of any changes in vision.

These teaching points are summarised in Box 17-4, which nurses can use for older adults or their carers.

In providing health education, it may be helpful to review the differences between **optical technicians**, **optometrists** and **ophthalmologists** and provide information about health insurance coverage for these services, as detailed in Box 17-5. Educational materials describing the scope of services of these eye care providers are distributed by eye care professionals and organisations listed in the resources section at the end of this chapter.

Older adults and their carers may also benefit from the many educational brochures that are available on the subjects of eye diseases, common vision problems, age-related eye changes and low-vision aids. Nurses can use these publications to supplement and reinforce the health education components of their care plans. National and local vision centres and other organisations provide these materials at little or no cost and some brochures are available in other languages. In addition, most of the information can be obtained and printed directly from these organisations' websites. One such organisation is the Macular Disease Foundation Australia. This organisation's website contains several resources which can be printed out about visual aids, coping strategies and strategies to minimise slips and falls.

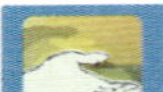

BOX 17-4
Health promotion teaching about visual wellness

Prevention and early detection of disease

- Minimise exposure to sunlight by using broad-brimmed hats and close-fitting sunglasses with UV-absorbing lenses.
- Have eyes examined annually or more frequently if you notice a change in vision; make sure the examination checks for glaucoma, cataracts and retinal disease.
- Use the appropriate eye care practitioner (ophthalmologist and optometrist) as described in Box 17-5.
- Because smoking is a risk factor for many eye diseases, stop smoking.
- Because diabetes and hypertension are risk factors for eye disease, make sure these conditions are managed optimally.

Nutritional considerations

- Include foods high in lutein, such as fruits, corn, spinach, green leafy vegetables, and egg yolks.
- Lutein supplements of 10 mg per day are safe and may be effective in preventing cataracts and age-related macular degeneration.
- People who have macular degeneration or risk factors for this condition are encouraged to take a daily supplement containing the following: 500 mg vitamin C, 400 IU vitamin E, 15 mg beta-carotene, 80 mg zinc oxide, and 2 mg cupric oxide (copper). However, people who smoke are advised to avoid beta-carotene because it can increase the risk of developing lung cancer.

BOX 17-5
Eye care practitioners

Practitioners

Ophthalmologists are licensed doctors of medicine (MD) who are trained to diagnose and treat diseases and conditions of the eye. Ophthalmological services include the following:

- Comprehensive eye examinations
- Diagnosis of eye diseases and disorders of the eye
- Prescription medications for eye problems (e.g. glaucoma)
- Eye surgery and postoperative care (e.g. cataracts)
- Laser treatments (e.g. retinopathy)
- Prescriptions for eyeglasses and contact lenses
- Prescriptions for low-vision aids
- Referrals for low-vision aids and training
- Medical referrals for diseases of the body that affect the eyes

Optometrists are not doctors, but are trained to examine eyes, screen for common eye problems, and prescribe eye exercises or corrective lenses. Optometrists use diagnostic medications, and they can prescribe certain therapeutic drugs for eye diseases. Optometric services include the following:

- Comprehensive eye examinations
- Eye refractions to determine the need for corrective lenses
- Prescriptions for eyeglasses, contact lenses, and low-vision aids
- Vision therapy to improve certain skills, such as tracking and focusing the eyes
- Referrals for low-vision aids and training
- Referrals to doctors for surgery, medication or further evaluation

Optical technicians are eye care practitioners who are trained to fit, adjust and dispense eyeglasses and contact lenses that have been prescribed by an optometrist or ophthalmologist. They do not perform eye examinations or refractions, and they cannot prescribe corrective lenses or medications.

Health insurance coverage

In New Zealand, there is government funding of some health services but it does not cover optometry. In Australia, a range of benefits are available to many optometry services. Some of these benefits are funded by the federal government's Medicare scheme, while others are covered by private health insurance. Benefits can include a direct payment to the optometrist, reimbursement to the person, or a reduction in initial costs.

WELLNESS OPPORTUNITY

Nurses promote self-care by encouraging older adults and their families to obtain information from reliable resources.

Comfort measures for dry eyes

If pertinent, simple measures to relieve dry eyes can be discussed. Use of over-the-counter artificial tears or ocular lubricants, especially before reading or engaging in other activities that require frequent eye movements, will usually relieve symptoms. People who use eye drops more frequently than every three hours should be advised to use preservative-free solutions to prevent any adverse effects from the preservatives. Other comfort measures, such as applying cold compresses or wearing wraparound glasses, are designed to prevent evaporation of tears. Maintenance of adequate environmental humidity, especially during the winter months or in dry climates, also decreases evaporation of eye moisture and adds to eye comfort. People who experience discomfort from dry eyes should avoid irritants, such as smoke and hairspray, and adverse environmental conditions such as hot rooms and high wind. People who are bothered by dry eyes and are taking a medication that might exacerbate the discomfort should be encouraged to discuss the problem with their medical practitioner.

Environmental modifications

Simple environmental modifications can improve the older person's safe performance of daily activities, thereby reducing risks of falls and accidents. Because older adults require more light for adequate vision, proper non-glare lighting is the single most important—as well as the easiest and the least costly—intervention to improve visual function (Box 17-6). Optimal illumination depends on both the quality and the quantity of lighting. For example, selection of broad-spectrum fluorescent lights and daylight-simulating lamps may be particularly beneficial in compensating for age-related vision changes.

Another important consideration in adapting the environment for optimal visual function is colour contrast. Appliances and other items such as ovens, irons, radios, thermostats and televisions may be difficult to use because of poor colour contrast around the control mechanisms. Modifications can easily be made to improve the older person's ability to use these items safely and accurately. For example, two dots of red nail polish can be used

BOX 17-6
Considerations for optimal illumination

- Older adults need at least three times as much light as younger people do.
- Older adults function best in environments with bright, broad-spectrum, non-glaring indirect sources of light.
- Sources of illumination should be placed about 30 cm to 60 cm away from the object to be viewed.
- The amount of light decreases fourfold when the distance is doubled.
- Flickering light, such as that generated by a single fluorescent tube, will cause fatigue and decreased visual performance.
- Light bulbs should be kept clean.
- Increased illumination has a greater positive effect on impaired vision than it does on normal vision.
- A gradual decrease in illumination from foreground to background is better than sharp contrasts in lighting.
- Moderate overhead lighting can be used to enhance brighter foreground lighting and prevent sharp contrasts.
- To reduce glare from reading material, place the light source to the left side of right-handed readers and to the right side of left-handed readers.
- Avoid glossy paper for reading materials.

to mark a designated and commonly used temperature setting and the older adult can be instructed to turn the dial above or below the matching dots for higher or lower settings.

Architectural designs and institutional constraints may limit the extent of environmental adaptations that nurses can implement, especially in institutional settings. In most settings, however, nurses can improve the visual abilities of older adults by using appropriate colours to enhance contrast, by using curtains to control light and glare and by placing chairs in positions that enhance illumination and avoid glare. Nurses have many opportunities to teach older adults and their carers about the environmental modifications that are most effective for optimal visual function. Box 17-7 summarises some environmental adaptations that can be used to compensate for deficits in visual skills and improve safety. All older adults can benefit from these environmental modifications, even in the absence of diagnosed eye disorders, because they are effective ways of improving vision for all people.

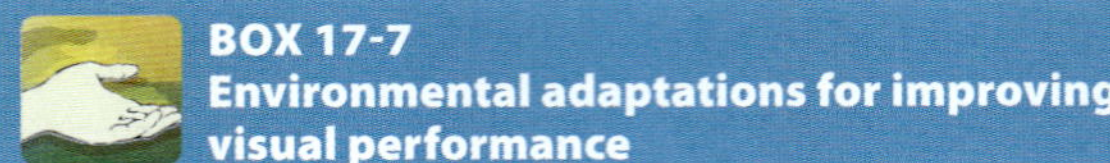

BOX 17-7
Environmental adaptations for improving visual performance

Illumination, glare control and dark/light adaptation

- Position a 60- or 75-watt soft-white light bulb or equivalent above and close to the head of the older person.
- Use a clear plastic shower curtain, rather than solid colours or printed curtains, for the tub or shower.
- Use light-coloured, sheer curtains to eliminate glare from windows.
- Place nightlights in hallways and bathrooms, or keep a high-intensity flashlight at the bedside.
- Use illuminated light switches.
- Provide good lighting in stairways and hallways.
- Use illuminated or magnifying mirrors.

Colour contrast

- Use brightly coloured tape or paint on the edges of stairs, especially on the top and bottom steps.
- Use light-coloured and dark-coloured cutting boards to contrast with dark and light foods.
- Use contrasting, rather than matching, colours for china, placemats and napkins.
- Use a toilet seat that contrasts with the bathroom walls and floor. Use coloured bars of soap on white sinks and tubs.
- Use utensils with brightly coloured handles.
- Place pillows of contrasting colours on stuffed furniture.
- Use decorative or lighted plates over light switches and wall sockets; avoid switch plates that blend in with the wallpaper or paint.
- Place decorative items of contrasting colours, such as plants and ceramics, on tables to provide cues to depth, especially on light-coloured furniture that is in a room with light-coloured walls.
- Use brightly coloured grooming utensils, such as combs, brushes and razors.
- Use pens with black ink rather than blue ink.

General adaptive measures and environmental modifications

- Do not rearrange furniture without informing or showing the older person.
- Advise older adults to pause in doorways when going from light to dark rooms (or vice versa) to allow time for their eyes to adjust to the light change.
- Teach older people to use their feet and hands as probes to feel for curbs, steps, edges of chairs, and the like.
- When walking with an older person, stop when necessary to allow a change in focus from near to far and from light to dark.

Low-vision aids

People with visual impairments can improve their safety and quality of life by using **low-vision aids** that improve focus, contrast, magnification or illumination (Box 17-8). Low-vision aids are most beneficial when used in conjunction with environmental modifications. For example, magnifiers are most effective when combined with measures that improve illumination and control glare. Reading glasses and other optical aids that magnify an image for visual tasks are available with or without a prescription. Low-vision aids also can be used to enhance contrast, reduce glare, improve lighting or enlarge the image. Printed and Internet catalogues with illustrations of low-vision aids are available through Vision Australia, the Macular Disease Foundation in Australia, the Blind Foundation in New Zealand, and other organisations. Also, local vision centres are good sources of low-vision aids, as well as training related to their use.

Although special low-vision aids can be obtained through catalogues and Internet sites, everyday items, if used advantageously, can serve as low-vision aids. An example of a low-vision aid that may be available to nurses is a photocopy machine that can be used to convert regular-print materials into large-print materials. Likewise, household lamps placed in the correct position and equipped with the right-wattage bulb can also serve as low-vision aids. Lighthouse International and the Centre for Eye Research Australia provide educational materials that illustrate examples of effective colour contrast and effective ways of making text legible. These free materials, which can be obtained from Lighthouse International (listed in the resources section at the end of this chapter), can be used as guides for developing more readable printed materials for signage, health education and other purposes.

Nurses can teach about the appropriate use of low-vision aids so that the most effective outcomes are achieved. For example, if people understand that halving the distance of a light source increases illumination by fourfold, they are more likely to place lights in the most effective positions. As an illustration of this principle, a light bulb that is 0.3 metres away from someone will

BOX 17-8
Low-vision aids for improving visual performance

Enlargement aids
- Microscopic spectacles
- Handheld or standing magnifiers
- Binoculars and handheld or spectacle-mounted telescopes
- Magnifying sheets
- Field expanders for diminished peripheral vision
- Large-print books, magazines and newspapers
- Photocopy machines or printers to enlarge print
- Telephones with enlarged letters and numbers, or a pad with enlarged letters and numbers designed to fit over rotary-dial or push-button phones
- Large numbers on rulers, playing cards and other items
- Thermometers with good colour coding and enlarged numbers
- Large-eye sewing needles

Illumination aids
- High-intensity lights
- Gooseneck lamps
- Floor or table lamps with three-way light bulbs

Contrast aids
- Use of broad-tipped felt markers in dark, yet bright, colours and coloured construction paper for making signs
- Red print on a yellow background or white letters on a green background
- Reading and signature guides (typoscopes)
- Clip-on yellow lenses

Glare control aids
- Sunglasses with UV-absorbing lenses
- Sun visors and broad-brimmed hats
- Non-glare (antireflective) coating on eyeglasses
- Yellow and pink acetate sheets
- Pinhole occluders

Other aids
Banknotes with larger, bold numerals, greater colour contrast, graduated note sizes and clearer backgrounds will be available in New Zealand from late 2015.

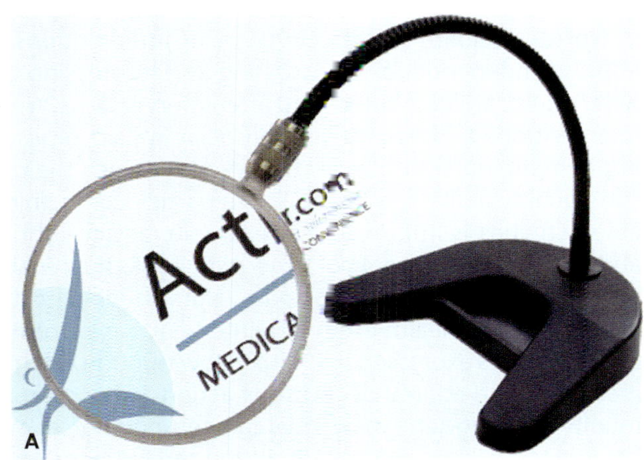

FIGURE A Examples of low-vision aids. (**A**) A combination of high-intensity lamp and magnifier.

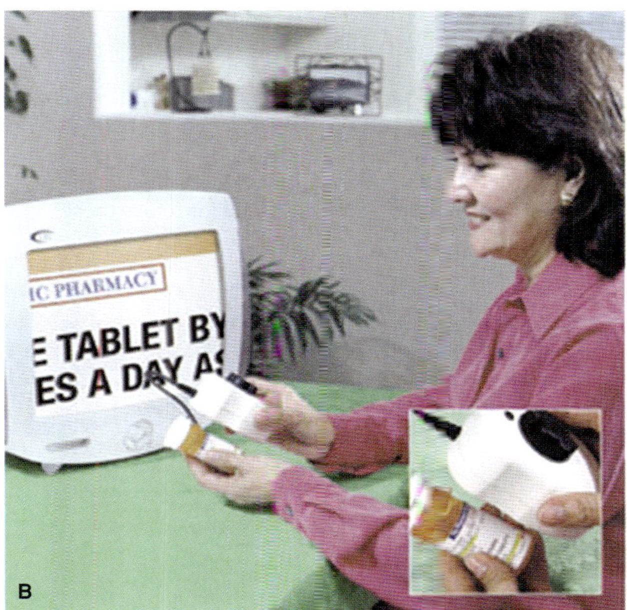

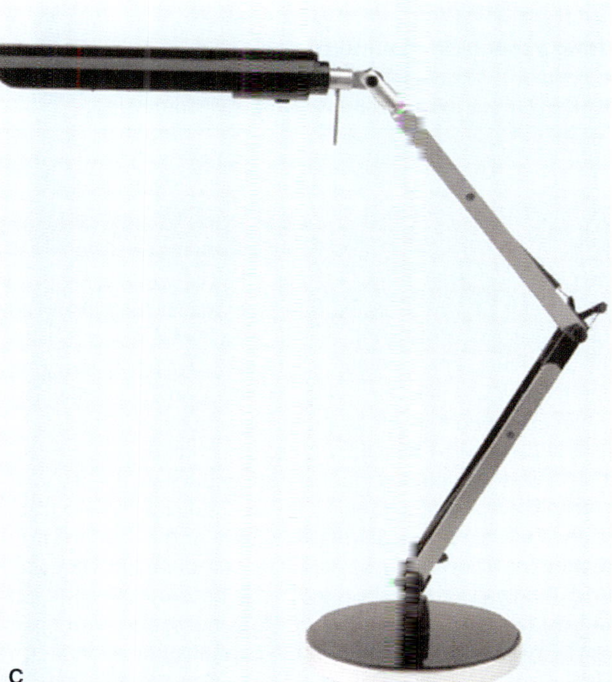

FIGURE B–C (**B**) A handheld digital magnifier that works with any television to magnify print. (**C**) A versatile lamp that uses an energy-efficient high-definition tube bulb for good contrast and brightness. (Photographs courtesy of ActiveForever.com.)

provide four times as much illumination as one that is 0.6 metres away. Nurses can use the information presented in Boxes 17-6 and 17-9 to teach about effective use of lights and magnification.

WELLNESS OPPORTUNITY

Nurses promote self-care for people who are visually impaired by facilitating referrals to local vision services and encouraging older adults and their families to use these resources.

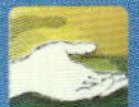

BOX 17-9
Guidelines for using magnifying aids

Using a handheld magnifier

- Begin by holding the magnifier close to the reading material.
- Slowly move the magnifier towards the face until the image totally fills the lens.
- For optimal focus, move the magnifier back towards the print about a distance of 2 cm.

Using a stand magnifier

- Rest the stand flat against the reading material.
- Do not move the stand.

Using a spectacle-mounted magnifier

- Begin with the reading material close to the nose.
- Slowly move the material away until it becomes clear.

UNFOLDING CASE STUDY

Part D

Mrs Fuller is now 81 years old. She had cataract surgery and an intraocular lens implanted in her left eye when she was 76 years old, and in her right eye when she was 77. Her vision was good until a year ago, when she developed macular degeneration. She knows this condition will be progressive, but she continues to drive and live alone. Her current medical conditions are osteoarthritis, hypertension and coronary artery disease. She stopped smoking several years ago after she was hospitalised for coronary artery disease. You are the practice nurse at the local medical centre that Mrs Fuller visits. During an appointment with you, Mrs Fuller confides that she is terrified of becoming totally blind and of losing her independence. Her grandmother went blind several years before she died and she had to go to a long-term care facility.

Thinking points

- What nursing issues apply to Mrs Fuller at this time?
- Which information in Boxes 17-4 through 17-9 might be appropriate for Mrs Fuller?
- What health promotion advice would you give?
- Would you suggest any referrals for information or community resources?
- What interventions would address Mrs Fuller's fear of becoming blind and losing her independence?

Maintaining and improving quality of life

As discussed earlier, the psychosocial consequences of impaired vision can be quite significant for older adults. Many of the interventions that help older adults compensate for visual deficits and function at their highest level will also improve their quality of life and address the psychosocial consequences of impaired vision. The use of appropriate reading glasses and good environmental lighting may enable the older adult to read books, newspapers and magazines. Subsequently, their quality of life may improve because they experience satisfying social interactions and increased intellectual stimulation. Nurses also encourage participation in support and educational groups because these interventions serve an important role in improving the quality of life for people with significant or progressive vision loss.

EVALUATING THE EFFECTIVENESS OF NURSING INTERVENTIONS

Nurses observe the compensatory behaviours of visually impaired older adults to evaluate the effectiveness of interventions for disturbed visual sensory perception. The following are indicators of successful interventions:

- Use of corrective lenses and low-vision aids to achieve the best possible visual function
- Adaptations of the environment for safety and improved visual function (e.g. bright, non-glare lighting, good colour contrast)
- Expressed feelings of safety in relation to visual function
- Maximum independence in activities such as dressing, personal care, using appliances and managing medications
- Expressed feelings of improved quality of life, despite visual impairments.

Nurses evaluate the effectiveness of interventions to improve independence by assessing and reassessing the older adult's abilities before and after interventions. When interventions address the psychosocial impact of visual impairment, nurses observe the extent to which the person's quality of life and the ability to participate in enjoyable activities is improved. For example, better lighting and the use of audiobooks or large-print books may enable someone to enjoy reading again. Nurses evaluate the effectiveness of health education interventions according to the person's expressed intent to follow through with the recommended referral or course of action. In home, community and long-term residential care settings, nurses may be able to facilitate referrals for vision screening or other vision care services. In these settings, nurses evaluate the effectiveness of interventions based on feedback from older adults or their carers about the actual use of suggested resources.

UNFOLDING CASE STUDY

Part E

Mrs Fuller is now 86 years old and is recovering from a recent fractured hip, which occurred when she fell while getting out of bed to go to the bathroom at night. After a brief hospitalisation for surgical repair of the fractured hip and a four-week period of rehabilitation, Mrs Fuller was assessed for community care for therapy, assessment, monitoring of her medical status, and evaluation of her ability to manage at home.

In addition to AMD, Mrs Fuller's current medical diagnoses include osteoarthritis, hypertension, coronary artery disease, and congestive heart failure. Mrs Fuller's medical conditions had been stable for several years, but during her hospitalisation for the fractured hip, she was started on oxygen and her medications were changed. Current medications are frusemide 40 mg daily, digoxin 0.125 mg daily, and enalapril 10 mg twice daily. A 2-g sodium diet has been prescribed, and she has been discharged with an order for oxygen per nasal cannula at a rate of 2 L/minute as needed.

Before her accident, despite the visual limitations from macular degeneration, Mrs Fuller had lived alone in her own home, but her daughter has become increasingly concerned about her mother's safety. Now Mrs Fuller's daughter is convinced that her mother should not remain in her own home but should instead move to a residential care facility. Mrs Fuller is adamant in her desire to stay in her own home and says the only reason she fell and broke her hip was because she was rushing to get to the bathroom. She says she has learned a lesson and will not hurry when she gets up at night. Furthermore, she says, she gave up driving to satisfy her daughter last year—now she is to give up her home, too? Mrs Fuller's daughter is staying with her mother for a couple of weeks until her mother regains her mobility to the point of independence. The daughter hopes that, in the interim, she will be able to convince her mother to move to a residential care facility. You are a community nurse working with Mrs Fuller in her home.

Nursing assessment

During your initial nursing assessment, you determine that Mrs Fuller is motivated to regain her mobility and manage her medical conditions, but she has difficulty reading small-print instructions because of poor vision. When you review Mrs Fuller's medications with her, you observe that she cannot read the labels on the bottles. You also observe that Mrs Fuller keeps her medications on the shelf above the kitchen counter, where the lighting is very dim. When you review the proper use of the oxygen, you note that she has difficulty seeing the markings on the flowmeter. Her daughter has been helping her with these regimens, but Mrs Fuller hopes to perform these activities independently so she can remain in her own home.

Mrs Fuller tells you that she is not concerned about falling because she walks slowly and carefully when she gets up during the night to go to the bathroom. She now uses a walker and says she feels safe. Her daughter expresses concern about her mother managing the oxygen and the walker when going to the bathroom. Mrs Fuller uses the oxygen when she sleeps and her daughter is sceptical about her ability to get to the bathroom without rushing.

You observe that the hallway between the bedroom and bathroom is dark and that the bedroom has an overhead light but no bedside lamp. The bathroom has a narrow doorway, and the toilet is at the other side of the sink. You assess the home for safety and determine that the pathways are clear and there is good lighting on the stairway and in the living areas. You identify no additional risks (e.g. throw rugs) to Mrs Fuller's safe mobility, but you do have concerns about Mrs Fuller's ability to navigate safely to the toilet with a walker.

When questioned about her vision problems, Mrs Fuller gives her history of successful cataract surgery and a diagnosis of AMD at the age of 80 years. She sees her ophthalmologist every year, and he has told her that her vision will get worse and that nothing can be done about it. He has mentioned that the local sight centre provides some rehabilitation services for people with low vision, but he told her that those services are mostly for "younger blind people". Also, she is concerned that the sight centre will suggest she purchase items that cost a lot of money, which she would not be able to afford anyway. She says her daughter got her a subscription for the large-print *Reader's Digest*, which she enjoys, and that she is not interested in reading the newspaper because she watches the news on television. She has an appointment to see her eye doctor next month.

Nursing issues

In addition to the nursing issues related to Mrs Fuller's medical condition, you identify a nursing issue of disturbed visual sensory perception related to age-related changes, sensory organ alterations and environmental factors. Supporting evidence for this issue can be found in Mrs Fuller's inability to read labels, instructions or the flowmeter markings, and the environmental factors that contribute to unsafe mobility. The nursing issues of anxiety, self-care deficit, and risk for injury might also be applicable. However, the issue of disturbed visual sensory perception addresses the source of Mrs Fuller's anxiety, risk for injury, and inability to perform her instrumental activities of daily living and, therefore, is probably the most comprehensive issue. Also, this issue prompts you to include a long-term goal of encouraging further evaluation and management of the visual impairments.

Nursing care plan for Mrs Fuller

Goals for wellness outcomes	Nursing interventions	Nursing evaluation
Mrs Fuller will manage her medication regimen accurately and independently.	• Print simplified medication instructions on large index cards by using a black felt-tip marker. • Use coloured dots to match pill bottles with instruction cards.	• Mrs Fuller demonstrates she can accurately fill the pill boxes. • Mrs Fuller takes her medications correctly.

Goals for wellness outcomes	Nursing interventions	Nursing evaluation
	• Establish a medication management system by using pill organiser boxes with markings that are bold and have good colour contrast. • Teach Mrs Fuller how to fill the pill boxes weekly, using the index cards you prepared for her. • Suggest that Mrs Fuller fill the pill boxes at the kitchen table during daylight hours while using an overhead light.	• Mrs Fuller's daughter observes that her mother follows the prescribed regimen.
Mrs Fuller will self-administer oxygen as needed.	• Use a copy machine to enlarge the small-print instructions for the oxygen equipment. • Place a coloured dot at the 2-L mark on the flowmeter. • Keep the oxygen tank in a well-lit location and suggest using a flashlight to help illuminate the flowmeter setting.	• Mrs Fuller demonstrates a safe and independent operation of the oxygen equipment. • Mrs Fuller's daughter observes that her mother administers her oxygen correctly.
Mrs Fuller will be able to use a commode safely and independently.	• Ask Mrs Fuller to use a bedside commode during the night; emphasise the importance of preventing another fall. • Work with a physiotherapist and occupational therapist to (1) evaluate the feasibility of installing grab bars or other devices that will assist Mrs Fuller in safely using the toilet, (2) identify a safe way for Mrs Fuller to use the bathroom during the daytime, (3) teach Mrs Fuller to transfer between the bed and commode for night-time use, (4) teach her to empty the bedside commode. • Place a lamp on the nightstand and make sure that Mrs Fuller can turn it on easily while in bed. Teach Mrs Fuller to turn on the bedside lamp and sit at the edge of the bed for a few minutes before getting up at night.	• Mrs Fuller demonstrates she safely use the bathroom during the day and a bedside commode at night. • Mrs Fuller is able to empty the commode independently. • Mrs Fuller has no further falls in the bathroom.
Mrs Fuller will compensate as much as possible for her progressive visual loss.	• Educate Mrs Fuller and her daughter about the services available online at the Centre for Eye Research Australia; emphasise that these services address the needs of older adults and people with recent and progressive visual loss. • Suggest that Mrs Fuller asks her eye doctor for a referral to the sight centre when she sees him next month. • Include Mrs Fuller's daughter in the discussion about these services, and ask her to assist with following through once a referral is obtained.	• Mrs Fuller makes and keeps an appointment for an initial evaluation at the sight centre. • Mrs Fuller uses low-vision aids to improve visual function

Thinking points

- How would you address concerns about Mrs Fuller living alone? What aspects of her safety and quality of life would you consider?
- How would you use any of the boxes in this chapter for health promotion teaching?
- What additional nursing issues and outcomes would you identify for Mrs Fuller?
- What additional interventions and referrals would you consider for Mrs Fuller?
- Identify at least one resource in your community that might provide help or information for Mrs Fuller. Call that agency to obtain information about their services.

CHAPTER HIGHLIGHTS

Age-related changes that affect vision

- Changes in appearance include arcus senilis, loss of orbital fat and diminished elasticity of eyelid muscles do not affect vision but can affect wellness by causing anxiety and discomfort
- Diminished tear production
- Degenerative changes affect all structures of the eye, the retinal–neural pathway and the visual cortex of the brain

Effects of age-related changes on vision

- Diminished ability to focus clearly on objects at various distances
- Diminished ability to detect details and discern objects
- Slower adaptive response to changes in lighting
- Increased sensitivity to glare
- Narrowed visual field
- Diminished depth perception
- Altered colour perception so objects look darker and whites appear more yellowed
- Diminished ability to perceive flashing lights
- Slower processing of visual information

Risk factors that affect visual wellness

- Environmental factors: glare, sunlight, poor lighting, low humidity
- Lifestyle factors: poor nutrition, cigarette smoking
- Chronic conditions: diabetes, hypertension, Alzheimer's or Parkinson's disease
- Adverse medication effects: oestrogen, corticosteroids, anticholinergics, beta-blockers and anti-parkinsonism agents

Functional consequences affecting visual wellness

- Presbyopia (diminished ability to focus on near objects)
- Need for three to five times more light than previously
- Difficulty with night driving
- Increased risk for unsafe mobility and falls
- Increased difficulty in performing usual activities
- Increased risk of visual disorders: cataract, AMD and glaucoma

Pathological conditions affecting vision

- Cataracts
- AMD
- Glaucoma

Nursing assessment of vision

- Vision screening tests
- Risk factors that affect vision
- Influence of vision changes on performance of activities of daily living
- Attitudes about eye examinations and preventive measures
- Attitudes regarding use of low-vision aids

Nursing issues

- Willingness for enhanced knowledge: improved vision
- Disturbed sensory perception: visual
- Additional issues that address the functional consequences of visual impairment include the following: anxiety, ineffective coping, self-care deficit, risk for injury, impaired social interaction, readiness for enhanced coping and readiness for enhanced self-care

Planning for wellness outcomes

- Improved visual function
- Increased safety
- Improved independence in activities of daily living
- Improved quality of life

Nursing interventions for visual wellness

- Prevention and detection of eye disease
- Comfort measures for dry eyes
- Environmental modifications (e.g. optimal illumination)
- Low-vision aids

Evaluating effectiveness of nursing interventions

- Use of corrective lenses and other aids that improve vision
- Environmental adaptations for optimal safety and visual function
- Improved independence in daily activities
- Expressed feelings of improved quality of life in relation to visual function

CRITICAL THINKING EXERCISES

1. Describe presbyopia and explain the functional consequences of this condition in the everyday life of an older adult.
2. What environmental factors are likely to interfere with the visual function of older adults?
3. Describe the specific effects of glaucoma, cataracts or AMD on one's ability to see a television program.
4. How would you assess the visual abilities of an older adult?
5. Explain the differences between optical technicians, optometrists and ophthalmologists.
6. List at least 10 adaptations that might be implemented to improve the visual function of older adults.

RESOURCES

For an extensive range of additional resources to enhance teaching and learning and to facilitate understanding of this chapter, please see the text's accompanying website located on thePoint at http://thepoint.lww.com.

Evidence-based practice

Australian Indigenous Health*InfoNet*, eye health: www.healthinfonet.ecu.edu.au/other-health-conditions/eye

Cacchione, P. Z. (2012). Sensory changes. In M. Boltz, E. Capezuti, T. Fulmer & D. Zwicker (Eds), *Evidence-based geriatric nursing protocols for best practice* (4th ed. pp. 48–73). New York: Springer.

Joanna Briggs Institute: http://connect.jbiconnectplus.org

Evidence summaries:

- Aziz Rahman, M. (2014). Visual assessment: Snellen chart.
- Campbell, J. (2014). Dual sensory loss (older people): Mental health.
- Hadwen, G. (2013). Eye irrigation: Clinician information.
- Krivan, S. (2014). Eye toilet.
- Khanh, L. (2013). Eye cleansing.
- Rathnayake, T. (2013). Eye irrigation.

Recommended practices:

- Eye irrigation (2013).
- Eye toilet (2013).
- Falls prevention: Correction of visual deficiency (2013) by T. McReynolds.
- Visual acuity testing.

National Guideline Clearinghouse: www.guideline.gov

Search for:

- Cataract in the adult eye.
- Dry eye syndrome.
- Glaucoma.
- Vision rehabilitation for adults.

Health education

Australian Indigenous Health*InfoNet*, eye health: www.healthinfonet.ecu.edu.au/other-health-conditions/eye

Blind Foundation (formally Royal New Zealand Foundation of the Blind): http://blindfoundation.org.nz

Glaucoma New Zealand: www.glaucoma.org.nz

Centre for Eye Research Australia (CERA): www.cera.org.au

Glaucoma Australia: www.glaucoma.org.au

Health Direct Australia, seniors' health: www.healthdirect.gov.au/eye-health-tips-for-over-60s

Lighthouse International: www.lighthouse.org

New Zealand Association of Optometrists: www.nzao.co.nz

Macular Disease Foundation Australia: www.mdfoundation.com.au

Optometry Australia: www.optometrists.asn.au

Read How You Want (large-print books: www.readhowyouwant.com

Save Sight Society, New Zealand: www.savesightsociety.org.nz/index.htm

Vision Australia: www.visionaustralia.org.au

Vision 20/20. The right to sight, Australia: www.vision2020australia.org.au

Vision 20/20. The right to sight, New Zealand: www.vision2020.net.nz

World Health Organization, *Universal eye health: A global action plan 2014–2019*: www.who.int/blindness/en

REFERENCES

Ackerman, M. L., Edwards, J. D., Ross, L. A., Ball, K. K. & Lunsman, M. (2008). Examination of cognitive and instrumental functional performance as indicators for driving cessation risk across 3 years. *Gerontologist, 48*(6), 802–810.

Australian Indigenous Health*InfoNet*. (2014). *Summary of Australian Indigenous health, 2013*. Viewed February 2015 at www.healthinfonet.ecu.edu.au/health-facts-summary.

Australian Institute Health and Welfare (AIHW). (2011). *Eye health in Aboriginal and Torres Strait Islander people*. Canberra: Author.

Australian Institute Health and Welfare (AIHW). (2013). *Eye health facts*. Accessed February 2015 at www.aihw.gov.au/eye-health-facts.

Baldock, M. R. J., Berndt, A. & Mathias, J. L. (2008). The functional correlates of older drivers' on-road driving test errors. *Topics in Geriatric Rehabilitation, 24*(3), 204–223.

Blind Foundation. (2011). *Clear focus: The economic impact of vision loss in New Zealand in 2009*. Available February 2015 via http://blindfoundation.org.nz/learn/blindness/clear-focus.

Cacchione, P. Z. (2008). Sensory changes. In E. Capezuti, D. Zwicker, M. Mezey & T. Fulmer (Eds), *Evidence-based geriatric nursing protocols for best practice* (3rd ed., pp. 477–502). New York: Springer.

Coleman, H. R., Chan, C. C., Ferris, F. L., III & Chew, E. Y. (2008). Age-related macular degeneration. *Lancet, 372*, 1835–1844.

Eichenbaum, J. W. (2012). Geriatric vision loss due to cataracts, macular degeneration, and glaucoma. *Mount Sinai Journal of Medicine, 79(2), 276–294.*

Fernandez, A., Sorokin, A. & Thompson, P. D. (2007). Corneal arcus as coronary disease risk factor. *Atherosclerosis, 193*(2), 235–240.

Ferrer-Blasco, T., Gonzalez-Meijome, J. M. & Montes-Mico, R. (2008). Age-related changes in the human visual system and prevalence of refractive conditions in patients attending an eye clinic. *Journal of Cataract Refractive Surgery, 34*, 424–432.

Gilbert, S. S. & Bassett, K. (2007, January). Bridging the gender gap. *Cataract & Refractive Surgery Today*, 65–67.

Hamilton, J. M., Salmon, D. P., Galasko, D., Raman, R., Emond, J., Hansen, L. A., . . . Thal, L. J. (2008). Visuospatial deficits predict rate of cognitive decline in autopsy-verified dementia with Lewy bodies. *Neuropsychology 22*(6), 729–737.

Jin, Y. P. & Wong, D. T. (2008). Self-reported visual impairment in elderly Canadians and its impact on healthy living. *Canadian Journal of Ophthalmology, 43*(4), 407–413.

Kalinowski, M. A. (2008). "Eye"dentifying vision impairment in the geriatric patient. *Geriatric Nursing, 29*(2) 125–132.

Mabuchi, F., Yoshimura, K., Kashiwagi, K. et al. (2012). Risk factors for anxiety and depression in patients with glaucoma. *British Journal of Ophthalmology, 96*(6), 821–825.

Mathew, R. S., Delbaere, K., Lord, S. R. et al. (2011). Depressive symptoms and quality of life in people with age-related macular degeneration. *Ophthalmic and Physiological Optics, 31*(4), 375–380.

Montgomery, M. P., Kamel, F., Pericak-Vance, M. A., Postel, E. A., Agarwal, A., Richards, M., . . . Schmidt, S. (2010). Overall diet quality and age-related macular degeneration. *Ophthalmic Epidemiology, 17*, 58–65.

Najm, W. & Lie, D. (2008). Dietary supplements commonly used for prevention. *Primary Care Clinics and Office Practice, 35*, 749–767.

Nassiri, N., Nassiri, N., Sadeghi Yarandi, S. H. & Rahnavardi, M. (2009). Immediate vs delayed sequential cataract surgery: A comparative study. *Eye, 23*(1), 89–95.

Norman, J. F., Norman, H. F., Craft, A. E., Walton, C. L., Bartholomew, A. N., Burton, C. L., . . . Crabtree, C. E. (2008). Stereopsis and aging. *Vision Research, 48*, 2456–2465.

Popescu, M. L., Boisjoly, H., Schmaltz, H. et al. (2012). Explaining the relationship between three eye diseases and depressive symptoms in older adults. *Investigative Ophthalmology & Visual Sciences,* 53(4), 2308–2313.

Ramulu, P. Y., van Landingham, S. W., Massof, R. W. et al. (2012). Fear of falling and visual field loss from glaucoma. *Ophthalmology, 119*(7), 1352–1358.

Ramulu, P. Y., West, S. J., Munoz, G., Jampel, H. D. & Friedman, D. S. (2009). Driving cessation and driving limitation in glaucoma: the Salisbury Eye Evaluation Project. *Ophthalmology, 116*, 1846–1853.

Tanabe, S., Yuki, K., Ozeki, N. et al. (2012). The association between primary open-angle glaucoma and fall. *Clinical Ophthalmology, 6*, 327–331.

Van Newkirk, M. R., Nanjan, M. D., Wang, J. J., Mitchell, P., Taylor, M. D., McCarty, C. A. (2000). The Prevalence of age-related maculopathy: The visual impairment project. *Ophthalmology* (107): 1593–1600.

Wang, M. Y., Rousseau, J., Boisjoly, H. et al. (2012). Activity limitation due to fear of falling in older adults with eye disease. *Investigative Ophthalmology & Visual Sciences, 53*(13), 7967–7972.

Wood, J. M., Lacherez, P. F., Black, A. A., Cole, M. H., Boon, M. Y. & Kerr, G. K. (2009). Postural stability and gait among older adults with age-related maculopathy. *Investigative Ophthalmology & Visual Science, 50*(1), 482–487.

Wysong, A., Lee, P. P. & Sloan, F. A. (2010). Longitudinal incidence of adverse outcomes of age-related macular degeneration. *Archives of Ophthalmology, 127*, 320–327.

Chapter 18

Digestion, nutrition and hydration

By Carol Miller and Sharyn Hunter

LEARNING OBJECTIVES

After reading this chapter, you should be able to:

1. Describe age-related changes that affect eating and hydration patterns and digestive processes.
2. List age-related changes in nutritional requirements.
3. Identify risk factors that affect the digestion, nutrition and hydration of older adults.
4. Explain the effects of age-related changes and risk factors on digestion, nutrition and hydration.
5. Assess aspects of digestion, nutrition and hydration behaviours that affect eating, food preparation and oral care pertinent to care of older adults.
6. Identify nursing interventions to promote optimal digestion, nutrition, hydration and oral care.

KEY POINTS

- body mass index (BMI) standards
- constipation
- dehydration
- dietary fibre
- dysphagia
- Nutrient Reference Values (NRVs)
- malnutrition
- Mini Nutritional Assessment (MNA)
- olfaction
- protein-energy undernutrition
- xerostomia
- undernutrition

Digestion of food and maintenance of nutrition and hydration are influenced by age-related gastrointestinal changes and by risk factors that commonly occur in older adulthood. Although older adults can usually easily compensate for age-related changes in the digestive tract, they have more difficulty compensating for the many factors that interfere with their ability to obtain, prepare and enjoy food. This chapter discusses age-related change, risk factors, functional consequences and nursing management in relation to digestion, eating patterns and nutritional requirements.

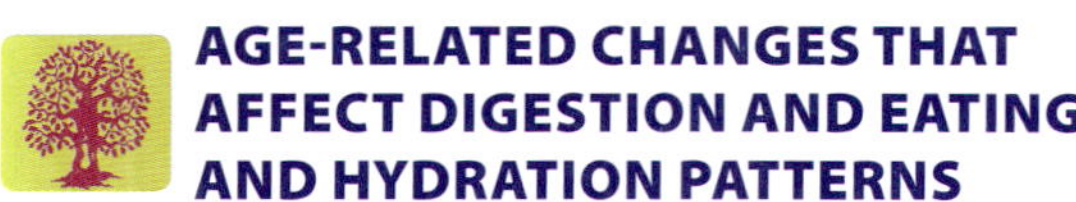

AGE-RELATED CHANGES THAT AFFECT DIGESTION AND EATING AND HYDRATION PATTERNS

Age-related changes affect the senses of smell and taste, thirst perception and all the organs of the digestive tract. These changes have very few functional consequences for healthy older adults, but they increase the vulnerability of older adults to risk factors.

Smell and taste

Both of the senses of smell and taste affect food enjoyment, and both of these senses decline in older adults because of a combination of age-related changes and risk factors. The ability to smell depends on the perception of odorants by the sensory cells in the olfactory mucosa, and on central nervous system processing of that information. The ability to detect and identify odours is optimal between the ages of 30 and 40 years, after which it gradually declines. Even in healthy older adults, age-related changes affect all of the structures involved in **olfaction** (i.e. the ability to smell odours), which begins in the nose and ends in the brain (Lafreniere & Mann, 2009). Prevalence rates for impaired sense of smell are between 1% and 5% in adults less than 35 years old, and between 14% and 25% for those 50 years or older (Huttenbrink et al., 2013; Schubert et al., 2012). Currently, researchers are exploring the relationship between impaired sense of smell as an early diagnostic marker for neurodegenerative diseases such as Parkinson's syndrome and Alzheimer's disease (Hummel, Landis & Huttenbrink, 2011). Additional conditions that can interfere with olfaction include smoking or chewing tobacco, viruses, poor oral health, periodontal disease, nasal sinus disease, trauma and medications. Medications that are associated with impaired olfactory function are angiotensin-converting enzyme (ACE) inhibitors, diuretics and antidepressants (Smoliner et al., 2013).

The ability to taste, called gustatory function, depends primarily on receptor cells in the taste buds, which are located on the tongue, palate and tonsils. Characteristics of taste sensation are measured according to the ability to perceive the intensity of taste, which diminishes with ageing, and the ability to identify different flavours. Although studies indicate that taste cells in the tongue papillae can regenerate and have a half-life of about 15 days, the sense of taste declines with increased age, but to a lesser degree than the sense of smell (Hummel, Landis & Huttenbrink, 2011). The most common causes of taste disorders are head trauma, radiation, upper respiratory tract infections, and medical conditions such as diabetes or hypothyroidism. Medications that can cause taste disorders include antibiotics, antimycotics, antiepileptics, antihistamines, immunosuppressants, antirheumatic drugs, corticosteroids, diuretics, antidiabetics, antihypertensives,

Digestive, nutritional and hydration wellness in older adults

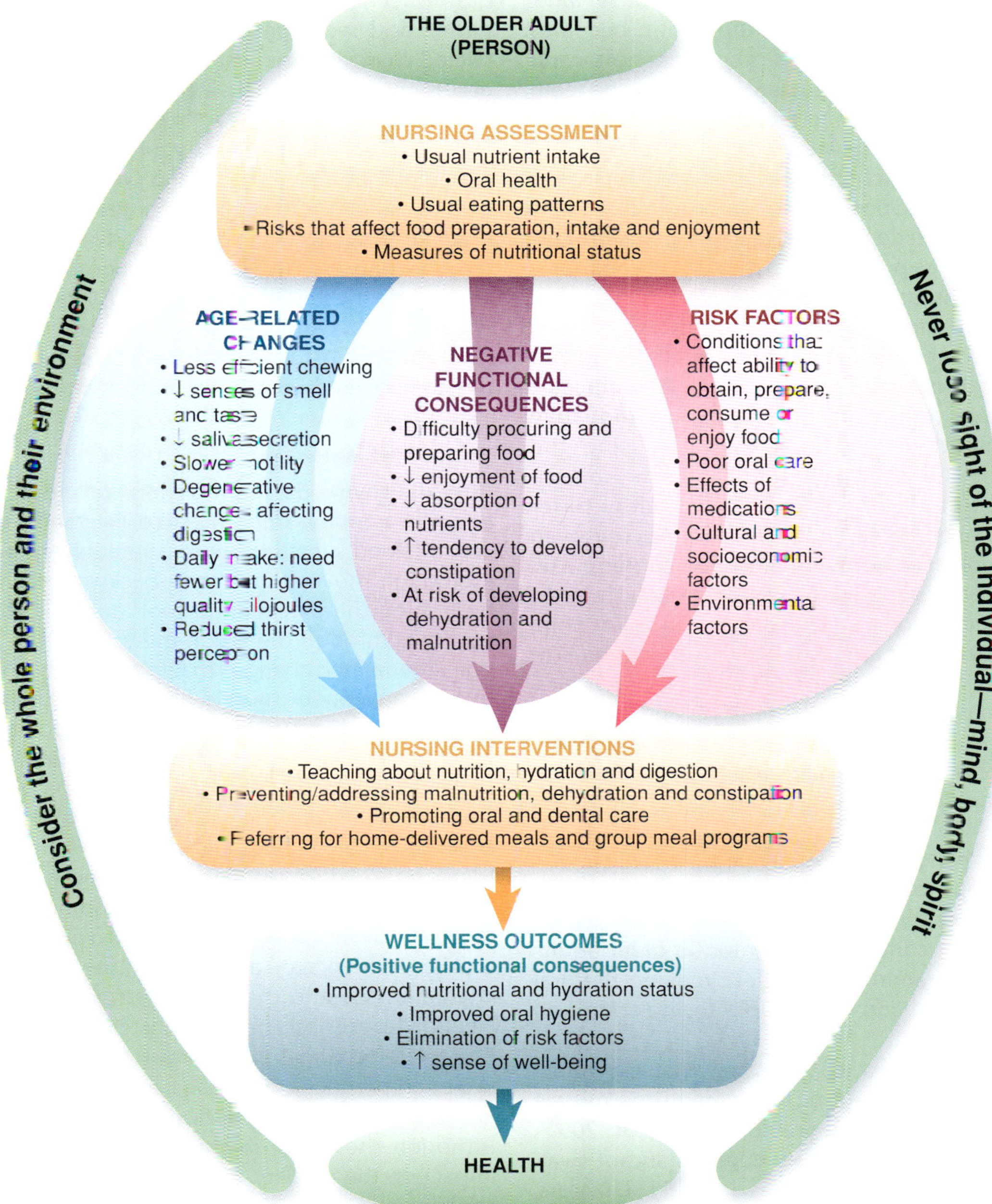

anti-parkinsonism drugs and vasodilators (Hummel, Landis & Huttenbrink, 2011).

Thirst perception

Diminished thirst perception is another age-related change that can affect homeostasis and level of hydration. Healthy older adults who are deprived of fluid do not sense thirst, experience discomfort from dry mouth or drink enough water to rehydrate themselves. With conditions that place additional demands on fluid and electrolyte balance, such as fever or infection, diminished thirst sensation can interfere with the mechanisms that normally compensate for these physiological stresses. Consequently, older people are likely to be at increased risk of dehydration.

Oral cavity

Digestion begins when food enters the mouth and is acted on by the teeth, saliva and neuromuscular structures responsible for mastication. Age-related changes in the teeth and support structures influence digestive processes and food enjoyment. With increased age, the tooth enamel becomes harder and more brittle, the dentin becomes more fibrous and the nerve chambers become shorter and narrower. Because of these age-related changes, the teeth are less sensitive to stimuli and more susceptible to fractures. These changes, along with decades of abrasive and erosive action, also cause a gradual flattening of the chewing cusps. The bones supporting the teeth of older adults diminish in height and density, and teeth may loosen or fall out, particularly in the presence of pathological conditions (e.g. periodontal disease).

Saliva and the oral mucosa play important roles in digestion. Saliva is essential for promoting chewing and swallowing, and for maintaining a moist oral mucosa. Saliva facilitates digestion by supplying digestive enzymes, regulating oral flora, re-mineralising the teeth, cleansing the taste buds, lubricating the soft tissue and preparing food for chewing. Healthy older adults do not experience any significant decreases in salivary flow; however, approximately 30% of people 65 years and older experience **xerostomia** (dry mouth) because of medications and diseases (Turner & Ship, 2007). Medications that are most likely to cause xerostomia are anticholinergics, antidepressants, antipsychotics, antiemetics, analgesics, antihypertensives and antihistamines (Lam et al., 2009; Ney et al., 2009; Uher et al., 2009). Other common causes are dehydration, diabetes and radiation therapy to the head and neck (Visvanathan & Nix, 2010).

Age-related changes of the oral mucosa include loss of elasticity, atrophy of epithelial cells and diminished blood supply to the connective tissue. These changes can be exacerbated by conditions common in older adults (e.g. xerostomia, vitamin deficiencies), making the oral mucosa more friable and susceptible to infection and ulceration.

Age-related neuromuscular changes that can affect mastication and swallowing include diminished muscle strength and reduced tongue pressure (Ney et al., 2009). Healthy older adults will not experience significant swallowing problems, unless there are additional risk factors, such as tooth loss or neurological conditions (as discussed in the section on risk factors).

Oesophagus and stomach

The second phase of digestion occurs when a combination of propulsive and non-propulsive waves propels food through the pharynx and oesophagus into the stomach. In older adults, the oesophagus stiffens and the peristaltic waves decrease (Gregersen, Pedersen & Drewes, 2008). *Presbyphagia* refers to the slowed swallowing that is associated with age-related changes and can increase the risk for aspiration (Ney et al., 2009).

After passing through the oesophageal sphincter, food enters the stomach, where gastric enzymes liquefy it and gastric action transforms it into chyme. Although reduced gastric acid secretions are sometimes attributed to age-related changes, recent studies suggest that this reduction occurs only in older adults who have atrophic gastritis or in the presence of *Helicobacter pylori* (Grassi et al., 2011). Reduced gastric acid, called hypochlorhydria, may interfere with absorption of nutrients and predispose the individual to bacterial overgrowth in the intestinal tract (Britton & McLaughlin, 2013). Studies have found a slight slowing of gastric emptying in older adults after ingestion of large meals, leading to early sensations of fullness (Morley, 2013; Rayner & Horowitz, 2013). Another age-related change that can lead to early sensation of fullness is slower postprandial peristalsis in the stomach (Bitar et al., 2011; Grassi et al., 2011).

Small and large tract

After the chyme passes into the *small intestine*, digestive enzymes from the small intestine, liver and pancreas convert the food substances into nutrients. A process of segmentation moves the chyme backwards and forwards, facilitating the digestion of food and the absorption of nutrients through the villi in the walls of the small intestine. Age-related changes that occur in the small intestine include atrophy of muscle fibres and mucosal surfaces; reduction in the number of lymphatic follicles; gradual reduction in the weight of the small intestine; and shortening and widening of the villi, which gradually form parallel ridges rather than finger-like projections. These structural changes do not significantly affect motility, permeability or transit time in the intestinal tract; however, they may affect immune function and absorption of some nutrients, such as folate, calcium and vitamins B_{12} and D.

After nutrients are absorbed in the small intestine, the chyme passes into the *large intestine*, where water and electrolytes are absorbed and waste products are expelled. Age-related changes in the large intestine include reduced secretion of mucus, decreased elasticity of the rectal wall and a diminished perception of rectal wall distension. Although these age-related changes have little or no impact on the motility of faeces through the bowel, they may predispose the older person to constipation.

Liver, pancreas and gallbladder

The liver assists in digestion by producing and secreting bile, which is essential for the utilisation of fats. It also plays an important role in the metabolism and storage of medications and nutrients. With increasing age, the liver becomes smaller and more fibrous, lipofuscin (a brown pigment) accumulates and blood flow to the liver decreases by approximately a third. However, some of these changes may be pathological, rather than age-related, in origin. Despite any age-related or pathological changes, the liver has an enormous regenerative and reserve capacity, which allows it to compensate for such changes without significantly affecting digestive function.

A primary digestive function of the pancreas is the secretion of enzymes essential for neutralising acids in the chyme and breaking down fats, proteins and carbohydrates in the small intestine. The pancreas also functions as an endocrine gland and produces insulin and glycogen, which are essential for glucose metabolism. Age-related changes in the pancreas include decreased weight, hyperplasia of the duct, fibrosis of the lobe and decreased responsiveness of pancreatic B cells to glucose. These changes do not directly affect digestive functioning; however, the effects on glucose metabolism can increase the susceptibility of older adults to the development of type 2 diabetes.

Age-related changes that affect the gallbladder and biliary tract include diminished bile acid synthesis, widening of the common bile duct and increased secretion of cholecystokinin, a peptide hormone that contracts the gallbladder and relaxes the biliary sphincter. These age-related changes can increase the susceptibility of older adults to the development of cholelithiasis (gallstones). In addition, a higher level of cholecystokinin can suppress the appetite.

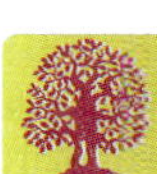

AGE-RELATED CHANGES IN NUTRITIONAL REQUIREMENTS

Since 1941, the Recommended Dietary Allowances (RDAs) had been the primary reference standard for measuring intake levels of essential nutrients that met the needs of healthy people. A major revision of the RDAs was published in 2006 for Australia and New Zealand (Australian Government Department of Health [AGDH], National Health and Medical Research Council [NHMRC] & New Zealand Ministry of Health [NZMOH], 2006). This revision produced a set of nutrient standards relevant for Australia and New Zealand, referred to as the **Nutrient Reference Values (NRVs)**.

An advantage of the NRVs is that they establish standards for meeting the basic nutrient needs of healthy adults according to specific age groups (e.g. adults aged 51 to 70 years and those 70 years and older), rather than generalising for all adults. In addition, the NRVs are applicable for health promotion because they include indicators for preventing chronic disease and avoiding the harmful effects of consuming too much of a nutrient. These standards need to be adjusted to compensate for people who have conditions such as nutrient deficiencies and medical conditions. In addition, adjustments for food and drug interactions may be necessary for people who take one or more medications. NRVs that increase with ageing are calcium (1100 mg/day for those 50 years and older) and vitamin D (10 and 15 mcg/day for those aged 51 to 70 years and those 70 years and older, respectively). The NRV for iron decreases to 5 mg/day in women 51 years and older as a result of menstruation cessation.

Kilojoules

In Australia and New Zealand, the energy-producing potential of food is measured in units called kilojoules (kJ). Kilojoule requirements are determined by a combination of factors, including height, weight, sex, body build, health–illness state and the usual level of physical activity.

Energy requirements gradually decrease throughout adulthood because of decreased physical activity and the decline in basal metabolic rate that is associated with diminished muscle mass. Thus, nutritional guidelines recommend a gradual reduction in kilojoules, beginning between the ages of 40 and 50 years. This decrease in kilojoule intake requires a proportionate increase in the quality of kilojoules (nutritional density) to meet minimal nutritional requirements. Thus, nutritional deficiencies will occur unless a reduced kilojoule intake is accompanied by an increased intake of foods with a high nutritional value, and a concomitant decrease in the intake of foods containing little or no nutrients.

DIVERSITY NOTE

Indigenous people who live in rural and remote areas of Australia have difficulties obtaining healthy food. The cost of food is higher in these communities and supply favours the metropolitan areas (Australian Institute of Health and Welfare [AIHW], 2010).

Protein

Protein provides the essential components for new tissue growth in the human body. Age-related changes, such as decreased lean body mass and muscle tissue, and decreased plasma albumin and total body albumin levels, may influence protein requirements in older adults. The recommended daily intake (RDI) for daily protein intake for all adults aged between 51 and 70 years and over is 0.64 g/kg of body weight and 0.81 g/kg of body weight (AGDH, NHMRC & NZMOH, 2006).

Women in the same age groups are recommended much less. This amount of protein is consumed when approximately 10% to 20% of the daily kilojoule intake is derived from protein. Although national surveys indicate that most adults exceed the RDI for protein, studies indicate that 11% of women 71 years and older have an intake less than the RDI (Furgoni, 2008). One review of studies concluded that the RDI for older adults should be increased to 1.0 to 1.2 g/kg protein for optimal muscle and bone health (Gaffney-Stomberg et al., 2009). Another study has emphasised that a dietary plan of 25 g to 30 g of high-quality protein at every meal would preserve muscle mass in older adults (Paddon-Jones & Rasmussen, 2009).

Carbohydrates and fibre

Carbohydrates provide an essential source of energy and fibre. Without an adequate intake of carbohydrates, the body will derive energy from fat and protein, causing an increase in serum cholesterol and triglyceride levels and a depletion of water, electrolytes and amino acids. **Dietary fibre** (i.e. the non-digestible carbohydrates and lignin in plants) has received much attention in recent years, primarily for its role in disease prevention, as an essential food component.

The RDI for fibre for Australasians is 25 g to 30 g/day for adult women and men, respectively (AGDH, NHMRC & NZMOH, 2006). However, around one-third of Australians aged 65 years and over have inadequate fruit consumption, and over two-thirds eat less than the recommended daily vegetable intake (AIHW, 2010), suggesting an inadequate consumption of fibre.

A review of studies found that dietary fibre intake from whole foods (12 g to 33 g/day) or supplements (42.5 g/day) may lower blood pressure, improve serum lipid levels and reduce indicators of inflammation. Studies found that dietary fibre may play a role in prevention and treatment of obesity, diabetes, cardiovascular disease and colorectal cancer (Dahm et al., 2010; Du et al., 2010; Hopping et al., 2010; Maki et al., 2010). Dietary guidelines suggest a daily intake of five to nine servings of fruits and vegetables, with at least 55% of the total kilojoules consumed derived from complex carbohydrates.

Fats

The primary functions of fat are to assist in temperature regulation, provide a reserve source of energy, facilitate the absorption of fat-soluble vitamins and reduce acid secretion and muscular activity of the stomach. Fats are also useful in providing a feeling of satiety and improving the taste of foods.

Fats are categorised according to their source. Saturated fats are derived from animals, whereas unsaturated fats are found in vegetables. Although either type of fat can meet nutritional needs, only the saturated fats are associated with the detrimental accumulation of serum cholesterol. Adults in most industrialised societies consume far more kilojoules in fats than is healthy or necessary. Because excessive fat intake is associated with harmful effects, such as hyperlipidaemia, fat should constitute no more than 10% to 30% of a person's daily kilojoule intake. Those fats that are consumed should be polyunsaturated and monounsaturated fatty acids, rather than cholesterol and saturated fats (see Chapter 20 for further discussion on types of fat).

Water

Water is so commonly available that it is often overlooked as a nutritional requirement. However, it is essential for all metabolic activities and must be consumed in adequate amounts for proper physiological performance. The functions of water include regulating the body temperature, maintaining a suitable metabolic environment, diluting water-soluble medications and facilitating renal and bowel excretion.

Potential consequences of reduced body water include decreased efficiency of thermoregulation, increased susceptibility to dehydration and increased concentrations of water-soluble medications in the body.

Throughout life, the proportion of total body water as a percentage of body weight gradually decreases. Whereas water constitutes approximately 80% of a newborn infant's weight, it represents 60% of a younger adult's weight, and approximately 50% or less of an older adult's weight. This decrease in total body water is associated with a loss of lean body mass and is influenced by sex and the degree of leanness, with women and obese people having a lower percentage of body water than do men and lean, muscular people.

In older adults, total body water may be further diminished by poor fluid intake. The recommended amount of water intake (in beverages, drinking water and food) is the same for adults of all ages: 3.4 L for men and 2.7 L for women (AGDH, NHMRC & NZMOH, 2006). Approximately 75% of total water intake comes from drinking water and beverages, and 25% comes from food.

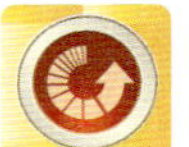

RISK FACTORS THAT AFFECT DIGESTION, NUTRITION AND HYDRATION

Certain behaviours and common disease processes are likely to interfere with nutrition, hydration and digestion in older adults. Some detrimental behaviour, such as limiting fluid intake and avoiding fresh fruit, may be based on myths and misconceptions. Although these conditions can create risks for people at any age, they occur more commonly in older adults, and the potential for harm is much greater than in other age groups because of the collective effects of risk factors and age-related changes.

Risk factors affect every phase of digestion, nutrition and hydration, and they can significantly influence eating patterns and nutritional intake. Functional and cognitive impairment are risk factors most closely associated with inadequate nutritional intake in older adults in community, acute care, and long-term care settings (Donini et al., 2013; Kiesswetter et al., 2013; Orsitto, 2012). Additional risks for poor nutritional status in older adults who live in long-term residential care facilities include polypharmacy, depression, recent hospitalisation, and presence of a wound or pressure ulcer (Verbrugghe et al., 2012). Risks that can cause specific nutrient deficiencies are listed in Table 18-1, along with the related functional consequences.

Conditions related to oral care

Oral health influences nutritional status because it affects chewing, eating, swallowing, speaking and social interaction. Lack of teeth and inadequate dental care are two conditions common in older adults that have detrimental effects on eating and nutrition. Some factors that contribute to inadequate dental care include low income, less education,

TABLE 18-1 Causes and consequences of nutrient deficiencies

Nutrient	Possible causes of deficiency	Functional consequences of deficiency
Kilojoules	Anorexia, depression, mental or physical impairments	Weight loss, lethargy, oedema, anaemia
Protein	Lack of teeth or dentures, anorexia, depression, dementia, high alcohol or carbohydrate consumption	Poor tissue healing, hypoalbuminaemia, reduced protein binding of drugs
Fat	Neomycin, phenytoin, laxatives, alcohol, colchicine, cholestyramine	Inability to absorb vitamins A, D, E and K
Vitamin A	Mineral oil, neomycin, alcohol, cholestyramine, aluminium antacids, liver disease	Dry skin and eyes, photophobia, night blindness, hyperkeratose
Thiamine (B_1)	High consumption of alcohol or caffeinated tea, pernicious anaemia, diuretics	Neuropathy, muscle weakness, heart disease, dementia, anorexia
Riboflavin (B_2)	Malabsorption syndromes, chronic diarrhoea, laxative abuse, alcoholism, liver disease	Cheilitis, glossitis photophobia, blepharitis, conjunctivitis
Niacin (B_3)	Poor dietary habits, diarrhoea, cirrhosis, alcoholism	Dermatitis, stomatitis, diarrhoea, dementia, depression
Pyridoxine (B_6)	Diuretics, hydralazine	Dermatitis, neuropathy
Folate (B_9)	Anticonvulsants, triamterene, sulfonamides, alcohol, smoking	Macrocytic anaemia, elevated levels of homocysteine
Vitamin B_{12}	Malabsorption syndrome, H2-receptor blockers, proton pump inhibitors, colchicine, oral hypoglycaemics potassium supplements, vegetarian diet	Pernicious anaemia, weakness, dyspnoea, glossitis, numbness, dementia depression
Vitamin C	Aspirin tetracycline, lack of fruits and vegetables in diet	Lassitude, irritability, anaemia, ecchymosis, impaired wound healing
Vitamin D	Phenytoin. mineral oil, phenobarbitone, sunlight deprivation	Muscle weakness and atrophy, osteoporosis, fractures
Vitamin E	Malabsorption syndromes	Peripheral neuropathy gait disturbance, retinopathy
Vitamin K	Mineral oil, warfarin sodium (Coumadin), antibiotics, cholestyramine, phenytoin	Ecchymosis; haemorrhage involving the gastrointestinal, urinary or central nervous system
Calcium	Phenytoin, aluminium-based antacids, laxatives, tetracycline, corticosteroids, frusemide, high intake of fibre or caffeine	Osteoporosis, fractures low back pain
Iron	Achlorhydria neomycin; aspirin; antacids; low intake of animal protein; high consumption of fibre, caffeine or tannic acid (contained in some teas)	Anaemia, weakness, lassitude, pallor
Magnesium	Alcohol. diuretics, diarrhoea, bulk-forming laxatives	Cardiac arrhythmias, neuromuscular and central nervous system irritability, disorientation
Zinc	Penicillamine, aluminium-based antacids, bulk-forming laxatives, high consumption of fibre	Poor wound healing. hair loss
Potassium	Laxatives, frusemide, antibiotics, corticosteroids, diarrhoea	Weakness, cardiac arrhythmias, digoxin toxicity
Water	Diuretics, laxatives, immobility, incontinence, diarrhoea	Dry skin and mouth, dehydration constipation
Fibre	Poor dietary habits	Constipation, haemorrhoids

lack of transportation, lack of dental insurance, high cost of dental services, more pressing health concerns and inaccessibility of services as a result of distance or environmental barriers, such as stairs to dental offices. In addition, because preventive dental care is a recent trend, older adults may believe that they should visit a dentist only when a toothache does not respond to home remedies.

Inadequate oral care is especially problematic for older adults in long-term residential care settings because many studies have documented the lack of oral healthcare for nursing home residents (Boczko, McKeon & Sturkie, 2009; Haumschild & Haumschild, 2009; Jablonski et al., 2009). Adverse effects of poor oral health include malnutrition, dehydration, periodontal disease, respiratory infections (e.g. pneumonia and aspiration pneumonia), joint infections, cardiovascular disease, poor glycaemic control in diabetes and increased risk of stroke (Haumschild & Haumschild, 2009; O'Connor 2012).

Until recently, tooth loss was so common among older people that it has been inaccurately viewed as a normal consequence of ageing; but the oral health of older people has improved in the past few decades so that older adults today are less likely to be edentulous (without any teeth). Tooth loss in older adulthood is often attributable to inadequate dental care, periodontal disease and other pathological conditions that occur with increasing frequency in later years.

DIVERSITY NOTE

Indigenous adult Australians have more than twice as many caries as non-Indigenous adults (Slade, Spencer & Roberts-Thomson, 2007). Indigenous adults also have much higher levels of endentulism and this occurs earlier in their life.

WELLNESS OPPORTUNITY

Nurses promote wellness by exploring reasons that older adults do not obtain dental care so they can address these barriers.

Functional impairments and disease processes

Functional impairments are strongly associated with poor nutrition, particularly with regard to dependence on others for assistance with eating (Oliveira, Fogaca & Leandro-Merhi, 2009). For example, mobility or visual impairments can interfere with the ability to procure and prepare food and fluids. In community settings, the extent to which functional impairments affect nutrition depends to a large degree on the availability of social supports, such as family, friends or agencies that assist with providing food.

Dysphagia (difficulty swallowing) is a functional impairment that can significantly affect chewing, safe swallowing and nutrition. More than 25% of community-living older adults and between 50% and 53% of residents in long-term care have dysphagia, which most commonly is caused by neurological and neuromuscular disorders (Clave et al., 2012; Park, Han, Oh et al., 2013). Because nurses caring for older adults are responsible for the assessment and interventions related to this common problem, the topic is addressed in the Evidence-based practice 18-1.

EVIDENCE-BASED PRACTICE 18-1
Dysphagia

Statement of the problem

- Dysphagia is defined as impairment of any part of the swallowing process.
- Prevalence of dysphagia ranges from 14% of community-residing older adults up to 60% of aged residents in long-term care.
- Dysphagia is common in older adults with neurological conditions, including stroke, dementia, multiple sclerosis and Parkinson's disease.
- In addition to neurological conditions, the following factors can increase the risk of dysphagia: absence of teeth, decreased saliva production, poorly fitting dentures, decreased level of consciousness, certain medications (e.g. anaesthetics, anticholinergics, sedatives, psychotropics, antihistamines, amiodarone).
- Dysphagia increases the risk of aspiration and aspiration pneumonia.
- Poor oral hygiene increases the risk for pneumonia.

Recommendations for nursing assessment

- Speech pathologists are responsible for performing comprehensive swallowing assessments, but nurses are responsible for identifying people who are at risk for dysphagia.
- Nursing assessment includes interview questions about difficulty with chewing or swallowing, avoidance of certain foods or beverages, sensation of food being stuck in throat, inability to handle secretions, voice changes, and so forth.
- A recommended three-step nursing assessment of swallowing is: (1) examine the level of consciousness, posture, voluntary cough, voice quality and saliva control; (2) have the patient/resident drink 1 teaspoon of water; (3) if the teaspoon of water clears safely, have the person drink a small glass of water.
- Signs and symptoms of dysphagia include drooling, coughing during meals, hoarse voice following meals, gurgling sounds in the throat, upper respiratory tract infection, wet lung sounds or packing food in the cheeks.
- Signs and symptoms of aspiration pneumonia include chills, cough, fever, elevated respiratory rate, pleuritic chest pain, rales, delirium.

Recommendations for nursing interventions

- Speech pathologists are the healthcare professionals who usually assume primary responsibility for recommendations, but nurses are responsible for initiating the referrals in a timely manner and implementing interventions.
- Interventions for prevention of aspiration during feeding of dysphagia individuals include the following: rest for 30 minutes before eating, sit upright, avoid rushing or forced feeding, alternate small amounts of solid and liquid foods, minimise distractions.
- Interventions for prevention of aspiration based on recommendations of speech pathologist include the following: nectar- or honey-thick liquids, chin-down position, head turned to one side, placement of food in one side of mouth, use of adaptive equipment, muscle strengthening exercises.
- Recognise that individuals with dysphagia require approximately 30 minutes for eating/assisted feeding.
- Good oral care is imperative for all older adults with dysphagia because it is associated with a lower incidence of pneumonia.
- Referrals for regular and "as-needed" dental care.
- Be prepared to perform the Heimlich manoeuvre.

Additional nursing interventions for preventing aspiration during tube feeding

- Keep head of bed or chair elevated to at least 30° during continuous feedings.
- Assess the following signs of gastrointestinal intolerance: nausea, feeling of fullness, abdominal pain or cramping.
- Measure gastric residual volumes every 4 to 6 hours during continuous feedings and immediately before each intermittent feeding.

Source: Metheny, N. A. (2012). Preventing aspiration in older adults with dysphagia. *Try This* series, issue 20. *Best Practices in Nursing Care to Older Adults*. Available 13 May 2013 at www.ConsultGeriRN.org; Nogueira, D. & Reis, E. (2013). Swallowing disorder in nursing home residents: How can the problem be explained? *Clinical Interventions in Aging, 8*, 221–227; Sura et al. (2012). Dysphagia in the elderly: Management and nutritional considerations. *Clinical Interventions in Aging, 7*, 287–298.

Disease processes also increase the risk for nutritional, hydration and digestive consequences. Vitamin B_{12} deficiency increases with increasing age and, in older adults, it is associated with malabsorption of foods resulting from atrophy of gastric mucosa (Allen, 2009). Other pathological conditions interfere with appetite and enjoyment of food in many ways. For example, infections, hyperthyroidism, hypoadrenalism and congestive heart failure are associated with anorexia, and rheumatoid conditions and chronic obstructive pulmonary disease (COPD) are associated with both decreased appetite and increased energy expenditure. Dementia and other neurodegenerative disorders often have serious negative effects on eating and nutrition related to procuring and preparing food, remembering to eat and drink, and chewing and swallowing food.

Medication effects

Medications can create risk factors for impaired digestion and inadequate nutrition through their effects on digestion, eating patterns and utilisation of nutrients. Adverse medication effects are more likely to occur in older adults because of the increased use of medications. Table 18-2 lists examples of medications and the related adverse effects on digestion and nutrition.

Medications can affect nutrition by interfering with the absorption and excretion of nutrients, as in the following examples:

- Broad-spectrum antibiotics can alter intestinal flora and impair nutrient synthesis.
- Medications and vitamins that are similar in chemical structure may compete at sites of action, thus altering their excretion pattern.
- Some medications bind to particular ions and form compounds that cannot be absorbed (e.g. tetracycline can bind to iron and calcium).
- Diuretics can interfere with the transport of water, sodium, glucose and amino acids.
- Nutritional supplements and herbal preparations also can affect nutrients (e.g. long-term use of beta-carotene supplements can cause a vitamin E deficiency).

Additional food, herb and medication interactions are discussed in Chapter 8.

Lifestyle factors

Alcohol and smoking can alter an older person's nutritional status in several ways. Alcohol has a high kilojoule content but a low nutrient value, so it provides empty kilojoules.

In addition, it interferes with the absorption of the B-complex vitamins and vitamin C. Alcoholism is often unrecognised and undertreated in older adults and may be a common contributing factor to nutritional disorders. Smoking diminishes the ability to smell and taste food and interferes with absorption of vitamin C and folic acid.

TABLE 18-2 Potential effects of medications on digestion and nutrition

Medication examples	Potential effect on digestion and nutrition
Digoxin, theophylline, fluoxetine, antihistamines	Anorexia
Anticholinergics, narcotics, calcium channel blockers, iron, aluminium- and calcium-based antacids	Constipation
Cimetidine, laxatives, antibiotics, cardiovascular drugs, cholinesterase inhibitors	Diarrhoea, nausea, vomiting
Non-steroidal anti-inflammatory drugs (NSAIDs), aspirin, corticosteroids	Gastric irritation
Phenytoin, nifedipine, diltiazem, cyclosporine	Gum hyperplasia
Anticholinergics, potassium-depleting medications	Paralytic ileus
Bulk-forming agents when taken before meals, anticholinergics	Early satiety
Potassium supplements, NSAIDs, bisphosphonates, prednisone	Dysphagia
Antihistamines, salicylates, hypoglycaemics, antiparkinsonism drugs, psychoactive drugs	Altered smell and taste sensations
Mineral oil, cholestyramine	Diminished absorption of vitamins A, D, E and K
Anticonvulsants	Diminished storage of vitamin K, decreased absorption of calcium
Aluminium- or magnesium-based antacids	Diarrhoea; decreased levels of calcium, fluoride and phosphorus
Ampicillin, amoxicillin, cephalosporins, clindamycin	*Clostridium difficile* diarrhoea
Products containing sodium bicarbonate	Sodium overload, water retention
Gentamicin and penicillin	Hypokalaemia
Tetracyclines	Diminished absorption of zinc, iron, calcium and magnesium
Neomycin	Diminished absorption of fat, iron, lactose, nitrogen, calcium, potassium and vitamin B_{12}
Aspirin	Gastrointestinal bleeding; decreased levels of iron, folate and vitamin C
Corticosteroids	Increased need for calcium, phosphorus, B vitamins, and vitamins C and D

Psychosocial factors

Psychosocial factors are likely to affect an older person's appetite and eating patterns. Any changes in mealtime companionship, as may occur through loss or disability of a spouse, are likely to have a negative impact on eating patterns. Eating alone is associated with poor nutritional status of older adults, particularly men (Hsieh, Sung & Wan, 2010). When older adults have established a long-term pattern of preparing meals for family and spouse, it may be especially difficult for the older adult to adjust to purchasing, preparing and eating food for just one person. Similarly, older adults who have never participated in the purchase or preparation of foods may have great difficulty assuming these tasks after the loss of a spouse or other person who performed them. If the older adult depends on others for assistance in procuring food, any factors that limit the availability of support resources may affect the older adult's ability to obtain food.

WELLNESS OPPORTUNITY

Nurses can work with older adults to identify ways of promoting positive social interaction during mealtimes.

Stress and anxiety affect digestive processes through their influence on the autonomic nervous system. Although stress-related effects on digestion are not unique to older adults, any alteration of the autonomic nervous system may compound age-related effects that otherwise would not have much effect.

Older adults who are depressed are likely to experience anorexia and loss of interest in food. Confusion, memory problems and other cognitive deficits may significantly interfere with eating patterns and the ability to prepare food. Studies indicate that cognitive impairment and depression are associated with poor nutritional status in older adults in community and long-term residential care settings (Grieger, Nowson & Ackland, 2009; Johansson et al., 2009; Sahyoun et al., 2010).

Cultural and socioeconomic factors

Ethnic background, religious beliefs and other cultural factors strongly influence the way people define, select, prepare and eat food and beverages. Cultural factors can also influence eating patterns and selection of food in relation to health status. For example, some Asian people may classify foods, beverages and medicines as hot or cold, and they may select a particular food on the basis of their belief that their illness would respond to warm, hot, cool or cold types of remedies. According to this health belief model, illnesses are caused by an imbalance between hot and cold, and so must be treated with substances that have the opposite characteristics. The characteristics of "hot" and "cold" are not related to temperature of the food but are culturally defined by different groups.

Cultural dietary customs are not usually detrimental for healthy older adults, as long as the diet includes essential nutrients and avoids extremes. However, for older adults with medical conditions that require diet modification (e.g. diabetes or hypertension), cultural food patterns may aggravate the person's condition and create barriers to nutritional therapy. Cultural considerations 18-1

CULTURAL CONSIDERATIONS 18-1
Cultural influences on eating patterns

Asians
- Common foods: rice, wheat, pork, eggs, chicken, soybean products and a variety of vegetables
- Methods of food preparation: stir-frying with lard, peanut oil or sesame oil; seasoning with ginger, soy sauce, sesame seeds and monosodium glutamate
- Beverages: green tea; rare use of milk products because lactose intolerance is common

Indonesians
- Rice is the main food
- Vegetables, fish, beef and chicken and hot sauces accompany the rice
- Tea and coffee are common drinks

Indian Hindus
- Orthodox Hindus do not drink alcohol
- Fasting occasionally is common. During fasting, only fruit and milk products are eaten

Italians
- Preferred foods are pasta, soups, fish, meat, salads and fruits
- Morning and afternoon tea/coffee is shared with others and is an important routine
- Older Italians prefer a glass of red wine with their meal and an espresso coffee after the meal
- Main meal of the day is dinner and this is consumed early in the evening

Māori
- Māori eat a mix of British and traditional foods. At large Māori gatherings, a *hāngi* still occurs. Two dishes regarded as Māori food that are still consumed are a meal of pork, potatoes, kumara and dumplings, and the other is pork and *puha* or sow thistle

Religious influences
- Some groups of Jews follow prescribed rules for preparing and serving foods (e.g. they eat only kosher meat and poultry and do not eat shellfish or any pork products)
- Mormons do not drink tea, coffee or alcohol
- Hindus may be vegetarians
- Seventh-Day Adventists may be lacto–ovovegetarians
- Many Catholics do not eat meat on Ash Wednesday or Good Friday

A comprehensive resource where information about cultures and food preferences for older Australians can be found is at the Centre for Cultural Diversity in Ageing website, www.culturaldiversity.com.au/resources/practice-guides/food-services.

summarises some of the food habits that are associated with major cultural and religious groups in Australia and New Zealand. Nurses should remember, though, that individual older adults vary in their eating patterns and may not adhere to the patterns of their cultural group. It is not usually necessary to try to change culturally influenced eating patterns, but it is important to recognise any cultural factors that may affect older adults' nutritional status.

WELLNESS OPPORTUNITY

Nurses address cultural needs by identifying food preferences and finding reasonable ways to provide these foods.

A person's past and present economic status also influences food choices. If nutrient intake has been inadequate because of long-standing financial limitations, the progressive effects of poor nutrition may precipitate new problems in some older adults, especially in combination with age-related changes in nutrient intake and utilisation. People of low socioeconomic status usually have a narrower selection of foods than do people of higher socioeconomic status. Lower socioeconomic status, including educational level, is also associated with lack of dental care and more tooth loss (Starr & Hall, 2010).

Environmental factors

Environmental factors affect the enjoyment of food and the ability to obtain and prepare it. Many barriers to food enjoyment have been identified in the dining environments of long-term residential care facilities and in other institutional settings. Older adults living in long-term residential care facilities may find it difficult to adjust to unfamiliar environments. Moreover, they may not desire the mealtime social interaction that is part of the institutional environment. A noisy or crowded dining room may have a negative impact on food enjoyment and consumption. Such an environment may be particularly stressful for older adults who use a hearing aid or who are accustomed to eating alone. The potential outcomes of a move to a new environment include poor nutrition and loss of interest in eating, particularly during the initial adjustment period.

Environmental influences, such as inclement weather conditions, particularly affect functionally impaired older adults who live in their own homes. For example, older persons who walk to the store or depend on public transportation may be unable or unwilling to obtain groceries in windy or rainy weather. Likewise, older adults may not be able to tolerate hot or sultry conditions. Older adults are particularly vulnerable to the development of dehydration when there occurs a short period of prolonged high temperatures, referred to as a "heat wave", which can occur during the Australian summer.

Older people who depend on others for transportation or who have difficulty manoeuvring in adverse weather conditions are likely to shop for groceries less frequently and to purchase their groceries at smaller convenience stores, where prices are higher and the selection is limited. The additional cost and limited selection may interfere with food intake and lead to nutrient deficiencies. Finally, environmental conditions and packaging trends in the grocery store may create additional difficulties for older people, especially those who are functionally impaired. For example, the combined glare of fluorescent lights; highly polished floors; shiny, clear wrappers; and white freezer cases often makes it extremely difficult, if not impossible, for older adults with vision challenges to read labels, especially when the print is small and contrasts poorly against the background.

Behaviours based on myths and misunderstandings

Myths and misunderstandings may be detrimental to a person's food intake and behaviours related to bowel function. For example, during the 1950s and 1960s, a widely held belief was that roughage and raw fruits or vegetables were harmful to the older person. It is now known that a lack of roughage in the diet and the consumption of only cooked fruits and vegetables are eating patterns that contribute to constipation by slowing the transit time of faeces through the large intestine.

Another commonly held belief is that a daily bowel movement is the norm for good digestive function. Rigid adherence to this standard may, in fact, lead to the unnecessary and detrimental use of laxatives. Advertisements have further reinforced this false belief by implying that daily bowel movements should be attained through medication. Although recent advertising trends emphasise the achievement of healthy bowel patterns through the ingestion of high-fibre food items, the negative impact of any long-term beliefs may be difficult to overcome.

Misunderstandings about fluid intake may also interfere with digestion, nutrition and hydration. Many older adults reduce the amount of liquids they consume in an attempt to decrease the incidence of urinary incontinence. Fluid intake may also be restricted if functional limitations, such as impaired mobility or manual dexterity, interfere with either the ability to obtain liquids or the ease of urinary elimination. Reduced fluid intake can have a number of detrimental consequences, such as constipation, xerostomia, diminished food enjoyment and dehydration.

WELLNESS OPPORTUNITY

Nurses identify myths and misunderstandings about constipation and teach older adults about habits that promote healthy elimination patterns.

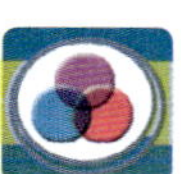

FUNCTIONAL CONSEQUENCES AFFECTING DIGESTION, NUTRITION AND HYDRATION

Functional consequences affect the following aspects of digestion and nutrition of older adults:

- Procurement, preparation and enjoyment of food
- Mastication and digestion of food
- Nutritional status
- Psychosocial function.

Negative functional consequences occur primarily because of the many risk factors that affect older adults, rather than because of age-related changes alone.

Ability to procure, prepare and enjoy food

Activities involved in procuring, preparing, consuming and enjoying food depend on the skills of cognition, balance, mobility and manual dexterity, as well as on the five senses.

Food procurement depends on getting to the supermarket, pushing a shopping trolley, reaching for food items on high shelves, reading the small print on shelves and food packages for cost and nutrition information, and coping with the glare of bright lights, especially in the frozen-food sections. Age-related changes and conditions that may interfere with these activities include vision impairments and any illness, such as arthritis, that limits mobility, balance or manual dexterity.

Food preparation activities that are likely to be more difficult for older adults include cutting food items, measuring ingredients accurately, carrying food and liquid without spilling, standing for long periods in the kitchen, reaching for items on high shelves and in cupboards, safely using the oven or stove and reading the temperature controls correctly. Impairments of vision, balance, cognition, mobility or manual dexterity are likely to cause difficulties in performing these tasks. Diminished sensory function can affect food enjoyment in all the following ways:

- Inaccurate perception of colour, taste or smell can interfere with appetite and food appeal.
- Diminished gustatory and olfactory sensitivity may lead to excessive use of condiments and seasonings, such as salt and sugar.
- Visual and olfactory impairments may make it difficult to detect spoiled food.

Moreover, food choices are influenced by the condition of the oral cavity and teeth, as well as by the quantity and the quality of natural or replacement teeth.

WELLNESS OPPORTUNITY

Nurses promote wellness through interventions that improve the older adult's independence in procuring and preparing satisfying meals.

Changes in oral function

Digestive processes in healthy older adults are not significantly affected by age-related changes, but older adults often have digestive complaints (e.g. "heartburn", constipation) caused by commonly occurring risk factors. For example, many negative functional consequences are associated with medications (see Table 18-2). Xerostomia causes negative functional consequences because it can interfere with oral comfort, food enjoyment and taste sensitivity. In addition, diminished saliva production makes it more difficult to chew food and increases the susceptibility of the teeth and tongue to bacterial action.

Older adults with poor oral health are likely to avoid eating whole fruits, raw vegetables and meat (Quandt et al., 2010). A review of studies identified the following consequences of impaired salivary function: gingivitis; oral lesions; dental caries; excessive plaque; periodontal disease; and impaired taste, speech, chewing and swallowing (Turner & Ship, 2007).

The functional consequences of being edentulous or using dentures include the avoidance of certain foods, decreased chewing efficiency and increased susceptibility to accidental choking from ineffective mastication. Because edentulous people tend to avoid meats, salads, fresh fruits and raw vegetables, they may be at risk for nutritional deficiencies (Savoca et al., 2010; Tsakos et al., 2010).

Nutritional status and weight changes

An older adult's nutritional status can also be altered when there is a decrease in the quantity of kilojoules without a corresponding increase in the quality of the food consumed. Older adults need fewer kilojoules and, as their intake decreases, if they do not increase the quality of food consumed then a deficiency of essential minerals or vitamins is likely to occur.

Risk factors (e.g. medications and pathological processes) that commonly occur in older adults can often cause nutrient deficiencies. For example, iron deficiency is associated with chronic diseases and low socioeconomic status. Other minerals and vitamins that are commonly deficient in older adults are zinc, calcium, most B vitamins and vitamins D and E. See Table 18-1 for examples of nutrient deficiencies and associated risk factors and functional consequences that are likely to affect older adults.

A number of other negative consequences are associated with older adults who have poor nutrition and these include increased mortality, prolonged and increased hospitalisation, institutional placement, increased falls, increased risk of osteoporosis and increased fracture risk (Australian and New Zealand Society for Geriatric Medicine [ANZSGM], 2007)

In older adults, there are two distinct phases of energy balance that impact on their nutritional status and weight changes. They are:

(a) A positive energy balance typically occurs between 40 and 65 years, causing an increase in body weight and fat stores (McLaren, 2006, p. 280).

(b) A negative energy balance typically begins in persons over 65 years, but mostly occurs in the 85 years and over age group (AIHW, 2010).

The first phase, the positive energy balance, occurs as a result of age-related changes in body composition, carbohydrate metabolism and a decrease in physical activity. The proportion of body fat to lean tissue begins to increase around 30 years of age and leads to disproportionately increased abdominal fat (commonly known as "middle age spread") during later adulthood. This pattern of fat distribution is associated with increased risk for diabetes, cardiovascular disease and other chronic conditions. In the second phase, the negative energy balance, there is a decrease in body weight and food intake, a decrease in muscle mass (sarcopenia), and an increase in the risk of malnutrition. Older people who experience a negative energy balance are at risk of two types of malnutrition: macronutrient and micronutrient malnutrition (refer to the next section for discussion about both types).

This pattern of energy balance is confirmed by reported prevalence rates. Prevalence of overweight and obesity among older adults between the ages of 65 and 74 years is approximately 75% (AIHW, 2014). However, the prevalence of obesity is reduced to below half for older people aged 85 years and over. Another consideration is that there is evidence the **body mass index (BMI) standards** should be increased for older adults. There is also evidence that waist circumference should be measured. The waist measure is a better indicator of a risk weight than abdominal obesity as it is recognised as an independent risk factor for many medical conditions, particularly type 2 diabetes (Houston, Nicklas & Zizza, 2009).

Quality of life

Good food and nutrition are important components of health-related quality of life in many ways. Food-related activities are often a focal point of celebrations, religious rituals or gatherings to share significant events. In addition, mealtimes are typically associated with caring, comfort, nurturing and social interaction. Thus, when mealtime enjoyment is affected in any way, the psychosocial aspects of eating are also affected. Older adults who enjoyed participating in family meals or eating in restaurants may withdraw from these activities if food is no longer enjoyable. Similarly, when these events are no longer part of life for older adults, they may lose interest in eating.

Perhaps even more detrimental than the psychosocial consequences of diminished food enjoyment are the psychosocial effects of inadequate nutrition. When fluid or nutrient intake is inadequate, older adults are likely to develop malnutrition and dehydration because of impaired homeostatic mechanisms. Changes in mental status, including memory impairment, are among the early signs of malnutrition, dehydration and electrolyte imbalance in older adults. Sometimes these mental changes are attributed incorrectly to irreversible conditions (e.g. dementia) rather than to a treatable and reversible metabolic imbalance. For example deficiencies of vitamins B_{12} or D are common nutritional causes of mental changes (Morley, 2010).

PATHOLOGICAL CONDITIONS AFFECTING DIGESTIVE WELLNESS: MALNUTRITION, DEHYDRATON AND CONSTIPATION

Malnutrition

Malnutrition is a state of abnormal nutrition caused by **undernutrition** or overnutrition or incorrect nutrition. All types of malnutrition produce observable adverse effects on the body's composition or function and result in poor health outcomes. Although studies related to specific nutritional deficits and undernutrition among older adults are confused by a lack of common definitions (ANZSGM, 2007), numerous studies conclude that dietary intake for most older adults does not meet recommended daily allowance standards. A review of studies concluded that the prevalence of undernutrition in older adults was 45% in the community, 50% to 84% in hospitals and between 84% and 100% in residential care facilities (Visvanathan & Chapman, 2009).

Two types of undernutrition can occur in older adults: *macronutrient* (lack of protein/energy) (ANZSGM, 2007), and *micronutrient* (vitamin deficiency; for example, calcium, vitamin D, folate, iron or vitamin B_{12}) (Biesalski et al., 2003).

The **protein-energy undernutrition** (PEU) is common in older people and its prevalence increases with increasing levels of frailty (ANZSGM, 2007). It occurs when the intake of kilojoules and protein is less than the amount required to meet daily needs. This condition is associated with a high-carbohydrate, low-protein diet, which often results from one or several of the risk factors (e.g. depression, loss of appetite, pathological conditions). Micronutrient undernutrition usually accompanies PEU (McLaren, 2006). Characteristics of mild or moderate protein-energy undernutrition include weakness, lethargy, unintentional weight loss, diminished muscle mass, a marked decrease in subcutaneous fat and an impaired ability to respond to physiological stresses (e.g. surgery, infection). If the condition progresses and becomes severe it is characterised by oedema and loss of visceral protein. In a study of patients between the ages of 65 and 99 years, negative consequences of protein-energy undernutrition included anaemia, decreased thyroid function, altered insulin production, anomalies in salt and water retention, loss of skeletal muscle mass, decreased glomerular filtration rate, decreased creatinine clearance and increased risk of pneumonia (Price, 2008).

Specific nutrients that are likely to be deficient in older adults include fibre, calcium, magnesium, potassium and vitamins C, D, E and K (Burnett-Hartman et al., 2009; Lichtenstein et al., 2008).

Diagnosis of undernutrition and PEU is made by physical examination, a health history that probes eating habits, anthropometric measurements (BMI, weight loss, skinfold thickness assessment) and haematology and biochemical assessment (hypoalbuminaemia, anaemia, hypocholesterolaemia, low lymphocyte counts) (ANZSGM, 2007).

Treatment of undernutrition and PEU focuses on providing adequate nutrition, restoring normal body composition and treating the conditions that caused the deficiency. Interventions are based on the level of the deficiency and the response of the individual.

Overnutrition

As mentioned previously overweight and obesity is prevalent in older adults aged 65 to 74 years. However, evidence supports significant decreases in BMI may not support wellness for obese older adults (National Health and Medical Research Council [NHMRC], 2013). Research suggests that addressing cardiovascular and diabetes risks are more appropriate goals than reducing weight alone as decreases in blood pressure and lipids are associated with a reduction in morbidity and mortality for older adults. Weight loss programs recommended for older adults include following a nutrient-dense diet and increasing physical activity.

UNFOLDING CASE STUDY

Part A

Mr and Mrs Donnelly, who are 71 and 72 years old, respectively, attend a local medical clinic. You are a practice nurse in this medical clinic. At an appointment, Mrs Donnelly tells you about her bowels, saying that she gets all "bound up" and she always feels "bloated". When you ask about her bowel patterns, she reports that she has a bowel movement "about every other day" and has to "sit on the commode for a good half-hour before anything happens". She has taken milk of magnesia every night for approximately 20 years, but "it doesn't seem to be any help anymore". She avoids fresh fruits and vegetables because her mother always told her that canned fruits and vegetables were easier to digest. She rarely eats cereal and uses white bread. Her weight is approximately 125% of her ideal body weight, and she does not walk often because of trouble with arthritis. She takes levothyroxine, 100 mcg once daily, and an over-the-counter generic calcium supplement that contains 500 mg calcium carbonate twice daily.

Thinking points

- Identify at least five risk factors that are likely to contribute to Mrs Donnelly's constipation.
- Describe how you would begin addressing one of these risk factors in health education.

Pharmacological interventions include nutritional supplements, multivitamin and mineral supplementation and orexigenic (appetite stimulant) and anabolic agents (ANZSGM, 2007). These are administered via either the oral or the enteral route. Supplementation is preferred via the oral route as this has been shown to promote weight gain and increase muscle mass in older adults with undernutrition in hospital (Joanna Briggs Institute [JBI], 2007) and other settings (ANZSGM, 2007). Orexigenic and anabolic agents are not recommended to be used routinely (ANZSGM, 2007). Enteral feeding (via nasogastric or percutaneous endoscopic gastrostomy) or parenteral (intravenous) feeding is used to supply nutrients to older adults who do not have the capacity to eat or won't eat protein-rich foods.

Nurses play a critical role in ensuring that the nutritional intervention prescribed is administered (JBI, 2007). Nurses are also involved in assessing the nutritional status of an older adult to identify those at risk of becoming undernourished or who are undernourished. Once assessment has been conducted, then nurses can initiate interventions to improve nutritional status, health or prevent undernutrition. These interventions are discussed in the sections in this chapter on nursing assessment and nursing interventions.

Dehydration

Dehydration is a condition where there is a depletion of body water and sodium (varies). This loss is not from vasculature but from intestines or as a result of reduced intake of water. Dehydration occurs when the osmotic pressure increases in the extracellular fluid drawing out and depleting the concentrations of water in the body's cells. The initial signs of dehydration relate to these physiological changes and not to hypovolaemia.

Older adults are at an increased risk of dehydration because of aged-related changes. Ageing changes alone do not cause dehydration. Aged-related changes that predispose older adults to dehydration include: the decrease in total body water, altered sense of thirst and the decreased ability of kidneys to concentrate urine as a result of decreased effectiveness of anti-diuretic hormone (ADH). Other risk factors include reduced mobility/functional status, female gender, incontinence, impaired cognitive status and some medications (sedatives, diuretics, laxatives (Mentes, 2006a). The functional consequences of dehydration include constipation, falls, medication toxicity, urinary tract and respiratory infections, delirium, renal failure, seizures, electrolyte imbalance, hyperthermia, and longer time for wounds to heal (Mentes, 2006a, p. 41). Dehydration has been found to increase mortality among hospitalised older adults.

There are three different categories of dehydration that can occur in older adults: isotonic, hypotonic and hypertonic. Table 18.3 illustrates the differences between these categories. There are also two types of dehydration that can develop in older adults: acute and chronic.

Acute dehydration occurs when there is a severe and rapid onset of loss of body fluids; for example, episodes of vomiting or diarrhoea, and other acute illness. Thirst is

TABLE 18-3 Classification of dehydration

Category	Description	Possible causes
Isotonic	Sodium loss = water loss	Complete fast Episodes of vomiting or diarrhoea
Hypotonic	Sodium loss > water loss Serum sodium <135 mmol/L	Overuse of diuretics
Hypertonic	Sodium loss < water loss Serum sodium >145 mmol/L	Fever Decreased fluid intake Fluid deprivation, possible neglect

Source: Joanna Briggs Institute (2001).

usually triggered by a loss of 1% to 2% of body weight, but because of an altered thirst perception by older adults, thirst may not be triggered by this loss.

When a loss of 2% to 3% of body weight occurs, clinical signs and symptoms begin to occur. Clinical signs and symptoms appear and progress if dehydration is not alleviated. Thirst develops first, followed by lethargy, dry mucosa and decreased urine output. As the degree of dehydration progresses, tachycardia and hypotension develop and finally shock occurs.

Acute dehydration can be recognised by the following signs and symptoms: dry mucosa, decreased skin turgor, high and increasing specific gravity usually greater than 1.029, increasingly darker urine (darker yellow-brown) and urine output approximately less than 30 mL/hour or less than 800 mL/day. Blood laboratory values include raised sodium, more than 145 mmol/L (note not in isotonic or hypotonic dehydration), haematocrit and blood urea and nitrogen (BUN). Weight may also be reduced.

The second type of dehydration, chronic dehydration, occurs in older adults when their daily fluid intake is inadequate over a longer period of time. Older adults who have chronic dehydration are often not diagnosed, and one study found only 26% were diagnosed (Bennett, Thomas & Riegel, 2004). This study found that of older adults who were chronically dehydrated, only 20% presented with dry mucous membranes, 3% presented with reduced skin turgor and there was no increase in specific gravity. Urine output was poor and sodium was often not raised. This study consistently found that blood urea and nitrogen (BUN) was raised. Frail older adults living in long-term residential care are at an increased risk of both types of dehydration (Mentes, 2006b). Tools have been developed to quantify the risk of dehydration for older adults living in long-term residential care (Mentes, 2006b; Mentes & Wang, 2011; see next section).

It is the role of nurses to screen and monitor older adults' hydration status to identify and treat factors contributing to dehydration. Nurses are also involved in initiating health promotion interventions to promote the hydration status of well older adults to prevent the development of dehydration, particularly when other risk factors occur such as an acute illness or environmental conditions change. These are discussed in the sections on nursing assessment and nursing interventions.

Constipation

Constipation, defined as a "decrease in normal frequency of defecation accompanied by difficult or incomplete passage of stool and/or passage of excessively hard, dry stool" (Herdman, 2012, p. 203), is one of the most common pathological conditions associated with digestion. The normal frequency for bowel movements, which shows significant individual variation but does not necessarily change with ageing, ranges from three times daily to once or twice weekly.

Another characteristic is that people experience a feeling of incomplete evacuation after a bowel movement. Approximately half of institutionalised older adults report problems with constipation, and three quarters use laxatives daily (Bouras & Tangalos, 2009). The prevalence of constipation in older adults is between 15% and 30% in those who live in the community and up to 75% to 80% of those who live in institutional settings (McKay, Fravel & Scanlon, 2012; Song, 2012).

Although constipation is a common complaint of older adults, it is caused by risk factors rather than age-related changes alone. Risk factors common in older adults include functional impairments (e.g. diminished mobility), pathological conditions (e.g. hypothyroidism), adverse medication effects (including long-term laxative abuse) and poor dietary habits (e.g. inadequate intake of bulk fibre and fluid). Table 18-2 lists common medications that contribute to constipation in older adults.

The management of constipation is based on the information obtained from a thorough assessment of the older adult's bowel risk factors, and history and physical assessment (JBI, 2008). The type of constipation will determine the treatment required. Management of constipation for older adults living in the community should follow the "Stepping out of Constipation" algorithm illustrated in Figure 18-1 (Home and Community Care [HACC]/Medical Aids Subsidy Scheme [MASS] Continence Project, 2010). Older adults are commenced on Step 1 of the ladder for the prevention or treatment of constipation, unless they have a recognised cause for constipation, such as drug therapies. Step 1 includes exercise, and increased fluid intake and fibre in the diet. Progression to Step 2, the introduction of bulk-forming laxatives and then the other

STEPPING OUT OF CONSTIPATION

Follow the "Stepping out of Constipation" algorithm for the management of constipation. Refer an individual wth recent, sudden onset of constipation or symptoms and signs such as blood in stools, pain associated with defecation etc., promptly to the general medical practitioner.

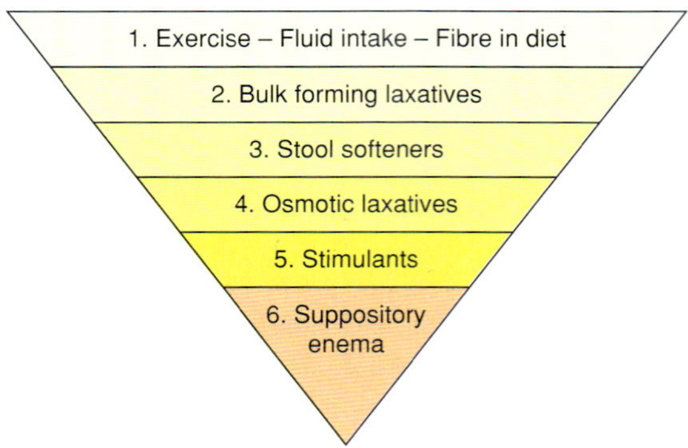

- Management of *simple* constipation starts at STEP 1, exercise, fluid intake and fibre in the diet. If constipation does not resolve in 3–4 days, compliance to recommendations should be checked. If compliance has been good, progress to STEP 2, non-prescription bulk-forming agent, if required.
- Management of *long-standing* constipation starts at STEP 1, exercise, fluid intake and fibre in the diet, and works through to STEP 3, stool softeners, if required.
- Management of *severe* constipation involves STEP 3, stool softeners, and STEP 4, osmotic laxatives, followed by STEP 1 and possibly STEP 2.

FIGURE 18-1 "Stepping out of Constipation" algorithm. (Home and Community Care/Medical Aids Subsidy Scheme Continence Project, 2010.)

steps, occurs only after an adequate trial is given for each step. If an older adult is acutely constipated, they are to commence at Step 5 or 6. Once constipation is alleviated, then they move back to Step 1, with one medication from Steps 2, 3 or 4.

A list of common medications used to manage constipation is listed in Table 18-4. If constipation is severe—that is, there has been a long history of infrequent bowel movements—faecal impaction can develop (HACC/MASS Continence Project, 2010). Faecal impaction can then lead to incontinence of solid or liquid stool. If faecal impaction develops, it is important for nurses to distinguish faecal incontinence due to impaction from other conditions. Faecal impaction requires special management, including suppositories, enemas and osmotic laxatives. Once the impaction is removed, nurses devise and implement a bowel management program to ensure it does not occur again.

Nurses also play an essential role in administering medications prescribed to treat and prevent constipation and monitor the effectiveness of these interventions. Nurses are involved in the prevention of constipation by assessing risk factors and initiating health promotion interventions, and these are discussed in the sections on nursing assessment and nursing interventions.

TABLE 18-4 Commonly used laxatives

Bulk-forming agents	These include methylcellulose, psyllium (Metamucil®) and dietary bran. Adequate fluid intake is required while taking these preparations otherwise they may contribute to constipation.
Stool softeners	Softeners moisten and soften hard dry stool and are used daily as needed. A common agent is docusate sodium.
Osmotic laxatives	Osmotive laxative agents include saline laxatives (milk of magnesia) and hyperosmotic agents (lactulose, sorbitol and glycerine suppository). These agents stimulate intestinal motility by attracting water into the bowel. Macrogol plus electrolytes (Movicol®) works differently to other osmotic laxatives. It belongs to a class of medications known as iso-osmotics. It does not cause dehydration or loss of electrolytes.
Stimulant agents	Agents include bisocodyl, cascara sagrada and senna. These should be used only for short-term management of constipation.

Source: Home and Community Care/Medical Aids Subsidy Scheme Continence Project, 2010.

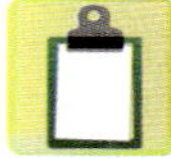

NURSING ASSESSMENT OF DIGESTION, NUTRITION AND HYDRATION

Nurses assess digestion and nutrition to identify: (1) the effects of age-related changes on digestion, nutrition, hydration and eating and drinking patterns; (2) risk factors that interfere with optimal nutrition and hydration; (3) cultural factors that influence eating patterns; (4) nutritional status and usual eating and drinking patterns; and (5) negative functional consequences of altered digestion or inadequate nutrition or hydration. On the basis of this assessment information, nurses identify opportunities for health promotion interventions.

Interviewing about digestion and nutrition and hydration

Nurses use an assessment interview to identify opportunities for health promotion by asking about the following information:

- Usual eating and drinking patterns and nutrient intake
- Health behaviours associated with oral care
- Age-related changes and risk factors that affect nutritional needs or digestive processes
- Environmental or social support factors that affect the procurement, preparation and enjoyment of food
- Symptoms of gastrointestinal dysfunction.

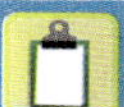

BOX 18-1
Guidelines for assessing digestion and nutrition

Assessing oral comfort and chewing ability
- Do you have any difficulty with soreness or bleeding in your mouth?
- Do you have any teeth that hurt, are loose or are sensitive to hot or cold temperatures?
- Do your gums bleed?
- Do you have any problems chewing or swallowing food or liquids? *If yes, ask about particular types of food or liquids that are problematic.*
- Are there foods you avoid because of problems with chewing or swallowing?
- Does your mouth or tongue ever feel dry?

Assessing dental habits and attitudes towards dental care
- How often do you see a dentist?
- When is the last time you had dental care?
- Where do you go for dental care?
- *If the person does not seek dental care at least once per year:* What prevents you from seeing the dentist?
- How do you care for your teeth?
- Do you use dental floss? *If yes:* How often? *If no:* Have you ever been taught to use dental floss?

Assessing nutritional needs
- Do you have diabetes, heart disease or any condition that requires dietary modifications?
- Do you have any food allergies?
- What medications do you take?
- What is your usual daily activity pattern?
- Do you drink fluids only when you are thirsty?

Identifying patterns of food procurement
- How do you get your grocery shopping done?
- Do you have any help getting to the store?
- Where and how often do you do your grocery shopping?
- What is your usual food budget?
- Do you have any difficulty getting food because of problems with vision, walking or transportation?

Identifying patterns of food preparation and consumption
- Where do you eat your meals?
- With whom do you eat?
- Does anyone help you prepare your meals?
- Do you have any trouble fixing your meals (e.g. difficulty opening containers)?
- Do you have any difficulties getting around your kitchen, using appliances or reaching the cupboards?
- Have there been recent changes in your eating or food preparation patterns (e.g. loss of eating companion or change in carer/caregiver situation)?
- When do you drink fluids (e.g. water)?
- Can you tell me how much fluid you drink in a day (e.g. how many cups)?

Assessing patterns of bowel elimination
- How often do you have a bowel movement?
- Have you noticed any recent changes in your pattern of bowel movements?
- Do you have any difficulty with your bowel movements? (e.g. Do you strain with bowel movements? or is the stool hard, dry or difficult to pass?)
- Do you ever have problems with loose stools or diarrhoea?
- Do you take laxatives or any other products to help you move your bowels?
- Do you ever have pain or bleeding when you move your bowels?

Nurses can assess the adequacy of nutrient intake by asking older adults to describe foods and beverages consumed during an average day. In addition, nurses follow a logical sequence for assessment questions by beginning with information about the oral cavity and ending with questions about bowel elimination. A major goal for assessing patterns of bowel elimination is to identify opportunities for health education about constipation. Box 18-1 summarises interview questions for a nursing assessment of nutrition, hydration and digestion in older adults.

WELLNESS OPPORTUNITY

Nurses promote personal responsibility by asking older adults to keep a 7-day diary of their food and beverage intake and eating and drinking patterns, and reviewing this to identify strengths and weaknesses of their diet.

Observing cues to digestion, nutrition and hydration

Nurses observe oral health indicators and eating patterns and environments for cues to digestion, nutrition and hydration. In addition, they consider social and cultural factors that influence eating, drinking and nutrition. Box 18-2 summarises observations and cultural considerations that are pertinent to nursing assessment of digestion, nutrition and hydration.

Nurses in institutional settings can assess behavioural cues to digestion, nutrition and hydration by observing older adults during meals and utilising Mentes' dehydration risk criteria (see later section on hydration). Nursing assessment of chewing and swallowing is especially important for older adults at risk for dysphagia, as described in Evidence-based practice 18-1.

WELLNESS OPPORTUNITY

Nurses observe environmental conditions to identify positive or negative effects on eating and drinking patterns.

Collecting cues using physical assessment and laboratory information

Physical assessment and laboratory data provide important additional information for assessing the older adult's

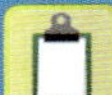

BOX 18-2
Behavioural cues to nutrition and digestion

Observations to assess oral health

- Condition of lips, teeth, gums, tongue and oral mucous membrane
- Number of teeth and use of full or partial dentures
- Fit of dentures
- Oral care items: condition of toothbrush, type of toothbrush or denture cleaning supplies, use of floss

Observations to assess eating and drinking patterns

- Does the person seem to enjoy eating meals with others, or does the presence of other people seem to interfere with mealtime enjoyment?
- If the person has dentures, are they worn at meals? If not, why not?
- What are the person's between-meal food and fluid consumption patterns?
- Are enjoyable non-caffeinated liquids readily available for between-meal fluid intake?
- Does the person drink fluid when offered, or only sips?
- What cultural influences affect the person's food preferences and preparation?

Observations to assess the eating environment

- Do environmental or social influences negatively affect mealtime enjoyment (e.g. a noisy dining room or disruptive mealtime companions)?
- If the person eats alone, is this the best arrangement, or should consideration be given to providing mealtime social interaction?

Cultural considerations that may influence nutrition and eating patterns

- What are the usual patterns of meals eaten (e.g. content, frequency, timing)? What is the usual social context of meals?
- Are there any culturally influenced food taboos or preferences? (Refer to Cultural considerations 18-1.)
- Are there any special foods that are important because of religious or cultural factors? (If yes, are they accessible to the older adult?)
- Are certain foods or beverages avoided or preferred in relation to an illness or chronic condition (e.g. foods or beverages that are considered yin and yang foods)?
- Is there a preference for the temperature of beverages (e.g. use of iced or heated beverages)?
- Is the person's ethnic background likely to increase his or her chance of being lactose intolerant? (Prevalence is highest among Asians and Africans; high among Hispanics; and lowest among white people of northern European descent.)

nutritional and hydration status. Height, weight, body mass index (BMI) and waist circumference provide important clues to nutritional status. The BMI—a measure of body composition related to body fat—is commonly used as an indicator of malnutrition. A healthy BMI is between 18.5 kg/m^2 and 24.9 kg/m^2 for adults. However, there is evidence to support a higher BMI for older adults. Studies indicate that a BMI of 30 or more may be healthy for adults older than age 65 (Bahat et al., 2012; Veronese et al., 2013). One review of studies found that optimal BMI for longer life expectancy in people older than age 70 is in the range of 25 to 30; however, this is higher than the ideal BMI associated with optimal function and lack of disability (Soenen & Chapman, 2013). Thus it is imperative to consider the BMI in relation to overall health and risk factors, additional assessment findings, and long-term patterns. Also, keep in mind that a high BMI does not eliminate the possibility of risk for malnutrition. For example, one study of community-living adults aged 75 and over found that one-third of those identified as at risk for malnutrition had a BMI of 25 or more and only 13% had a BMI in the underweight category (Winter et al., 2013).

Recommended BMI classifications for older adults are as follows:

- Underweight <23 kg/m^2
- Healthy weight 24–30 kg/m^2
- Overweight >30 kg/m^2. (Queensland Government, 2014)

The waist circumference has been recommended to be considered alongside BMI when determining optimal nutrition. Waist measures of 94 cm or under for men, and 80 cm or under for women, are considered optimal for health (NARI, 2014).

Standardised tables do not necessarily provide the most realistic or appropriate goal for older adults and nurses need to consider individual circumstances including BMI, waist circumference and other observable and measureable cues. For many older adults, maintenance of a stable weight may be more important as patterns of weight loss and gain are important indicators of overall health condition.

Weight loss is considered in relation to percentage of loss, which is calculated by subtracting current weight from usual weight, and dividing that by the usual weight. For example, (73 kg – 55 kg)/73 kg = 18 kg/73 kg, or approximately 25% weight loss. An unintentional weight loss of more than 5% of body weight in 1 month, or more than 10% in 6 months, is considered a significant indicator of poor nutrition (Kruizenga et al., 2010).

Laboratory data can also provide clues to nutritional deficiencies, even before any clinical signs are evident; however, test results must be evaluated in relation to the person's overall health status. For instance, low serum albumin is an indicator of poor nutrition, but it also occurs with trauma, oedema, infection and neoplasm. Box 18-3 summarises information about physical assessment indicators and laboratory values that are especially important in assessing the nutritional status of older adults. Additional indicators of nutrient deficiencies are listed in Table 18-1 in the column describing functional consequences.

Although there are many indicators of dehydration, one study suggests tongue dryness is strongly associated with

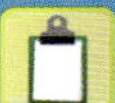

BOX 18-3
Physical assessment and laboratory data

Examination of the oral cavity
- Inspect the oral cavity by using a tongue depressor and a light
- Observe for evidence of oral disease, including pain, lumps, soreness, bleeding, swelling, loose teeth and abraded areas
- Note the presence or absence of teeth, dentures and partial bridges

Normal findings
- Lips: pink, moist, symmetrical
- Teeth intact, without cavities or tartar
- Gums: pink, no bleeding
- Mucous membranes: pink, moist
- Tongue: pink, moist, presence of numerous varicosities on undersurface
- Pharynx: soft palate rises slightly when 'ahh' is vocalised

Indicators of nutritional deficiency
- Lips: dry, fissured, cracked at corners
- Teeth: decayed or missing
- Gums: red, swollen, recessed, spongy or prone to bleeding
- Mucous membranes: dry, ulcerated, inflamed, bleeding, white patches
- Tongue: dry, swollen, reddened or very smooth

Examination of the abdomen and rectum
- Examine the abdomen with the person lying comfortably in the supine position.
- Perform a rectal examination with the person in the side-lying position.

Normal findings
- Symmetrical, soft abdomen that moves with respirations
- Audible bowel sounds (heard through the diaphragm of a stethoscope) occurring at irregular intervals (5 to 15 seconds apart)
- Smooth skin around anus; no evidence of haemorrhoids, fissures, inflammation or rectal prolapse
- Soft, brown stool that tests negative for occult blood
- Waist circumference less than 94 cm for men and 80 cm for women.

Indicators of nutritional deficiency
- Swollen abdomen
- Stool that tests positive for occult blood

General physical assessment indicators of malnutrition
- Weight loss
- Lack of subcutaneous fat
- Diminished size and strength of muscles
- Skin that is dry, rough or tissue thin
- Abnormal pulse or blood pressure
- Oedema, especially in the face or lower extremities
- Hair that is dry, dull, thin, brittle or sparse
- Dry or dull-looking eyes
- Listless, apathetic or depressed mood
- Difficulty with walking or maintaining balance
- BMI less than 23 kg/m^2

General physical assessment indicators of dehydration
- Lethargy and changes in mental state
- Dry mucosa
- Decreased urine output
- Decreased skin turgor

Laboratory data
- Biochemical data that will provide information about nutritional status: serum ferritin; serum or red blood cell folate and vitamin B_{12}; complete lipid profile; and serum albumin, glucose, sodium and potassium levels
- Urinalysis results should be within the normal adult range, except for a slight decrease in the upper limit for specific gravity
- Biochemical data that will provide information about hydration status: sodium, haemoglobin, creatinine, osmolality and BUN

Indicators of nutritional deficiency
- Anaemia
- Lymphocytopenia
- Serum albumin level of less than 35 mg/L
- Serum 25(oh)D less than 30 nmol/L
- Cholesterol levels of less than 5.5 mmol/L
- Total iron-binding capacity less than 45 mmol/L

poor hydration status in older adults (Vivanti, Harvey & Ash, 2010). Another indicator is the skin turgor, but only if the skin on the forehead or over the anterior chest wall is assessed in older adults. These areas are less affected by age-related skin changes, unlike the skin on the back of the hands and wrists. Orthostatic hypotension, oliguria or anuria, changes in mental status and dry mucous membranes are considered common manifestations of dehydration in older adults. Urinalysis can also indicate the hydration status. Highly concentrated urine (i.e. specific gravity above 1.029) can indicate dehydration. In addition, a sudden loss of body weight may indicate dehydration. Blood values that may be altered in dehydration include haematocrit, haemoglobin, creatinine, osmolality and blood urea nitrogen (BUN), all of which may be elevated. Sodium may also increase, but this is dependent on the type of dehydration. Biochemical measures for the assessment of acute and chronic dehydration in older adults, especially the BUN, are considered the most accurate methods to determine hydration status of an older adult (Bennett, Thomas & Riegel, 2004; JBI, 2001).

Using assessment tools

There are a number of assessment tools that nurses use to assess digestion, nutrition and hydration.

Oral assessment

For oral assessment, the Hartford Institute for Geriatric Nursing recommends the use of the Kayser-Jones Brief Oral Health Status Examination, an evidence-based tool to evaluate the oral health status of older adults in a variety of settings. An oral health assessment and care planning tools are also available for older adults who are functionally

EVIDENCE-BASED PRACTICE 18-2
Oral healthcare for older adults

Statement of the problem

- Oral health is essential for promoting overall health, preventing disease, maintaining speech and alimentary functioning, and preserving quality of life.
- Even though regular oral care is essential for good health, it is often neglected as an aspect of care for older adults.
- Oral hygiene declines as older adults experience cognitive and functional impairments and become increasingly dependent in daily activities.
- Oral problems are not the direct result of ageing and can be prevented or at least detected at an early stage.
- Medications and medical conditions can increase the risk for oral problems, even when good oral care is provided.
- Dental caries and periodontal disease are plaque-related and preventable oral diseases that are likely to develop from poor oral hygiene.
- When untreated, poor oral health leads to malnutrition, dehydration, pneumonia, cardiovascular disease, joint infections and poor diabetic control.

Recommendations for nursing assessment

- Make use of the 10-item Kayser-Jones Brief Oral Health Status Examination, an evidence-based tool for assessing and rating the following aspects of oral health in older adults: lymph nodes, lips, tongue, mouth and cheek tissue, gums, saliva, condition of natural and artificial teeth, chewing position of teeth, and oral cleanliness (available at http://consultgerirn.org).
- Immediately arrange for a dental evaluation if any of the following occur: enlarged and tender lymph nodes; lips red at corners; discolouration, break in integrity or any abnormality of any oral tissue that has been present for 2 weeks or more; more than one loose, broken or missing tooth; redness at borders around teeth; redness or soreness under artificial teeth; fewer than four teeth in either jaw; seven or fewer pairs of teeth in chewing position; dentures missing, not being worn, or damaged.
- Assess self-care ability of older adults related to effective oral care, and involve occupational therapy services as appropriate.

Recommendations for nursing interventions

- Use a toothbrush with soft nylon bristles and toothpaste with fluoride.
- Provide oral care (for teeth and dentures) morning, evening and as needed.
- Brush teeth, dentures and tongue.
- Plain foam swabs can be used for cleaning oral mucous membrane of an edentulous adult, but they are not as effective as toothbrushes for cleaning teeth.
- Never use lemon–glycerin swabs because they dry the mucous membrane and erode tooth enamel.
- Mouth rinses that contain alcohol dry the mucous membrane and should be diluted in half with water if they are used.
- Use chlorhexidine and only if it is prescribed by a dentist.
- Brush dentures before placing them in a denture cup.
- Arrange for at least annual dental evaluations and more frequent evaluations if problems are identified.

Additional recommendations for nursing interventions for people with dementia

- If the person resists oral care, consider that oral pain is the cause of the resistance.
- Develop an individualised oral care plan that includes specific communication techniques (e.g. approach person at eye level) and care strategies (e.g. demonstrating, task segmentation) for each person.
- Teach all nursing staff about the individualised care plan and involve family carers as appropriate.
- Arrange for more frequent dental examinations if it is difficult to provide adequate oral hygiene.

Source: Johnson, V. B. & Schoenfelder, D. P. (2012). Evidence-based practice guideline: Oral hygiene care for functionally dependent and cognitively impaired older adults. *Journal of Gerontological Nursing, 38*(11), 11–19; Legg, T. J. (2012). Oral care in older adults with dementia: Challenges and approaches. *Journal of Gerontological Nursing, 38*(8), 10–13; O'Connor. L. J. (2012). Oral health care. In M. Boltz, E. Capezuti, T. Fulmer & D. Zwicker (Eds), *Evidence-based practice protocols for best practice* (4th ed., pp. 409–418). New York: Springer; Taub, L.-F. (2012). Oral health assessment of older adults: The Kayser-Jones Brief Oral Health Status Examination (BOHSE). *Try This* series, issue 18. *Best Practices in Nursing Care to Older Adults.* Accessed 13 May 2013 via www.Consult-GeriRN.org.

or cognitively impaired (Chalmers & Johnson, 2004). An overview of evidenced-based practice for oral care for older adults is contained in Evidence-based practice 18-2.

Bowel assessment

There exists many bowel continence assessment tools but none of them is currently recommended specifically for older adults. All collect information about:

- Presenting bowel problems, duration and triggers
- Previous investigations, treatment and management strategies
- The effect of bowel problem on person's life
- Medical/surgical history
- Medications (particularly opiates, antidiarrhoeal, anticholinergic)
- Cognitive and functional abilities
- Level of exercise and fibre and fluid intake. (Home and Community Care [HACC]/Medical Aids Subsidy Scheme [MASS] Continence Project, 2010)

Information gathered from a Bowel Diary is also required. A 5- to 7-day bowel diary is completed and then this information is used to assess for pattern and types of bowel movements. A useful assessment tool is the Seven Day Bowel Chart (see Figure 18-2). This chart enables both the recording of bowel motions for seven days and contains the Bristol Stool Form Scale to describe the stool type. The Bristol Stool Form Scale assists in the determination of constipation (types 1–2) and diarrhoea (types 5–7).

Nutrition assessment

Nutrition assessment tools are used for identifying people at risk of nutritional problems so that preventive and

Seven Day Bowel Chart

Document No: ______________

ID LABEL

Please complete details for each time the resident has a bowel movement.

Date	Shift	Time	Type of bowel movement refer to Bristol Stool Form Scale)	Incontinent of stool Yes/No	Number of pad/ clothing changes (identify pads or clothing or both)	Comments (associated circumstances/effects on daily activities/laxative use)
	am					
	pm					
	night					
	am					
	pm					
	night					
	am					
	pm					
	night					
	am					
	pm					
	night					
	am					
	pm					
	night					
	am					
	pm					
	night					
	am					
	pm					
	night					

The Bristol Stool Form Scale *(Use this as a guide to the stool type)*

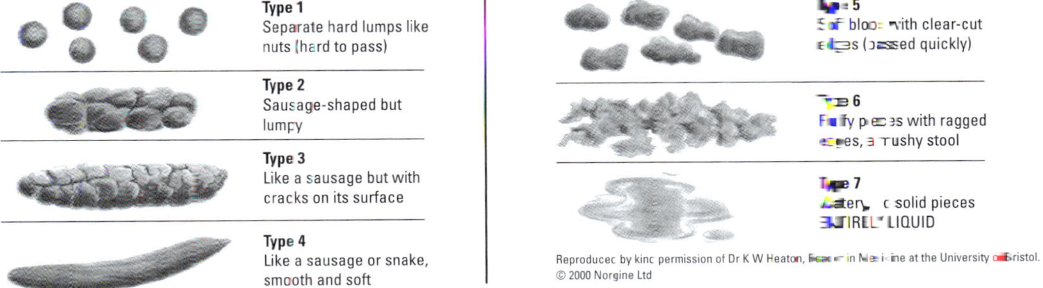

Developed by Deakin University and funded under the National Continence Management Strategy

FIGURE 18-2 Seven Day Bowel Chart. (From *Continence Tools for Residential Aged Care: An education guide*. Developed by Deakin University, Melbourne, and funded under the Australian Government's National Continence Management Strategy. Accessible via www.bladderbowl.gov.au. Permission granted from the Australian Government Department of Social Services. Go to www.dss.gov.au for more information.)

Mini Nutritional Assessment MNA®

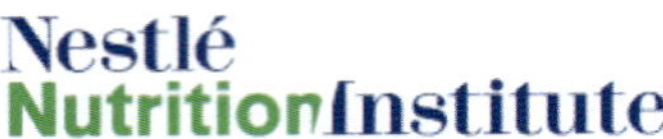

Last name: First name:

Sex: Age: Weight, kg: Height, cm: Date:

Complete the screen by filling in the boxes with the appropriate numbers. Total the numbers for the final screening score.

Screening

A Has food intake declined over the past 3 months due to loss of appetitie, digestive problems, chewing or swallowing difficulties?

0 = severe decrease in food intake
1 = moderate decrease in food intake
2 = no decrease in food intake ☐

B Weight loss during the last 3 months

0 = weight loss greater than 3 kg (6.6 lbs)
1 = does not know
2 = weight loss between 1 and 3 kg (2.2 and 6.6 lbs)
3 = no weight loss ☐

C Mobility

0 = bed or chair bound
1 = able to get out of bed / chair but does not go out
2 = goes out ☐

D Has suffered psychological stress or acute disease in the past 3 months?

0 = yes 2 = no ☐

E Neuropsychological problems

0 = severe dementia or depression
1 = mild dementia
2 = no psychological problems ☐

F1 Body Mass Index (BMI) (weight in kg) / (height in m²)

0 = BMI less than 19
1 = BMI 19 to less than 21
2 = BMI 21 to less than 23
3 = BMI 23 or greater ☐

IF BMI IS NO AVAILABLE, REPLACE QUESTION F1 WITH QUESTION F2.
DO NOT ANSWER QUESTION F2 IF QUESTION F1 IS ALREADY COMPLETED.

F2 Calf circumference (CC) in cm

0 = CC less than 31
3 = CC 31 or greater ☐

Screening score (max. 14 points)

12 - 14 points: Normal nutritional status
8 - 11 points: At risk of malnutrition
0 - 7 points: Malnourished ☐☐

References

1. Vellas, B., Villars, H., Abellan, G. et al. (2006). Overview of MNA®: Its history and challenges. *Journal of Nutrition, Health & Aging, 10*, 456–465.
2. Rubenstein, L. Z., Harker, J. O., Salva, A., Guigoz, Y., Vellas, B. (2001). Screening for undernutrition in geriatric practice: Developing the Short-Form Mini Nutritional Assessment (MNA-SF). *Journal of Gerontology, 56A*, M366–M377.
3. Guigoz, Y. (2006). The Mini-Nutritional Assessment (MNA®) review of the literature: What does it tell us? *Journal of Nutrition, Health & Aging, 10*, 466–487.
4. Kaiser, M. J., Bauer, J. M., Ramsch, C. et al. (2009). Validation of the Mini Nutritional Assessment Short-Form (MNA®-SF): A practical tool for identification of nutritional status. *Journal of Nutrition, Health & Aging, 13*, 782–788.

For more information: www.mna-elderly.com.

FIGURE 18-3 The Mini Nutritional Assessment—Short Form (MNA-SF). (From Nestlé Nutrition Institute, Vevey, Switzerland. Copyright Nestle, 1994, revision 2009. Available at www.mna-elderly.com.)

therapeutic interventions can be implemented. The **Mini Nutritional Assessment (MNA)** is an evidence-based tool that has been widely used since 1990 in a variety of settings. Advantages of this tool include validation and reliability, ease of use, low cost, acceptability, effectiveness and availability in many languages (Skates & Anthony, 2009).

The MNA consists of 6 screening and 12 assessment questions and takes approximately 15 minutes to complete. Additional information about this tool is available at http://consultgerirn.org or www.nursingcenter.com (DiMaria-Ghalili & Guenter, 2008). Figure 18-3 illustrates a six-item short form, which can be administered in 5 minutes and has been validated as a first-step screening process for identifying older adults who should be assessed further for poor nutrition (Kaiser et al., 2009). Another tool, the Malnutrition Universal Screening Tool (MUST), was designed to identify malnourished adults, those at risk of malnutrition and obese adults. It has been used successfully to identify older adults with malnutrition (Stratton et al., 2006). This tool is easy and quick to use, reproducible and internally consistent. The MUST is a good alternative when height and weight are not obtainable.

Hydration assessment

There is no screening tool available for nurses to measure the risk of the dehydration status of older adults in community and hospital settings. A careful history of oral intake is required, as well as the collection of physical signs and symptoms mentioned in the previous section. A quick guide to level of hydration is the colour of urine. (See an example in Figure 18-4.) Despite being useful, nurses need to be aware that this is not a precise measure of the level of hydration.

Another tool, the Mentes' Typology of Oral Hydration, categorises frail older adults in different risk groups for dehydration. Those who can drink independently but forget to drink, those who can't drink independently and require one-to-one assistance, and those who have a swallowing problem and do not tolerate thin fluids, are classified as a medium risk for dehydration (Mentes, 2006b). Those older adults who are at a high risk are those who won't drink much

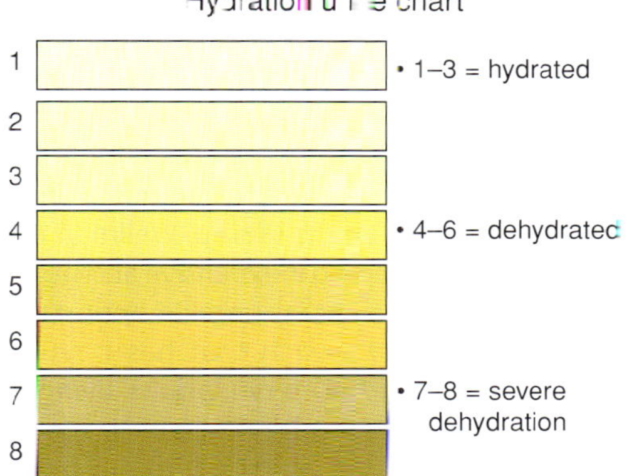

FIGURE 18-4 Level of hydration as determined by the urine colour.

> **BOX 18-4**
> **Dehydration Risk Appraisal Checklist (Mentes & Wang, 2010*)**
>
> The greater the number of characteristics present, the greater the risk for hydration problems. Please tick all that apply
>
> - ☐ >85 years
> - ☐ Female
>
> **Significant health conditions**
>
> - ☐ MMSE score <24 (indicating cognitive impairment)
> - ☐ Dementia diagnosis
> - ☐ GDS score ≥6 (indicating depression)
> - ☐ Semi-dependent in ADLs
> - ☐ Repeated infections
> - ☐ History of dehydration
> - ☐ Urinary incontinence
>
> **Medications**
>
> - ☐ Laxatives
> - ☐ Diuretics
> - ☐ Psychotropics: Antipsychotics, Antidepressants, Anxiolytics
>
> **Intake behaviours**
>
> - ☐ BMI <21 or >27
> - ☐ Requires assistance to drink
> - ☐ Has difficulty swallowing
> - ☐ Can drink independently but forgets
> - ☐ Poor eater
>
> *This 2010 material was published in the following journal: Mentes, J. & Wang, J. (2011). Measuring risk for dehydration in nursing home residents: Evaluation of the Dehydration Risk Appraisal Checklist. *Research in Gerontological Nursing, 4*(2), 148–156. MMSE: Mini Mental State Exam; GDS: Geriatric Depression Scale 15.

and will only sip and those who limit intake to reduce incontinence. Mentes advocated that both the medium- and high-risk groups require strategies to prevent the development of dehydration. Those at risk require the offering of fluids regularly; every one to two hourly.

The other tool that can be used to screen for dehydration is the Dehydration Risk Appraisal Checklist (DRAC) (Mentes & Wang, 2011). The DRAC identifies 17 characteristics that provide an indication of dehydration. The more these characteristics are present, the greater risk for dehydration. The DRAC is presented in Box 18-4. It is important that the long-term residential care staff receive education about dehydration so they are alert to the risk and have an understanding of the importance of the interventions in preventing dehydration.

Fluid balance charts can be used to assess hydration status when the older adult is receiving care in a hospital or long term care facility. However, caution is required when interpreting fluid balance charts. An accurate fluid record can be difficult to obtain because of a number of factors. These may include a reduced ability to measure urinary output because of incontinence and impaired cognition of an older adult. Impaired cognition may contribute to the recording of an inaccurate fluid intake. Older people, even those without cognitive impairment, may overestimate the amount they drink.

> **UNFOLDING CASE STUDY**
>
> **Part B**
>
> Recall that you are a practice nurse at the local medical centre attended by Mr and Mrs Connelly, who now are 75 and 76 years old, respectively. At an appointment, Mrs Donnelly asks your advice

about her gradual unintended weight loss over the past few months. Although Mrs Donnelly continues to cook meals because her husband enjoys eating, she states that food no longer appeals to her. You notice that her mouth is very dry and her teeth are in poor condition. She had a stroke 2 years ago and recovered well except for some dysphagia and right-sided weakness. She takes an antidepressant and two blood pressure medications but does not know the names of the pills. She asks what she can do about the weight loss.

Thinking points

- What risk factors are likely to be contributing to Mrs Donnelly's weight loss?
- Make a list of assessment questions you would use with Mrs Donnelly. Select applicable questions from Box 18-1 and list any additional questions that you would use for further assessment.
- What would you ask Mrs Donnelly to do to provide additional assessment information so that you can plan some teaching interventions?

NURSING ISSUES

The nursing assessment may identify problems related to nutrition, hydration, digestion or oral health.

If nutritional deficits are identified, a pertinent nursing issue is imbalanced nutrition: less than body's metabolic requirements. Related factors that may affect older adults include medications, anorexia, depression, chewing or swallowing difficulties, social isolation and an inability to procure or prepare food.

If a hydration deficit is identified, a pertinent nursing issue is fluid volume deficit: less than body's metabolic requirements. Related factors that may affect an older adult's hydration status include anorexia, depression, swallowing difficulties, inability to procure fluids, being acutely ill, especially fever and infection, and environmental conditions.

If the nursing assessment identifies constipation or risks for constipation, the applicable nursing issue is: constipation. The nursing assessment may also identify certain oral health problems that are common in older adults. These include xerostomia, medication effects, chewing difficulties, periodontal disease, diminished taste sensation, ill-fitting dentures, inadequate oral hygiene and broken or missing teeth. A relevant nursing issue to address these problems would be impaired oral mucous membrane.

WELLNESS OPPORTUNITY

A nursing wellness issue of willingness for enhanced nutrition is applicable for those older adults who express an interest in improving nutritional patterns.

GOAL PLANNING FOR WELLNESS OUTCOMES

Nursing goals that address risk factors and promote nutrition and hydration wellness outcomes in older adults are improved: appetite, bowel elimination, knowledge about diet, nutritional status, hydration status, oral hygiene; self-care: eating; sensory function: taste and smell, swallowing status; and weight: body mass. The following nursing goals that are related to constipation include improved hydration, bowel elimination, the response to medication and control of symptoms.

WELLNESS OPPORTUNITY

A nursing wellness outcome for older adults who are ready to improve their nutrition to protect themselves from illness is knowledge: health promotion.

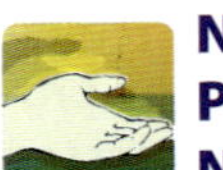

NURSING INTERVENTIONS TO PROMOTE HEALTHY DIGESTION, NUTRITION AND HYDRATION

The following nursing interventions focus on the areas of bowel management, environmental management, health education, nutrition management, nutritional counselling, oral health, hydration management, maintenance/promotion, referral, self-care assistance and weight management. Nursing interventions to promote healthy digestion, nutrition and hydration in older adults include health education about optimal nutrition, hydration and disease prevention. Nurses also direct interventions to eliminate risk factors that interfere with digestion, nutrition, hydration and oral health.

Addressing risk factors that interfere with digestion, nutrition and hydration

Nursing interventions may be needed to address functional consequences of age-related changes, even in healthy older adults. For example, if older adults experience early satiety during meals, they may benefit from eating five smaller meals a day, rather than the customary three meals a day. Similarly, nurses can encourage older adults to maintain a sitting or upright position during eating, and for 30 minutes to 1 hour after eating, to compensate for any effects of slowed swallowing.

When functional limitations interfere with the activities involved in procuring, preparing and enjoying food, interventions focus on improving the person's access to palatable and nutritious meals. For the community-living older adults, this may involve identifying resources that offer assistance in obtaining food. Home-delivered meal programs, "Meals on Wheels", may be available to older adults at minimal cost, and group meal programs are available in almost all community day centres. Studies found that formal meal programs are effective in reducing nutritional risk for community-living older adults (Kamp, Wellman & Russell, 2010). In addition to providing inexpensive and nutritionally balanced meals, these programs provide opportunities for social interaction. An approach that has been used to improve functioning in frail older adults living in their homes is to provide a commercially available protein-energy supplement containing 1680 kcal of energy, 25 g of protein, 9.4 g of essential amino acids, and 400 mL of water daily (Kim & Lee, 2013).

In Australia, community aged care programs funded by the federal government can assist older people with transportation or grocery shopping, and they are an excellent source of information about group and home-delivered meal programs. When environmental barriers, such as high cupboards, interfere with older adults' ability to prepare meals safely, environmental modifications can be made. Nurses can apply many of the environmental adaptations suggested in the chapters on vision (see Chapter 17) and mobility (see Chapter 22) to improve the ability of older persons to prepare meals. When older adults have functional impairments, nurses can suggest specially adapted items for improving independence in eating and food preparation, such as those illustrated in Figure 18-5. Another useful online resource for assistive devices is the Independent Living Centre, available at www.ilc.com.au.

In aged care settings, nurses can use the following interventions to address risk factors:

- Plan seating arrangements in the dining area to improve social interaction and to minimise the negative effects of disruptive people.
- Use low- or no-sodium flavour enhancers (e.g. herbs and lemon).
- Provide good oral hygiene before meals.
- Provide easy access to fluids and nutritious snacks.
- Prompt the older adult to drink, offering fluids regularly. Adjust the fluid schedule to suit the seasons. Increase prompting and offering of fluids during hot weather.

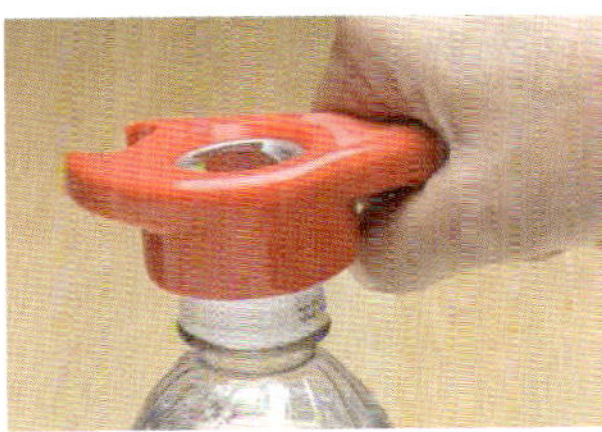

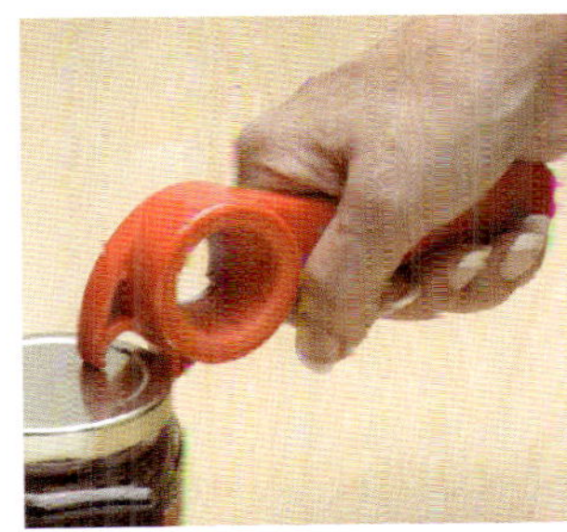

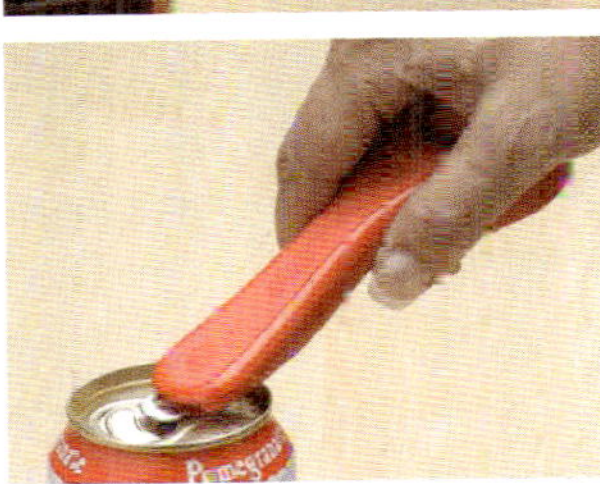

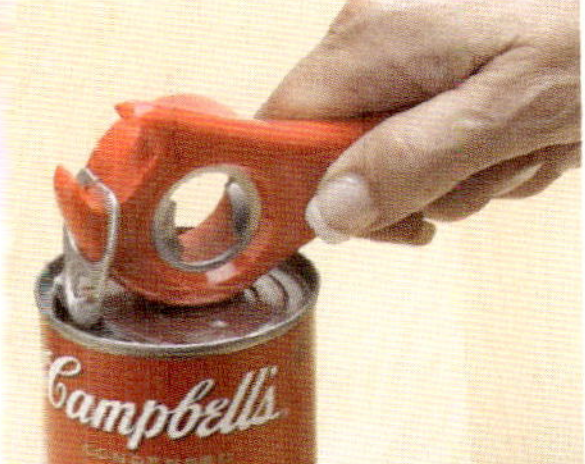

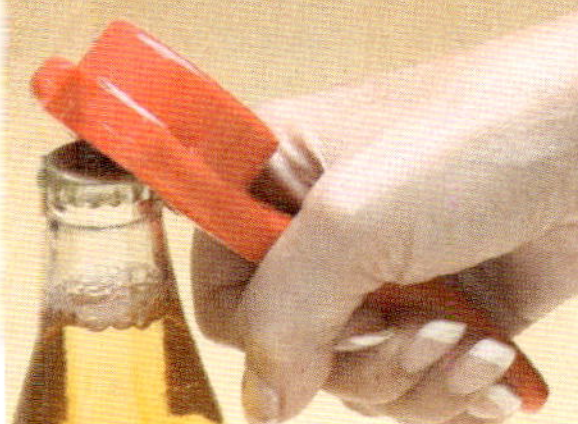

FIGURE 18-5 Adaptive devices. (Reprinted with permission from www.ActiveForever.com.)

- Ensure fluid consistency is correct and adequate time is scheduled for assisting those with dysphagia.

When older adults are misinformed about constipation, or when other risk factors (e.g. a low-fibre diet) interfere with good bowel function, nursing interventions are directed towards education. Daily use of bran cereals or bran mixed with other foods is a common and effective strategy for preventing constipation. Box 18-5 identifies some of the foods and other interventions that aid in preventing constipation.

WELLNESS OPPORTUNITY

Nurses try to find "teachable moments" so they can correct any myths or misconceptions associated with unhealthy eating patterns.

When medication affect nutrition and digestion, nurses, carers or older adults can discuss this problem with prescribing medical practitioners to identify ways of alleviating this risk or addressing the consequences. If over-the-counter medications have a detrimental effect on nutrition, hydration or digestion, nurses educate older adults about medication–nutrient interactions and discuss ways of addressing the negative effects. Pharmacists help by suggesting interventions that will compensate for, or minimise, the effects of both prescription and over-the-counter medications on nutrition, hydration and digestion.

When alcohol consumption interferes with nutrition, interventions might address the potential problem of alcoholism, or they may be aimed at compensating for the detrimental effects on nutrition. Nurses can recommend vitamin supplementation for people with a history of alcoholism after a medical evaluation has been performed to identify any underlying conditions, such as pernicious anaemia.

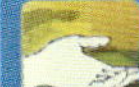

BOX 18-5
Health education regarding constipation

- A bowel movement every day is not necessarily the norm for every adult.
- Each adult has an individual pattern of bowel regularity, with the normal range varying from 3 times a day to 2 times a week.
- Include several portions of the following high-fibre foods in your daily diet: fresh uncooked fruits and vegetables; bran and other cereal products made from whole grains.
- Drink 8 to 10 glasses of non-caffeinated liquid, including fruit juices, every day.
- Avoid laxatives and enemas.
- If medication is needed to promote bowel regularity, a bulk-forming agent (e.g. psyllium or methylcellulose) is least likely to have detrimental effects, especially if fluid intake is adequate.
- Do not ignore the urge to defecate; try to respond as soon as you feel the urge.
- Exercise regularly.

Promoting oral and dental health

Nurses have important responsibilities in implementing interventions to promote oral and dental health. If older adults have avoided dental care because of resignation to poor oral health or a poor understanding of the need for preventive dental care, nurses attempt to change these attitudes through education.

Nurses also emphasise the importance of obtaining dental care every 6 months and, if appropriate, facilitate referrals for dental care. For housebound older adults, some dentists offer limited services by visiting homes. For those older Australians who are eligible, dental services are available at no or little cost through Medicare. In New Zealand some older people may be eligible for assistance from Work and Income New Zealand (WINZ) or other organisations (New Zealand Dental Association, 2010). Some District Health Boards (DHBs) have oral health services and they may provide some care for older people.

Nurses need to be familiar with local resources, so that they can inform older adults and their carers about the dental services that are available in their community. In long-term residential care settings, nurses are usually responsible for facilitating referrals for dental care every 6 to 12 months. For older adults in any setting, if xerostomia interferes with digestion or nutrition, nurses may suggest or facilitate a referral for a medical evaluation to identify disease processes or medication effects that may be contributing factors.

Good oral care is an essential, but often overlooked component of daily nursing care for dependent older adults. In institutional settings, staff education about oral care, including information about the myths related to oral health and ageing, is imperative (O'Connor, 2012). Evidence-based recommendations related to oral care are described in Evidence based practice 18-2.

For independent older adults, nurses provide health education about oral care, including alleviation of dry mouth if this is pertinent, as described in Box 18-6. Older adults who have any impairment of manual dexterity can adapt handles of toothbrushes for ease of use, or obtain specially designed brushes to increase the self-care abilities. Nurses can also suggest the use of battery-operated brushes, which are effective, easy to use and relatively inexpensive. Child-size toothbrushes (manual or automatic) may be easier to use for dependent older adults, especially if access to all their teeth is limited.

WELLNESS OPPORTUNITY

Nurses promote independence and self-care in oral hygiene by facilitating referrals for occupational therapy for older adults with functional impairments.

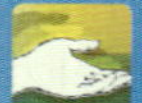

BOX 18-6
Health education regarding oral and dental care

Health education regarding care of the teeth and gums

- Oral care should include daily use of dental floss and twice-daily brushing of all tooth surfaces.
- Use a soft-bristled toothbrush and fluoridated toothpaste.
- If you have any limitations that interfere with your ability to use a regular toothbrush, you may benefit from using an electric or battery-powered brush or a brush with a specially designed handle (available where medical supplies are sold).
- Easy-to-use floss aids are inexpensive and widely available for facilitating dental flossing; they are especially helpful for people with any limitations in manual strength or dexterity or limited range of motion in the upper extremities.
- Some mouth rinses have cleansing, antimicrobial and moisturising effect, but they are used in conjunction with, not instead of, brushing.
- Avoid using alcohol-containing mouthwashes because of their drying effect.
- Because sugar is a major contributing factor to tooth decay, it is important to limit the intake of sugary substances, especially substances that are kept in the mouth for long periods (e.g. gum, hard candy).
- After eating sugar-containing foods, rinse your mouth or brush your teeth.
- Visit a dentist every 6 months for regular oral care.
- If partial or complete dentures are worn, remove them at night, keep them in water and clean them before placing them back in your mouth.

Health education regarding dry mouth

- Excessive dry mouth may be caused by medical conditions or medication effects and should be evaluated before symptomatic treatment is initiated.
- Drink at least 10 to 12 glasses of non-caffeinated fluid during the day, and drink sips of water at frequent intervals.
- Suck on xylitol-flavoured fluoride tablets or sugar-free hard lollies to stimulate saliva flow.
- Chew sugar-free gum with xylitol for 15 minutes after meals to stimulate saliva flow and promote oral hygiene.
- Try using one of the many brands of saliva substitutes available at pharmacies, but avoid those that contain sorbitol because this can worsen the condition.
- Avoid sucking lozenges containing citric acid because of their detrimental effects on tooth enamel.
- Avoid alcohol, alcohol-containing mouthwashes and highly acidic drinks (e.g. orange or grapefruit juice) because these tend to exacerbate the condition.
- Avoid smoking because this exacerbates the symptoms and further irritates the oral mucous membranes.
- Pay particular attention to oral hygiene because a dry mouth increases the risk for gum and dental diseases.
- Maintain optimal room humidity, especially at night.

Promoting optimal nutrition and preventing disease

Therapeutic diets have long been recognised as essential interventions for diseases such as diabetes and cardiovascular conditions, and in recent years, there is increasing recognition of the role nutrients play in preventing disease.

Nutritional interventions for healthy ageing emphasise the inclusion of foods containing antioxidants and other nutrients that may play a protective and preventive role. For example, there is strong support from longitudinal studies that a diet rich in antioxidants and omega-3 fatty acids prevents age-related macular degeneration (Montgomery et al., 2010; Raniga & Elder, 2009; Parekh et al., 2009).

In analysing information about nutrients as preventive interventions, distinctions must be made between nutrients obtained from foods and those that are found in supplements. For example, a high dietary intake of a particular nutrient (e.g. carotenoids) may be beneficial in health promotion or disease prevention, but a dietary supplement product with the same nutrient may not necessarily have the same beneficial effects. Thus nurses need to educate older adults about the importance of obtaining nutrients from food sources rather than relying primarily on dietary supplements.

Nurses teach older adults about basic nutritional requirements, using easy-to-understand educational materials. Current recommendations for older adults are that they need to:

- Increase their intakes of whole grains, dried peas and beans, all types of fruits and vegetables (especially dark green and orange vegetables), fat-free or low-fat milk and milk products, and water
- Replace solid fats with oils, including those in fish, nuts and seeds
- Consume less sodium and saturated fat
- Ensure adequate fluid intake of 1.6 L to 3.5 L/day and
- Consume less food and beverages with added sugar, solid fats and alcohol (Nutrition Australia, 2013; Dietitians NZ, 2011)

Healthy older adults generally maintain optimal nutritional status through the daily intake of the foods listed in Box 18-7 and illustrated in Figure 18-6. In Figure 18-6 a circle is located at the top of the plate, which represents the need by older adults to supplement their diets with calcium, vitamin D and vitamin B_{12}, all of which are absorbed less with ageing. This supplementation can be achieved either by supplements usually prescribed by a medical practitioner or in fortified foods.

If older adults have any illness or take any medications or chemicals that interfere with homeostasis, digestion, nutrition or hydration, their daily intake will have to be modified to compensate for these effects. If, for any reason, the food intake is inadequate to meet daily nutritional requirements, older adults can be encouraged to use a broad-spectrum vitamin and mineral supplement. Studies indicate that older adults who take multivitamin/mineral supplements are less likely to be deficient in the following nutrients: vitamins B_6 and C, folate, zinc and magnesium (men and women); and vitamins A and E (men only) (Marra & Boyar, 2009).

BOX 18-7
Guidelines for daily food intake for older adults

- Because older adults need fewer kilojoules but the same amount of nutrients, it is important to select a variety of high-quality foods and avoid empty kilojoules.
- Use salt, sugar sodium only in moderation.
- Avoid saturated fats and replace solid fats with oils, including those in fish, nuts, seeds.
- Choose foods rich in fibre.
- Drink plenty of liquids without added sugars.
- Basic nutritional requirements will be met if the daily diet includes at least the minimum number of servings from each food group listed below, and if it includes complex carbohydrates and high-fibre foods.

Servings and food group

6–9	Bread, rice, pasta cereal
3–4	Vegetables
2–3	Fruits
2–3	Meat, fish, poultry, or legumes (dried peas and beans, lentils, nut butters, soy products)
2–3	Non-fat or low-fat milk, cheese, yoghurt dairy desserts
8+	8 or more 250 mL glasses of water or other fluids that are low in added sugars

Healthy older adults generally maintain optimal hydration status through the daily fluid intake. Adults require at least 1600 mL/day (JBI, 2001) although there is no standard recommended daily intake (RDI) of fluid. RDI can be calculated by three different methods and each calculates a different RDI. The three methods are:

1. 30 mL/kg body weight;
2. 1 mL fluid/kcal (or 4.18 kJ) consumed; and
3. 100 mL/kg for the first 10 kg, then 50 mL for the next 10 kg, and then 15 mL/kg for the remainder of weight. (JBI, 2001, p. 3)

For example, if the third method is used to calculate the fluid requirements of a 65 kg person, the calculation would be as follows:

$$(100 \times 10 = 1000) + (50 \times 10 = 500) + (15 \times 45 = 675) = 2175$$

Therefore, the total fluid intake required for a 65 kg resident would be 2175 mL fluid/day.

Nurses need to explain to older adults that they often do not experience a sensation of thirst and even in the presence of dehydration, their intake of liquids may be inadequate if they drink fluids only when thirsty. Interventions to promote adequate fluid intake will include identifying non-alcoholic, non-caffeinated and non-carbonated beverages that the

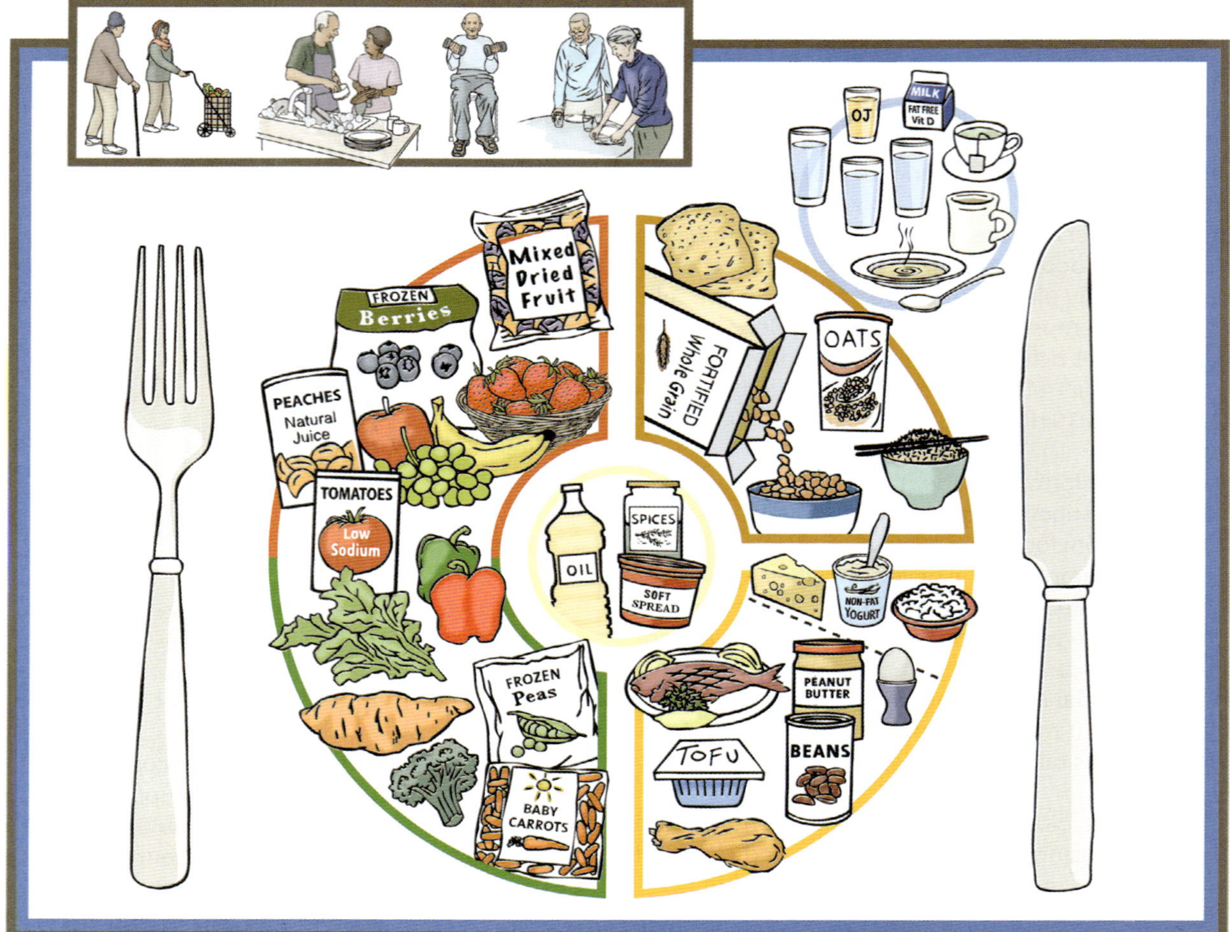

FIGURE 18-6 MyPlate for older adults. (Reprinted with permission from Tufts University.)

older adult will drink at appropriate intervals, even in the absence of a thirst sensation. Nurses can explain to older adults that they should monitor their daily fluid intake. One method they can use is to fill a jug of water at the beginning of the day and consume it during the day, thus monitoring and ensuring an adequate daily fluid intake.

WELLNESS OPPORTUNITY

Nurses promote personal responsibility by suggesting that older adults use the modified food guide shown in Figure 18-6 to identify beneficial and detrimental eating patterns.

Nutrition education can be provided on an individual basis or in group settings, perhaps with registered dietitians. In acute care settings, registered dietitians are usually available, but their services are often limited to people who have special dietary needs or an identified nutritional problem. In long-term residential care settings, a registered dietitian can assess the nutritional needs and usual eating patterns of older adults to establish a plan of care aimed at attaining and maintaining optimal nutrition. In community settings, nurses sometimes provide nutrition education to groups of older adults. Community nurses making home visits include nutrition education in their health teaching, make referrals for registered dietitian assessment and recommendations, and use available community resources to supplement these interventions. Nurses can use the Transtheoretical Model (discussed in Chapter 5) as an effective approach to working with older adults towards improved nutrition and changes in eating patterns (Wright, Velicer & Prochaska, 2009).

UNFOLDING CASE STUDY

Part C

Mrs Donnelly returns to the medical clinic and presents you with a 7-day diet history and a list of her medications, as you requested. You review the diet history and find that in response to your previous health education about constipation, Mrs Donnelly now uses whole-wheat bread instead of white and eats more fresh fruits and vegetables. You assess that her daily intake is only approximately 3300 kilojoules, of which pastries account for a high percentage. She rarely eats meat, perhaps because of the poor condition of her teeth. Her medications include citalopram 20 mg daily; clonidine 0.2 mg daily; and triamterene 37.5 mg/hydrochlorothiazide 25 mg daily.

Thinking points

- What specific risk factors do you address in your health teaching interventions?
- What health teaching would you give about alleviating risk factors?
- What interventions would you suggest to improve Mrs Donnelly's nutrition?
- What interventions would you suggest to help address Mrs Donnelly's dry mouth (which you noticed during Mrs Donnelly's last visit)?
- What health teaching would you provide about oral and dental care?

EVALUATING EFFECTIVENESS OF NURSING INTERVENTIONS

Nursing care for older adults with imbalanced nutrition: less than body requirements is evaluated by determining whether older adults have a daily nutrient intake that corresponds with metabolic needs and by older adults achieving a body weight within 10% of their ideal body weight.

The nursing care for fluid volume deficit or potential for fluid volume deficit can be evaluated by the older adult's intake of at least 1600 mL/day, and maintaining adequate urine output, specific gravity within normal range (if previously identified as abnormal, and a range of blood pathology values within normal values. For older adults with constipation, or risks for constipation, evaluation criteria would depend on their verbalising accurate information about constipation, identifying the factors that contribute to constipation and reporting that they pass soft stools on a regular basis without any straining or discomfort.

UNFOLDING CASE STUDY

Part D

Mr Donnelly is an 85-year-old widower who was referred for home care after a hospitalisation for congestive heart failure. During the hospitalisation, the geriatric assessment team diagnosed protein-energy undernutrition because Mr Donnelly's weight (58 kg) is only 75% of his ideal body weight (70.5 kg). In addition, laboratory work revealed the following abnormal values: haemoglobin, 11%; haematocrit, 35%; and serum albumin, 32 mg/L. Mr Donnelly's congestive heart failure is stable, and he ambulates with a walker but is very weak. In addition to orders pertaining to assessment and management of the newly diagnosed congestive heart failure, home care orders include nursing assessment of his home situation, nutrition education, and monitoring of weight. The geriatric assessment team in the medical unit which included a registered dietitian, recommended that Mr Donnelly have a daily intake of 6700 kilojoules, including a minimum of 60 g of protein (1000 kilojoules). Mr Donnelly could meet this goal if his daily intake included the minimum number of servings from each food group as listed in Box 18-7.

Nursing assessment

Mr Donnelly lives alone in a high-rise apartment and, until recently, participated in social activities and took advantage of van transportation to get to medical appointments and the grocery store. He used to prepare his own meals and shop for his groceries once a week but has not been out of his apartment in the past month because of gradually increasing weakness, shortness of breath and swelling in his legs. After his health began declining, a neighbour began doing his grocery shopping. Typical meals are toast and coffee for breakfast; canned soup, a luncheon meat sandwich and cookies for lunch; and a Budget Gourmet entree for supper. Mr Donnelly says that he never really learned to cook very well but that he got along "well enough for a man my age". He says that he does not particularly enjoy the convenience foods that he eats but states, "They sure are easy to fix, even if they are boring. Besides, I'm never very hungry because food just doesn't interest me the way it used to when I had Magda's good Hungarian cooking." Mr Donnelly reports a gradual weight loss of approximately 23 kilograms since his wife died 2 years ago. He says that he was too heavy when his wife used to do the cooking, so he is not concerned about his weight loss. He has full dentures but has not used them for the past year because they do not fit well anymore. He has not done anything about his dentures because he manages to chew the kinds of food he buys. In addition, his dentist retired 2 years ago, and he has not considered going to a new one.

Nursing issues

One issue that you address in your home care plan is altered nutrition: less than body requirements, related to social isolation, declining health, ill-fitting dentures and lack of enjoyment of food. You also question whether depression may be a contributing factor. Evidence comes from his low body weight, laboratory data consistent with poor nutritional status and his descriptions of his eating and food preparation patterns.

Nursing care plan for Mr Donnelly

Goals for wellness outcomes	Nursing interventions	Nursing evaluation
Mr Donnelly will state what his daily needs are for each food group	• Give Mr Donnelly a copy of Box 18-7 and use it as a basis for teaching about daily nutrient requirements	• Mr Donnelly describes an eating pattern that meets his daily nutritional needs
Mr Donnelly will identify a method for meeting his nutrient needs	• Gain Mr Donnelly's permission to arrange for home health aide assistance three times weekly for meal preparation and grocery shopping	• Mr Donnelly describes an acceptable plan for meeting his nutritional needs
	• Explore with Mr Donnelly various options for broadening his food selection to improve his nutritional intake (e.g. including dairy products and more fruits and vegetables)	• Mr Donnelly gains between 0.25 kg and 0.6 kg weekly until he reaches the goal of 68 kg.
	• Develop a meal plan with Mr Donnelly that includes foods that he enjoys but are not currently part of his diet. Discuss the nutritional value of these foods and suggest that he add new food items in each of the food group categories in which he is deficient	
Mr Donnelly will have his dentures evaluated and modified or replaced	• Discuss with Mr Donnelly the importance of dentures in chewing efficiency and food enjoyment	• Mr Donnelly has dentures that fit so he can chew his food.
	• Discuss the long-term detrimental effects of lack of dentures	
	• Explore ways of obtaining a dental evaluation	

Thinking points

- What risk factors are likely to be contributing to Mr Donnelly's gradual weight loss during the past 2 years?
- What further assessment information would you want to have?

CHAPTER HIGHLIGHTS

Age-related changes that affect digestion and eating and drinking patterns

- Diminished senses of smell and taste
- Altered thirst perception
- Less efficient chewing
- Decreased saliva secretion
- Degenerative changes in all structures of the gastrointestinal tract

Age-related changes in nutritional requirements

- Kilojoules: need less quantity, better quality
- Protein: minimum daily intake of 1.0 g to 1.2 g/kg of body weight
- Fibre: 25 g to 38 g/day
- Fat: no more than 10% to 30% of daily kilojoule intake
- Fluid at least 1.6 L/day of clear fluids

Risk factors that affect digestion, nutrition and hydration

- Poor oral care
- Conditions that can lead to nutritional deficiencies
- Functional impairments and disease processes
- Dysphagia (Evidence-based practice 18-1)
- Effects of medications
- Psychosocial factors (e.g. dementia, depression, loneliness)
- Cultural and socioeconomic factors (Cultural considerations 18-1)
- Environmental factors (e.g. noisy or unpleasant environment in institutional setting)
- Behaviours based on myths and misunderstandings (e.g. overuse of laxatives)

Functional consequences affecting digestion, nutrition and hydration

- Diminished ability to procure, prepare and enjoy food
- Changes in oral function
- Changes in nutrition needs and weight changes
- Effects on quality of life

Pathological conditions affecting digestive wellness

- *Malnutrition*: state of abnormal nutrition caused by undernutrition or overnutrition or incorrect nutrition
- *Dehydration*: depletion of body water and sodium (varies), not from vasculature but from intestines or reduced intake of water
- *Constipation*: two or fewer bowel movements weekly, or hard, dry faeces

Nursing assessment of digestion, nutrition and hydration

- Usual nutrient intake and eating and drinking patterns
- Risks that interfere with any aspect of obtaining, preparing, eating and enjoying food
- Physical examination and laboratory data regarding nutritional status
- Kayser-Jones Brief Oral Health Status Examination
- Seven Day Bowel Chart with the Bristol Stool Chart
- Mini Nutritional Assessment Tool and Malnutrition Universal Screening Tool
- Urine colour chart and Mentes' Typology of Oral Hydration
- Dehydration Risk Appraisal Checklist (DRAC)

Nursing issues

- Willingness for enhanced nutrition
- Altered nutrition: less than body requirements
- Constipation
- Impaired oral mucous membrane
- Fluid volume deficit

Goal planning for wellness outcomes

- Improved appetite, nutritional status, hydration status, oral hygiene, depression level
- Improved self-care about eating, drinking and oral hygiene
- Increased knowledge about diet and hydration, improved health beliefs about constipation

Nursing interventions to promote healthy digestion, nutrition and hydration

- Teaching older adults about nutrition, hydration and digestion
- Applying daily food and fluid guide to older adults
- Promoting oral and dental health
- Referring for community resources (e.g. home-delivered meals, group meal programs)

Evaluating effectiveness of nursing interventions

- Daily nutrient intake corresponds to metabolic needs
- Achieving/maintaining body weight within 10% of ideal body weight for the individual
- Achieving/maintaining regular bowel elimination
- Daily fluid intake that corresponds to metabolic needs; at least 1500 mL
- Maintaining an adequate urine output
- Range of blood values within normal limits

CRITICAL THINKING EXERCISES

1. Discuss specific ways in which each of the following conditions might influence the eating patterns of older adults: depression, medications, sensory changes, cognitive impairments, functional impairments, economic factors, social circumstances and oral health factors.
2. Describe at least three characteristics of eating patterns for each of the following cultural groups: Asians, Aboriginals and Torres Strait Islanders, Pacific people and Māori people.
3. How would you assess digestion and nutrition for an older adult in each of the following settings: at home, a long-term care facility and hospital?
4. Outline a health education plan for teaching older adults about constipation. Include the following points: definition of constipation, risk factors for constipation, and interventions to prevent and address constipation.
5. Outline a health education plan for teaching older adults about oral and dental care.

RESOURCES

For an extensive range of additional resources to enhance teaching and learning and to facilitate understanding of this chapter, please see the text's accompanying website located on thePoint at http://thepoint.lww.com

Clinical tools

Hartford Institute for Geriatric Nursing, ConsultGeriRN.org: http://consultgerirn.org/resources

Assessment tools *Try This*® series and *How to Try This* resources

General assessment series:

- *Try This*, issue 9: Assessing nutrition in older adults. DiMaria-Ghalili, R. A. & Amella, E. J. (2012). *Best Practices in Nursing Care to Older Adults*.
- *How to Try This* (article): The Mini Nutritional Assessment. DiMaria-Ghalili, R. A. & Guenter, P. A. (2008). *American Journal of Nursing*, *108*(2), 50–59. (Updated May 2015.)
- *How to Try This* (video): *Assessing nutrition in older adults*.
- *Try This*, issue 20: Preventing aspiration in older adults with dysphagia. Metheny, N. A. (2012). *Best Practices in Nursing Care to Older Adults*.
- *How to Try This* (article): Preventing aspiration in older adults with dysphagia. Palmer, J. L. & Metheny, N. A. (2008). *American Journal of Nursing*, *108*(2), 40–48. (Updated May 2015.)
- *How to Try This* (video): *Preventing aspiration in older adults with dysphagia*.

Dementia series:

- *Try This*, issue D11.1: Eating and feeding issues in older adults with dementia, Part I: Assessment. Amella, E. (2007). *Best Practices in Nursing Care to Older Adults*.
- *Try This*, issue D11.2: Eating and feeding issues in older adults with dementia, Part II: Interventions. Amella, E. (2007). *Best Practices in Nursing Care to Older Adults*.
- *How to Try This* (video): *Eating and feeding issues in older adults with dementia*.
- *How to Try This* (article): The Edinburgh Feeding Evaluation in Dementia Scale: Determining how much help people with dementia need at mealtime. Stockdell, R. & Amella, E. (2008). *American Journal of Nursing*, *108*(8), 46–54. (Updated May 2015.)

Evidence-based practice

Amella, E. J. & Aselage, M. B. (2012). Mealtime difficulties. In M. Boltz, E. Capezuti, T. Fulmer & D. Zwicker (Eds), *Evidence-based geriatric nursing protocols for best practice* (4th ed. pp. 453–468). New York: Springer.

DiMaria-Ghalili, R. A. (2012). Nutrition. In M. Boltz, E. Capezuti, T. Fulmer & D. Zwicker (Eds), *Evidence-based geriatric nursing protocols for best practice* (4th ed. pp. 439–452). New York: Springer.

Joanna Briggs Institute: http://connect.jbiconnectplus.org

Evidence summaries:

Hydration and nutrition

- Campbell, J. (2013). Ensuring hydration: Older people.
- Chu, V. (2014). Risk assessment of malnutrition: Older people.
- Dao Le, L. (2013). Malnutrition risk (elderly): Protein and energy supplementation.
- D'Arcy, M. (2013). Reducing nutritional risk in hospital: The Red Tray System.
- Kunde, L. (2014). Advanced dementia: Clinical care with eating and drinking.
- Kunde, L. (2014). Nutritional screening: Community settings.
- Kunde, L. (2014). Oral hydration for the older person.
- Tolu Feyissa, G. (2014). Dementia: Oral hygiene care.
- Rahman, M. (2013). Risk assessment of malnutrition in inpatient facilities.
- Sharma, L. (2014). Older adults: Oral hydration.

Continence care

- D'Arcy, M. (2013). Urinary and fecal incontinence: Absorbent products.
- D'Arcy, M. (2014). Continence care.
- Slade, S. (2013). Urinary and fecal incontinence (older person): Assessment.
- Slade, S. (2014). Constipation management.
- Jayasekara, R. (2013). Effective management of fecal impaction for older people in community settings.

Recommended practices:

- Bowel charting and reporting. (2013).
- Continence care. (2014).
- Constipation management. (2013).
- Feeding assistance and older people. (2013).
- Munn, Z. (2013). Nutrition screening: Community settings.
- Oral hygiene. (2013).
- Patient nutrition. (2013).

Systematic reviews:

- Fallon, A., Westaway, J. & Moloney, C. (2008). A systematic review of psychometric evidence and expert opinion regarding the assessment of faecal incontinence in older community-dwelling adults. *Joanna Briggs Institute Library of Systematic Reviews, 6*(11), 367–431.
- Whitelock, G. & Aromataris, E. (2013). Effectiveness of mealtime interventions to improve nutritional intake of adult patients in the acute care setting: A systematic review. *Joanna Briggs Library of Systematic Reviews, 11*(3), 263–305.
- Mentes, J. C. (2012). Managing oral hydration. In M. Boltz, E. Capezuti, T. Fulmer & D. Zwicker D. (Eds), *Evidence-based geriatric nursing protocols for best practice* (4th ed. pp. 419–438). New York: Springer.
- O'Connor, L. J. (2012). Oral health care. In M. Boltz, E. Capezuti, T. Fulmer & D. Zwicker (Eds), *Evidence-based geriatric nursing protocols for best practice* (4th ed. pp. 409–418). New York: Springer.

Health education

Academy of Nutrition and Dietetics: www.eatright.org

Australian Dietary Guidelines (adults): eatforhealth.gov.au

Centre for Cultural Diversity and Ageing, food services: www.culturaldiversity.com.au

Dietitians Association of Australia (DAA): www.daa.asn.au

Dietitians NZ: www.dietitians.org.nz

Food and Nutrition Information Center (US): http://fnic.nal.usda.gov/

Independent Living Centre (ADL tools, aids): www.ilc.com.au

National Dairy Council: www.nationaldairycouncil.org

NIHSenior Health: nihseniorhealth.gov/category/healthy-aging.html

Nestlé Nutrition: www.nestlenutrition.com

New Zealand Ministry of Health, nutrition: www.health.govt.nz/our-work/preventative-health-wellness/nutrition

Nutrition Australia, older adults: www.nutritionaustralia.org/national/resources/older-adults

REFERENCES

Allen, L. H. (2009). How common is vitamin B-12 deficiency? *American Journal of Clinical Nutrition, 89*(Suppl.), 693S–696S.

Australian & New Zealand Society for Geriatric Medicine (ANZSGM). (2007). Under-nutrition and the older person. Position statement no. 6. Available February 2015 via www.anzsgm.org/posstate.asp.

Australian Government Department of Health (AGDH), National Health and Medical Research Council (NHMRC) & New Zealand Ministry of Health (NZMOH). (2006). *Nutrient reference values for Australia and New Zealand*. Canberra: NHMRC.

Australian Government Department of Social Services. (n.d.). Seven Day Bowel Chart. In *Continence tools for residential aged care: An education guide*. Accessible April 2015 via www.bladderbowl.gov.au.

Australian Institute of Health and Welfare (AIHW). (2010). *Australia's health 2010.* Australia's health series no. 12. Cat. no. AUS 122. Canberra: AIHW.

Australian Institute of Health and Welfare (AIHW). (2014). *Australia's health 2014.* Australia's health series no. 14. Cat. no. AUS 178. Canberra: AIHW.

Bahat, G., Tufan, F., Saka, B. et al. (2012). Which body mass index (BMI) is better in the elderly for functional status? *Archives of Gerontology and Geriatrics, 54*(1), 78–81.

Bennett, J. A. Thomas, V. & Riegel, B. (2004). Unrecognized chronic dehydration in older adults: Examining prevalence rate and risk factors. *Journal of Gerontological Nursing, 30*(11), 22–28.

Biesalski, H. K., Brummer, R. J., Koenig, J., O'Connell, M. A., Ovesen, L. Rechkemmer, G., Stos, K. & Thurnham, D. . (2003). Micronutrient deficiencies: Hohenheim Consensus Conference. *European Journal of Nutrition, 42*, 353–363.

Bitar, K., Greenwood-Van Meerveld, B., Saad, R. et al. (2011). Aging and gastrointestinal neuromuscular function. *Neurogastrointestinal Motility, 23*(6), 490–501.

Boczko, F., McKeon, S. & Sturkie, D. (2009). Long-term care and oral health knowledge. *Journal of American Directors Association, 10*, 204–206.

Bouras, E. P. & Tangalos, E. G. (2009). Chronic constipation in the elderly. *Gastroenterological Clinics of North America, 38*, 463–480.

Bowman, S. A. (2009). Socioeconomic characteristics, dietary and lifestyle patterns, and health and weight status of older adults in NHANES, 1999–2002: A comparison of Caucasians and African Americans. *Journal of Nutrition and the Elderly, 28*(1), 30–46.

Britton, E. & McLaughlin, J. T. (2013). Ageing and the gut. *Proceedings of the Nutrition Society, 72*(1), 173–177.

Burnett-Hartman, A. N., Fitzpatrick, A. L., Gao, K., Jackson, S. A. & Schreiner, P. J. (2009). Supplement use contributes to meeting recommended dietary intakes for calcium, magnesium, and vitamin C in four ethnicities of middle-aged and older Americans: The Multi-Ethnic Study of Atherosclerosis. *Journal of the American Dietetic Association, 109*, 422–429.

Chalmers, J. & Johnson, V. (2004). Evidence-based protocol: Oral hygiene care for functionally dependent and cognitively impaired older adults. *Journal of Gerontological Nursing, November*, 5–12.

Clave, P., Rofes, L., Carrion, S. et al. (2012). Pathophysiology, relevance and natural history of oropharyngeal dysphagia among older people. *Nestle Nutrition Institute Workshop Service, 72*, 57–66.

Dahm, C. C., Keogh, R. H., Spencer, E. A., Greenwood, D. C., Key, T. J., Fentiman, I. S., . . . Rodwell Bingham, S. A. (2010). Dietary fibre and colorectal cancer risk: A nested case-control study using food diaries. *Journal of the National Cancer Institute, 102*(9), 614–626.

Dietitians NZ. (2011) Healthy eating for older people. Viewed February 2015 at http://dietitians.org.nz/nutrition-resources/aged-care.

DiMaria-Ghalili, R. A. & Guenter, P. A. (2008). The Mini Nutritional Assessment. *American Journal of Nursing, 108*(2), 50–54.

Donini, L. M., Scardella, P., Piombo, L. et al. (2013). Malnutrition in the elderly: Social and economic determinants. *Journal of Nutrition, Health and Aging, 17*(1), 9–15.

Du, H., Van Der A, D. L., Boshuizen, H. C., Forouhi, N. G., Wareham, N. J., Halkjaer, J., . . . Feskens, E. J. (2010). Dietary fiber and subsequent changes in body weight and waist circumference in European men and women. *American Journal of Clinical Nutrition, 91*(2), 329–336.

Fulgoni, V. L., III. (2008). Current protein intake in America: Analysis of the National Health and Nutrition Examination Survey, 2003–2004. *American Journal of Clinical Nutrition, 87*(Suppl.), 1554S–1557S.

Gaffney-Stomberg, E., Insogna, K. L., Rodriguez, N. R. & Kerstetter, J. E. (2009). Increasing dietary protein requirements in elderly people for optimal muscle and bone health. *Journal of the American Geriatrics Society, 57*(6), 1073–1079.

Grassi, M., Petraccia, L., Mennuni, G. et al. (2011). Changes, functional disorders, and diseases in the gastrointestinal tract of elderly. *Nutricion Hospitalaria, 26*(4), 659–668.

Gregersen, H., Pedersen, J. & Drewes, A. M. (2008). Deterioration of muscle function in the human esophagus with age. *Digestive Diseases and Sciences, 53*(12), 3065–3070.

Grieger, J. A., Nowson, C. A. & Ackland, L. M. (2009). Nutritional and functional status indicators in residents of a long-term care facility. *Journal of Nutrition and the Elderly, 28*(1), 47–60.

Guigoz, Y. (2006). The Mini-Nutritional Assessment (MNA®) review of the literature: What does it tell us? *Journal of Nutrition, Health & Aging, 10*, 466–487.

Haumschild, M. S. & Haumschild, R. J. (2009). The importance of oral health in long-term care. *Journal of American Medical Directors Association, 10*, 667–671.

Herdman, T. H. (Ed.). (2012). *NANDA International nursing diagnoses: Definitions and classification 2012–2014*. Oxford: Wiley-Blackwell.

Home and Community Care (HACC)/Medical Aids Subsidy Scheme (MASS) Continence Project. (2010). *First steps in the management of urinary incontinence in community-dwelling older people: A clinical practice guideline for primary level clinicians (registered nurses and allied health professionals)*. Revised version 2010. Brisbane: Queensland Health. Available for download February 2015 at www.health.qld.gov.au/mass/documents/clinical-guide-continence-first-1.pdf.

Hopping, B. N., Erber, E., Grandinetti, A., Verheus, M., Kolonel, L. N. & Maskarinec, G. (2010). Dietary fiber, magnesium, and glycemic load alter risk of type 2 diabetes in a multiethnic cohort in Hawaii. *Journal of Nutrition, 140*(1), 68–74.

Houston, D. K., Nicklas, B. J. & Zizza, C. A. (2009). Weighty concerns: The growing prevalence of obesity among older adults. *Journal of the American Dietetic Association, 109*, 1886–1895.

Hsieh, Y. M., Sung, T. S. & Wan, K. S. (2010). A survey of nutrition and health status of solitary and non-solitary elders in Taiwan. *Journal of Nutrition and Health and Ageing, 14*(1), 11–14.

Hummel, T., Landis, B. & Huttenbrink, K.-B. (2011). Smell and taste disorders. *GMS Current Topics in Otorhinolaryngology, 10*. ISSN 1865-1011.

Huttenbrink, K.-B., Hummel, T., Berg, D. et al. (2013). Olfactory dysfunction: Common in later life and early warning of neurodegenerative disease. *Deutsches Ärzteblatt International, 110*(1–2), 1–7.

Jablonski, R. A., Munro, C. L., Grap, M. J., Schubert, C. M., Ligon, M. & Spigelmyer, P. (2009). Mouth care in nursing homes: Knowledge, beliefs, and practices of nursing assistants. *Geriatric Nursing, 30*(2), 99–106.

Joanna Briggs Institute. (2007). Effectiveness of interventions for undernourished older patients in the hospital setting. *Best practice: Evidence-based information sheets for health professionals*, *11*(2), 1–4.

Joanna Briggs Institute. (2001). Maintaining oral hydration in older people. *Best practice: Evidence-based information sheets for health professionals*, *5*(1), 1–6.

Joanna Briggs Institute. (2008). Management of constipation in older adults. *Best practice: Evidence-based information sheets for health professionals*, *12*(7), 1–4.

Johansson, L., Sidenvall, B., Malmberg, B. & Christensson, L. (2009). Who will become malnourished? A prospective study of factors associated with malnutrition in older persons living at home. *Journal of Nutrition and Health and Ageing, 13*(10), 855–861.

Johnson, V. B. & Schoenfelder, D. P. (2012). Evidence-based practice guideline: Oral hygiene care for functionally dependent and cognitively impaired older adults. *Journal of Gerontological Nursing, 38*(11), 11–19.

Kaiser, M. J., Bauer, J. M., Ramsch, C. et al. (2009). Validation of the Mini Nutritional Assessment Short-Form (MNA®-SF): A practical tool for identification of nutritional status. *Journal of Nutrition, Health & Aging*, *13*, 782–788.

Kamp, B. J., Wellman, N. S. & Russell, C. (2010). Position of the American Dietetic Association, American Society for Nutrition, and Society for Nutrition Education: Food and nutrition programs for community-residing older adults. *Journal of the American Dietetic Association, 110*(3), 463–472.

Kiesswetter, E., Pohlhausen, S., Uhlig, K., et al. (2013). Malnutrition is related to functional impairment in older adults receiving home care. *Journal of Nutrition, Health and Aging, 17*(4), 345–350.

Kim, C.-O. & Lee, K.-R. (2013). Preventive effect of protein-energy supplementation on the functional decline of frail older adults with low socioeconomic status: A community-based randomized controlled study. *Journals of Gerontology: Medical Sciences, 68*(3), 300–316.

Kruizenga, H. M., de Vet, H. C., Van Marissing, C. M., Stassen, E. E., Strijk, J. E., Van Bokhorst-de Van Der Schueren, M. A., . . . Visser, M. (2010). The SNAQ(RC), an easy traffic light system as a first step in the recognition of undernutrition in residential care. *Journal of Nutrition and Health, and Ageing, 14*(2), 83–89.

Lafreniere, D. & Mann, N. (2009). Anosmia: Loss of smell in the elderly. *Otolaryngology Clinics of North America, 42*, 123–131.

Lam, A., Kiyak, A., Gossett, A. M. & McCormick, L. (2009). Assessment of the use of xerogenic medications for chronic medical and dental conditions among adult day health participants. *Consultant Pharmacist: Journal of the American Society of Consultant Pharmacists, 24*(10), 755–764.

Legg, T. J. (2012). Oral care in older adults with dementia: Challenges and approaches. *Journal of Gerontological Nursing, 38*(8), 10–13.

Lichtenstein, A. H., Rasmussen, H., Yu, W. W., Epstein, S. R. & Russell, R. M. (2008). Modified MyPyramid for older adults. *Journal of Nutrition, 138*, 5–11.

Maki, K. C., Beiseigel, J. M., Jonnalagadda, S. S., Gugger, C. K., Reeves, M. S., Farmer, M. V., . . . Rains, T. M. (2010). Whole-grain ready-to-eat oat cereal, as part of a dietary program for weight loss, reduces low-density lipoprotein cholesterol in adults with overweight and obesity more than a dietary program including low-fiber control foods. *Journal of the American Dietetic Association, 110*(2), 205–214.

Marra, M. V. & Boyar, A. P. (2009). Position of the American Dietetic Association: Nutrient supplementation. *Journal of the American Dietetic Association, 109*(12), 2073–2085.

McKay, S. L., Fravel, M. & Scanlon, C. (2012). Evidence-based practice guideline: Management of constipation. *Journal of Gerontological Nursing, 38*(7), 9–15.

McLaren, S. M. (2006). Eating and drinking. In Redfern, S. J. & Ross, F. M (Eds), *Nursing older people* (4th ed., pp. 279–314). Sydney: Elsevier.

Mentes, J. C. (2006a). Oral hydration in older adults. *American Journal of Nursing, 106*(6), 40–49.

Mentes, J. C. (2006b). A typology of oral hydration: Problems exhibited by frail nursing home residents. *Journal of Gerontological Nursing, 32*(1), 13–19.

Mentes, J. C. & Wang, J. (2011). Measuring risk for dehydration in nursing home residents: Evaluation of the Dehydration Risk Appraisal Checklist. *Research in Gerontological Nursing*, *4*(2), 148–156.

Metheny, N. A. (2012). Preventing aspiration in older adults with dysphagia. *Try This* series, issue 20. *Best Practices in Nursing Care to Older Adults*. Accessed 13 May 2013 via www.ConsultGeriRN.org.

Montgomery, M. P., Kamel, F., Pericak-Vance, M. A., Haines, J. L., Postel, E. A. & Agarwal, A. (2010). Overall diet quality and age-related macular degeneration. *Ophthalmic Epidemiology, 17*(1), 58–65.

Morley, J. E. (2010). Nutrition and the brain. *Clinics in Geriatric Medicine, 26*, 89–98.

Morley, J. E. (2013). Pathophysiology of the anorexia of aging. *Current Opinion in Clinical Nutrition and Metabolic Care, 16*, 27–32.

National Ageing Research Institute (NARI). (2014). Healthy Ageing Quiz. Accessed February 2015 at www.mednwh.unimelb.edu.au/nari_tips_for_healthy_ageing/nari_healthy-ageing-quiz.html.

Nestlé Nutrition Institute. (2009). Mini Nutritional Assessment—Short Form. Vevey, Switzerland: Nestle Inc.

National Health and Medical Research Council (NHMRC). (2013). *Australian dietary guidelines*. Canberra: National Health and Medical Research Council.

New Zealand Dental Association. (2010). Healthy mouth, healthy ageing: Oral health guide for caregivers of older people. Available February 2015 via www.healthysmiles.org.nz/default,228,public-resources.sm.

Ney, D., Weiss, J., Kind, A. & Robinson, J. A. (2009). Senescent swallowing: Impact, strategies and interventions. *Nutrition in Clinical Practice, 24*(3), 395–413.

Nogueira, D. & Reis, E. (2013). Swallowing disorder in nursing home residents: How can the problem be explained? *Clinical Interventions in Aging, 8*, 221–227.

Nutrition Australia. (2013). Nutrition and older adults. Available February 2015 via www.nutritionaustralia.org/national/resource/nutrition-and-older-adults#attachments.

Oliveira, M. R. M., Fogaca, K. C. P. & Leandro-Merhi, V. A. (2009). Nutritional status and functional capacity of hospitalized elderly. *Nutrition Journal, 8*(11), 54–62.

O'Connor, L. J. (2012). Oral health care. In M. Boltz, E. Capezuti, T. Fulmer & D. Zwicker (Eds), *Evidence-based practice protocols for best practice* (4th ed., pp. 409–418). New York: Springer.

Orsitto, G. (2012). Different components of nutritional status in older inpatients with cognitive impairment. *Journal of Nutrition, Health and Aging, 16*(5), 468–471.

Paddon-Jones, D. & Rasmussen, B. B. (2009). Dietary protein recommendations and the prevention of sarcopenia: Protein, amino acid metabolism and therapy. *Current Opinion in Clinical Nutrition and Metabolic Care, 12*(1), 86–90.

Palmer, J. L. & Metheny, N. A. (2008). Preventing aspiration in older adults with dysphagia. *How to Try This* series. *American Journal of Nursing, 108*(2), 40–48.

Parekh, N., Voland, R. P., Moeller, S. M., Blodi, B. A., Ritenbaugh, C., Chappell, R. J., . . . Mares, J. A. (2009). Association between dietary fat intake and age-related macular degeneration in the Carotenoids in Age-Related Eye Disease Study (CAREDS): An ancillary study of the Women's Health Initiative. *Archives of Ophthalmology, 127*(11), 1483–1493.

Park, Y.-H., Han, H.-R., Oh, B.-M. et al. (2013). Prevalence and associated factors of dysphagia in nursing home residents. *Geriatric Nursing, 34*(3), 212–217.

Price, D. M. (2008). Protein-energy malnutrition among the elderly: Implications for nursing care. *Holistic Nursing Practice, 22*(6), 355–360.

Quandt, S. A., Chen, H., Bell, R. A., Savoca, M. R., Anderson, A. M., Leng, X., . . . Arcury, T. A. (2010). Food avoidance and food modification practices of older rural adults: Association with oral health status and implications for service provision. *Gerontologist, 50*(1), 100–110.

Queensland Government Health Department. (2014). Dietitian/nutritionists from the nutrition education materials online. Accessed at www.health.qld.gov.au/nutrition/resources/hphe_usingbmi.pdf.

Raniga, A. & Elder, M. J. (2009). Dietary supplement use in the prevention of age-related macular degeneration progression. *New Zealand Medical Journal, 122*(1299), 32–38.

Rayner, C. K. & Horowitz, M. (2013). Physiology of the ageing gut. *Current Opinion in Clinical Nutrition and Metabolic Care, 16*, 33–38.

Rubenstein, L. Z., Harker, J. O., Salva, A., Guigoz, Y., Vellas, B. (2001). Screening for undernutrition in geriatric practice: Developing the Short-Form Mini Nutritional Assessment (MNA-SF). *Journal of Gerontology, 56A*, M366–M377.

Sahyoun, N. R., Anyanwu, U. O., Sharkey, J. R. & Netterville, L. (2010). Recently hospital-discharged older adults are vulnerable and may be underserved by the Older American Act Nutrition Program. *Journal of Nutrition for the Elderly, 29*(2), 227–240.

Savoca, M. R., Arcury, T. A., Leng, X., Bell, R. A., Anderson, A. M., Anderson, A. M., . . . Quandt, S. A. (2010). Severe tooth loss in older adults as a key indicator of compromised dietary quality. *Public Health Nutrition, 13*(4), 466–474.

Schubert, C. R., Cruickshanks, K. J., Fischer, M. E. et al. (2012). Olfactory impairment in an adult population. *Chemical Senses, 37*(4), 325–334.

Skates, J. J. & Anthony, P. (2009). The Mini Nutritional Assessment: An integral part of geriatric assessment. *Nutrition Today, 44*(1), 21–28.

Slade, G. D., Spencer, A. J. & Roberts-Thomson, K. F. (2007). *Australia's dental generations: The national survey of adult oral health 2004–06*. Canberra: Australian Institute of Health and Welfare.

Smoliner, C., Fischedick, A., Sieber, C. et al. (2013). Olfactory function and malnutrition in geriatric patients. *Journals of Gerontology: Medical Sciences, 68*(12), 1582–1588.

Soenen, S. & Chapman, I. M. (2013). Body weight, anorexia, and undernutrition in older people. *Journal of the American Medical Directors Association, 14*(9), 642–648.

Song, H. J. (2012). Constipation in community-dwelling elders: Prevalence and associated factors. *Journal of Wound, Ostomy, and Continence Nursing, 39*(6), 640–645.

Starr, J. M. & Hall, R. (2010). Predictors and correlates of edentulism in healthy older people. *Current Opinion in Clinical Nutrition and Metabolic Care, 13*(1), 19–23.

Stratton, R., King, C., Stroud, M., Jackson, A. & Elia, M. (2006). Malnutrition Universal Screening Tool predicts mortality and length of hospital stay in acutely ill elderly. *British Journal of Nutrition*, *95*, 325–330.

Sura, L., Madhavan, A., Carnaby, G. et al. (2012). Dysphagia in the elderly: Management and nutritional considerations. *Clinical Interventions in Aging, 7,* 287–298.

Tanner, D. C. (2010). Lessons from nursing home dysphagia malpractice litigation. *Journal of Gerontological Nursing, 36*(3), 41–46.

Taub, L.-F. (2012). Oral health assessment of older adults: The Kayser-Jones Brief Oral Health Status Examination (BOHSE). *Try This* series, issue 18. *Best Practices in Nursing Care to Older Adults*. Available 13 May 2013 via www.ConsultGeriRN.org.

Tsakos, G., Herrick, K., Sheiham, A. & Watt, R. G. (2010). Edentulism and fruit and vegetable intake in low-income adults. *Journal of Dental Research, 89*(5), 462–467.

Turner, M. D. & Ship, J. A. (2007). Dry mouth and its effects on the oral health of elderly people. *Journal of the American Dental Association, 138*(9, Suppl.), 15S–20S.

Uher, R., Farmer, A., Henigsberg, N., Rietschel, M., Mors, O., Maier, W., . . . McGuffin, P. (2009). Adverse reactions to antidepressants. *British Journal of Psychiatry, 195*(3), 202–210.

Vellas, B., Villars, H., Abellan, G. et al. (2006). Overview of MNA®: Its history and challenges. *Journal of Nutrition, Health & Aging*, *10,* 456–465.

Verbrugghe, M., Beeckman, D., Van Hecke, A. et al. (2013). Malnutrition and associated factors in nursing home residents. *Clinical Nutrition. 32*(3), 438–443.

Veronese, N., De Rui, M., Toffanello, E. D. et al. (2013). Body mass index as a predictor of all-cause mortality in nursing home residents during a 5-year follow-up. *Journal of the American Medical Directors Association, 14*, 53–57.

Visvanathan, R. & Chapman, I. M. (2009). Undernutrition and anorexia in the older person. *Gastroenterology Clinics of North America, 38*, 393–409.

Visvanathan, V. & Nix, P. (2010). Managing the patient presenting with xerostomia: A review. *International Journal of Clinical Practice, 64*(3), 404–407.

Vivanti, A., Harvey, K. & Ash, S. (2010). Developing a quick and practical screen to improve the identification of poor hydration in geriatric and rehabilitative care. *Archives of Gerontology and Geriatrics, 50*(2), 156–164.

Winter, J., Flanagan, D., McNaughton, S. A. et al. (2013). Nutrition screening of older people in a community general practice using the MNA-SF. *Journal of Nutrition, Health and Aging, 17*(4), 322–325.

Wright, J. A., Velicer, W. F. & Prochaska, J. O. (2009). Testing the predictive power of the transtheoretical model of behavior change applied to dietary fat intake. *Health Education Research, 24*(2), 224–236.

Chapter 19

Urinary function

By Carol Miller and Sharyn Hunter

LEARNING OBJECTIVES

After reading this chapter, you should be able to:

1. List age-related changes that affect the complex processes involved in urinary elimination.
2. Describe risk factors that influence kidney function and urinary elimination
3. Describe the functional consequences of age-related changes and risk factors related to each of the following aspects of urinary function: the elimination of medications and metabolic wastes; patterns of urinary elimination; and consequences of incontinence for older adults and their carers.
4. Define urge, stress, overflow, and functional and mixed incontinence.
5. Propose interview questions, and describe observations and laboratory data used in the nursing assessment of urinary function in older adults.
6. Identify interventions for addressing risk factors that influence urinary elimination and for alleviating and managing incontinence.

KEY POINTS

- benign prostatic hyperplasia
- bladder diary
- catheter-associated urinary tract infection (CAUTI)
- continence training
- creatinine clearance
- functional urinary incontinence
- mixed urinary incontinence
- nocturia
- overactive bladder (OAB)
- overflow urinary incontinence
- pelvic floor disorders
- pelvic floor muscle exercise (PFME)
- prompted voiding
- stress urinary incontinence
- urge urinary incontinence
- urinary incontinence (UI)
- urinary tract infection (UTI)

The primary function of urinary elimination is the excretion of water and chemical wastes, such as metabolic and pharmacological by-products, that would become toxic if allowed to accumulate. Efficient urinary excretion depends on renal blood flow, filtering activities within the kidneys, good functioning of the urinary tract muscles, and nervous system control over voluntary and involuntary mechanisms of elimination. Control of urinary elimination also depends on ambulatory and sensory abilities and on social, emotional, cognitive and environmental factors.

Healthy older adults experience very few functional consequences affecting urinary elimination, but when risk factors are present, negative functional consequences, such as **urinary incontinence (UI)**, are common. Urinary incontinence is defined as any involuntary leakage of urine. An important risk factor—and one that can be alleviated through health education interventions—is the false belief that urinary incontinence is an inevitable part of ageing. Nurses have many opportunities to improve quality of life for older adults by addressing the risk factors that contribute to urinary incontinence.

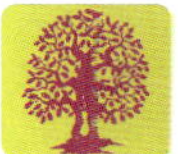

AGE-RELATED CHANGES THAT AFFECT URINARY WELLNESS

Age-related changes in the kidneys, bladder, urethra and control mechanisms in the nervous and other body systems affect the physiological processes that control urinary elimination. In addition, any age-related change that interferes with the skills involved in socially appropriate urinary elimination can interfere with urinary control. Age-related changes that directly or indirectly affect urinary function and control are discussed in the next two sections.

Changes in the kidneys

The complex process of urinary excretion begins in the kidneys with the filtering and removal of chemical wastes from the blood. Blood circulates through the glomeruli, where liquid wastes, called *glomerular filtrate*, pass through Bowman's capsule and the renal tubules to the collecting ducts. During this process substances needed by the body (such as water, glucose and sodium) are retained and waste products are excreted in the urine. These functions are important for maintaining *homeostasis* and excreting many medications. Excretory function, which is measured by the *glomerular filtration rate* (GFR), depends on the number and efficiency of nephrons and on the amount and rate of renal blood flow.

The kidney increases in weight and mass from birth until early adulthood, when the number of functioning nephrons begins to decline, particularly in the cortex, where the glomeruli are located. This decline continues throughout life, and results in an approximately 25%

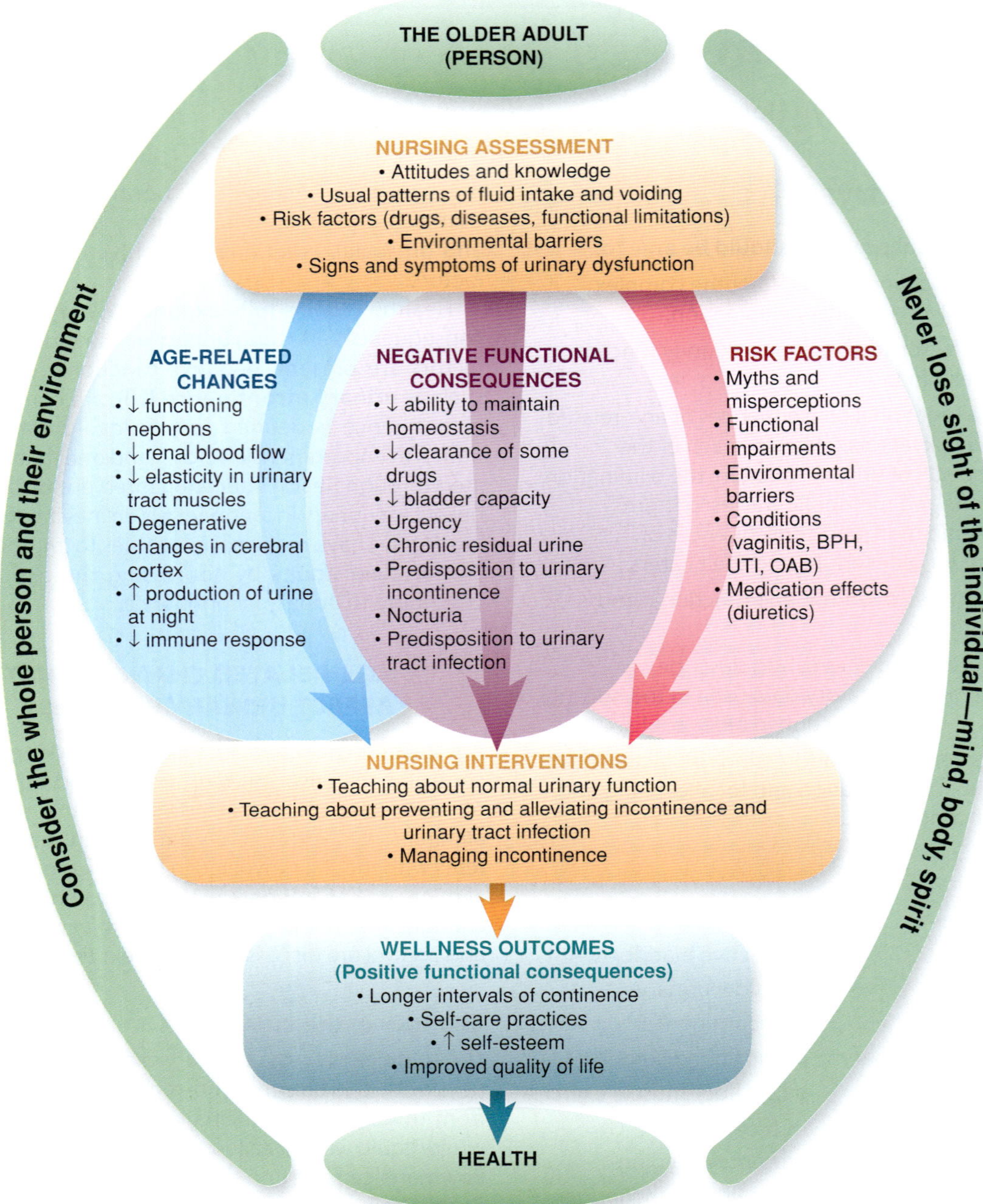

decrease in kidney mass by the age of 80 years. The remaining kidney glomeruli undergo various age-related changes such as increased size, diminished lobulation and thickened basement membrane. In addition, the proportion of sclerotic glomeruli increases from fewer than 5% at the age of 40 years to 35% by the age of 80 years. Beginning in the fourth decade, renal blood flow gradually diminishes, particularly in the cortex, at a rate of 10% per decade.

An average decline in renal function of 1% per year has been widely accepted since the 1970s as a hallmark of ageing that begins between the ages of 30 and 40 years. Most studies indicate that a gradual decline in renal function is a normal age-related change and any *substantial* decline in renal function is associated with common pathological conditions such as hypertension (Glassock & Winearls, 2009; Lerma, 2009).

Renal tubules regulate the dilution and concentration of urine and subsequent excretion of water from the body, in a diurnal rhythm. The physiological processes responsible for urine concentration and water excretion are influenced by the following factors:

- The amount of fluid in the body
- Reabsorption of water through and transport of substances across the tubular membrane
- Osmoreceptors in the hypothalamus, which regulate the level of circulating *antidiuretic hormone* (ADH) according to plasma–water concentration
- Substances and activities that influence ADH secretion, such as caffeine, medications, alcohol, pain, stress and exercise
- The concentration of sodium in the glomerular filtrate.

Normally, production of ADH is stimulated by haemorrhage, dehydration and other conditions that affect plasma volume or osmolality. This physiological protective mechanism helps to maintain plasma volume and conserve fluid and sodium under conditions of water or sodium deprivation.

Many age-related changes affect the renal tubules and thereby affect the dilution and concentration of urine. These changes include fatty degeneration, diverticula, a loss of convoluted cells and alterations in the composition of the basement membranes. Functionally, the renal tubules in older adults are less efficient in the exchange of substances, the conservation of water and the suppression of ADH secretion in the presence of hypo-osmolality. Age-related changes also decrease the ability of the older kidney to conserve sodium in response to salt restriction. These age-related changes predispose healthy older adults to hyponatraemia and other fluid and electrolyte imbalances, particularly in the presence of any condition that alters renal circulation, water or sodium balance, or plasma volume or osmolality.

Changes in the bladder and urinary tract

After being filtered by the kidneys, liquid wastes pass through the ureters into the bladder for temporary storage. The bladder is a balloon-like structure composed of collagen, smooth muscle (called *detrusor*) and elastic tissue. Liquid wastes are eliminated from the bladder through a complex physiological process involving the following mechanisms:

- The ability of the bladder to expand for adequate storage and to contract for complete expulsion of liquid wastes
- The maintenance of higher urethral pressure relative to intravesicular pressure
- Regulation of the lower urinary tract through autonomic and somatic nerves
- Voluntary control of urination (micturition) through the cerebral centres.

Age-related changes alter each of these mechanisms and affect urinary function in older adults. In younger adults, the bladder stores 350 to 450 mL of urine before the person experiences sensations of fullness and discomfort. With increasing age, hypertrophy of the bladder muscle and thickening of the bladder wall interfere with the bladder's ability to expand, limiting the amount of urine that can be stored comfortably to approximately 200 to 300 mL.

As urine flows into the bladder, the smooth muscle expands without increasing intravesical pressure and the urethral pressure increases to the point that it is slightly higher than the intravesical pressure. As long as the volume of urine does not rise above 500 to 600 mL, this balance can be maintained and urination can be controlled voluntarily. If the volume rises above this level or if the detrusor muscle contracts involuntarily, the intravesical pressure will exceed the urethral pressure and leakage of urine is likely to occur. In addition to the amount of urine in the bladder, the following factors influence the balance between intravesical and urethral pressure:

- Abdominal pressure
- Thickness of the urethral mucosa
- Tone of the pelvic, detrusor, urethral and bladder neck muscles
- Replacement of the smooth muscle tissue in the bladder and urethra with less elastic connective tissue.

Internal and external sphincters regulate urine storage and bladder emptying (see Figure 19-1). The internal sphincter is part of the base of the bladder and is controlled by autonomic nerves; however, the parasympathetic nerves control the contractions of the detrusor muscle and inhibit the internal urethral sphincter.

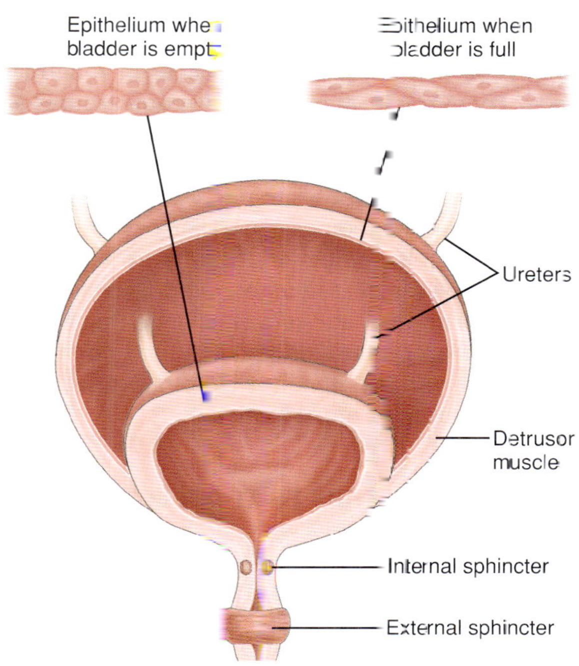

FIGURE 19-1 Structure of the bladder and internal and external sphincters. (From Farrell, M. & Dempsey, J. [Eds]. [2014]. *Smeltzer & Bare's textbook of medical-surgical nursing* [3rd Australian & New Zealand ed.]. Sydney: Lippincott Williams & Wilkins.)

The external sphincter is part of the pelvic floor musculature and is controlled by the pudendal nerve. When urination takes place, the detrusor and abdominal muscles contract and the perineal and external sphincter muscles relax. When necessary, the external sphincter contracts to inhibit or interrupt voiding and to compensate for sudden surges in abdominal pressure. Age-related changes involving the loss of smooth muscle in the urethra and the relaxation of the pelvic floor muscles reduce the urethral resistance and diminish the tone of the sphincters.

Additional aged-related changes that affect urinary function

Changes in the nervous system and other regulatory systems affect urinary function. For example, motor impulses in the spinal cord control urination, but higher centres in the brain are responsible for detecting the sensation of bladder fullness, for inhibiting bladder emptying when necessary and for stimulating bladder contractions for complete emptying. As the bladder fills, sensory receptors in the bladder wall send a signal to the sacral spinal cord. In healthy older adults, degenerative changes in the cerebral cortex may alter both the sensation of bladder fullness and the ability to empty the bladder completely. In younger adults, a sensation of fullness begins when the bladder is about half full. This sensation occurs at a later point for older adults, so the interval between the initial perception of the urge to void and the actual need to empty the bladder is shortened, which may trigger an episode of incontinence.

Many urinary tract structures involved in urination contain oestrogen receptors and are affected by hormonal changes, particularly those that occur in menopausal women. For example, diminished oestrogen causes a loss of tone, strength and collagen support in the urogenital tissues and can contribute to a decrease in urethral closure pressure, which predisposes to urinary leakage problems. Also, because nerve endings depend on oestrogen, diminished oestrogen increases sensitivity to irritating stimuli, which leads to an increased urge to void. Diminished thirst perception is another age-related change that can affect urinary function because underhydration or dehydration can interfere with maintenance of homeostasis, which is necessary for optimal urinary function.

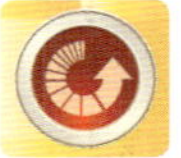

RISK FACTORS THAT AFFECT URINARY WELLNESS

As with many other areas of functioning, risk factors play a more significant role than age-related changes in causing negative functional consequences for urinary function. Because urinary incontinence is a fundamental aspect of urinary wellness for older adults—and an aspect that is affected by many risk factors—this section discusses risks in relation to both overall urinary wellness and urinary incontinence.

Fluid intake and dietary factors

Limited fluid intake, which often is perceived as a method of maintaining continence, can unintentionally have the opposite effect and lead to lower urinary tract symptoms (Lukacz et al., 2011). Inadequate fluid intake causes urine to be more concentrated and this leads to increased bladder irritability and subsequent difficulty maintaining continence. In addition, limited fluid intake is a risk factor for urinary incontinence because perception of the need to void depends on adequate bladder fullness. Inadequate fluid intake also is important for clearance of pathological organisms from the bladder and prevention of bacteriuria (Lin, 2013).

Dietary factors can affect urinary wellness, particularly with regard to foods and beverages that irritate the bladder or increase the risk for urinary incontinence. The following relationships between dietary factors and urinary wellness have been identified in studies:

- Caffeine, carbonated beverages, and artificial sweeteners stimulate diuresis and cause urinary urgency or other symptoms (Lukacz et al., 2011)
- Tea, coffee, soda, alcohol, artificial sweeteners, citrus products and hot peppers are common bladder irritants (Lukacz et al., 2011)
- Daily caffeine intake of 204 mg or more for women and 250 mg or more for men was associated with higher prevalence of urinary incontinence (Davis et al., 2012; Gleason et al., 2013)
- Consumption of green tea is associated with lower risk for urinary incontinence in middle-aged and older women (Hirayama & Lee, 2011).

Medication effects

Medications influence urinary function in a number of ways and are common risk factors in the development of urinary incontinence. For example, loop diuretics increase urinary output, placing additional demands on the urinary system and compounding the effects of an age-related decrease in bladder capacity. Older adults with other urinary tract conditions may be particularly susceptible to adverse medication effects. Two examples are:

- Men with prostatic hyperplasia are at increased risk for urinary retention when they take an adrenergic or anticholinergic agent.
- Medications that are used to treat incontinence can also cause incontinence. Terazosin, which is used for benign prostatic hyperplasia, can cause urethral relaxation and stress incontinence.

Thus, it is imperative that causes of incontinence be identified accurately before treatment is initiated.

In addition to causing incontinence through their direct effects on the urinary tract, medications can cause incontinence through their effects on functional abilities. Anticholinergics (including those in over-the-counter agents) can cause cognitive and other functional impairments

TABLE 19-1 Medications that can cause urinary incontinence

Medication type	Examples	Mechanism of action
Diuretics	Frusemide, bumetanide	Increased diuresis can cause urinary urgency, frequency and polyuria
Anticholinergic agents	Antihistamines, antipsychotics, antidepressants, antispasmodics, anti-parkinsonism agents	Decreased bladder contractility and relaxed bladder muscle can cause urinary retention, frequency and incontinence
Adrenergics (alpha-adrenergic agonists)	Decongestants	Decreased bladder contractility and increased sphincter tone can cause urinary retention, frequency and incontinence
Alpha-adrenergic blockers	Prazosin, terazosin, doxazosin	Decreased urethral and internal sphincter tone can cause leakage and stress incontinence
Calcium channel blockers	Nifedipine, nicardipine, isradipine, felodipine, nimodipine	Decreased bladder contractility can cause urinary retention, frequency, nocturia and incontinence
Angiotensin-converting enzyme inhibitors	Captopril, enalapril, lisinopril	Can cause chronic cough, which precipitates or exacerbates stress incontinence
Hypnotics and antianxiety agents	Benzodiazepines	Can interfere with voluntary control over urination by causing sedation, delirium and cognitive impairments
Alcohol	Wine, beer, liquor	Can interfere with voluntary control over urination by causing sedation, delirium, increased diuresis and cognitive impairment

which can interfere with voluntary control over urination. Many medications cause constipation, which is a causative factor for incontinence. This adverse effect may be particularly detrimental in the presence of prostatic hyperplasia or weakened pelvic floor muscles.

In addition to creating risk factors for incontinence, medications can increase ADH secretion, which may compound age-related effects that predispose older adults to hyponatraemia. Medications that stimulate ADH secretion include aspirin, narcotics, Panadol, antidepressants, barbiturates, chlorpropamide, fluphenazine and haloperidol. Table 19-1 presents some types and examples of medications that can cause incontinence in older adults.

Myths and misperceptions

Attitudes based on myths or lack of knowledge about urinary function can have a detrimental effect on the behaviour of older adults and their carers/caregivers. Despite the fact that increased age is a risk factor for urinary incontinence, it is a major mistake to perceive incontinence as an inevitable consequence of ageing that cannot be reversed. This commonly held misperception can lead to underdiagnosis and mismanagement of urinary incontinence, which causes serious functional consequences. Studies consistently find that assessment of urinary incontinence is often delayed until symptoms progress to the point that they significantly affect quality of life, and at least some of the delay is caused by myths about ageing (Adedokun et al., 2012; Rios et al., 2011; Welch, Taubenberger & Tennstedt, 2011).

Cultural factors may also influence perceptions and help-seeking behaviours. Approximately 80% of women from a Middle Eastern culture did not seek help for incontinence because of embarrassment and because they assumed that this was a normal part of ageing (El-Azab & Shaaban, 2010). In New Zealand and Australia it has also been reported that Indigenous older people who have urinary incontinence are less likely to seek health professional assistance because of shyness, embarrassment and resignation (Quintal, 2003; New Zealand Continence Association, 2009). Indigenous Australians regard incontinence as "women's business" or "men's business" and this means women only talk to women and men only to men about their problems (Home and Community Care [HACC]/Medical Aids Subsidy Scheme [MASS] Continence Project, 2010). These cultural factors contribute to poor management and outcomes: the early signs and symptoms of urinary dysfunction may be missed and the problem progresses.

Influence of carers

Behaviours of carers based on misperceptions or lack of information can affect the care of older adults. For instance, if an episode of incontinence occurs soon after an older adult is admitted to an acute-care or long-term residential care facility, nursing staff may falsely assume that this has been an ongoing symptom. Subsequent behaviours of nursing staff, such as using absorbent products rather than initiating an appropriate care plan, may give the message that voluntary control over urination is not expected. Similarly, carers in institutional and home-care settings may promote the use of absorbent products as a substitute for more time-consuming interventions, such as providing assistance with toileting. When incontinence products are used for ease or convenience, incontinence is likely to develop unnecessarily (Zisberg et al., 2011).

WELLNESS OPPORTUNITY

Nurses should examine their own attitudes and behaviours about incontinence to be sure they are based on accurate information rather than on misperceptions or ageist perspectives that could blind them to opportunities to promote urinary wellness.

Functional impairments and environmental conditions

Control over urination is affected not only by age-related changes that directly affect urinary function but also by many conditions that affect socially appropriate urinary elimination. All the following conditions can affect one's ability to identify and use appropriate toilet facilities in a timely manner:

- Cognition, balance, mobility, coordination, visual function and manual dexterity
- Identification of a designated receptacle in a private area
- Accessibility and acceptability of toilet facilities
- Ability to get to and use a suitable receptacle
- Amount of time between the perception of the urge to void and the actual need to empty the bladder
- Ability to voluntarily control the urge to void.

Functional impairments are a major risk factor for the development of incontinence because they can interfere with the ability to recognise and respond to the urge to void in a timely manner. Because older adults have a shorter interval between the perception of the urge to void and the actual need to empty the bladder, any delay in reaching an appropriate receptacle can result in incontinence. Thus, dependency in performing activities of daily living (ADLs) for any reason is strongly associated with incontinence. Conditions, such as arthritis or Parkinson's disease, may slow the ambulation of older adults as well as their ability to manipulate clothing. Likewise, dementia and other conditions that impair cognitive abilities can interfere with the timely processing of information that is necessary for maintaining voluntary control over urination. Finally, restraints can cause significant functional limitations and increase the risk for developing incontinence.

People with limited mobility or impaired vision encounter many environmental factors that can interfere with their ability to get to accessible toileting facilities in home, public and institutional settings. Examples of environmental obstacles include stairs, inadequate signage, lack of grab bars, and toilet seats that are too low. Box 19-1 summarises some environmental risk factors that may contribute to the incidence of incontinence in older adults.

BOX 19-1
Environmental factors that can contribute to urinary incontinence

- Stairways between the bathroom level and the living or sleeping areas
- A distance to the bathroom that is more than 12 metres
- Living arrangements where several or many people share a bathroom
- Small bathrooms and narrow doors and hallways that do not accommodate walkers or wheelchairs
- Chair designs and bed heights that hinder mobility
- Poor colour contrast, as between a white toilet and seat and light-coloured floor or walls
- Public settings with poorly visible or poorly colour-contrasted signs designating gender-specific bathroom facilities
- Public settings with dim lighting and out-of-the-way bathroom facilities
- Very bright environments, where glare interferes with the perception of signs for bathrooms
- Mirrored walls, which reflect bright lights and create glare

Pathological conditions and other factors

An increased risk for urinary incontinence is associated with many pathological conditions including all the following: stroke, arthritis, dementia, delirium, depression, diabetes mellitus, metabolic syndrome, Parkinson's disease, faecal impaction, and COPD (Devore et al., 2012; Dowling-Castronovo & Bradway, 2012; Kupelian et al., 2013). In addition, any acute illness or surgical intervention that temporarily limits mobility or compromises cognition also represents a risk factor for urinary incontinence. Constipation and low stool frequency (i.e. fewer than three bowel movements weekly) are other conditions that increase the risk for urinary incontinence and other urinary tract symptoms in men and women (Carter & Beer-Gabel, 2012; Thurmon, Breyer & Erickson, 2012). A urinary tract infection (UTI) is a common cause of incontinence in older adults, with an annual incidence of 10% (Mohsin & Siddiqui, 2010). Urinary incontinence is also a risk factor for UTI in older adults (Hu et al., 2004). It is important to regularly screen for UTI in older adults with incontinence.

Although dementia is strongly associated with urinary incontinence, the relationship between these two conditions is complex and episodes of incontinence can often be prevented or minimised, particularly during early and middle stages. For example, older adults with dementia may lack the perceptual abilities that are necessary for finding and using appropriate facilities, but they may be able to maintain continence when given appropriate cues and reminders.

Obesity and smoking are conditions that are strongly associated with urinary incontinence and urinary tract symptoms (Tahtinen et al., 2011; Vaughan et al., 2012). Other risk factors associated with urinary incontinence that commonly occur in older adults include hearing and/or vision impairment, radiation or surgical treatments for prostate cancer, and residence in a long-term residential care facility (Dowling-Castronovo & Bradway, 2012). Researchers also are investigating a potential link between vitamin D and urinary incontinence, with emphasis on its influence on pelvic floor muscle functioning (Parker-Autry et al., 2012).

Gender-specific conditions

Gender-specific conditions of the genitourinary tract commonly occur in older adults and increase the risk for urinary incontinence and other lower urinary tract symptoms, including pain and infection. Although these conditions are generally addressed by a gynaecologist or urologist, they are discussed in relation to urinary wellness because of their direct effects on control over urination in older men and women.

DIVERSITY NOTE

Women are more likely than men to have a urinary tract infection (Jeoson, Mihaljevic & Craig, 2008).

The term **pelvic floor disorders** (also called pelvic support problems) refers to a group of medical conditions in which a pelvic organ prolapses into the vagina due to weakness or injury involving muscles and connective tissue of the pelvic floor and related structures. These conditions, which sometimes occur together, can involve any of the following structures:

- Urinary bladder (cystocele)
- Bladder and urethra (cystourethrocele)
- Bladder neck (urethrocele)
- Uterus (uterine prolapse)
- Part of the small bowel and peritoneum (enterocele)
- Rectum (rectocele or rectal prolapse).

Sometimes such terms as "dropped", "sagging" or "fallen" are used in reference to the involved structure (e.g. "dropped bladder").

In addition to increased age and postmenopausal status, factors that increase the risk for pelvic floor disorders include smoking, obesity, surgery, pelvic radiation, genetic predisposition, chronic constipation, high number of vaginal births, and fractures of the pelvis or lower vertebrae. Pelvic floor disorders can lead to urinary frequency and incontinence because these conditions interfere with the complete emptying of the bladder, resulting in residual urine and an increased risk for bacteriuria. Atrophy of the vaginal and trigonal tissue with subsequent diminished resistance to pathogens is another condition that can affect urinary wellness in older women because vaginitis and trigonitis can cause urinary urgency, frequency and incontinence.

Benign prostatic hyperplasia (also called benign prostatic hypertrophy) is a common cause of voiding problems in older men because the enlarged prostate compresses the urethra, which leads to obstruction of the vesical neck. As the condition progresses the bladder wall becomes thinner and less elastic and urinary retention occurs, increasing the risk for bacteriuria and infection. Men with prostatic hyperplasia may experience decreased urine flow, incomplete bladder emptying, and urinary urgency and frequency. Eventually the ureters and kidneys are affected, and hydroureter, hydronephrosis, diminished GFR and uraemia may develop.

WELLNESS OPPORTUNITY

Nurses holistically assess older adults by recognising that urinary incontinence can be an indicator of physiological disturbances (e.g. urinary tract infection), psychosocial conditions (e.g. dementia or depression) or a combination of functional limitations and environmental barriers.

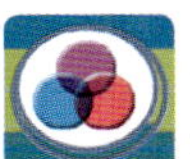

FUNCTIONAL CONSEQUENCES AFFECTING URINARY WELLNESS

Despite the many age-related changes in the urinary tract, the elimination of wastes is not significantly affected in healthy, non-medicated older adults. However, with any unusual physiological demands, such as those that occur with medications or disease conditions, older adults are likely to experience functional consequences affecting homeostatic mechanisms and urinary control. Age-related changes and risk factors also cause functional consequences in patterns of urinary elimination and predispose older adults to incontinence. When incontinence occurs, additional functional consequences, particularly psychosocial effects, can be quite serious.

Effects on renal function

Functional consequences related to renal function in healthy older adults include impaired absorption of calcium and a predisposition to hyponatraemia and hyperkalaemia. Age-related changes in the kidney and in aldosterone secretion interfere with compensatory mechanisms that maintain fluid and electrolyte balance, so older adults have a delayed and less effective response to variations in sodium intake than younger individuals. Similarly, diminished renal function lengthens the time needed for pH imbalances to be corrected in older adults. Even with normal states of hydration, a decrease in GFR delays water excretion and may lead to hyponatraemia in healthy older adults. Likewise, even routine daily activities can challenge the renal function of older adults because of diminished renal efficiency. For example, when older adults perspire during exercise, they may tire easily because of age-related delays in the mechanisms controlling water and sodium conservation.

With increasing age, the kidneys become less responsive to ADH and are less able to concentrate urine, causing a decrease in the maximal urinary concentration. Age-related changes also increase urine production at night in older adults compared with younger adults, even in the absence of pathological factors. This may result in **nocturia**, which is when older adults wake to pass urine one or more times during the night.

Older adults who take certain medications or have medical conditions are likely to experience functional consequences such as the following:

- Diuretics are more likely to cause hypervolaemia and dehydration in older adults than in younger people.
- Under conditions of physiological stress (e.g. surgery, infection or excessive fluid loss), older adults are likely to develop dehydration, volume depletion and other fluid and electrolyte imbalances.
- Volume depletion may occur soon after the onset of fever-producing illnesses because of the inability to compensate for insensible fluid losses.
- Any condition or medication that stimulates ADH secretion, such as pneumonia or chlorpropamide, is likely to cause water intoxication and hyponatraemia in older adults because of their diminished ability to compensate for excessive levels of ADH.

Diminished renal function contributes to the increased incidence of drug interactions and adverse medication reactions in older adults. These age-related changes are most likely to affect water-soluble medications that are highly dependent on GFR (e.g. digoxin, cimetidine and aminoglycoside antibiotics) or renal tubular function (e.g. penicillin and procainamide). Unless medication doses are adjusted to account for age-related changes in GFR and renal tubular function, excretion may be delayed and toxic substances are likely to accumulate. These adverse medication effects can significantly impair physical and mental abilities and have profound functional consequences, as discussed in Chapter 8.

Effects on voiding patterns

Because of age-related changes, the bladder of the older adult has a smaller capacity, empties incompletely and contracts during filling. Thus, older adults experience shorter intervals between voiding and they have less time between the perception of the urge to void and the actual need to empty the bladder. Older adults often describe this by saying, "When you gotta go, you gotta go." Another consequence is that the bladder retains up to 50 mL of residual urine after voiding, causing symptomatic or asymptomatic bacteraemia and predisposing older adults to urinary tract infections.

Age-related changes in the diurnal production of urine in the kidneys cause a shift in voiding pattern to more urinary output at night than during the day. Pathological conditions (e.g. hypothyroidism, heart failure, venous insufficiency) and certain medications (e.g. calcium channel blockers) are risk factors that lead to urinary frequency and nocturia associated with a supine position (Rahn & Roshanravan, 2009). In addition, an overactive bladder and pathological conditions (e.g. pelvic floor dysfunction in women and benign prostatic enlargement in men) are common causes of nocturia in older adults (van Kerrebroeck et al., 2010). Functional consequences of nocturia include disturbed sleep, increased risk for night time falls and decreased quality of life (Bliwise et al., 2009; Endeshaw 2009; Vaughan, Brown, Goode et al., 2010).

Urinary incontinence

As stated, age-related changes alone do not cause urinary incontinence; they predispose older adults to it, making it the most commonly occurring condition associated with the urinary tract in older adults. The estimated prevalence of incontinence for older adults ranges from 38% for community-dwelling older adults to 60% for those in long-term residential care facilities and up to 90% for people with dementia (Dowling-Castronovo & Bradway, 2012; French et al., 2009; Griebling, 2009). In Australia older adults are 12 times more likely to experience severe incontinence than other adults (Australian Institute of Health and Welfare, 2014). Studies identify all the following risk factors for urinary incontinence: increased age, functional limitations, impaired cognition, obesity, smoking, white race, constipation, vaginal delivery, low vitamin D levels, medications (e.g. oral oestrogen, antipsychotics) and pathological conditions (diabetes, stroke, arthritis, Parkinson's disease) (Amselem et al., 2010; Badalian & Rosenbaum, 2010; Byles et al., 2009; Menezes, Hashimoto & de Gouveia Santos, 2009).

Urinary incontinence is a focus of much attention among healthcare consumers and practitioners, particularly with regard to its effects on quality of life (Botlero et al., 2010; Tennstedt et al., 2010). Urinary incontinence is categorised according to signs and symptoms as follows:

- **Functional urinary incontinence** is characterised by the inability to reach or use a toilet due to a physical, mental or environmental problem. This results in not getting to the toilet in time or passing urine in inappropriate places.
- **Overflow urinary incontinence** is caused by urinary retention due to an obstruction of urine flow. This results in poor urinary flow, increased frequency of urination and dribbling of urine after voiding.
- **Stress urinary incontinence** is characterised by an involuntary leakage of urine as a result of an activity that increases abdominal pressure (e.g. lifting, coughing, sneezing, laughing or exercise).
- **Urge urinary incontinence** is characterised by involuntary urinary leakage due to the inability to hold urine long enough to reach a toilet after perceiving the urge to void (Australian Government Department of Social Services, 2014).
- **Mixed urinary incontinence** is a mix of usually two types of urinary incontinence, stress and urge. This type of urinary incontinence is therefore characterised by leakage of urine with both the sensation of urgency and activities such as coughing, sneezing or exertion (HACC/MASS Continence Project, 2010).

When any type of urinary incontinence develops, nurses are required to conduct a comprehensive assessment to identify the causes and risk factors that can be addressed through interventions, which are discussed later in this chapter.

Overactive bladder (OAB) is a syndrome characterised by bothersome urgency, usually accompanied by nocturia and daytime frequency, and sometimes accompanied by urge urinary incontinence. In recent years, OAB has become widely recognised because of advertisements related to prescription medications for the treatment of this condition. By definition, OAB is not always accompanied by incontinence, but in reality, many people with this condition also experience incontinence. One study of 311 adults between the ages of 18 and 97 years found a prevalence of OAB in 60.5% of men and 48.3% of women, with 37% and 92% of the men and women, respectively, also experiencing incontinence (Cheung et al., 2009). In this study, obesity was a major risk factor for OAB, particularly in premenopausal women. Other studies have found that diuretics, particularly loop diuretics, are associated with OAB (Ekundayo et al., 2009).

Urinary incontinence can negatively affect an older adult's quality of life through both physical and psychosocial consequences. Physical consequences of incontinence include a predisposition to falls, fractures, pressure ulcers, skin infections or irritations, urinary tract infections and limitation of functional status (Dowling-Castronovo & Bradway, 2012; Hasegawa, Kuzuya & Iguchi, 2010). Psychosocial consequences associated with urinary incontinence include significantly decreased quality of life, shame or embarrassment, anxiety, depression, social isolation and loss of self-confidence. Another consequence is that people who have experienced episodes of incontinence may become preoccupied with covering up any evidence of wetness or urinary odours, so they can avoid social stigma.

Negative psychosocial consequences can arise when carers communicate infantilising attitudes and behaviours, such as unnecessarily using incontinence products rather than providing assistance with toileting. These attitudes and behaviours can have a devastating effect on the older adult's dignity and self-esteem. In addition, older adults who do not understand age-related changes may have exaggerated fears of progressive incontinence, triggered by the onset of urgency or frequency. Even in older adults who are not incontinent, the experience of urinary urgency and frequency can cause psychosocial consequences such as anxiety, restricted activity, feelings of insecurity and powerlessness, and embarrassment about frequent trips to the bathroom.

DIVERSITY NOTE

One study reported a prevalence rate of 34% for urinary incontinence in community-based women in New Zealand. Different cultural groups' prevalence rates were also reported: 47% for Māori women, 31% for European and 29% for Pacific Island women (New Zealand Continence Association, 2009).

PATHOLOGICAL CONDITIONS AFFECTING URINARY FUNCTION: URINARY TRACT INFECTIONS

A **urinary tract infection (UTI)** is one of the most common bacterial infections experienced by older adults (Lutters & Vogt, 2002). Incidence of UTI in older adults is between 12% and 29% for those in community settings and 44% and 58% for residents of long-term residential care facilities (Caljouw, den Elzen, Cools et al., 2011). UTIs develop in older adults because of a variety of factors. These include reduced immune function, dehydration, hormonal changes, changes in urinary and vaginal pH, poor hygiene practices and changes in the ability to empty bladder properly (HACC/MASS Continence Project, 2010). Symptoms, which may associated with a UTI, include dysuria, urgency, haematuria, fever, vaginitis, lower abdominal pain, nausea and vomiting (Bent & Saint, 2002), nocturia, and urinary incontinence (HACC/MASS Continence Project, 2010). The void may be described as a slow, intermittent stream with some straining to void and the older adult my feel their bladder is not completely empty after voiding. However, it is not uncommon that urinary tract infections in older adults may be without symptoms. This is referred to as an asymptomatic UTI. Symptomatic UTIs require medical review; however medical treatment for an asymptomatic UTI is not recommended (Nicolle et al., 2005).

Instead the older person is encouraged to increase their fluid intake and to void regularly, with bladder emptying. Cranberry juice has been recommended for many years as a treatment to reduce the incidence of UTI in older adults and evidence is now available to support its use (Jepson, Mihaljevic & Craig, 2008). Symptoms of atrophic urethritis have a similar presentation as a UTI and it is important to screen for this condition in older women when a UTI is suspected.

In older adults urinary incontinence may be an initial or *primary* indication of a UTI. A change in behaviour or level of functioning may also be another indication of a UTI, particularly in people with dementia. The presence of fever may exist but may be overlooked in older adults. For instance 37°C may be a normal temperature for younger adults but for an older adult whose normal temperature is normally much lower, for example 35.5°C, then a temperature of 37°C represents a fever. Table 19-2 delineates different manifestations of UTI in adult age groups identified in a cross-sectional analysis of adults diagnosed in emergency rooms. Older adults are also at increased risk of developing chronic bacteraemia, a condition characterised as 10^5 or more colony-forming units that is asymptomatic. One study reported a prevalence of chronic bacteraemia in aged residents in long-term care of 25% to 50% of women and 15% to 40% of men (Nicolle, 2009).

TABLE 19-2 Manifestations of urinary tract symptoms (according to adult age groups, cross-sectional analysis of adults diagnosed in emergency rooms)

Manifestation	18 to 64 years old	65 to 84 years old	85 years and older
Fever	13%	21%	13%
Altered mental status	1%	7%	13%
Urinary tract symptoms	32%	24%	17%

Source: Caterino, J. M., Ting, S. A., Sisbarro, S. G. et al. (2012). Age, nursing home residence, and presentation of urinary tract infection in U. S. emergency departments, 2001–2008. *Academic of Emergency Medicine, 19*(10), 1173–1180.

In institutional settings, the use of indwelling catheters increases the risk for developing **catheter-associated urinary tract infections (CAUTIs)**. Since 2008, there has been increasing attention about CAUTIs and it has been identified as the single most common cause of preventable healthcare-associated infections. Evidence-based practice 19-1 summarises the current guidelines for the prevention, diagnosis and management of CAUTIs.

WELLNESS OPPORTUNITY

Nurses address the person's relationships with others by being sensitive to the psychosocial responses of family carers who are dealing with incontinence.

UNFOLDING CASE STUDY

Part A

Mr and Mrs Chung, who are 69 and 68 years old, respectively, attend the local medical centre where you provide monthly health checks. During a recent health check, Mrs Chung confided that she does not know what to do about her husband's "smelly dribbling" and that she worries that he has prostate problems. She has perceived a strong odour of urine and has noticed yellow stains on his clothing when she does the laundry. Even their children have mentioned the odour to her, but when she tries to discuss it with her husband, he changes the subject. She says that he will not talk with his doctor about it because he "hears so much about prostate cancer, and he's afraid that he has an untreatable condition". She asks your advice about this and asks if you would talk with him

EVIDENCE-BASED PRACTICE 19-1
Prevention of catheter-associated urinary tract infections

Statement of the problem

- Catheter-associated urinary tract infections (CAUTIs) account for 34% to 40% of healthcare-associated infections, which are considered largely preventable adverse events that occur during hospitalisation.
- Between 21% and 54% of indwelling urinary catheters (IUCs) (also called Foley catheters) are used inappropriately when they are not medically necessary.
- IUCs are frequently left in longer than necessary.
- IUCs significantly increase the risk for urinary tract infection, delirium, local trauma and encrustation.
- The risk for developing a CAUTI is directly related to the duration of IUC use, beginning at 48 hours after insertion and increasing at the rate of 5% per day and reaching almost 100% by day 30.
- Adherence to recommended infection control measures (as described in the recommendations for care section) would prevent 17% to 69% of CAUTI.

Recommendations for nursing assessment

- Identify appropriate indications for use of an IUC: perioperative care, prolonged surgery, operative patients with urinary incontinence, monitoring during surgery or critical illness, major trauma patients, urinary retention or obstruction, pressure ulcer management, and comfort care during terminal illness.
- Recognise the definition of a CAUTI, which is a UTI that occurs while a person has an IUC or within 48 hours of its removal.
- Assess for the following indicators of CAUTI: suprapubic tenderness, costovertebral angle pain or tenderness, fever over 38°C without another identifiable cause, positive blood culture with the same organisms as in the urine.
- Recognise the definition of a positive urine culture as (1) 10^5 or more microorganisms/cc of urine with no more than two species of microorganisms, or (2) 10^3 microorganisms/cc of urine with no more than two species of microorganisms and a positive urinalysis involving dipstick, pyuria and organisms seen on the Gram stain of unspun urine.

Recommendations for nursing care

- Avoid use of IUC: adhere to criteria and protocols for medically necessary use; incorporate alternative methods for urinary elimination in the care plan (e.g. toileting program, collecting devices, absorbent products and intermittent straight catheterisation).
- Recommended care strategies for IUC: smallest effective size for catheter, use aseptic technique for insertion, provide routine meatal care, prevent reflux, maintain closed system, keep catheter secure in place.
- Nurses have essential roles in ensuring the timely removal of IUCs by frequently reassessing the need for keeping the catheter inserted.

Source: Andreessen, L., Wilde, M. H. & Herendeen, P. (2012). Preventing catheter-associated urinary tract infections in acute care: The bundle approach. *Journal of Nursing Care Quarterly, 27*(3), 209–217; Wald, H. L., Fink, R. M., Makic, M. B. F. & Oman, K. S. (2012). Catheter-associated urinary tract infection prevention. In M. Boltz, E. Capezuti, R. Fulmer & D. Zwicker (Eds), *Evidence-based geriatric nursing protocols for best practice* (4th ed., pp. 388–408). New York: Springer. Modified version is available online via http://consultgerirn.org.

when he comes to see you next week. At your next session you decide to discuss this sensitive topic.

Thinking points

Decide what information you would discuss with Mr and Mrs Chung about the following topics:

- What can older men (women) expect of their urinary tract?
- What factors increase the risk of having problems with urinary control in older men (women)?
- Are there any cultural considerations required in this discussion?

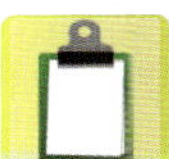

NURSING ASSESSMENT OF URINARY FUNCTION

Nurses can identify opportunities for health promotion interventions by assessing all of the following aspects of urinary function:

- Risk factors that influence overall urinary function
- Risk factors that increase the potential for incontinence
- Signs and symptoms of any dysfunction involving urinary elimination
- Fears and attitudes about urinary dysfunction
- Psychosocial consequences of incontinence.

Nurses obtain most of this information by interviewing older adults and carers of dependent older adults. In addition, the nurse obtains objective data from laboratory tests and by observing behaviours, behavioural cues and environmental influences.

Talking with older adults about urinary function

Because urinary elimination is associated with certain social expectations, discussion of this topic may be particularly influenced by a person's attitudes and feelings. Although nurses usually learn to discuss urinary elimination with relative ease, older adults may feel uncomfortable with the topic, particularly if there are gender or age differences between the older person and the nurse or if a communication barrier, such as a hearing impairment, exists. In addition, if older adults accept urinary leakage as an inevitable consequence of ageing, they may not volunteer information.

Terminology related to urinary elimination presents further difficulties in interviewing older adults. In social settings, people commonly use euphemisms to avoid directly discussing urination (e.g. "I'm going to the powder room", "I'm going to take a leak", "I have to use the john"). Even the sounds associated with urinary elimination may be viewed as embarrassing, so people may run the tap or flush the toilet to disguise the sound of urination when others are present. Because of this social context, successful interviewing about urinary elimination and incontinence depends on identifying the terms that are least embarrassing and most understandable to the older adult. If any hearing impairment is present, a term such as "urinate", which is not used in everyday social language, or a one syllable word like "pee" may be difficult to understand or may be misinterpreted. Although phrases like "use the toilet" and "go to the bathroom" are not specific to urinary elimination, they may prove to be acceptable, particularly if additional questions are asked in order to distinguish between urinary and bowel elimination. Similarly, the term "incontinence" may be problematic for people who may not be familiar with this term. Hearing impairments, if present, may further interfere with the comprehension of this word. Rather than referring to incontinence, it may be more acceptable to older adults to discuss "trouble holding their water". Older adults may tend to use words such as "accidents", "leaking", "weak kidneys", or "bladder trouble" to describe incontinent episodes.

The nurse can set the stage for direct questions about urinary elimination by focusing initial questions on risk factors. Nurses can indirectly assess the perception of and attitudes about urinary incontinence by observing responses to the interview questions. If the older adult acknowledges incontinence, the nurse asks about any actions the person has taken and what impact the incontinence has had on their daily activities and social life.

WELLNESS OPPORTUNITY

Nurses show respect for older adults by using terms such as "briefs" rather than terms such as diapers, which are associated with infants.

Collecting cues for urinary wellness

Begin a nursing assessment by asking about risk factors and observing the person's responses. If the older adults acknowledge incontinence, ask about any actions they have taken and about any effects on their daily activities and social life. Box 19-2 presents interview questions related to urinary elimination. Check other parts of their records for pertinent information (e.g. medication use and medical history) and incorporate it into the assessment of urinary elimination. There are two mnemonics that may be useful when assessing for potentially reversible/treatable causes of urinary incontinence (HACC/MASS Continence Project, 2010). DIAPPERS refers to:

D—Delirium
I—Infection of urinary tract (UTI)
A—Atrophic urethritis/vaginitis
P—Pharmaceuticals
P—Psychological
E—Excessive urine output, endocrine disorders (e.g. diabetes)
R—Reduced mobility
S—Stool impaction.

The other mnemonic that could be used instead of DIAPPERS is TOILETED and it refers to:

T—Thin and dry vagina and urethral epithelium
O—Obstruction (of bowels)

BOX 19-2
Guidelines for assessing urinary elimination

Interview questions to assess risk factors influencing urinary elimination

- (*Men*) Have you had any surgery for prostate or bladder problems?
- (*Men*) Have you ever been told you had prostate problems? (or Do you think you have prostate problems?)
- (*Women*) Have you had any children? (If yes, ask about the number of pregnancies and any problems with childbirth.)
- (*Women*) Have you had any surgery for pelvic, bladder or uterine disorders?
- (*Women*) Have you had any infections in your vaginal area?
- Do you have any pain, burning or discomfort when you urinate (pass water)?
- Have you had any urinary tract infections? If so, when?
- Do you have any chronic illnesses?
- What medications do you take?
- Do you have any problems with your bowels?
- How much water and other liquids do you drink during the day? (Ask for details about timing and the amount of alcoholic, carbonated and caffeinated beverages consumed.)
- Do you get up during the night to go to the toilet? If so, how often?

Interview questions to assess risk factors for socially appropriate urinary elimination

- Do you have any trouble walking or any difficulty with balance?
- Do you have any trouble reading signs or finding restrooms when you are in public places?

Interview questions to assess signs and symptoms of urinary dysfunction

- Do you ever leak urine?
- Do you ever wear pads or protective garments to protect your clothing from wetness?
- Do you ever have difficulty holding your urine (water) long enough to get to the toilet? (or How long can you hold your urine after you first feel the need to go to the bathroom?)
- Do you have trouble holding your urine (water) when you cough, laugh or make sudden movements?
- Do you wake up at night because you have to go to the bathroom to urinate (pass water)? (If the person's response is affirmative, try to differentiate between this symptom and the habit of going to the bathroom after waking up for some other reason.)
- Immediately after urinating (passing your water), does it feel like you have not emptied your bladder completely?
- Do you have to exert pressure during urination to feel like your bladder is being completely emptied?
- (*Men*) When you urinate (pass water), do you have any difficulty starting the stream or keeping the stream going?
- Do you get any pain when urinating?

Interview questions if incontinence has been acknowledged

- When did your incontinence begin?
- What have you done to manage the problem? (Have you cut down on the amount of liquids you drink? Do you empty your bladder at frequent intervals as a precautionary measure?)
- Are there certain things that make the problem worse or better?
- Does it happen all the time, or just at certain times?
- Do you have any pain when you urinate (pass water)?
- (*Women*) Do you feel any pressure in your pelvic area?

Interview questions to assess fears, attitudes and psychosocial consequences of incontinence

- Have you ever sought help or talked to your doctor or other healthcare professional about this problem?
- Have you changed any of your activities because you need to stay near a toilet?
- Do you avoid going to certain places because of difficulty holding your urine (water)?

I—Infection (urinary tract)
L—Limited mobility
E—Emotional or psychological factors
T—Therapeutic medications
E—Endocrine disorders
D—Delirium.

Further information about the person's patterns of urinary elimination and by assessing environmental factors that may interfere with control over urinary elimination is also required in the assessment interview. A **bladder diary** (also called a bladder record, or voiding or urinary diary) can be used to obtain information about fluid intake, the times of urinations, and other factors that can affect continence (Figure 19-2). Use the information from the bladder diary to identify potential causes of and interventions for incontinence, particularly with regard to identifying opportunities for health education.

WELLNESS OPPORTUNITY

Nurses promote self-care by encouraging older adults to assess their patterns of urinary elimination in relation to factors such as food and fluid intake.

A bowel diary (see Chapter 18) may also be required if constipation is identified as a possible contributor of incontinence. Many tools exist for urinary continence assessment, but none is currently recommended specifically for older adults. All collect information about:

- Presenting bladder problems, symptoms, duration and triggers
- Previous investigations, treatment and management strategies
- Effect of bladder problem on person's life
- Medical/surgical, obstetric/gynaecological history
- Medications (diuretics and anticholinergics)

Your daily bladder diary

This diary will help you and your health care team figure out the causes of your bladder control trouble. The "sample" line shows you how to use the diary.

Your name: ______________________________

Date: ______________

Time	Drinks: What kind?	Drinks: How much?	Trips to the toilet: How many times?	Trips to the toilet: How much urine? (circle one)	Accidental leaks: How much? (circle one)	Did you feel a strong urge to go? Circle one	What were you doing at the time? Sneezing, exercising, having sex, lifting, etc.
Sample	Coffee	2 cups	✓✓	sm med lg (sm circled)	sm med lg (med circled)	Yes No (No circled)	Running
6–7 a.m.				sm med lg	sm med lg	Yes No	
7–8 a.m.				sm med lg	sm med lg	Yes No	
8–9 a.m.				sm med lg	sm med lg	Yes No	
9–10 a.m.				sm med lg	sm med lg	Yes No	
10–11 a.m.				sm med lg	sm med lg	Yes No	
11–12 noon				sm med lg	sm med lg	Yes No	
12–1 p.m.				sm med lg	sm med lg	Yes No	
1–2 p.m.				sm med lg	sm med lg	Yes No	
2–3 p.m.				sm med lg	sm med lg	Yes No	
3–4 p.m.				sm med lg	sm med lg	Yes No	
4–5 p.m.				sm med lg	sm med lg	Yes No	
5–6 p.m.				sm med lg	sm med lg	Yes No	
6–7 p.m.				sm med lg	sm med lg	Yes No	
7–8 p.m.				sm med lg	sm med lg	Yes No	
8–9 p.m.				sm med lg	sm med lg	Yes No	
9–10 p.m.				sm med lg	sm med lg	Yes No	
10–11 p.m.				sm med lg	sm med lg	Yes No	
11–12 midnight				sm med lg	sm med lg	Yes No	
12–1 a.m.				sm med lg	sm med lg	Yes No	
1–2 a.m.				sm med lg	sm med lg	Yes No	
2–3 a.m.				sm med lg	sm med lg	Yes No	
3–4 a.m.				sm med lg	sm med lg	Yes No	
4–5 a.m.				sm med lg	sm med lg	Yes No	
5–6 a.m.				sm med lg	sm med lg	Yes No	

FIGURE 19-2 Example of a bladder diary. (Adapted from Let's Talk About Bladder Control for Women, National Kidney and Urologic Diseases Information Clearinghouse. Accessible via www.kidney.niddk.nih.gov.)

Continence Screening Form

Document No: ____________

ID LABEL

To be completed within 48 hours of resident's admission or if there is a change in their continence status.

If the resident is unable to answer these questions, please complete using your observations or by asking a family member or other staff member.

Date: ____/____/____

Bladder Health

1. Does the resident go to the toilet more than 6 times in the day to pass urine?
☐ Yes ☐ No ☐ Don't know

2. Does the resident get up more than once during the night to pass urine?
☐ Yes ☐ No ☐ Don't know

3. Does the resident leak urine?
☐ Yes ☐ No ☐ Don't know

4. Does the resident have any other bladder problems (ie. difficulties passing urine and/or pain)?
☐ Yes ☐ No ☐ Don't know

Bowel Health

5. Has the resident lost control of or leaked bowel motions?
☐ Yes ☐ No ☐ Don't know

6. Does the resident have any other bowel difficulties (ie. constipation or diarrhoea)?
☐ Yes ☐ No ☐ Don't know

Pad Usage

7. Does the resident wear pads?
☐ Yes ☐ No ☐ Don't know

8. Does the resident have to change his/her underclothes or wear protection because of bladder or bowel leakage or soiling?
☐ Yes ☐ No ☐ Don't know

If you ticked YES or DON'T KNOW to any of these questions, please:

- **Complete Bladder Chart and Bowel Chart**

Developed by Deakin University and funded under the National Continence Management Strategy

FIGURE 19-3 Continence Screening Form. (From *Continence Tools for Residential Aged Care: An education guide.* Developed by Deakin University, Melbourne, and funded under the Australian Government's National Continence Management Strategy. Accessible via www.bladderbowl.gov.au. Permission granted from the Australian Government Department of Social Services. Go to www.dss.gov.au for more information.)

- Cognitive and functional abilities
- Fluid intake (HACC/MASS Continence Project, 2010)

An example of a useful urinary screening continence tool has been developed for those living in long-term residential care in Australia. The Australian Government recommends using this tool to screen for urinary and bowel continence when older adults are newly admitted into long-term residential care and if there is a change in the older adults' continence status. See Figure 19-3.

Older adults who are cognitively impaired or dependent on others for their care may not be able to keep a bladder diary. In these situations or when incontinence is an unacknowledged problem, observations on patterns of urinary elimination are particularly important. In long-term residential care facilities and other institutional settings, nurses have many opportunities to observe behavioural cues to incontinence. In home settings, carers of dependent older adults may observe behavioural cues and provide valuable information about urinary elimination patterns. Box 19-3 summarises specific observations that may yield important assessment information.

Home environments are assessed for barriers that might interfere with the quick performance of urinary elimination (refer to Box 19-1). Stairways, long hallways, poor lighting and cluttered surroundings can lengthen the time needed to get to the toilet, particularly for people who have a functional impairment or use assistive devices, such as a walker. Also, it is important to assess the environment for safety and assistive devices or their potential benefit to the individual. For instance, an elevated toilet seat, grab bars near the toilet and grab bars on the walls leading to the toilet may improve the person's ability to urinate safely.

See Box 19-3 for specific environmental factors that can affect socially appropriate urinary elimination.

Using laboratory information

Data from urinalysis and blood chemistry tests contribute important information to the assessment of urinary elimination. A midstream or second-void specimen is the best type of sample for a urinalysis. The dipstick (reagent strip) test has a high sensitivity and specificity for screening for UTIs and is considered an adequate method for screening for UTIs (Deville, Yzermans, van Duijin et al., 2004). A negative nitrate and leucocyte result from dipstick urinalysis rules out a UTI, whereas a positive nitrate with/without leucocytes present indicates a UTI. At the age of 80 years, the normal upper limit for specific gravity is 1.024 and slight proteinuria is considered normal in older adults. Other than these two variations, the urinalysis results should be within the normal range for healthy older adults.

Blood chemistry values that may be helpful in assessing renal function include the following: electrolyte level, creatinine level, creatinine clearance, non-protein nitrogen level and blood urea nitrogen level. In older adults, the serum creatinine may not be an accurate indicator of the GFR, but a 24-hour urine collection for **creatinine clearance** may have greater value as an indicator of renal functioning. Another more convenient method used to calculate creatinine clearance is the Cockcroft-Gault equation. This equation calculates plasma creatinine (umol/L) and considers the older person's weight (kg), gender and age.

BOX 19-3
Guidelines for assessing behavioural cues to and environmental influences on incontinence

Behavioural cues

- Does the older adult use disposable or washable pads or products?
- Is there an odour of urine on clothing, floor coverings or furniture (particularly couches and stuffed chairs)?
- Has the older adult withdrawn from social activities, particularly those held away from home?

Environmental influences

- Where are the bathroom facilities located in relation to the older adult's usual daytime and night time activities?
- Does the person have to go up or down stairs to use the toilet at night or during the day?
- Are there any grab bars or other aids in, near or on the way to the bathroom?
- Would the person benefit from using an elevated toilet seat?
- Does the person use a urinal or other aid to cut down on the number of trips to the bathroom?
- How many people share the same bathroom facilities?
- Is privacy ensured?

UNFOLDING CASE STUDY

Part B

Recall that you are the nurse at the local medical centre attended by Mr and Mrs Chung. Mr Chung schedules an appointment for a follow-up session after your previous discussion. He tells you that he has a "little dribbling" problem but has ignored it because it did not bother him very much. He has not talked with any doctor about this because he thought it was "to be expected", but since thinking about the talk he and his wife had with you, he thinks that maybe he should have the problem evaluated and wants further information from you. During other sessions with Mr Chung, he has told you that he is taking medications for hypertension and Parkinson's disease.

Thinking points

- What risk factors are likely to be contributing to Mr Chung's problems with urinary control?
- Make a list of assessment questions that you would use with Mr Chung. (Use applicable questions from Box 19-2 and any additional questions that might be appropriate.)
- What observations would you make as part of your assessment?
- What would you teach Mr Chung about filling out the voiding diary (see Figure 19-2)?

NURSING ISSUES

When the nursing assessment identifies any risk factors for incontinence or any complaints about or evidence of incontinence, a nursing issue would be impaired urinary elimination. Major defining characteristics commonly found in older adults include urgency, frequency, dribbling, nocturia, hesitancy and incontinence. When nurses identify negative functional consequences related to urinary problems, the following nursing issues might be applicable: anxiety, social isolation, disturbed body image, disturbed sleep pattern, impaired skin integrity or carer role strain (or risk for).

WELLNESS OPPORTUNITY

The nursing issue of willingness for enhanced urinary elimination for older adults is applicable for those older adults who are interested in learning self-care practices such as pelvic floor muscle training.

GOAL PLANNING FOR WELLNESS OUTCOMES

Nursing care plans are directed towards preventing, minimising or compensating for the negative functional consequences that affect urinary elimination. Specific goals that achieve wellness outcomes for urinary elimination include improved kidney function (maintenance of homeostasis) and prevention of adverse medication effects or the effects of other risk factors. Goals for older adults who have urinary incontinence include achieving continence and preventing negative consequences; initial goals would focus on controlling and alleviating, rather than simply managing, incontinence.

The goals pertinent to older adults who experience urinary incontinence and related consequences are: improved urinary continence; improved urinary elimination; improved self-care: toileting; reduced fear level; improved health beliefs: perceived control; and improved tissue integrity: skin.

In addition, other goals that may be pertinent to carers, particularly family members, who are caring for someone with urinary incontinence are: reduction in carer stressors; improved carer well-being; improved carer performance: direct care; reduced disruption in carer lifestyle; improved carer emotional health; and improved carer endurance potential.

WELLNESS OPPORTUNITY

Quality of life is an outcome that can be achieved for older adults and their carers through nursing interventions that are effective in alleviating or managing urinary incontinence.

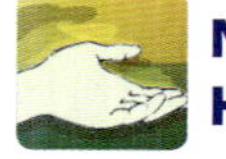

NURSING INTERVENTIONS TO PROMOTE HEALTHY URINARY FUNCTION

Nurses have numerous opportunities to promote wellness in relation to urinary function, particularly for older adults who have difficulty maintaining urinary control. For example, nurses can challenge myths about urinary incontinence, address attitudes of resignation and teach self-care interventions. The following nursing interventions pertinent to promoting urinary continence and addressing the associated psychosocial consequences are: biofeedback; emotional support; environmental management; exercise promotion; fluid management; health education; pelvic muscle exercise; perineal care; prompted voiding; referral; self-esteem enhancement; teaching: individual; urinary bladder training; urinary elimination management; and urinary habit training.

Health promotion: Teaching about urinary wellness

Healthy older adults are not significantly affected by age-related kidney changes during normal activities; however, under conditions of physiological stress, such as exercise, homeostasis can be affected unless the older adult initiates compensatory actions. Thus, nurses teach older adults about functional consequences affecting homeostasis and inform them of self-care actions to prevent problems. For example, nurses can explain that exercising in a cool (rather than hot) environment and increasing one's fluid intake prior to exercise may compensate for the age-related diminished ability to conserve water and sodium. Nurses can also suggest that older adults take protective measures when they are in very hot and humid environments. Examples of appropriate protective measures are the use of fans and air conditioners; an increase in fluid intake; and avoidance of alcoholic, carbonated and caffeinated beverages. If an older adult is at risk of recurrent UTI, nurses can promote the inclusion of cranberry juice as part of their daily intake to reduce the risk of future episodes of UTI. The nurse can also assess for the causal factors of UTI and either address them, in the instance of poor hygiene practices, or refer the older person to their medical practitioner for further investigations.

Older adults taking normal doses of water-soluble medications may experience adverse medication effects because of diminished renal function. Therefore, when water-soluble medications are prescribed for older adults, dose adjustments should be based on an accurate assessment of kidney function and serum drug levels. Nurses need to be aware of and teach older adults about the increased potential for adverse medication effects, particularly when the older adult is taking more than one medication. Further information about adverse medication effects and interventions for medication management is discussed in Chapter 8.

Perhaps the risk factor most amenable to nursing interventions is the false perception of incontinence as an inevitable effect of ageing for which nothing can be done. Because this attitude is based on myths or a lack of information, it can be changed through education. Nurses can emphasise the need for a comprehensive evaluation of urinary incontinence so that risk factors can be alleviated

Teaching older adults the rationale for maintaining adequate fluid intake as a means of preventing incontinence and maintaining good urinary function is a simple but important intervention. Older adults may be more willing to consume adequate amounts of fluid if they understand that concentrated urine can cause incontinence by stimulating bladder contractions and also increase the risk of a UTI. Teaching about normal age-related changes, such as a decreased sensation of thirst, can help to challenge ageist beliefs that negative functional consequences are inevitable. (Chapter 18 also discusses hydration.) Health education about appropriate management strategies for urinary incontinence is an important nursing intervention because studies indicate that some modifying strategies are detrimental to health over the long term (St John et al., 2010).

When a risk factor contributes to incontinence or otherwise interferes with normal urinary elimination, interventions focus on optimal management of the precipitating factor. For example, if postmenopausal oestrogen depletion leads to vaginitis and trigonitis, health education is directed towards encouraging the older woman to seek medical treatment for the underlying condition. When faecal impaction or chronic constipation are risk factors for urinary incontinence, interventions are aimed at attaining and maintaining good bowel function, as discussed in Chapter 18. *Pelvic floor muscle exercise (PFME)*, as discussed in the next section, is another health promotion intervention that can be performed by men and women who are at increased risk of developing, or are already experiencing, urinary incontinence.

In Australia there is a national continence helpline (phone 1800 33 00 66) which provides a free advisory service about all aspects of urinary and bowel continence. Resources are also available via the Australian Government Department of Social Services' website www.bladderbowel.gov.au, while in New Zealand the Continence Association (phone 0800 650 659) provides comprehensive support as well as resources via www.continence.org.nz. Box 19-4 summarises teaching points about self-care activities that promote optimal overall urinary function and help older adults maintain continence.

WELLNESS OPPORTUNITY

Nurses promote personal responsibility by encouraging older adults to talk with their healthcare practitioner about identifying risk factors for urinary incontinence that can be addressed through self-care measures.

BOX 19-4 Health education to promote urinary wellness

Promoting good urinary function

- Drink 8 to 10 glasses of non-caffeinated liquid every day.
- Do not depend on thirst sensation as an accurate indicator for adequate fluid intake—drink liquids even if you do not feel thirsty.
- Avoid excessive use of alcoholic, caffeinated or carbonated beverages, particularly before bedtime.
- Avoid foods and beverages that can irritate the bladder (e.g. sugar, caffeine, alcohol, chocolate, artificial sweeteners and spicy and acidic foods).
- Drink 1 or 2 glasses of fluid before, and every 15 minutes during, periods of sweat-producing exercise or activity.
- Avoid smoking.
- Maintain ideal body weight and good physical fitness.
- Take steps to prevent constipation.
- Practise pelvic muscle exercises.
- Seek medical advice from a knowledgeable practitioner about any difficulties with urinary continence.
- If at risk of recurrent UTI then advise to include cranberry juice to intake daily.

Understanding why incontinence may occur

- If incontinence occurs, a pathological condition or other influencing factor can usually be identified through a comprehensive evaluation.
- A requirement for voluntary control over urination is the signal of the need to void because of a full bladder. Restricting fluid intake interferes with this signal.
- Highly concentrated urine, from inadequate fluid intake, will stimulate involuntary bladder contractions and may lead to incontinence.
- Consistently emptying the bladder at intervals of less than 1 or 2 hours may contribute to problems with incontinence.

Correcting myths about incontinence

- Incontinence is not an inevitable age-related change.
- Normal age-related changes affecting urination include a shortened interval between the perception of the urge to void and the actual need to empty the bladder, an increased frequency of voiding and the need to get up to urinate several times during the night.
- Nocturia, urgency and frequency do not necessarily lead to total incontinence.

Using support services

- Australia: The Continence Foundation of Australia helpline is a free service providing advice, referrals and leaflets on many aspects of incontinence for older adults, carers and health professionals (free call 1800 33 00 66).
- New Zealand: The NZ Continence Association has a helpline that posts information on incontinence and makes referrals (free phone 0800 650 659).

Interventions for urinary incontinence

Interventions for urinary incontinence are initially directed towards the resolution of any conditions that affect control over urination. Nursing interventions directly related to this goal are as follows:

- Facilitating referrals to appropriate professionals
- Utilising indwelling catheters long term
- Being knowledgeable about medical and surgical interventions
- Teaching about pelvic floor muscle exercises (PFME)
- Initiating continence training programs
- Suggesting environmental modifications.

When incontinence cannot be alleviated, nursing responsibilities include using appropriate continence aids, being knowledgeable about commonly used medications and medical and surgical interventions, and promoting wellness for carers of dependent older adults in home settings.

Facilitating referrals

Nurses facilitate referrals for medical professionals and specialised advance practice nurses who can perform comprehensive evaluations and prescribe medications or medical devices or perform surgical procedures. An important nursing role is to encourage older adults who experience urinary incontinence to explore options for treatment rather than only self-managing their symptoms. Studies consistently find that lack of knowledge about available options is a major barrier to obtaining treatment for urinary incontinence (Berger et al., 2011).

WELLNESS OPPORTUNITY

Nurses promote self-care by encouraging older adults to seek further evaluation by qualified healthcare professionals rather than relying solely on the reported experiences of friends.

A resource that is available in some healthcare settings is a continence nurse. Continence nurses are able to provide expert assessment and management of older adults with urinary and faecal incontinence. Continence nurses are effective in achieving the important health outcomes, including the improved resolution and prevention of urinary incontinence and UTI (Bliss, Westra et al., 2013).

Medical and surgical interventions

It is important for nurses to be knowledgeable about the safe and effective options for treatment. A variety of intravaginal or intraurethral devices are available for resolving stress incontinence. For many decades, pessaries have been used as an inexpensive, low-risk and conservative treatment for pelvic organ prolapse in women. These simple devices are placed in the vagina to support the bladder, compress the urethra, or both. They are available in many sizes and shapes and are individually fitted by a primary care practitioner (Figure 19-4). Pessaries need to be removed and reinserted at intervals ranging from nightly to once every few months, depending on the type that is used.

In recent years, many urinary control devices have become available or are used in clinical trials for self-insertion into the urethra. For example, one type of device controls urination through the inflation and deflation of a small balloon that rests at the bladder neck. Other currently available devices for women include urethral plugs; intraurethral catheters with unidirectional valves; and external occlusive devices, which cover the external urinary meatus and provide a watertight seal to prevent leakage. For men, foam-cushioned penile clamps with compression mechanisms are available. Interventions for urinary incontinence are developing rapidly and evidence-based and up-to-date information is available at websites listed in the resources section at the end of the chapter. Use Evidence-based practice 19-2 to teach

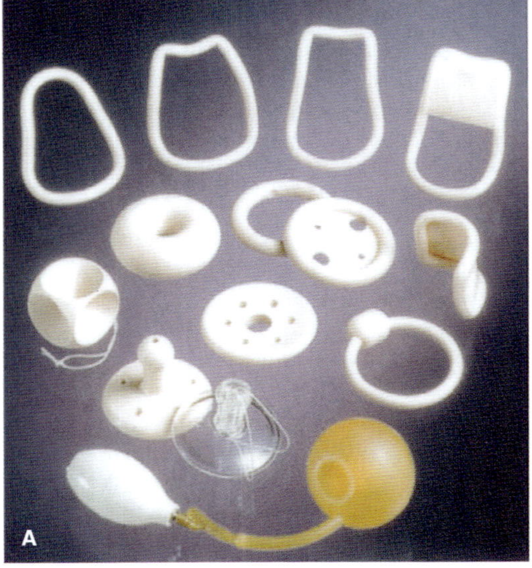

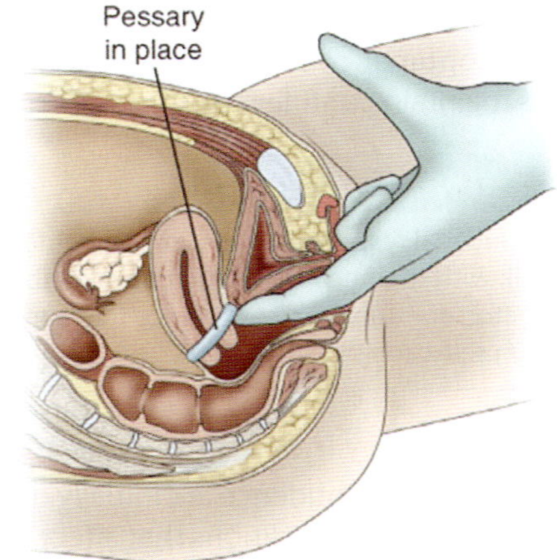

FIGURE 19-4 (**A**) Examples of various shapes and sizes of pessaries available. (**B**) Insertion of one type of pessary. (From Farrell, M. & Dempsey, J. [Eds]. [2014]. *Smeltzer & Bare's textbook of medical-surgical nursing* [3rd Australian & New Zealand ed.]. Sydney: Lippincott Williams & Wilkins.)

EVIDENCE-BASED PRACTICE 19-2
Interventions for urinary incontinence

Non-pharmacological interventions effective for men and women
- Pelvic floor muscle exercises
- Achieving and maintaining healthy weight
- Behavioural techniques: fluid management (i.e. intake of adequate amounts of fluids until several hours before bedtime), timed voiding; prompted voiding (i.e. gradually lengthening the interval between urination)

Medical and surgical treatment for men and women
- Antimuscarinic (anticholinergic) medications for overactive bladder: darifenacin, oxybutynin, solifenacin, tolterodine. MOA relax the bladder and inhibit uncontrolled contractions.
- Biofeedback to enhance performance of pelvic floor muscle exercises through the use of a simple probe placed in the vagina (women) or rectum (men) to measure physiological processes involved in pelvic muscle contractions
- Neuromodulation (i.e. stimulation of nerves through the use of an implantable device)
- Injection of bulking agent (e.g. collagen, carbon spheres) into tissues around the bladder neck and urethra

Specific for women
- Vaginal oestrogen (cream or intravaginal ring)
- Pessary (i.e. ring or other device inserted into the vagina to place pressure on the urethra)
- Surgery for pelvic floor disorders (e.g. retropubic suspension or sling procedure)

Specific for men
- Alpha-blockers or 5-alpha reductase inhibitors for prostate enlargement and bladder outlet obstruction: alfuzosin, doxazosin, dutasteride, finasteride, tamsulosin, terazosin. MOA relax the smooth muscle of the urethra and prostate capsule
- Surgical implantation of an artificial urinary sphincter to keep the urethra closed
- Male sling surgery to provide support for the urethra
- Urinary diversion surgery

about types of options that older adults can discuss with a healthcare professional. Also listed in Evidence-based practice 19-2 are the pharmacological interventions that may be used to treat urinary conditions.

Utilising indwelling catheters long term

Indwelling catheters are an intervention that until recently was commonly used for long-term management of urinary incontinence. However, because they are associated with a high rate of serious UTIs (as discussed in Box 19-1 about CAUTI), their use is limited primarily to short term. Indwelling catheters are an indicator of quality of care, with lower numbers of indwelling catheters being associated with better quality of care. However, indwelling catheters are used long term for stage III or IV pressure sores when urine impedes healing, urinary retention that cannot be treated medically or surgically, or for comfort during terminal illness. Intermittent clean catheterisation is sometimes used as a self-care or carer-administered intervention for some types of incontinence.

Teaching about PFME

Pelvic floor muscle exercise (PFME) is an evidence-based practice that is effective as a first-line intervention for men and women with stress, urge and mixed incontinence and in women with pelvic organ prolapse (Bo & Hilde, 2012; Hagen & Stark, 2011; Hay-Smith, Herderschee, Dumoulin et al., 2012; Tienforti, Sacco, Marangi et al., 2012). These exercises were first promoted for postpartum therapy by an American gynaecologist named A. H. Kegel and they are now widely used for control of urinary incontinence. Other terms used interchangeably with PFME include Kegels, pelvic muscle exercise, pelvic floor training, and pelvic muscle rehabilitation. The goal of PFME is the improvement of urethral resistance through active exercise of the pubococcygeal muscle. There are no contraindications to or negative effects of these exercises, which can be initiated by any motivated person who is able to learn the technique. Nurses can use the information in Box 19-5 to teach older men and women to perform PFME, which is a nursing intervention recognised by NANDA. A related nursing intervention is to facilitate referrals to physiotherapists who are skilled in teaching about these exercises.

Initiating continence training programs

Continence training is a nursing intervention that can be categorised as (1) methods that are self-directed by motivated and cognitively intact people or (2) methods that are directed by motivated carers of cognitively impaired people. The goal of continence training is to achieve a continent interval of 2 to 4 hours between voiding. These intervals will not necessarily be equal and will usually be longer during the night. In self-directed programs, the person hopes to regain voluntary urinary control, whereas in carer-directed programs, the carer hopes to reduce the episodes of incontinence. Self-directed continence training, alone or in combination with biofeedback or medications, is most successful with urge incontinence.

Although specific techniques vary, essential elements of any continence training program include motivation, an assessment of voiding patterns, an individualised and carefully timed intake of approximately 1500–2000 mL of fluid per day, timed voiding in the most appropriate place, methods of reinforcing expected behaviours, and

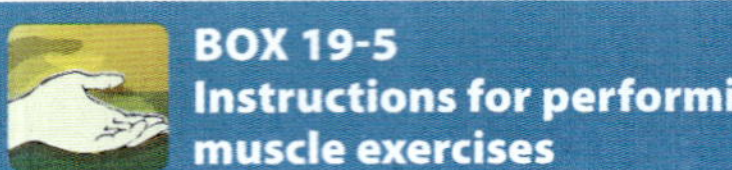

BOX 19-5
Instructions for performing pelvic muscle exercises

Purpose: To prevent the involuntary loss of urine by strengthening the pelvic floor muscles

Frequency: Minimum of 3 sets of 10 contractions/relaxations daily, continued indefinitely

Position: Lying, sitting, walking or standing with the muscles of your thighs, buttocks and abdomen relaxed

Results: Most people begin to notice an improvement in urinary control after 3 to 6 weeks, but some will not notice the improvement until several months later

Techniques to identify the pubococcygeal muscle

- Contract the muscle that stops the flow of urine. Do NOT do this regularly when urinating.
- (*Women*) Imagine that you are sitting on a marble and trying to suck it up into your vagina.
- (*Women*) Lie down and insert a finger about three quarters of the way up your vagina. Squeeze the vaginal wall so you feel pressure on your finger and a sensation in your vagina.
- (*Men*) Stand in front of a mirror and try to make the base of your penis move up and down without moving the rest of your body.
- Biofeedback, weighted vaginal cones or a perineometer (a balloon-like device that is placed in the vagina) can be used to assist in identifying the pubococcygeal muscle and in measuring the strength of the contraction.

Method

- Tighten your pubococcygeal muscle and hold for a period of at least 3 seconds; gradually increase the contraction time by 1 second per week until you can do a 10-second squeeze
- Relax this muscle for an equal period; rest and take deep breaths between contractions
- Do 10 sets of a contraction–relaxation cycle (one exercise) 3 times daily
- Breathe normally during these exercises and do NOT tighten other muscles at the same time. Be careful not to contract your legs, buttocks or abdominal muscles while you are contracting your pubococcygeal muscle.
- For each of the daily sessions, vary your position (e.g. perform the exercise while lying down in the morning, standing in the afternoon and sitting in the evening).

Additional information: You can ask your medical practitioner for a referral to a physiotherapist or continence advisor who can teach you to do these exercises.

ongoing monitoring. During the initial assessment, diaries are used to record times and circumstances of toileting, as well as times of and reasons for any episode of incontinence. After the usual voiding pattern is identified, the older adult is encouraged to resist the sensation of urgency and to postpone voiding rather than responding immediately to an urge.

With carer-directed methods the carer uses the initial assessment of voiding patterns to establish a schedule for assisting with voiding. All these programs are most successful when the timed intervals are based on a good assessment of the person's needs and voiding patterns. There are three types of supportive toileting programs:

- *Scheduled voiding* where assisted toileting is to a fixed schedule, for example, 2-hourly. This program is appropriate for those who are cognitively impaired and have an erratic voiding pattern.
- *Habit training* where assisted toileting occurs to an individual's assessed toileting pattern. This program is appropriate for those who have a predictable voiding pattern.
- ***Prompted voiding*** is supplemental to a fixed or individualised schedule. This program is appropriate for those who require to prompting additional to a schedule to remain continent. This type of program is usually implemented with older adults with cognitive impairment.

Carer-directed programs include the use of behaviour modification techniques, such as praising the person for staying dry between scheduled trips to the bathroom and self-initiating requests to use the toilet. Box 19-6 identifies some of the terms used for and the general principles of continence training programs.

WELLNESS OPPORTUNITY

Using biofeedback and other devices acknowledges the connection between the person's body and mind and may enhance self-care abilities.

Suggesting environmental modifications

When incontinence is associated with the inability to reach an appropriate receptacle after perceiving the need to

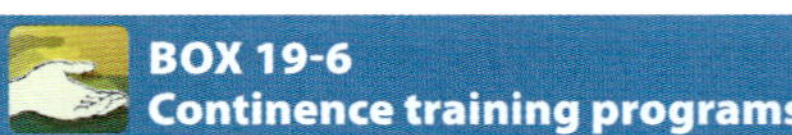

BOX 19-6
Continence training programs

Goal of programs: To achieve voluntary control over urination at intervals of 2 to 4 hours

Terminology

- *Terms used for self-directed programs:* bladder training, bladder retraining, bladder exercise, bladder retention exercise
- *Terms used for carer-directed programs:* scheduled toileting, prompted voiding, habit training

Method

- *Step 1:* Identify the usual voiding pattern, noting the times of incontinence and information about fluid intake. During the first few days, keep a diary to record the following information at hourly intervals: dry or wet, amount voided, place of voiding, fluid intake and sensation and awareness of need to void.
- *Step 2:* Using information from the voiding diary, establish a schedule that allows for emptying of the bladder before incontinence is likely to occur.
- *Step 3:* Provide the equipment and assistance necessary for optimal voiding at scheduled times.
- *Step 4:* Provide 2000 mL of non-caffeinated liquids per day for liquid intake. Consume the largest amounts during the early part of the day, and limit fluid intake at about 2 to 4 hours before bedtime.

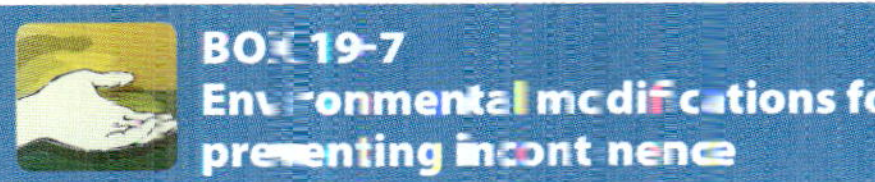

BOX 19-7
Environmental modifications for preventing incontinence

Modifications to enhance visibility of facilities

- Use contrasting colours for the toilet seat and surroundings.
- Provide adequate lighting in and near toilet areas, but avoid creating glare.
- Use nightlights in the pathway between the bedroom and bathroom.

Modifications to improve the ability to use the toilet in time

- Encourage the use of chairs or beds that are designed to help the person arise unaided after sitting or lying.
- Install handrails in the hallway(s) leading to the bathroom.
- Make sure the pathway to the bathroom is safe and uncluttered.

Modifications to improve the ability to use the toilet

- Place grab bars at appropriate places to facilitate getting on and off the toilet and to assist them in maintaining their balance when standing at the toilet.
- Use elevated toilet seats, or an over-the-toilet chair, to compensate for any functional limitations of the lower extremities.
- If the person has functional limitations involving the upper extremities, clothing for the lower body should feature easy-open closures such as Velcro or elastic waistbands.

void, interventions are directed toward modifying the environment and improving functional abilities. If environmental adaptations cannot be made, as in public places, older adults are encouraged to become familiar with the location and arrangement of the bathroom facilities before the need to urinate is imminent. In home and institutional settings, the provision of bedside commodes and privacy can be an effective intervention. If space is limited or privacy cannot be assured, however, bedside commodes may not be acceptable. Box 19-7 lists environmental modifications for preventing incontinence when functional limitations are a contributing factor. Interventions discussed in chapters on vision (Chapter 17) and mobility (Chapter 22) can address functional limitations that can contribute to incontinence.

Using appropriate continence aids

When incontinence cannot be alleviated, it can be managed with the use of various aids and equipment, such as incontinence products and collecting devices. When used in conjunction with environmental modifications to increase the accessibility of toilet facilities, such equipment usually has beneficial effects. However, when aids and equipment are used by carers as substitutes for other methods of promoting continence, they are beneficial only to the carer and are detrimental to the older adult. For example, if protective products are used to manage incontinence, the positive effect for the carer may be the ease of care; however, the negative effects for the older adult include the likelihood of skin breakdown and decreased self-esteem. Because continence aids can be beneficial as well as detrimental, they should be used only after careful evaluation of all contributing factors, including the needs of family carers in home settings.

The selection of the most appropriate products for managing incontinence depends on such factors as cost, convenience, preference and effectiveness. Economic considerations are particularly important because disposable incontinence products can be quite expensive, particularly if used daily. The initial and periodic cost of reusable products also needs to be considered, as does the time and expense of laundering. In Australia there is a federal government scheme, the Continence Aids Payment Scheme (CAPS, www.bladderbowel.gov.au/caps) which assists eligible older adults with the costs of incontinence products who have permanent or severe incontinence. In New Zealand, if a person is assessed by a continence advisor as requiring continence aids, then these are free (New Zealand Continence Association, 2014).

Many products are designed specifically for either male or female incontinence. Product absorbency is affected by such variables as the size, shape, depth and the location and type of absorbent material (e.g. gel, pulp, polymer). Keep in mind that someone may need several types of products for different activities (e.g. light protection during the day and heavy protection during the night). Ease of use is a major consideration, particularly for people who are independent and can manage incontinence with little or no supervision. "Pull-ups" now provide a convenient alternative to the products with tabs that cannot be easily removed before and reapplied after toileting. Box 19-8 lists factors to be considered in selecting and using various types of aids and equipment for managing urinary incontinence.

WELLNESS OPPORTUNITY

Nurses promote self-care by helping older adults to identify ways of improving their functional abilities that can affect urinary control.

UNFOLDING CASE STUDY

Part C

Mr and Mrs Chung are now 73 and 72 years old, respectively, and continue to attend the local medical centre where you are the nurse. Mr Chung has been under the care of a urologist for 3 years and has been taking terazosin for prostatic hyperplasia. Until recently, he was able to maintain urinary continence, but lately his Parkinson's has worsened. Then a month ago he started taking 80 mg of frusemide daily for congestive heart failure. He makes an appointment to ask your advice about incontinence products that would be best for him because "it's just hopeless to get to the toilet on time because our only bathroom is upstairs, and I like to be downstairs during the day". He reports that he limits his fluid intake to 4 cups of liquid daily, which includes 2 cups of black coffee. Because of his Parkinson's disease, he has trouble standing at the toilet and usually sits down; however, he is "slow and clumsy" in managing his clothing. His son bought him some "jogging" outfits with elastic waists, but he does not wear them because he prefers to "dress up" when he goes out, so he wears trousers with belts.

Thinking points with regard to Mr Chung

- What risk factors are likely to be contributing to Mr Chung's incontinence, and which factors might be alleviated with interventions?
- What environmental modifications might be helpful when addressing her incontinence?
- What health education would you give about alleviating risk factors?
- What health education would you give about incontinence products?

UNFOLDING CASE STUDY

Part D

Mrs Chung also makes an appointment to see you to discuss her recent problem with incontinence. She tells you that for several years she has been wearing "light-days pads" because "I have trouble holding my water whenever I sneeze or cough". In the past few months, she notices that she has to go to the bathroom every hour or two and is reluctant to be away from her house for more than an hour at a time. Her health has been good overall, but her arthritis has been getting worse, and she is very slow in her mobility, particularly when she needs to go up and down stairs. She drinks about 6 cups of liquid daily, consisting mostly of tea and coffee. She has heard some of her friends talking about "those exercises, we had to do when we had our babies". One friend even talked about having some "cones she puts in to help her with exercises".

Thinking points with regard to Mrs Chung

- What risk factors are likely to be contributing to Mrs Chung's incontinence?
- What environmental modifications might be helpful when addressing her incontinence?
- What health education would you give about alleviating risk factors?
- What health education would you give about exercises?
- What health education would you give about incontinence products?

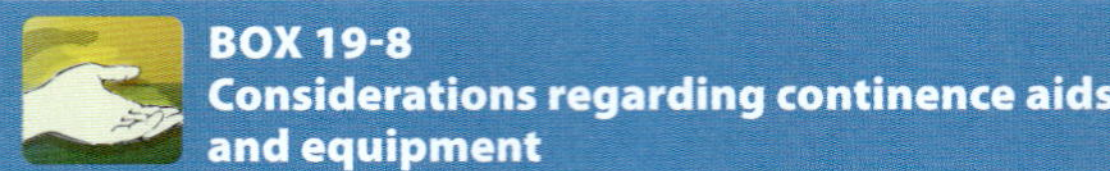

BOX 19-8 Considerations regarding continence aids and equipment

Assessment considerations

- What are the costs of various disposable and washable products, both initially and over a period of time? (Include the time and expense of laundry when considering costs of washable products.)
- What are the preferences of the incontinent person? (e.g. Is a "brief" or "pull-up" style garment more acceptable than a "nappy" style product? Also, how much noise a product makes when the person is walking or moving around in social settings may influence the acceptability of a product.)
- What level of absorbency is appropriate for different circumstances?
- What are the needs and abilities of the carers of dependent older adults in home settings? (Can the carer manage the tasks involved in toileting?)
- What are the consequences if the incontinence cannot be managed in the home setting? (For example, will the older adult need to be in a long-term care setting?)

Teaching related to aids and equipment

- Many types of external collecting devices are available for men and women (e.g. male or female urinals, condom catheters, retracted penis pouches and bedside urinals with attached drainage bags).
- An elevated toilet seat with rails can be used to increase safety and transfer mobility.
- Commodes are useful in diminishing the distance between the place of usual activities and toilet facilities.
- A variety of commodes are available and can be selected according to needs and preferences of the dependent person.
- If commodes are viewed as socially unacceptable, measures can be taken to ensure privacy and increase their social acceptability. Privacy can be ensured by placing an attractive screen around the commode.
- Commodes are now available that are attractively designed to resemble normal furniture items.
- A bedpan can be placed on a regular chair, particularly in the bedroom, and removed when not in use.

EVALUATING THE EFFECTIVENESS OF NURSING INTERVENTIONS

Nursing care for older adults with urinary incontinence is evaluated by measuring the extent to which the person can achieve periods of continence that are as long as possible. When older adults attribute incontinence to ageing processes, nurses evaluate the effectiveness of their teaching by the degree to which the person verbalises accurate information and understands the importance of identifying treatable causes. Another measure of the effectiveness of nursing interventions in such cases would be that the person seeks evaluation for his or her incontinence, rather than accepting this condition as inevitable.

If incontinence cannot be resolved, nursing care is directed towards managing urinary elimination in such a way as to maintain the dignity of the older adult and to prevent negative consequences. In these situations, the effectiveness of nursing interventions might be measured by the extent to which the person maintains daily activities. For example, if older adults restrict their social activities because of incontinence, a measure of the success of nursing interventions might be that they begin using incontinence products to permit them to be away from their home for 4 hours at a time. For people with total incontinence, a measure of the effectiveness of nursing interventions would be the absence of skin irritation and breakdown.

UNFOLDING CASE STUDY

Part E

Mrs Chung, who is now 79 years old, is being transferred to a rehabilitation unit after sustaining a hip fracture. An indwelling catheter was inserted before her hip surgery 7 days ago, and it was removed two days after surgery. She is ambulating with a walker but needs one-person assistance. The discharge summary describes her as incontinent of urine. Mrs Chung hopes to regain her independence in performing ADLs so that she can return to her own home, where she lives with her husband.

Nursing assessment

During your functional assessment, Mrs Chung tells you she has had "trouble holding her water" since they removed the catheter. She is quite embarrassed about this and has not discussed it with any other healthcare practitioner. She says that she had too many other questions to discuss with her orthopaedic surgeon and states that the nurses kept a large absorbent pad on her bed so that she would not have to walk to the bathroom. When she went to physiotherapy she used sanitary napkins that her friend brought to her. She limited her fluid intake to a cup of coffee with each meal and a few sips of water with her pills.

Further assessment of Mrs Chung's incontinence reveals that, for many years, she has had difficulty with "leaking", particularly when she coughs, sneezes or exercises. Also, she gets up to urinate about four to five times nightly. It was during one of these trips to the bathroom that she tripped and fractured her hip. She says that she wakes up a lot during the night and goes to the bathroom because she is afraid of wetting the bed. She does not feel the need to urinate every time she wakes up but goes to the bathroom to prevent any leakage. She limits her fluid intake to 6 glasses per day and does not drink anything after 5 p.m. A few years ago, a nurse taught her "how to do exercises and they helped for a couple of years, but I don't bother to do them anymore". She tearfully confides that she thinks that the orthopaedic surgeon damaged a nerve in her bladder, which she believes is the reason she has such little control over urination since the surgery. She thinks that the hospital staff inserted the catheter because she has "weak kidneys". She states, "Before I had this fractured hip, I just had the usual problems holding water like all my friends have, but now it's really bad and I'll probably never be able to hold my water again. I wish you'd just put that tube back in me, so I can go home again and not worry about accidents."

Nursing issues

In addition to the nursing issues related to Mrs Chung's impaired mobility, you address her problem with urinary incontinence. In deciding which type of urinary incontinence to include in your nursing issue, you conclude that both stress incontinence and functional incontinence are appropriate because of the combination of long-term and recent factors that contribute to her incontinence. Your nursing issue is stress/functional incontinence related to limited mobility, recent indwelling catheter and insufficient knowledge of normal urinary function and pelvic muscle exercises. Evidence for this issue can be found in Mrs Chung's statements reflecting misconceptions and lack of information and in her description of current and past problems with incontinence. Evidence is also derived from your observations that she needs one-person assistance for walking and that she uses sanitary napkins and bed pads for urinary incontinence.

Nursing care plan for Mrs Chung

Goals for wellness outcomes	Nursing interventions	Nursing evaluation
Mrs Chung's knowledge of normal urinary function will increase.	• Discuss normal urinary function using a balloon partially filled with water and a simple illustration of the female urinary tract. • Emphasise the relationship between adequate fluid intake and continence.	• Mrs Chung describes normal urinary function and the mechanisms involved in maintaining continence.
Mrs Chung's knowledge about causative factors for incontinence will increase.	• Describe age-related changes that contribute to incontinence using the information in Box 19-4. • Discuss the effects of frequent bladder emptying and limited fluid intake on the maintenance of continence. • Discuss the relationship between limited mobility and urinary incontinence.	• Mrs Chung describes age-related changes that influence urinary elimination. • Mrs Chung identifies risk factors that contribute to her incontinence.
Mrs Chung's misconceptions about her urinary incontinence will be corrected.	• Emphasise that as Mrs Chung regains her mobility, she will regain continence. • Emphasise that urinary incontinence is not an inevitable consequence of ageing.	• Mrs Chung states correct information about the relationship between her hip surgery and her incontinence. • Mrs Chung expresses confidence in regaining urinary control.

Nursing care plan for Mrs Chung

Goals for wellness outcomes	Nursing interventions	Nursing evaluation
	• Explain that the orthopaedic surgeon was not operating on or near her bladder or urinary tract. • Explain that the Foley catheter probably contributed to her current incontinence, but that this is a temporary situation that will resolve with proper interventions. • Emphasise that the nursing home staff will work with her to improve or alleviate her incontinence.	
The factors that contribute to Mrs Chung's functional incontinence will be eliminated.	• Provide a bedside commode for Mrs Chung's use until she is able to walk to the bathroom without assistance. • Work with the physiotherapy staff to teach Mrs Chung a proper technique for independent transfer to the commode. • The nursing and dietary staff will provide 2000 mL of fluids per day, taking into consideration Mrs Chung's preferences. • The nursing and dietary staff will work with Mrs Chung to schedule her fluid intake at acceptable times of the day with minimal intake in the evening. • Talk with Mrs Chung about eliminating the bed pads as soon as she feels confident about maintaining continence.	• Mrs Chung is continent of urine, except for stress incontinence.
Mrs Chung will regain full control over urination.	• Suggest that Mrs Chung seek a comprehensive assessment of her urinary incontinence. • Give Mrs Chung a copy of Box 19-5 as a guide for performing PFMT. • Emphasise the need to perform PFMT on an ongoing basis for the alleviation of stress incontinence. • Give Mrs Chung information about health education that may be helpful for her.	• Mrs Chung reports a reduction in or elimination of her stress incontinence.

Thinking points

- What myths and misunderstandings affect Mrs Chung's attitude about urinary incontinence?
- What risk factors are contributing to Mrs Chung's urinary incontinence?
- What additional assessment information would you want to obtain?

CHAPTER HIGHLIGHTS

Age-related changes that affect urinary wellness

- Kidney: degenerative changes, decreased blood flow, decreased number of functioning nephrons
- Urinary tract muscles: hypertrophy of bladder muscle, replacement of smooth muscle with connective tissue, relaxation of pelvic floor muscles
- Voluntary control mechanisms: central nervous system, urinary tract, age-related changes of other systems (e.g. increased postural sway)
- Decreased immune response

Risk factors that affect urinary wellness

- Misperceptions and attitudes (e.g. resignation, viewing urinary incontinence as "normal", staff and carer attitudes that interfere with maintaining continence)
- Functional impairments that affect control over socially appropriate urinary elimination (e.g. dependency in ADLs)
- Gender-specific conditions (e.g. pelvic floor dysfunction, benign prostatic hyperplasia)
- Other conditions (e.g. dementia, Parkinson's, constipation, OAB and UTI

- Medication effects
- Dietary and lifestyle factors (e.g. obesity, tobacco smoking, intake of caffeinated beverages)
- Environmental factors

Functional consequences affecting urinary wellness

- Effects on homeostasis: diminished ability to maintain electrolyte balance, and changes in diurnal pattern of urine production, can lead to nocturia
- Delayed excretion of water-soluble medications and increased risk of drug interactions and adverse effects
- Diminished bladder capacity; urinary urgency and frequency
- Decrease in the interval between the signal of the need to void and the actual need to empty the bladder

Pathological condition affecting urinary function

- Urinary tract infection

Nursing assessment of urinary function

- Talking with older adults about urinary function (finding appropriate terminology)
- Identifying usual voiding patterns and influencing factors
- Identifying risk factors for urinary tract infection
- Identifying risk factors for urinary incontinence
- Identifying risk factors that influence renal function and homeostasis
- Identifying symptoms of impaired urinary elimination
- Being alert to misunderstandings about urinary elimination
- Psychosocial consequences of incontinence (e.g. anxiety, depression, social isolation)

Nursing issues

- Willingness to improve urinary elimination
- Impaired urinary elimination
- Social isolation
- Carer role strain (or risk for)

Goal planning for wellness outcomes

- Urinary continence
- Urinary elimination
- Health beliefs: perceived control
- Carer stressors
- Carer endurance potential

Nursing interventions to promote healthy urinary function

- Teaching older adults about age-related changes and preventing urinary incontinence and UTI
- Promoting continence and alleviating incontinence (pelvic floor muscle training, urinary control devices, continence training, environmental modifications, medications and surgical or minimally invasive procedures)
- Managing urinary incontinence

Evaluating effectiveness of nursing interventions

- Longer intervals of continence
- Accurate understanding of normal urinary function and risks for incontinence
- Self-care practices to promote continence and urinary wellness
- Use of resources for further evaluation of incontinence when appropriate

CRITICAL THINKING EXERCISES

1. Describe how each of the following age-related changes or risk factors might influence urinary function in older adults: medications, renal function; functional abilities; environmental conditions; altered thirst perception; changes in the urinary tract and nervous system; and myths and misunderstandings on the part of older adults, their carers and healthcare professionals.
2. What are the psychosocial consequences of urinary incontinence for older adults and their carers?
3. Describe how you would address the following statement made by a 74-year-old woman: "Of course I have to wear pads all the time, just like when I was a teenager. I haven't talked to the doctor because I figured this was pretty normal at my age."
4. Describe the nursing assessment, with regard to urinary elimination, for a 75-year-old man and a 75-year-old woman.

RESOURCES

For an extensive range of additional resources to enhance teaching and learning and to facilitate understanding of this chapter, please see the text's accompanying website located on thePoint at http://thepoint.lww.com.

Clinical tools

Hartford Institute for Geriatric Nursing, ConsultGeriRN.org: http://consultgerirn.org/resources

Assessment tools *Try This*® series and *How to Try This* resources

General assessment series:

- *Try This*, Issue 11.1: Urinary incontinence assessment in older adults, Part I: Transient urinary incontinence. Dowling-Castronovo, A. (2013). *Best Practices in Nursing Care to Older Adults*.
- *How to Try This* (article): Assessment of transient urinary incontinence in older adults. Dowling-Castronovo, A. & Specht, J. K. (2009). *American Journal of Nursing*, 109(2), 62–71.
- *How to Try This* (video): *Transient urinary incontinence in older adults*

- *Try This*, issue 11.2: Urinary incontinence assessment in older adults, Part II: Persistent urinary incontinence. Dowling-Castronovo, A. (2013). *Best Practices in Nursing Care to Older Adults*.

Evidence-based practice

Dowling-Castronovo, A. & Bradway, C. (2012). Urinary incontinence. In M. Boltz, E. Capezuti, T. Fulmer & D. Zwicker D. (Eds), *Evidence-based geriatric nursing protocols for best practice* (4th ed. pp. 363–387). New York: Springer.

Joanna Briggs Institute: http://connect.jbiconnectplus.org

Evidence summaries:

- Chu, V. (2014). Urinary incontinence: Prompted voiding.
- D'Arcy, M. (2013). Urinary and fecal incontinence: Absorbent products.
- D'Arcy, M. (2014). Continence management.
- Slade, S. (2013). Urinary and fecal incontinence (older person): Assessment.

Recommended practice:

- Continence care. (2013).

Systematic review:

- Hodgkinson, B., Josephs, K., Leira, E., Synnott, R. & Hegney, D. (2008). A systematic review of the effect of educational interventions for urinary and faecal incontinence by healthcare staff/carers/clients in aged care, on level of knowledge, frequency of incontinence episodes and hours spent on the management of incontinence episodes. *Joanna Briggs Institute Library of Systematic Reviews, 6*(1), 1–66.

National Guideline Clearinghouse: www.guideline.gov

Search for: Urinary incontinence

- Urinary incontinence in older adults admitted to acute care. In *Evidence-based geriatric nursing protocols for best practice*. (2003; revised 2012).
- Urinary incontinence in the long term care setting. (1996; revised 2012).
- Urinary incontinence in women. (2005; reaffirmed 2009).
- Urinary incontinence: The management of urinary incontinence in women. (2006; revised Sept. 2013).

National Health and Medical Research Council (NHMRC) (Australia), clinical practice guidelines search portal: www.clinicalguidelines.gov.au

- First steps in the management of urinary incontinence in community-dwelling older people. A clinical practice guideline for primary clinicians (registered nurses and allied health professionals) (2010).

Health education

Australian Government Department of Health, continence: www.health.gov.au//internet/main/publishing.nsf/Content/Home

Bladder and Bowel Australia: www.bladderbowel.gov.au

Continence Foundation of Australia: www.continence.org.au

International Continence Society: www.icsoffice.org

Master Locksmiths Access Key (MLAK), Australia (enables people with disabilities to gain 24/7 access to a network of public facilities, including toilets): www.masterlocksmiths.com.au/mlak.php

National Association for Continence (NAFC) (U.S.): www.nafc.org

National Toilet Map, Australia: https://toiletmap.gov.au

New Zealand Continence Foundation: www.continence.org.nz

TENA: www.tena.com.au

Toilet Map, New Zealand: www.toiletmap.co.nz

REFERENCES

Adedokun, B. O., Morhason-Bello, I. O., Ojengbede, O. A. et al. (2012). Help-seeking behavior among women currently leaking urine in Nigeria. *Patient Preference and Adherence, 2*(6), 815–819.

Amselem, C., Puigdollers, A., Azpiroz, F., Sala, C., Videla, S., Fernandez-Fraga, X., … Malagelada, J. (2010). Constipation: A potential cause of pelvic floor damage? *Neurogastroenterology and Motility: The Official Journal of the European Gastrointestinal Motility Society, 22*(2), 150–153.

Andreessen, L., Wilde, M. H. & Herendeen, P. (2012). Preventing catheter-associated urinary tract infections in acute care: The bundle approach. *Journal of Nursing Care Quarterly, 27*(3), 209–217.

Australian Government Department of Social Services. (2014). Incontinence. At myaged*care* portal, viewed March 2015 at www.myagedcare.gov.au/health-conditions/incontinence.

Australian Institute of Health and Welfare (2014). *Australia's health 2014*. Australia's health series no. 14. Cat. no. AUS 178. Canberra: Author.

Badalian, S. S. & Rosenbaum, P. F. (2010). Vitamin D and pelvic floor disorders in women: Results from the National Health and Nutrition Examination Survey. *Obstetrics and Gynecology, 115*(4), 795–803.

Bent, S. & Saint, S. (2002). The optimal use of diagnostic testing in women with acute uncomplicated cystitis. *The American Journal of Medicine, 113*, 20–28.

Berger, M. B., Patel, J. M., Miller, J. M. et al. (2011). Racial differences in self-reported healthcare seeking and treatment for urinary incontinence in community-dwelling women from the EPI study. *Neurourology and Urodynamics, 30*(8), 1442–1447.

Bliss, D. Z., Westra, B. L., Savik, K. et al. (2013). Effectiveness of wound, ostomy and continence-certified nurses on individual patient outcomes in home health care. *Journal of Wound, Ostomy, and Continence Nursing, 40*(2), 135–142.

Bliwise, D. L., Foley, D. J., Vitiello, M. V., Ansari, F. P., Ancoli-Israel, S. & Walsh, J. K. (2009). Nocturia and disturbed sleep in the elderly. *Sleep Medicine, 10*(5), 540–548.

Bo, K. & Hilde, G. (2012). A systematic review on pelvic floor muscle training for female stress urinary incontinence. *Neurology and Urodynamics, 32*(3), 215–223.

Botlero, R., Bell, R. J., Urquhart, D. M. & Davis, S. R. (2010). Urinary incontinence is associated with lower psychological general well-being in community-dwelling women. *Menopause, 17*(2), 332–337.

Byles, J., Millar, C. J., Sibbritt, D. W. & Chiarelli, P. (2009). Living with urinary incontinence: A longitudinal study of older women. *Age and Ageing, 38*, 333–338.

Caljouw, M. A., den Elzen, W., Cools, H. et al. (2011). Predictive factors of urinary tract infections among the oldest old in the general population. *BMC Medicine, 9*, 57. Available at www.biomedcentral.com/1741-7015/9/57.

Carter, D. & Beer-Gabel, M. (2012). Lower urinary tract symptoms in chronically constipated women. *International Urogynecology Journal, 23*(12), 1785–1789.

Caterino, J. M., Ting, S. A., Sisbarro, S. G. et al. (2012). Age, nursing home residence, and presentation of urinary tract infection in U. S. emergency departments, 2001–2008. *Academic of Emergency Medicine, 19*(10), 1173–1180.

Cheung, W. W., Khan, N. H., Choi, K. K., Bluth, M. H. & Vincent, M. T. (2009). Prevalence, evaluation and management of overactive bladder in primary care. *BMC Family Practice, 10*(8), 1–7.

Davis, N. J., Vaughan, C. E., Johnson, T. M. et al. (2012). Caffeine intake and its association with urinary incontinence in US men. *Journal of Urology, 189*(6), 2170–2174.

Deville, W., Yzermans, J., van Duijn, N., Bezemer, P., van der Windt, D. & Bouter, L. (2004). The urine dipstick test useful to rule out infections. A meta-analysis of the accuracy. *BMC Urology, 4*(4), 1–14.

Devore, E. E., Townsend, M. K., Resnick, N. M. et al. (2012). The epidemiology of urinary incontinence in women with type 2 diabetes. *Journal of Urology, 188*(5), 1816–1821.

Dowling-Castronovo, A. & Bradway, C. (2012). Urinary incontinence. In M. Boltz, E. Capezuti, R. Fulmer & D. Zwicker (Eds), *Evidence-based geriatric nursing protocols for best practice* (4th ed., pp. 363–386). New York: Springer. Modified version is available online at http://consultgerirn.org.

Dumoulin, C. & Hay-Smith, J. (2010). Pelvic floor muscle training versus no treatment or inactive control treatments for urinary incontinence in women. *Cochrane Database of Systematic Reviews, 1*. Article no. CD005654. doi:10.1002/14651858.CD005654.pub2.

Ekundayo, O. J., Markland, A., Lefante, C., Sui, X., Goode, P. S., Allman, R. M., … Ahmed, A. (2009). Association of diuretic use and overactive bladder syndrome in older adults: A propensity score analysis. *Archives of Gerontology and Geriatrics, 49*(1), 64–68.

El-Azab, A. S. & Shaaban, O. M. (2010). Measuring the barriers against seeking consultation for urinary incontinence among Middle Eastern women. *BMC Women's Health, 10*(3), 1–6.

Endeshaw, Y. (2009). Correlates of self-reported nocturia among community-dwelling older adults. *Journal of Gerontology: A Biological Sciences Medical Sciences, 64A*(1), 142–148.

Farrell, M. & Dempsey, J. (Eds). (2014). *Smeltzer & Bare's textbook of medical-surgical nursing* (3rd Australian & New Zealand ed.). Sydney: Lippincott Williams & Wilkins.

French, L., Phelps, K., Pothula, N. R. & Mushkbar, S. (2009). Urinary problems in women. *Primary Care: Clinics in Office Practice, 36*, 53–71.

Glassock, R. J. & Winearls, C. (2009). Ageing and the glomerular filtration rate: Truths and consequences. *Transactions of the American Clinical and Climatological Association, 120*, 419–423.

Gleason, J. L., Richter, H. E., Redden, D. T. et al. (2013). Caffeine and urinary incontinence in US women. *International Urogynecology Journal, 24*(2), 295–302.

Griebling, T. L. (2009). Urinary incontinence in the elderly. Clinics in Geriatric Medicine, 25, 445–457.

Hagen, S. & Stark, D. (2011). Conservative prevention and management of pelvic organ prolapse in women. *Cochrane Database Systematic Reviews, 12*. Art. no. CD003882.

Hasegawa, J., Kuzuya, M. & Iguchi, A. (2010). Urinary incontinence and behavioral symptoms are independent risk factors for recurrent and injurious falls, respectively, among residents in long-term care facilities. *Archives of Gerontology and Geriatrics, 50*(1), 77–81.

Hay-Smith, J., Herderschee, R., Dumoulin, C. et al. (2012). Comparison of approaches to pelvic floor muscle training for urinary incontinence in women. *European Journal of Physical and Rehabilitation Medicine, 48*(4), 689–705.

Hirayama, F. & Lee, A. H. (2011). Green tea drinking is inversely associated with urinary incontinence in middle-aged and older women. *Neurourology and Urodynamics, 30*(7), 1262–1265.

Home and Community Care (HACC)/Medical Aids Subsidy Scheme (MASS) Continence Project (2010). First steps in the management of urinary incontinence in community-dwelling older people: A clinical practice guideline for primary level clinicians: registered nurses and allied health professionals). Revised version 2010. Brisbane: Queensland Health. Accessed March 2015 at www.health.qld.gov.au/mass/docs/resources/continence/firststepscompanion.pdf

Hu, K., Boyko, E., Scholes, D., Normand, E., Chen, C., Grafton, J. et al. (2004). Risk factors for urinary tract infections in postmenopausal women. *Archives of Internal Medicine, 164*, 989–993.

Jepson, R., Mihaljevic, L. & Craig, J. (2008). Cranberries for preventing urinary tract infections (review). *Cochrane Database of Systematic Reviews, 1*, Art. no: CD001321.

Kupelian, V., McVary, K. T., Kaplan, S. A. et al. (2013). Association of lower urinary tract symptoms and the metabolic syndrome. *Journal of Urology, 189*(1 Suppl.), S107–S114.

Lerma, E. V. (2009). Anatomic and physiologic changes of the aging kidney. *Clinics in Geriatric Medicine, 25*, 325–329.

Lin, S. Y. (2013). A pilot study: Fluid intake and bacteriuria in nursing home residents in southern Taiwan. *Nursing Research, 62*(1), 66–72.

Lukacz, E. S., Sampselle, C., Gray, M. et al. (2011). A health bladder: Consensus statement. *International Journal of Clinical Practice, 65*(10), 1026–1036.

Lutters, M. & Vogt, N. (2002). Antibiotic duration for treating uncomplicated, symptomatic lower urinary tract infections in elderly women (review). *Cochrane Database of Systematic Reviews, 3*. Art. no.:CD001535.

Menezes, M. A. J., Hashimoto, S. Y. & de Gouveia Santos, V. L. C. (2009). Prevalence of urinary incontinence in a community sample from the city of Sao Paulo. *Journal of the Wound, Ostomy and Continence Nurses Society, 36*(4), 436–440.

Mohsin, R. & Siddiqui, K. M. (2010). Recurrent urinary tract infections in females. *The Journal of the Pakistan Medical Association, 60*(1), 55–59.

New Zealand Continence Association. (2009). Continence services in New Zealand: History, services, costs and impacts. Accessed March 2015 at www.continence.org.nz/user_files/Continence_Services_in_New_Zealand_FINAL_Oct_2009.pdf.

New Zealand Continence Association. (2014). Continence products. Accessed March 2015 www.continence.org.nz/index.php?mode=display_content&page_id=19.

Nicolle, L. E. (2009). Urinary tract infections in the elderly. *Clinics in Geriatric Medicine, 25*, 423–436.

Nicolle, L. E., Bradley, S., Colgan, R. et al. (2005). IDSA Guidelines for asymptomatic bacteriuria. *Clinical Infectious Diseases, 40*, 643–654.

Parker-Autry, C. Y., Markland, A. D., Ballard, A. C. et al. (2012). Vitamin D status in women with pelvic floor disorder symptoms. *International Urogynecology Journal, 23*(12), 1699–1705.

Quintal, E. (2003). Minding our own business: How Indigenous communities are dealing with incontinence. *The Continence Advisor, 2*.

Rahn, D. D. & Roshanravan, S. M. (2009). Pathophysiology of urinary incontinence, voiding dysfunction and overactive bladder. *Obstetrics and Gynecology Clinics of North America, 36*, 463–474.

Rios, A. A., Cardoso, J. R. & Rodriques, M. A. (2011). The help-seeking by women with urinary incontinence in Brazil. *International Urogynecology Journal, 22*(7), 879–884.

St John, W., Wallis, M., Griffiths, S. & McKenzie, S. (2010). Daily-living management of urinary incontinence: A synthesis of the literature. *Journal of the Wound, Ostomy and Continence Nurses Society, 37*(1), 80–90.

Smeltzer, S. C., Bare, B. G., Hinkle, J. E. & Cheever, K. (2008). *Brunner and Suddarth's textbook of medical-surgical nursing* [11th ed.]. Philadelphia: Lippincott Williams & Wilkins.

Tahtinen, R. M., Auvinen, A., Cartwright, R. et al. (2011). Smoking and bladder symptoms in women. *Obstetrics & Gynecology, 118*(3), 643–648.

Tennstedt, S. L., Chiu, G. R., Link, C. L., Litman, H. J., Kusek, J. W. & McKinlay, J. B. (2010). The effects of severity of urine leakage on quality of life in Hispanic, white and black men and women: The Boston Community Health Survey. *Urology, 75*(1), 27–28.

Thurmon, K. L., Breyer, B. N. & Erickson, B. A. (2012). Association of bowel habits with lower urinary tract symptoms in men. *Journal of Urology, 189*(4), 1409–1414.

Tienforti, D., Sacco, E., Marangi, F. et al. (2012). Efficacy of an assisted low-density programme of perioperative pelvic floor muscle training in improving recovery after radical prostatectomy. *BJU International, 110*(7), 1004–1010.

van Kerrebroeck, P., Hashim, H., Holm-Larsen, T., Robinson, D. & Stanley, N. (2010). Thinking beyond the bladder: Antidiuretic treatment of nocturia. *International Journal of Clinical Practice, 64*(6), 807–816.

Vaughan, C. P., Auvinen, A., Cartwright, R. et al. (2012). Impact of obesity on urinary storage symptoms. *Journal of Urology, 189*(4), 1377–1382.

Vaughan, C. P., Brown, C. J., Goode, P. S., Burgio, K. L., Allman, R. M. & Johnson, T. M. II. (2010). The association of nocturia with incident falls in an elderly community-dwelling cohort. *International Journal of Clinical Practice, 64*(5), 577–583.

Wald, H. L., Fink, R. M., Makic, M. B. F. & Oman, K. S. (2012). Catheter-associated urinary tract infection prevention. In M. Boltz, E. Capezuti, R. Fulmer & D. Zwicker (Eds), *Evidence-based geriatric nursing protocols for best practice* (4th ed., pp. 388–408). New York: Springer. Modified version is available online at http://consultgerirn.org.

Welch, L. C., Taubenberger, S. & Tennstedt, S. L. (2011). Patients' experiences of seeking health care for lower urinary tract symptoms. *Research in Nursing & Health, 34*(6), 496–507.

Zisberg, A., Sinoff, G., Gur-Yaish, N. et al. (2011). In-hospital use of continence aids and new-onset urinary incontinence in adults aged 70 and older. *Journal of the American Geriatrics Society, 59*(6), 1099–1104.

Chapter 20

Cardiovascular function

By Carol Miller and Sharyn Hunter

LEARNING OBJECTIVES

After reading this chapter, you should be able to:

1. Describe age-related changes that affect cardiovascular function.
2. Identify risk factors for cardiovascular disease and orthostatic and postprandial hypotension.
3. Describe the functional consequences of age-related changes and risk factors related to cardiovascular function.
4. Assess cardiovascular function and risks for cardiovascular disease with emphasis on those that can be addressed through health promotion interventions.
5. Teach older adults and their carers about health interventions to reduce the risk for cardiovascular disease.

KEY POINTS

abdominal obesity
adaptive response
atherosclerosis
atypical presentation
baroreflex mechanisms
cardiovascular disease
chronic heart failure
DASH dietary pattern
home blood pressure monitoring
hypertension
lipid disorders
Mediterranean dietary pattern
metabolic syndrome
obesity
orthostatic hypotension
physical deconditioning
physical inactivity
plaques
postprandial hypotension
pseudohypertension
stepped-care approach
white coat hypertension

The cardiovascular system helps maintain homeostasis by bringing oxygen and nutrients to organs and tissues, and by transporting carbon dioxide and other waste products to other body systems for removal. Because the cardiovascular system has a tremendous adaptive capacity, healthy older adults will not experience any significant change in cardiovascular performance because of age-related changes alone. However, in the presence of risk factors, the cardiovascular system is less efficient in performing life-sustaining activities and serious negative functional consequences can occur.

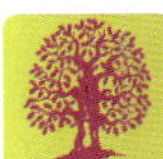

AGE-RELATED CHANGES THAT AFFECT CARDIOVASCULAR FUNCTION

As with many aspects of physiological function, it is difficult to determine whether cardiovascular changes are attributable to normal ageing or other factors. Knowledge about distinct age- or disease-related changes in cardiovascular function is confounded by the fact that, until recently, there was no technology to detect asymptomatic pathological cardiovascular processes, such as the occlusion of a major coronary artery. Some conclusions from earlier studies may have attributed pathological changes to normal ageing. A study using newer diagnostic techniques found that 36% and 39% of men and women, respectively, have subclinical coronary heart disease and only 12.6% of people aged 85 years or older have neither clinical nor subclinical disease (Cademartiri et al., 2008). Currently, many studies of age-related changes are longitudinal and include subjects who have been carefully screened for asymptomatic cardiovascular disease.

In addition, because sociocultural factors affect cardiovascular function, it is difficult to draw conclusions about lifestyle factors that affect entire societies. Systolic blood pressure, for example, increases gradually in adults who live in Western societies but not in those from less industrialised societies. Therefore, changes that have been attributed to increased age may, in fact, be related to lifestyle, sociocultural factors or pathological conditions. Cross-cultural studies are now being used to identify the effects of lifestyle and other sociocultural factors that affect cardiovascular function. A major focus of research is on identifying those risk factors that are most amenable to interventions so that evidence-based interventions can be recommended.

Myocardium and neuroconduction mechanisms

Age-related changes of the myocardium include amyloid deposits, lipofuscin accumulation, basophilic degeneration, myocardial atrophy or hypertrophy, valvular thickening and stiffening and increased amounts of connective tissue. The left ventricular wall becomes slightly enlarged in healthy older adults, but any significant myocardial atrophy that occurs is due to pathological processes. In addition, the left atrium enlarges, even in healthy older adults. Other age-related changes include thickening of the atrial endocardium, thickening of the atrioventricular valves and calcification of at least part of the mitral

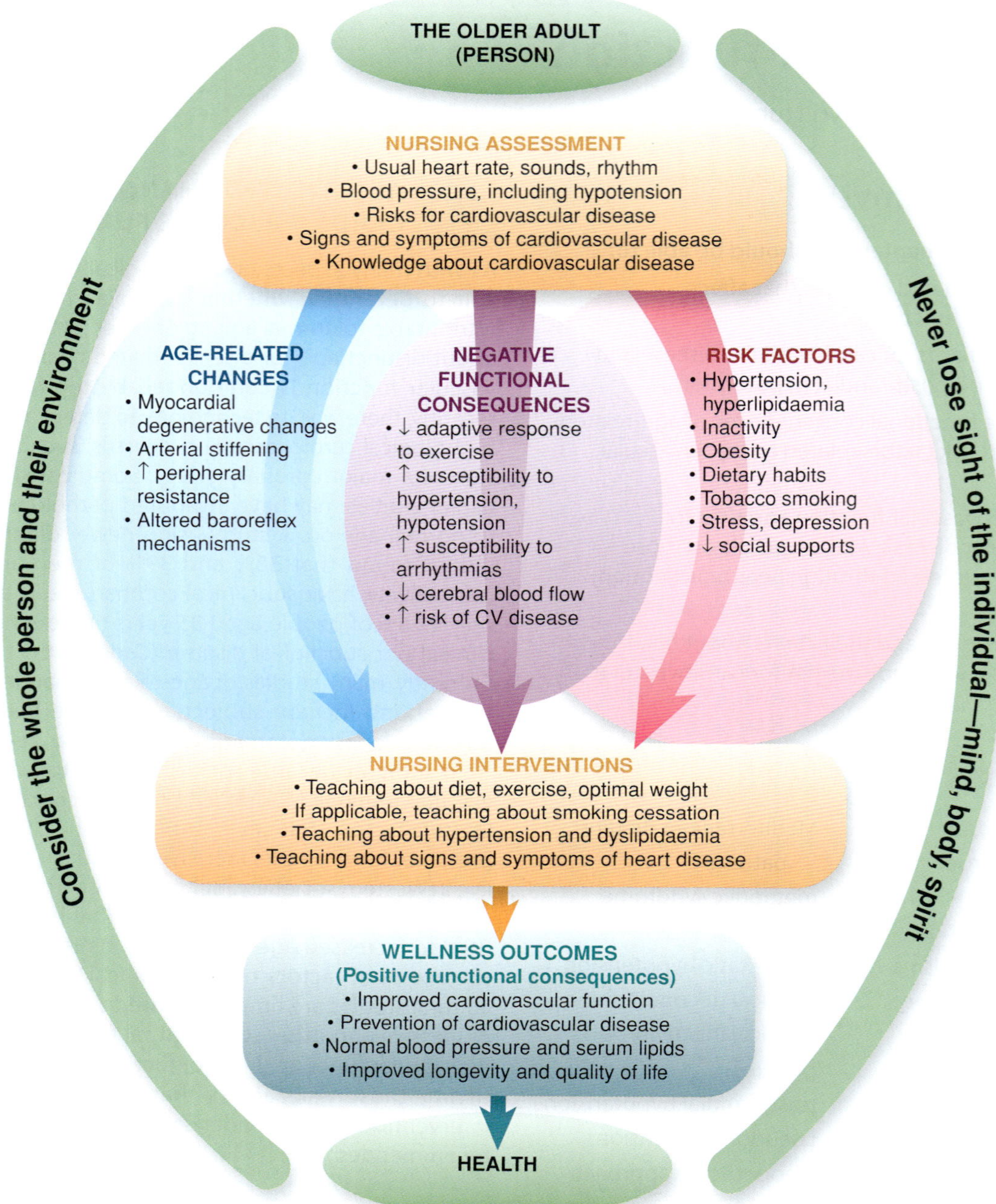

annulus of the aortic valve. These changes interfere with the ability of the heart to contract completely. With less effective contractility, more time is required to complete the cycle of diastolic filling and systolic emptying. In addition, the myocardium becomes increasingly irritable and less responsive to the impulses from the sympathetic nervous system.

Age-related changes in cardiac physiology are minimal and the changes that do occur affect cardiac performance only under conditions of physiological stress. Even under stressful conditions, the heart in healthy older adults is able to adapt, but the adaptive mechanisms may differ from those of younger adults or be slightly less efficient. The age-related changes that cause functional consequences primarily involve the electrophysiology of the heart (i.e. the neuro-conduction system) and these include a decrease in the number of pacemaker cells; increased irregularity in the shape of pacemaker cells; and increased deposits of fat, collagen and elastic fibres around the sinoatrial node.

Vasculature

Age-related changes affect two of the three vascular layers and functional consequences vary, depending on which layer is affected. For example, changes in the tunica intima (innermost layer) have the most serious functional consequences in the development of atherosclerosis, whereas changes in the tunica media (middle layer) are associated with hypertension. The tunica externa (outermost layer) does not seem to be affected by age-related changes. This layer, composed of loosely meshed adipose and connective tissue, supports nerve fibres and the vasa vasorum, the blood supply for the tunica media.

The tunica intima consists of a single layer of endothelial cells on a thin layer of connective tissue. It controls the entry of lipids and other substances from the blood into the artery wall. Intact endothelial cells allow blood to flow freely without clotting; however, when the endothelial cells are damaged, they function in the clotting process. With increasing age, the tunica intima thickens because of fibrosis, cellular proliferation and lipid and calcium accumulation. In addition, the endothelial cells become irregular in size and shape. These changes cause the arteries to dilate and elongate. As a result, the arterial walls are more vulnerable to atherosclerosis (see section on risk factors).

The tunica media is composed of single or multiple layers of smooth muscle cells surrounded by elastin and collagen. The smooth muscle cells are involved in the tissue-forming functions of producing collagen, proteoglycans and elastic fibres. Because it provides structural support, this layer controls arterial expansion and contraction. Age-related changes that affect the tunica media include an increase in collagen and a thinning and calcification of elastin fibres, resulting in stiffened blood vessels. These changes are particularly pronounced in the aorta, where the diameter of the lumen increases to compensate for the age-related arterial stiffening. Although these changes are viewed as age related, longitudinal and cross-cultural studies are raising questions about the impact of lifestyle variables on arterial stiffness.

Age-related changes in the tunica media cause increased peripheral resistance, impaired baroreceptor function and diminished ability to increase blood flow to vital organs. Although these changes do not cause serious consequences in healthy older adults, they increase the resistance to blood flow from the heart so that the left ventricle is forced to work harder. Moreover, the baroreceptors in the large arteries become less effective in controlling blood pressure, especially during postural changes. Overall, the increased vascular stiffness causes a slight increase in the systolic blood pressure.

Veins undergo changes similar to those affecting the arteries, but to a lesser degree. Veins become thicker, more dilated and less elastic with increasing age. Valves of the large leg veins become less efficient in returning blood to the heart. Peripheral circulation is further influenced by an age-related reduction in muscle mass and a concurrent reduction in the demand for oxygen.

Baroreflex mechanisms

Baroreflex mechanisms are physiological processes that regulate blood pressure by increasing or decreasing the heart rate and peripheral vascular resistance to compensate for transient decreases or increases in arterial pressure. Age-related changes that alter baroreflex mechanisms include arterial stiffening and reduced cardiovascular responsiveness to adrenergic stimulation. These changes cause a blunting of the compensatory response to both hypertensive and hypotensive stimuli in older adults, so the heart rate does not increase or decrease as efficiently as in younger adults.

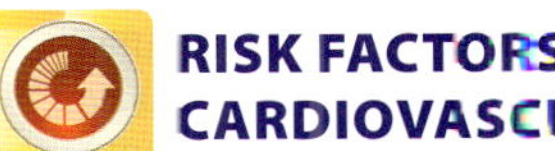

RISK FACTORS THAT AFFECT CARDIOVASCULAR FUNCTION

Many factors affect cardiovascular function by increasing the risk for heart disease, which has been the leading cause of death in Australia and New Zealand for almost a century. Heart disease, or **cardiovascular disease**, refers to all pathological processes that affect the heart and circulatory system, including specific disease entities such as coronary heart disease (also called coronary artery disease), arrhythmias, atherosclerosis, heart failure, myocardial infarction, peripheral vascular disease, venous thromboembolism, stroke and transient ischaemic attacks. Stroke (also called "brain attack" or cerebrovascular disease) and transient ischaemic attacks are not considered cardiovascular diseases in this text. Rather, they are considered neurovascular diseases and, as a consequence, are not addressed in this chapter.

Researchers, health planners and healthcare providers are concerned about risks for cardiovascular disease not only because of its significant prevalence and mortality rate but also because it poses a heavy economic burden. Most importantly from a wellness perspective, there is mounting evidence that most cardiovascular disease is preventable through modification of risk factors (Foxcy, 2008). Therefore, this is a major focus of health promotion efforts, including education and motivation for behaviour change.

Modifiable conditions associated with the highest risk for cardiovascular disease include physical inactivity, elevated blood pressure, obesity, tobacco smoking, dyslipidaemia and excessive alcohol consumption (Smith, Collins, Ferrari et al., 2012). These conditions can be addressed through medical management and health promotion interventions, as discussed in this chapter and in Chapters 21 (smoking cessation) and 27 (diabetes). In addition, evidence-based dietary measures include limited intake of foods with sodium or saturated fats and increased intake of fruits, vegetables and all plant-based foods.

Some risk factors such as age, race, gender and heredity cannot be modified, but it is important to consider their influence on the overall risk profile. In recent years there is increasing recognition that race and gender can affect both the risk for developing cardiovascular disease and the chance of having adverse outcomes. For example, there is strong evidence of health inequalities associated with increased prevalence and poorer management of heart disease and related risk factors in women (Weiss, 2009), Indigenous Australians (Heart Foundation, 2015) and Māori and Pacific people (Jayathissa et al., 2010). Socioeconomic and psychosocial factors, which are particularly relevant to a holistic health promotion approach to care of older adults, also affect the risk profile for heart disease.

DIVERSITY NOTE

The average age of a person having a first major cardiovascular event is 65.8 years in men and 70.4 years in women (Berra, 2008). At age 40, the lifetime risk for cardiovascular disease in men is 67% and for women it is 50%. By the age of 85 years, the risk is equal in men and women (Berra, 2008).

Atherosclerosis

Atherosclerosis is a disorder of the medium and small arteries in which patchy deposits of lipids and atherosclerotic **plaques** reduce or obstruct blood flow. It is the major cause of cardiovascular deaths (Lewis, 2009). Because atherosclerosis is the underlying pathological process associated with most cardiovascular disease, the term *atherosclerotic cardiovascular disease* is sometimes used (see discussion on pathological conditions for details). Several theories about the pathophysiology of atherosclerosis have been proposed since the mid-1970s and our understanding of atherosclerosis has increased significantly in recent years due to the use of more sophisticated imaging techniques. It is now understood that atherosclerosis is a pathological condition that begins during childhood with asymptomatic but identifiable changes and progresses through adulthood to the point that it is found in 80% to 90% of adults aged 30 years and older (Lewis, 2009).

Atherosclerosis involves a continuum of changes in the arterial wall that develop in the following sequence (Insull, 2009):

1. *Early fatty streak development during childhood and adolescence:* low-density lipoprotein (LDL) cholesterol particles accumulate in the arterial intima and initiate an inflammatory response.
2. *Early fibroatheroma phase during teens and 20s:* (a) macrophage "foam cells" and other inflammatory cells accumulate; (b) some protective responses are initiated but necrotic debris causes further inflammation; (c) extracellular lipids accumulate and form lipid-rich necrotic cores that occupy 30% to 50% of the arterial wall volume; (d) a fibrous cap, called a plaque, forms over the necrotic core under the endothelium.
3. *Advancing atheroma at 55 years and older:* (a) fibrous cap in a few sites becomes thin and weakened; (b) the thin-capped fibroatheroma is susceptible to rupturing and causing a life-threatening thrombosis; (c) if fibroatheroma does not rupture, it may enlarge and further reduce the arterial lumen; (d) as long as the plaque does not occupy more than 40% of the lumen, the arterial walls can expand to compensate, but if the plaque occupies more arterial space, symptoms result; (e) diseased artery may leak within the arterial wall and provoke further fibrous tissue.

In summary, atherosclerotic changes begin in childhood and can progress to plaque formation. Atherosclerosis is a systemic disease process that develops in many arteries but may be more concentrated in some parts of the body, such as the coronary or carotid arteries (Go, Mozaffarian, Roger et al., 2014). Plaque lesions, which can rupture, remain stable or continue to grow, are the underlying cause of most cardiovascular disease. When coronary arteries are affected, sudden death is the primary consequence in 50% of men and 64% of women (Castellon & Bogdanova, 2013). It is important to identify and address risk factors before symptoms are experienced. All the risk factors associated with cardiovascular disease, as described in this section, are risks for the development and progression of atherosclerosis. In Australia, high cholesterol levels were reported for 6% in the year 2007–08 with the prevalence highest for those in the 65 age groups (19% and 16% respectively) (Australian Bureau of Statistics [ABS], 2012).

Physical inactivity

Physical inactivity (also called **physical deconditioning**) is a factor that not only increases the risk for cardiovascular disease for all people but also diminishes cardiovascular function in healthy older adults. Even in the absence of pathological processes, inadequate patterns of physical activity will interfere with the ability of older adults to adapt to age-related cardiovascular changes. Evidence-based guidelines state that the risk for cardiovascular disease is increased in people who have fewer than 30 minutes of moderate physical activity at least 5 days weekly or 20 minutes of vigorous physical activity at least 3 days weekly. Although older adults are likely to have conditions that make it difficult to obtain adequate physical activity, even 75 minutes a week of light physical activity can reduce cardiovascular risk by as much as 14% (Barnes, 2012). Conditions that often occur in older adults and contribute to physical deconditioning include acute illness, a sedentary lifestyle, mobility limitations, any chronic condition that interferes with physical activity, and psychosocial influences such as depression or lack of motivation.

National data indicate that 72% of Australians aged 15 years and over did not participate in sufficient physical activity. Physical inactivity was lowest in younger adults, 65%, and highest in older adults aged 75 years and over, 84% (Australian Institute Health & Welfare [AIHW], 2011). Data also suggest that the proportions of people who are physically inactive are increasing. An international survey about physical activity revealed that the Australian population scored similarly to the U.S., but that New Zealand was significantly lower, at 40%. There are 14 risk factors for cardiovascular disease, and physical activity is ranked the fourth highest and contributes to 10% of the total burden of this disease in Australia.

DIVERSITY NOTE

Physical inactivity is higher in women than in men across all age groups (AIHW, 2011)

Tobacco smoking and second-hand smoke

Tobacco smoking is a major avoidable cause of cardiovascular disease, and there is indisputable evidence that all forms of tobacco (i.e. smoking tobacco, using smokeless tobacco products, or exposure to second-hand smoke) increase the risk for cardiovascular disease and mortality (Go, Mozaffarian, Roger et al., 2014):

- There is a dose-dependent relationship between increased risk for cardiovascular disease and exposure to cigarette smoke.
- Current smokers have a two to four times increased risk of stroke compared with non-smokers or those who have quit for more than 10 years.
- Risk ratio for smokers to non-smokers for developing coronary heart disease was 25% higher for women than men.
- Non-smokers exposed to second-hand smoke increased their risk of developing coronary heart disease by 25% to 30%.
- Male and female smokers shorten their average life expectancy by 13.2 and 14.5 years, compared with non-smokers.

Tobacco smoking was responsible for 8% of the burden of cardiovascular disease in Australia (AIHW, 2011). Heart, stroke and vascular disease was also more prevalent in Australian adults who had ever smoked (8%) than those who had never smoked (5%) (ABS 2012).

Australia is ranked second and New Zealand third lowest percentage of population who smoke daily compared with other developed countries. There have been significant declines in older adults who smoke in the last decade (ABS, 2013a; New Zealand Ministry of Health, 2014). Effects of smoking on the cardiovascular system include acceleration of atherosclerotic processes, increased systolic blood pressure, elevated LDL cholesterol level, and decreased high-density lipoprotein (HDL) cholesterol level. Even short exposures to second-hand smoke increase the risk of a heart attack because of immediate adverse effects on the heart, blood and vascular systems. These cardiovascular effects are in addition to the effects of nicotine on respiratory function (see Chapter 21) and other aspects of health (e.g. increased risk for development of cataracts and many cancers).

Dietary habits

Randomised controlled trials confirm that dietary habits can increase many risk factors for cardiovascular disease, including weight, blood pressure, glucose levels, and lipoprotein and triglyceride levels. A review of studies summarised the following findings related to dietary habits and cardiovascular health (Go, Mozaffarian, Roger et al., 2014):

- Replacing saturated fat with polyunsaturated fat reduced cardiovascular risk by 10% for each 5% reduction in energy exchange.
- Each 2% of kilojoules from trans fats was associated with a 23% higher risk of coronary heart disease.
- Intake of 2.5 servings daily of whole grains was associated with a 21% lower risk of cardiovascular disease when compared with 0.2 servings daily.
- When compared with little or no consumption of fish or fish oil, consumption of one to two servings per week of oily fish was associated with a 36% lower risk of cardiovascular mortality.
- Each daily serving of fruits or vegetables was associated with a 4% lower risk of coronary heart disease and 5% lower risk of stroke.
- Low-sodium interventions were associated with a 25% lower risk of cardiovascular disease after 10 to 15 years of follow-up.

The section on nursing interventions provides teaching information about dietary patterns that are most effective for preventing cardiovascular disease.

Obesity

Obesity in adults, which is defined by body mass index (BMI) ≥ 30 kg/m^2, is associated with increased risk for many pathological conditions including stroke, diabetes, lipid disorders, atherosclerosis, hypertension and coronary heart disease. In recent years, increasing attention is being paid to **abdominal obesity** (also called *abdominal adiposity*) as an independent risk factor for cardiovascular disease. Abdominal obesity, defined as a waist circumference more than 102 cm and 88 cm or waist-to-hip ratio of 0.95 and 0.88 for men and women, respectively, can occur even in people with normal BMI. Significant evidence indicates that abdominal adipose tissue is biologically and metabolically different from subcutaneous fat and a risk factor for mortality from cardiovascular disease, even among normal-weight women.

Rates of overweight and obesity in Australia generally increased with age, peaking at 65–74 years for both men and women (see Figure 20-1) (ABS, 2013b). Box 20-1 contains information about older adults and obesity in New Zealand.

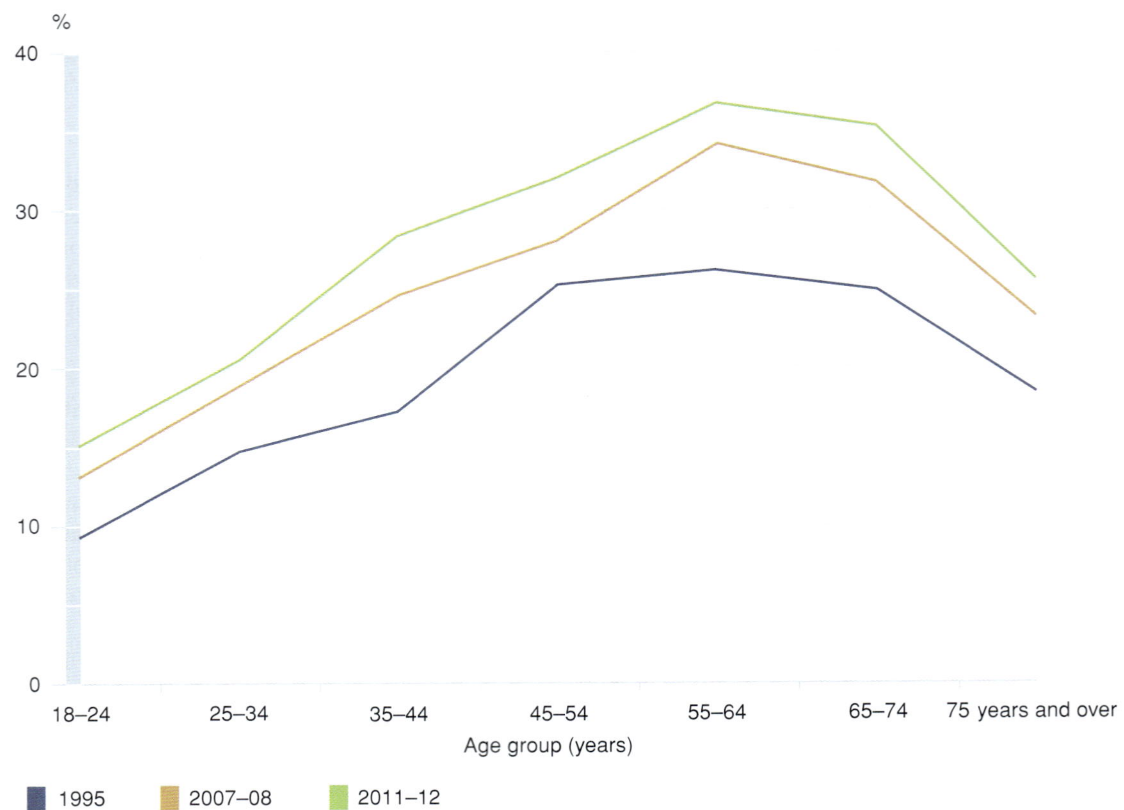

FIGURE 20-1 Rates of obesity in Australia for age over time. (Australian Bureau of Statistics. [2013b]. Overweight and obesity. In Australian Health Survey: Updated results, 2011–2012. Cat. no. 4364.0.55.003. Canberra: Author. Permission granted under a Creative Commons BY 2.5 [CC BY 2.5 AU] licence.)

> **BOX 20-1**
> **Obesity and older adults in New Zealand**
>
> Prevalence of obesity among community-living older adults in New Zealand is the highest for the 65–74 age group. The 75-and-over age group is lower but it has the greatest gender difference, with 29.7% for women and 25.8% for men (Statistics New Zealand, 2014).

Hypertension

Hypertension is a disease of the cardiovascular system, and it is also an independent risk factor for additional cardiovascular diseases, including coronary artery disease, ischaemic stroke, peripheral arterial disease and heart failure.

Risk factors for the development of hypertension include age, ethnicity, genetic factors, overweight, physical inactivity, sleep apnoea, psychosocial stressors, and lower education and socioeconomic status. In addition, dietary patterns that increase the risk for hypertension include higher intake of fats and sodium, lower potassium intake, and excessive alcohol consumption (Go, Mozaffarian, Roger et al., 2014).

The latest Australian Heart Foundation's guide to management of hypertension 2008 (revised 2010) recommends a classification of hypertension by stages to emphasise the risk of any degree of high blood pressure as a factor in cardiovascular disease (Heart Foundation, 2010). The following list describes some blood pressure classifications for adults (Heart Foundation, 201), but the complete guide can be accessed via www.heartfoundation.org.au. These guidelines are also currently in use in New Zealand (New Zealand Guidelines Group, 2012):

- *Normal:* <120 mm Hg systolic; <80 mm Hg diastolic
- *Grade 1 (mild) hypertension:* 140–159 mm Hg systolic; 90–99 mm Hg diastolic
- *Grade 2 (moderate) hypertension:* 160–179 mm Hg systolic; 100–109 mm Hg diastolic
- *Grade 3 (severe) hypertension:* ≥180 mm Hg systolic; ≥110 mm Hg diastolic
- *Isolated systolic hypertension:* ≥140 mm Hg systolic; <90 mm Hg diastolic.

However, new Australian guidelines for the management of hypertension are expected that will incorporate the latest guideline from the European organisation, the National Institute for Health and Care Excellence (NICE) (Box 20-2). The NICE guideline supports the reduction in target blood-pressure levels. This is consistent with the research findings about treatment thresholds for adults older than 80 years, which suggest a target of

BOX 20-2
BP targets and recommendations for older adults

- Aim for a target clinic blood pressure below 140/90 mm Hg in people aged under 80 years, with treated hypertension.
- Aim for a target clinic blood pressure below 150/90 mm Hg in people aged 80 years and over, with treated hypertension.
- When using ABPM or HBPM to monitor response to treatment (e.g. in people identified as having a "white coat effect" and people who choose to monitor their blood pressure at home), aim for a target average blood pressure during the person's usual waking hours of:
  - below 135/85 mm Hg for people aged under 80 years
  - below 145/85 mm Hg for people aged 80 years and over.

Source: National Institute for Health and Care Excellence (NICE) (2011). *Hypertension: Clinical management of primary hypertension in adults.* London: Author. Accessed via www.nice.org.uk.

150/90 mm Hg or less (Oliva & Bakris, 2012; Weber, Schiffrin, White et al., 2014).

Lipid disorders

Lipid disorders (also called *dyslipidaemias* or *hyperlipidaemias*) is a broad term that encompasses all abnormalities of lipoprotein metabolism, including low levels of HDLs (often referred to as "good cholesterol") and elevated levels of total cholesterol, triglycerides or LDL (often referred to as "bad cholesterol"). Public awareness of the importance of testing for lipid disorders has increased since the early 1980s, when *cholesterol* and *saturated fat* became household words. By the 1990s numerous studies began confirming a positive association between lipoprotein levels and coronary heart disease and there was widespread support for cholesterol screening for all adults.

The latest guidelines about risk assessment for lipids and lipid management have been produced by the National Vascular Disease Prevention Alliance (NVDPA) (2012). This evidence-based guideline emphasises the value of screening for and treating lipid disorders in adults.

Although there is much scientific support for addressing lipid disorders as a risk for cardiovascular disease, questions have been raised about the value of cholesterol screening and treatment for older adults, particularly for those older than 80 years and those who have no cardiovascular disease. According to guidelines, screening for lipid disorders is appropriate for older people who had never been evaluated, but repeated screening is less important for older adults who have normal levels because lipid levels are not likely to change after age 65 (National Heart Foundation of Australia [NHFA] and the Cardiac Society of Australia and New Zealand [CSANZ], 2005). For adults over 74 years it is recommended that clinical judgement be utilised in deciding if treatment is suitable. Consideration of the older adult's risks and benefits of treatment, comorbidities and lipid values is required (NVDPA, 2012).

See the Evidence-based practice 20-1 that summarises pertinent information about preventing cardiovascular disease.

Metabolic syndrome

Metabolic syndrome (also called insulin resistance syndrome) refers to a group of clinically identifiable conditions that double the risk of cardiovascular disease and increase

EVIDENCE-BASED PRACTICE 20-1
Practices related to the prevention of cardiovascular disease

Statement of the problem
- Significant advances have been made in preventing and treating cardiovascular disease through medical interventions. However, diet and lifestyle therapies—which are commonly neglected—remain the foundation of clinical intervention for prevention.

Recommendations for nursing assessment
- Assess health-related behaviours pertinent to cardiovascular health: dietary patterns, weight, level of physical activity and smoking.

Recommendations for nursing care
- Calculate BMI and discuss with the person.
- Advocate a healthy dietary pattern consistent with recommendations.
- Encourage regular physical activity.
- Discourage smoking among non-smoking adults and encourage smoking cessation among those who do smoke.

Health promotion: Teaching points for older adults and carers/caregivers
- Consume an overall healthful diet: variety of fruits, vegetables and grains, especially whole grains; choose fat-free and low-fat dairy products, legumes, poultry and lean meats; eat fish, preferably oily fish at least twice weekly; limit intake of saturated and trans fat and cholesterol; limit intake of foods and beverages that have added sugar; select nutrient-dense foods.
- Aim for a healthy BMI of 18.5 to 26 kg/m^2.
- Aim for optimal lipid profile: TC <4.0 mmol/L, HDL-C ≥1.0 mmol/L; LDL-C <2.0 mmol/L; Non HDL-C <2.5 mmol/L and TG <2.0 mmol/L.
- Aim for normal blood pressure: systolic blood pressure, 120 mm Hg and diastolic blood pressure, <80 mm Hg.
- Adopt dietary modifications that lower blood pressure: reduced salt intake, increased potassium intake, kilojoule deficit to induce weight loss, moderation of alcohol intake for those who drink.
- Aim for fasting blood glucose level 5.5 mmol/L.
- Be physically active: accumulate 30 minutes of physical activity most days of the week and at least 60 minutes most days of the week for people attempting to lose weight or maintain weight loss.
- Avoid use of and exposure to tobacco products.

Sources: National Vascular Disease Prevention Alliance (NVDPA) (2012). Quick reference guide for health professionals: Absolute cardiovascular disease risk management. Accessed via http://strokefoundation.com.au.

the risk of diabetes by fivefold regardless of ethnic diversity (Setayeshgar, Whiting & Vatanparast, 2013). The presence of at least three of the following five metabolic risk factors constitutes the diagnosis of metabolic syndrome:

- Abdominal obesity, defined as waist circumference of over 102 cm in men or 88 cm in women from European/North American descent (see the diversity note regarding ethnic groups and waist circumference).
- Blood pressure equal to or higher than 130/85 mm Hg;
- HDL cholesterol level less than 1.0 mmol/L in men or equal to or lower than 1.3 mmol/L in women, or drug treatment for a lipid disorder;
- Triglyceride levels of 1.7 mmol/L or more, or specific treatment for hypertriglyceridaemia;
- Fasting blood glucose level of 5.5 mmol/L or more, or drug treatment for increased glucose levels.

This combination of conditions is a "call to action" to address underlying lifestyle-related risks factors and manage all contributing factors (Go, Mozaffarian, Roger et al., 2014).

DIVERSITY NOTE

Recommended waist circumference varies with ethnic group as a criterion for the metabolic syndrome:

Ethnic group	Men	Women
European/North American	≥102 cm	≥88 cm
Asian	≥90 cm	≥80 cm
Central and South American	≥90 cm	≥80 cm
Middle Eastern/Mediterranean	≥94 cm	≥80 cm
Sub-Saharan African	≥94 cm	≥80 cm

(Harris, 2013)

Psychosocial factors

Psychosocial factors that are associated with increased risk for developing cardiovascular disease include stress, anxiety, depression, social isolation, poor social supports, and personality characteristics such as higher anger and hostility indices. A review of studies found that one-third of the attributable risk of acute myocardial infarction is associated with psychosocial factors such as major life events or depression, or stress related to work, family or finances (Prata, Ramos, Martins et al., 2014). Studies have identified the following associations between psychosocial factors and risk for cardiovascular disease:

- Stress, anger, anxiety and depressed mood are modifiable risk factors for both acute and chronic cardiovascular conditions (Kim & Cho, 2013; Thurston, Rewak & Kubzansky, 2013).
- Loneliness, depression, social isolation and work-related stress are specific stressors linked to increased risk of coronary heart disease (Neylon, Canniffe, Anand et al., 2013; Steptoe & Kivimaki, 2013).
- Chronic feelings of anger, cynical distrust and antagonistic behaviour may increase the risk of onset and progression of cardiovascular disease (Suls, 2013).
- Poor social support increases the risk for depression in people with heart failure, which affects up to 50% of these people (Friedmann, Son, Thomas et al., 2014; Graven & Grant, 2012).

Researchers have explored the relationship between depression and cardiovascular disease but the cause-effect relationship remains unclear, particularly with regard to whether depression is a risk for first-time coronary events. Many studies show there is a high prevalence of depression in people with symptomatic cardiovascular disease and that it is an independent risk for recurrent cardiovascular events and poorer prognosis after the first coronary event (Colquhoun, Bunker, Clarke et al., 2013). For example, prevalence of depression in people hospitalised with acute coronary syndrome is three times higher than in the general population (Frazier, Sanner, Yu et al., 2013). Moreover, depression after cardiac surgery is a major cause of death and decreased functional status and its effects are long lasting, with deaths increasing for up to 10 years after surgery (Doering, Chen, Bodan et al., 2013). Because of the close association between depression and chronic cardiovascular disease (e.g. heart failure) or a history of a major cardiovascular event (e.g. myocardial infarction), it is important to routinely screen for depression in this population.

Heredity and socioeconomic factors

Heredity plays a significant role in the risk for developing cardiovascular disease. Large population-based studies show a strong link between reported history of premature parental coronary heart disease and cardiovascular disease, including atherosclerosis and myocardial infarction, in offspring (Lloyd-Jones et al., 2009). Although inherited conditions cannot be changed, people who are aware of having these risk factors may be more motivated to address modifiable risks.

The relationship between socioeconomic status and cardiovascular disease has been a focus of research for several decades. Australians in the lowest socioeconomic groups had a higher prevalence of cardiovascular disease than those in the highest socioeconomic groups (AIHW, 2011). Although income and education are not easily modified, it is important to recognise that these conditions influence not only the risk for cardiovascular disease but also the use of preventive and interventional measures. From a holistic perspective, nurses need to consider these factors when planning health education interventions to address individualised needs of older adults.

Risk for cardiovascular disease in women and minority groups

Because cardiovascular disease was viewed as a disease of middle-aged men, early research focused primarily or exclusively on men. This perspective began changing during the 1990s when studies showed that, although the prevalence of cardiovascular disease is lower in younger women than younger men, it increases dramatically after the age of 50 years in women.

There has also been an increasing focus on the disproportionate burden of cardiovascular-related death and disability among minority populations. National data from Australia and New Zealand show that Indigenous Australians and Māori and Pacific people experience higher rates of hypertension and have a higher risk of heart disease than other Australians and New Zealanders (Heart Foundation, 2015; Jayathissa et al., 2010). In addition, Indigenous Australians, Māori and Pacific people are more likely than other groups to have risk factors such as diabetes, obesity, hypertension and lipid disorders. For these ethnic groups it is recommended that risk assessment be commenced 10 years earlier than for others; that is, at 35 years rather than 45 years.

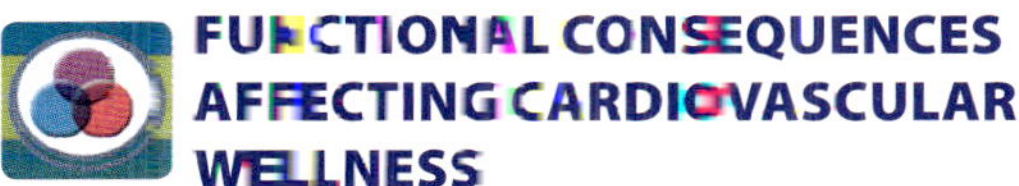

FUNCTIONAL CONSEQUENCES AFFECTING CARDIOVASCULAR WELLNESS

Healthy older adults experience no significant cardio-vascular effects when they are resting, but, when they engage in exercise, their cardiovascular function is less efficient. However, older adults who have risk factors for cardiovascular disease are likely to experience negative functional consequences associated with pathological processes. This section reviews the functional consequences in older adults who have no risk factors and then examines nursing assessment and interventions that focus on preventable risk factors that commonly affect cardiovascular function. It is not the intention of this chapter to address the functional consequences of all cardiovascular disease. Only two cardiovascular conditions are discussed here in this section because nurses have a key role in the identification and management of hypotension and heart failure for older adults.

Effects on cardiac function

Cardiac output, the amount of blood pumped by the heart per minute, is an important measure of cardiac performance because it represents the heart's ability to meet the oxygen requirements of the body. Although reduced cardiac output is common in older adults, it is associated primarily with pathological, rather than age-related, conditions. With the exception of a slight decrease in cardiac output at rest in older women, healthy older adults do not experience any decline in cardiac output.

Effects on pulse and blood pressure

Normal pulse rate for healthy older adults is slightly lower than that for younger adults, but older adults are likely to have harmless ventricular and supraventricular arrhythmias because of age-related changes that affect cardiac conduction mechanism. *Atrial fibrillation*—a more serious arrhythmia—commonly occurs in older adults, but this is associated with pathological conditions (e.g. hypertension, coronary artery disease) rather than with age-related changes. In most populations across the world, there is an age-related linear increase in systolic blood pressure from age 30 to 40 years and this change is steeper for women than for men. There is also a progressive decrease in diastolic pressure beginning around age 60 years (Williams, Lindholm & Sever, 2008).

Effects on the response to exercise

A negative functional consequence that affects cardiovascular performance in healthy older adults is a blunted **adaptive response** to physical exercise. Physiological stress, such as that associated with exercise, increases the demands on the cardiovascular system by four to five times the basal level. The adaptive response involves many aspects of physiological function, including the respiratory, cardiovascular, musculoskeletal and autonomic nervous systems. The maximum heart rate achieved during exercise is markedly decreased and the peak exercise capacity and oxygen consumption decline in older adults. Physical deconditioning and other risk factors account for some of this decline. Similarly, studies confirm that maximum oxygen uptake during exercise decreases with ageing but are affected to a greater extent by risk factors, such as prolonged bed rest (McGavock et al., 2009).

Effects on circulation

Functional consequences can also affect circulation to the brain and the lower extremities. For example, age-related changes in cardiovascular and baroreflex mechanisms can reduce cerebral blood flow to some extent in healthy older adults and to a greater extent in older adults who have diabetes, hypertension, lipid disorders and heart disease. In addition, increased tortuosity and dilation of the veins, along with decreased efficiency of the valves, lead to impaired venous return from the lower extremities. Consequently, older adults are prone to developing stasis oedema of the feet and ankles and they are more likely to develop venous stasis ulcers.

UNFOLDING CASE STUDY

Part A

Mr Constantine is a 6[illegible]-year-old Italian immigrant. He has been taking hydrochlorothiazide, 25 mg, and verapamil, 120 mg, every morning, and his blood pressures range between 126/80 and 130/84 mm Hg. Mr Constantine sees his medical practitioner monthly for health check-ups. Mr Constantine's 86-year-old mother recently died of a cerebrovascular accident, and his father died in his early 50s of a heart attack. Mr Constantine has had hypertension since he was 24, and both of his daughters have high blood pressure as well. Neither Mr Constantine nor anyone in the household smokes tobacco. He gets very little exercise and weighs 95 kilograms, about 14 kilograms more than his ideal weight. He reports that he "gets winded easily" when walking up or down a flight of steps or when he has to walk "a long distance" (which he defines as the distance across the car park to the medical centre). He attributes this to "getting old".

Thinking points

- What age-related changes in cardiovascular function is Mr Constantine likely to be experiencing?
- What risk factors are likely to be contributing to Mr Constantine's experience of "getting winded"?
- What risk factors does Mr Constantine have for cardiovascular disease?
- What further information would you want to obtain for assessing his risk for cardiovascular disease?

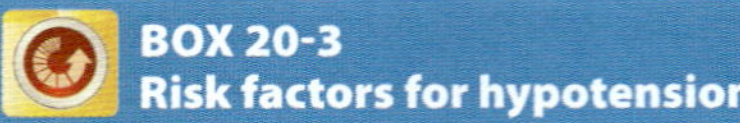

BOX 20-3
Risk factors for hypotension

Risks for orthostatic hypotension

Pathological processes

- Hypertension, including isolated systolic hypertension
- Parkinson's disease
- Cerebrovascular disorders
- Diabetes
- Anaemia
- Autonomic dysfunction
- Arrhythmias
- Volume depletion (e.g. dehydration)
- Electrolyte imbalances (e.g. hyponatraemia, hypokalaemia)

Medications

- Antihypertensives
- Anticholinergics
- Phenothiazines
- Antidepressants
- Anti-parkinsonism agents
- Vasodilators
- Diuretics
- Alcohol

Risks for postprandial hypotension

Pathological processes

- Systolic hypertension
- Diabetes mellitus
- Parkinson's disease
- Multisystem atrophy

Medications

- Diuretics
- Antihypertensive medications ingested before meals

PATHOLOGICAL CONDITIONS AFFECTING CARDIOVASCULAR WELLNESS: ORTHOSTATIC POSTPRANDIAL HYPOTENSION AND CHRONIC HEART FAILURE

Hypotension

Orthostatic and postprandial hypotension are conditions that occur in older adults due to a combination of age-related changes (e.g. decreased baroreflex sensitivity) and risk factors (e.g. hypertension and antihypertensive medications). These conditions may be symptomatic or asymptomatic and it clearly is within the realm of nursing to identify hypotension in older adults by assessing lying and standing blood pressure as discussed in the section on nursing assessment. Assessing for these conditions is important because orthostatic and postprandial hypotension occur more frequently in older adults and they can lead to serious consequences, including falls and fall-related injuries.

Orthostatic hypotension (also called postural hypotension) is a reduction in both systolic blood pressure and diastolic blood pressure of at least 20 or 10 mm Hg, respectively, within 3 minutes of standing after being recumbent for at least 5 minutes. Prevalence of orthostatic hypotension ranges from 6% in healthy older adults to 68% of hospitalised older adults (Aung, Corcoran, Nagalingam et al., 2012; Pepersack, Gilles, Petrovic et al., 2013). Orthostatic hypotension is often associated with the risk factors listed in Box 20-3, with an underlying impairment in autonomic response being the most likely common denominator (Aung, Corcoran, Nagalingam et al., 2012; Lagro et al., 2013). The risk can be increased by a combination of conditions such as Parkinson's disease and anti-parkinsonism medications.

Orthostatic hypotension can be asymptomatic (identified by physical assessment) or it can be accompanied by symptoms such as fatigue, lightheadedness, blurred vision, or syncope upon standing. Whether orthostatic hypotension is symptomatic or asymptomatic, it can affect the safety and quality of life and lead to serious negative functional consequences such as increased risk for falls, and the development of cardiovascular problems such as heart failure (van Hateren et al., 2012; Xin, Lin & Li, 2013).

Postprandial hypotension, defined as a systolic blood pressure reduction of 20 mm Hg or more within 2 hours of eating a meal, affects up to two-thirds of older adults and as many as 72.8% of older adults with hypertension (Zanasi, Tincani, Evandri et al., 2012). Impaired autonomic function is the pathophysiological mechanism responsible for postprandial hypotension. Contributing factors include gastrointestinal vasoactive peptides and impaired glucose metabolism, which is often associated with diabetes (Abdel-Rahman, 2012; Fukushima, Asahina, Fujinuma et al., 2013). It is recommended that nurses assess for postprandial hypotension, even in older adults who are in bed, as an important intervention for reducing the incidence of falls, syncope, strokes and other complications (Son & Lee, 2012, 2013).

Promoting wellness for older adults with orthostatic or postprandial hypotension

Interventions aimed at preventing orthostatic and postprandial hypotension can be initiated as health measures for older adults who have any of the risk factors listed in Box 20-3. For older adults with symptomatic orthostatic hypotension, interventions to alleviate the problem are important for maintaining quality of life and preventing serious consequences. In addition, nurses address safety issues by implementing interventions that are directed towards preventing falls and fractures, as discussed in Chapter 22.

For older adults with postprandial hypotension, interventions can be implemented around mealtimes. In institutional or home care settings, registered dietitians may be helpful in developing a plan for addressing postprandial hypotension, but in any setting, nurses assume responsibility for health education about interventions. In older adults with postprandial hypotension, low-carbohydrate meals may be effective in addressing postprandial hypotension. Additional interventions are summarised in Box 20-4, which can be used as a tool for educating older adults about orthostatic and postprandial hypotension.

Chronic heart failure

Chronic heart failure (CHF) "... is a complex clinical syndrome with typical symptoms (e.g. dyspnoea, fatigue) that can occur at rest or on effort, and is characterised by objective evidence of an underlying structural abnormality or cardiac dysfunction that impairs the ability of the ventricle of the heart to fill with reject blood (particularly during physical activity)" (NHFA & CSANZ, 2011, p. 4). The most common causes of heart failure are ischaemic heart disease and hypertension. Heart failure is diagnosed on the presence of clinical features (exertional dyspnoea, dry cough and fatigue), chest x-ray and ventricular function by echocardiography. An individual's blood level of B-type natriuretic peptide (BNP) has a role in diagnosis, but also assists with the determination of the severity of heart failure, the risk of hospitalisation, and survival. Diagnosis may be confirmed by the improvement in symptoms in response to treatment.

The incidence and prevalence of CHF increases with age. For example, prevalence of CHF has been reported at about 1% for those aged 50, about 10% for those age 65 years and older, and over 50% in people aged 85 years and older (NHFA & CSANZ, 2011). Heart failure in older adults over 70 years is one of the most common reasons for medical consultation, admission and readmission into hospitals. It has been estimated that heart failure affects 1.5% to 2% of Australians, and its prevalence is increasing in both Australia and New Zealand (NHFA & CSANZ, 2011). There is also a concern that a significant number of people with heart failure remain undiagnosed.

It is now understood that many of the admissions are potentially preventable with adequate self-care, including medication adherence and monitoring of symptoms (Jurgens et al., 2009). In addition to recurrent hospitalisations, other common consequences of heart failure in older adults include the following:

- Increased likelihood for developing arrhythmias, which can threaten life or cause syncope episodes
- Increased risk for hypotension and falls because of compromised cardiovascular function and adverse medication effects

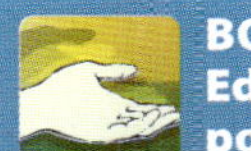

BOX 20-4
Education regarding orthostatic and postprandial hypotension

Preventing and managing orthostatic and postprandial hypotension

- Maintain adequate fluid intake (i.e. eight glasses of non-caffeinated beverages daily).
- Eat five or six smaller meals daily, rather than large meals.
- Avoid excessive alcohol consumption.
- Avoid sitting or standing still for prolonged periods, especially after meals.

Health promotion measures specific to orthostatic hypotension

- Change your position slowly, especially when moving from a sitting or lying position to a standing position.
- Before standing up, sit at the side of the bed for several minutes after rising from a lying position.
- Maintain good physical fitness, especially good muscle tone, and engage in regular, but not excessive exercise. (Swimming is an excellent form of exercise because the hydrostatic pressure prevents blood from pooling in the legs.)
- Wear a waist-high elastic support garment or thigh-high elastic stockings during the day, and put them on before getting out of bed in the morning.
- Sleep with the head of the bed elevated on blocks.
- During the day, rest in a recliner chair with your legs elevated.
- Take measures to prevent constipation and avoid straining during bowel movements.
- Avoid medications that increase the risk for orthostatic hypotension, particularly if additional risk factors are present (refer to Box 20-3).
- Avoid sources of intense heat (e.g. direct sun, electric blankets and hot baths and showers) because these cause peripheral vasodilation.
- If taking glyceryl trinitrate, do not take it while standing.

Health promotion measures specific to postprandial hypotension

- Minimise the risk for postprandial hypotension by taking antihypertensive medications (if prescribed) 1 hour after meals rather than before meals.
- Eat small, low-carbohydrate meals.
- Avoid alcohol consumption.
- Avoid strenuous exercise, especially for 2 hours after meals.

Safety precautions if hypotension cannot be prevented

- Reduce the potential for falls and other negative functional consequences of postprandial hypotension by remaining seated (or by lying down) after meals
- Call for assistance if help is needed with walking.
- Adapt the environment to minimise the risk and consequences of falling (e.g. ensure good lighting, install grab bars, keep pathways clear).

- Increased risk for hospital-acquired iatrogenic conditions
- Increased risk for drug interactions and adverse medication effects, especially if the older adult has concomitant conditions and requires several types of medications
- High incidence of sleep disorders
- Shorter life expectancy.

Because of consequences such as these—which make it a major source of chronic disability, increased mortality and impaired quality of life—heart failure in older adults has emerged as a major focus of health promotion interventions.

Nursing assessment

Nurses assess for signs and symptoms of heart failure in older adults using the same assessment techniques that apply to adults of any age. However, older adults are more likely to have concomitant conditions that can affect the assessment. For example, because older adults with mobility limitations may not exert themselves enough to experience dyspnoea, nurses need to consider other limiting factors when they assess the effects of heart failure on respirations. Nurses need to ask very direct assessment questions about signs and symptoms because older adults have poor symptom recognition and are likely to attribute early symptoms such as fatigue and shortness of breath to normal ageing (Riegel et al., 2010; Jurgens et al., 2009).

Another assessment consideration is that older adults with heart failure are likely to have some degree of chronic renal failure, which often fluctuates within an abnormal range. Thus, nurses need to identify and document the older adult's usual indicators of renal function (i.e. ranges of blood urea nitrogen and creatinine that are typical for that individual). Because older adults with heart failure and renal failure are at increased risk for electrolyte imbalance and adverse medication effects, nurses need to assess for these and other consequences. For example, hyperkalaemia, which can be life-threatening in people with heart failure, can be caused by cardiovascular medications such as angiotensin-converting enzyme (ACE) inhibitors, angiotensin II receptor blockers, and aldosterone antagonists (Poggio, Grancelli & Miriuka, 2010).

In addition to assessing signs and symptoms of heart failure, nurses assess risk factors, paying particular attention to those that can be addressed through health promotion interventions. Factors that increase the risk for heart failure include hypertension, coronary artery disease, myocardial infarction, family history of heart failure, hyperthyroidism, diabetes, smoking and obesity. Even though older adults may have long-term patterns of behaviour that affect disease management (e.g. smoking, inadequate physical activity or high-sodium diets), nurses need to assess attitudes about changing these behaviours so that they can address this in health promotion teaching. Additional wellness-focused assessment considerations that are important for older adults who have heart failure are outlined in Box 20-5.

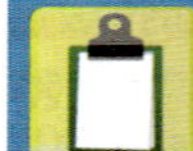

BOX 20-5
Assessment guidelines for older adults with heart failure

Considerations about the meaning of heart failure
- What is the older adult's understanding of heart failure?
- What terminology is appropriate for discussing the condition? Does the term *failure* cause anxiety or fear?
- What personal experiences or those of significant others are influencing the older adult's response to cardiovascular disease? (For example, how life-threatening does the person perceive this to be?)

Considerations regarding the influence of ageist attitudes
- Do ageist attitudes interfere with health promotion interventions? (For example, do healthcare providers avoid teaching about smoking cessation because they think the person is too old to quit or to benefit from quitting?)

Considerations regarding disease management
- Does the older adult have questions or fears about engaging in therapeutic or enjoyable activities (e.g. exercise, swimming, sexual relationships)? If so, would he or she benefit from health education about this?
- Do socioeconomic factors affect disease management (e.g. limited income that interferes with ability to purchase needed medications or healthy foods)?

Wellness nursing issues and wellness outcomes

Nurses can use the wellness nursing issue of willingness for enhanced therapeutic regimen management to promote increased personal responsibility/involvement for management of heart failure, prevention of hospitalisations and other complications. The wellness nursing issue of willingness for enhanced fluid balance might be applicable when older adults with heart failure are interested in learning about actions they can take to improve and maintain fluid and electrolyte balance.

Outcomes that are pertinent to promoting wellness in older adults with heart failure include cardiac disease self-management, energy conservation, health-promoting behaviour, and knowledge about cardiac disease management, avoidance of complications and hospitalisation.

Nursing interventions

Wellness-oriented care plans for older adults with heart failure focus on teaching about actions the person can take to achieve the best possible level of functioning and quality of life despite the chronic condition. For example, nurses can teach older adults about planning appropriate rest and "energy management" techniques to achieve optimum quality of life with limited energy. A systematic review found that health education interventions provided by nurses were beneficial for secondary prevention in heart failure, with regard to lipids, blood pressure, weight loss, physical activity, dietary intake, cigarette smoking psychosocial measures, quality of life and mortality (Allen & Dennison, 2010).

Teaching about symptom recognition is an important aspect of self-care because older adults may not associate signs and symptoms with heart failure. One study found that teaching older adults to keep a symptom diary, including documentation of daily body weights, can be helpful for symptom recognition and self-care (White et al., 2010). From a holistic perspective, nurses also need to address psychosocial consequences associated with heart failure such as fear, anxiety, loneliness and depression (discussed in Chapters 12, 13 & 15).

In addition to providing the usual teaching about medications, nurses caring for older adults with heart failure must monitor signs and symptoms of digoxin toxicity (because there is a very narrow therapeutic range) and provide education about drug interactions and the effect of drugs and other concomitant conditions. For example, non-steroidal anti-inflammatory drugs, including over-the-counter ones, are associated with development of heart failure and can interfere with antihypertensives and ACE inhibitors. One study found that use of non-steroidal anti-inflammatory agents is common among older people with heart failure and may lead to hospitalisations (Muzzarelli et al., 2009).

WELLNESS OPPORTUNITY

Because stress-reduction activities are especially important when older adults have chronic conditions such as heart failure, nurses can suggest relaxation and health promotion activities such as deep breathing, meditation and guided imagery.

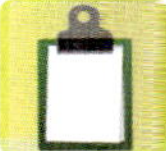

NURSING ASSESSMENT OF CARDIOVASCULAR FUNCTION

From a wellness perspective, nursing assessment of cardiovascular function focuses on identifying risks for cardiovascular disease and the older adult's knowledge about his or her risk profile. Many of these risks can be addressed through health education interventions. Moreover, when older adults would benefit from improving their health-related behaviours (e.g. diet, exercise), nurses need to assess their readiness for changing behaviours, as discussed in Chapter 5. Assessment of physical aspects of cardiovascular function (e.g. heart rate, blood pressure) is similar in older and younger adults, but nurses also need to assess for hypotension. In addition, nursing assessment needs to consider that older adults may have atypical manifestations of cardiovascular disease (e.g. a heart attack).

WELLNESS OPPORTUNITY

Nurses address body–mind–spirit interconnectedness by identifying stress-related factors that increase the risk for cardiovascular disease and encouraging the use of stress management methods, such as meditation.

Assessing baseline cardiovascular function

Physical assessment indicators of cardiovascular function (e.g. peripheral pulses and heart rhythm and sounds) are the same for all healthy adults. Nurses must keep in mind, however, that older adults are more likely to have chronic conditions that affect cardiovascular function. The following findings are common in older adults, but in the absence of symptoms or other abnormal findings, they are usually not indicative of any serious pathological process:

- Auscultation of a fourth heart sound
- Auscultation of short systolic ejection murmurs
- Difficulty percussing heart borders
- Diminished or distant-sounding heart sounds
- Electrocardiographic changes such as arrhythmias, left axis deviation, bundle branch blocks, ST-T wave changes and prolongation of the P-R interval.

If a murmur, arrhythmia or any other unusual finding is detected, it is important to determine whether it reflects a new development, a pre-existing but previously unidentified condition or a pre-existing condition that has already been evaluated. The nurse asks questions to determine the person's awareness of such abnormal findings. Any of the following terms might be used by older adults to describe arrhythmias: fluttering, palpitations, skipped beats, extra beats or flip-flops. It is advisable to ask the older person about a history of arrhythmias before auscultation, because asking immediately after auscultation could cause undue concern.

Arrhythmias may be caused by cardiac diseases, electrolyte imbalances, physiological disturbances or adverse medication effects; alternatively, they may be harmless manifestations of age-related changes. Likewise, murmurs may be caused by age- or disease-related conditions. Therefore, when murmurs or arrhythmias are detected, their significance is assessed in relation to the person's history as well as in relation to the potential underlying causes. It is also important to find out the date of the person's last electrocardiogram because this may provide baseline information regarding the duration of asymptomatic or unrecognised changes.

Assessing blood pressure

Although only a few nurses have primary responsibility for medical management of blood pressure all nurses are responsible for accurate assessment of blood pressure and for decisions regarding the implications of these findings. All nurses need to be familiar with the most current guidelines for detection of hypertension so that health promotion efforts can be directed towards interventions. Despite mounting medical evidence that the identification and management of hypertension has important health benefits, fewer than 40% of people with hypertension achieve good control in community settings (Banegas et al., 2008). Nurses are in a key position to detect hypertension, provide health education and refer older adults for further medical evaluation and treatment.

Accurately assessing blood pressure in older adults may be more difficult than in younger adults for several reasons.

First, blood pressure in older adults is more variable and has an increased tendency to fluctuate in response to postural changes and other factors. In addition, older adults commonly have **pseudohypertension**, which is the phenomenon of elevated systolic blood pressure readings that result from the inability of the external cuff to compress the arteries in older people with arteriosclerosis. This phenomenon explains the finding of extremely elevated systolic blood pressure readings in people without any evidence of end-organ damage and with normal diastolic blood pressure readings. Another assessment consideration is the common occurrence of **white coat hypertension** (also called *isolated office hypertension*), which is the phenomenon of blood pressure readings being high during office visits to a medical practitioner but normal when self-assessed at home.

In recent years, **home blood pressure monitoring**, which is the practice of self-measurement of blood pressure, has been endorsed by national and international guidelines, including those posted by the Australian Heart Foundation and New Zealand Heart Foundation. Self-monitoring provides a more accurate assessment base of information, which is particularly important for older adults because they are more susceptible to white coat hypertension and their systolic readings are more variable. Moreover, self-measurement of blood pressure can also be used to detect orthostatic or postprandial hypotension if readings are taken in both sitting and standing positions. In addition, studies suggest that home blood pressure monitoring can lead to better control of hypertension if healthcare professionals use the information and take appropriate action (Mallick, Kanthety, & Rahman, 2009).

Assessment of blood pressure in older adults is aimed at detecting not only hypertension but also orthostatic and postprandial hypotension. Box 20-6 summarises guidelines

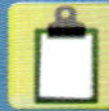

BOX 20-6
Guidelines for assessing blood pressure

For accurate blood pressure measurement in older adults

- Recognise that blood pressure readings are likely to vary, particularly in response to external factors (e.g. meals or postural changes).
- Blood pressure measurements are likely to have diurnal variations, with lowest levels during the night and highest levels after rising in the morning.
- The person should wait 1 hour after eating to have his or her blood pressure checked, except when checking for postprandial hypotension.
- The person should not have ingested caffeine or smoked a cigarette within 30 minutes before having his or her blood pressure checked.
- The person should be seated and resting for 5 minutes before having his or her blood pressure checked.

For assessment of orthostatic hypotension

- Maintain the person's arm in the same position (either parallel or perpendicular to the torso) during supine and standing positions.
- Obtain initial blood pressure reading after the person has been in a sitting or lying position for at least 5 minutes.
- Obtain second blood pressure reading after the person has been standing for 1 to 3 minutes.

For assessment of postprandial hypotension

- Obtain initial blood pressure reading before a meal.
- Obtain second and third reading at 15-minute intervals after the meal is completed.

Method of assessing blood pressure

- The person should be seated with arm bared and feet flat on the floor.
- Support the person's arm as near to the heart level as possible.
- Ask the person to refrain from talking while you check his or her blood pressure.
- Use a sphygmomanometer that has been checked for accuracy.
- Use an appropriate-sized cuff (i.e. the length of the cuff bladder should be at least 80% of the circumference of the arm, and the width should be 20% wider than the diameter of the arm).
- Record the cuff size that is used. (Cuffs that are too small will yield falsely high readings, whereas cuffs that are too large will yield falsely low readings.)
- Fit the deflated cuff firmly around the upper arm, with the centre of the cuff bladder over the brachial artery and the bottom of the cuff about 2.5 to 3.8 centimetres above the bend of the arm.
- Inflate the cuff to 20 or 30 mm Hg above the palpated systolic blood pressure.
- Deflate the cuff at a rate of 2 to 3 mm Hg per second.
- Measure systolic blood pressure at the first sound and diastolic blood pressure at the onset of silence.
- If auscultatory gaps are heard, estimate the systolic blood pressure by applying the cuff, palpating the radial pulse and inflating the cuff until the pulse is no longer felt.
- Record the magnitude and range of the gap (e.g. 184/82 mm Hg, auscultatory gap 176–148).
- If a very low diastolic blood pressure is heard, record the onset of Korotkoff phases IV and V (e.g. 138/72/10 mm Hg). Also, be sure not to press too hard on the stethoscope.
- Measure blood pressure in both arms the first time it is assessed, then measure it in the arm with the higher reading on subsequent determinations.
- If sounds are difficult to auscultate, support the person's arm above his or her head for 30 seconds. Then inflate the cuff, have the person lower the arm and measure the blood pressure.
- If it is necessary to recheck the blood pressure in the same arm, deflate the cuff fully before reinflating it and wait at least 2 minutes before taking another measurement.

Normal findings

- Normal blood pressure is less than 120 mm Hg systolic blood pressure, and less than 80 mm Hg diastolic blood pressure.
- The normal difference between lying/sitting and standing systolic blood pressure is 20 mm Hg or less after standing for 1 minute.
- The normal difference between lying/sitting and standing diastolic blood pressure is 10 mm Hg or less after standing for 1 minute.

for accurate assessment of blood pressure in older adults, including the technique for assessing for orthostatic and postprandial hypotension.

Identifying risks for cardiovascular disease

The assessment of risks for cardiovascular disease, with emphasis on identifying modifiable risk factors, provides a basis for health promotion interventions. Hypertension, lipid disorders and smoking cessation (further discussed in Chapter 21) are important remediable conditions for older adults who have these risks. In addition, obesity, physical inactivity and certain dietary habits are risk factors that can be addressed through improved health-related behaviours. It is especially important to identify older adults who have several risk factors because the co-occurrence of several risks can amplify the effect of individual risk factors (Berry, Dyer, Cai et al., 2012; Kariuki et al., 2013).

An Australian Absolute Cardiovascular Risk Calculator is available at www.cvdcheck.org.au. This online tool calculates heart and stroke risk within the next 5 years (NVDPA, 2012). Other risk assessment tools are available online, including the Framingham Risk Score available at www.mdcalc.com/framingham-coronary-heart-disease-risk-score; the QRISK®2 calculator available at http://qrisk.org; and ASSIGN calculator available at www.assign-score.com.

Additional tests, including electrocardiogram, exercise-stress testing and ankle-brachial index, are not currently recommended for routine screening. However, a one-time screening for abdominal aortic aneurysm is recommended for men aged 65 to 75 years who are current or past smokers (Lim, Hag, Mahmood et al., 2011). In 2003, the American Heart Association and the CDC recommended that C-reactive protein levels be tested in people with moderate risk for cardiovascular disease. In recent years, questions have been raised about this recommendation and a recent review of studies indicates that it may be useful in men, but not in women (Emerging Risk Factors Collaboration Coordination, 2012). Nurses can use Box 20-7 as a guide for nursing assessment of risks.

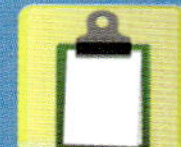

BOX 20-7
Guidelines for assessing risks for cardiovascular disease in older adults

Questions to identify risk factors for cardiovascular disease

- Do you have, or have you ever had, any heart or circulation problems (e.g. stroke, angina, heart attack, blood clots or peripheral vascular disease)? *If yes, ask the usual questions about type of therapy, and so on.*
- When was the last time you had an electrocardiogram?
- What is your normal blood pressure? Have you ever been told that you have high blood pressure, or borderline high blood pressure?
- Do you take, or have you ever taken, medications for heart problems or blood pressure? *If yes, ask the usual questions about type, dose, duration of therapy, and the like.*
- Do you smoke, or have you ever smoked? *If yes, ask additional questions, such as those appropriate for assessing respiratory function, Chapter 21.*
- Do you know what your cholesterol levels are? When was the last time you had your cholesterol checked?
- Do you have diabetes? When was the last time you had your blood sugar (glucose) level checked and what was the result?
- What is your usual pattern of exercise?

Additional considerations regarding risk factors

- Calculate BMI and compare the person's ideal weight to his or her present weight.
- Determine usual dietary habits, paying particular attention to the person's intake of sodium, fibre and types of fat. (This information is usually obtained during the nutritional assessment.)

WELLNESS OPPORTUNITY

Nurses promote personal responsibility and self-awareness by teaching older adults to use self-assessment tools to identify their risks for heart disease.

Assessing signs and symptoms of heart disease

Assessment of older adults for heart disease is complicated by the fact that the symptoms often differ from the expected manifestations. Congestive heart failure, for example, often begins very subtly and the early manifestations may be mental changes secondary to the physiological stress. Therefore, older adults are likely to be in more advanced stages of heart failure before an accurate diagnosis is made. Likewise, older people with angina and acute myocardial infarctions are likely to have subtle and unusual manifestations, called **atypical presentation**, rather than the classic symptom of chest pain. Between a quarter and two-thirds of all myocardial infarctions are not clinically recognised as such, with women and older adults having a higher rate of atypical presentation. Studies also indicate that women and older adults are more likely to seek help for atypical symptoms during the months before they experience an acute coronary event (Graham et al., 2008). Atypical signs and symptoms include fatigue; nausea; anxiety; headache; cough; visual disturbance; shortness of breath; and pain in the jaw, neck or throat.

An important nursing assessment consideration is that older adults as well as healthcare professionals are likely to attribute atypical symptoms to other conditions, such as arthritis or indigestion or even to "normal ageing". Therefore, nurses need to keep in mind that complaints about fatigue, digestion, respiration, or pain in the arms, shoulders or upper trunk can be indicators of cardiac disease. Assessment is further complicated by the fact that older adults often have more than one underlying condition that could be responsible for these symptoms. It is not unusual, for example, for an older person to have an oesophageal reflux disorder as well as a history of ischaemic heart disease. Nurses also need to consider that older adults who have mobility impairments or other functional limitations may not be active enough to experience exertion-related symptoms. Therefore, in addition to focusing the assessment on the usual manifestations of cardiovascular function, the nurse must incorporate information about other systems and overall functioning. In addition, a baseline electrocardiogram is helpful in establishing the possibility of silent or atypical myocardial ischaemia.

Assessing knowledge about heart disease

In addition to assessing signs and symptoms, nurses need to assess the older adult's knowledge about manifestations of heart disease. This is particularly important because immediate medical attention is a major factor in determining outcomes of heart attacks and all people need to be aware of the warning signs so that they can initiate appropriate help-seeking actions. Nurses should ask at least one question to determine the older adult's knowledge about the signs and symptoms of a heart attack. Nurses can also include a question about what the person would do and whom they would call if they thought they were experiencing a heart attack. Box 20-8 summarises the guidelines for assessing cardiovascular function and detecting cardiovascular disease in older adults. It emphasises the assessment components that are unique to older adults and refers to additional assessment components that apply to adults in general.

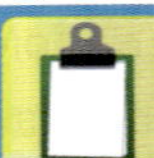

BOX 20-8
Guidelines for assessing cardiovascular function in older adults

Questions to assess for cardiovascular disease

- Do you ever have chest pain or tightness in your chest? *If yes, ask the usual questions to explore the type, onset, duration and other characteristics.*
- Do you ever have difficulty breathing? *If yes, ask the usual questions regarding onset and other characteristics.*
- Do you ever feel lightheaded or dizzy? *If yes, ask about specific circumstances, medical evaluation and methods of dealing with symptoms and ensuring safety.*
- Do you ever feel like your heart is racing, is irregular or has extra or skipped beats? *If yes, ask about any prior medical evaluation.*
- Have you ever been told that you had a heart murmur? *If yes, ask about any prior medical evaluation.*

Information obtained during other portions of an assessment that may be useful in assessing cardiovascular function

- Do you tire easily or feel you need more rest than is ordinarily required?
- Do you have any problems with indigestion?
- Do your feet or ankles ever get swollen?
- Do you wake up at night because of difficulty breathing or because of any other discomfort? Have you made any adjustments in your sleeping habits because of difficulty breathing (e.g. do you use more than one pillow or sleep in a chair)?
- Do you have any pain in your upper back or shoulders?

Interview questions to assess for postural hypotension

- Do you ever feel lightheaded or dizzy, especially when you get up in the morning or after you've been lying down?
- *If yes:* Is this feeling accompanied by any additional symptoms, such as sweating, nausea or confusion?
- *If yes:* Do any of the risks listed in Box 20-3 apply to you? *If yes, ask about any prior medical evaluation.*

NURSING ISSUES

If the nursing assessment identifies risks for cardiovascular disease, a health issue for the older person may be an inability to identify, manage and/or seek out help to maintain health. Related factors common in older adults include lack of physical activity and insufficient knowledge about preventive measures. For older adults with impaired cardiovascular function, other problems may include activity intolerance, decreased cardiac output and ineffective tissue perfusion (cardiopulmonary).

WELLNESS OPPORTUNITY

Nurses can use the wellness nursing issues, willingness for enhanced nutrition or willingness for enhanced knowledge for older adults who are interested in developing heart-healthy dietary habits or learning about health-promoting behaviours to prevent heart disease.

GOAL PLANNING FOR WELLNESS OUTCOMES

When older adults have risks for cardiovascular disease, goals are developed to achieve wellness outcomes. These include developing health-promoting behaviour such an increased knowledge of diet and weight control, and controlling the risks of cardiovascular health such as reduced tobacco use. Goals for older adults with cardiovascular disease include cardiac disease self-management, improved circulation status, development of health-seeking behaviour, knowledge of cardiac disease management, improved tissue perfusion: cardiac, and improved tissue perfusion: peripheral.

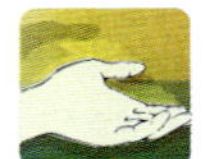

NURSING INTERVENTIONS TO PROMOTE HEALTHY CARDIOVASCULAR FUNCTION

From a wellness perspective, nursing interventions to promote healthy cardiovascular function focus on primary and secondary prevention of cardiovascular disease. Although pharmacological and medical interventions are often used to reduce risk factors, teaching about health promotion actions is a nursing intervention that is appropriate in almost all situations. In addition to addressing risks for cardiovascular disease, nurses can address orthostatic or postprandial hypotension and the related functional consequences, such as falls and fractures.

Nurses can also include interventions that are focused on improving level of coping providing counselling, exercise promotion, health education, meditation facilitation, nutritional counselling, self-responsibility enhancement, simple guided imagery, simple relaxation therapy and individual teaching.

Role of nurses in teaching about cardiovascular disease

In recent years, there is increasing emphasis on the importance of health promotion for prevention of cardiovascular disease, with particular attention to teaching women and members of minority groups about this leading cause of morbidity and mortality. There are many resources available for health professionals and older adults and carers. These are listed at the end of the chapter. Box 20-9 can be used for health promotion to teach older adults about steps they can take to reduce their risk for cardiovascular disease.

Addressing risks through nutrition and lifestyle interventions

Nutritional interventions are particularly important for prevention or management of obesity, hypertension and lipid disorders. Research reviews related to dietary influences on cardiovascular disease support the following evidence-based recommendations (Go, Mozaffarian, Roger et al., 2014; Miller, Stone, Ballantyne et al., 2011; Miuri, Stamler, Brown et al., 2013; Scholl, 2012; Weihua, Yougang & Jing, 2013):

- Type and quality of fats consumed is more important than total fat content or relative percentage of fat, with polyunsaturated and monounsaturated fatty acids (e.g. olive oil, oleic acid from vegetable sources) being the most beneficial, and trans fats and saturated fats being the most detrimental.
- Heart-healthy diets include high intake of nuts, fish, fruits, vegetables and fibre-rich whole grains; less than 1500 mg of sodium a day, and no more than 1 litre of sugar-sweetened beverages a week.
- Although one alcoholic beverage a day for women and two for men may reduce the risk for cardiovascular disease, excessive use increases the risk and alcohol consumption is contraindicated in some conditions (e.g. cardiomyopathy, risk for alcoholism). Australian guidelines (2013) to reduce health risks from drinking alcohol are available via www.alcohol.gov.au.
- Current evidence does not support the use of dietary supplements, but diets should include fruits and vegetables that are rich in essential nutrients, including antioxidants.

Many studies have looked at the effects of a **Mediterranean dietary pattern**, which is characterised by higher intakes of fish, poultry, nuts, fruits, legumes and vegetables, and a lower intake of red and processed meats (Go, Mozaffarian, Roger et al., 2014). Overall, the Mediterranean dietary pattern involves lower intake of saturated and trans fats, higher intake of monounsaturated and polyunsaturated fats, and complex carbohydrates as the main type of carbohydrates. There is much evidence-based support for benefits of this dietary pattern both for primary prevention of coronary heart disease in the general population and for secondary prevention for people who already have pathological changes (e.g. Estruch, Ros, Salas-Salvado et al., 2013; Rees, Hartley, Flowers et al., 2013).

The **DASH dietary pattern**, which refers to the Dietary Approaches to Stop Hypertension, is an evidence-based eating plan promoted by many organisations. This dietary pattern—widely recognised as a primary and secondary preventive intervention for hypertension—is characterised by a high intake of fruits, vegetables and plant proteins from grains, nuts and legumes; moderate intake of low-fat or non-fat dairy foods and low intake of sodium and animal protein. Beneficial effects of DASH-type diets include

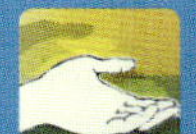

BOX 20-9
Health promotion activities to reduce the risks for cardiovascular disease

Detection of risks

- Have blood pressure checked annually.
- If the total serum cholesterol level is less than 5 mmol/L, have it rechecked every 5 years. If the total serum cholesterol level is between 5 and 6 mmol/L, follow dietary measures to reduce it and have it rechecked annually. If the total serum cholesterol level is 6 mmol/L or more, obtain a further medical evaluation.

Reduction of risks

- Give high priority to smoking cessation, if you smoke.
- Avoid passive smoking (i.e. inhaling smoke from other people's cigarettes).
- Maintain weight within normal limits.
- Exercise daily, and engage in aerobic exercise (i.e. exercise that increases the pulse rate) several times weekly for 30 to 45 minutes each time.
- Avoid foods that are high in sodium, and follow dietary measures to reduce serum cholesterol levels.
- Discuss with your medical practitioner the use of low-dose aspirin therapy as a preventive measure, particularly if there is any history of coronary artery disease or cerebrovascular events.

Heart-healthy eating pattern

- Consume at least 3 to 5 servings of fruits daily, especially the deeply coloured ones.
- Consume at least 3 to 5 servings of vegetables daily, especially the deeply coloured ones.
- Include 2 to 3 servings of low-fat or non-fat dairy products.
- Choose whole-grain products as sources of carbohydrates and fibre (e.g. rye, barley, oats, whole wheat).
- Aim for at least 25 g of fibre daily.
- Choose only the leanest meats, poultry, fish and shellfish.
- Avoid foods high in kilojoules, trans fats and refined sugars.
- Use oils that are least saturated (e.g. canola, safflower, sunflower, corn, olive, soybean and peanut oils) and use margarine that is soft and free of trans fats.
- Limit salt intake to no more than 2300 mg daily.

lowered blood pressure, decreased LDL and triglyceride levels, and lower mortality rates. Studies have confirmed a strong association between a DASH-like diet and reduced incidence of cardiovascular diseases by at least 20% (Fitzgerald, Chiuve, Buring et al., 2012; Go, Mozaffarian, Roger et al., 2014; Salehi-Abargouei et al., 2013).

Another focus of nutrition-related research is on the potential benefits of commonly consumed foods and beverages that are rich in polyphenols. Although there is increasing evidence that cocoa and dark chocolate have cardioprotective effects (e.g. antioxidant, anti-inflammatory, antiplatelet and vasodilation actions), larger randomised trials are required to establish a cause–effect relationship (Arranz et al., 2013; Ellam & Williamson, 2013). Similarly, although there is increasing evidence that both green and black tea may reduce the risk for cardiovascular disease, research is not sufficient to support an evidence-based recommendation (Hartley, Flowers, Holmes et al., 2013).

Addressing risks through lifestyle interventions

Lifestyle interventions that are a mainstay of interventions for preventing cardiovascular disease include remaining physically active, managing stress, refraining from smoking, and maintaining ideal body weight. There is strong evidence supporting the importance of physical activity as an intervention for preventing cardiovascular disease and improving life expectancy (see Figure 20-2). For example, a meta-analysis of studies concluded that high levels of leisure time physical activity reduced the risk of cardiovascular disease by 20% to 30%, whereas moderate leisure or occupational physical activity reduced the risk by 10% to 20% (Li & Siegrist, 2012). Specific positive effects on cardiovascular function include weight loss; reduced blood pressure; improved overall cardiac function; lower rates of cardiovascular disease; improved lipid, glucose and triglyceride levels; and decreased risk of developing diabetes and cardiovascular disease. There also is abundant evidence that aerobic exercise is a "decisive factor in reducing cardiovascular morbidity and mortality" (Nilsson, Boutouyrie, Cunha et al., 2013). Positive effects of exercise on other aspects of health are noted throughout this text, and nurses can incorporate this information when they teach about the many positive functional consequences of regular physical exercise.

Smoking is a major risk factor for cardiovascular disease, and quitting smoking is beneficial for people at any age. A longitudinal study found that smoking cessation was the most important independent predictor of mortality in people who had coronary artery bypass graft surgery, with a 30-year survival rate of 29% in people who quit smoking and 14% in those who continued to smoke (de Boer et al., 2013). The benefits of smoking cessation as a secondary prevention intervention begin immediately and are as effective in older adults as they are in younger people. An important nursing responsibility is to provide health education regarding smoking cessation, and is further discussed in Chapter 21.

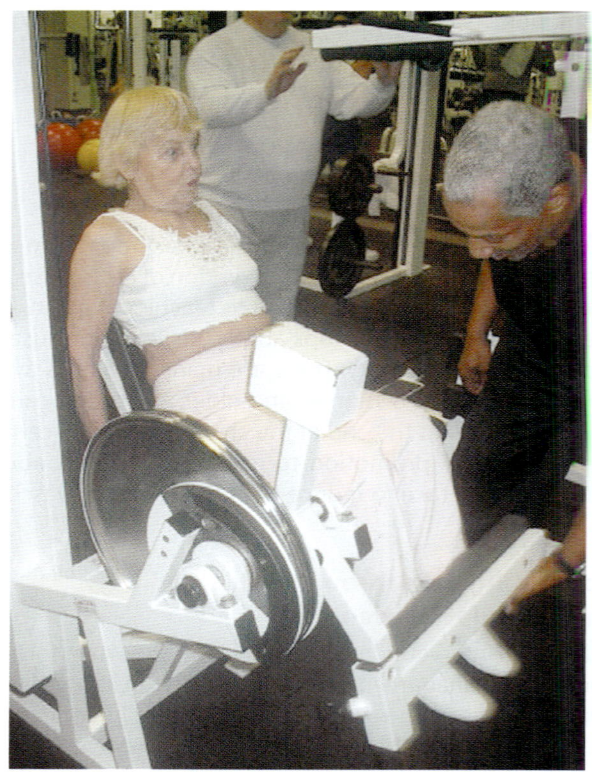

FIGURE 20-2 Exercise is an important preventive intervention. (Courtesy of Monte Unetic.)

Teaching about stress reduction is an important health promotion intervention for reducing risks related to cardiovascular disease. An evidence-based review found that mind–body therapies have positive effects on cardiovascular function by improving stress management and coping skills and influencing physiological stress mechanisms (Rabito & Kaye, 2013). For example, many studies indicate that yoga can reduce cardiovascular risk factors, including obesity, hypertension, high cholesterol, and high blood glucose (e.g. Hagins, States, Selfe et al., 2013; Okonta, 2012). Studies also have found that tai chi may prevent and reverse the progression of cardiovascular disease (Dalusung-Angosta, 2011; Lo, Yeh, Chang et al., 2012; Ng, Wang, Ho et al., 2012). Nurses can encourage older adults to participate in mind–body activities, which community- or hospital-based senior centres offer.

WELLNESS OPPORTUNITY

Nurses address body–mind–spirit interconnectedness by including stress level as an outcome directed towards reducing the risk for cardiovascular disease.

Secondary prevention

When nurses care for older adults who have cardiovascular disease, referrals for secondary prevention programs such as cardiac rehabilitation are an important part of care.

Evidence-based guidelines recommend cardiac rehabilitation programs as a comprehensive approach to reducing mortality by nearly 25% and restoring individuals to their optimal physiological, psychosocial, nutritional and functional status (Arena, Williams, Forman et al., 2012). Despite this evidence of efficacy and cost-effectiveness, referral and participation rates for cardiac rehabilitation programs are low. Although referrals need to be initiated by medical practitioners, nurses have important roles in encouraging participation when these referrals are made. Nurses also can suggest referrals for additional preventive services that address stress management, smoking cessation, or diet or exercise counselling.

WELLNESS OPPORTUNITY

Nurses communicate positive attitudes about ageing by talking with older adults about personal responsibility for addressing risks for cardiovascular disease and communicating that it's never too late to incorporate healthy behaviours into daily life.

Addressing risks through pharmacological interventions

Before and during the 1990s, hormonal replacement therapy was recommended for menopausal women as an intervention for preventing cardiovascular disease. This recommendation was based on epidemiological studies, but it was reversed in 2002 when longitudinal and large-scale investigations concluded that risks outweighed the benefits as a preventive intervention. The use of low-dose aspirin is another pharmacological intervention that has been investigated for the prevention of cardiovascular disease, with emphasis on determining whether the potential benefits outweigh the increased risks for gastrointestinal bleeding and haemorrhagic stroke. Studies conclude that the use of low-dose aspirin is most favourable in people with a high risk for, or a history of, cardiovascular disease:

- Men aged 45 to 79 years and women aged 55 to 79 years: encourage aspirin use when potential cardiovascular benefit outweighs potential harm of gastrointestinal haemorrhage or ischaemic strokes.
- Men less than age 45 and women less than age 55 years: do not encourage aspirin use.
- Men and women aged 80 years and older: no recommendation due to insufficient evidence. (U.S. Preventive Services Task Force [USPTF], 2012)

Preventing and managing hypertension

Although relatively few nurses prescribe medications for hypertension, all nurses need to apply current guidelines and recommendations for management of hypertension when caring for older adults. Nursing interventions for people with hypertension include evaluating a person's response to prescribed medications and teaching about interventions for hypertension. In addition, nurses can promote wellness by teaching about self-care measures for preventing and treating hypertension. This is particularly important because lifestyle interventions—including diet, weight loss, physical activity, stress-reduction techniques, and moderation of alcohol—are an integral component of effective hypertension management (Brook, Appel, Rubenfire et al., 2013).

The **stepped-care approach** to management of hypertension recommends that lifestyle modifications be tried initially, followed by pharmacological interventions to achieve target blood pressure. Lifestyle interventions that have the most significant impact on hypertension are substantial weight loss and a dietary pattern that includes low-sodium and high-potassium foods. Guidelines from major organisations, such as the Heart Association, emphasise that sodium intake of 2300 mg/day (or salt intake of 6 grams) or less is associated with greater reductions in blood pressure (2010). If the older adult is at risk of heart disease or has been diagnosed with heart disease then salt intake should be reduced to less than 4 g/day. Nurses have important responsibilities with regard to teaching older adults and their carers about sodium intake.

Many medications are used for treating hypertension, and selection of the best medication is based on variables such as therapeutic effectiveness, presence of concomitant conditions, and the avoidance of adverse effects. Current emphasis is on the need for individualised treatment options, particularly for certain groups, such as those with the conditions of diabetes or chronic kidney disease. Also for older adults aged over 74 years, it is recommended that clinical judgement be utilised, which considers the benefits and risks of treatment and comorbidities, before commencing treatment (NLDPA, 2012). Box 20-10 summarises guidelines for interventions for hypertension and includes health education information about nutrition and lifestyle interventions. Resources for evidence-based practice and health education for hypertension are listed at the end of this chapter.

WELLNESS OPPORTUNITY

Nurses promote personal responsibility for managing hypertension by talking with older adults about self-monitoring of blood pressure.

UNFOLDING CASE STUDY

Part B

Mr Constantine is now 70 years old and his blood pressure fluctuates between 130/88 and 146/94 mm Hg. He continues to take hydrochlorothiazide, 25 mg, and verapamil 120 mg, every morning. Mr Constantine and his wife live with their daughter and her teenage children. Mr and Mrs Constantine usually do the family grocery shopping, and his wife and daughter prepare the family meals. A diet history reveals that the family usually eats fried food about four times a week and pasta dishes for the other main meals. Mr Constantine enjoys a glass or two of red wine every night. For cooking, the family uses lard, salt pork or bacon drippings. He also drinks coffee with sugar and cream. The family generally has cereal and toast for breakfast, but they have bacon and eggs on Saturdays and Sundays. Mr Constantine's weight is still about 14 kilograms more than his ideal weight. He gets little exercise and continues to complain of "getting winded" when he walks across the car park.

Thinking points

- What additional information would you obtain for further assessment of Mr Constantine's cardiovascular status?
- What nutritional and lifestyle interventions would you discuss with Mr Constantine regarding his hypertension?
- What teaching materials would you use for health education with Mr Constantine?

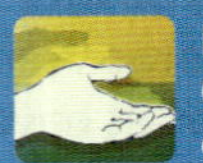

BOX 20-10
Guidelines for nursing management of hypertension

Health promotion interventions

The following lifestyle modifications are recommended for all people with hypertension:

- Avoidance of tobacco
- Weight reduction when appropriate (i.e. when the person weighs more than 110% of his or her ideal weight)
- 30 to 45 minutes of exercise, such as brisk walking, at least five times weekly
- Limitation of alcohol intake to two or less standard drinks per day (e.g. 60 mL of 40% alcoholic spirit, 300 mL of wine, or 550 mL of full-strength beer).

The following nutritional interventions are recommended for all people with hypertension:

- Sodium intake limited to 2 to 3 g daily
- Avoidance of processed foods
- Daily intake of 7 to 8 servings of grains and grain products, and 8 to 10 servings of fruits and vegetables

Considerations regarding the treatment of hypertension

- Risks from and definitions of hypertension apply to all age categories (refer to www.heartfoundation.org.au for criteria).
- A person's blood pressure should be measured at least three times before making any decisions about treatment.
- Home blood pressure monitoring is recommended for initial and ongoing assessment.
- The safety of antihypertensive agents is improved by carefully selecting the medication, starting with low doses, and changing the medication regimen gradually, in small increments, if necessary.
- The goals of hypertensive treatment are to control blood pressure by the least intrusive means and to prevent cardiovascular morbidity and mortality.
- Treatment is directed towards achieving and maintaining a systolic blood pressure of less than 139/89 mm Hg if this can be achieved without compromising cardiovascular function.

Preventing and managing lipid disorders

Although nurses usually do not prescribe medications for treatment of lipid disorders, they are responsible for teaching about preventing and managing lipid disorders. Nurses need to be familiar with lipid disorders treatment guidelines such as those by the National Heart Foundation of Australia and the NVDPA. See the section, risk factors affecting cardiovascular function, for targets for lipids. The guidelines identify different ethnic groups that are of a higher risk. They are adults with clinical evidence of:

- Vascular disease, including coronary heart disease, stroke, peripheral arterial disease
- Diabetes mellitus (including diagnostic biochemical criteria)
- Chronic kidney disease
- Familial hypercholesterolaemia
- Aboriginal and Torres Strait Islander people
- Those with absolute risk of ≥15% risk of a CVD event in the next 5 years using the 1991 Framingham equation
- Those with absolute risk of 10% to 15% of a CVD event in the next 5 years when any of the following is present: family history of premature CHD (first degree relative who developed CHD before age 60) or the metabolic syndrome. (NVDPA, 2012, p. 2)

As with treatment of hypertension, nutrition and lifestyle interventions are the first-line approaches, and medications (e.g. statins) are prescribed if goals are not achieved with non-pharmacological interventions. Essential nutrition and lifestyle interventions for lipid disorders include dietary modifications, maintenance of ideal body weight and incorporation of regular exercise in one's daily routine. Nutrition interventions focus on dietary fat intake with emphasis on limiting foods containing saturated fats and trans fatty acids and increasing foods that are high in polyunsaturated and monounsaturated fats. Box 20-11 summarises health education interventions for prevention and management of lipid disorders in older adults.

EVALUATING EFFECTIVENESS OF NURSING INTERVENTIONS

One measure of the effectiveness of health promotion interventions is the extent to which the older adult verbalises correct information about the risks. Also, the older adult may verbalise intent to change or eliminate the lifestyle factors that increase the risk of impaired cardiovascular function. For example, the older adult may agree to join an exercise program and follow dietary measures to reduce serum cholesterol levels. Effectiveness of interventions can also be measured by determining the actual reduction in risk factors. For example, the person's serum cholesterol level may decrease from 6 mmol/L to 3.5 mmol/L after 6 months of regular exercise and dietary modifications. For older adults with impaired cardiovascular function, nurses evaluate the extent to which the signs and symptoms are alleviated and the extent to which older adults verbalise correct information about managing their condition.

BOX 20-11
Nutritional interventions for people with high cholesterol

Dietary measures to promote a healthy lipid profile

- Include foods that are high in fibre content in your daily diet (e.g. whole grains).
- Include soy proteins in your daily diet (e.g. tofu, soy milk).
- Eat a minimum of two servings of fatty fish weekly.
- Limit total fat intake to less than 30% of your total daily kilojoule intake.
- Limit total daily cholesterol intake to 200 mg.
- Use non-fat or low-fat dairy desserts.
- Consumption of butter or margarine should be limited, but margarines that contain stanols are beneficial (e.g. Benecol).
- Use egg whites, omega-3 eggs or egg substitutes.
- Limit consumption of lean meats to five or fewer 85 - to 140-gram servings per week. Trim fat off meats and the skin off poultry.
- Avoid eating processed meats (e.g. bacon, bologna, sausage, hot dogs).
- Avoid gravies, fried foods and organ meats.

Guide to types of fats

Type of fat	*Sources*	*Examples*	*Effect on lipid profile*
Saturated fatty acids	Animal fats and some vegetable oils (usually solid at room temperatures)	Meat, poultry, butter and lauric and palm oils	Negative: increases LDL and total cholesterol
Trans fatty acids	Vegetable oils that are processed into margarine or shortening	Dairy products, baked goods, snack foods	Negative: increases LDL cholesterol and lowers HDL cholesterol
Monounsaturated fatty acids	Vegetable oils (usually liquid at room temperatures)	Olive, peanut and canola oils	Positive: decreases LDL
Polyunsaturated fatty acids	Seafood and vegetable oils (soft or liquid at room temperatures)	Corn, sunflower, safflower, canola and linoleic oils	Positive: decreases LDL
Omega-3 fatty acids	Fatty fish	Tuna, salmon, herring, mackerel	Positive: decreases LDL cholesterol and triglycerides

LDL, low-density lipoprotein; HDL, high-density lipoprotein.

UNFOLDING CASE STUDY

Part C

Mr Constantine is now 74 years old. You are the practice nurse at his medical centre. He reports that his doctor recently started him on a medication for high cholesterol and told him to "watch my diet", but gave no further information or educational materials about what to do about his cholesterol.

Nursing assessment

Mr Constantine has no knowledge about dietary sources of cholesterol, and is unaware that his diet, which he terms "soul food", is high in cholesterol. Although he says he has heard a lot about "good and bad cholesterol" in the news, he does not know which foods are good or bad. He tries to buy foods that say "no cholesterol" on the label, but says the labels are too confusing about the different kinds of fats.

Nursing issues

Your nursing issue is altered health maintenance related to lack of regular exercise, dietary habits that contribute to hyperlipidaemia and insufficient information about lifestyle factors that increase the risk of cardiovascular disease. Evidence of these risk factors comes from Mr Constantine's inactivity, eating patterns, history of hypertension and family history of cardiovascular disease. Also, Mr Constantine has verbalised insufficient information about the relationship between exercise and cardiovascular function and about dietary measures to control cholesterol.

Nursing care plan for Mr Constantine

Goals for wellness outcomes	Nursing interventions	Nursing evaluation
Mr Constantine's knowledge of risk factors for cardiovascular impairment will increase	• Discuss the risk factors for impaired cardiovascular function, using information from Box 20-7.	• Mr Constantine describes his risk factors for cardiovascular disease.

Goals for wellness outcomes	Nursing interventions	Nursing evaluation
	• Emphasise the risk factors that can be addressed through life style modifications (e.g. exercise, weight loss and dietary measures to control cholesterol levels).	• Mr Constantine identifies those risk factors that he can address through lifestyle changes.
Mr Constantine's knowledge of the relationship between diet and serum cholesterol levels will increase.	• Use teaching materials obtained from the Heart Foundation to illustrate the relationship between diet and serum cholesterol levels. Provide a copy of these pamphlets for Mr Constantine to take home. • Suggest that Mr Constantine discusses the information in the pamphlets with his wife and daughter. • Ask Mr Constantine to bring his wife to the clinic next month so that you can talk with both of them about dietary measures to control cholesterol.	• Mr Constantine accurately describes the relationship between food intake and cholesterol levels. • Mr Constantine identifies family eating habits contributing to his elevated serum cholesterol level.
Mr Constantine will modify one dietary habit that contributes to his high cholesterol level.	• Work with Mr Constantine to make a list of the foods associated with high cholesterol levels (e.g. fried foods, bacon and eggs). • Give Mr Constantine a copy of Box 20-11 and use it to discuss dietary measures to reduce cholesterol. • Ask Mr Constantine to select one change in dietary habits that will have a positive effect on his cholesterol level.	• Mr Constantine states that he is willing to change one eating habit that contributes to his high cholesterol level. • Next month, Mr Constantine reports that he has changed one eating pattern that contributes to high cholesterol levels.
Mr Constantine will increase his knowledge about the relationship between exercise and cardiovascular function.	• Use pamphlets from the Heart Foundation to teach about the effects of aerobic exercise on cardiovascular function. • Review information together about the relationship between exercise and weight.	• Mr Constantine describes the beneficial effects of regular aerobic exercise.
Mr Constantine will begin exercising on a regular basis.	• Discuss ways in which Mr Constantine can incorporate regular exercise into his daily activities. • Invite Mr Constantine and his wife to walk daily for 30 minutes at the local park.	• Mr Constantine verbalises a commitment to perform 30 minutes of exercise 3 days a week.
Mr Constantine will eliminate lifestyle factors that increase the risk for cardiovascular disease.	• Ask Mr Constantine to invite his wife to your monthly appointments so that she can also receive important health education. • Identify a plan that will enable Mr and Mrs Constantine to gradually incorporate additional dietary measures aimed at reducing cholesterol into the family meal plans. • Identify a plan that will enable Mr and Mrs Constantine to include 30 minutes of exercise 5 times a week. • Discuss weight reduction with Mr Constantine and emphasise that dietary modifications and regular exercise are interventions that should facilitate weight loss.	• Mr Constantine's total cholesterol level is ≤5.5 mmol/L at the end of 6 months. • Mr Constantine's serum cholesterol level remains below 5.5 mmol/L. • Mr Constantine reports that he engages in 30 minutes of exercise 5 times weekly. • Mr Constantine reports that he follows the dietary measures presented in Box 20-11. • Mr Constantine's weight is reduced to between 80 and 90 kilograms, and he maintains that weight.

Thinking points

- What factors affect Mr Constantine's ability to manage his cardiovascular condition and address his risk factors, and how would you address these factors in your interventions?
- Explore some of the health education listed at the end of this chapter to find teaching tools that would be appropriate for Mr Constantine.

CHAPTER HIGHLIGHTS

Age-related changes that affect cardiovascular function

- Degenerative changes of myocardium
- Arterial stiffening
- Thicker, less-elastic, more dilated veins
- Increased peripheral resistance
- Altered baroreflex mechanisms

Risk factors that affect cardiovascular function

- Atherosclerosis
- Physical inactivity
- Tobacco smoking
- Dietary habits
- Obesity, especially abdominal obesity
- Hypertension
- Lipid disorders
- Metabolic syndrome
- Psychosocial factors
- Heredity and socioeconomic factors
- Special considerations for women and minority groups

Functional consequences affecting cardiovascular wellness

- Effects on cardiac function
- Effects on pulse and blood pressure
- Effects on response to exercise
- Effects on circulation
- Increased risk of CV disease

Pathological conditions affecting cardiovascular function

- Orthostatic and postprandial hypotension
- Chronic heart failure

Nursing assessment of cardiovascular function

- Baseline cardiovascular function (heart rate, sounds and rhythm)
- Blood pressure, including hypertension and orthostatic or postprandial hypotension
- Risks for cardiovascular disease, with emphasis on modifiable conditions
- Signs and symptoms of heart disease
- Knowledge about heart disease

Nursing issues

- Ineffective maintenance of health
- Decreased cardiac output
- Inadequate tissue perfusion (cardiopulmonary)
- Willingness for enhanced knowledge; enhanced nutrition; weight control; smoking cessation; enhanced exercise; stress reduction

Goal planning for wellness outcomes

- Health-promoting behaviours
- Control of risk of cardiovascular health
- Control of risk of tobacco use and weight control
- Cardiac disease self-management

Nursing interventions to promote healthy cardiovascular function

- Addressing risks through nutritional interventions
- Addressing risks through lifestyle interventions (exercise, heart-healthy diet, optimal body weight, cessation of smoking if applicable)
- Secondary prevention programs for older adults who have cardiovascular disease
- Pharmacological interventions for prevention of cardiovascular disease
- Preventing and managing hypertension
- Preventing and managing lipid disorders

Evaluating effectiveness of nursing interventions

- Verbalisation of correct information about risks
- Reported participation in health promotion interventions (e.g. heart-healthy diet, regular exercise, weight reduction and smoking cessation when applicable)
- Indicators of cardiovascular function within normal range (e.g. blood pressure, serum lipids)
- If applicable, alleviation of signs and symptoms of cardiovascular disease

CRITICAL THINKING EXERCISES

1. Discuss how each of the following factors influences cardiovascular function, including orthostatic hypotension: lifestyle, medications, age-related changes and pathological conditions.
2. Demonstrate how you would teach a home health aide to assess blood pressure and orthostatic hypotension correctly.
3. Describe the questions and considerations you would include in an assessment of cardiovascular function in an older adult who has no complaint of heart problems, but who has a history of falling twice in the past month and who has not been evaluated by a medical practitioner in the past year.
4. You are asked to give a health education talk entitled "Keeping Your Heart Healthy" at a senior day care centre. What information would you include in the presentation? What local resources (i.e. specific contact information for agencies or organisations in your area) would you suggest for your audience to contact for further information? What audiovisual aids would you use? How would you involve the participants in the discussion?
5. You are working in a long-term residential care facility in which several of the residents have orthostatic hypotension. What would you include in their health education regarding the management of their orthostatic hypotension?

RESOURCES

For an extensive range of additional resources to enhance teaching and learning and to facilitate understanding of this chapter, please see the text's accompanying website located on thePoint at http://thepoint.lww.com.

Clinical tools

American Heart Association: www.heart.org/HEARTORG
- My Life Check: Interactive self-assessment tools related to blood pressure and cardiovascular risks.
- Interactive cardiovascular library, *Watch, learn and live*: Animations that help explain high blood pressure and many other cardiovascular diseases.

Hartford Institute for Geriatric Nursing, ConsultGeriRN.org: http://consultgerirn.org/resources
Try This specialty practice series:
- Issue SP3: Cardiac Risk Assessment of the Older Cardiovascular Patient: The Framingham Global Risk Assessment Tools. Coke, L. A. (2010). *Best Practices in Nursing Care to Older Adults.*
- View topic-related resources from Preventive Cardiovascular Nurse's Association (PCNA).
- Issue SP4: Vascular risk assessment of the older cardiovascular patient: The Ankle-Brachial Index (ABI). Coke, L. A. (2010). *Best Practices in Nursing Care to Older Adults.*

Heart Foundation Australia: www.heartfoundation.org.au
- Search: Absolute risk (videos and health calculator); health risks and BMI calculator.

National Heart Lung and Blood Institute (US): www.nhlbi.nih.gov
- Search: Health-risk calculators (related to blood pressure, BMI and cardiovascular risks factors).

Evidence-based practice

American College of Cardiology and American Heart Association (ACC/AHA) Task Force on Practice Guidelines. (2013). ACC/AHA guideline on the treatment of blood cholesterol to reduce atherosclerotic cardiovascular risk in adults.

Briffa, T., Maiorana, A., Allan, R. et al. (2006). *National Heart Foundation of Australia physical activity recommendations for people with cardiovascular disease*. Sydney: National Heart Foundation of Australia.

James, P. A., Oparil, S., Carter, B. L. et al. (2014). Evidence-based guideline for the management of high blood pressure in adults: Report from the panel members appointed to the Eighth Joint National Committee (JNC 8). *Journal of the American Medical Association, 311*(5), 507–520.

Jensen, M. D., Ryan, D. H., Apovian, C. M., Ard, J. D, Comuzzie, A. G., Donato, K. A., . . . Yanovski, S. Z. (2014). AHA/ACC/TOS guideline for the management of overweight and obesity in adults: A report of the American College of Cardiology/American Heart Association Task Force on Practice Guidelines and The Obesity Society. *Circulation, 129*, S102–S138.

Joanna Briggs Institute: http://connect.jbiconnectplus.org
Evidence summary: D'Arcy, M. (2013). Chronic heart failure: Self-care.

Mosca, L., Benjamin, E. J., Berra, K., Bezanson, J. L., Dolor, R. J., Lloyd-Jones, D, M., . . . Wenger, N. K. (2011). Evidence-based guidelines for cardiovascular disease prevention in women: 2011 update. *Circulation, 123*(11), 1243–1262.

National Heart Foundation of Australia: www.heartfoundation.org.au
- Information for professionals/clinical information.
- National Heart Foundation of Australia. (2014). *Blueprint for an active Australia* (2nd ed.). Melbourne: Author.
- Reducing risk in heart disease guide (2012).
- Physical activity in patients with cardiovascular disease: Management algorithm and information for general practice (2006).
- Promoting physical activity: Ten recommendations from the Heart Foundation.

National Guideline Clearinghouse: www.guideline.gov
Search for: Cardiovascular and/or exercise, hypertension, lipids
- Clinical practice guideline on the management of lipids as a cardiovascular risk factor (2008, revised 2013).
- AHA/ACC guideline on lifestyle management to reduce cardiovascular risk: A report of the American College of Cardiology/American Heart Association Task Force on Practice Guidelines (2013).
- AHA/ACC/TOS guideline for the management of overweight and obesity in adults: A report of the American College of Cardiology/American Heart Association Task Force on Practice Guidelines and The Obesity Society (2013).
- Exercise promotion: Walking in elders.
- Lipid disorders.
- Lipid management in adults (1997, revised 2013).
- Hypertension.

National Health and Medical Research Council (NHMRC) Clinical Practice Guidelines Portal (Australia): National Vascular Disease Prevention Alliance (NVDPA) (2012). Guidelines for the management of absolute cardiovascular disease risk. Accessed February 2015 at www.clinicalguidelines.gov.au/search.php?pageType=2&fldglrID=2079&.

Health education

American Heart Association: www.heart.org

Centers for Disease Control and Prevention, Division for Heart Disease and Stroke Prevention: www.cdc.gov/dhdsp/data_statistics/fact_sheets/fs_stroke.htm

Australia New Zealand Obesity Society: www.anzos.com

DASH diet (U.S.): http://dashdiet.org

Health Direct Australia, seniors' health: www.healthdirect.gov.au/how-to-lower-blood-pressure

Heart Foundation (Australia): www.heartfoundation.org.au

Heart Foundation (New Zealand). A guide to heart-healthy eating and The Pacific Heartbeat Programme (healthy lifestyle materials): www.heartfoundation.org.nz
National Heart, Lung and Blood Institute (U.S.): www.nhlbi.nih.gov
National Stroke Association (U.S.): www.stroke.org
Obesity Australia: www.obesityaustralia.org
Stroke Foundation (Australia): www.strokefoundation.com.au
Stroke Foundation of New Zealand: www.stroke.org.nz

REFERENCES

Abdel-Rahman, T. A. (2012). Orthostatic hypotension before and after meal intake in diabetic patients and healthy elderly people. *Journal of Family & Community Medicine, 19*(1), 20–25.

Allen, J. K. & Dennison, C. R. (2010). Randomized trials of nursing interventions for secondary prevention in patients with coronary artery disease and heart failure. *Journal of Cardiovascular Nursing, 25*(3), 207–220.

Arena, R., Williams, M., Forman, D. E. et al. (2012). Increasing referral and participation rates to outpatient cardiac rehabilitation: The valuable role of healthcare professionals in inpatient and home health settings. *Circulation, 125*, 1321–1329.

Arranz, S., Valderas-Martinez, P., Chiva-Blanch, G. et al. (2013). Cardioprotective effects of cocoa: Clinical evidence from randomized clinical intervention trials in humans. *Molecular Nutrition & Food Research, 57*(6), 936–947.

Aung, A. K., Corcoran, S. J., Nagalingam, V. et al. (2012). Prevalence, associations, and risk factors for orthostatic hypotension in medical, surgical, and trauma patients. *Ochsner Journal, 12*(1), 35–4 .

Australian Bureau of Statistics (ABS). (2012). Health risk factors. *Year book Australia, 2012*. Cat. no. 1301. Accessed February 2015 at www.abs.gov.au/ausstats/abs@.nsf/Lookup/1301.0Main+Features2332012.

Australian Bureau of Statistics (ABS). (2013a). Smoking. Cat. no. 4125.0. *Gender indicators, Australia, Jan. 2013*. Accessed February 2015 at www.abs.gov.au/ausstats/abs@.nsf/Lookup/4125.0main+features3320Jan%202013.

Australian Bureau of Statistics. (2013b). Overweight and obesity. Australian Health Survey: Updated results, 2011–2012. Cat. no. 4364.0.55.003. Canberra: Author. Accessed March 2015 via www.abs.gov.au/ausstats/abs@.nsf/lookup/33C64022ABB5ECD5CA257B8200179437?opendocument.

Australian Institute of Health and Welfare (AIHW). (2011). *Cardiovascular disease: Australian facts 2011*. Cardiovascular disease series no. 35. Cat. no. CVD 53. Canberra: Author.

Banegas, J. R., Segura, J., de la Sierra, A., Gorostidi, M., Rodriguez-Artalejo, F., Sobrinho, J., . . . Spanish Society of Hypertension ABPM Registry Investigators. (2008). Gender differences in office and ambulatory control of hypertension. *American Journal of Medicine, 121*, 1078–1084.

Barnes, A. S. (2012). Obesity and sedentary lifestyles risk for cardiovascular disease in women. *Texas Heart Institute Journal, 39*(2), 224–227.

Berra, K. (2008). Lipid-lowering therapy today. *Journal of Cardiovascular Nursing, 23*(5), 414–421.

Berry, J. D., Dyer, A., Cai, X. et al. (2012). Lifetime risks of cardiovascular disease. *New England Journal of Medicine, 366*(4), 321–329.

Brook, R. D., Appel, L. J., Rubenfire, M. et al. (2013). Beyond medications and diet: Alternative approaches to lowering blood pressure. A scientific statement from the American Heart Association. *Hypertension, 61*(6), 1360–1383.

Cademartiri, F., LaGrutta, L. ., de Feyter, P. J. & Kresstin, G. P. (2008). Physiopathology of the aging heart. *Radiology Clinics of North America, 46*, 653–662.

Castellon, X. & Bogdanova, V. (2013). Screening for subclinical atherosclerosis by noninvasive methods in asymptomatic patients with risk factors. *Clinical Interventions in Aging, 8*, 573–580.

Colquhoun, D. M., Bunker, S. J., Clarke, D. M. et al. (2013). Screening, referral and treatment of depression in patients with coronary heart disease. *Medical Journal of Australia, 198*(9), 483–484.

Dalusung-Angosta, A. (2011). The impact of tai chi exercise on coronary heart disease: A systematic review. *Journal of the American Academy of Nurse Practitioners, 23*(7), 376–381.

de Boer, S. P., Serruys, P. W., Valstar, G. et al. (2013). Life-years gained by smoking cessation after percutaneous coronary intervention. *American Journal of Cardiology, 112*(9), 1311–1314.

Doering, L. V., Chen, B., Bodar, R. C. et al. (2013). Early cognitive behavioral therapy for depression after cardiac surgery. *Journal of Cardiovascular Nursing, 28*(4), 370–379.

Ducharme, N. & Radhamma, R. (2008). Hyperlipidemia in the elderly. *Clinics in Geriatric Medicine, 24*, 471–487.

Ellam, S. & Williamson, G. (2013). Cocoa and human health. *Annual Review of Nutrition, 33*, 105–128.

Emerging Risk Factors Collaboration (2012). C-Reactive protein, fibrinogen, and cardiovascular disease prediction. *New England Journal of Medicine, 367*(14), 1310–1320.

Estruch, R., Ros, E., Salas-Salvado, J. et al. (2013). Primary prevention of cardiovascular disease with a Mediterranean diet. *New England Journal of Medicine, 368*(14), 1279–1290.

Fitzgerald, K. C., Chiuve, S. E., Buring, J. E. et al. (2012). Comparison of associations of adherence to a DASH-style diet with risks of cardiovascular disease and venous thromboembolism. *Journal of Thrombosis and Haemostasis, 10*(2), 189–198.

Foody, J. M. (2008). Prevention as the intervention. *Cardiology Clinics, 26*, xiii–xv.

Frazier, L., Sanner, J., Yu, E. et al. (2013). Using a single screening question for depressive symptoms in patients with acute coronary syndrome. *Journal of Cardiovascular Nursing*, 29(4), 347–353.

Friedmann, E., Son, H., Thomas, S. et al. (2014). Poor social support is associated with increases in depression but not anxiety over 2 years in heart failure outpatients. *Journal of Cardiovascular Nursing, 29*(1), 20–28.

Fukushima, T., Asahina, M., Fujinuma, Y. et al. (2013). Role of intestinal peptides and the autonomic nervous system in postprandial hypotension in patients with multiple system atrophy. *Journal of Neurology, 260*(2), 475–483.

Go, A. S., Mozaffarian, D., Roger, V. L. et al. (2014). Heart disease and stroke statistics: 2014 update. A report from the American Heart Association. *Circulation, 128*, e1–e267.

Graham, M. M., Westerhout, C. M., Kaul, P., Norris, C. M. & Armstrong, P. W. (2008). Sex differences in patients seeking medical attention for prodromal symptoms before an acute coronary event. *American Heart Journal, 156*(6), 1210–1216.

Graven, L. J. & Grant, J. (2012). The impact of social support on depressive symptoms in individuals with heart failure. *Journal of Cardiovascular Nursing, 28*(5), 429–443.

Hagins, M., States, R., Selfe, T. et al. (2013). Effectiveness of yoga for hypertension: Systematic review and meta-analysis. *Evidence-Based Complementary and Alternative Medicine,* article ID 649836. Accessed February 2015 at http://dx.doi.org/10.1155/2013/649836.

Harris, M. F. (2013). The metabolic syndrome. *Australian Family Physician, 42*(8), 524–527.

Hartley, L., Flowers, N., Holmes, J. et al. (2013). Green and black tea for the primary prevention of cardiovascular disease. *Cochrane Database of Systematic Reviews*, 18(6). Article no. CD009934.

Heart Foundation. (2010). Guide to management of hypertension 2008: Assessing and managing raised blood pressure in adults (Table 2, p. iii) (updated December 2010). Accessed March 2015 at www.heartfoundation.org.au/SiteCollectionDocuments/Guide-to-management-hypertension-2008.pdf.

Heart Foundation. (2015). Indigenous health. Information for professionals. Accessed February 2015 via www.heartfoundation.org.au.

Jayathissa, S., Mann, J., Mann, S. & Sharpe, N. (2010). Assessing cardiovascular risk: What the experts think. *Best Practice Journal, 33*. Accessed online February 2015 at www.bpac.org.nz/BPJ/2010/December/cvra.aspx.

Insull, W. (2009). The pathology of atherosclerosis: Plaque development and plaque responses to medical treatment. *American Journal of Medicine, 122*, S3–S14.

Jurgens, C. Y., Hoke, L., Byrnes, J. & Riegel, B. (2009). Why do elders delay responding to heart failure symptoms? *Nursing Research, 58*(4), 274–282.

Kariuki, J. K., Stuart-Shor, E. M. & Hayman, L. L. (2013). The concept of risk as applied to cardiovascular disease. *Journal of Cardiovascular Nursing, 28*(3), 201–203.

Kim, H. S. & Cho, K. I. (2013). Impact of chronic emotional stress on myocardial function in postmenopausal women and its relationship with endothelial dysfunction. *Korean Circulation Journal, 43*, 295–302.

Lagro, J., Meel-van den Abeelen, A., de Jong, D. L. et al. (2013). Geriatric hypotensive syndromes are not explained by cardiovascular autonomic dysfunction alone. *Journals of Gerontology: Medical Sciences, 68*(5), 581–589.

Lewis, S. J. (2009). Prevention and treatment of atherosclerosis: A practitioner's guide for 2008. *American Journal of Medicine, 122*, S38–S50.

Li, J. & Siegrist, J. (2012). Physical activity and risk of cardiovascular disease: A meta-analysis of prospective cohort studies. *Indian Journal of Environmental Research and Public Health, 9*, 391–407.

Lim, L. S., Hag, N., Mahmood, S. et al. (2011). Atherosclerotic cardiovascular disease screening in adults: American College of Preventive Medicine position statement on preventive practice. *American Journal of Preventive Medicine, 40*(3), 381, e1–10.

Lloyd-Jones, D., Adams, R., Carnethon, M., DeSimone, G., Ferguson, B., Flegal, K. & American Heart Association Statistics Committee and Stroke Statistics Subcommittee. (2009). Heart disease and stroke statistics—2009 update. *Circulation, 119*, e1–e161.

Lo, H. M., Yeh, C. Y., Chang, S. C. et al. (2012). A tai chi exercise programme improved exercise behaviour and reduced blood pressure in outpatients with hypertension. *International Journal of Nursing Practice, 18*(6), 545–551.

Mallick, S., Kanthety, R. & Rahman, M. (2009). Home blood pressure monitoring in clinical practice: A review. *American Journal of Medicine, 122*, 803–810.

McGavock, J. M., Hastings, J. L., Snell, P. G., McGuire, D. K., Pacini, E. L., Levine, B. D. & Mitchell, J. H. (2009). A forty-year follow-up of the Dallas bed rest and training study: The effect of age on cardiovascular response to exercise in men. *Journal of Gerontology: Medical Sciences, 64A*, 293–299.

McSweeney, J. C., Cleves, M. A., Zhao, W., Lefler, L. L. & Yang, S. (2010). Cluster analysis of women's prodromal and acute myocardial infarction symptoms by race and other characteristics. *Journal of Cardiovascular Nursing, 25*, 311–322.

Miller, M., Stone, N. J., Ballantyne, C. et al. (2011). Triglycerides and cardiovascular disease: A scientific statement from the American Heart Association. *Circulation, 123*, 2292–2333.

Miuri, K., Stamler, J., Brown, I. et al. (2013). Relationship of dietary monounsaturated fatty acids to blood pressure: The international study of macro/micronutrients and blood pressure. *Journal of Hypertension, 31*(6), 1144–1150.

Mosca, L., Hammond, G., Mochari-Greenberger, H. et al. (2013). Fifteen-year trends in awareness of heart disease in women. *Circulation, 127*(11), 1254–1263, e1-29.

Muzzarelli, S., Tobler, D., Leibundgut, G., Schindler, R., Buser, P., Pfisterer, M. E. & Brunner-La Rocca, H. P. (2009). Detection of intake of nonsteroidal anti-inflammatory drugs in elderly patients with heart failure. How to ask the patient? *Swiss Medicine Weekly, 139*(33–34), 481–485.

National Heart Foundation of Australia (NHFA) and the Cardiac Society of Australia and New Zealand (CSANZ). (2005). Position statement on lipid management 2005. *Heart Lung and Circulation, 14*(4), 275–297. Viewed February 2015 at www.heartfoundation.org.au/SiteCollectionDocuments/The-lipid-position-statement.pdf.

National Heart Foundation of Australia and the Cardiac Society of Australia and New Zealand. (2011). Guidelines for the prevention, detection and management of chronic heart failure in Australia. Sydney: National Heart Foundation of Australia.

National Institute for Health and Care Excellence (NICE). (2011). *Hypertension: Clinical management of primary hypertension in adults*. London: NICE. Available via www.nice.org.uk.

National Vascular Disease Prevention Alliance (NVDPA). (2012). Quick reference guide for health professionals: Absolute cardiovascular disease risk management. Available February 2015 via http://strokefoundation.com.au.

New Zealand Guidelines Group. (2012). *New Zealand primary care handbook 2012* (3rd ed.). Wellington: Author. Available February 2015 via www.health.govt.nz.

New Zealand Ministry of Health. (2014). Tobacco use 2012/13: New Zealand Health Survey. Wellington: Author.

Neylon, A., Canniffe, C., Anand, S. et al. (2013). A global perspective on psychosocial risk factors for cardiovascular disease. *Progress in Cardiovascular Disease, 55*(6), 574–581.

Ng, S. M., Wang, C. W., Ho, R. T. et al. (2012). Tai chi exercise for patients with heart disease: A systematic review of controlled clinical trials. *Alternative Therapies in Health and Medicine, 18*(3), 16–22.

Nilsson, P., Boutouyrie, P., Cunha, P., et al. (2013). Early vascular ageing in translation: From laboratory investigations to clinical applications in cardiovascular prevention. *Journal of Hypertension, 31*(8), 1517–1526.

Okonta, N. R. (2012). Does yoga therapy reduce blood pressure in patients with hypertension? *Holistic Nursing Practice*, 137–141.

Oliva, R. V. & Bakris, G. L. (2012). Management of hypertension in the elderly population. *Journals of Gerontology: Medical Sciences, 67*(12), 1343–1351.

Pepersack, T., Gilles, C., Petrovic, M. et al. (2013). Prevalence of orthostatic hypotension and relationship with drug use amongst older patients. *Acta Clinica Belgica, 68*(2), 107–112.

Poggio, R., Grancelli, H. C. & Miriuka, S. G. (2010). Understanding the risk of hyperkalaemia in heart failure: Role of aldosterone antagonism. *Postgraduate Medical Journal, 86*(1013), 136–142.

Prata, J., Ramos, S., Martins, A. et al. (2014). Women with coronary artery disease: Do psychosocial factors contribute to a higher cardiovascular risk? *Cardiology in Review, 22*(1), 25–29.

Rabito, M. J. & Kaye, A. D. (2013). Complementary and alternative medicine and cardiovascular disease: An evidence-based review. *Evidence-Based Complementary and Alternative Medicine*, 8. Article ID 672097.

Rees, K., Hartley, L., Flowers, N. et al. (2013). “Mediterranean” dietary pattern for the primary prevention of cardiovascular disease. *Cochrane Database of Systematic Reviews*, 8. Article no. CD009824.

Riegel, B., Dickson, V. V., Cameron, J., Johnson, J. C., Bunker, S., Page, K. & Worrall-Carter, L. (2010). Symptom recognition in elders with heart failure. *Journal of Nursing Scholarship, 42*(1), 92–100.

Salehi-Abargouei, A., Maghsoudi, Z., Shirani, Z., Shirani, F. et al. (2013). Effects of dietary approaches to stop hypertension (DASH)-style diet on fatal or nonfatal cardiovascular diseases—Incidence: A systematic reviews and meta-analysis on observational prospective studies. *Nutrition, 29*(4), 611–618.

Scholl, J. (2012). Traditional dietary recommendations for the prevention of cardiovascular disease: Do they meet the needs of our patients? *Cholesterol*, article ID 367898. Viewed February 2015 at http://dx.doi.org/10.1155/2012/367898.

Setayeshgar, S., Whiting, S. J. & Vatanparast, H. (2013). Prevalence of 10-year risk of cardiovascular diseases and associated risks in Canadian adults: The contribution of cardiometabolic risk assessment introduction. *International Journal of Hypertension*, article ID 276564. Accessed February 2015 at http://dx.doi.org/10.1155/2013/276564.

Smith, S. C., Collins, A., Ferrari, R. et al. (2012). Our time: A call to save preventable death from cardiovascular disease (heart disease and stroke). *Circulation, 126*, 2769–2775.

Son, J. T. & Lee, E. (2012). Postprandial hypotension among older residents of a nursing home in Korea. *Journal of Clinical Nursing, 21*(23–24), 3565–3573.

Son, J. T. & Lee, E. (2013). Comparison of postprandial blood pressure reduction in elderly by different body position. *Geriatric Nursing, 34*, 282–288.

Statistics New Zealand. (2014). NZ social indicators: Obesity. Accessed February 2015 at www.stats.govt.nz/browse_for_stats/snapshots-of-nz/nz-social-indicators/Home/Health/obesity.aspx.

Steptoe, A. & Kivimaki, M. (2013). Stress and cardiovascular disease: An update on current knowledge. *Annual Review of Public Health, 34*, 337–254.

Suls, J. (2013). Anger and the heart: Perspectives on cardiac risk, mechanisms and interventions. *Progress in Cardiovascular Disease, 55*(6), 538–547.

Thurston, R. C., Rewak, M. & Kubzansky, L. D. (2013). An anxious heart: Anxiety and the onset of cardiovascular diseases. *Progress in Cardiovascular Disease, 55*(6), 524–537.

U.S. Preventive Services Task Force. (2012). *The guide to clinical preventive services 2012*. Recommendations of the U.S. Preventive Services Task Force. Agency for Healthcare Research and Quality. Publication no. 12-05154. Available 2 January 2014 via www.ahrq.gov.

van Hateren, K. J., Kleefstra, N., Blanker, M. H. et al. (2012). Orthostatic hypotension, diabetes, and falling in older patients. *British Journal of General Practice, 62*(603), e696–e702.

Weber, M. A., Schiffrin, E. L, White, W. B. et al. (2014). Clinical practice guidelines for the management of hypertension in the community. A statement by the American Society of Hypertension and the International Society of Hypertension. *Journal of Hypertension, 32*(1), 3–15.

Weihua, L., Yougang, W. & Jing, W. (2013). Reduced or modified dietary fat for preventing cardiovascular disease. *Journal of Cardiovascular Nursing, 28*(3), 204–205

Weiss, A. M. (2009). Cardiovascular disease in women. *Primary Care Clinics: Office Practice, 36*, 73–102.

White, M. M., Howie-Esquivel, J. & Caldwell, M. A. (2010). Improving heart failure symptom recognition: A diary analysis. *Journal of Cardiovascular Nursing, 25*(1), 7–12.

Williams, B., Lindholm, L. H. & Sever, P. (2008). Systolic pressure is all that matters. *Lancet, 371*, 2219–2221.

Xin, W., Lin, Z. & Li, X. (2013). Orthostatic hypotension and the risk of congestive heart failure: A meta-analysis of prospective cohort studies. *PLoS One, 8*(5), e63169.

Zanasi, A., Tincani, E., Evandri, V. et al. (2012). Meal-induced blood pressure variation and cardiovascular mortality in ambulatory hypertensive elderly patients. *Journal of Hypertension*, *30*(11), 2125–2132.

Chapter 21

Respiratory function

By Carol Miller and Sharyn Hunter

LEARNING OBJECTIVES

After reading this chapter, you should be able to:

1. Describe age-related changes that affect respiratory function.
2. Identify the risk factors that interfere with respiratory wellness for older adults.
3. Discuss the functional consequences that affect respiratory function in older adults.
4. Assess respiratory function, with emphasis on identifying opportunities for health promotion.
5. Identify nursing interventions to improve respiratory function and reduce risk factors that interfere with respiratory wellness.

KEY POINTS

aspiration pneumonia
chronic obstructive pulmonary disease (COPD)
detection
elastic recoil
involuntary smoking
kyphosis
lung parenchyma
pneumonia
second-hand smoke
smokeless tobacco

The primary functions of respiration are to supply oxygen to and remove carbon dioxide from the blood. Adequate respiratory performance is essential to life because all body organs and tissues need oxygen. Thus, it is noteworthy that the respiratory system shows less age-related decline than other body systems in healthy, non-smoking, older adults. The age-related changes that do affect respiratory performance are subtle and gradual and healthy older adults are able to compensate for these changes. However, when illness, anaesthesia or another complicating factor places extraordinary demands for oxygen on the body, age-related respiratory changes can influence the overall function of the older adult.

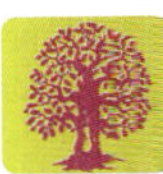

AGE-RELATED CHANGES THAT AFFECT RESPIRATORY FUNCTION

It is difficult to distinguish the effects of age-related changes from those caused by disease processes and external influences, such as tobacco smoking. Although these influences occur throughout the life span, their cumulative effects become more pronounced in older adults because they interact with age-related changes, such as diminished immune response, or with risk factors, such as diminished mobility.

Upper respiratory structures

The nose and other upper respiratory structures are affected by age-related changes that can affect comfort and function in the following ways:

- Degenerative changes in connective tissue causing the nose to have a retracted columella (the lower edge of the septum) and a poorly supported, downwardly rotated tip
- Diminished blood flow to the nose, causing the nasal turbinates to become smaller
- Thicker mucus in nasopharynx due to degenerative changes in submucosal glands
- Stiffening of trachea due to calcification of cartilage
- Blunted cough and laryngeal reflexes
- Atrophy of the laryngeal nerve endings.

Chest wall and musculoskeletal structures

The chest wall and lungs function like a bellows, with the chest expanding outwards in relation to lung expansion. The rib cage and the vertebral musculoskeletal structures are affected by the same kind of age-related changes that affect other musculoskeletal tissue: the ribs and vertebrae become osteoporotic, the costal cartilage calcifies and the respiratory muscles weaken. Because of these age-related processes, the following structural changes, which can affect respiratory performance, occur: **kyphosis** (i.e. an increased curvature of the spine), shortened thorax, chest wall stiffness and increased anteroposterior diameter of the chest. As a result of these changes, older adults experience diminished respiratory efficiency and reduced maximal inspiratory and expiratory force. Because older adults compensate for age-related changes by increased use of the diaphragm and other accessory muscles, they are more sensitive to any changes in intra-abdominal pressure. In summary, older adults expend more energy to achieve the same respiratory efficiency as younger adults, but the overall effects on healthy older people are minimal.

Lung structure and function

Even in healthy older adults, the lungs become smaller and flabbier, and age-related changes affect the **lung**

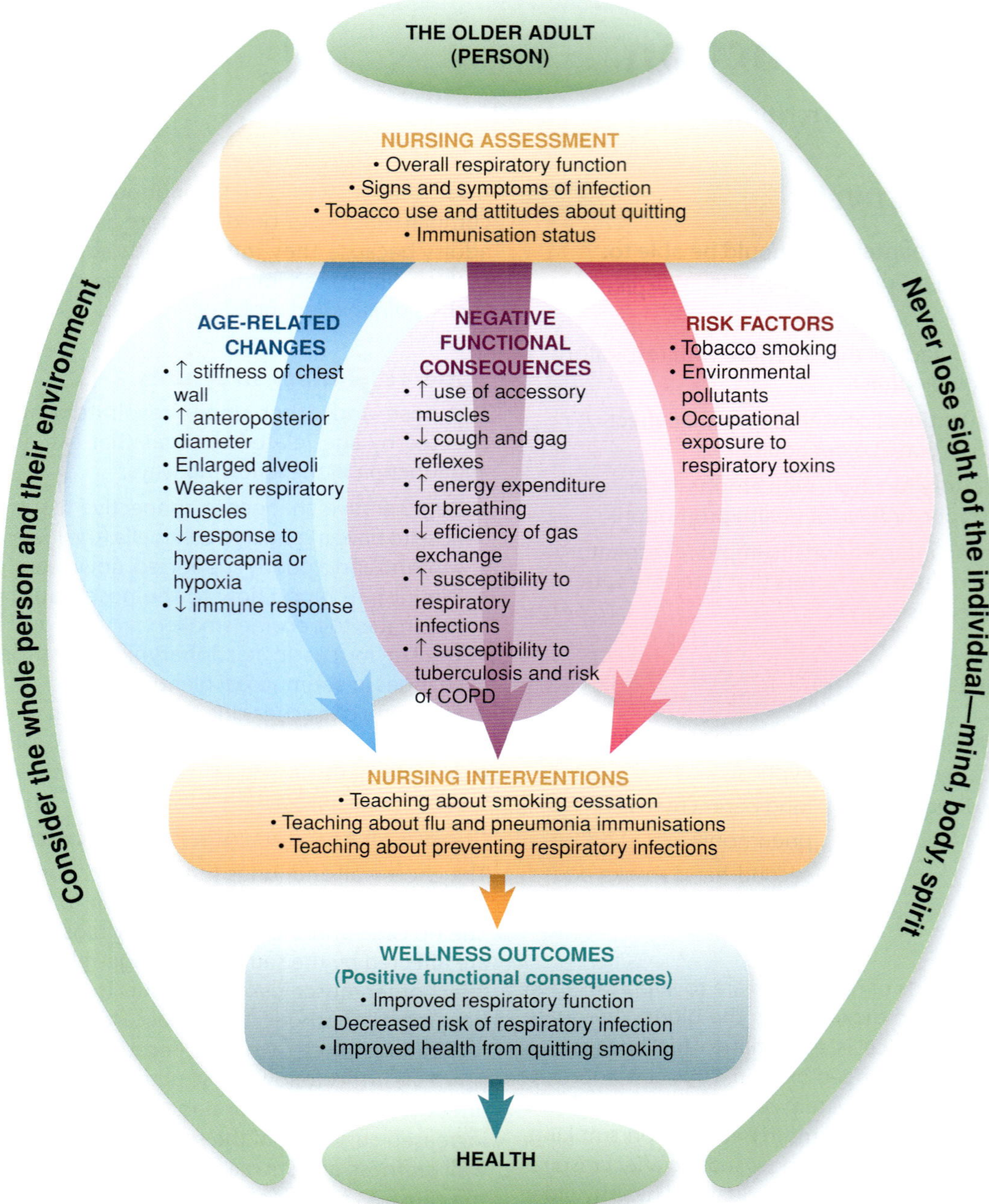

parenchyma, which is the part of the respiratory system where gas exchange takes place. Changes that have the most effect on respiratory function are as follows:

- Ductectasia (i.e. the alveoli enlarge and their walls become thinner) begins around the age of 20 or 30 years and continues throughout adulthood, resulting in a gradual increase in the amount of anatomical dead space.
- The pulmonary artery becomes wider, thicker and less elastic.
- The number of capillaries diminishes.
- The pulmonary capillary blood volume decreases.
- The mucosal bed, where diffusion occurs, thickens.

Elastic recoil is the characteristic that keeps the airways open during inspiration by resisting expansion and maintaining a positive pressure across the lung surface. If the airways close prematurely, air is trapped and the lungs cannot expire to their maximum capacity. A combination of age-related changes in the parenchyma and elastic fibres interferes with elastic recoil, which results in early airway closure. Because of this and other age-related changes, gas exchange is compromised in the lower lung regions and inspired air is preferentially distributed in the upper regions. Effects of these changes include decreased arterial oxygen pressure (PaO_2) and changes in airflow rates.

Compensatory changes in respiratory rate are made under conditions of hypercapnia or hypoxia. The response to hypercapnia is initiated by a central chemoreceptor, located in the medulla, whereas the response to hypoxia is initiated by peripheral chemoreceptors, located in the carotid and aortic bodies. Age-related changes reduce the ventilatory response to both hypoxia and hypercapnia, so instead of—or in addition to—experiencing breathlessness or other respiratory symptoms when blood gases are abnormal, older adults are likely to develop mental changes.

Changes in immune function

Age-related changes in the immune system affect respiratory function, even in healthy older adults. For example, studies confirm that age-related alterations of T cells (i.e. a component of the immune system that is essential for protecting against infections and malignancies) are a major factor contributing to the increased prevalence of lung diseases among older adults (Lee, Shin & Kang, 2012).

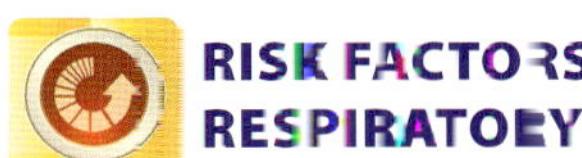

RISK FACTORS THAT AFFECT RESPIRATORY WELLNESS

For people of any age, tobacco smoking is the single most important risk factor for lung disease and impaired respiratory function. These risks are both immediate and cumulative. Other risks are mentioned because, particularly for non-smokers, they can be addressed through health promotion interventions to improve respiratory function. For smokers, however, these other risks are of minimal importance and attention must be focused on the serious negative consequences of smoking.

Tobacco use

Tobacco smoking causes detrimental effects through multiple heat and chemical actions on the respiratory system. Harmful physiological effects on the respiratory system include bronchoconstriction, impaired air flow, inflammation of the mucosa throughout the respiratory tract, and inhibited ciliary action, leading to increased coughing and mucous secretions and diminished protection from harmful organisms. The most serious consequence of smoking is a significantly increased risk of developing diseases of the lungs, cardiovascular system, and many other systems. Thus, smoking-related diseases are considered the world's most preventable cause of death. Even though pipes, cigars and **smokeless tobacco** products (such as electronic cigarettes and chewing tobacco or gum) are sometimes viewed as safer than cigarettes, all forms and doses of tobacco are associated with serious health consequences, which are similar to those of cigarette smoking (American Cancer Society, 2013). Examples of the serious risks and detrimental effects are as follows:

- Lung cancer is responsible for almost one in five cancer deaths in Australia of which smoking is a major cause. Lung cancer in New Zealand is the leading cause of cancer death and smoking was the contributor in about 85% (New Zealand Ministry of Health [NZMOH], 2012a).
- Smoking increases the risk for developing all the following types of cancers: paranasal sinus, nasopharynx, nasal cavity, lip, oral cavity, larynx, pharynx, oesophagus, lung, kidney, bladder, stomach, pancreas, colorectum, ovary, uterine cervix, and acute myeloid leukaemia. There is limited evidence of the link between smoking and breast cancer in women.
- Smoking is a major cause of heart disease, cerebrovascular disease (including stroke), chronic bronchitis, and emphysema (chronic obstructive pulmonary disease); it also is associated with gastric ulcers.

Researchers also are identifying links between smoking and conditions that disproportionately affect older adults, including all of the following: cognitive impairment (Okusaga, Stewart, Butcher et al., 2013; Rincon & Wright, 2013); osteoporosis (Ni, Glavin & Power, 2013); cataracts (Richter, Choudhury, Torres et al., 2012); age-related macular degeneration (Willeford & Rapp, 2012); and hearing loss (Yamasoba, Lin, Someya et al., 2013). Studies especially relevant to health promotion for older adults focus on beneficial effects of quitting during older adulthood. For example, Gellert and colleagues (2013) compared the new onset of cardiovascular events in 8807 current, never and former smokers aged from 50 to 74 years for a mean follow-up of 9.1 years and concluded that smoking cessation was highly and rapidly beneficial for older adults.

> **DIVERSITY NOTE**
>
> Studies suggest that men and women are genetically predisposed to respond differently to tobacco smoke, with men being more likely to develop emphysema-like manifestations and women experiencing more airway affectation (Carrasco-Garrido et al., 2009).

> **DIVERSITY NOTE**
>
> Prevalence of cigarette smoking is higher for Indigenous Australians than other Australians (Cancer Council NSW, 2013).

Another potentially detrimental health effect related to smoking that has implications for care of older adults is the potential for altering the effects of medications. Interactions can occur in people who smoke or use nicotine products (including smokeless tobacco) and in people who have recently quit smoking. Interactions can be due directly to the physiological effects of nicotine or they may be caused by the hydrocarbons in tobacco smoke, which can affect hepatic metabolism of some medications.

Additional information and examples of drug–nicotine interactions are discussed in Chapter 8.

WELLNESS OPPORTUNITY

Nurses need to be aware of opportunities to teach older adults about potential interactions between medications and nicotine products, which are often overlooked.

Second-hand smoke and other environmental factors

Second-hand smoke (also called passive smoke or environmental tobacco smoke) is a mixture of smoke that comes primarily from the end of lighted cigarettes, cigars or pipes (called *sidestream smoke*) and secondarily from smoke that is exhaled by the smoker (called *mainstream smoke*). The Environment Protection Agency classifies second-hand smoke as a carcinogen because it contains hundreds of carcinogenic chemical compounds.

The terms ***involuntary smoking*** and *passive smoking* refer to the involuntary exposure and breathing in of second-hand smoke. Although the negative effects of second-hand smoke were viewed with scepticism when they were first reported in the 1972 Surgeon General's Report, increasing evidence indicates that there is no safe level of exposure to second-hand smoke. The following evidence-based statistics substantiate strong links between second-hand smoke and disease and mortality for adults (Llewellyn et al., 2009; Shafey et al., 2009):

- Even brief exposure to second-hand smoke can cause immediate cardiovascular and respiratory damage.
- There is sufficient evidence that non-smokers exposed to second-hand smoke at home or work increase their risk for lung cancer and coronary artery disease risk by at least 20% to 30%.
- There is suggestive evidence that second-hand smoke increases the risk for stroke, atherosclerosis, breast cancer, nasal sinus cancer, COPD, asthma, chronic respiratory symptoms and impaired lung function.
- A longitudinal study found that non-smoking subjects with high salivary cotinine levels from second-hand smoke had increased odds of cognitive impairment.

Another environmental risk factor that can lead to negative functional consequences is the inhalation of air pollutants. Like the effects of cigarette smoking, the effects of air pollution are cumulative over many years and, therefore, have an increased impact on older adults who have been exposed to air pollutants for as many as eight or nine decades.

As well as being exposed to general air pollutants, older adults who worked in occupations such as mining and firefighting might experience the cumulative and long-term effects of occupational exposure to toxic substances. Because hazards in the workplace were largely unregulated before the 1970s, many older people never benefited from the protections enforced under the various Occupational Safety and Health Acts in Australia.

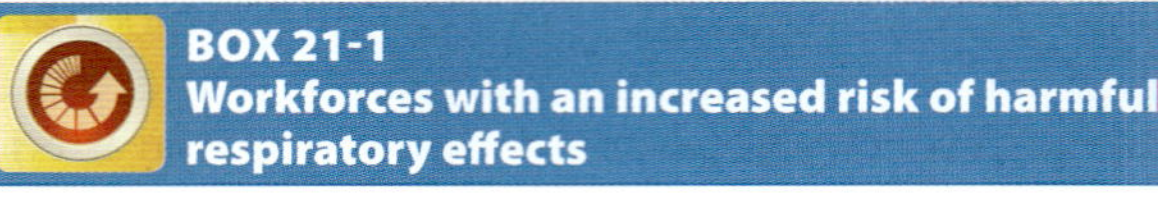

BOX 21-1
Workforces with an increased risk of harmful respiratory effects

Firefighters
Miners
Traffic controllers
Shipyard workers
Rubber workers
Aluminium workers
Iron and steel foundry workers
Tunnel and street repair workers
Asbestos workers
Quarry workers
Farmers, agricultural workers, grain handlers
Construction workers
Paper mill workers
Workers exposed to the following: dust, fumes, gases, nickel, arsenic, beryllium, chromium or radiation

In addition, much of the information now available on the harmful effects of certain chemicals was not widely available when these older adults were working. Even though the exposure to harmful substances may have occurred long ago, the signs and symptoms may not manifest until later adulthood. Box 21-1 lists some job categories that are associated with an increased risk of respiratory disease.

The level of humidity is another environmental condition that can affect respiratory function. For example, dry air can affect the upper airway by further drying the nasal secretions, causing them to be thicker and more difficult to remove. Environmental humidity does not have serious detrimental effects, but it should be considered as a condition that affects overall respiratory wellness.

Additional risk factors

Older adults are likely to have additional risks associated with conditions (e.g. obesity or chronic illness) that interfere with their usual ability to obtain adequate physical activity, which is necessary to maintain optimal respiratory function. In addition, even brief periods of bed rest during acute illnesses can increase the risk for developing pneumonia or exacerbate the effects of chronic lung conditions. Kyphosis is associated with poor posture and shallow breathing patterns, which can diminish the respiratory function in older adults. Lack of vaccinations increases the risk for pneumonia and influenza, as discussed in the section on preventing lower respiratory infections.

Medications increase the risk for impaired respiratory function in several ways. For example, sedatives and anticholinergic medications can affect upper airway function by drying the mucus. Medications may also influence cough reflexes or cause a persistent dry cough (e.g. angiotensin-converting enzyme inhibitors).

A student's perspective

I was glad to interact with someone who has emphysema and to learn about her struggles and about how care needs to be specialised for her because of her condition. Listening to E. A.'s breath sounds was frightening to me. I knew she was unable to breathe well, but I had no idea it was that obstructed. The struggle and stress her condition puts on her body to breathe is saddening. I really am amazed she is able to function as well as she does with her decreased level of oxygen.

I really enjoyed how talkative E. A. was. I had no problem getting information from her to complete her functional health assessment. It really hit me after I walked out of the nursing home on Friday that she literally talked to me for 3 hours. She was absolutely beside herself just to have someone there to listen and to interact with. I was glad I was able to give that to her. I believe this experience with E. A. will help me in the future to remember to give the emotional care as well as the physical. In the next week, the things I would like to improve include supporting and promoting E. A. to get up and get dressed. I would like to help her with performing ADLs and help make her morning more worthwhile. I think helping E. A. become a little more productive could also help improve her social interactions. This is an area she needs a lot of help with and I hope this week I will be able to give her support in doing so.

Jenna W.

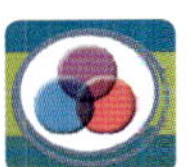

FUNCTIONAL CONSEQUENCES AFFECTING RESPIRATORY WELLNESS

In the absence of smoking and other risk factors, healthy older adults do not experience any significant functional consequences related to respiratory function when performing ordinary activities. Under conditions of physical stress, however, older adults may experience dyspnoea and fatigue because their respiratory system is less efficient in gas exchange. Similarly, age related changes in the respiratory system do not affect exercise capacity, but deconditioning and risk factors can compromise it. Table 21-1 summarises the functional consequences of age-related changes that affect respiratory wellness. Older adults who smoke or have other risk factors experience the same negative consequences as younger adults, but the effects are cumulative and the consequences are likely to be more serious.

Increased susceptibility to lower respiratory infections

Even for healthy non-smoking older adults, the most important functional consequence related to respiratory wellness is due to a combination of age-related changes in the respiratory tract and the immune system. Because of this combination of age-related changes, older adults have higher rates of illness and death due to all types of lower respiratory infections, including pneumonia and influenza (Goldstein, 2012). **Pneumonia** and influenza are one of the leading causes of death among older adults. Additional factors that commonly occur in older adults to increase their risk for lower respiratory infections, even for non-smokers, include age-related diminished physiological reserve and cumulative effects of exposure to toxins, including tobacco smoke, occupational dusts, and indoor and outdoor air pollution (Fragoso & Gill, 2012). Additional factors that further compromise the ability of older adults to defend against respiratory infections include frailty, malnutrition, dysphagia, serious illness and diminished functional status. Poor oral care in hospitalised people and long-term care residents is another condition that increases the risk for pneumonia (Tada & Miura, 2012). Another complicating factor is the difficulty of diagnosing lower respiratory infections during early stages because the manifestations are subtle and non-specific, as discussed in the section on nursing assessment of respiratory function.

Aspiration pneumonia, defined as an inflammation of the lungs caused by food or secretions entering into the bronchial tree, is a serious respiratory condition that is common in older adults with risk factors. One major risk factor for aspiration pneumonia is *dysphagia* (swallowing difficulties), which affects 25% of independently living older adults and more than 50% of those in long-term residential care homes (Clave, Rofes, Carrion et al., 2012; Serra-Prat et al., 2012). Other factors that increase the risk for aspiration pneumonia include achlorhydria, general debility, tube feeding, malnutrition and dehydration, decreased cough reflex, diminished salivary flow, compromised immune function, and diminished level of consciousness.

TABLE 21-1 Functional consequences of age-related changes affecting respiratory function

Change	Consequence
Upper airway changes: calcification of cartilage, altered neuromuscular function and reflexes	Snoring, mouth breathing, diminished cough reflex, decreased efficiency of gag reflex
Increased anteroposterior diameter, chest wall stiffness, weakened muscles and diaphragm	Increased use of accessory muscles, increased energy expended for respiratory efficiency
Enlargement of alveoli, thinning of alveolar walls, diminished number of capillaries	Diminished efficiency of gas exchange, decreased arterial oxygen pressure (PaO_2)
Decreased elastic recoil and early airway closure	Changes in lung volumes, slight decrease in overall efficiency
Tidal volume unchanged or slightly diminished, increased residual volume, decreased vital capacity	Total lung capacity unchanged

Increased susceptibility to tuberculosis

Older adults are also at increased risk for tuberculosis because of changes in immunity. Additionally, those born before 1950, and who are now older, have a higher rate of TB infection and are at an increased risk of progressing to active disease due to immunosuppression caused by risk factors (Australian Government Department of Health [AGDH], 2012). Risk factors include smoking, diabetes, malnutrition and debilitating conditions as well as immunosuppressant medications. Moreover, altered and more subtle disease manifestations interfere with identification and treatment of tuberculosis in older adults. The incidence of tuberculosis has not decreased in recent years in either Australia (AGDH, 2012) or New Zealand (Immunisation Advisory Centre, 2013). Immigration is a major contributor to the incidence of tuberculosis in both countries. In Australia, 80% to 90% of Australia's new cases are immigrated (AGDH, 2012). In New Zealand, those 70 years and older were in the second highest age group for tuberculosis notifications in New Zealand (Immunisation Advisory Centre, 2013).

DIVERSITY NOTE

Tuberculosis is more prevalent in people who have migrated to Australia from India, Vietnam, the Philippines and China than other migrant populations (AGDH, 2012).

PATHOLOGICAL CONDITION AFFECTING RESPIRATORY FUNCTION: COPD

Chronic obstructive pulmonary disease (COPD) is a group of diseases, including emphysema, chronic bronchitis and a subset of asthma, characterised by chronic airflow obstruction that interferes with normal breathing. In addition to tobacco smoking as the primary risk factor, conditions that increase the risk for developing COPD include genetic predisposition, low socioeconomic status, exposure to secondary smoke and other air pollutants and a history of significant childhood respiratory disease.

The most common manifestations of COPD are cough, dyspnoea, wheezing and increased sputum production. The condition is progressive and its cumulative effects become more disabling as the person ages. Functional consequences of COPD for older adults include longer and more frequent hospitalisations, an increased risk for being discharged to nursing facilities and impaired health-related quality of life. Studies indicate that 80% of older adults with COPD have concurrent disease and are likely to attribute dyspnoea to other conditions, including ageing (Akgun, Crothers & Pisani, 2012). People with COPD are more likely to have several coexisting conditions, including (in order of prevalence) arthritis, depression, osteoporosis, cancer, coronary heart disease, heart failure and stroke (Schnell, Weiss, Lee et al., 2012).

COPD is the fifth leading cause of death in Australia (Australian Bureau of Statistics [ABS], 2012) and fourth in New Zealand (Asthma Foundation, 2012). Up to 14.5% of Australians 40 years or over have COPD, and this increases to 29.2% in Australians 75 years or over (Toelle, Xuan, Bird et al., 2011). In New Zealand approximately 15% of those over the age of 45 years have COPD (Asthma Foundation, 2012).

An important health promotion implication when caring for older adults with COPD is to encourage participation in pulmonary rehabilitation programs (Bolton et al., 2013). These programs aim to improve exercise capacity, dyspnoea and psychological well-being, while supporting self-management of the disease process. Participation in physical activity is considered an essential self-management intervention for improving symptoms in people with COPD (Thorpe & Kumar, 2012). It is recommended that the older adult participate in a supervised program with a "... combination of progressive muscle resistance and aerobic training" (Bolton et al., 2013, p. ii). These exercise programs may be interval or continuous training, depending on their assessed condition and preference. Pulmonary rehabilitation also offers smoking cessation advice. Evidence-based practice recommendations for people living with COPD in Australia and New Zealand have been released in 2014, and continues to be updated quarterly (Lung Foundation Australia and the Thoracic Society of Australia and New Zealand, 2014). These guidelines, The COPD-X concise guide for primary care, can be accessed via http://lungfoundation.com.au. Evidence-based practice 21-1 summarises recommendations for nursing assessment and care for people with dyspnoea, which is also called the sixth vital sign in people with COPD (Registered Nurses Association of Ontario, 2010).

DIVERSITY NOTE

The rate of death among Indigenous Australians from respiratory disease between 2006 and 2010 was about twice that of the non-Indigenous population (Australian Health Ministers' Advisory Council, 2012). COPD was responsible for 55% of these deaths.

COPD hospitalisation and mortality rates for Māori aged 65+ years were significantly higher than for non-Māori (NZMOH, 2012b). Māori females in the 65+ years' age group had a COPD hospitalisation rate almost five times higher than non-Māori, and the death rate was three times higher. Smoking is the major cause of COPD in Māori, with Māori adults twice as likely to smoke as other populations in New Zealand.

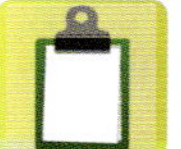

NURSING ASSESSMENT OF RESPIRATORY FUNCTION

With the exception of minor differences in physical assessment of the respiratory system, nursing assessment of respiratory function is similar for younger and older adults.

EVIDENCE-BASED PRACTICE 21-1
Nursing care of dyspnoea

Statement of the problem

- Dyspnoea is the sixth vital sign in people with chronic obstructive pulmonary disease (COPD).

Recommendations for nursing assessment

- Assess all the following vital signs: pulse oximetry, lung sounds, chest wall shape and movement, accessory muscle use, productive or non-productive cough, peripheral oedema, ability to complete a full sentence, level of consciousness.
- Assess current level of dyspnoea and usual breathing pattern.
- Assess for hypoxaemia/hypoxia.
- Identify signs and symptoms of stable and unstable dyspnoea and acute respiratory failure.
- Screen for COPD in adults older than 40 years who have a history of smoking by asking each person these three questions: (1) Do you have progressive activity-related shortness of breath? (2) Do you have a persistent cough and sputum production? (3) Do you experience frequent respiratory tract infections?
- Advocate for spirometry testing for people who have a history of smoking and are older than 40 years.
- If inhaler is used, assess self-administration technique.

Recommendations for nursing interventions

- Acknowledge and accept the person's self-report of dyspnoea.
- Administer prescribed oxygen therapy, ventilation modalities and medications (e.g. bronchodilators, corticosteroids, antibiotics and psychotropics).
- Implement smoking cessation strategies: consider nicotine replacement and other smoking cessation modalities during hospitalisation.
- Remain with the person during episodes of acute respiratory distress.

Recommendations for teaching older adults and carers about dyspnoea

- Prescribed medications, including correct technique for inhaler use.
- Administration of oxygen therapy if prescribed.
- Strategies for secretion clearance, energy conservation, relaxation techniques, nutrition and breathing retraining.
- Influenza and pneumococcal vaccinations.
- Pulmonary rehabilitation and exercise training as appropriate.
- Smoking cessation strategies if appropriate.
- Disease self-management strategies, including development of action plan and decision-making regarding advanced directives.

Source: Registered Nurses Association of Ontario (RNAO). (2010). *Nursing care of dyspnea: The 6th vital sign in individuals with chronic obstructive pulmonary disease.* Toronto, ON: RNAO. Accessible March 2015 via www.rnao.ca.

However, nurses must be aware of variations in the manifestations of lower respiratory infections when they occur in older adults. Another difference is that nurses assess the different life experiences of older adults with regard to their exposure to environmental toxins and attitudes about tobacco use when identifying opportunities for health promotion. From a wellness perspective, nursing assessment of respiratory function focuses on identifying opportunities for health promotion, detecting lower respiratory infections, assessing smoking behaviours and identifying other risk factors.

Identifying opportunities for health promotion

Nurses interview older adults or their caregivers, to identify the risk factors that can be addressed through health promotion activities. Because tobacco smoking is the risk factor that has serious detrimental effects on lung health as well as many other aspects of health, nurses assess the potential for influencing all smokers, even older adults, to quit. Health education is based on assessment information about health-related behaviours, such as smoking and avoidance of second-hand smoke, as well as preventive interventions, such as influenza and pneumonia vaccinations. Nurses also assess the attitudes of older adults about these preventive measures, so they can plan appropriate educational approaches. Last, nurses ask older adults about their overall respiratory function to identify respiratory problems that can be addressed in the nursing care plan. Box 21-2 presents an interview format that nurses can use to assess risk factors, overall respiratory function and opportunities for health education.

WELLNESS OPPORTUNITY

One question a nurse can ask to identify the person's health-promoting behaviours is "What do you do to avoid environmental tobacco smoke?"

Detecting lower respiratory infections

The term **detection** is more accurate than assessment with regard to lower respiratory infections because these conditions commonly present atypically in older adults and treatment may be delayed, increasing the risk for serious complications, including death. Rather than presenting with a fever, cough and purulent sputum, older adults are more likely to have subtler and non-specific disease manifestations. Even initial chest radiography may not provide accurate diagnostic information. A review of studies by Akgun and colleagues (2012) summarised the following manifestations of several types of pneumonia in older adults:

- Bacterial pneumonia: tachypnoea, delirium, failure to thrive, malaise and falls
- Viral pneumonia: bronchospasm and recent-onset dyspnoea
- Aspiration pneumonia: gradual course and low-grade fevers.

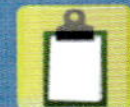

BOX 21-2
Guidelines for assessing respiratory function

Questions to identify risk factors for respiratory problems

- Have you had any respiratory problems, such as asthma, chronic lung disease, pneumonia or other infections?
- Do you have a family history of chronic lung disease?
- Have you ever had tuberculosis?
- Have you ever worked in a job where you were exposed to dust, fumes, smoke or other air pollutants (e.g. in mining, farming or any of the occupations listed in Box 21-1)?
- Have you lived in neighbourhoods where there was a lot of pollution from traffic or factories?
- Do you smoke now, or have you ever smoked? (If yes, continue with the questions in Box 21-3.)
- Have you been exposed to passive smoke in home, work or social environments?

Questions to identify opportunities for education about disease prevention and health promotion

- Have you ever had a pneumonia vaccination? *If yes*, when was the vaccination administered and was a booster ever given?
- Do you get annual influenza vaccinations?

Questions to assess overall respiratory function

- Do you have any problems with breathing?
- Do you have any wheezing?
- Do you have spells of coughing? *If yes*, When do they occur? How long do they last? What brings them on? Are they dry or productive? Does the phlegm come from your throat or lungs? What does the phlegm look like?
- Do you ever have trouble getting enough air during any particular activities or when you lie down at night?
- Have you stopped doing any particular activities because of problems breathing? For example, have you stopped going up or down stairs, or have you limited the amount of walking you do? (For people with mobility limitations, this question might not be relevant.)
- Do you ever have any chest pain or feelings of heaviness or tightness in your chest?
- Do you use more than one pillow at night, or make any other adjustments, because of trouble with breathing?
- Do you wake up at night because of coughing or difficulty with breathing?
- Do you ever feel as though you can't catch your breath?
- Do you have trouble breathing when the weather is hot, cold or humid?
- Do you tire easily?

An important assessment consideration is to recognise that older adults do not necessarily exhibit the expected manifestations of pneumonia. The most significant finding on physical assessment of the lungs may be a diminished intensity of lung sounds or the presence of abnormal sounds, which are very non-specific findings. In addition, a change in mental status or another alteration in functional status, such as falls or incontinence, may be a major clue to pneumonia. Thus, an important nursing responsibility is to detect non-specific manifestations of pneumonia and collect additional information. This is essential for ensuring a timely diagnosis and preventing complications.

As with other lower respiratory infections, non-specific assessment findings can delay and complicate the diagnosis of tuberculosis in older adults. The atypical presentation of tuberculosis in older adults can lead to delayed diagnosis and treatment and a higher rate of serious consequences, including death. The common occurrence of false-negative tuberculin skin test reactions in older adults is another reason that tuberculosis may be undetected; however, the two-step Mantoux test with tuberculin purified protein derivative (PPD) is the recommended method of assessing for previous exposure to tuberculosis. Because tuberculosis often occurs as a reactivation of dormant disease, nurses must be particularly alert for manifestations of this disease in older adults who have a history of tuberculosis.

Assessing smoking behaviours

Although smoking affects all people, regardless of age, some aspects of smoking behaviours differ according to age cohorts. Therefore, an assessment of smoking as a risk factor must address the age-related factors that affect these behaviours. The cohort of people born between 1910 and 1930, for example, is the first age group to be exposed to the social pressures that encouraged smoking without knowing about its detrimental effects. As a result, people who began smoking in the early 1920s, when it became a popular habit for men, may have smoked for four or five decades before finding out that smoking is harmful. For women, smoking was not socially acceptable until the mid-1940s. Thus, today's generation of older adults has smoking rates among the highest in history.

Over the last decade the number of Australians aged 15 years and over who smoke has decreased by 28% (Heart Foundation, 2012). In New Zealand, it has been reported that cigarette consumption among adults has almost halved since 1991 (New Zealand Ministry of Social Development, 2010). Despite this decrease, older smokers may have an outlook reflected in statements such as, "If I've smoked this long and am still alive, why should I quit now?"

In addition to assessing attitudes about smoking, nurses should assess past and present smoking patterns. Frequency of smoking and type of tobacco smoked are important determinants of the relative risk of smoking. Smokeless tobacco, for example, is not as detrimental to respiratory and cardiovascular function as cigarette smoking, but it increases the risk for oral cancer and other types of cancer. Cigarettes vary in the amount of nicotine they contain and this variable influences the degree of risk associated with a particular type of cigarette. In contrast to younger adults, who began smoking when cigarettes had filters and were lower in nicotine, older adults began smoking when cigarettes had no filters and contained greater amounts of tar and nicotine. Older adults, therefore, are likely to smoke cigarettes that have higher and more harmful nicotine levels. Some older adults, in fact, may still roll their own cigarettes using loose tobacco.

For older adults who smoke, nurses ask questions to determine their readiness to consider quitting smoking as well as their knowledge about the health effects of smoking. This is important because older adult smokers may falsely believe that there are no health benefits to quitting, so they are likely to respond positively to health education about smoking cessation. Nurses also assess the older adult's perception of smoking as a manifestation of his or her rights and autonomy. For example, long-term care residents may view smoking as the one remaining indicator of their former life and the one pleasurable activity that they can control. As with other healthcare decisions, adults are entitled to make decisions about their health-related behaviours, but these decisions should be based on full knowledge of the benefits and risks of their choices.

Nurses may need to examine their own attitudes about smoking, especially in relation to older adults. For example, it is important to identify ageist influences that can lead to the view that smoking cessation would not be beneficial for older adults. Similarly, although it is important to respect the rights of older adults who choose to smoke, healthcare professionals should not exclude older adults from health promotion interventions about smoking simply because they are old. Assessment questions designed to help determine smoking habits and attitudes about smoking are included in Box 21-3.

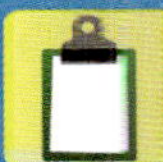

BOX 21-3
Guidelines for nursing assessment of older adults who smoke

Questions to assess smoking behaviours

- How long have you smoked?
- How much do you smoke?
- What do you smoke?
- Have you smoked other types of tobacco in the past?

Questions to assess knowledge of the risk from smoking

- Do you think there are any harmful effects of smoking for people in general?
- Do you think you are at risk for any harmful effects from smoking?
- Do you think there are any benefits to quitting smoking?

Questions to assess attitudes towards smoking

- Have you ever thought about quitting smoking?
- Has any health professional ever talked to you about quitting smoking?
- What do you think about the idea of quitting smoking?
- Have you ever tried to quit? *If yes:* What was your experience with the attempt?
- Would you be interested in finding out information about quitting smoking now?

WELLNESS OPPORTUNITY

To assess smoking behaviours from a whole-person perspective, nurses need to ask questions about the older adults' knowledge of the detrimental effects of smoking as well as their perception of smoking as an expression of autonomy.

Identifying other risk factors

In addition to assessing tobacco use as a risk factor, nurses identify other factors that affect respiratory function in less significant ways. Because maximum respiratory function is attained by early adulthood, nurses assess factors that may have influenced respiratory development in early life. For example, questions about nutrition, respiratory infections and exposure to cigarette smoke may provide information about the person's vulnerability to the effects of age-related changes and risk factors. For this reason, nurses incorporate questions about exposure to environmental tobacco smoke and harmful air pollutants in their assessments.

Occupational exposure to certain harmful substances is particularly important for smokers because the risk of either one of these factors is compounded when the other factor is present. Nurses also assess the person's level of activity and identify factors that interfere with mobility or routine activities because these conditions can influence the degree to which the person can improve his or her level of activity. If, for example, people have limited mobility because of arthritis, they may not be able to engage in vigorous physical exercise, but they might benefit greatly from water exercises. Box 21-2 summarises guidelines for assessing respiratory function in older adults.

WELLNESS OPPORTUNITY

To set the stage for health education about preventive measures, nurses assess the older adult's understanding of influenza and pneumonia vaccinations.

Physical assessment findings

Nurses use the usual methods of inspection, palpation, percussion and auscultation to evaluate respiratory performance in both younger and older adults. Minor differences in assessment findings for healthy older adults include:

- Slight increase in the normal respiratory rate, which ranges from 16 to 24 respirations per minute
- Increased anteroposterior diameter
- Forward-leaning posture because of kyphosis
- Increased resonance on percussion
- Diminished intensity of lung sounds
- Increased presence of adventitious sounds in the lower lungs.

Begin the assessment of respiratory function by observing the person's breathing pattern in different positions, such as walking or sitting. To facilitate auscultation, ask the older adult to sit upright, cough before auscultation, and breathe with mouth open. When observing respirations in a sleeping older adult, assess for brief periods of apnoea, which are associated with sleep problems. This is further discussed in Chapter 24, Sleep and rest.

Specific aspects of lung function, such as air volumes and airflow rates, can be measured by pulmonary function tests, spirometry, and peak flow. Of the two, nurses commonly measure peak flow to assess respiratory function. Nurses are required to have an understanding of the spirometry values in relation to respiratory function. Older adults do experience alterations in air volumes because of age-related changes in the chest wall and in lung elastic recoil, and these are additional to the changes caused by the risk factors. However, because various air volumes are interrelated and compensatory mechanisms, the aged related changes have limited effect on the total lungs' airflow. Airflow rates are only affected to a small degree by age-related changes, but are affected to a greater degree by additional variables such as height and gender. Pulse oximetry is another common assessment performed by nurses to determine respiratory function. There is a small but not significant decline with ageing. Overall, there is an age-related decline in all airflow rates, but because of the many interacting variables and a wide range of normal values, these declines are usually minor. The most significant decline is demonstrated with peak flow. From approximately 35 years peak flow will decline. However, this decline increases for older adults over 60 years; approximately 0.5% to 1% per decade. Table 21-2 summarises the age-related changes of some lung function parameters.

UNFOLDING CASE STUDY

Part A

Mr Rein is 65 years old and comes with his wife to the local medical centre. Both Mr and Mrs Rein smoke one to two packs of cigarettes a day. Mr Rein has mild COPD and Mrs Rein has hypertension and coronary artery disease. Every year the medical centre provides flu shots for anyone older than 65 years. You are the practice nurse and as you are preparing to give flu shots, Mr and Mrs Rein come to you and ask, "Is this the shot that takes care of pneumonia? Our daughter said we should get a pneumonia shot every year, but we don't want a flu shot because our friend says she got the flu from one of those shots and she'll never get a shot again. Can you just give us the pneumonia shot today? We got one from the doctor last year."

Thinking points

- What myths and misunderstandings do Mr and Mrs Rein express?
- What further assessment questions would you ask?
- What health promotion teaching would you do?

NURSING ISSUES

The nursing issue of ineffective breathing pattern would be applicable when the nursing assessment identifies factors that may impair the older adult's respiratory function. Defining characteristics include bradypnoea, dyspnoea, orthopnoea, tachypnoea, altered chest excursion, use of accessory muscles to breathe and alterations in depth of breathing. If impaired respiratory function interferes with activities of daily living, a nursing issue of activity intolerance might be appropriate. Debilitated or chronically ill older adults who live in group settings may be at risk for

TABLE 21-2 Age-related changes in indicators of lung function

Indicator	Definition	Age-related change
Tidal volume	Amount of air moved in and out during a normal breath	Slight decrease
Residual volume	Amount of air left in the lungs after a forced expiration	Increases by 5%–10% per decade
Forced expiratory volume	Amount of air expelled within 1 second after a maximum inspiration	Decreases 23–32 mL/year in men, 19–26 mL/year in women
Forced inspiratory volume	Maximum volume of air that can be inhaled in addition to tidal volume	Decreases
Forced vital capacity	Maximum volume of air that can be expelled following a maximum inspiration	Decreases 14–30 mL/year in men, 14–24 mL/year in women
Total lung capacity	Amount of air that can be held in the lungs after a maximum inspiratory effort	Unchanged, as a result of compensatory mechanisms
Diffusing capacity	Ability of lungs to transfer gases between the lungs and blood	Declines 2.03 mL/min/mm Hg per decade in men and 1.47 mL/min/mm Hg in women
Peak expiratory flow	Peak speed of airflow from lungs during one expiration	Declines in men and women from age 35 years
Arterial oxygen pressure (PaO_2)	Amount of oxygen in arteries	Declines 0.3% per year or 4 mm Hg per decade but remains stable after the age of 75

infections, particularly pneumonia, influenza and tuberculosis. For example, if a long-term care resident has active tuberculosis, the nursing staff might address the nursing issue of risk for transmission of infection for the affected resident and the nursing issue of risk for infection for all other residents. Likewise, when influenza affects one or more residents or staff of a long-term care facility, the same nursing issue may be applicable. Ineffective health maintenance is a nursing issue that may be used for older adults who have insufficient knowledge about the detrimental effects of active or passive smoking.

WELLNESS OPPORTUNITY

When nurses provide pneumonia or influenza immunisations for older adults, they can use the wellness nursing issue of willingness for enhanced immunisation status.

GOAL PLANNING FOR WELLNESS OUTCOMES

When caring for older adults with respiratory problems, nurses develop goals that achieve wellness outcomes as an essential part of the planning process. The following nursing goals apply to the nursing issue of ineffective breathing pattern: improved vital signs, and ventilation and airway patency.

For most older adults who have adequate respiratory function, nurses plan for wellness outcomes by addressing their increased vulnerability to pneumonia, influenza and tuberculosis. Pertinent goals for the nursing issue of risk for infection include improved immune status and development of proactive behaviour towards immunisation and prevention of community transmission of a communicable disease. An appropriate wellness goal for older adults who lack knowledge about preventing respiratory infections would be knowledge about health behaviours.

WELLNESS OPPORTUNITY

Nurses promote wellness when their care plans address the immunisation status of older adults.

Because tobacco smoking is the most important factor that influences respiratory function, nurses working with older adults who smoke should always consider the possibility of identifying and working towards a goal of reducing or eliminating tobacco use. Thus, for older adults who smoke applicable outcomes include the control of tobacco use and knowledge about substance use control

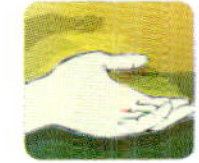

NURSING INTERVENTIONS FOR RESPIRATORY WELLNESS

For all older adults, nursing interventions to promote respiratory wellness focus on protection from second-hand smoke and prevention of respiratory infections. For those who smoke, teaching about smoking cessation is the most important intervention for respiratory wellness. Nursing interventions would focus on the promotion of respiratory wellness through environmental risk protection, health education, immunisation/vaccination management, infection control, infection protection, referral and smoking cessation assistance.

Promoting respiratory wellness

Smoking is the single most important preventable cause of disease and therefore should be a major target of disease prevention activities for all people who smoke tobacco. Because older smokers are likely to have smoking-related functional consequences, smoking cessation will address secondary or tertiary prevention rather than primary prevention. Smoking cessation is widely recognised as a cost-effective health promotion activity that healthcare professionals should routinely address (Wilkinson, Bass, Diem et al., 2012). Many health promotion materials are available in Australia and New Zealand. A recent smoking cessation campaign has been launched in New Zealand (2014) that features the logo "Ask about the Elephant!", which provides information about effective and affordable stop smoking interventions. The information is contained in guidelines released by the New Zealand Ministry of Health. These guidelines advocate using the revised pathway the steps of which include:

- Ask about and document every person's smoking status.
- Give brief advice to stop to every person who smokes.
- Strongly encourage every person who smokes to use cessation support (a combination of behavioural support and stop-smoking medicine works best) and offer to help them access it. Refer to, or provide, cessation support to everyone who accepts your offer. (NZMOH, 2014a, p. 1)

In Australia it is recommended that the "5As" approach be utilised by health professionals for structuring smoking cessation support (Royal Australian College of General Practitioners, 2011). The 5As is a five-components counselling program that includes: ask, assess, advise, assist and arrange follow-up.

For all older adults, disease prevention and health promotion interventions related to respiratory function include pneumonia and influenza vaccinations and education about the importance of avoiding environmental tobacco smoke. These intervention are discussed in the following sections and are summarised in Boxes 21-4 and 21-5. In addition, numerous educational materials are available for use in disease prevention and health promotion interventions, and many use languages other than English. (See the resources section at the end of this chapter.)

BOX 21-4 Health promotion teaching about respiratory problems

Factors that increase the risk of pneumonia and influenza

- Diabetes or any chronic lung, heart or kidney disease
- Hospitalisation within the past year for heart or lung diseases
- Severe anaemia or a debilitating condition
- Confinement to bed or very limited mobility
- Residence in a nursing home or other group living setting
- Immunosuppressive medications

Preventing respiratory infection

- Wash your hands frequently with an antibacterial soap or hand sanitiser.
- Avoid hand-to-mouth and hand-to-eye contact.
- Avoid inhaling air that has been contaminated with particles from the cough or sneeze of someone with an infection.
- Avoid crowds during the flu season.
- Be sure that influenza and pneumonia vaccinations are up to date.

Information about influenza vaccinations

- New vaccinations are developed every year, based on information about the strains of viruses that are most likely to affect people during the influenza season.
- Vaccines are made from inactivated viruses and, therefore, should have few or no side effects.
- People who are allergic to eggs and egg products should NOT receive influenza immunisations.
- Immunisations do not offer immediate protection because there is a 2- to 3-week delay in developing an antibody response.
- Every year, the manufacturers of the influenza vaccination provide recommendations as to the best time for administering the immunisations for optimal effectiveness. The best time is during the late autumn, but the exact time period will vary slightly from year to year.
- Vaccines are not 100% effective, but they are helpful for most older people.
- Influenza immunisations provide protection against the most serious viruses but not against all types of respiratory infections.
- The duration of effectiveness of vaccinations may be shorter than 6 months in some older people; therefore, one vaccination might not protect the person through the entire season.
- Influenza immunisation in Australia and New Zealand is free for older adults.

Information about pneumonia vaccinations

- Pneumonia vaccinations are recommended for people older than 65 years of age.
- Pneumonia vaccinations are recommended for older adults every 5 years.
- Side effects, if they occur, are not serious and will subside within a few days.
- Common side effects include a slight fever accompanied by pain, redness or tenderness at the injection site.
- Pneumonia vaccinations are covered by Medicare.

Nutritional considerations

- Include foods high in zinc and vitamins A, B-complex, C and E.

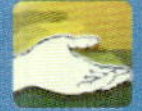

BOX 21-5 Health promotion teaching about cigarette smoking

Attitudes about smoking

- Stopping smoking at any age is more beneficial than continuing to smoke.
- Many of the harmful effects of smoking are reversed once the smoker quits.
- Although some of the effects of past smoking are irreversible, all of the harmful effects of future smoking can be avoided by quitting now.
- Smoking is a major risk factor for many cancers, including those of the lung, head, stomach, kidney and pancreas.
- Smoking is a major risk factor for lung and heart disease, including high blood pressure and heart attacks.
- Passive smoking (inhaling smoke from the air) is associated with an increased risk for many diseases.

Type of tobacco

- The lower the tar and nicotine content of cigarettes, the less harmful the effects. However, many cigarettes with lower tar and nicotine levels have additional chemical additives that can be harmful.
- Pipe and cigar smokers are at a higher risk for chronic lung disease than non-smokers, just as cigarette smokers are.
- The harmful effects of tobacco use on the mouth and upper respiratory tract are equal for all types of tobacco, including smokeless tobacco. All smokers have the same risk for developing cancer of the mouth and upper respiratory tract.

Approaches to quitting

- Any reduction in present tobacco use is better than maintaining the current level. The negative effects of smoking are directly proportional to the number of cigarettes inhaled.
- Various forms of prescription and over-the-counter nicotine substitutes (e.g. gum, skin patches and nasal sprays) are available and may be helpful, especially when used in conjunction with counselling and self-help techniques.
- Besides nicotine substitutes, some non-nicotine prescription medications and over-the-counter products may be effective as a component of a smoking cessation program.
- People who are trying to quit smoking should discuss their goals with a healthcare professional to identify the methods that might be most effective.
- Many self-help programs are available for support and education regarding quitting smoking.
- Information about group programs can be obtained on the Internet

Non-pharmacological practices to help quit smoking

- Exercise, music, imagery, massage, meditation, affirmations, deep breathing, stress reduction, social support or individual or group counselling.

WELLNESS OPPORTUNITY

Nurses promote self-care behaviours by encouraging older adults to use teaching materials. Materials are available at the end of the chapter in the resources section.

Preventing lower respiratory infections

Interventions which prevent pneumonia and influenza are particularly important. Adults 65 years or over are at an increased risk of contracting pneumococcal disease and influenza than other adults. The majority of deaths from this disease occur in this age group (Immunisation Advisory Centre, 2011). During 2014, adults 80 years and over were the age group with the highest number of notifications of all types of influenza (AGDH, 2014). In New Zealand in 2013, notifications from pneumococcal disease were the highest for adults aged 70 years and over (Institute of Environmental Science and Research, 2013). Importantly, pneumonia and influenza are the only diseases of all the leading causes of death in older adults that can be prevented through immunisations. Nurses also have important roles in addressing tuberculosis, particularly for medically compromised older adults in long-term and residential care facilities. The following sections discuss the role of the nurse in preventing these types of lower respiratory infections, with emphasis on health education interventions.

The influenza and pneumococcal vaccines are safe and well tolerated by older adults and studies indicate that these measures reduce morbidity and mortality and decrease hospitalisation admission rates for respiratory infections (AGDH, 2013). In Australia, the National Pneumococcal Vaccination Program for Older Australians commenced in 2005 and provides free pneumococcal polysaccharide vaccine to older aged adults every 5 years. In Australia and New Zealand a free annual influenza vaccination is available for all older adults (AGDH, 2013; NZMOH, 2014b). The influenza vaccine has been found to be very effective in reducing mortality and morbidity in older adults. The influenza vaccine is 30% to 70% effective in preventing all hospitalisations for pneumonia and influenza for older adults living outside long-term residential care (AGDH, 2013). For those who live in residential care, the influenza vaccine assists with the prevention of severe illness, secondary complications and deaths. The vaccine can be 50% to 60% effective in preventing hospitalisation or pneumonia, and 80% effective in preventing death for these older adults.

Long-term residential care facilities have standing orders for influenza and pneumonia vaccinations and nurses play a primary role in implementing this health promotion intervention in community, residential and other institutional settings. In addition, all healthcare workers who care for older adults should receive annual influenza vaccinations to prevent transmission, thereby indirectly reducing mortality from influenza in the older population. Box 21-4 summarises current information about influenza and pneumonia immunisations, along with information about risk factors for these illnesses.

DIVERSITY NOTE

In Australia, Indigenous people aged 55 years and over in remote areas were more likely than those in non-remote areas to have been recently vaccinated for influenza. They were also twice as likely to have received a vaccination against pneumonia in the last 5 years (ABS, 2007).

In addition to promoting pneumonia and influenza immunisations, nurses need to promote adequate nutrition and hydration as preventive measures for all older adults. Nurses who care for long-term care residents and older adults with compromised functioning need to implement direct nursing interventions to prevent pneumonia, including aspiration pneumonia. Studies have found that good oral hygiene—including measures to prevent the accumulation of plaque on teeth and dentures—is important for reducing the risk for pneumonia (Johnson, 2012). Additional nursing interventions for preventing lower respiratory infections include meticulous attention to hand washing and optimal positioning and turning of older adults who have limited mobility.

Nurses working in long-term care or other healthcare facilities are responsible for implementing programs to detect and address tuberculosis. Guidelines are available from the Australian Department of Health, Victorian Department of Health and the New Zealand Ministry of Health. All provide information about interventions for people with tuberculosis and prevention of its spread. The web addresses are available in the resources section at the end of the chapter. Any nurse or direct-care staff member working with older adults should undergo periodic skin testing to screen for exposure to tuberculosis.

Eliminating the risk from smoking

Educational interventions for older smokers begin by addressing attitudes that influence health-related behaviours. For example, if an older person expresses an "I'm-too-old-to-change" attitude, an initial step is to explore the older adult's understanding of his or her ability to change behavioural patterns. Even though older adults may be long-term smokers, their success rate for quitting is higher than that of younger adults. Information about models of behaviour change (discussed in Chapter 5) is applicable to help smokers to quit.

Another commonly expressed belief that nurses can address through health education is "It's too late to do any good". When nurses encounter this type of attitude, they can emphasise that the substantial health benefits derived from quitting smoking are both immediate and long term. Benefits from smoking cessation for people of any age include improved quality of life, decreased susceptibility to smoking-related illnesses (e.g. heart disease and cancer), and a more rapid recovery from illnesses that usually are exacerbated by smoking. Health benefits of quitting smoking occur at any age, and people who quit at the age of 65 or older increase their life expectancy by 2 to 3 years (van Meijgaard & Fielding, 2012).

Evidence-based guidelines emphasise the importance of nurses and other healthcare providers initiating the topic of tobacco dependence and routinely identifying and intervening with all tobacco users—including light smokers and smokeless tobacco users—at every opportunity (Sarna, Bialous, Ong et al. 2012; Wilkinson, Bass, Diem et al., 2012). Additional points of evidence-based guidelines are as follows:

- Tobacco dependence is a chronic disease that may require repeated interventions; however, effective treatments can significantly increase rates of long-term abstinence.
- Individual, group and telephone counselling methods are effective; problem solving and social support as part of treatment are especially effective counselling interventions.
- Nicotine-based medications that reliably increase long-term smoking abstinence are nicotine gum, inhaler, lozenge, patch and nasal spray.

Non-nicotine medications that are effective for smoking cessation include sustained-release bupropion and varenicline; however, warnings have been issued about serious cardiovascular and neuropsychiatric symptoms that can occur with varenicline. Both drugs are listed in the Pharmaceutical Benefits Scheme in Australia and therefore available at a reduced cost (iCanQuit, 2014). Both drugs are available for use in New Zealand but the costs are not subsidised (Pharmac, 2014).

Counselling and medication are effective for treating tobacco dependence, but the combination of these methods is more effective than either alone in quitting. Three in four smokers would like to quit. Smokers reported they were more likely to quit if they had a health scare than any other reason (Heart Foundation, 2012).

Non-pharmacological interventions that are effective for smoking cessation include exercise, guided imagery, breathing techniques, positive self-talk, journaling, integration of rewards, and identification of habit breakers for events that trigger smoking (Jackson, 2012). Box 21-5 can be used as a guide to teaching older adults about quitting smoking.

WELLNESS OPPORTUNITY

Nurses support wellness in older adults by communicating that old age is not an inevitable barrier to changing health-related behaviours: it's never too late to quit.

UNFOLDING CASE STUDY

Part B

Mr Rein is now 70 years old and attends the local medical centre. During one of his visits he says while you, the practice nurse, are checking his blood pressure that he is thinking about quitting smoking, but that his son just quit and gained a lot of weight and had a lot of trouble sleeping. He's not sure if quitting smoking is worth the effort, especially because his son has been so miserable since he quit. Also, at his age, it probably won't do any good to quit now, he says.

Thinking points

- What further questions would you ask to assess Mr Rein's readiness to discuss quitting smoking?
- What health promotion teaching would you do?
- What would your response be if you determine that Mr Rein is not ready to consider quitting smoking?

EVALUATING EFFECTIVENESS OF NURSING INTERVENTIONS

Measuring the effectiveness of interventions for the nursing issue of ineffective breathing pattern is based on a reassessment of subjective indicators such as ease of breathing and objective indicators such as lung sounds and respiratory rate and rhythm. An indicator of successful health education interventions for older adults with ineffective breathing pattern is that they can accurately identify factors that can be addressed to improve their respiratory function. Disease prevention interventions for the nursing issue of risk for infection could be documented on a record of the person's history of immunisations for pneumonia and influenza. For older adults who smoke and are willing to address this risk factor, effectiveness of interventions would be measured by the person's increased knowledge about the detrimental effects of smoking and by his or her willingness to develop a plan to stop smoking. Long-term effectiveness would be evaluated by the person's successful participation in the smoking cessation program.

UNFOLDING CASE STUDY

Part C

Mr Rein is now 72 years old and recently moved into a long-term residential facility where you are employed as the nurse. One day he asks you how he can get some nicotine gum because he has heard that this is a good way to cut down on cigarettes. Now that he lives in the facility, he can't smoke in the dining room, and he'd like to chew nicotine gum before and after he eats. He admits that he smokes a pack of cigarettes every day but denies having experienced any bad effects from smoking. Mr Rein sees his doctor for COPD and takes Flixotide, two puffs twice a day, and Serevent, two puffs twice a day.

Nursing assessment

You begin your nursing assessment by exploring Mr Rein's attitudes about smoking and ascertaining his knowledge about the harmful effects of cigarette smoking. Mr Rein says he thought about quitting smoking many times but never actually tried to quit because his wife smoked even more than he did until she died a few months ago. He felt it would be too hard to quit as long as she was smoking two packs per day. He also states that he's heard a lot about passive smoking and he figured it wasn't worth trying to quit as long as he was around his wife's cigarette smoke. He states that he's been smoking for 50 years, and if he hasn't got lung cancer by now, he's not going to get it at his age. To comply with the rules in the facility, Mr Rein says he plans to chew nicotine gum when he can't smoke cigarettes, but he sees no reason to quit.

In assessing Mr Rein's knowledge about the effects of cigarette smoking, you determine that he is aware of some of the harmful effects of passive smoking but has very little information about the detrimental effects of cigarette smoking. He relates that his wife died of lung cancer, but he attributes her death to a history of breast cancer, which she had 10 years before the lung cancer. Mr Rein has no knowledge about cigarette smoking as a risk factor for cardiovascular disease, nor does he realise that his hypertension poses an additional risk. Mr Rein reports that he has experienced no ill effects from cigarette smoking, but when you ask about his history of respiratory infections, he admits he had pneumonia 3 years ago. He says that he received a pneumonia shot 2 years ago, so he doesn't have to worry about getting pneumonia again, and that he has had bronchitis several times, so he doesn't worry about getting any lung infections, either.

Nursing issue

Based on the assessment findings, an appropriate nursing issue would be ineffective health maintenance, related to insufficient knowledge about the effects of tobacco use and self-help resources. Some of Mr Rein's statements reflect a lack of accurate information about the harmful effects of cigarette smoking, particularly regarding risks for respiratory infections and impaired cardiovascular function. Other statements probably reflect an intellectualisation of his continued smoking. Your intuition tells you that, with some education and support, he may be willing to quit smoking.

Nursing care plan for Mr Rein

Goals for wellness outcomes	Nursing interventions	Nursing evaluation
Mr Rein will increase his knowledge about the harmful effects of cigarette smoking.	• Give Mr Rein brochures and illustrations provided by the Office on Smoking and Health and use them to discuss the effects of cigarette smoking. • Use brochures from the Heart Foundation to discuss the risk factors for cardiovascular disease. • Discuss cigarette smoking as a risk factor for respiratory infections. • Give Mr Rein a copy of Box 21-5 and discuss the immediate and long-term benefits of quitting smoking.	• Mr Rein verbalises correct information about the risks of cigarette smoking. • Mr Rein describes the benefits derived from quitting smoking.
Mr Rein will be knowledgeable about techniques for quitting smoking.	• Using information from the Heart Foundation, discuss some of the strategies for quitting smoking (e.g. quitting cold turkey, using nicotine substitutes, participating in self-help groups).	• Mr Rein describes the advantages and disadvantages of the various methods of quitting smoking.
Mr Rein will quit smoking.	• Identify the method Mr Rein prefers for quitting smoking. • Emphasise the importance of nutrition, exercise, and adequate fluid intake. • Agree on realistic goals for smoking cessation. • Discuss supportive resources. Set up weekly appointments at the local medical centre for support and further discussions.	• Mr Rein reports he has stopped or significantly reduced his smoking.

Thinking points

- How would you assess Mr Rein's readiness and motivation to quit smoking?
- What health education approach would you take with Mr Rein?
- What additional interventions or health education points would you use for Mr Rein?

CHAPTER HIGHLIGHTS

Age-related changes that affect respiratory wellness

- Upper airway changes (e.g. calcification of cartilage)
- Increased anteroposterior diameter
- Chest wall stiffness, weakened muscles
- Alveoli enlarged and have thinner walls
- Alterations in lung volumes and airflow
- Decreased compensatory response to hypercapnia and hypoxia
- Decreased immune response

Risk factors that affect respiratory wellness

- Tobacco smoking
- Environmental factors (e.g. pollution, dry air, second-hand smoke)
- Occupational hazards

Functional consequences affecting respiratory wellness

- Mouth breathing, diminished cough reflex, less efficient gag reflex
- Increased use of accessory muscles, increased energy expended for breathing
- Diminished efficiency of gas exchange, decreased PaO_2 levels
- Decreased vital capacity, slight decrease in overall efficiency
- Increased susceptibility to lower respiratory infections
- Increased susceptibility to tuberculosis
- Increased risk of COPD

Pathological condition affecting respiratory wellness: COPD

- COPD: a group of diseases, including emphysema, chronic bronchitis and a subset of asthma, characterised by chronic airflow obstruction

Nursing assessment of respiratory function

- Overall respiratory function
- Detection of lower respiratory infections
- Tobacco use and attitudes regarding smoking

Nursing issues

- Health-seeking behaviours
- Ineffective breathing pattern
- Risk for infection

Goal planning for wellness outcomes

- Improved vital signs and ventilation, airway patency
- Improved immune status and immunisation behaviour and community risk control
- Knowledge about health behaviours
- Risk control of tobacco use and knowledge about substance use

Nursing interventions for respiratory wellness

- Prevention and detection of pneumonia and influenza
- Health education about smoking cessation

Evaluating effectiveness of nursing interventions

- Ease of breathing
- Up-to-date status for pneumonia immunisation
- Influenza immunisation every year
- For older adults who smoke: active participation in smoking cessation behaviours

CRITICAL THINKING EXERCISES

1. What will a healthy, non-smoking, 83-year-old person experience in his or her daily life with regard to respiratory function?
2. What would you include in a health education program which is designed for older adults, on the prevention of pneumonia and influenza?
3. How would you address the following statement made by a 71-year-old person: "I've lived this long and don't have lung cancer. Why should I start worrying now?"
4. Find the names, addresses and phone numbers of local agencies that would be appropriate resources for someone interested in quitting smoking. Contact at least one of these organisations to find out specific information about support groups, written materials and other resources.

RESOURCES

For an extensive range of additional resources to enhance teaching and learning and to facilitate understanding of this chapter, please see the text's accompanying website located on thePoint at http://thepoint.lww.com.

Clinical tools

Hartford Institute for Geriatric Nursing, ConsultGeriRN.org: http://consultgerirn.org/resources

General assessment series:

- *Try This*, issue 21: Immunizations for the older adult. Greenberg, S. (2012). *Best Practices in Nursing Care to Older Adults.*

Evidence-based practice

Joanna Briggs Institute: http://connect.jbiconnectplus.org

Evidence summaries:

- Krivan, S. (2014). Influenza vaccination of healthcare workers: Older people's health.
- Krivan, S. (2014). Influenza vaccination: Older people.

Recommended practices:

- Pneumococcal infection: Adult vaccination, by Chronic Disease Node Group. V. H. Wong (2013).

National Guideline Clearinghouse: www.guideline.gov

Search for:

- Chronic obstructive pulmonary disease (COPD).
- Clinical guideline for the evaluation, management and long-term care of obstructive sleep apnea in adults (2013).

- Nursing care of dyspnea: The 6th vital sign in individuals with chronic obstructive pulmonary disease (2010).
- Tobacco treatment (2012).

Health education

American Lung Association: www.lungusa.org
Australian immunisation handbook (10th ed.) (2013): www.immunise.health.gov.au
Cancer Council NSW: www.cancercouncil.com.au
Department of Health, Victoria, tuberculosis guidelines: www.health.vic.gov.au
Immunisation Advisory Centre, New Zealand: www.influenza.org.nz
Lung Foundation Australia COPD-X concise guide for primary care: www.lungfoundation.com.au
National Heart, Lung and Blood Institute (U.S.): www.nhlbi.nih.gov/health-pro
Office on Smoking and Health, Centers for Disease Control and Prevention (U.S.): www.healthfinder.gov/orgs/HR0049.htm

REFERENCES

Akgun, K. M., Crothers, K. & Pisani, M. (2012). Epidemiology and management of common pulmonary diseases in older persons. *Journals of Gerontology: Biological Sciences, 67A*(3), 276–291.

American Cancer Society. (2013). *Cancer facts & figures 2013.* Atlanta, GA: American Cancer Society.

Asthma Foundation. (2012). COPD in NZ. Accessed March 2015 at asthmafoundation.org.nz/your-health/living-with-copd/copd-in-nz.

Australian Bureau of Statistics. (2007). *Older Aboriginal and Torres Strait Islander people: A snapshot, 2004–05.* Cat. no. 4722.0.55.002. Viewed March 2015 at www.abs.gov.au/AUSSTATS/abs@.nsf/mf/4722.0.55.002.

Australian Bureau of Statistics. (2012). *Causes of death, 2012.* Cat. no. 3303.0. Viewed March 2015 via www.abs.gov.au.

Australian Government Department of Health. (2012). Strategic Plan for Control of Tuberculosis in Australia: 2011–2015. Accessed March 2015 at www.health.gov.au/internet/main/publishing.nsf/Content/cda-cdi3603i.htm.

Australian Government Department of Health. (2013). Immunise Australia Program: Older Australians. Accessed March 2015 at www.immunise.health.gov.au/internet/immunise/publishing.nsf/Content/older-aust.

Australian Government Department of Health. (2014). Australian Influenza Surveillance Report No. 8. Accessed March 2015 via www.health.gov.au/flureport#current.

Australian Health Ministers' Advisory Council (AHMAC). (2012). Aboriginal and Torres Strait Islander Health Performance Framework 2012 Report. Canberra: Author.

Bolton, C. E., Bevan-Smith, E. F., Blakey, J. D. et al. (2013). British Thoracic Society guideline on pulmonary rehabilitation in adults. *Thorax, 68*, ii1–ii30.

Cancer Council NSW. (2013). How many people smoke? Accessed March 2015 at www.cancercouncil.com.au/79096/reduce-risks/smoking-reduce-risks/tobacco-statistics/how-many-people-smoke-in-nsw.

Carrasco-Garrido, P., Miguel-Diez, J., Rejas-Gutierrez, J., Martin-Centeno, A., Gobartt-Vasquez, E., Hernandez-Barrera, V., . . . Jimenez-Caterino, J. M. (2008). Evaluation and management of geriatric infections in the emergency department. *Emergency Medicine Clinics of North America, 26*, 319–343.

Clave, P., Rofes, L., Carrion, S. et al. (2012). Pathophysiology, relevance and natural history of oropharyngeal dysphagia among older people. *Nestlé Nutrition Institute Workshop Series, 72*, 57–66.

Fragoso, C. A. V. & Gill, T. M. (2012). Respiratory impairment and the aging lung. *Journals of Gerontology: Medical Sciences, 67A*(3), 264–275.

Gellert, C., Schottker, B., Muller, H. et al. (2013). Impact of smoking and quitting on cardiovascular outcomes and risk advancement periods among older adults. *European Journal of Epidemiology, 28*(8), 649–658.

Goldstein, D. R. (2012). Role of aging on innate responses to viral infections. *Journals of Gerontology: Biological Sciences, 67A*(3), 242–246.

Heart Foundation. (2012). Smoking statistics. Accessed March 2015 at www.heartfoundation.org.au/SiteCollectionDocuments/Factsheet-Smoking.pdf.

iCanQuit. (2014). Using prescribed quit smoking medication. Accessed March 2015 at www.icanquit.com.au/quit-guide/methods-to-quit/prescribed-medicines.

Immunisation Advisory Centre, New Zealand. (2013). Tuberculosis. Accessed www.immune.org.nz/diseases/tuberculosis.

Institute of Environmental Science and Research. (2013). Surveillance Report: Notifiable and Other Diseases in New Zealand. Accessed March 2015 at https://surv.esr.cri.nz/surveillance/annual_surveillance.php?we_objectID=3962.

Jackson, C. (2012). Smoking cessation. In B. Dossey & L. Keegan (Eds), *Holistic nursing: A handbook for practice* (6th ed., pp. 513–538). Boston, MA: Jones & Bartlett.

Johnson, V. B. (2012). Evidence-based practice guideline: Oral hygiene care for functionally dependent and cognitively impaired older adults. *Journal of Gerontological Nursing, 38*(11), 11–19.

Lee, N., Shin, M. S. & Kang, I. (2012). T-Cell biology in aging, with a focus on lung disease. *Journals of Gerontology: Biological Sciences, 67A*(3), 254–263.

Llewellyn, D. J., Lang, I. A., Naughton, F. & Matthews, F. E. (2009). Exposure to second-hand smoke and cognitive impairment in non-smokers: National cross sectional study with cotinine measurement. *British Medical Journal, 338*, 632–634.

Lung Foundation Australia and the Thoracic Society of Australia and New Zealand. (2014). The COPD X Plan: Australian and New Zealand guidelines for the management of chronic obstructive pulmonary disease. Accessed March 2015 at http://lungfoundation.com.au/health-professionals/guidelines/copd/copd-x-concise-guide-for-primary-care.

New Zealand Ministry of Health. (2012a). Lung cancer. Accessed March 2015 at www.health.govt.nz/your-health/conditions-and-treatments/diseases-and-illnesses/lung-cancer.

New Zealand Ministry of Health. (2102b). Respiratory disease (50+ years). Accessed March 2015 at www.health.govt.nz/nz-health-statistics/health-statistics-and-data-sets/maori-health-data-and-stats/tatau-kura-tangata-health-older-maori-chart-book/nga-mana-hauora-tutohu-health-status-indicators-50-years/respiratory-disease-50-years.

New Zealand Ministry of Health. (2014a). New Zealand guidelines for helping people to stop smoking. Accessed March 2015 at www.health.govt.nz/publication/new-zealand-guidelines-helping-people-stop-smoking.

New Zealand Ministry of Health. (2014b). New Zealand Immunisation Schedule. Accessed March 2015 at www.health.govt.nz/our-work/preventative-health-wellness/immunisation/new-zealand-immunisation-schedule.

New Zealand Ministry of Social Development. (2010). The Social Report. Available March 2015 via www.socialreport.msd.govt.nz/index.html.

Ni, C., Glavin, P. & Power, D. (2013). Awareness of osteoporosis, risk and protective factors and own diagnostic status. *Archives of Osteoporosis, 8*(1–2), 117.

Okusaga, O., Stewart, M. C., Butcher, I. et al. (2013). Smoking, hypercholesterolaemia and hypertension as risk factors for cognitive impairment in older adults. *Age and Ageing, 42*(3), 306–311.

Pharmac. (2014). Online pharmaceutical schedule. Accessed www.pharmac.govt.nz/Pharmaceutical Schedule/Schedule.

Registered Nurses Association of Ontario (RNAO). (2005). *Nursing care of dyspnea: The 6th vital sign in individuals with chronic obstructive pulmonary disease*. Toronto, ON: Author.

Registered Nurses Association of Ontario (RNAO). (2010). *Nursing care of dyspnea: The 6th vital sign in individuals with chronic obstructive pulmonary disease*. Supplement 2010. Toronto, ON: Author.

Richter, G. M., Choudhury, F., Torres, M. et al. (2012). Risk factors for incident cortical, nuclear, posterior subcapsular, and mixed lens opacities. *Ophthalmology, 119*(10), 2040–2047.

Rincon, F. & Wright, C. B. (2013). Vascular cognitive impairment. *Current Opinion in Neurology, 26*(1), 29–36.

Royal Australian College of General Practitioners (RACGP) (2011). Supporting smoking cessation: A guide for health professionals (updated 2014). Accessed March 2015 at www.racgp.org.au/your-practice/guidelines/smoking-cessation.

Sarna, L., Bialous, S. A., Ong, M. K. et al. (2012). Increasing nursing referral to telephone quitlines for smoking cessation using a web-based program. *Nursing Research, 61*(6), 433–440.

Schnell, K., Weiss, C. O., Lee, T. et al. (2012). The prevalence of clinically-relevant comorbid conditions in patients with physician-diagnosed COPD. *BMC Pulmonary Medicine, 12*, 26.

Serra-Prat, M., Palomera, M., Gomez, C. et al. (2012). Oropharyngeal dysphagia as a risk factor for malnutrition and lower respiratory tract infection in independently living older persons. *Age and Ageing, 41*(3), 376–381.

Shafey, O., Eriksen, M., Ross, H. & Mackay, J. (2009). *The tobacco atlas* (3rd ed.). Atlanta, GA: American Cancer Society and World Lung Foundation.

Tada, A. & Miura, H. (2012). Prevention of aspiration pneumonia with oral care. *Archives of Gerontology and Geriatrics, 55*(1), 16–21.

Thorpe, O. & Kumar, S. (2012). Barriers and enables to physical activity participation in patients with COPD: A systematic review. *Journal of Cardiopulmonary Rehabilitation and Prevention, 32*, 359–369.

Toelle, B., Xuan, W., Bird, T. et al. (2011). COPD in the Australian burden of lung disease (BOLD) study. *Respirology, 16*(Suppl. 1), 12.

Van Meijgaard, J. & Fielding, J. E. (2012). Estimating benefits of past, current, and future reductions in smoking rates using a comprehensive model with competing causes of death. *Preventing Chronic Disease, 9*, 110295. doi:10.5888/pcd9.110295.

Wilkinson, J., Bass, C., Diem, S. et al. (2012). Preventive services for adults. Bloomington, MN: Institute for Clinical Systems Improvement. Viewed March 2015 at www.icsi.org/_asset/gtjr9h.

Willeford, K. T. & Rapp, J. (2012). Smoking and age-related macular degeneration. *Optometry and Vision Science, 89*(11), 1662–1666.

Yamasoba, T., Lin, F. R., Someya, S. et al. (2013). Current concepts in age-related hearing loss: Epidemiology and mechanistic pathways. *Hearing Research, 303*, 30–38.

Chapter 22

Mobility and safety

By Carol Miller and Sharyn Hunter

LEARNING OBJECTIVES

After reading this chapter, you should be able to:

1. Delineate age-related changes that affect mobility and safety.
2. Identify risk factors that increase the risk of osteoporosis and influence the safety and mobility of older adults.
3. Discuss the following functional consequences: diminished musculoskeletal function, increased susceptibility to fractures and increased susceptibility to falls.
4. Discuss the psychosocial and long-term consequences of falls, fractures and osteoporosis.
5. Conduct a nursing assessment of musculoskeletal performance and risks for falls and osteoporosis.
6. Identify interventions directed towards safe mobility and the elimination of risks for falls and osteoporosis.

KEY POINTS

bone densitometry	osteoarthritis
exercise programs	osteopenia
fall risk assessment tools	osteoporosis
fear of falling	sarcopenia
fragility fracture	

Mobility is one of the most important aspects of physiological function because it is essential for maintaining independence and because serious consequences occur when independence is lost. For older adults, mobility is influenced by age-related changes to some extent, but risk factors play a much larger role. Because of the many risks that affect mobility, falls and fractures are an unfortunately common occurrence in old age. Older adults, then, have the dual challenge of maintaining mobility skills and avoiding falls and fractures. For these reasons, safety is an integral aspect of mobility.

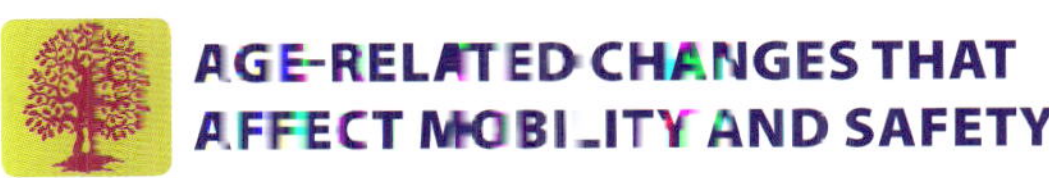

AGE-RELATED CHANGES THAT AFFECT MOBILITY AND SAFETY

The bones, joints and muscles are the body structures most closely associated with mobility, but many additional functional aspects are involved in *safe* mobility. Neurological function, for example, influences all facets of musculoskeletal performance and visual function influences the ability to interact safely with the environment. In the musculoskeletal system, osteoporosis is the age-related change that has the most significant overall impact, has been studied the most and is most amenable to interventions aimed at prevention and management.

Bones

Bones provide the framework for the entire musculoskeletal system and work in conjunction with the muscular system to facilitate movement. Additional functions of bone in the human body include storing calcium, producing blood cells and supporting and protecting body organs and tissues. Bone is composed of a hard outer layer, called cortical or compact bone and an inner, spongy meshwork, called trabecular or cancellous bone. The proportion of cortical to trabecular components varies according to bone type. Long bones, such as the radius and femur, are composed of as much as 90% cortical cells, whereas flat and vertebral bones are composed primarily of trabecular cells. Both cortical and trabecular bone components are affected by age-related changes, but the rate and impact of age-related changes differ in the two types of bone.

Bone growth reaches maturity in early adulthood, but bone remodelling continues throughout one's lifetime. The following age-related changes affect this remodelling process in all older adults

- Increased bone reabsorption (i.e. breakdown of bone that is necessary for remodelling)
- Diminished calcium absorption
- Increased serum parathyroid hormone
- Impaired regulation of osteoblast activity
- Impaired bone formation secondary to reduced osteoblastic production of bone matrix
- Fewer functional marrow cells due to replacement of marrow with fat cells
- Decreased oestrogen in women and testosterone in men.

Muscles

Skeletal muscles, which are controlled by motor neurons, directly affect all activities of daily living (ADLs). Age-related changes that have the greatest impact on muscle function include:

- Decreased size and number of muscle fibres
- Loss of motor neurons

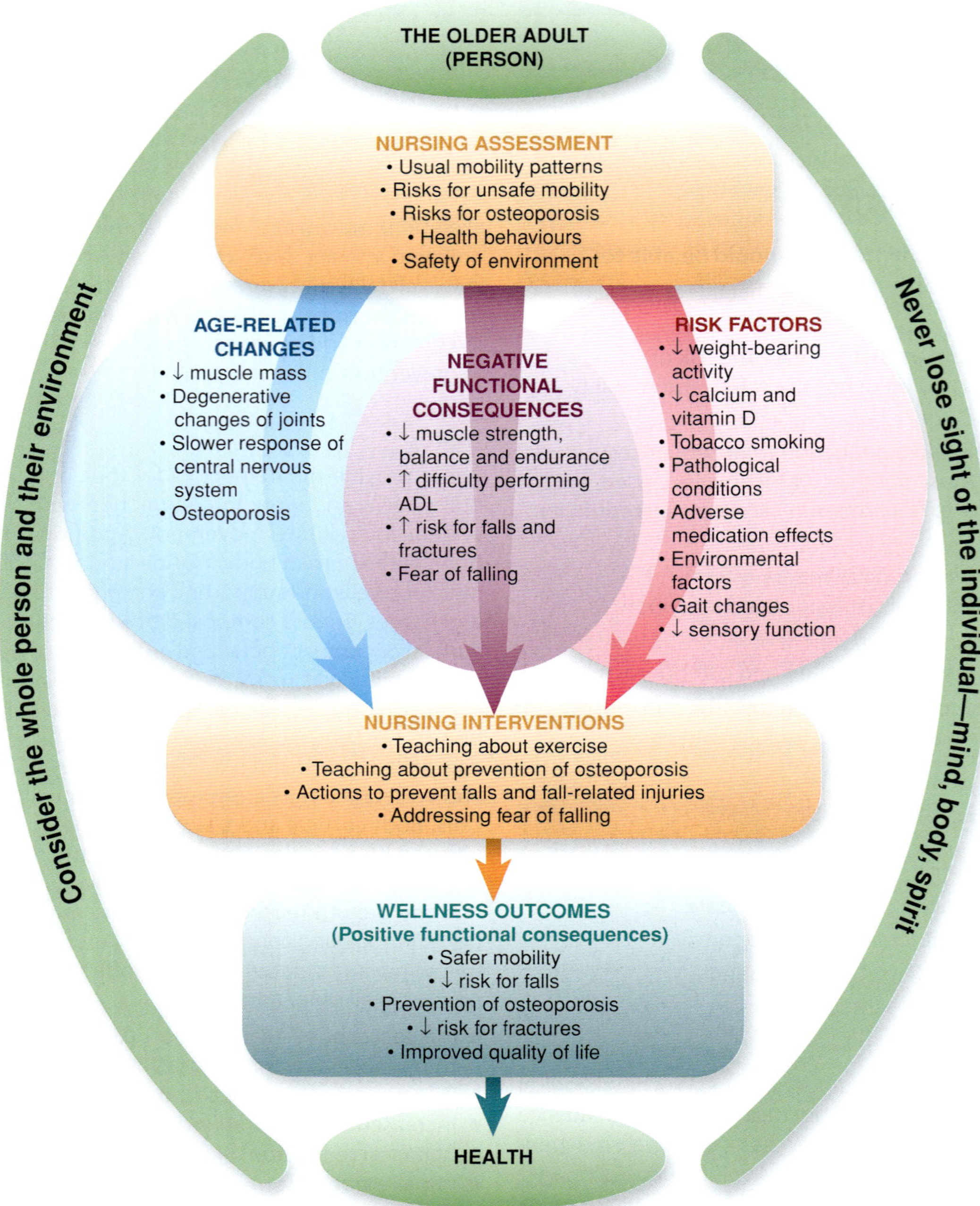

- Replacement of muscle tissue by connective tissue and, eventually, by fat tissue
- Deterioration of muscle cell membranes and a subsequent escape of fluid and potassium
- Diminished protein synthesis.

The overall effect of these age-related changes is a condition called **sarcopenia**, which is a loss of muscle mass, strength and endurance.

Joints and connective tissue

Numerous age-related changes affect the function of all musculoskeletal joints, including non–weight-bearing joints. In contrast to the bones or muscles, which benefit from exercise, the joints are harmed by continued use and begin to show the effects of wear and tear during early adulthood. In fact, degenerative processes begin to affect the tendons, ligaments and synovial fluid during early adulthood, even before skeletal maturity is reached. Some of the most significant age-related joint changes include the following:

- Diminished viscosity of synovial fluid
- Degeneration of collagen and elastin cells
- Fragmentation of fibrous structures in connective tissue
- Outgrowths of cartilaginous clusters because of continuous wear and tear
- Formation of scar tissue and areas of calcification in the joint capsules and connective tissue
- Degenerative changes in the articular cartilage resulting in extensive fraying, cracking and shredding, in addition to a pitted and thinned surface.

Consequences of these changes include impaired flexion and extension, decreased flexibility of the fibrous structures, diminished protection from forces of movement, erosion of the bones underlying the outgrowths of cartilage and diminished ability of the connective tissue to transmit the tensile forces that act on it.

Nervous system

Maintenance of balance in an upright position is a complex skill affected by the following age-related changes of the nervous system: altered visual abilities; a decline in the righting reflex; impaired proprioception, particularly in women; and diminished vibratory sensation and joint position sense in the lower extremities. In addition, age-related changes in postural control cause an increase in body sway, which is a measure of the motion of the body while standing. Finally, because of the age-related slowing in reaction time, older adults walk more slowly and are less able to respond in a timely manner to environmental stimuli. Researchers have found that older adults can learn to compensate for age-related changes in the central nervous system to avoid falls (Doumas, Rapp & Krampe, 2009).

Osteopenia and osteoporosis

Loss of bone mass is an age-related change that affects all adults as they age. The extent to which it occurs, however, is affected by many variables and emphasis needs to be placed on health promotion interventions that limit the extent and consequences of bone loss (Horan & Timmins, 2009). Because of the widespread availability of simple imaging techniques, called **bone densitometry**, in recent years, bone mineral (mass) density (BMD) is now routinely evaluated in adults beginning around their sixth decade. Bone mass density is scored according to standard deviations below that of healthy young adults, called a T-score. When a T-score is between 1 and 2.5 standard deviations below this range, the condition is called **osteopenia**; when a T-score is lower than this, the condition is called **osteoporosis**.

Osteoporosis is called a silent disease because it is usually asymptomatic and the first sign may be a fracture that occurs with little or no trauma. This type of fracture is called a **fragility fracture** or an osteoporotic fracture. As osteoporosis progresses, it can cause pain, loss of height, dowager's hump and an increased risk of fractures.

Prevalence of osteoporosis increases with age in both men and women, but it increases at an earlier age in men and is higher in women at all ages. Although osteoporosis has been recognised as a common condition among post-menopausal women for many decades, only in recent decades has it been recognised as a condition that also affects men. This increased attention is warranted because 20% to 25% of men and 50% of women aged 50 years and older will have a fracture due to osteoporosis during their lifetime (National Osteoporosis Foundation, 2013).

DIVERSITY NOTE

Prevalence of osteoporosis in Australians by age and gender (Watts, Abimanyi-Ochom & Sanders, 2013):

- 50–69 years: Men 3.2% and women 13%
- 70+ years: Men 12.9% and women 43.2%

Prevalence of osteoporosis in New Zealand by race for older people (New Zealand Ministry of Health, 2008):

- Males: Māori 1.4% and non-Māori 2.7%
- Females: Māori 10.1% and non-Māori 18.4%

Gender differences in age-related changes account for the relatively higher rate of osteoporosis among women compared with men. Both men and women reach peak bone mass in their mid-30s, then there are significant difference in rates of bone loss. Men experience about 1% annual bone loss after peak bone mass has been reached, and this bone loss is steady across their remaining lifetime. In contrast, women experience a rapid period of bone loss beginning during the transition to and early phase of menopause, which is more than they will experience in their remaining lifetime (McClung, 2012). During the first decade after the onset of menopause, the annual rate of bone loss may be as great as 7%, but after menopause, it is between 1% and 2%. In summary, osteoporosis occurs in both men and women, but women have a much greater percentage of bone loss over their lifetime and experience greater bone loss at an earlier age.

DIVERSITY NOTE

Osteoporosis affects both men and women, but the onset is about a decade earlier in women. Another difference is that men are more likely to have heterogeneous risk factors rather than age-related changes primarily (Herrera et al., 2012).

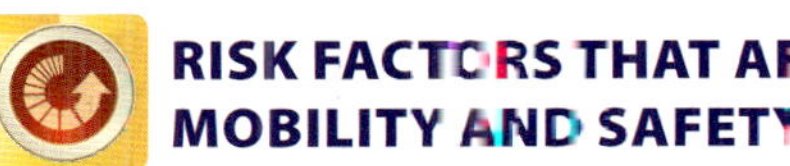

RISK FACTORS THAT AFFECT MOBILITY AND SAFETY

The risk factors for safe mobility that are of greatest concern are those that contribute to osteoporosis, fractures and falls. These risks are of particular importance to nurses because health promotion interventions can be used to address many of the risk factors. In addition, eliminating or minimising the risks is likely to prevent the serious functional consequences.

Risk factors that affect overall musculoskeletal function

Physical inactivity and nutritional deficits are major risk factors for diminished musculoskeletal function in older adults. Low level of physical activity (i.e. lack of exercise) is the most commonly occurring risk for poor musculoskeletal function across the full spectrum of health and functioning, ranging from healthy older adults to those who are frail or seriously ill. This is particularly pertinent to health promotion because interventions to improve physical activity in older adults have extensive benefits, not only for improving overall musculoskeletal function and preventing falls and fractures, but also for many other aspects of functioning, as discussed throughout this text.

Nutritional deficits are important risk factors for diminished musculoskeletal performance. For example, researchers have focused on vitamin D deficiency because this vitamin is essential for absorption of calcium and bone health. Studies in many countries find a strong association between low serum levels of vitamin D (also called 25[OH] D) and low bone density, and increased risk for fragility fractures and mobility limitations in otherwise healthy older adults (e.g. Houston, Neiberg, Tooze et al., 2013; Mosele, Coin, Manzato et al., 2013; Narula, Tauseef, Ahmad et al., 2013). Adequate dietary intake of calcium is also strongly associated with good musculoskeletal function; however, excessive calcium intake in the form of dietary supplements is associated with adverse effects, as discussed in the section on health education about osteoporosis. Other dietary factors that increase the risk for poor overall musculoskeletal function include low intake of high-quality proteins (i.e. less than 1 g/kg of body weight daily from sources such as soy and whey) and inadequate food sources of vitamin B_{12} and folic acid (Mithal, Bonjour, Boonen et al., 2013; Reidy, Walker, Dickinson et al., 2013).

WELLNESS OPPORTUNITY

Many lifestyle, environmental and other reversible factors can be addressed for preventing falls and fractures.

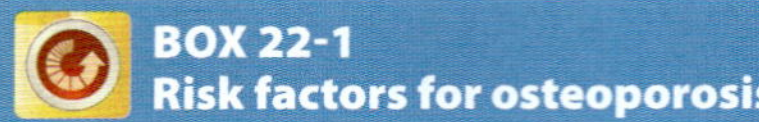

BOX 22-1
Risk factors for osteoporosis

Factors that increase the risk for osteoporosis

- Age 65 or 70 years or older for women and men, respectively
- Family history of osteoporosis or osteoporotic fracture
- Low calcium intake, both past and current
- Vitamin D deficiency
- Lack of weight-bearing activity
- Hormonal deficiency from age-related changes or pathological conditions
- Cigarette smoking
- Excessive alcohol intake
- Pathological conditions (e.g. hypogonadism, hyperparathyroidism, thyrotoxicosis, malabsorption, low gastric acid, pre- or postsolid organ transplant, low gastric acid)
- Medications (e.g. corticosteroids, anticonvulsants, anticoagulants, aromatase inhibitors, cancer chemotherapeutic agents)

Additional factors that increase the risk for fragility fracture

- Postmenopausal status for women
- 75 years or older for men
- Female sex
- Multiple risk factors for osteoporosis
- Previous fragility fracture, especially in combination with under-treatment of osteoporosis
- Family history of hip fracture
- Body mass index less than 18.5 kg/m^2
- Current or previous use of oral or systemic glucocorticoids
- Falling
- Rheumatoid arthritis

Source: Levis & Theodore (2012); National Clinical Guideline Centre (2012); Yurgin et al. (2013).

Risk factors for osteoporosis and fragility fractures

In addition to risks that affect overall musculoskeletal function, some conditions increase the risk for osteoporosis and osteoporotic fractures, as listed in Box 22-1. Although some risk factors such as age, ethnicity and family history cannot be changed, other conditions can be addressed through health promotion interventions. Current emphasis is on modifiable risk factors, including low level of weight-bearing activity, cigarette smoking, excessive alcohol consumption, and inadequate intake of calcium and vitamin D. Hormonal changes also affect the risk for osteoporosis, particularly with regard to oestrogen in women which has been the focus of research for many decades. For example, a 34-year longitudinal study found that menopause before 47 years is associated with increased risk of osteoporosis and fragility fractures (Svejme, Ahlborg, Nilsson et al., 2013). When medications or pathological conditions are a primary underlying cause, the condition is referred to as secondary osteoporosis.

In recent years there is increasing attention to identifying risks for fragility fractures with an emphasis on preventing hip fractures as they are strongly associated with serious and permanent negative consequences. In particular, a major focus of hospital quality and safety initiatives is the prevention of fractured hips that result from in-hospital falls in medical and postsurgical patients. Common risk factors for in-hospital hip fractures from falls include dementia, increased age, altered mental status, and adverse medication effects (Zapatero, Barba, Canora et al., 2013).

Since 2012 the International Osteoporosis Foundation has been promoting the Capture the Fracture campaign, with the goal of implementing best practices to reduce the incidence of fragility fractures, which occur every 3 seconds worldwide (Akesson, Marsh, Mitchell et al., 2013). A major focus of this initiative is to prevent hip fractures in people who have already had a fracture because a history of any prior fracture almost doubles the risk for another fracture (International Osteoporosis Foundation, 2012). Conditions that increase the risk for fragility fractures are listed in Box 22-1. It is imperative to consider that a combination of risk factors significantly increases the risk for fragility fractures. One study found that more than one-half of people who sustained a fragility fracture had low levels of serum vitamin D and nearly one-third had another underlying condition (Bogoch et al., 2012).

UNFOLDING CASE STUDY

Part A

Mrs Mayo is 55 years old and works as the secretary in the community nursing centre where you are a nurse. Ms Mayo's responsibilities include finding and organising health education materials under the direction of the nurses. You often go to lunch with her and discuss social and health-related topics. Ms Mayo has always been inquisitive about health-related concerns, and one day she asks your advice about osteoporosis. She says that both she and her mother, who is 83 years old, have been receiving flyers about getting a bone density test, and that her mother asked if she would go with her so that they could both be tested. You know from past conversations that Ms Mayo's mother fractured her wrist a long time ago, but otherwise is relatively healthy. Ms Mayo is fairly healthy, although she admits that she "could stand to lose a little weight". You also know from previous discussions that Ms Mayo was using hormone therapy for 3 years but stopped about 4 years ago. In your work as a community nurse, you have developed and presented several health education programs about osteoporosis and are fairly familiar with recent literature on osteoporosis.

Thinking points

- Based on what you know about Ms Mayo, what would you tell her about her risk factors for osteoporosis?
- Based on what you know about Ms Mayo's mother, what additional information would you want to know before advising her about a test for her mother?
- How would you answer Ms Mayo's inquiry?
- What suggestions would you make to help Ms Mayo become more knowledgeable about osteoporosis?

Risk factors for falls

Falling is unfortunately very common among older adults and it has been the focus of attention by health professionals for decades. More than a half century ago, an article titled "On the Natural History of Falls in Old Age" began with the following declaration: "The liability of old people to tumble and often to injure themselves is such a commonplace of experience that it has been tacitly accepted as an inevitable aspect of ageing, and thereby deprived of the exercise of curiosity" (Sheldon, 1960, p. 1685). In recent years, geriatricians and gerontologists have challenged this view that falls are a normal consequence of ageing or are accidental or random events. There is now wide agreement that falls and mobility problems result from multiple, diverse and interacting risk factors. The current clinical approach is to identify the most likely causes and contributing conditions and to plan interventions to prevent falls.

Numerous studies have been published about risks for falls, with variable conclusions. Systematic reviews identify a history of falls and use of walking aids as the strongest predictors of falls in hospitals, nursing homes and community settings (Deandrea, Bravi, Turati et al., 2013). Deandrea and colleagues suggest that these two conditions are not causal factors, but are indicators of underlying problems that need to be addressed. A consistent research finding is that falls are the result of a combination of risk factors, rather than one isolated risk factor. Moreover, the risk of falls increases in proportion to the number of fall risk factors. Current emphasis is on preventing serious fall-related injuries such as fractures and traumatic brain injury, because up to one-fifth of falls in older adults results in injury, hospitalisation or death (Moller Midlov, Kristensson et al., 2013). Risk factors for falls can be categorised according to their origin as follows: age-related changes, common pathological conditions and functional impairments, medication effects, and environmental factors (Box 22-2).

The many studies of reasons for falling in older adults have identified different underlying causes in different age groups. Falls in older adults who are younger than 75 years are often associated with trips and slips that are predominantly attributable to a combination of age-related changes and unfavourable environmental conditions. By contrast, falls in people older than 75 years are usually associated with a combination of disease- and medication-related factors.

Pathological conditions and functional and cognitive impairments

Nocturia, sleep problems, gait changes, sensory changes, orthostatic hypotension, decreased muscle strength, and central nervous system changes are conditions that can increase the risk of falls in older adults. In addition, vision impairment is an independent risk for falls in older adults because of its effects on mobility, balance, safety, fear of falling, and ability to perform daily activities (Aartolahti, Hakkinen, Lonnroos et al., 2013; Reed-Jones et al., 2013). In general, commonly occurring pathological conditions can increase the risk for falls in older adults in all of the following ways:

- Pathological conditions can cause functional impairments that affect vision, balance or mobility.
- Pathological conditions may be treated with medications that create risks for falling.
- Chronic conditions often interfere with optimal exercise and other health practices that are important in promoting safe mobility.

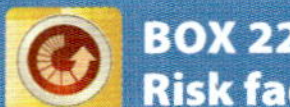

BOX 22-2
Risk factors for falls

Pathological conditions and functional impairments

- Age-related conditions (e.g. nocturia, osteoporosis, gait changes, postural hypotension, sensory deficits)
- Cardiovascular diseases (e.g. arrhythmias or myocardial infarction)
- Respiratory diseases (e.g. chronic obstructive pulmonary disease [COPD])
- Neurological disorders (e.g. parkinsonism, cerebrovascular accident [CVA])
- Metabolic disturbances (e.g. dehydration, electrolyte imbalances)
- Musculoskeletal problems (e.g. osteoarthritis)
- Transient ischaemic attack (TIA)
- Vision impairments (e.g. cataracts, glaucoma, macular degeneration)
- Cognitive impairments (e.g. dementia, confusion)
- Psychosocial factors (e.g. depression, anxiety, agitation)

Medication effects and interactions

- Antiarrhythmics
- Anticholinergics, including ingredients in over-the-counter products (e.g. diphenhydramine)
- Anticonvulsants
- Diuretics
- Benzodiazepines and other hypnotics
- Antipsychotics
- Antidepressants
- Alcohol

Environmental factors

- Inadequate lighting
- Lack of handrails on stairs
- Slippery floors
- Throw rugs
- Cords or clutter
- Unfamiliar environments
- Highly polished floors
- Improper height of beds, chairs or toilets
- Physical restraints, including bedrails

Depression and other cognitive impairments can increase the risk for falls, especially in combination with other risk factors. For example, both dementia and depression diminish one's awareness of the environment and can interfere with the ability to process information about environmental stimuli. Older adults with dementia have at least a twofold fall risk, which is associated with slowed gait and executive dysfunction (Kearney, Harwood, Gladman et al., 2013). The following combination of factors is likely to increase the risk for falls in people living with dementia: concurrent conditions, vision impairment, impaired balance, and slowed psychomotor speed (Chen, Peronto & Edwards, 2012; Martin, Blizzard, Srikanth et al., 2013). Depressed older adults are at increased risk for falls secondary to gait changes, adverse medication effects, and a diminished ability to concentrate on and respond to environmental factors. One study found that antidepressant medications increased the risk of outdoor falls by 70% (Quach, Yang, Berry et al., 2013). Considering all of these possible associations, it is not surprising that most falls resulting in injuries occur in people who have functional impairments and multiple, chronic medical problems.

Medication effects

Numerous studies have identified hundreds of medications that can contribute to falls and attempts have been made to identify those medications that are associated with the highest risk of falls. Central nervous system drugs such as hypnotics, antipsychotics and antidepressants are medications most often identified as independent and significant risks for falls in institutional and community-based settings (Costa-Dias et al., 2013; Lamis, Kramer, Hale et al., 2012; Van Strein et al., 2013; Whitney, Close, Lord et al., 2012). Central nervous system drugs with long half-lives are associated with the highest risk for falls (Obayashi, Araki, Nakamura et al., 2013; Olazaran, Valle, Serra et al., 2013). Diuretics also are associated with increased risk for falls and fractures, particularly during the first week after initiation of the drug (Berry, Zhu, Choi, et al., 2013). The use of more than four medications is another commonly identified risk for falls (Damian et al., 2013; Freeland, Thompson, Zhao et al., 2012).

Studies also identify medication-related factors that increase the risk of fall-related injuries. For example, anticoagulant medications, which are commonly used for stroke prevention, increase the risk for serious bleeding if a fall occurs. Dosing of medications also can affect the risk for fall-related injuries. Studies indicate that the risk for hip fractures for long-term care residents may be especially high soon after a hypnotic is initiated or when the dose of an antipsychotic is adjusted (Berry, Lee, Cai et al., 2013; Rigler et al., 2013).

Although most studies have focused on prescription medications, over-the-counter medications also can create risks for falls through their adverse effects on psychomotor function. Many over-the-counter preparations for pain, colds and insomnia contain alcohol or anticholinergics. These ingredients may themselves pose risks or may interact with other medications to increase the risk for falls. The adverse effects of diphenhydramine, a widely used ingredient in over-the-counter products for sleep, colds and allergies, have received much attention in the media and medical literature. Diphenhydramine has been associated with significant adverse effects on the psychomotor skills necessary for safe driving, and many states include this and other over-the-counter agents in laws pertaining to driving while impaired.

The following adverse medication effects can increase the risk for falls: confusion, depression, sedation, arrhythmias, hypovolaemia, orthostatic hypotension, delayed reaction time, diminished cognitive function, and changes in gait and balance (e.g. ataxia, decreased proprioception and increased body sway). Thus, any medication that has one or more of these adverse effects may increase the risk for falls. Other considerations that influence the risk of falls include medication–disease interactions, medication–medication interactions and medication–alcohol interactions.

An approach to identifying the relationship between medications and an increased risk for falls is to consider the underlying mechanism of the medication action, as well as the pathological condition and the potential interactions among various factors. For example, orthostatic hypotension can result from pathological conditions, age-related changes, or adverse medication effects and can increase the risk for falls. If an 80-year-old person has a pathological condition (e.g. Parkinson's disease) that may cause orthostatic hypotension, and if the person is taking a medication (e.g. a vasodilator) that causes orthostatic hypotension, the risk for falls significantly increases. Therefore, rather than memorising all of the medications known to increase the risk for falls, nurses can focus their attention on the underlying mechanisms that increase the risk for falls. Some medications that are likely to increase the risk for falls are listed in Box 22-2.

Environmental factors

Some environmental hazards were discussed in Chapter 7, but additional environmental influences must be considered specifically in relation to falls. In institutional settings, for example, falls are most likely to occur in the bedroom and bathroom. In the bedroom, most falls occur while the person is getting into or out of bed and some falls are related to climbing over side rails or bed ends. In the bathroom, falls generally occur while transferring on or off toilet seats or while hurrying to urinate or defecate. In community settings, most falls occur in the home, particularly in stairways, bedrooms and lounge rooms. Environmental hazards that increase the risk of falls in homes include clutter, poor lighting and lack of handrails on stairs or grab bars in bathrooms. Ill-fitting footwear is also a common cause of falls in all settings.

Physical restraints

Physical restraints have been used since the 1960s in institutional settings with the intent of protecting impaired people from injury and reducing staff workload. Historically, the belief that using physical restraints protects vulnerable people from falls and shields the institution from liability was widespread.

However, questions about using physical restraints and bedrails were first raised during the 1980s and many studies have addressed the safety and effectiveness of these measures. In recent decades, there has been increasing evidence that restraints (including bedrails) increase the risk for falls as well as additional problems, including pressure ulcers, contractures, more serious injury from falls and increased dependency in ADLs (Castle & Engberg, 2009; Fonad et al., 2009). Studies have also found that there is no significant increase in number of falls or use of psychotropic medications after restraint-reduction interventions were implemented (Pellfolk et al., 2010).

It is best practice, when a restraint is required, to use the least-restrictive device (Joanna Briggs Institute, 2002a, 2002b). The Australian Government Department of Social Services (DSS) (2012a, 2012b) has provided comprehensive best practice guides for restraint minimisation in the community, titled, Supporting a restraint free environment in community aged care, and for long-term residential care, Supporting a restraint free environment in residential aged care. Both of these documents are accessible via the website www.dss.gov.au.

Further information about the use of restraints is contained in Chapter 9.

UNFOLDING CASE STUDY

Part B

Ms Mayo is now 67 years old and has retired from her secretarial job. One day she comes to the medical centre where you work as a practice nurse with a cast on her left wrist and reports that she fractured her wrist when she slipped and fell on ice in her driveway. You know from prior conversations with her that she stopped taking hormone therapy many years ago because she had been on it for over three years and was concerned about long-term effects. You also know that she takes medications for arthritis, hypertension and depression and that she self-monitors her blood pressure. In the past 10 years, she has gradually gained "a little weight every year" and her current height/weight is 162 cm/79 kilograms. She participates in the weekly "walkers" exercise program but does not often exercise independently. She says that "my housework is enough exercise" and that the weekly group exercise activity is "as much as my arthritis will tolerate". She lives in a small, single-storey house. Although Ms Mayo says she is not really concerned about sustaining any more fractures because she views the recent fall as a "fluke of bad winter luck", she makes an appointment to talk with you. During the appointment, she reports that she is a "little concerned about osteoporosis".

Thinking points

- What risk factors for osteoporosis can you identify from what you already know about Ms Mayo?
- What risk factors for falls and fall-related injuries can you identify from what you already know about Ms Mayo?
- Can you identify any factors that diminish her risk for falls or fractures?
- What additional information about Ms Mayo would be helpful in identifying additional risks for osteoporosis?
- What additional information would be helpful in identifying additional risks for falls and fractures?

PATHOLOGICAL CONDITION AFFECTING MUSCULOSKELETAL FUNCTION: OSTEOARTHRITIS

Osteoarthritis is a degenerative inflammatory disease affecting joints and attached muscles, tendons and ligaments. It is characterised by pain, swelling and limited

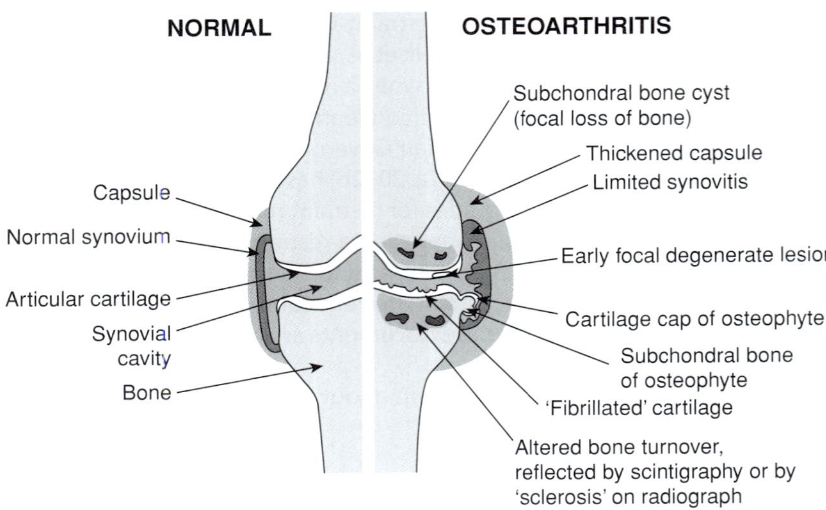

FIGURE 22-1 Effects of osteoarthritis on a joint. (Moskowitz, R. W., Altman, R. D., Buckwalter, J. A., Goldberg, V. M. & Hochberg, M. C. [2006]. *Osteoarthritis: Diagnosis and medical surgical management*. Philadelphia PA: Lippincott, Williams & Wilkins.)

movement in joints and it is the major cause of disability and chronic pain in Australia. Figure 22-1 describes the effects of osteoarthritis on a joint. It occurs more commonly in people over 55 years, affecting more females than males. Osteoarthritis is a very complex disease process that results from the interplay of risk factors such as trauma, genetics, obesity and age-related changes. In Australia approximately 25% of males and 45% of females aged 65 to 79 years have the disease, and the prevalence increases between genders for those aged 80+ years: 35% of males and 50% of females (Australian Institute of Health and Welfare [AIHW], 2013a). In New Zealand approximately 34% of males and 50% of females who are 65 years and over report they have osteoarthritis (New Zealand Ministry of Health [NZMOH], 2011).

DIVERSITY NOTE

In Australia, Aboriginal and Torres Strait Islanders are 1.1 times more likely than non-Indigenous people to report having osteoarthritis (AIHW, 2013a).

Because self-care is an important aspect of managing osteoarthritis, nurses focus on health education interventions. Nurses can encourage participation in self-management programs, which are effective for the management of pain and prevention of disability in osteoarthritis (Shelton, 2013). See Chapter 28 for a discussion about self-management programs. In addition, nurses can teach older adults with osteoarthritis about the following self-care practices that are recommended in evidence-based guidelines (Davies, 2011; Moskowitz, 2013):

- Participating in aerobic, resistance, land-based and aquatic **exercise programs** that focus on improving musculoskeletal strength, balance and endurance (e.g. yoga, aquatherapy, tai chi)
- Avoiding high-impact activities
- Wearing good shock-absorbing shoes
- Balancing weight-bearing activities with rest periods
- Losing weight if appropriate
- Using orthotics, supports, brace or shoe inserts as appropriate
- Using canes, walkers and other assistive devices as appropriate to relieve weight-bearing joints, improve balance, or achieve independent functioning
- Using moist heat and analgesics for pain.

Care plans for managing osteoarthritis are most effective when they are based on an interdisciplinary approach that includes medicine, nursing and physical and occupational therapy. Because there are many medical and surgical interventions for osteoarthritis, nurses should emphasise the importance of obtaining regular medical care for ongoing evaluation and treatment as this condition changes. Nurses can also encourage older adults to ask for a referral for physical therapy to learn effective muscle strengthening strategies for lower-limb osteoarthritis (Bennell et al., 2005). Self-care practices recommended by evidence-based guidelines include aqua therapy, balance training exercise, land-based exercise, tai chi, cold therapy and weight reduction (if applicable) (Royal Australian College of General Practitioners, 2009; Williams et al., 2010).

Increasing numbers of older adults are receiving surgical interventions for osteoarthritis. It has been estimated that 90% of the joint replacement surgery performed in New Zealand is because of osteoarthritis (Hooper, 2013). In Australia there has been a 54% increase in total knee replacements and 20% increase in hip replacements for osteoarthritis in the period 2002–03 to 2011–12 (Arthritis & Osteoporosis NSW, 2014).

WELLNESS OPPORTUNITY

Older adults with osteoarthritis need to engage in self-management of their disease, including making informed decisions about medication and activities that promote optimal comfort and functioning.

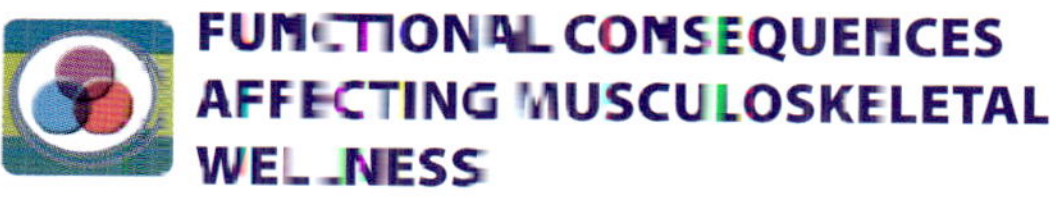

FUNCTIONAL CONSEQUENCES AFFECTING MUSCULOSKELETAL WELLNESS

Older adults can partially compensate for age-related changes that affect musculoskeletal function through health promotion interventions, such as good nutrition and physical activity. The functional consequences of osteoporosis, however, are quite serious, as are the functional consequences that result from the many risk factors that contribute to falls and fractures in older adults. As with many other aspects of function in older adulthood, cumulative and interacting effects of risk factors rather than age-related changes most significantly affect function and quality of life.

Effects on musculoskeletal function

Muscle strength, endurance and coordination are affected to some extent by age-related changes, even in the absence of risk factors. Beginning around the age of 40 years, muscle strength declines gradually, resulting in an overall decrease of 30% to 50% by the age of 80 years, with a greater decline in muscle strength in the lower extremities than in the upper extremities. Diminished muscle strength is attributed primarily to age-related loss of muscle mass. In addition, a person's current level of activity and lifelong patterns of exercise can influence muscle strength at any age. Muscle endurance and coordination diminish as a result of age-related changes in the muscles and central nervous system. Because of these changes, older adults experience muscle fatigue after shorter periods of exercise compared with their younger counterparts.

Joint function begins to decline during early adulthood and progresses gradually to cause the following changes in range of motion:

- Decreased range of motion in the upper arms
- Decreased lower back flexion
- Decreased external rotation of the hip
- Decreased hip and knee flexion
- Decreased dorsiflexion of the foot.

These changes result in slowed performance of daily activities such as writing, eating, grooming and putting on socks and shoes; difficulty climbing stairs and kerbs; and an overall diminished ability to respond to environmental stimuli.

Gait changes, which differ in men and women, are one of the more noticeable functional consequences that occur after the age of 75 years. Women have less muscle control, develop a narrower standing and walking gait and develop bowlegged-type changes that affect the lower extremities and alter the angle of the hip. Older men develop a wider walking and standing gait, characterised by less arm swing, a shorter stride, decreased height of steps and a more flexed position of the head and trunk than when they were younger. The overall impact of these changes is that older men and women have a slower walking speed and spend more time in the support phase of gait than in the swing phase. Any significant gait changes that occur are not due to ageing alone but are the consequences of other conditions, such as osteoarthritis or neurological disorders (e.g. dementia, Parkinson's disease).

Susceptibility to falls and fractures

Older adults are at an increased risk of falling. It has been reported that more than one in four people 65 years and over fall at least once per year and many fall more than once (New South Wales Department of Health, 2011). The risk of falling also increases with increasing levels of frailty where up to 50% of older adults in long-term residential care may fall once a year. For instance, in 2009, 26% of people 65 years and over, living in the state of New South Wales, fell at least once. These falls led to approximately 27,000 admissions to hospital and at least 400 deaths in older people. It has been calculated that hospitalisations for falls for older adults in New South Wales is over three times higher for residents of long-term care facilities than other older adults. A study in New Zealand reported that over one-third of older adults (Māori aged over 80 years and non-Māori aged over 85 years) had fallen in the last 12 months (Kerse, 2014). Of those who had fallen, one person in five required hospital care. An alarming trend noted is that falls-related admissions to hospital among older people have been increasing for more than 10 years.

The combination of age-related changes and multiple interacting risk factors increase the risk of fall-related fractures. Fractures are not unique to older adults, but they do differ in many respects from those that occur in younger populations. First, bones of older adults can be fractured with little or no trauma, whereas bones of healthy children and younger adults are usually fractured in response to a forceful impact. Fractures that result from an impact that is no more severe than that which results from falling to the floor from a standing position. Second, the risk of fractures increases in direct relation to age. Third, it is more likely that fractures in older adults, particularly hip fractures, will have serious consequences affecting independence, quality of life and morbidity and mortality. Studies show that older adults who have had fractures are at increased risk for functional decline, recurrent falls, permanent admission to a long-term residential care and shortened life expectancy (Frost, Nguyen, Center et al., 2013; Gill, Murphy, Gahbauer et al., 2013; Tajeu, Delzell, Smith et al., 2013).

In Australia, it is estimated that 24% of individuals will die within 12 months after fracturing a hip. Of those remaining, half will be placed in a long-term residential care facility, with the other half no longer able to walk unaided and the majority requiring assistance with everyday activities of living (Australian Bureau of Statistics [ABS], 2011). In New Zealand falls have been estimated to account for 75% of injury-related hospital admissions for older adults (Accident Compensation Corporation [ACC], 2014).

Further, falls statistics for New Zealand include 22% to 60% of older people suffer injuries from falls; 10% to 15% suffer serious injuries; 2% to 6% suffer fractures; and 0.2% to 1.5% suffer hip fractures.

Fear of falling

Since the early 1990s there has been increasing attention to **fear of falling**, which is excessive anxiety about falling that leads to activity avoidance and decline in functioning. It is considered a major problem that affects between 40% and 75% of long-term care residents and up to 76.6% of community-dwelling older adults (Kim & So, 2013; Lach & Parsons, 2013). Rather than leading to a cautious awareness of actions to prevent falls, fear of falling increases the risk for falling and leads to additional serious negative consequences. Studies have found that fear of falling can lead to functional decline, increased dependency, significant activity restrictions, depression, social isolation and increased risk for falling (Huang, Chi & Hu, 2013; Lach & Parsons, 2013).

Another concern is that carers/caregivers of older adults may be quite anxious about potential falls, and this can lead to increased carer burden and increased vigilance (Dow, Meyer, Moore et al., 2013). In some cases, carers restrict the older adult's activities or decide to move the person to a setting that provides a greater level of assistance or supervision than the older person desires. Although a move to more restrictive environment will not necessarily protect the person from falls, and may even increase the risk of falls, carers may derive some peace of mind because they perceive the older person is safer. Similarly, carers may begin using restraints or otherwise limiting the person's mobility; however, as already discussed, restraints do not prevent falls and are likely to contribute to more serious fall-related injuries. Nurses have important roles in addressing carers' fear of falls by teaching about fall-prevention interventions, as discussed in the section on promoting carer wellness.

DIVERSITY NOTE

Studies have found that fear of falling is more common in women than men (Filiatrault, Desrosiers & Trottier, 2009; Kempen et al., 2009).

WELLNESS OPPORTUNITY

Nurses respect older adults' autonomy and involve them in decisions by creatively finding ways to promote safety while also allowing as much freedom of movement as possible.

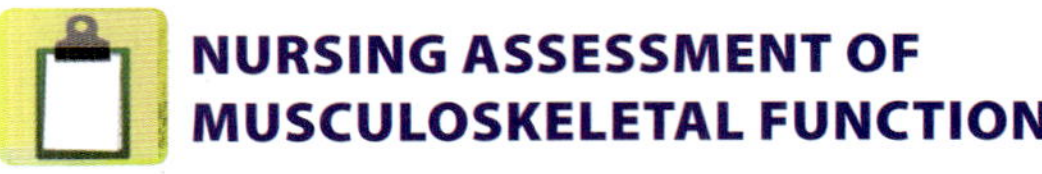

NURSING ASSESSMENT OF MUSCULOSKELETAL FUNCTION

Nursing assessment of musculoskeletal function focuses on identifying risks for falls, fractures and osteoporosis, with particular attention to those factors that can be modified or alleviated through nursing interventions. Nurses can use a **fall risk assessment tool** to identify older adults who might benefit from appropriate preventive interventions.

Assessing musculoskeletal performance

Assessment of overall musculoskeletal performance begins with observation of the person's mobility and activities. In addition to watching the person walk, it is especially important to observe the person getting up from a chair. The Timed Up and Go (TUG) test is an evidence-based and simple-to-use tool for assessing gait speed and balance that has been widely used since the early 1990s in many healthcare and home settings. The test is a reliable measure of gait speed, as well as an indicator of fall risk and ability to safely perform ADLs. The TUG, which is illustrated in Figure 22-2, can be administered in 5 minutes or less and it can be used repeatedly to identify declines or improvements over time. Higher scores (i.e. longer time to complete the tasks) are associated with increased risk for falls. Cut-off scores between 12 and 14 seconds are discussed in the literature, but a score of 12.47 seconds is recommended in a review of studies (Murphy & Lowe, 2013). Before administering this test it is important to explain and demonstrate the procedure, have the person wear regular footwear, and use usual assistive devices.

Assessment information also is obtained by asking questions about the person's ability to perform ADLs. When limitations are identified, it is important to find out if the older adult is using assistive devices to improve safety, mobility, balance, independence or overall function. If the person is not using such devices—and may benefit from them—it is important to assess the person's knowledge about the availability of such devices. It also is important to assess the person's attitude about using assistive devices because attitudes are likely to influence the acceptability of using recommended aids. Nurses can use the criteria for the functional assessment of all ADLs provided in Chapter 7, together with the assessment information in this chapter.

In addition to experiencing minor changes in performing ADLs, older adults experience diminished height and changes in posture. Older adults may or may not be concerned about or aware of a loss of height; however, a loss of about 2 to 4 cm per decade is normal, owing to osteoporosis and other age-related changes. Including a question about the person's usual height and any noticeable loss of height will give the nurse an opportunity to assess the older adult's awareness of this change. Although the functional consequences of decreased height are minimal, older people who never were very tall may experience increased difficulty performing activities that depend on height. In these

Patient: Date: Time: AM/PM

The Timed Up and Go (TUG) Test

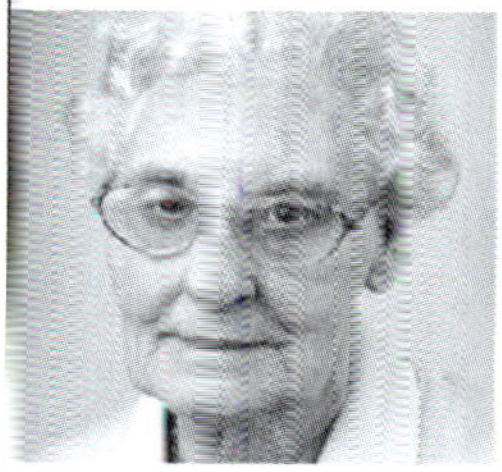

Purpose: To assess mobility

Equipment: A stopwatch

Directions: Patients wear their regular footwear and can use a walking aid if needed. Begin by having the patient sit back in a standard arm chair and identify a line 3 meters or 10 feet away on the floor.

Instructions to the patient:

When I say **"Go,"** I want you to:

1. Stand up from the chair
2. Walk to the line on the floor at your normal pace
3. Turn
4. Walk back to the chair at your normal pace
5. Sit down again

On the word **"Go"** begin timing.

Stop timing after patient has sat back down and record.

Time: ________ **seconds**

An older adult who takes ≥12 seconds to complete the TUG is at high risk for falling.

Observe the patient's postural stability, gait, stride length, and sway.

Circle all that apply: ■ Slow tentative pace ■ Loss of balance ■ Short strides ■ Little or no arm swing ■ Steadying self on walls ■ Shuffling ■ En bloc turning ■ Not using assistive device properly

Notes:

For relevant articles, go to: **www.cdc.gov/injury/STEADI**

Centers for Disease Control and Prevention
National Center for Injury Prevention and Control

STEADI Stopping Elderly Accidents, Deaths & Injuries

FIGURE 22-2 The Timed Up and Go (TUG) Test. (Reprinted from the Centers for Disease Control and Prevention [CDC]; www.cdc.gov/homeandrecreationalsafety/pdf/steadi/timed_up_and_go_test.pdf.)

situations they may find it is safer and more effective to use assistive devices such as long-handled reachers. They may also need encouragement to rearrange cupboards so that the most frequently used items are accessible. Another assessment implication of decreased height is that the pants legs of older adult's clothing may be too long, especially if the person also has lost weight. Therefore, nurses observe if the length of clothing increases the risk for falls because this risk can be alleviated through relatively simple interventions.

Box 22-3 summarizes guidelines for assessing overall musculoskeletal performance in older adults.

Identifying risks for osteoporosis

Nurses assess risks for osteoporosis in all older adults because some health promotion interventions for osteoporosis—such as adequate intake of calcium and vitamin D, and participation in regular weight-bearing exercise—are universally applicable. Nurses also identify modifiable risk factors, such as smoking and drinking excessive

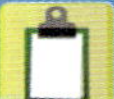

BOX 22-3
Guidelines for assessing overall musculoskeletal function and risks for falls and osteoporosis

Questions to assess overall musculoskeletal performance

- Do you have any trouble performing your usual activities because of joint limitations?
- Do you have any pain or discomfort in your joints?
- Do you ever feel like you are losing your balance?
- Do you have any trouble walking or getting around?
- Do you use any assistive devices (e.g. a walker, quad cane or reaching devices) to help you do things?

Questions to assess risks for osteoporosis

Questions to ask all older adults

- Do you know of any blood relatives who have had osteoporosis or who have sustained fractures late in life?
- Have you sustained any fractures during your adult years? (If yes, ask additional questions regarding age at the time, type, location, circumstances, treatment, and so on.)
- Do you take any calcium or vitamin D supplements?
- Have you ever had your bone density measured?
- Have you ever talked with your medical practitioner about prevention of osteoporosis?
- Do you take any medications for osteoporosis?

Questions to ask women

- When did you begin menopause?
- Do you take, or have you ever taken, oestrogen or other hormone therapy? (If yes, ask additional questions regarding type, dose, duration, and so on.)

Questions to assess risk for falls and fear of falling

- Have you had any falls in the past few years? (If yes, ask additional questions about the circumstances and ask about pertinent risk factors as summarised in Box 22-2.)
- Are you afraid of falling? (If yes, ask additional questions about specific fears, such as, *What do you think might happen if you were to fall?*)
- Are there any activities you would like to do, but do not do, because of any difficulty moving or getting around? (If yes, ask about specific activities, such as shopping, using public transportation, and so on.)
- Are there any activities you would like to do, but do not do because you are afraid of falling? (If yes, ask about specific activities, such as going up or down stairs, taking a bath or shower and so on.)

Observations regarding overall musculoskeletal performance

- Measure and record the person's present height and stated peak height.
- Observe the individual's walking and gait pattern.
- Observe the person rising from a chair.

Information from the overall assessment that is also useful in assessing musculoskeletal function

- Observe and document a functional assessment, as described in Chapter 7.
- How much exercise does the person get on a regular basis? In particular, how much weight-bearing exercise?
- Does the person smoke cigarettes?
- How much alcohol does the person consume?
- What is the person's usual daily intake of calcium and vitamin D?
- Does the person have any medical conditions that are associated with falls or osteoporosis (as summarised in Boxes 22-1 and 22-2)?
- Is the person taking any medications that might create risks for falls (including over-the-counter medications)?
- Does the person have postural hypotension?
- Is the person moderately or seriously visually impaired?
- Does the person have any cognitive impairments or other psychosocial impairments that diminish his or her attention to the environment or interfere with the ability to respond to environmental stimuli?

amounts of alcohol that can be alleviated through lifestyle interventions. If the nursing assessment identifies risk factors that cannot be modified (e.g. long-term use of corticosteroids), this information may be used to motivate the person to take action to eliminate the risks that can be modified. Nurses obtain much of the information regarding risks for osteoporosis during an overall assessment or health history and they consider this information in relation to mobility and safety.

Evidence-based guidelines recommend that people at risk for osteoporotic fractures are best identified through a combination of bone density measurement and an assessment of clinical risk factors (Sanders, Nowson, Kotowicz et al. 2009). Nurses need to be knowledgeable about BMD tests so that they can encourage older adults to talk with their medical practitioners about these tests. Two fracture risk calculators have been developed using BMD information and other risk factors. The FRAX® WHO Fracture Risk Assessment Tool and the Garvan Institute's Bone Fracture Risk Calculator are available via their respective addresses, www.sheffield.ac.uk and http://garvan org.au.

See Box 22-3 for assessment questions and considerations relating to osteoporosis.

WELLNESS OPPORTUNITY

From a holistic perspective, nurses ask older adults to identify enjoyable ways of engaging in weight-bearing activities.

Identifying risks for falls and injury

Identifying fall risks is an essential and multidimensional part of healthcare for all older adults because it is imperative to initiate preventive interventions. The best assessment information is obtained by observing the person in his or her environment and paying particular attention to the person's awareness of and attention to unsafe conditions.

Observations also provide information about adaptive behaviours that otherwise might not be acknowledged. For example, a person might state that he or she has no difficulty with stair climbing, but observations might reveal that the person performs this activity in a highly unsafe manner. When nurses do not have the opportunity to observe home environments directly, they can observe the person in the immediate environment and ask the person or carers about the older adult's ability to function safely in that setting. They can also consider referrals to homecare agencies for home assessment as part of the discharge plan.

WELLNESS OPPORTUNITY

Whenever possible, nurses actively involve the older adult and family members in identifying environmental factors that either support or create risks for safe mobility.

Another important aspect of assessing the environment in any setting is identifying the factors likely to cause serious injury if a fall does occur. For example, stationary objects such as bathroom sinks or heavy wooden furniture can cause serious head injuries if someone falls near the object. The guidelines summarised in Chapter 7 can be used to assess the safety of any environment and can be applied to all older adults, particularly those who have intrinsic risk factors for falls.

Important assessment information can be obtained simply by asking one or two questions. For example, a nursing study found that asking people hospitalised what they would do if they need to go to the toilet helped identify who was at high risk for falls (Ko, Van Nguyen, Chan et al., 2012). It is recommended that health practitioners ask all older adults if they have fallen or experienced difficulty walking during the past year (Ambrose, Paul & Hausdorff, 2013). Box 22-3 includes assessment questions applicable to older adults who are independent or relatively independent.

Many fall risk assessment tools are used to identify people who are at risk for falls so that preventive measures can be implemented. Two types of fall risk assessment tools are *functional assessment scales* and nursing *fall risk tools*. Functional assessment scales focus on the person's gait and balance and are used by rehabilitation therapists. Nurses can informally assess gait and balance by asking the person to sit in a firm, straight-backed chair with armrests, stand up from the chair and walk a few steps, then turn around and return to the chair. Nurses also can observe the usual walking pattern of the person, paying particular attention to any gait or balance unsteadiness or unusual patterns. If any abnormalities are noted, nurses can facilitate referrals for further evaluation by a physical therapist.

Nursing fall risk assessment tools

There are numerous nursing fall risk assessment tools available, and each organisation will have chosen the tool with the best utility for their care context. Two examples are the Hendrich II Fall Risk Model (Hendrich, 2013) available via the Hartford Institute for Geriatric Nursing website, and the Falls Risk Assessment Tool (FRAT) (for example, Figure 22-3), both of which can be used in institutional settings, the home and other community-based settings.

Although fall risk assessment tools are useful in identifying people who are at high risk for falls, they do not address the underlying causes. When older adults have several risk factors or have already had fall-related injuries, a comprehensive fall assessment should be performed in a multidisciplinary setting, such as a geriatric assessment program. A comprehensive fall assessment addresses the following: mental status, nutrition, environment, medications, pathological conditions, functional assessment, usual footwear, and a complete physical examination (including visual acuity, musculoskeletal function, neurological function and cardiovascular status).

Because fear of falling has negative functional consequences in addition to those associated with actual falls, nurses include at least one question about fear of falling in any assessment of falls and fall risk. If the older person expresses a fear of falling, it is important to ask additional questions in relation to specific activities that may be associated with fears or falls. If the older person relies on family or other carers for assistance, it is important to assess carer concerns and observations. Assessment questions aimed at identifying fear of falling and related negative functional consequences are included in Box 22-3.

UNFOLDING CASE STUDY

Part C

Ms Mayo is now 75 years old. At a recent medical appointment she sees you, the practice nurse, for a blood pressure check. She tells you that she has significantly cut down on her exercise because she experienced pain in one knee about a month ago after she took a long walk in the park with her dog. She talked with her doctor about this and was told to start taking ibuprofen, but she has not started taking it because she is not sure how much to take and her knee does not bother her except when she takes a long walk. She used to take her dog for daily walks, but now ties him up so she does not have to go out. Current prescription medications are enalapril, 5 mg twice daily, and hydrochlorothiazide, 25 mg daily. She also takes a multiple vitamin daily and paracetamol 1000 mg every 6 hours as needed. She continues to live in her single-storey house and is independent in doing all of her household chores. She is also responsible for all year-round outdoor maintenance activities, including mowing the lawn and raking leaves.

Thinking points

- What assessment questions from Box 22-3 would you ask Ms Mayo at this time?
- Would you use any information from Box 22-1 or Box 22-2 at this time?
- What myths or misunderstandings related to mobility and exercise might be influencing Ms Mayo?
- Would you take any steps to assess Ms Mayo's home environment for fall risks?

Peninsula Health

FALLS RISK ASSESSMENT TOOL (FRAT)

(see instructions for completion of FRAT in the FRAT PACK - Falls Resource Manual)

UR NUMBER..

SURNAME..

GIVEN NAMES..

DATE OF BIRTH ....
Please fill in if no Patient Label available

App.23/04/15 Print Code:15665

PHF574526 5

PART 1 - FALL RISK STATUS

RISK FACTOR	LEVEL	RISK SCORE	Ward............ ....../....../......	Ward............ ....../....../......	Ward............ ....../....../......	Ward............ ....../....../......
RECENT FALLS	none in last 12 months	2				
	one or more between 3 + 12 months ago	4				
	one or more in last 3 months	6				
	one or more in last 3 months whilst inpatient/resident	8				
MEDICATIONS (Sedatives, Anti-Depressants Anti-Parkinson's, Diuretics Anti-Hypertensives, hypnotics)	not taking any of these	1				
	taking one	2				
	taking two	3				
	taking more than two	4				
PSYCHOLOGICAL (Anxiety, Depression ↓Cooperation, ↓Insight or ↓ Judgement exp. re mobility)	does not appear to have any of these	1				
	appears mildly affected by one or more	2				
	appears moderately affected by one or more	3				
	appears severely affected by one or more	4				
COGNITIVE STATUS (m-m: Hodkinson Abbreviated Mental Score)	m-m score 9 or 10/10 OR intact	1				
	m-m score 7 - 8 mildly impaired	2				
	m-m score 5 - 6 mod impaired	3				
	m-m score 4 or less severely impaired	4				
Low Risk: 5-11	**Medium Risk: 12-15 High Risk: 16-20**	**RISK SCORE** /20	/20	/20	/20	/20
		Nurse Initials				

AUTOMATIC HIGH RISK STATUS: *(Clinical assessment)*

☐ Impaired mobility / poor balance

☐ Dizziness / postural hypotension

FALL RISK STATUS: *(circle)* **LOW / MEDIUM / HIGH**

➔ List Fall status on Care Plan

IMPORTANT: IF HIGH, record details on Clinical Information System (Clover) and Patient Administration System (iPM)

INTERVENTION PLAN ALWAYS ENSURE – CALL BELL HANDY, REMOVE CLUTTER, ADEQUATE NIGHT LIGHTING, BED/CHAIR APPROPRIATE HEIGHT, ORIENTATE TO ENVIRONMENT

PART 2 - RISK FACTORS	PART 3 - INTERVENTIONS	Start date & initial	End date & initial
VISION ☐ Changes in vision, difficulty seeing objects, finding way around, reading signs ☐ Hearing Impairment	☐ Clean and current prescription glasses ☐ Appropriate hearing aid with working battery		
MOBILITY AND TRANSFERS ☐ Muscle weakness, poor balance, coordination, fatigue, pain affecting safe mobility	☐ Document transfer/mobility requirements		
	☐ Physio ☐ OT Assessment ☐ RAD Assessment ☐ Gait aid within reach		
BEHAVIOURS ☐ Delirium, confusion, depression	☐ Move within view of nurses station		
	☐ Lo-Lo bed		
☐ Aggression, restlessness impulsive	☐ Bed rails down		
☐ Reduced insight into safe mobility	☐ Bed/chair sensor		
☐ Difficulty following instructions	☐ Cognition CNC ☐ Refer Falls CNC		
☐ Drug and alcohol withdrawal	☐ Hip Protectors - complete over page ☐ Do not leave unattended in bathroom or toilet ☐ 30 minute visual observations		
ADLS	☐ Falls prevention information supplied		
☐ Observed risk taking behaviour ☐ Observed unsafe use of gait aid	☐ Promote safe footwear use – complete over page		
☐ Unable to use call bell	☐ Do not leave unattended in bathroom or toilet		
☐ Unsafe footwear	☐ High falls risk alert card and sticker		
ENVIRONMENT ☐ Difficulty with orientation to the environment	☐ OT PADLS assessment ☐ Communication aids including picture signage		
NUTRITION ☐ Underweight / low appetite / dehydration	☐ Referral to a dietitian ☐ Check Vitamin D levels		
CONTINENCE ☐ Urgency / frequency / nocturia / constipation / diarrhoea	☐ Urinal/commode handy ☐ Toileting regime		
	☐ Continence aids as appropriate		
MEDICAL ☐ Anticoagulant therapy, previous fracture, osteoporosis diabetes, strokes, seizures, respiratory disease	☐ Lying and standing BP ☐ Medication review		

.... Signature .... Print Name .... Designation .... Date/Time

FALLS RISK ASSESSMENT TOOL (FRAT)

MR/574526

23/04/15 Print Code:15665 page 1 of 2

FIGURE 22-3 The Falls Risk Assessment Tool (FRAT) (page 1 of 2). (Research conducted by Falls Prevention Service, Peninsula Health, Victoria, Australia. Not to be used without permission.)

Peninsula Health

FALLS RISK ASSESSMENT TOOL cont. (FRAT)

UR NUMBER..

SURNAME..

GIVEN NAMES..

DATE OF BIRTH ....
Please fill in if no Patient Label available

USE OF BEDRAILS RISK ASSESSMENT

Date / Time	**Bedrails to be used:**	**Bedrails NOT to be used:**
	a) Transporting patients b) Patient with capacity requests c) Risk of injury falling from bed outweighs the risks of bedrails	a) Risk of climbing over and falling from a greater height b) Risk of entrapment in bedrails outweighs risks of falling c) Patient is independent d) Patient with capacity refuses
	.... Signature / Print Name / Designation	.... Signature / Print Name / Designation
	.... Signature / Print Name / Designation	.... Signature / Print Name / Designation

REVIEW

Review Date	Risk Status	New Risk Factors Identified	Signature Print Name	Review Date	Risk Status	New Risk Factors Identified	Signature Print Name

HIP PROTECTOR USE Patient ☐ Accepted ☐ Declined

....
Signature *Print Name* *Designation* *Date/Time*

Date of Issue: .... Date Ceased: ....

Reason for ceasing use: ....

....
Signature *Print Name* *Designation* *Date/Time*

FOOTWEAR Appropriate Footwear (please tick): ☐ Yes ☐ No

....
Signature *Print Name* *Designation* *Date/Time*

FALLS PREVENTION ☐ Group Attended ☐ Provided with opportunity to ask questions ☐ Provided with falls prevention brochure

....
Signature *Print Name* *Designation* *Date/Time*

FALLS SINCE ADMISSION - Record summary of details of falls as an inpatient here

Date / Time of Fall		Date / Time of Fall		Date / Time of Fall	
Activity at time of fall		Activity at time of fall		Activity at time of fall	
Incident Report No		Incident Report No		Incident Report No	
Signature Print Name Designation		Signature Print Name Designation		Signature Print Name Designation	

23/01/15 Print Code 15665 page 2 of 2

FIGURE 22-3 The Falls Risk Assessment Tool (FRAT) (*continued*) (page 2 of 2).

NURSING ISSUES

Impaired physical mobility is a nursing issue that is applicable when the assessment identifies limitations in mobility of an older adult. Related factors common in older adults include arthritis, depression, chronic pain, fractured hip and neurological disorders (e.g. dementia or Parkinson's disease). If the nursing assessment identifies a history of falls or any risks for falls, the nursing issue of risk for falls would be applicable. Related factors common in older adults include all those factors listed in Box 22-2.

In long-term residential care and rehabilitation settings, nurses frequently address the needs of older adults who have a diagnosis of osteoporosis or a history of fractures. In these situations, as well as in any situation where someone has several risk factors for osteoporosis, a nursing issue of an inability to identify, manage and/or seek out help to maintain health is applicable.

WELLNESS OPPORTUNITY

Nurses can use the nursing issue willingness for enhanced self-health management for older adults who are willing to explore opportunities for improving musculoskeletal function and preventing falls and fractures.

GOAL PLANNING FOR WELLNESS OUTCOMES

When planning care for older adults who are at risk for osteoporosis, nurses develop goals to achieve wellness outcomes that focus on primary and secondary prevention. In these situations, the following nursing goals may apply: the development of health-promoting behaviour, increased knowledge of health behaviour, prevention of risk of osteoporosis or detection of risks.

Nursing outcomes for an older adult with an issue of impaired physical mobility would focus on optimising functional abilities, preventing further loss of function and preventing falls and injuries. Goals applicable to an older adult with this issue include improved muscle strength, balance, endurance, mobility, activity tolerance or decreased pain level.

Care of older adults with a nursing issue of risk for falls focuses on preventing the occurrence of falls and fall-related injuries by implementing fall-prevention programs. The following goals with regard to safety and fall prevention are: detection of risk, minimisation of risk fall prevention behaviour, development of safe behaviour at home or other environments, development of safe behaviour by the individual and prevention of physical injury or falls.

WELLNESS OPPORTUNITY

Wellness outcomes that address the body–mind–spirit interrelatedness for people who are afraid of falling include coping, fear control, comfort level, anxiety control and quality of life.

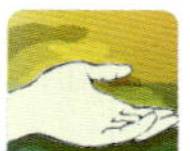

NURSING INTERVENTIONS FOR MUSCULOSKELETAL WELLNESS

Nurses have numerous opportunities to promote musculoskeletal wellness because most older adults can benefit from learning about health promotion interventions for improved musculoskeletal function and prevention of osteoporosis, falls and fractures. Thus, interventions focus not only on direct actions to prevent falls but also on teaching about eliminating or addressing risks. Some nursing interventions that would be applicable would focus on: environmental management, exercise promotion, fall prevention, health education, risk identification and individual teaching.

Promoting healthy musculoskeletal function and preventing falls

Healthy older adults experience only a slight decline in overall musculoskeletal function, but they can compensate for these minor functional consequences by maintaining an active lifestyle. Various types of exercise are beneficial in promoting healthy musculoskeletal function and nurses can encourage older adults to incorporate several exercise strategies into their regular health-behaviour routines. An exercise program that maintains musculoskeletal function should include progressive resistance, flexibility and balance activities (New Zealand Ministry of Health, 2013). The positive effects of these types of programs include increased muscle and bone strength, and increased flexibility and endurance, leading to improved functioning and prevention of falls and disability. Additionally, flexibility exercises are an essential intervention for osteoporosis. Moderate aerobic exercise can also assist with intentional weight loss. Thus, an important nursing intervention is to help older adults identify ways in which they can incorporate physical activity as a daily health-promoting practice. For example, using an exercise DVD is an effective approach to improving musculoskeletal function in community-living older adults (McAuley, Wojcicki, Gothe et al., 2013). Because promotion of physical activity is a wellness outcome that affects many aspects of functioning, this topic is addressed in Chapter 5.

In recent years, there has been increasing attention to holistic types of exercise that address balance, mobility and the mind–body connection. Tai chi, which is a traditional Chinese martial art and a mind–body exercise that involves focused attention and a series of fluid and continuous movements, has been used in Asian countries for centuries and is now widely available in Western countries. Many studies and systematic reviews have confirmed the following beneficial effects of tai chi related to musculoskeletal function (Huang, Yang & Liu, 2011; Tousignant, Corriveau, Roy et al., 2013; Wei, Xu, Fan et al., 2013):

- Improved balance and neuromuscular coordination
- Increased muscle strength, flexibility and endurance
- Improved postural stability

- Decreased risk of falls and fractures
- Reduced fear of falling.

Studies also found that long-term participation in tai chi has beneficial effects, including fall prevention, for older adults with chronic conditions that affect musculoskeletal function, such as osteoarthritis, Parkinson's disease, and peripheral neuropathy (Lauche, Langhorst, Dobos et al., 2013; Manor, Lipsitz, Wayne et al., 2013; Tsang, 2013; Yan, Gu, Sun et al., 2013).

Yoga is another body–mind therapy that is effective for improving balance and mobility in older adults (Tiedemann, O'Rourke, Sesto et al., 2013). Recent studies identify positive outcomes of dancing as an intervention for improving balance and preventing falls in older adults, including those aged 85 and older and those with dementia (e.g. Abreu & Hartley, 2013; Hackney, Hall, Echt et al., 2013). The advantages of dance-type exercises are that they are safe, feasible, enjoyable and have a high adherence rate (Granacher, Muehlbauer, Bridenbaugh et al., 2012). The Feldenkrais method is another holistic form of exercise found to improve balance and mobility and decrease fear of falling in older adults (Connors, Galea, Said, 2011).

WELLNESS OPPORTUNITY

Walking, dancing, swimming, tai chi and bicycle riding are examples of wellness intervention that are enjoyable and have positive effects on one's body, mind and spirit.

Health promotion: Teaching about osteoporosis

Interventions for prevention and treatment of osteoporosis need to be an integral part of fracture prevention regimens for older adults, particularly in healthcare settings where a major focus of care is on chronic conditions (e.g. homecare and long-term care settings). Although primary care practitioners are responsible for diagnosing and treating osteoporosis, nurses are responsible for health education about osteoporosis interventions and prevention of fractures. Because awareness about osteoporosis in men is just beginning to develop, nurses have a particular responsibility for teaching older men about screening for osteoporosis. It also is important to focus health education on older adults who already have had fractures because secondary prevention measures are often overlooked.

Health education includes information about risk factors with emphasis on developing a plan to address the modifiable risk factors. Nurses can encourage older adults with risk factors to ask their primary care practitioner about screening tests and interventions. All adults can benefit from lifestyle interventions for osteoporosis, and teaching about these self-care activities is well within the realm of nursing responsibilities. Important self-care interventions for osteoporosis include daily weight-bearing activities, quitting smoking, and limiting alcohol intake.

Nurses can also teach older adults and their carers about the importance of adequate intake of calcium and vitamin D. A registered dietitian, if available, can evaluate a food journal to determine the usual intake of calcium and vitamin D. If intake does not provide at least 1000 to 1200 mg of calcium and 800 to 2000 IU of vitamin D, then health teaching focuses either on increasing dietary intake to the recommended amount or on taking a daily supplement. In long-term care residential facilities, all care plans should include a review of nutritional interventions for osteoporosis, particularly in relation to preventing fractures. Nurses can take the lead in involving dietitians and primary care providers in developing and implementing appropriate preventive interventions. Box 22-4 summarises health promotion information that can be used as a guide for teaching older adults about osteoporosis.

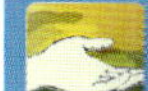

BOX 22-4
Health promotion teaching about osteoporosis

Health promotion interventions for early detection and treatment

- Review risk factors for osteoporosis, as summarised in Box 22-1.
- Plan interventions for modifiable risk factors using Box 22-1 and Box 22-3 as guides.
- Encourage discussion with the primary care provider about:
  - Bone density tests
  - Medical interventions for osteoporosis if risk factors are present
  - Prevention of fractures if osteoporosis is diagnosed.

Lifestyle interventions

- Implement weight-bearing exercise regimen for one half-hour daily.
- Engage in activities such as yoga, swimming, massage, acupressure and tai chi.
- Wear supportive shoes.
- Discontinue cigarette smoking.
- Maintain ideal body weight.
- Avoid excessive alcohol intake.

Nutritional interventions

- A daily intake of at least 1000 mg of calcium from food sources is recommended, rather than using calcium supplements that may have adverse effects.
- Foods that are high in calcium include milk, cheese, yogurt, custard, ice cream, raisins, tofu, canned salmon or sardines, and broccoli and other dark green vegetables.
  - If a higher dose of calcium is required, for example, for osteoporosis, this should be under the direction of a primary care practitioner.
- Provide adequate dietary intake of vitamin D and use supplement if needed to assure daily intake of at least 800 to 2000 IU vitamin D.
  - People with low serum vitamin D levels may require higher daily doses, which should be taken under the direction of a primary care practitioner.

A student's perspective

This past week, I chose to do the water aerobics with the older adults at the swimming centre. I was encouraged by the vitality and general zest for life that these older women showed. I was enlightened by their sense of pride in their health and level of activity. I left with the impression that this group activity was something that each of them attributed her good health to. I also noted that they got more out of this activity than just physical exercise. The social connection that these women had was truly admirable. They were constantly encouraging each other and me during the class. They also used the time just to connect with each other and discuss normal life events.

My take-away lesson from this experience was the importance of having opportunities like this for older adults to exercise their muscles as well as their social personalities. Older adults are often portrayed as socially inferior in today's popular culture, but I felt these older women were living truly balanced lives, maybe more so than me in some respects. I think that often I find myself so busy that I do not take time to invest myself in more meaningful relationships—something that these people are obviously benefiting from.

Clint H.

WELLNESS OPPORTUNITY

Promoting self-care practices to prevent osteoporosis is particularly important when working with older adults who have a history of falls or fractures.

Pharmalogical interventions for osteoporosis

A major goal of pharmacological interventions for osteoporosis is prevention of osteoporotic fractures, which are associated with serious consequences, including chronic pain, decreased quality of life, and significant morbidity and mortality. In recent years, many types of medications have been approved for prevention of fragility fractures, which are in addition to the menopausal hormonal therapy that was widely used until the mid-1990s. A systematic review of 567 clinical studies published between 2005 and 2011 identified the following pharmaceutical agents as effective for preventing fragility fractures in postmenopausal women with osteoporosis (Agency for Healthcare Research and Quality Effective Health Care Program, 2012):

- Bisphosphonates: alendronic acid, risedronate, zoledronic acid, ibandronate
- Menopausal hormone therapy (e.g. oestrogen conjugated—Premarin)
- Selective oestrogen receptor modulator—raloxifene
- Parathyroid hormone (e.g. anabolic drug—teriparatide).

The effectiveness of bisphosphonates has been shown to be associated with adequate vitamin D and calcium levels (Australian Commission on Safety and Quality in Health Care [ACSQHC], 2009a). It is recommended that vitamin D and calcium be prescribed, together with bisphosphonates. Oral bisphosphonates can also cause upper gastrointestinal injury, particularly when taken daily or when there are acidic conditions or pre-existing oesophageal irritation (Recker et al., 2009). Measures to prevent potential adverse effects on the gastrointestinal tract include taking the medication in the morning with a full glass of water (not mineral water) at least half an hour before any food. In addition, the person must be in an upright position when taking this medication and avoid lying down for half an hour after the dose. Because of the adverse effects associated with daily oral dosing, newer bisphosphonates have been developed for weekly, monthly or even annual dosing to increase compliance. Annual dosing of bisphosphonates is administered intravenously. The most commonly prescribed intravenous bisphosphonates are pamidronate and zoledronate (trade names Aredia and Aclasta).

It is important to note that all types of osteoporosis medications have been shown to reduce the incidence of vertebral fractures; however, the only ones that reduced the risk for hip fracture were alendronic acid, risedronate, zoledronic acid, and denosumab. Because all these medications are associated with various adverse effects, including serious ones, such as thromboembolic events and increased risk for breast cancer, it is imperative to advise older women to discuss the benefits and risks with their primary care practitioners so they can make informed decisions about this important preventive intervention.

Because most clinical trials of medical interventions for osteoporosis focus primarily on women, much less evidence is available about safe and effective pharmacological treatments for men with the disease. Based on a systematic review of studies, the Endocrine Society Task Force on Osteoporosis in Men (Watts, Adler, Bilezikian et al., 2012) recommended that men at high risk for fracture be treated with one of the following medications: alendronic acid, risedronate, zoledronic acid, or parathyroid hormone. The Task Force emphasised that selection of a pharmaceutical agent should be individualised based on factors such as fracture history, severity of osteoporosis, and risk for hip fracture. In summary, there is sound evidence that pharmacological treatment of osteoporosis can improve bone density, reduce the rate of bone loss, and decrease the risk for fragility fractures, including hip fracture. Evidence is less clear about pharmacological interventions for older adults who do not have osteoporosis but have risks for it. Decisions about preventive pharmacological interventions for people at risk for osteoporosis and fractures must be based on an appraisal of the relative risks and benefits of any particular intervention. Pharmacological treatment is just one component of a comprehensive management plan that must also include nutritional intake of calcium and vitamin D, physical activity to maintain musculoskeletal function and reduce the risk of falls, and education regarding osteoporosis and fall prevention.

UNFOLDING CASE STUDY

Part D

Recall that you are the practice nurse at the medical clinic where Ms Mayo, who is 75 years old, regularly attends. Based on additional assessment information, you know that Ms Mayo does not take any calcium or vitamin D supplements because she drinks milk twice daily and believes that this should be sufficient. She stopped having menstrual periods when she was 50 years old and began hormone therapy at that time. She stopped taking oestrogen after a few years because she began "hearing too many bad things about oestrogen". When she fractured her wrist 8 years ago, the orthopaedic surgeon said that her x-rays showed that her "bones were pretty good for her age". She has not had any further x-rays or any BMD tests and says her doctor has never brought up the subject of osteoporosis because "I guess he's too worried about my heart problems to be concerned about my bones". Although she fell once when she was raking leaves last autumn and tripped over a small tree stump, she has had no serious fall-related injuries since she fractured her wrist. She does not smoke and drinks alcohol only on major social occasions. When you assessed her blood pressure, you found that her blood pressure while standing was 146/88 mm Hg and while lying was 128/78 mm Hg. Her record of self-monitored blood pressure readings indicates that her usual blood pressure is around 134/82 mm Hg. Her vision is adequate, but she has stopped driving at night and is being monitored by her ophthalmologist for progression of bilateral cataracts. Her eye doctor told her that she is likely to need cataract surgery sometime during the next 2 to 3 years.

Thinking points

- What further assessment information would you want to have?
- What health promotion interventions would you advise for Ms Mayo? Specifically, what health teaching would you do with regard to further assessment, lifestyle interventions, nutrition, and nutritional supplements and pharmalogical interventions?
- What educational materials would you use for Ms Mayo?
- What follow-up health promotion would you consider for Ms Mayo? Specifically, how would you work with Ms Mayo to develop long-term health promotion interventions?

Preventing falls and fall-related injuries

Evidence-based guidelines have been developed about preventing falls in older adults in a range of Australian settings. These guidelines provide a comprehensive fall-prevention program for older adults in hospital, in long-term residential care and in the community (ACSQHC, 2009a, 2009b, 2009c). These guidelines address conditions in a particular setting, factors that are unique to each at-risk person and provide multidisciplinary fall-prevention programs. Because falls are multifaceted in their causes, it is recognised that multidisciplinary fall-prevention programs are required. These guidelines are also endorsed by the Australian and New Zealand Falls Prevention Society.

Comprehensive programs focus on reducing the occurrence of falls and preventing fall-related injuries as well as addressing intrinsic and extrinsic risk factors. Key aspects of fall prevention programs are the identification of people who are at risk for falls and the consistent implementation of preventive actions by all staff. An important part of these programs is the education of all professional and non-professional staff members who have contact with the person who is at risk for falls. Education may involve strategies to heighten staff awareness of the importance of reducing fall risks. For example, posters and brochures may be used initially and periodically as reminders. Also, some form of person or chart identification can be used to draw attention to those people who have an increased risk for falls. Box 22-5 describes a fall-prevention program that could be adapted for use in institutional settings. An excellent website that contains a comprehensive list of fall prevention resources is located at http://fallsnetwork.neura.edu.au/resources.

Addressing intrinsic risk factors

Because any gait and balance impairment increases the risk for falls, interventions that improve mobility are likely to be beneficial in preventing falls. Interventions for improving mobility are implemented primarily by therapists, nurses and nursing staff, often through an interdisciplinary approach. Teaching about the proper use of mobility aids and other assistive devices is an important part of fall-prevention programs (Figure 22-4). Nurses are responsible for raising questions about whether an older adult may benefit from the use of mobility aids or assistive devices and facilitating a referral to a physical therapist for evaluation and teaching regarding their use. In community settings, nurses can teach older adults and their carers about the availability of various mobility aids, transfer assistance devices and other aids that might improve safety. Nurses can suggest that older adults seek professional help with selecting appropriate mobility aids and assistive devices. Some suppliers of home healthcare equipment have therapists or a staff member who can provide advice and assist with processing claims if the aids are covered by insurance. When mobility aids are prescribed, nurses are responsible for encouraging the person to use the aids and making sure the aids are accessible. Nurses are responsible for facilitating referrals for reassessment if questions arise about the safety or effectiveness of mobility aids that are being used.

Because proper footwear is essential to prevent slips and falls, nurses can advise older adults about wearing non-slip footwear for safety. Walking outdoors can be particularly hazardous, especially when wet conditions create a very dangerous environment for older people who have a predisposition for falls. Nurses can emphasise the importance of removing slip hazards from paths and help older adults explore resources for assistance with this. In addition, a simple gait-stabilising device, such as the Yaktrax Walker (Figure 22-5), may help prevent outdoor falls when applied and worn properly.

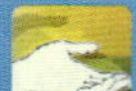

BOX 22-5
A fall-prevention program for older adults being cared for in hospitals or long-term residential care

Identification of people who are at risk for falling

- Use a nursing judgement and a fall risk assessment tool to identify any risks for falling and fall-related injuries (e.g. medications, osteoporosis, medical conditions, history of falls, impaired cognition, diminished alertness, impaired mobility, age 75 years or older).
- Document the risk factors on the designated fall assessment guide.
- Address any risk factors for falls, osteoporosis or fall-related injuries that can be modified; this often requires a multidisciplinary approach.
- Reassess the risks for falls and fall-related injuries at predetermined times (e.g. every shift, every day, whenever there is a change in the person's functional status).
- Use colour-coded items (e.g. brightly coloured stickers for the chart, a brightly coloured identification band for the person's wrist and signs near the person's bed and outside the room) to identify those who are included in the fall-prevention program.

Education of the staff, person and family

- Instruct the person and family about the fall-prevention program and provide written information about preventing falls and obtaining help if falls occur.
- Provide staff education about the fall-prevention program and the risk factors for falls, especially those factors that the staff influences (e.g. use of restraints, selection of footwear).
- Use posters and fliers to heighten staff awareness of the fall-prevention program.

Interventions to be implemented for all high-risk people

- Keep the call light within reach at all times.
- Make sure that ambulatory the person wears sturdy, non-slip footwear when out of bed.
- Offer assistance with activities of daily living (ADLs) and try to anticipate the person's needs before help is needed.
- Encourage the person to call for help when needed.
- Frequently check all people who cannot be relied on to call for help.
- Make sure the bed is in the lowest position possible and the wheels are locked.
- Carefully and frequently assess the environment for factors that increase the risk for either falls or fall-related injuries; address all modifiable risk factors.
- Consider the use of a movement detection device.
- Adhere to institutional policies about use of physical restraints, including bedrails.
- If appropriate, orient the person to person, place and time every shift and as needed.
- Document fall-prevention interventions on the person's chart.

It has been recognised that older adults' feet also require particular care so that safe mobilisation is supported and falls are prevented. Box 22-6 lists major practice points about foot care for older adults. Box 22-7 is a practice guide for cutting older adults' toenails.

In recent years, fall-prevention literature has emphasised the effectiveness of various exercise routines as an intervention for reducing intrinsic fall risk. An important role for nurses is to identify those older adults who may benefit from gait and balance training programs and to facilitate referrals for physical therapy when appropriate. Nurses are also responsible for encouraging adequate and consistent follow-through with recommended exercise programs. In long-term residential aged care settings, nurses generally oversee restorative nursing programs in which nursing assistants help residents with walking and other exercise regimens established by physical therapists or physiotherapists. These restorative nursing routines are essential aspects of fall-prevention programs. Group exercise programs are also widely used as fall-prevention

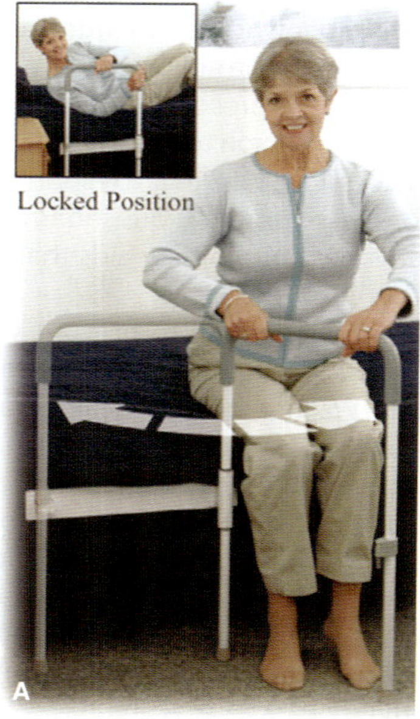

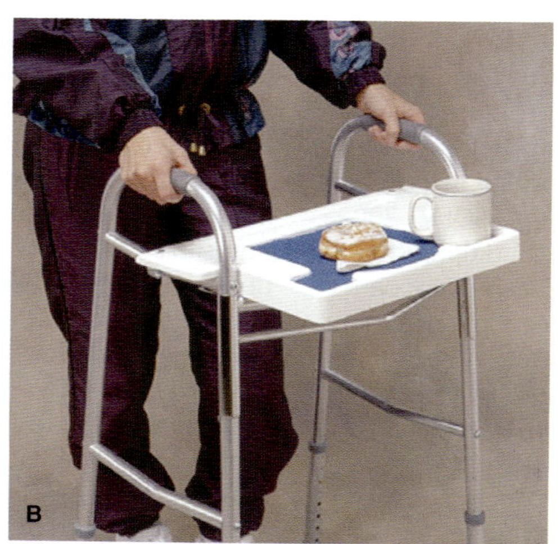

FIGURE 22-4 The use of assistive devices can help reduce the risk of falls. (**A**) Transfer assistive devices are used to facilitate safer transfer in and out of beds. (**B**) Walkers are available in various styles with wheels, brakes, baskets, seats and other features to improve safety and mobility. (Photographs courtesy of ActiveForever.com.)

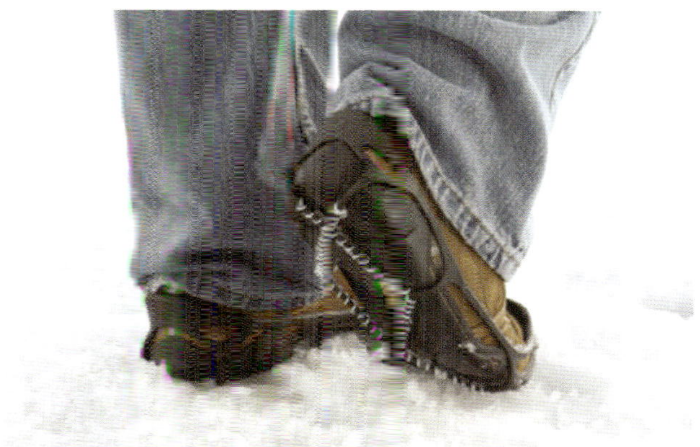

FIGURE 22-5 The Yaktrax Walker is an example of a gait-stabilising device that can be used to prevent falls on slippery outdoor surfaces. (Photograph courtesy of Yaktrax, LLC.)

interventions that are beneficial to all at-risk people. Many programs incorporate exercises that are aimed specifically at improving gait, balance, ankle strength or other aspects of fall prevention.

Fall-prevention programs also include multidisciplinary interventions to address medication effects and pathological conditions that increase the risk for falls. Nurses are responsible for knowing the common adverse effects of medications and raising questions about any effects that increase the risk for falls. Nurses should assess for postural hypotension, for example, as a potential adverse medication effect and as a risk factor for falls. Medication regimens should be reviewed periodically and nurses can take the lead in suggesting that pharmacists and also prescribing practitioners evaluate medications in relation to fall risks.

Addressing extrinsic risk factors

Interventions for addressing extrinsic risk factors, such as environmental conditions and use of restraints, are applicable for older adults in any setting. Hospital in-patients who are at risk for falls should receive referrals for environmental home assessments when they are discharged. Environmental assessment guidelines provided in Chapter 7 can help with planning interventions that may eliminate or reduce environmental risks. In addition, environmental modifications to improve a person's vision, as discussed in Chapter 17, are applicable to fall prevention.

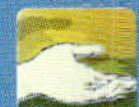

BOX 22-6
Practice points about foot care and older adults

- Many older people are unable to care for their own feet.
- Common disorders associated with the feet for older adults include hardened or ingrown toenails, toe deformities such as overlapping toes, corns and calluses, bunions and fungal infections. These disorders interfere with mobility and the wearing of safe supportive non-slip shoes.
- It has been estimated that three-quarters of older adults have foot problems and about one-third are unable to cut their own toenails.
- It is recommended that nurses provide basic foot care and know when to refer on to specialised podiatry services.

Source: Soliman, A. & Brogan, M. (2014). Foot assessment and care for older people. *Nursing Times, 110*(50), 12–15.

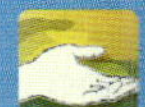

BOX 22-7
Practice guide for cutting older adults' toenails

- Toenails are best cut after a bath when the nails are slightly softer and easier to cut.
- Use a pair of nail clippers to cut straight across (do not cut nails too short or cut down the sides).
- Gently file away any rough or sharp edges using a nail file or large emery.
- To prevent cross infection all older adults should have their own board or foot file, nail clippers and a nail file.
- Nail clippers should be cleaned with detergent and dried after each use.

Source: Soliman, A. & Brogan, M. (2014). Foot assessment and care for older people. *Nursing Times, 110*(50), 12–15.

WELLNESS OPPORTUNITY

Fall-prevention interventions that address the person–environment relationship can be as simple and effective as involving older adults in decisions about removing or replacing slippery throw rugs.

Using monitoring devices

Monitoring devices can be useful in alerting staff to potentially unsafe movement by the person; however, concerns have been raised about the overuse and negative consequences of some types of devices. All monitoring devices contain a mechanism for transmitting a signal to a remote location (e.g. a nursing station) when activated by certain levels of movement by the person. Some devices, such as a pad, are applied to the bed or chair, whereas others are attached to the person's clothing. Less restrictive devices are programmed specifically for the person's movement in a confined environment, such as his or her room. Because alarm-type devices emit a loud signal, these are associated with negative consequences, such as (1) staff responding to the alarm rather than the person, (2) disruptive noise, which can be confusing when more than one alarm is sounding, (3) provision of a false sense of security for staff, and (4) decreased overall mobility for the person who is being monitored (Crogan & Dupler, 2014).

Most movement-detection devices were originally designed for institutional use, but simplified monitoring and signal systems have now been developed for home use by family carers. In home settings, a simple auditory room-monitoring device (i.e. a "baby room monitor") may be useful when carers need to detect the sound of someone moving around in another room. A major limitation of any movement-detection device is that its effectiveness depends on the timely response of someone who is able to prevent the fall. These devices are not useful for people living alone or for people without responsible and responsive carers.

Providing assistance in independent settings

For people living alone and at risk for falls, it is important to consider interventions for summoning help in a timely manner if falls occur. Many types of personal emergency response systems are available and these involve the use of a small portable transmitter that is worn on the person's body or clothing. When the person falls, he or she can summon help by using the transmitter to signal a receiver unit attached to the telephone. In turn, a call is automatically made to the personal emergency response system provider, who then checks in with the person on a speaker-phone system and calls the local emergency response team or a contact person such as a neighbour or family member if the person needs help. Some of these devices are set up so that a monitoring call is made to the person once a day if the person does not push a reset button or otherwise notify the company that he or she is well.

The effectiveness of personal emergency response system depends on the ability of the fallen person to signal for help and on the availability of a helping person. A major limitation of such devices is that cognitively impaired people may not be able to learn to use them. Hospitals, homecare agencies and other organisations for older people provide information about local personal emergency response system programs, and information about national programs is available on the Internet. Cordless phones, especially if pre-programmed for emergency help and placed within reach where someone might fall, can also be used for obtaining help.

Interventions in the older adult's physical environment

When falls cannot be prevented, interventions are directed towards reducing the risk of fractures and other serious fall-related injuries. Two interventions for preventing fall-related injuries that should be used for all people who are at risk for falls are (1) to implement evidence-based measures for osteoporosis (discussed previously) and (2) to adapt the environment as much as possible to reduce the risk for fall-related injuries. Heavy furniture that is in a pathway where a fall is likely to occur can be moved out of the way or replaced with items that would move easily if the person falls into them. Also, hard edges of furniture and built-in cabinets can be padded. Particular attention should be paid to padding hard edges of bathroom cabinets and either padding or removing swinging shower doors. Using a bed that can be adjusted to a very low position can reduce risk of injury from falling out of bed. Soft mats can be placed near beds and in other locations where people are likely to fall, but caution must be used so that these pads do not become fall risks.

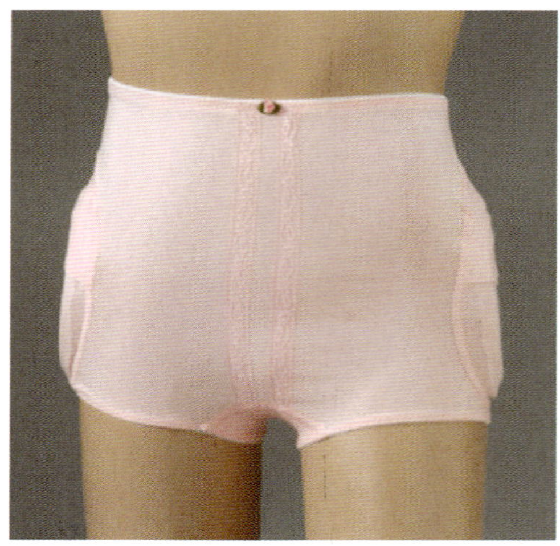

FIGURE 22-6 Hip protectors come in a variety of styles, such as the Posey Community Hipsters (Photograph courtesy of Posey Company, Arcadia, CA).

External hip protectors have been available since the 1990s and many types of hip protectors are used internationally (Figure 22-6). Hip protectors, which are designed to decrease the impact of a fall, consist of pads with or without hard shells that are placed over the hips and worn under garments. Studies have found that hip protectors represent a "promising strategy" for reducing the risk of hip fracture if they are positioned properly; however, not all studies have demonstrated clinical effectiveness (Cameron et al., 2010; Choi, Hoffer & Robinovitch, 2010a). Some studies suggest that hip protectors are effective in preventing fractures in people who have low body mass index (BMI) and other risk factors (e.g. previous falls) (Choi, Hoffer & Robinovitch, 2010b; Koike et al., 2009). Another study, a systematic review, provides evidence that hip protectors may reduce the rate of hip fractures in older people receiving nursing care and living in long-term residential care but it is not conclusive for older adults who live in the community (Santesso, Carrasco-Labra & Brignardello-Petersen, 2014). Another intervention, the training in martial arts about proper fall techniques, has been trialled. One study found this intervention prevented fall-related injuries and reduced the impact on hips (Groen et al., 2010).

Finally, nurses need to recognise that bedrails and other types of restraints do not necessarily reduce the risk of falls and are associated with more serious fall-related injuries (Gray-Miceli & Quigley, 2012). In recent years the Australian Government has encouraged healthcare institutions to develop policies for restraint reduction or restraint-free care. Bed rails are considered a high risk restraint and are recommended for use only after a thorough process of

EVIDENCE-BASED PRACTICE 22-1
Prevention of falls

Statement of the problem

- About 30% of community-dwelling older adults fall each year.
- Many studies in recent years have identified evidence-based interventions that are effective for reducing falls, risks for falls and fall-related injuries.

Recommendations for screening and assessment

- Ask older adults if they have had a fall during the past year.
- Find out details about circumstances of each fall.
- Ask about gait and balance problems.
- Perform simple test for gait and balance (e.g. Timed Get Up and Go).
- Arrange for multifactorial fall risk assessment including comprehensive physical examination, functional assessment, environmental assessment, medical history and medication review.

Evidence-based fall-prevention interventions

- Implementation of interventions for individual fall risks identified during multifactorial assessment.
- Participation in a multiple component group or home-based exercise program that includes balance, strength and gait-training exercises.
- Optimal management of all medical conditions, especially cardiac arrhythmias and postural hypotension.
- Modification of prescription medication regimens, including gradual withdrawal of psychotropic medication.
- Treatment of vision impairment: cataract surgery as needed, not using multifocal lenses while walking.
- Management of foot problems and footwear.
- Vitamin D supplementation for people with lower serum vitamin D levels.
- Home safety assessment and modification, which is particularly effective for people who are visually impaired and when delivered by an occupational therapist.

Recommendations for nursing interventions

- Facilitate implementation of applicable evidence-based interventions.
- Teach about recommended level of physical activity for older adults: 2.5 hours of moderate-intensity or 1.25 hours of vigorous-intensity aerobic physical activity every week, plus muscle-strengthening activities twice weekly, and balance training 3 or more days per week for those with risks for falls.
- Teach about self-care actions, including using appropriate assistive devices and safety measures (e.g. antislip shoe devices in icy conditions).

Source. American Geriatrics Society and British Geriatrics Society (2010); Gillespie, Robertson, Gillespie et al. (2012); U.S. Preventive Services Task Force (2012).

assessment and clinical collaborative consultation has occurred (DSS, 2012b). Evidence-based guidelines emphasise the need for individualised care plans to prevent falls and for education of the older adult, family members and all care staff members about the concept of restraint-free care as well as fall-prevention measures. Nurses play an extremely important role in decisions about using restraints, the education about their associated risks and the implementation and monitoring of restraint. Evidence-based practices for prevention of falls are summarised in Evidence-based practice 22-1.

WELLNESS OPPORTUNITY

Health promotion interventions need to be broad and include precautions to minimise the risk of injury if falls do occur.

Addressing fear of falling

Any interventions that reduce the risk of falls are also likely to reduce a person's fear of falling, but some people may need additional interventions to address this problem. The "Falls and Feelings" discussion group is a nursing model that was designed to facilitate discussion of feelings related to falling experiences. The goal for group members was "to enhance self-confidence and life satisfaction, resulting in empowerment of the individual to handle fear of falling" (Gentleman & Malozemoff, 2001, p. 36). Themes of the sessions included risks for falls, the prevention of falls, falls and feelings, and fear as a consequence of falls (Gentleman & Malozemoff, 2001). Nurses can address fear of falling in the same way they address other fears: encourage the expression of feelings and provide education and reassurance about interventions that are being implemented as part of an individualised fall prevention care plan. Family members and carers should be included in nursing interventions and health education to address fear of falling. For people living alone, a PERS may be very reassuring and at least alleviate the fear of being helpless if a fall occurs.

Promoting carer wellness

In home and community settings, preventing falls and fall-related injuries are major responsibilities for the carers of people who have risks for falls or a history of falls. This responsibility can significantly increase the stress for families as they try to balance the desire of the older adult to have privacy and independence against the risk of the person falling and incurring significant, or even fatal, injuries. Nurses working in home care settings often address this issue and weigh the responsibility to respect autonomy versus the responsibility to assure safety. Information in Chapters 9 and 10 is applicable to ethical issues when working with carers to address these questions.

On the practical side, nurses can address carer stress related to their concerns about falls by arranging for a multidisciplinary approach to risk assessment and interventions for preventing falls and fall-related injuries. These

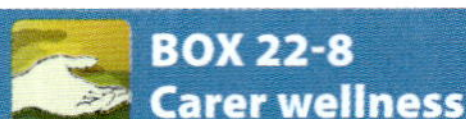

BOX 22-8
Carer wellness

Family carers often experience stress because their older relative desires to remain independent even though he or she is at risk for falls, has already had a fall, or even is a "frequent faller". In these situations carers weigh the right of the older adult to take risks versus the need for safety and protection. When faced with this situation, it is important to use professional resources for promoting as safe and independent functioning as possible for the older person and peace of mind for concerned relatives. Implementing some strategies that promote safety and prevent injuries and thereby help to relieve carer stress follow.

Strategies for preventing falls and fall-related injuries in home settings

Interventions to reduce the risk for falls

- Obtain a comprehensive fall risk assessment to identify and address risks related to medical conditions, medication effects, and functional limitations.
- Obtain ophthalmological evaluation to assure optimal visual function (e.g. cataract surgery may improve safety).
- Arrange for a home visit by a physical therapist or other qualified professional to identify and address environmental risks.
- Modify the home for safety by installing grab bars, handrails, good lighting, and other appropriate modifications for safe and independent mobility.

Actions to promote safe and independent functioning

- Arrange for occupational and physical therapy evaluations and recommendations for assistive devices, home modification for safety, and therapeutic exercises.
- Encourage frequent participation in enjoyable and beneficial physical activity programs, such as dancing, tai chi, water exercises.
- Encourage the person to engage in home-based physical activity by using videos, Wii Fit, and simple exercise equipment; consider doing these activities with them.

Actions to assure timely response for assistance

- Arrange for personal emergency response system.
- Place cordless phones in strategic locations in the home.
- Encourage the person to keep a cell phone handy at all times.
- If the person has memory problems, frequently remind him about the importance of calling for help when needed.

Resources for information about fall prevention in home settings

- Australian Commission on Safety and Quality in Health Care: www.safetyandquality.gov.au
- Clinical Excellence Commission, falls prevention (number of languages available): www.cec.health.nsw.gov.au
- Victorian Government: www.health.vic.gov.au

assessments are available at outpatient geriatric assessment programs and through skilled homecare agencies for people who are homebound. Nurses also can teach carers about fall-prevention strategies and resources for additional information, as described in Box 22-8.

WELLNESS OPPORTUNITY

Nurses address body–mind–spirit interrelatedness by talking with older adults about ways of diminishing their fear of falling and identifying ways of improving their safety.

EVALUATING EFFECTIVENESS OF NURSING INTERVENTIONS

Nursing care for older adults with impaired musculoskeletal function is evaluated by the degree to which the person achieves and maintains the highest possible level of independence and safe mobility. Nursing care of older adults who are at high risk for osteoporosis is evaluated according to the degree to which the older adult incorporates preventive measures in his or her daily life. For example, older adults might begin a regimen of three half-hour periods of weight-bearing exercise weekly. The nursing care of older adults who are at high risk for falls and fall-related injuries is evaluated according to the extent to which falls and serious injuries are prevented. Nurses cannot, of course, measure the number of falls that do not occur, but they can measure the risk factors that have been addressed in the care plan. Evaluation of these risk factors is facilitated by careful documentation of interventions, such as environmental modifications and fall prevention programs.

UNFOLDING CASE STUDY

Part E

Ms Mayo is now 89 years old and has been admitted to the hospital for heart failure. Additional medical problems include osteoarthritis, osteoporosis, recurrent depression, early-stage dementia and history of fractured hip. Current medications include frusemide, 40 mg twice daily; enalapril, 10 mg twice daily; digoxin, 0.125 mg daily; calcitonin nasal spray daily; calcium 500 mg with D 200 units; and sertraline, 50 mg at bedtime. Ms Mayo lives in a long-term residential care facility, where she receives help with her medications and goes to the dining room for meals. You are the nurse on the acute care floor assigned to her care on the day of admission.

Nursing assessment

During your initial nursing assessment, Ms Mayo is quiet and withdrawn. When you ask about her living situation, she says she moved to the residential care facility 2 years ago, after she was hospitalised for treatment of a fractured hip. At the time of the injury, she had been living alone. She had fallen while making her way to the bathroom at night and remained lying on the floor until her daughter came to visit her the next morning. During the past year, Ms Mayo reports that she has fallen twice in her room, but that she has been able to call for help and has not had any serious injuries. You determine that Ms Mayo will need help in ambulating to the bathroom and that she should be supervised whenever she gets out of bed.

Ms Mayo confides that she is very unhappy about her lack of energy and her hospitalisation for congestive heart failure. A mental status assessment indicates that Ms Mayo is alert and oriented but that her short-term memory is impaired. She has a great deal of difficulty with abstract ideas, such as learning to use the call button. You check her vital signs, which are within normal range, with no evidence of postural hypotension.

Nursing issues

In addition to the nursing issues related to Ms Mayo's medical condition, you identify a nursing issue of risk for falls. Related factors include weakness, diuretic and cardiovascular medications, a history of falls, a risk of depression and impaired cognition. You are concerned about preventing falls during her hospitalisation.

Nursing care plan for Ms Mayo

Goals for wellness outcomes	Nursing interventions	Nursing evaluation
Ms Mayo will ambulate safely and avoid falls during her hospitalisation.	• Identify Ms Mayo as a participant in the fall-prevention program by using an orange wrist bracelet, posting a Fall Alert sign near her bed and placing an orange Fall Alert sticker on her chart. • Reassess fall risks every shift and document these on the Fall Assessment form included in Ms Mayo's chart. • Talk with Ms Mayo's doctor about a referral for physiotherapy. • Keep the call light button within her reach and review instructions for its use every shift. • Make sure that the bed is in the lowest possible position with the wheels locked. • Use a movement detection bed pad and explain to Ms Mayo that the purpose of the pad is to ensure that the staff knows when she needs to get out of bed. • Every 2 hours, when Ms Mayo is awake, the nursing staff will ask her if she needs to go to the bathroom.	• Ms Mayo receives assistance with ambulation every time she is out of bed. • Ms Mayo has not fallen during her hospitalisation.

Thinking points

- If you were the nurse on the acute care floor where Ms Mayo was an in-patient, what concerns would you address in a discharge plan? Would you identify any additional nursing issues related to safe mobility and musculoskeletal function? What additional nursing interventions would you plan to supplement the care plan described in this chapter?
- If you were a nurse in the residential care facility where Ms Mayo lives, what concerns would you have about her care? How would you address these concerns in a care plan?

CHAPTER HIGHLIGHTS

Age-related changes that affect mobility and safety

- Degenerative changes in bones, muscles, joints and connective tissue
- Central nervous system changes: slowed reaction time, body sway
- Diminished bone density: osteopenia and osteoporosis

Risk factors that affect mobility and safety

- Risk factors for impaired musculoskeletal function: inactivity, inadequate protein and vitamin D intake
- Risk factors for osteoporosis and fractures: inadequate calcium and vitamin D intake, lack of weight-bearing activity, female gender, small bones, increased age, tobacco smoking, excessive alcohol consumption, certain medications (e.g. corticosteroids)
- Risk factors for falls: pathological conditions and functional impairments, medication effects, environmental factors, physical restraints

Functional consequences affecting musculoskeletal wellness

- Diminished muscle strength, balance, endurance and coordination
- Increased difficulty performing ADLs
- Increased susceptibility to falls
- Increased susceptibility to fall-related injuries, including death
- Fear of falling

Pathological condition affecting musculoskeletal wellness

- Osteoarthritis

Nursing assessment of musculoskeletal function

- Assessment of overall musculoskeletal performance
- Risks for osteoporosis (e.g. intake of calcium and vitamin D, history of fractures)
- Identifying risks for falls and injury
- Assessing for safety of the environment

Nursing issues

- Wellness nursing issue: willingness for enhanced self-health management
- Related to osteoporosis: health-seeking behaviours, ineffective health maintenance
- Related to fall risks: impaired physical mobility, risk for falls
- Another issue would be fear of falling

Goal planning for wellness outcomes

- Improved balance, endurance, mobility, activity tolerance
- Risk detection
- Safety behaviour: fall prevention at home or other environments
- Increased level of coping, reduced fear and increased comfort level
- Prevention of injury or falls

Nursing interventions for musculoskeletal wellness

- Promoting healthy musculoskeletal function
- Teaching about osteoporosis (e.g. early detection and treatment, lifestyle interventions, nutritional interventions, medications) (Box 22-4)
- Preventing falls and fall-related injuries by addressing intrinsic and extrinsic risk factors in institutional and community settings (Box 22-5; Figures 22-4, 22-5 and 22-6)
- Using monitoring devices in institutional settings and personal emergency response systems in home settings
- Addressing fear of falling
- Promoting carer wellness (Box 22-8)

Evaluating effectiveness of nursing interventions

- Maintenance of highest level of safe mobility
- Incorporation of preventive measures in daily life to ensure safety and prevent osteoporosis
- Expressed feelings of safety and improved quality of life

CRITICAL THINKING EXERCISES

1. Identify factors that increase or reduce the risk for osteoporosis.
2. Describe how each of the following age-related changes or risk factors might increase an older person's risk for falls and fractures: nocturia, osteoporosis, medications, altered gait, pathological conditions, sensory impairments, cognitive impairments, functional impairments, slowed reaction time.
3. Describe the environmental factors you would assess, in both home and institutional settings, to identify potential risks for falls.
4. Describe how you would design and implement a fall-prevention program in a long-term residential care facility.
5. How would you deal with a daughter who demanded that restraints be used whenever her 84-year-old mother, an in-patient on your acute care unit, is sitting in a chair?
6. What information would you include in health education about osteoporosis?
7. Use the Internet to find information about fall-prevention products that you might use in clinical practice.

RESOURCES

For an extensive range of additional resources to enhance teaching and learning and to facilitate understanding of this chapter, please see the text's accompanying website located on thePoint at http://thepoint.lww.com.

Clinical tools

Hartford Institute for Geriatric Nursing, ConsultGeriRN.org: http://consultgeri.org/resources

Assessment tool - *Try This®* series and *How to Try This* resources

General assessment series:

- *Try This*, issue 3: Fall risk assessment for older adults: The Hendrich II Fall Risk Model™. Hendrich, A. (2013). *Best Practices in Nursing Care to Older Adults.*
- *How to Try This* (article): Predicting patient falls. Hendrich, A. (2007). *American Journal of Nursing, 107*(11), 50–58.
- *How to Try This* (video): *The Hendrich II Fall Risk Assessment.*

Evidence-based practice

Bradas, C. M., Sandhu, S. K. & Mion, L. C. (2012). Physical restraints and side rails in acute and critical care settings. In M. Boltz, E. Capezuti, T. Fulmer & D. Zwicker (Eds), *Evidence-based geriatric nursing protocols for best practice* (4th ed., pp. 229–245). New York: Springer.

Gray-Miceli, D. & Quigley, P. A. (2012). Fall prevention: Assessment, diagnoses and intervention strategies. In M. Boltz, E. Capezuti, T. Fulmer & D. Zwicker (Eds), *Evidence-based geriatric nursing protocols for best practice* (4th ed., pp. 268–297). New York: Springer.

Joanna Briggs Institute: http://connect.jbiconnectplus.org

Best practice information sheets:

- Joanna Briggs Institute. (2010). Interventions to reduce the incidence of falls in older adult patients in acute care hospitals. *Evidence-Based Practice information Sheets for Health Professionals, 14*(15), 1–4.

Evidence summaries:

- Baker, S. (2013). Falls: Risk factors in the elderly.
- Campbell, J. (2014a). Osteoporosis: Risk factors and diagnosis.
- Campbell, J. (2014b). Technologies for falls prevention and detection: Older people's experience.
- Chen, Z. (2013). Osteoporosis: Exercise therapy.
- Chen, Z. (2014). Falls prevention strategies: Acute in-hospital setting.
- Dao Le, L. K. (2014a). Residential aged care: Physical restraint.
- Dao Le, L. K. (2014b). Tai chi: Benefits for the older person.
- D'Arcy, M. (2014a). Falls (older people): Assessment and prevention.
- D'Arcy, M. (2014b). Fracture (leg—older people): Management.
- Fong, E. (2013). Fracture (hip—older people): Prevention.
- Jayasekara, R. (2014). Osteoporosis in adults: Intervention.
- Kunde, L. (2014a). Falls: Assessment and prevention (community setting).
- Kunde, L. (2014b). Falls (older people): Observation.
- Kunde, L. (2014c). Muscle strength and physical function in older people: Dehydroepiandrosterone (DHEA).
- Kunde, L. (2014d). Physical activity programs: Older adults.
- Psalios, S. (2014). Injury reduction: Home environment modification.
- Slade, S. (2013). Walking frames and sticks.
- Slade, S. (2014). Progressive resistance training: Efficacy in the elderly.
- Stanhope, J. (2014). Fracture (hip): Acute management and immediate rehabilitation.
- Yusof, N. M., McNamara, K. & Khalil, H. (2013). Deprescribing interventions: Reducing falls among the elderly.

Recommended practice:

- Campbell, J. (2013a). Hip fracture management: Older people.
- Campbell, J. (2013b). Hip fracture recovery: Dietary supplementation.
- Campbell, J. (2013c). Observation following falls in acute care: Older people.
- Campbell, J. (2013d). Observation following falls in the community: Older people.
- Campbell, J. (2013e). Observation following falls in residential aged care: Older people.
- JBI. (2013). Fall prevention: Interventions.
- JBI. (2013). Restraint standards.
- JBI. (2013). Walking frames and sticks.
- McReynolds, T. (2013a). Falls prevention: Correction of visual deficiency.
- McReynolds, T. (2013b). Falls prevention: Exercise/physical therapy interventions.

Systematic reviews:

- Sze, T. W., Leng, C. Y. & Lin, S. K. S. (2012). The effectiveness of physical restraints in reducing falls among adults in acute care hospitals and nursing homes: A systematic review. *Joanna Briggs Institute Library of Systematic Reviews, 10*(5), 307–351.
- Oh, E. G., Lee, J. E. & Yoo, J. Y. (2012). A systematic review of the effectiveness of lifestyle interventions for improving bone health in women at high risk of osteoporosis. *Joanna Briggs Institute Library of Systematic Reviews, 10*(30), 1732–1784.

National Guideline Clearinghouse: www.guideline.gov

Search for: Falls or osteoporosis

- Prevention of falls.
- Prevention of falls and fall injuries in older adults (2011).
- Falls: Assessment and prevention of falls in older people (revised 2013).
- Fall prevention. In *Evidence-based geriatric nursing protocols for best practice.* (2013).
- Prevention of falls in community-dwelling older adults: U.S. Preventive Services Task Force recommendation statement. (2012).
- Osteoporosis.
- Osteoarthritis.

National Health and Medical Research Council (NHMRC), Clinical practice guidelines (Australia): www.clinicalguidelines.gov.au

- Australian and New Zealand Society for Geriatric Medicine. Position statement 22: Frailty in older people (2013).

Health education

Age Concern New Zealand Inc: www.ageconcern.org.nz
Aged Care in Victoria: www.health.vic.gov.au/agedcare/maintaining/falls_dev
Arthritis Australia: www.arthritisaustralia.com.au
Arthritis New Zealand: www.arthritis.org.nz
Australian and New Zealand Falls Prevention Society (ANZFPS): www.anzfallsprevention.org
Australian Commission on Safety and Quality in Health Care: www.safetyandquality.gov.au/search/falls
Australian Menopause Society: www.menopause.org.au/health-professionals
Fall Prevention Center of Excellence (U.S.): www.stopfalls.org
Health Direct Australia, seniors' health: www.healthdirect.gov.au/healthy-bones
Health*Insite*: www.healthinsite.gov.au/topics/Falls_Prevention
Independent Living Centre (ADL tools): www.ilc.com.au
myaged*care* (portal of the Australia Government Department of Social Services): www.myagedcare.gov.au/healthy-and-active-living/falls-prevention
NIH Senior Health (U.S.): http://nihseniorhealth.gov/falls/toc.html
North American Menopause Society: www.menopause.org
NSW Falls Prevention Network: http://fallsnetwork.neura.edu.au
NZ Menopause Institute: www.nzmenopause.co.nz
Osteoporosis Australia: www.osteoporosis.org.au
Osteoporosis New Zealand: www.bones.org.nz

REFERENCES

Aartolahti, E., Hakkinen, A., Lonnroos, E. et al. (2013). Relationship between functional vision and balance and mobility performance in community-dwelling older adults. *Aging Clinical and Experimental Research, 25*(5), 545–552.

Abreu, M. & Hartley, G. (2013). The effects of Salsa Dance on balance, gait, and fall risk in a sedentary patient with Alzheimer's dementia, multiple comorbidities, and recurrent falls. *Journal of Geriatric Physical Therapy, 36*(2), 100–107.

Accident Compensation Corporation (ACC). (2014). Preventing injuries at home: Older people. Accessed March 2015 at www.acc.co.nz/preventing-injuries/at-home/older-people/information-for-health-professionals/index.htm.

Agency for Healthcare Research and Quality, Effective Health Care Program. (2012). Clinician summary: Treatment to prevent osteoporotic fractures: An update. Accessed March 2015 at www.effectivehealthcare.ahrq.gov/ehc/index.cfm/search-for-guides-reviews-and-reports/?pageAction=displayProduct&productID=1048#5268.

Akesson, K., Marsh, D., Mitchell, P. J. et al. (2013). Capture the fracture: A best practice framework and global campaign to break the fragility fracture cycle. *Osteoporosis International, 24*, 2135–2152.

Ambrose, A. F., Paul, G. & Hausdorff, J. (2013). Risk factors for falls among older adults: A review of the literature. *Maturitas, 75*(1), 51–61.

American Geriatrics Society and British Geriatrics Society (2010). AGS/BGS clinical practice guideline: Prevention of falls in older persons. Available March 2015 at www.guideline.gov/content.aspx?id=37707.

Arthritis & Osteoporosis NSW. (2014). Latest statistics. Accessed March 2015 at http://arthritisnsw.org.au/arthritis/research/latest-statistics.

Australian Bureau of Statistics. (2011). *Arthritis and osteoporosis in Australia: A snapshot, 2007–08*. Cat. no. 4843.0.55.001. Canberra: Author.

Australian Commission on Safety and Quality in Health Care. (2009a). *Guidebook for preventing falls and harm from falls in older people: Australian hospitals*. Canberra: Commonwealth of Australia. Accessed www.safetyandquality.gov.au/our-work/falls-prevention.

Australian Commission on Safety and Quality in Health Care. (2009b). Preventing falls and harm from falls in older people: Best practice guidelines for Australian residential aged care facilities. Canberra: Commonwealth of Australia.

Australian Commission on Safety and Quality in Health Care. (2009c). Preventing falls and harm from falls in older people: Best practice guidelines for Australian community care 2009. Canberra: Commonwealth of Australia.

Australian Government Department of Social Services (DSS). (2012a). Decision-Making Tool: Supporting a restraint free environment in community aged care. Available March 2015 via www.dss.gov.au.

Australian Government Department of Social Services (DSS). (2012b). Decision-Making Tool: Supporting a restraint free environment in residential aged care. Available March 2015 via www.dss.gov.au.

Australian Institute of Health and Welfare (AIHW). (2013a). Who gets osteoarthritis? Accessed March 2015 at www.aihw.gov.au/osteoarthritis/who-gets-osteoarthritis.

Australian Institute of Health and Welfare (AIHW). (2013b). *Australia's welfare, 2013*. Australia's welfare series no.11. Cat. no. AUS 174. Canberra: Author.

Bennell, K. L., Hunt, M. A., Wrigley, T. V., Lim, B.-W. & Hinman, R. S. (2009). Muscle and exercise in the prevention and management of knee osteoarthritis: An internal medicine specialist's guide. *Medical Clinics of North America, 93*(1), 161–177.

Berry, S. D., Lee, Y., Cai, S. et al. (2013). Non-benzodiazepine sleep medications and hip fractures in nursing home residents. *Journal of the American Medical Association Internal Medicine, 173*(9), 754–761.

Berry, S. D., Zhu, Y., Choi, H. et al. (2013). Diuretic initiation and the acute risk of hip fracture. *Osteoporosis International, 24*(2), 689–695.

Bogoch, E. R., Elliot-Gibson, V., Wang, R. Y. et al. (2012). Secondary causes of osteoporosis in fracture patients. *Journal of Orthopaedic Trauma, 26*(9), e145–e152.

Cameron, I. D., Robinovitch, S., Birge, S., Kannus, P., Khan, K., Lauritzen, J., . . . Kiel, D. P. (2010). Hip protectors: Recommendations for conducting clinical trials: An international consensus statement (part II). *Osteoporosis International, 21*(1), 1–10.

Castle, N. G. & Engberg, J. (2009). The health consequences of using physical restraints in nursing homes. *Medical Care, 47*(11), 1164–1173.

Chen, T. Y., Peronto, C. L. & Edwards, J. D. (2012). Cognitive function as a prospective predictor of falls. *Journals of Gerontology: Psychological Sciences and Social Sciences, 67*(6), 720–728.

Choi, W. J., Hoffer, J. A. & Robinovitch, S. N. (2010a). The effect of positioning on the biomechanical performance of soft shell hip protectors. *Journal of Biomechanics, 43*(5), 818–825.

Choi, W. J., Hoffer, J. A. & Robinovitch, S. N. (2010b). Effect of hip protectors, falling angle and body mass index on pressure distribution over the hip during simulated falls. *Clinical Biomechanics, 25*(1), 63–69.

Connors, K. A., Galea, M. P. & Said, C. M. (2011). Feldenkrais method balance classes improve balance in older adults: A controlled trial. *Evidence-Based Complementary and Alternative Medicine*. Article ID 873672. Viewed March 2015 at http://dx.doi.org/10.1093/ecam/nep055.

Costa-Dias, M. J., Oliveira, A. S., Martins, T. et al. (2013). Medication fall risk in old hospitalized patients: A retrospective study. *Nurse Education Today, 34*(2), 171–176.

Crogan, N. L. & Dupler, A. E. (2014). Quality improvement in nursing homes. *Journal of Nursing Care Quality, 29*(1), 60–65.

Damian, J., Pastor-Barriuso, R., Valderrama-Gama, E. et al. (2013). Factors associated with falls among older adults living in institutions. *BMC Geriatrics*. doi:10.1186/1471-2318-13-6.

Davies, P. S. (2011). New developments in the treatment of osteoarthritis: A focus on women. *Pain Management Nursing, 12*( ), S17–S22.

Deandrea, S., Bravi, F., Turati, F. et al. (2013). Risk factors for falls in older people in nursing homes and hospitals: A systematic review and meta-analysis. *Archives of Gerontology and Geriatrics, 56*, 407–415.

Doumas, M., Rapp, M. A. & Krampe, R. T. (2009). Working memory and postural control: Adult age differences in potential for improvement, task priority and dual tasking. *Journal of Gerontology. Psychological Sciences, 64B*(2), 193–201.

Dow, B., Meyer, C., Moore, K. J. et al. (2013). The impact of care recipient falls on caregivers. *Australian Health Review, 37*(2), 152–157.

Filiatrault, J., Desrosiers, J. & Trottier, L. (2009). An exploratory study of individual and environmental correlates of fear of falling among community-dwelling seniors. *Journal of Aging & Health, 21*(6), 881–894.

Fonad, E., Emami, A., Wahlin, T. B., Winblad, B. & Sandmark, H. (2009). Falls in somatic and dementia wards at community care units. *Scandinavian Journal of Caring Sciences, 2*(10), 2–10.

Freeland, K. N., Thompson, A. N., Zhao, Y. et al. (2012). Medication use and associated risk of falling in geriatric outpatient population. *Annals of Pharmacotherapeutics, 46*(9), 1188–1192.

Frost, S. A., Nguyen, N. D., Center, J. R. et al. (2013). Excess mortality attributable to hip-fracture: A relative survival analysis. *Bone, 56*(1), 23–29.

Gentleman, B. & Malozemoff, W. (2001). Falls and feelings: Description of a psychosocial group nursing intervention. *Journal of Gerontological Nursing, 27*(10), 35–39.

Gill, T. M., Murphy, T. E., Gahbauer, E. A. et al. (2013). Association of injurious falls with disability outcomes and nursing home admission in community-living older persons. *American Journal of Epidemiology, 178*(3), 418–425.

Gillespie, L. D., Robertson, M. C., Gillespie, W. J. et al. (2012). Interventions for preventing falls in older people living in the community. *Cochrane Database of Systematic Reviews, 9*. Article no. CD007614. doi:10.1002/14651858.CD007146.pub3.

Granacher, U., Muehlbauer, T., Bridenbaugh, S. A. et al. (2012). Effects of salsa dance training on balance and strength performance in older adults. *Gerontology, 58*(4), 305–312.

Gray-Miceli, D. & Quigley, P. A. (2012). Fall prevention: Assessment, diagnoses, and intervention strategies. In M. Boltz, E. Capezuti, T. Fulmer & D. Zwicker (Eds.), *Evidence-based practice protocols for best practice* (4th ed., pp. 268–297). New York: Springer.

Groen, B. E., Smulders, E., deKam, D., Duysens, J. & Weerdesteyn, V. (2010). Martial arts fall training to prevent hip fractures in the elderly. *Osteoporosis International, 21*(2), 215–221.

Hackney, M. E., Hall, C. D., Echt, K. V. et al. (2013) Dancing for balance: Feasibility and efficacy in oldest-old adults with visual impairment. *Nursing Research, 62*(2), 138–143.

Hanlon, J. T., Boudreau, R. M., Roumani, Y. F., Newman, A. B., Ruby, C. M., Wright, R. M., . . . for the Health ABC study (2009). Number and dosage of central nervous system medications on recurrent falls in community elders: The health, aging and body composition study. *Journal of Gerontology Series A: Biological Sciences and Medical Sciences, 64A*(4), 492–498.

Hendrich, A. (2013). Fall risk assessment for older adults: The Hendrich II Fall Risk Model. *Try This* series, issue 8. The Hartford Institute for Geriatric Nursing, New York University, College of Nursing. Accessed March 2015 at http://consultgerirn.org/uploads/File/trythis/try_this_8.pdf.

Herrera, A., Lobo-Escolar, A., Mateo, J. et al. (2012). Male osteoporosis: A review. *World Journal of Orthopedics, 3*(12), 223–234.

Horan, A. & Timmins, F. (2009). The role of community multidisciplinary teams in osteoporosis treatment and prevention. *Journal of Orthopaedic Nursing, 13*, 85–96.

Hooper, G. (2013). Editorial: The ageing population and the increasing demand for joint replacement. *New Zealand Medical Journal, 126*(1377), 1–2.

Houston, D. K., Neiberg, R. H., Tooze, J. A. et al. (2013). Low 25-hydroxyvitamin D predicts onset of mobility limitation and disability in community-dwelling older adults: The Health ABC Study. *Journals of Gerontology: Biological Sciences and Medical Sciences, 68*(2), 181–187.

Huang, T. T., Yang, L. H. & Liu, C. Y. (2011). Reducing the fear of falling among community-dwelling elderly adults through cognitive-behavioural strategies and intense tai chi exercise: A randomized controlled trial. *Journal of Advances in Nursing, 67*(5), 961–971.

Huang, W.-N., Chi, W.-C. & Hu, L.-J. (2013). Associations between fear of falling and functional balance in older adults. *International Journal of Therapy and Rehabilitation*, *20*(2), 101–106.

International Osteoporosis Foundation. (2012). *Capture the fracture: Report 2012.* Viewed March 2015 via www.iofbonehealth.org/capture-fracture-report-2012.

Joanna Briggs Institute (JBI). (2002a). Best practice: Physical restraint, part 1: Use in acute and residential care facilities. *Best Practice: Evidence-Based Practice Information Sheets for Health Professionals, 6*(3), 1–5.

Joanna Briggs Institute (JBI). (2002b). Best practice: Physical restraint, part 2: Minimisation in acute and residential care facilities. *Best Practice: Evidence-Based Practice Information Sheets for Health Professionals, 6*(4), 1–5.

Kearney, F. C., Harwood, R. H., Gladman, J. R. et al. (2013). The relationship between executive function and falls and gait abnormalities in older adults: A systematic review. *Dementia and Geriatric Cognitive Disorders, 36*(1–2), 20–35.

Kempen, G. I. J. M., van Haastreg, J. C. M., McKee, K. J., Delbaere, K. & Zijlstra, G. A. R. (2009). Socio-demographic, health-related and psychosocial correlates of fear of falling and avoidance of activity in community-living older persons who avoid activity due to fear of falling. *BioMed Central Public Health, 9*(170).

Kerse, N. (2014). Falls in advanced age: Findings from LiLACS NZ. Auckland: School of Population Health, The University of Auckland. Available March 2015 via www.fmhs.auckland.ac.nz/en/faculty/lilacs/research/publications.html.

Kim, S. & So, W. Y. (2013). Prevalence and correlates of fear of falling in Korean community-dwelling elderly subjects. *Experimental Gerontology, 48*(11), 1323–1328.

Ko, A., Van Nguyen, H., Chan, L. et al. (2012). Developing a self-reported tool on fall risk based on toileting responses on in-hospital falls. *Geriatric Nursing, 33*(1), 9–16.

Koike, T., Orito, Y., Toyoda, H., Tada, M., Sugama, R., Hosino, M., . . . Takaoka, K. (2009). External hip protectors are effective for the elderly with higher-than-average risk factors for hip fractures. *Osteoporosis International, 20*(9), 1613–1620.

Lach, H. W. & Parsons, J. L. (2013). Impact of fear of falling in long-term care: An integrative review. *Journal of the American Medical Directors Association, 14*(8), 573–577.

Lamis, R. L., Kramer, J. S., Hale, L. S. et al. (2012). Fall risk associated with inpatient medications. *American Journal of Health Systems Pharmacy, 69*(1), 1888–1894.

Lauche, R., Langhorst, J., Dobos, G. et al. (2013). A systematic review and meta-analysis of tai chi for osteoarthritis of the knee. *Complementary Therapies in Medicine, 21*(4), 396–406.

Levis, S. & Theodore, G. (2012). Summary of AHRQ's comparative effectiveness review of treatment to prevent fractures in men and women with low bone density or osteoporosis. Update of 2007 report. *Journal of Managed Care Pharmacy, 18*(Suppl. B), S1–S15.

Manor, B., Lipsitz, L. A., Wayne, P. M. et al. (2013). Complexity-based measures inform tai chi's impact on standing postural control in older adults with peripheral neuropathy. *BMC Complementary and Alternative Medicine, 13*, 87.

Martin, K. L., Blizzard, V. K., Srikanth, V. K. et al. (2013). Cognitive function modifies the effects of physiological function on the risk of multiple falls: A population-based study. *Journals of Gerontology: Biological Sciences and Medical Sciences, 68*(9), 1091–1097.

McAuley, E., Wojcicki, T. R., Gothe, N. P. et al. (2013). Effects of a DVD-delivered exercise intervention on physical function in older adults. *Journals of Gerontology: Biological Sciences and Medical Sciences, 68*(9), 1076–1082.

McClung, M. R. (2012). Revisiting the prevention of bone loss at menopause. *Menopause: Journal of the North American Menopause Society, 19*(11), 1173–1175.

Mithal, A., Bonjour, J. P., Boonen, S. et al. (2013). Impact of nutrition on muscle mass, strength, and performance in older adults. *Osteoporosis International, 24*(5), 1555–1566.

Moller, U. O., Midlov, P., Kristensson, J. et al. (2013). Prevalence and predictors of falls and dizziness in people younger and older than 80 years of age—A longitudinal cohort study. *Archives of Gerontology and Geriatrics, 56*, 160–168.

Mosele, M., Coin, A., Manzato, E. et al. (2013). Association between serum 25-hydroxyvitamin D levels, bone geometry, and bone mineral density in healthy older adults. *Journals of Gerontology: Biological Sciences and Medical Sciences, 68*(8), 992–998.

Moskowitz, R. W., Altman, R. D., Buckwalter, J. A., Goldberg, V. M. & Hochberg, M. C. (2006). *Osteoarthritis: Diagnosis and medical/surgical management*. Philadelphia PA: Lippincott, Williams & Wilkins.

Moskowitz, R. W. (2013). The 2012 ACR guidelines for osteoarthritis: Not a cookbook. *Cleveland Clinic Journal of Medicine, 80*(1), 26–32.

Murphy, K. & Lowe, S. (2013). Improving fall risk assessment in home care: Interdisciplinary use of the Timed Up and Go (TUG). *Home Healthcare Nurse, 31*(7), 389–396.

Narula, R., Tauseef, M., Ahmad, I. A. et al. (2013). Vitamin D deficiency among postmenopausal women with osteoporosis. *Journal of Clinical and Diagnostic Research, 7*(2), 336–338.

National Clinical Guideline Centre. (2012). Osteoporosis: Assessing the risk of fragility fractures. Guideline summary. Accessed March 2015 at www.guideline.gov/content.aspx?id=38410&search=osteoporosis.

National Osteoporosis Foundation. (2013). Debunking the myths. Accessed March 2015 at www.nof.org/articles/4.

New South Wales Department of Health. (2011). Prevention of falls and harm from falls among older people 2011–2015. Policy directive. Viewed March 2015 at www.health.nsw.gov.au/policies/pd/2011/pdf/PD2011_029.pdf.

New Zealand Ministry of Health (NZMOH). (2008). The 2006/07 New Zealand Health Survey. Accessed March 2015 via www.health.govt.nz.

New Zealand Ministry of Health. (2011). *Tatau Kura Tangata: Health of older Māori chart book 2011*. Wellington: Author.

New Zealand Ministry of Health. (2013). Guidelines on physical activity for older people (aged 65 years and over). Wellington: Author. Accessed March 2015 at www.health.govt.nz/your-health/healthy-living/food-and-physical-activity/physical-activity/physical-activity-older-people-aged-65-years-and-older.

Obayashi, K., Araki, T., Nakamura, K. et al. (2013). Risk of falling and hypnotic drugs: Retrospective study of inpatients. *Drugs in R&D, 13*, 159–164.

Olazaran, J., Valle, D., Serra, J. A. et al. (2013). Psychotropic medications and falls in nursing homes: A cross-sectional study. *Journal of the American Medical Directors Association, 14*, 213–217.

Pellfolk, T. J., Gustafson, Y., Bucht, G. & Karlsson, S. (2010). Effects of a restraint minimization program on staff knowledge, attitudes and practice: A cluster randomized trial. *Journal of American Geriatric Society, 58*(1), 62–69.

Quach, L., Yang, F. M., Berry, S. D. et al. (2013). Depression, antidepressants, and falls among community-dwelling elderly people: The MOBILIZE Study. *Journals of Gerontology: Biological Sciences and Medical Sciences, 68*(12), 1575–1581.

Recker, R. R., Lewiecki, E. M., Miller, P. D. & Reiffel, J. (2009). Safety of bisphosphonates in the treatment of osteoporosis. *American Journal of Medicine, 122*, S22–S32.

Reed-Jones, R. J., Solis, G. R., Lawson, K. A. et al. (2013). Vision and falls: A multidisciplinary review of the contributions of visual impairment to falls among older adults. *Maturitas, 75*(1), 22–28.

Reidy, P. T., Walker, D. K., Dickinson, J. M. et al. (2013). Protein blend ingestion following resistance exercise promotes human muscle protein synthesis. *Journal of Nutrition, 143*(4), 410–416.

Rigler, S. K., Shireman, T. I., Cook-Wiens, G. J. et al. (2013). Fracture risk in nursing home residents initiating antipsychotic medications. *Journal of the American Geriatrics Society, 61*(5), 715–722.

Royal Australian College of General Practitioners. (2009). Guidelines for the non-surgical management of hip and knee osteoarthritis. East Melbourne: Royal Australian College of General Practitioners.

Sanders, K. M., Nowson, C. A., Kotowicz, M. A. et al. (2009). Calcium and bone health: Position statement for the Australian and New Zealand Bone and Mineral Society, Osteoporosis Australia and the Endocrine Society of Australia. *Medical Journal of Australia, 190*(6), 316–320.

Santesso, N., Carrasco-Labra, A. & Brignardello-Petersen, R. (2014). Hip protectors for preventing hip fractures in older people. *Cochrane Database of Systematic Reviews, 3*. Art. no. CD001255. doi:10.1002/14651858.CD001255.pub5.

Sheldon, J. H. (1960). On the natural history of falls in old age. *British Medical Journal, 2*, 1685–1690.

Shelton, L. R. (2013). A closer look at osteoarthritis. *Nurse Practitioner, 38*(7), 30–36.

Soliman, A. & Brogan, V. (2014). Foot assessment and care for older people. *Nursing Times, 110*(50), 12–15.

Svejme, O., Ahlborg, H. G., Nilsson, J.-A. et al. (2013). Low BMD is an independent predictor of fracture and early menopause of mortality in post-menopausal women: A 34-year prospective study. *Maturitas, 74*, 341–345.

Tajeu, G. S., Delzell, E., Smith, W. et al. (2013). Death, debility, and destitution following hip fracture. *Journals of Gerontology: Biological Sciences and Medical Sciences, 69*(3), 346–353.

Tiedemann, A., O'Rourke, S., Sesto, R. et al. (2013). A 12-week Iyengar Yoga program improved balance and mobility in older community-dwelling people: A pilot randomized controlled trial. *Journals of Gerontology: Biological Sciences and Medical Sciences, 68*(9), 1068–1075.

Tousignant, M., Corriveau, H., Roy, P. M. et al. (2013). Efficacy of supervised tai chi exercises versus conventional physical therapy exercises in fall prevention for frail older adults: A randomized controlled trial. *Disability and Rehabilitation, 35*(17), 1429–1435.

Tsang, W. W. (2013). Tai chi is effective in reducing balance impairments and falls in patients with Parkinson's disease. *Journal of Physiotherapy, 59*(1), 55.

U.S. Preventive Services Task Force. (2012). Prevention of falls in community-dwelling older adults: U.S. Preventive Services Task Force recommendation statement. *Annals of Internal Medicine, 157*(3), 197–204.

Van Strein, A. M., Koek, H. L., Van Marum, R. J. et al. (2013). Psychotropic medications, including short acting benzodiazepines, strongly increase the frequency of falls in elderly. *Maturitas, 74*(4), 357–362.

Victorian State Government Department of Health (2011). FRAT: Falls Risk Assessment Tool. Accessed March 2015 at www.health.vic.gov.au/agedcare/maintaining/falls_dev/Section_b2b_1.htm.

Watts, N. B., Adler, R. A., Bilezikian, J. P. et al. (2012). Osteoporosis in men: An Endocrine Society clinical practice guideline. *Journal of Endocrinology and Metabolism, 97*(6), 1802–1822.

Watts, J. J., Abimanyi-Ochom, J. & Sanders, K. M. (2013). Osteoporosis costing all Australians: A new burden of disease analysis 2012 to 2022. Accessed March 2015 at www.osteoporosis.org.au/statistics-burden-disease.

Wei, G.-X., Xu, T., Fan, F.-M. et al. (2013). Can tai chi reshape the brain? A brain morphometry study. *PLoS One, 8*(4), e61038.

Whitney, J., Close, J. C., Lord, S. R. et al. (2012). Identification of high risk fallers among older people living in residential care facilities: A simple screen based on easily collectable measures. *Archives of Gerontology and Geriatrics, 55*(3), 690–695.

Williams, S. B., Brand, C. A., Hill, K. D., Hunt, S. B. & Moran, H. (2010). Feasibility and outcomes of a home-based exercise program on improving balance and gait stability in women with lower-limb osteoarthritis or rheumatoid arthritis: A pilot study. *Archives of Physical Medicine and Rehabilitation, 91*(1), 106–114.

Yan, J. H., Gu, W. J., Sun, J. et al. (2013). Efficacy of tai chi on pain, stiffness and function in patients with osteoarthritis: A meta-analysis. *PLoS One, 8*(4), e61672. Available at www.plosone.org.

Yurgin, N., Wade, S., Satram-Hoang, S. et al. (2013). Research article: Prevalence of fracture risk factors in postmenopausal women enrolled in the POSSIBLE US Treatment cohort. *International Journal of Endocrinology*. Article ID 715025. Available March 2015 at http://dx.doi.org/10.1155/2013/715025.

Zapatero, A., Barba, R., Canora, J. et al. (2013). Hip fracture in hospitalized medical patients. *BMC Musculoskeletal Disorders*. Available March 2015 at www.biomedcentral.com/1471-2474/14/15.0.

Chapter 23

Integument

By Carol Miller and Sharyn Hunter

LEARNING OBJECTIVES

After reading this chapter, you should be able to:

1. Delineate age-related changes that affect the skin, hair, nails and glands.
2. Describe risk factors that can affect skin wellness for older adults.
3. Discuss the functional consequences of age-related changes and risk factors that affect the skin, hair, nails and glands.
4. Assess skin in older adults and recognise normal and pathological skin changes.
5. Describe the assessment, prevention and management of skin tears.
6. Describe the assessment, prevention and management of pressure ulcers.
7. Describe the assessment, prevention and management of chronic wounds.
8. Implement nursing interventions to address the following aspects of skincare: maintenance of healthy skin, prevention of xerosis and referrals for the treatment of pathological skin lesions.

KEY POINTS

basal cell carcinoma	pressure ulcer
bacterial burden	skin tears
chronic wounds	squamous cell carcinoma
melanoma	staging system
photoageing	xerosis
photosensitivity	

For many people, and particularly for older adults, skin is the most visible indicator of the combined effects of biological ageing, lifestyle and environment. Thus, the skin, hair and nails have not only physiological functions but also many social functions. Physiologically, the skin directly affects all of the following processes:

- Thermoregulation
- Excretion of metabolic wastes
- Protection of underlying structures
- Synthesis of vitamin D
- Maintenance of fluid and electrolyte balance
- Sensation of pain, touch, pressure, temperature and vibration.

The social functions of the skin include facilitating communication and serving as an indicator of race, gender, work status and other personal characteristics.

Hair serves to protect underlying organs, primarily the skin, from injury and adverse temperatures. In addition, in social contexts, the length and style of one's hair can reflect certain characteristics such as age, gender and personality. Although hair is one of the most visible manifestations of ageing, hair colour can easily be altered if grey is viewed as an undesirable indicator of age. Like the skin and hair, nails have both a physiological and social capacity. Physiologically, nails protect the underlying tissue from injury. In social contexts, nails can reflect personal characteristics such as grooming and occupational activities.

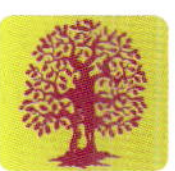

AGE-RELATED CHANGES THAT AFFECT THE SKIN

The skin is the largest, as well as the most visible, body organ. Structurally, the skin comprises three layers: the epidermis, the dermis and the subcutaneous tissue. Hair, nails and sweat glands are also parts of the integumentary system. As with many other aspects of functionality, it is difficult to distinguish between changes that are strictly attributable to ageing and those that occur because of risk factors. Genetics, lifestyle and environmental factors exert a significant effect on skin throughout the life span and have a cumulative effect in older adults.

Epidermis

The epidermis is the relatively impermeable outer layer of skin that serves as a barrier, preventing both the loss of body fluids and the entry of substances from the environment. The density of the epidermis varies, depending on the part of the body it covers. The epidermis comprises layers of cells that undergo a continual cycle of regeneration, cornification and shedding. Epidermal cells develop in the innermost layer of the epidermis and continually migrate to the surface of the skin where they are shed. With increasing age, these cells become larger and more variable in shape and the rate of epidermal turnover gradually decreases.

Melanocytes are epidermal cells that give the skin its colour and provide a protective barrier against ultraviolet radiation. Beginning around the age of 25 years, the

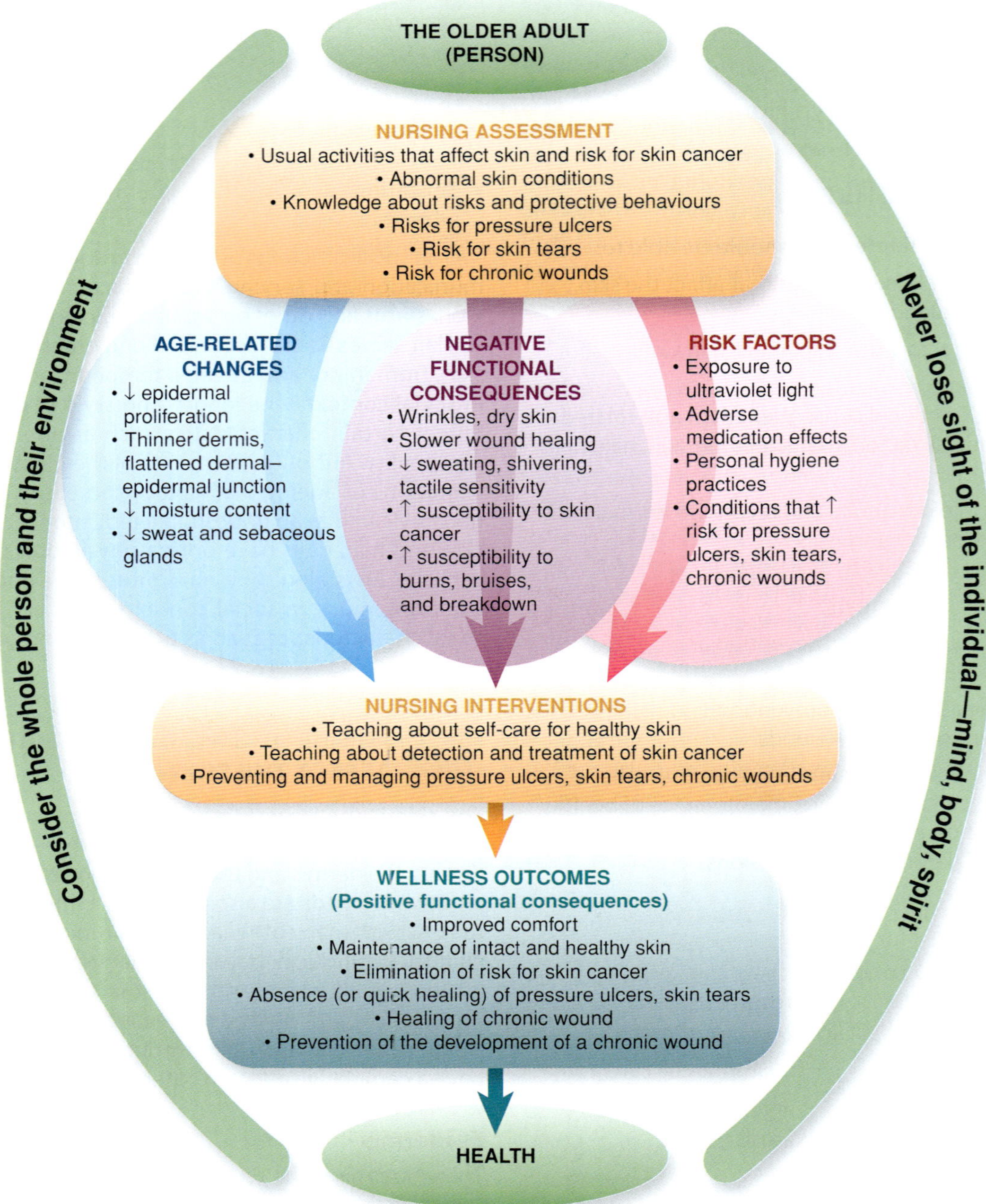

number of active melanocytes decreases by 10% to 20% each decade. Although this decline occurs in both sun-exposed and unprotected skin, the density of melanocytes in exposed skin is double or triples that in unexposed skin. With increased age, the number of Langerhans cells, which serve as macrophages, also decreases in both sun-exposed and sun-protected skin; the decrease ranges from 50% to 70% in sun-exposed skin. Another age-related change is a decrease in the moisture content of the outer epidermal layer.

Papillae give the skin its texture and connect the epidermis to the underlying dermis at the dermal–epidermal junction. With increased age, the papillae retract, causing a flattening of the dermal–epidermal junction and diminishing the surface area between the epidermis and dermis. This age-related change slows the transfer of nutrients between the dermis and epidermis. In contrast to other epidermal changes that are more prominent on exposed skin surfaces, this change occurs to some degree on all skin surfaces.

Dermis

The primary functions of the dermis are:

- Provision of support for structures within and below this layer
- Nourishment of the epidermis which has no blood supply of its own
- Colouration
- Sensory perception
- Temperature regulation.

Collagen, which constitutes 80% of the dermis, confers elasticity and tensile strength, which help to prevent tearing and overstretching of the skin. Elastin, which constitutes 5% of the dermis, maintains skin tension and allows for stretching in response to movement. The dermal ground substance, which has a water-binding capacity, determines skin turgor and elastic properties. Blood vessels in the deep plexus play a role in thermoregulation, and those in the superficial plexus supply nutrients to the epidermal layer. Cutaneous nerves in the dermis receive information from the environment regarding pain, pressure, temperature, and deep and light touch.

Beginning in early adulthood, dermal thickness gradually diminishes, with collagen thinning at a rate of 1% per year. Elastin increases in quantity and decreases in quality because of age-related and environmentally induced changes. The dermal vascular bed decreases by approximately one-third with increased age; this contributes to the atrophy and fibrosis of hair bulbs, sweat and sebaceous glands. Additional age-related changes in the dermis include a decrease in the number of fibroblasts and mast cells.

Subcutaneous tissue and cutaneous nerves

The subcutis is the inner layer of fat tissue that protects the underlying tissues from trauma. Additional functions include the storage of kilojoules, insulation of the body and regulation of heat loss. With increased age, some areas of subcutaneous tissue atrophy, particularly in the plantar foot surface and in sun-exposed areas of the hands, face and lower legs. Other areas of subcutaneous tissue hypertrophy, however, with the overall effect being a gradual increase in the proportion of body fat between the third and eighth decades. This increased body fat is more pronounced in women than in men and is most noticeable in the waists of men and the thighs of women. Age-related changes also affect the cutaneous nerves responsible for sensations of pressure, vibration and light touch.

Sweat and sebaceous glands

Eccrine and apocrine sweat glands originate in the dermal layer and are most abundant in the palms of the hands, soles of the feet and axillae. Eccrine glands, which are important for thermoregulation, open directly onto the skin surface and are most abundant on the palms, soles and forehead. Apocrine glands are larger than eccrine glands and open into hair follicles, primarily in the axillae and genital area. The sole function of these glands is to produce secretions, which create a distinctive body odour when they decompose. Both eccrine and apocrine glands decrease in number and functional ability with increased age.

Sebaceous glands are present in the dermal skin layer over every part of the body except the palms of the hands and the soles of the feet. These glands continually secrete sebum—a substance that combines with sweat to form an emulsion. Functionally, sebum prevents the loss of water and serves as a mild retardant of bacterial and fungal growth. The secretion of sebum begins to diminish during the third decade, with women having a greater decline than men. In younger adults, sebum production is closely related to the size of the sebaceous glands; however, in older adults, the sebaceous glands increase in size but produce less sebum.

Nails

The rate of nail growth is influenced by many factors including age, climate, state of health, circulation to and around the nails and activity of the fingers and toes. Nail growth begins to slow in early adulthood, with a gradual decrease of 30% to 50% over the individual's life span. Other age-related changes affecting the nails include the development of longitudinal striations and a decrease in lunula size and nail plate thickness. Because of these changes, the nails become increasingly soft, fragile and brittle and are more prone to splitting. In appearance, the older nail is dull, opaque, longitudinally striated and yellow or grey.

Hair

Hair colour and distribution change to some degree in all older adults, with the most noticeable changes being baldness and grey hair. By the age of 50 years, approximately 50% of people have greying hair and approximately 60% of white men have a noticeable degree of baldness. Hair that is greying results from a decline in melanin production and the gradual replacement of pigmented hairs by non-pigmented ones. Age-related changes also affect hair distribution, with patches of coarse terminal hair developing over the upper lip and lower face in older women and in the ears, nares and eyebrows of older men. Another age-related change is a progressive loss of body hair, initially in the trunk, then in the pubic area and axillae. In addition, some men are genetically predisposed to baldness, which is attributable to a change in production from coarse terminal hair to fine vellus hair.

DIVERSITY NOTE

Caucasians have earlier onset and greater skin wrinkling than other groups, whereas Asians experience more problems related to skin pigmentation (Vierkotter & Kurtmann, 2012).

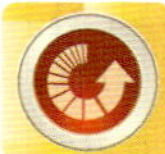

RISK FACTORS THAT AFFECT SKIN WELLNESS

The risk factors that influence the skin and hair of older adults include heredity, lifestyle and environmental factors and adverse medication effects. Lifestyle and environmental factors have a cumulative effect that manifests more fully during later adulthood, but it is important to identify the risk factors that nurses can address through health education. Risk factors associated with skin tears, pressure ulcers, chronic wounds and skin cancer are addressed in the section on pathological conditions affecting the skin.

Genetic influences

Heredity plays an important role in the development of skin and hair changes. People with fair skin, light hair and light eyes are more sensitive to the effects of ultraviolet radiation than people with dark skin, as evidenced by the fact that skin cancers are common in light-skinned people of northern European ancestry but rare in Africans.

Health behaviour and environmental influences

Smoking, sun exposure, emotional stress, and substance or alcohol abuse are the health behaviours and environmental factors that significantly affect skin wellness. Exposure to ultraviolet radiation is the most significant environmental factor, but adverse climate conditions can also cause negative functional consequences. For example, because the water content of the stratum corneum is influenced by relative humidity, **xerosis** (dry skin) is exacerbated when the relative humidity is below 30%.

Cigarette smoking is another factor that has been associated with detrimental skin changes, as well as with faster rates of developing baldness and grey hair (Gatherwright, Liu, Amirlak et al., 2013; Gatherwright, Liu, Gliniak et al., 2012). Effects of smoking on the skin include all of the following:

- More wrinkles
- Greyish discolouration
- Diminished ability to protect against ultraviolet radiation damage
- Increased risk of skin cancer.

WELLNESS OPPORTUNITY

From a holistic perspective, nurses need to non-judgementally consider the influence of cultural and societal attitudes on personal care practices and address any factors that negatively affect self-esteem.

Sociocultural influences

Cultural factors, societal attitudes and advertising trends influence hygiene and skin care practices. People in industrialised societies place a high value on frequent bathing and the use of commercial products for hygienic and cosmetic purposes. Although most of the personal practices associated with these values are desirable or harmless in younger adults, they may adversely affect older adults. For example, frequent bathing with deodorant soaps may cause or exacerbate dry skin problems in an older person.

Medication effects

Common adverse medication effects involving the skin include pruritus, dermatoses and photosensitivity reactions. Less common adverse medication effects on the skin and hair include alopecia and pigmentation changes of the skin or hair. Cytotoxic agents are the type of drug most commonly associated with hair loss, but other drugs that can cause alopecia include anticoagulants, non-steroidal anti-inflammatory agents, and cardiovascular medications.

Dermatoses, or rashes, are the most frequently cited adverse medication effect, and they can be caused by virtually any medication. Medication-related skin eruptions vary widely in their manifestations, including their onset. Drug rashes can occur from 1 day to 4 weeks after initiating or discontinuing the causative medication; the most common type of drug-related skin reaction is maculopapular eruptions. Antibiotics are the type of medication most often associated with skin eruptions; however, any medication can cause skin reactions. Medications that commonly cause dermatitis include antibiotics, non-steroidal anti-inflammatory drugs, anticonvulsants and antihypertensive agents (Turk, Gunaydin, Ertam et al., 2013).

Photosensitivity is an adverse medication effect that causes an intensified response to ultraviolet radiation. The inflammatory reaction is initially distributed over sun-exposed areas, but it may spread to non-exposed areas and persist even after the medication is discontinued. Photosensitivity may begin during a seasonal exposure to bright sunlight or during a vacation in an unusually hot climate. Amiodarone, frusemide, naproxen, phenothiazines, sulfonamides, tetracyclines and thiazides are examples of medications that can cause photosensitivity reactions. St John's wort and other herbal preparations may also increase the risk of photosensitivity.

In addition to causing adverse effects, medications can indirectly cause skin problems by exacerbating age-related changes. For example, fluid loss from diuretics can exacerbate xerosis and cause further discomfort or skin problems for the older adult. Another example of the combined effects of ageing and medications is that older adults taking anticoagulants are likely to bruise easily, and bruising may become extensive.

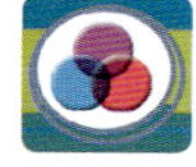

FUNCTIONAL CONSEQUENCES AFFECTING SKIN WELLNESS

Age-related changes and risk factors negatively affect many functions of the skin, including thermoregulation, tactile sensitivity and response to injury. Age-related changes do not interfere with the protective function of the nails; however the nails in older persons are brittle and more likely to split.

Psychosocial consequences may result when changes in the appearance of the skin and hair are associated with negative attitudes about visible indicators of ageing.

Delayed wound healing and increased susceptibility to skin problems

The regeneration of healthy skin takes twice as long for an 80-year-old as for a 30-year-old person. In perfectly intact skin, this slowed regeneration has no noticeable effects. When skin integrity is compromised, however, this age-related change contributes to delayed wound healing, even for superficial wounds. The consequences of age-related changes that affect the healing of deep wounds include an increased risk for postoperative wound disruption, decreased tensile strength of healing wounds, and increased risk of secondary infections.

Age-related changes in all layers of the skin combine with the effects of long-term exposure to the sun and other risk factors to increase the susceptibility of older adults to many types of problems (e.g. skin tears, pressure ulcers, stasis dermatitis), as delineated in Table 23-1 and described in the section on pathological conditions affecting skin. In addition, the age-related diminished immune function increases older adults' susceptibility to skin cancers, cutaneous fungal infections, and herpes zoster (commonly called *shingles*) (Chang, Wong, Endo et al., 2013).

DIVERSITY NOTE

Risk factors for skin tears include female sex and white race (LeBlanc & Baranoski, 2009).

Photoageing

Photoageing is the term used to describe skin changes that occur because of exposure to ultraviolet radiation, even at levels that do not cause any detectable sunburn. These changes are sometimes viewed as premature ageing; however, they are biologically distinct processes that occur independently and are superimposed on normal ageing changes. One reason for the misconception that photoageing is an age-related change is that the cumulative effects of ultraviolet radiation may not be evident until later adulthood. Common characteristics of photoageing are as follows:

- Coarse, leathery and ruddy or yellowed appearance
- Deep wrinkles, particularly on the face and neck
- Pathological lesions and seborrhoeic and actinic keratoses
- Thickened epidermis
- Enlarged sebaceous glands
- Marked loss of elasticity
- Dilated and tortuous blood vessels
- Numerous freckles.

Smoking is another condition that contributes to the development of photoageing (Durai, Thappa, Kumari et al., 2012). Recent studies are focusing on factors that counteract the effects of sun exposure and reduce the risk for photoageing. For example, a survey of dietary intake of 2920 adults in France found that healthy dietary habits and higher consumption of olive oil were associated with reduced evidence of facial photoageing (Latreille et al., 2012).

Comfort and sensation

Dry skin is one of the most universal complaints of older adults; indeed, it has been observed in up to 85% of non-institutionalised older people. Age-related changes, such as diminished output of sebum and eccrine sweat,

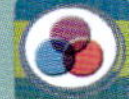

TABLE 23-1 Age-related changes and the respective functional consequences affecting skin and appendages

Age-related change	Consequence
Decreased rate of epidermal proliferation	Delayed wound healing; increased susceptibility to infection
Flattened dermal–epidermal junction; thinning of dermis and collagen; increased quantity, but decreased quality, of elastin	Decreased resiliency; increased susceptibility to injury, bruising, mechanical stress, ultraviolet radiation and blister formation
Reductions in dermal blood supply and the number of melanocytes and Langerhans cells	Decreased intensity of tanning; irregular pigmentation; increased susceptibility to skin cancer; diminished dermal clearance, absorption and immunological response
Reductions in eccrine sweat, subcutaneous fat, and dermal blood supply	Decreased sweating and shivering; increased susceptibility to hypothermia or hyperthermia
Decreased moisture content	Dry skin; discomfort
Decreased number of Meissner's and Pacinian corpuscles	Diminished tactile sensitivity; increased susceptibility to burns
Slowed nail growth	Increased susceptibility to cracking and injury; delayed healing
Changes in hair colour, quantity and distribution	Negative impact on self-esteem in proportion to negative attitudes

contribute to a decrease in the moisture content of the skin. Risk factors that may contribute to dry skin include stress, smoking, sun exposure, dry environments, excessive perspiration, adverse medication reactions, excessive use of soap and certain medical conditions (e.g. hypothyroidism).

Tactile sensitivity begins to decline around the age of 20 years, eventually causing older adults to have a diminished and less intense response to cutaneous sensations. This decline is attributable, at least in part, to age-related changes in Pacinian and Meissner's corpuscles, which are the skin receptors that respond to vibration. Other contributing factors include lower body temperature and functional alterations in the central nervous system. Functionally, older adults are more susceptible to scald burns because of their diminished ability to feel dangerously hot water temperatures.

Thermoregulation is also affected by age-related reductions in eccrine sweat, subcutaneous fat and dermal blood supply. These age-related changes interfere with sweating, shivering, peripheral vasoconstriction and vasodilation and insulation against adverse environmental temperatures. Thus, older adults are more at risk for the development of hypothermia and heat-related illnesses, as discussed in Chapter 25.

Cosmetic effects

The overall cosmetic effect of age-related skin changes is that the skin looks paler, thinner, more translucent and is irregularly pigmented. Additional indicators of age-related skin changes include sagging, wrinkling and various growths and lesions. Skin colouration changes are attributable to decreased melanocytes and dermal circulation. Wrinkling and sagging of the skin are caused by age-related changes in the epidermis and dermis, particularly those changes that affect the collagen fibres. Decreased subcutaneous tissue contributes to the sagging of the skin, particularly over the upper arms, by allowing gravity to pull the skin downwards.

Although these changes in appearance are gradual and do not interfere significantly with physiological function, the psychosocial consequences of these changes can be significant because of the social value placed on personal appearance and negative attitudes that may be held about growing old. Regardless of age, one's physical appearance has been shown to be an important determinant of self-perception and modern societies associate attractiveness with young-looking skin.

WELLNESS OPPORTUNITY

Nurses can promote positive attitudes about ageing by challenging societal perspectives that associate beauty only with youth.

Because of the high visibility of the face and neck, any signs of increased age that are prominent around the eyes and mouth may be particularly bothersome to the person who wants to avoid visible indications of age. Characteristic signs of advanced age that are evident around the eyes include increased pigmentation, crow's-feet wrinkles and fat and fluid accumulation in the upper lid and under the eye. Also, because of diminished skin elasticity and the loss and shifting of subcutaneous fat, the neck skin sags and a double chin may develop.

Table 23-1 summarises the functional consequences resulting from age-related changes of the skin, hair, nails and glands.

PATHOLOGICAL CONDITIONS AFFECTING SKIN: SKIN CANCER, SKIN TEARS, PRESSURE ULCERS AND CHRONIC WOUNDS

Skin cancer

Skin cancer, defined as an abnormal growth of skin cells, is the most common—as well as the most preventable—type of cancer. Older adults are highly vulnerable to the two most common types of skin cancer, primarily because of the cumulative effects of sun exposure. **Basal cell carcinoma**, which is the most common type, occurs most often on the head and neck (Figure 23-1A). If diagnosed and treated during its early stage, the cure rate for basal cell carcinoma is close to 100%; however, if left untreated, it invades the surrounding tissue. **Squamous cell carcinoma**, the second most common type, occurs most commonly on the head, neck, forearms and dorsal hands (Figure 23-1B).

Melanoma, which is the most serious type of skin cancer, originates in the melanocytes (see Figure 23-1C). The incidence of melanoma has been gradually increasing in recent decades, with older men accounting disproportionately for the increase (Tucker, 2009). Men aged 60 and 70 years have experienced more than a fourfold and fivefold increase, respectively, in incidence between 1975 and 2005 (Geller, 2009). Melanoma is the skin cancer most likely to metastasise and cause death, with nearly three-quarters of all melanoma deaths occurring in people aged 55 years and older (Geller, 2009).

DIVERSITY NOTE

Twice as many men as women die from melanoma each year in Australia (Australian Institute Health and Welfare, 2010).

Early detection and treatment are imperative for improving the outcomes of all types of skin cancer, and nurses have an essential role in assessing and teaching older adults about skin cancer, as discussed in the sections on nursing assessment and nursing interventions. Nurses also need to be alert to risk factors, so they consider these in their assessments and address them in health promotion. Advanced age increases the risk for all types of skin lesions, including skin cancers. Exposure to

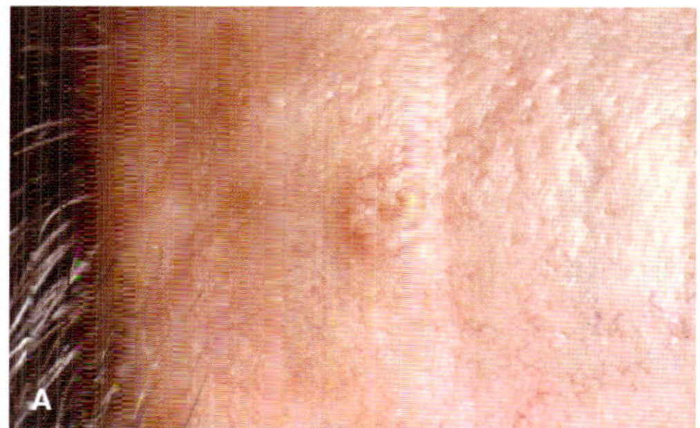

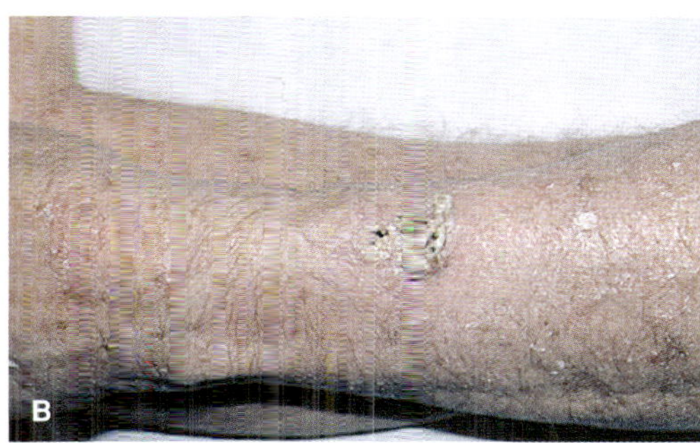

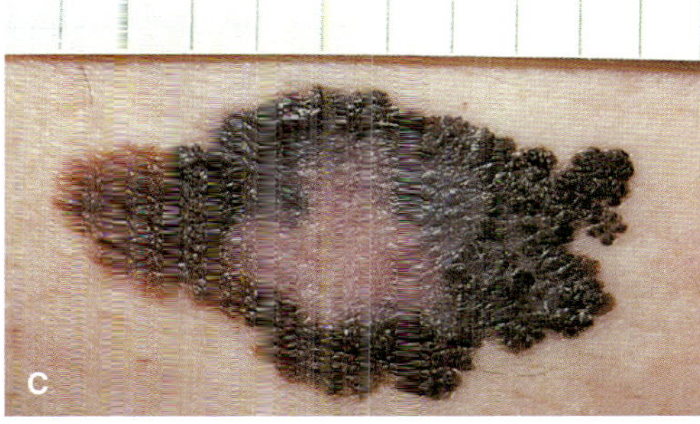

FIGURE 23-1 Common types of skin cancer. (**A**) Basal cell carcinoma (**B**) Squamous cell carcinoma. (**C**) Melanoma. (A & B, Reprinted with permission from Rosenthal, T. C., Williams, M. E. & Naughton, B. J. [2007]. *Office care geriatrics*. Philadelphia: Lippincott Williams & Wilkins; and C, from Goodheart, H. P. [2009]. *Goodheart's photoguide of common skin disorders*. Philadelphia: Lippincott Williams & Wilkins.)

ultraviolet rays, including those from tanning booths, is a risk factor that is highly associated with skin cancers and most amenable to protective measures. Studies indicate that chronic sun exposure, which is the type that one receives during usual daily outdoor activities, is less of a risk for melanoma than intermittent excessive exposure (Berwick & Erdei, 2009). Additional risk factors for melanoma include a personal or family history of melanoma and fair skin that burns easily and has many large or irregular moles.

WELLNESS OPPORTUNITY

Nurses promote self-care for wellness by teaching older adults to examine their skin for suspicious changes once a month.

Skin tears

Skin tears are traumatic wounds involving the dermal and/or epidermal layers of the skin and usually caused by friction, rubbing or a shearing force. Skin tears commonly occur in older adults because of a combination of age-related skin changes and such risk factors as frailty, limited mobility and poor nutrition. In addition to advanced age, risk factors associated with skin tears include immobility; polypharmacy; poor nutrition; and sensory, cognitive or functional impairment (LeBlanc & Baranoski, 2009). Skin tears usually occur on an older adult's extremities (Xu et al., 2009).

A risk assessment tool for predicting skin tears in older adults, called the Skin Tear Risk Assessment Pathway (LeBlanc, Baranoski, Christensen et al., 2013), is available via www.skintears.org. It has three categories of assessment, which include:

- General health: chronic/critical disease, polypharmacy, impaired sensory, cognitive, visual, auditory, nutrition
- Mobility: history of falls and/or impaired mobility, dependent activities of daily living (ADLs)
- Skin: extremes of age, fragile skin, previous skin tears.

If a person has one or more of the above risk factors they are considered at risk. Those who are classified at high risk require a risk reduction program. Older adults with identified ageing skin changes are at an increased risk of developing a skin tear. Consequently all older adults require education about skincare and this increased risk. Although skin tears are considered to be minor wounds, if they are not cared for appropriately they can become infected or develop into a chronic wound.

In Australia skin tear prevalence is not well reported, although some data are available. It was found that in public hospitals skin tears were the third-largest group of wounds treated, and most of these wounds were acquired while in care (WoundsWest, 2009). In another study, in a Western Australian community, 20% of adults over 70 years had sustained a skin tear (Carville & Smith, 2004).

The assessment of the type of skin tear must be conducted before wound management. There are a number of skin tear classification systems. However, in December 2011, the International Skin Tear Advisory Panel (ISTPA) proposed a Skin Tear Classification System (STCS) to establish a common language for documenting skin tears to facilitate research and development of best practices (LeBlanc, Baranoski, Holloway & Langemo, 2013). The ISTPA system is based on the original system developed by Payne and Martin (1993). The ISTPA categories of skin tear are as follows:

- Category I is a skin tear without tissue (flap) loss
- Category II is a skin tear with partial tissue (flap) loss
- Category III is a skin tear with complete tissue loss (flap), where the epidermal flap is absent.

Silver Chain

STAR Skin Tear Classification System

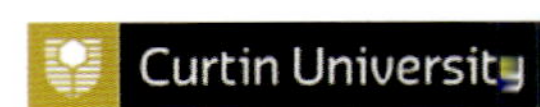

STAR Skin Tear Classification System Guidelines

1. Control bleeding and clean the wound according to protocol.
2. Realign (if possible) any skin or flap.
3. Assess degree of tissue loss and skin or flap colour using the STAR Classification System.
4. Assess the surrounding skin condition for fragility, swelling, discolouration or bruising.
5. Assess the person, their wound and their healing environment as per protocol.
6. If skin or flap colour is pale, dusky or darkened, reassess in 24–48 hours or at the first dressing change.

STAR Classification System

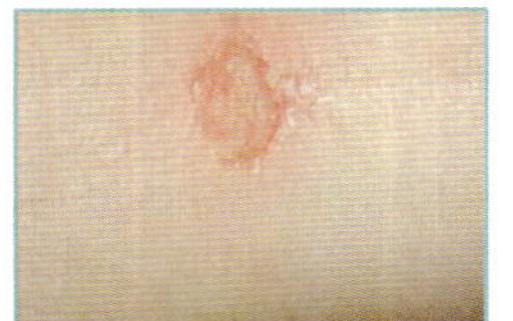

Category 1a
A skin tear where the edges **can** be realigned to the normal anatomical position (without undue stretching) and the skin or flap colour **is not** pale, dusky or darkened.

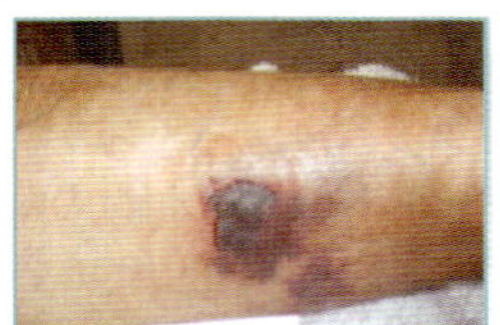

Category 1b
A skin tear where the edges **can** be realigned to the normal anatomical position (without undue stretching) and the skin or flap colour **is** pale, dusky or darkened.

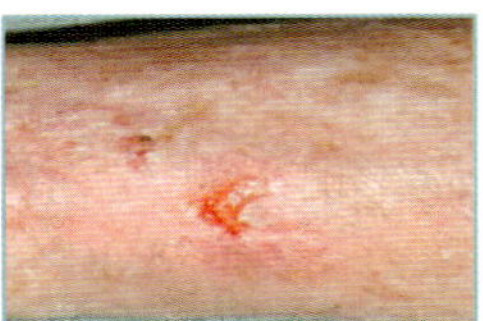

Category 2a
A skin tear where the edges **cannot** be realigned to the normal anatomical position and the skin or flap colour **is not** pale, dusky or darkened.

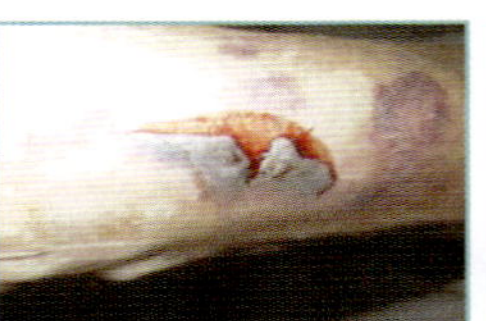

Category 2b
A skin tear where the edges **cannot** be realigned to the normal anatomical position and the skin or flap colour **is** pale, dusky or darkened.

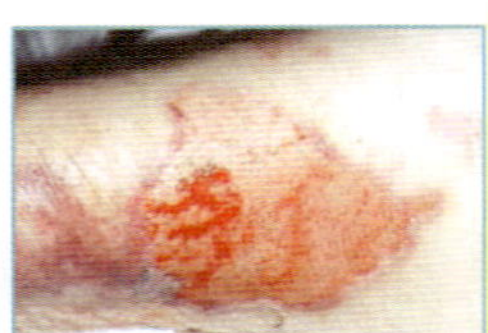

Category 3
A skin tear where the skin flap is completely absent.

FIGURE 23-2 STAR Skin Tear Classification System. Used with permission. (Skin Tear Audit Research [STAR]. Silver Chain Group Limited, Curtin University, Australia. Revised 4 February 2010. Reprinted August 2012. Accessed June 2015 at www.silverchain.org.au/assets/group/research/STARSkin-Tear-tool-04022010.pdf.)

Another tool developed and used in Australia is the STAR (Skin Tear Classification System) (Payne & Martin, 1993; Carville et al., 2007; Silver Chain Nursing Association & School of Nursing & Midwifery, Curtin University of Technology, 2012). The STAR also has three categories, as well as subcategories, which consider important skin and flap colour changes (see Figure 23-2).

Once the skin tear has been classified then the appropriate wound care can be conducted. Those with a skin flap require a different approach to those without. Where possible the aim of wound care when a skin flap is still evident is to maintain the viability of the flap. Usually dry non-stick wound management is required for this type of skin tear. When the skin tear does not have a flap then wound management using the moist wound healing approach is required. Selection of a moist wound dressing is dependent on the wound assessment. All wound management of a skin tear should also include: minimising any further trauma to the skin, promoting an optimal wound-healing environment and minimising the risk of infection (Xu et al., 2009). The interventions for treating skin tears with a flap are summarised in Box 23-1. The nursing interventions that may assist with the prevention of skin tears in older adults are summarised in Box 23-2.

Pressure ulcers

In recent years the focus on the development, prevention and management of pressure ulcers has increased significantly. Although pressure ulcers have been a topic of concern since the 1970s, it is now being addressed as an essential aspect of in-patient safety.

Definition and overview

A **pressure ulcer** is a "localised injury to the skin and/or underlying tissue, usually over a bony prominence, as a result of pressure, or pressure in combination with shear" (National Pressure Ulcer Advisory Panel [NPUAP], 2009). Many factors contribute to the development of pressure ulcers, but the immediate determinant is the degree to

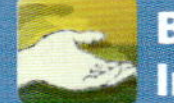

BOX 23-1
Interventions for treating skin tears with a flap

- Gently clean the skin tear with normal saline.
- Let the area air dry or pat dry carefully.
- Approximate the skin tear flap with an appropriate wound product.
- Skin sealants, petroleum-based products and other water-resistant products such as protective barrier ointments or liquid barriers may be used to protect the surrounding skin from wound drainage or dressing/tape removal trauma.
- Always assess the size of the skin tear; consider doing a wound tracing.
- Document assessment and treatment findings.

Source: Ayello, E. A. & Sibbald, R. G. (2012). Preventing pressure ulcers and skin tears. In M. Boltz, E. Capezuti, T. Fulmer & D. Zwicker (Eds), *Evidence-based geriatric nursing protocols for best practice* (4th ed., pp. 403–429). New York: Springer.

BOX 23-2
Preventions of skin tears

Perform an assessment of skin

- Collect information about skin history, current medications and skin care.
- Observe for signs of adequate hygiene, variations in skin colouring, bruising, inflammation, scratch marks, jaundice, swelling, breaks, sores and lesions.
- Assess skin texture, moisture, turgor and temperature.

Provide a safe environment

- Do a skin tear risk assessment of all older adults on admission.
- Implement prevention protocol for older adults identified as at risk for skin tears.
- Have older adults wear long sleeves or pants to protect their extremities.
- Have adequate light to reduce the risk of bumping into furniture or equipment.
- Provide a safe area for wandering.
- Educate the older adult about their increased risk of skin tears.
- Educate staff or family carers in the correct way of handling the older adult to prevent skin tears.

General skin care

- Use warm rather than hot water and do not soak skin to reduce risk of dehydrating skin.
- Use lotion, especially on dry skin on arms and legs, twice daily.
- Use no-rinse soapless bathing products.
- Keep skin from becoming dry; apply moisturiser.

Maintain nutrition and hydration

- If necessary, obtain a dietary consultation.

Protect from self-injury or injury during routine care

- Use a slide sheet to move and turn the person.
- Use transfer techniques that prevent friction or shear.
- Pad bedrails, wheelchair arms, and leg supports.
- Support dangling arms and legs with pillows or blankets.

General wound care principles

- Use non-adherent dressings on frail skin.
- If you must use tape, be sure it is made of paper, and remove it gently. Also, you can apply the tape to hydrocolloid strips placed strategically around the wound rather than taping directly onto fragile surrounding skin around the skin tear.
- Use gauze wraps, stockinettes, flexible netting or other wraps to secure dressings rather than tape.

Source: Adapted from Lurde, L. (2014). Skin tears: Prevention. Evidence summary. Joanna Briggs Institute.

which tissues can tolerate the intensity and duration of pressure. People who are unable to move around independently, even for short periods (e.g. during surgery), are most vulnerable. Figure 23-3 illustrates areas of the body that are most susceptible to development of pressure ulcers, with sacrum/coccyx and heel being the first and second most common sites.

Medical devices also can be a source of pressure to cause *medical device-related pressure ulcers*. Device-related pressure ulcers account for 9.1% of ulcers, with the ears being the most common location (Ayello & Sibbald, 2012). Medical devices commonly associated with increased risk for pressure ulcers include masks, orthotics, tubing, immobilisers, stockings or boots, nasogastric tubes, cervical collars or braces, and tracheostomy tubes and ties (Apold & Rydrych, 2012; Coyer, Stotts & Blackman, 2013).

Since the early 2000s there has been increasing attention to the incidence, prevalence and serious consequences of pressure ulcers. This increased attention is due to the steadily growing awareness of safety issues in people hospitalised with pressure ulcers being identified as one of the top three concerns (Gadd, 2012). In Australia and New Zealand there is an increase in pressure area prevention measures in hospitals and long-term residential care. All hospital in-patients and residents in long-term residential care facilities are required to be risk assessed for pressure areas and a plan of care created and implemented based on the assessment findings.

DIVERSITY NOTE

Analysis of data related to pressure ulcers across the skin pigmentation spectrum shows that people with darkly pigmented skin have a higher incidence of serious pressure ulcers. Clinicians need to pay particular attention to a variety of indicators for detection of early-stage pressure ulcers (Ayello & Sibbald, 2012).

Functional consequences

Pressure ulcers are associated with many serious functional consequences, including pain, loss of function, and decreased quality of life. The NPUAP emphasises the important role of nurses in assessing and intervening for pain in older adults with pressure ulcers. This emphasis is warranted because older adults with pressure ulcers report that pain is their most distressing symptom and pressure-related pain is often experienced even before skin breakdown is evident (Briggs, Collinson, Wilson et al., 2013). Studies have identified *hospital-acquired pressure ulcers* (HAPUs) as a major risk for all the following: doubling the length of stay, increased rates of mortality during the hospitalisation or within 30 days of discharge, and increased rates of bacteraemia with multidrug-resistant organisms with a poor outcome (Braga, Pirett, Ribas et al., 2013; Lyder, Wang, Metersky et al., 2012; Theisen, Drabik & Stock, 2012).

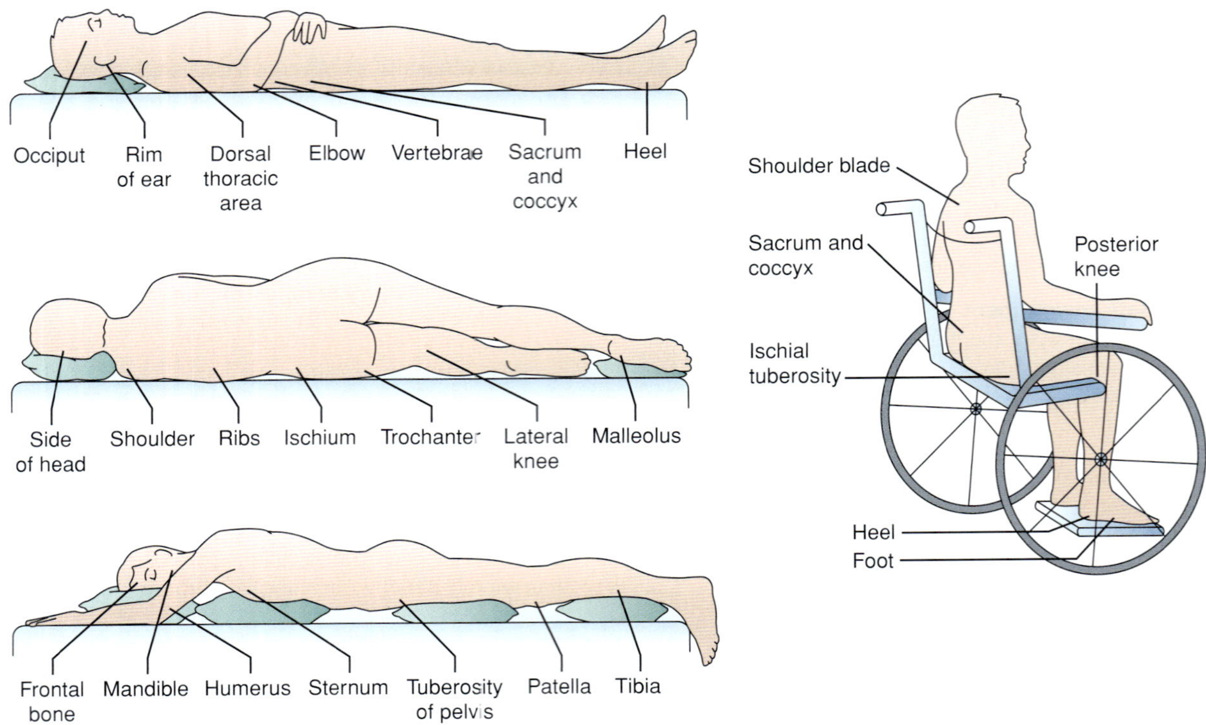

FIGURE 23-3 The risk of developing pressure ulcers is higher at these points.

Risk identification

Evidence-based tools are used to identify and rate risk factors for pressure ulcer development. The Braden Scale (Figure 23-4) is commonly used as a screening tool for older adults, and the Hartford Institute for Geriatric Nursing recommends this tool as a best practice for identifying older adults at risk for the development of pressure ulcers. Other tools used are the Norton Scale and Waterlow Scale. Reviews of studies indicate that all three of these scales can help identify people at risk for pressure ulcers who might benefit from targeted interventions (Chou, Dana, Bougatsos et al., 2013). However, it is important to recognise that these tools are not necessarily predictive of pressure ulcers, but their major purpose is to provide the initial step in pressure ulcer prevention programs (Kelechi, Arndt & Dove, 2013; Kelleher, Moorer & Makic, 2012).

A current focus of research is on the reliability of the Braden Scale in predicting pressure ulcers in specific groups of hospitalised in-patients. These studies emphasise the need to focus on specific subscale scores (e.g. friction/shear subscale) to implement preventive plans that address individual needs (Tescher, Brand, Byrne et al., 2012). A comprehensive research review of the predictive power of the Braden Scale in adult critical care patients found that the subscales for Sensory perception, Mobility, Moisture and Friction/Shear were more predictive of pressure ulcer development than the subscales for Activity and Nutrition (Cox, 2012).

Current research is focusing on critically ill patients who develop HAPU and have multiple risk factors, including ones that are not identified on risk assessment tools. For example, Bry and colleagues (2012) reported a study of 82 patients who had at least 1 HAPU and found that all had multiple risk factors, yet almost one-quarter of the Braden scores were graded as low risk. Similarly, Black and colleagues (2012) found that critically ill in-patients shared a unique pattern of pressure ulcer risk with the following characteristics: elderly, immobile, inactive, dehydrated, undernourished, anaemic, moist skin, sedated or unconscious, and mechanically ventilated and requiring head-of-the-bed elevation. Studies of HAPU in postsurgical patients have identified the following risk factors: diabetes, longer operative time, recurrent surgeries, and low body mass index (Liu, He & Chen, 2012; Tschannen, Bates, Talsma et al., 2012). Studies such as these underscore the importance of using evidence-based tools in conjunction with clinical judgement as components of a comprehensive assessment of all factors that increase the risk for pressure ulcers.

Staging classifications

Since 1975, the NPUAP has promoted the use of a **staging system**, which is an assessment system that classifies pressure ulcers according to the anatomical depth of soft-tissue damage. In 2009, the NPUAP and the European Pressure Ulcer Advisory Panel jointly issued a revised classification system, as described, illustrated and summarised in Table 23-2.

Once a pressure ulcer is identified according to the defined stages, it must be frequently reassessed to evaluate the effectiveness of interventions. Since 1996, the NPUAP has encouraged the use of a standardised tool for assessing changes in pressure ulcers called the Pressure Ulcer Scale for Healing (PUSH) tool. The PUSH tool scores

BRADEN SCALE FOR PREDICTING PRESSURE SORE RISK

Patient's Name ______________ Evaluator's Name ______________ Date of Assessment

SENSORY PERCEPTION ability to respond meaningfully to pressure-related discomfort	**1. Completely Limited** Unresponsive (does not moan, flinch, or grasp) to painful stimuli, due to diminished level of consciousness or sedation. OR limited ability to feel pain over most of body.	**2. Very Limited** Responds only to painful stimuli. Cannot communicate discomfort except by moaning or restlessness OR has a sensory impairment which limits the ability to feel pain or discomfort over 1/2 of body.	**3. Slightly Limited** Responds to verbal commands, but cannot always communicate discomfort or the need to be turned. OR has some sensory impairment which limits ability to feel pain or discomfort in 1 or 2 extremities.	**4. No Impairment** Responds to verbal commands. Has no sensory deficit which would limit ability to feel or voice pain or discomfort.				
MOISTURE degree to which skin is exposed to moisture	**1. Constantly Moist** Skin is kept moist almost constantly by perspiration, urine, etc. Dampness is detected every time patient is moved or turned.	**2. Very Moist** Skin is often, but not always moist. Linen must be changed at least once a shift.	**3. Occasionally Moist** Skin is occasionally moist, requiring an extra linen change approximately once a day.	**4. Rarely Moist** Skin is usually dry, linen only requires changing at routine intervals.				
ACTIVITY degree of physical activity	**1. Bedfast** Confined to bed.	**2. Chairfast** Ability to walk severely limited or non-existent. Cannot bear own weight and/or must be assisted into chair or wheelchair.	**3. Walks Occasionally** Walks occasionally during day, but for very short distances, with or without assistance. Spends majority of each shift in bed or chair.	**4. Walks Frequently** Walks outside room at least twice a day and inside room at least once every two hours during waking hours.				
MOBILITY ability to change and control body position	**1. Completely Immobile** Does not make even slight changes in body or extremity position without assistance.	**2. Very Limited** Makes occasional slight changes in body or extremity position but unable to make frequent or significant changes independently.	**3. Slightly Limited** Makes frequent though slight changes in body or extremity position independently.	**4. No Limitation** Makes major and frequent changes in position without assistance.				
NUTRITION usual food intake pattern	**1. Very Poor** Never eats a complete meal. Rarely eats more than 1/2 of any food offered. Eats 2 servings or less of protein (meat or dairy products) per day. Takes fluids poorly. Does not take a liquid dietary supplement. OR is NPO and/or maintained on clear liquids or IV's for more than 5 days.	**2. Probably Inadequate** Rarely eats a complete meal and generally eats only about 1/2 of any food offered. Protein intake includes only 3 servings of meat or dairy products per day. Occasionally will take a dietary supplement. OR receives less than optimum amount of liquid diet or tube feeding	**3. Adequate** Eats over half of most meals. Eats a total of 4 servings of protein (meat, dairy products per day. Occasionally will refuse a meal, but will usually take a supplement when offered. OR is on a tube feeding or TPN regimen which probably meets most of nutritional needs.	**4. Excellent** Eats most of every meal. Never refuses a meal. Usually eats a total of 4 or more servings of meat and dairy products. Occasionally eats between meals. Does not require supplementation.				
FRICTION & SHEAR	**1. Problem** Requires moderate to maximum assistance in moving. Complete lifting without sliding against sheets is impossible. Frequently slides down in bed or chair, requiring frequent repositioning with maximum assistance. Spasticity, contractures or agitation leads to almost constant friction.	**2. Potential Problem** Moves feebly or requires minimum assistance. During a move skin probably slides to some extent against sheets, chair, restraints or other devices. Maintains relatively good position in chair or bed most of the time but occasionally slides down.	**3. No Apparent Problem** Moves in bed and in chair independently and has sufficient muscle strength to lift up completely during move. Maintains good position in bed or chair.					
				Total Score				

FIGURE 23-4 The Braden Scale is a widely used screening tool to identify people at risk for pressure ulcers. Scores – 15–18, at risk; 13–14, moderate risk; 10–12, high risk; <9, very high risk. (From Bergstrom, N. & Braden, B. et al. [1987]. Reprinted with permission. Permission to use this tool should be sought at www.bradenscale.com.)

TABLE 23-2 Stages of pressure ulcer development

Stage	Description
0	Normal skin 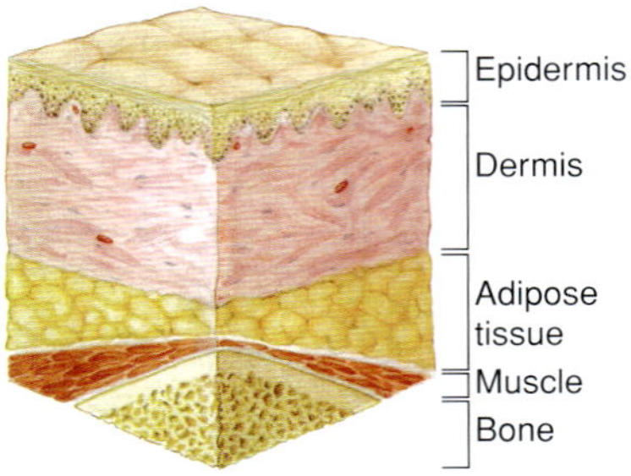
I	**Non-blanchable erythema.** Intact skin with non-blanchable redness of a localised area usually over a bony prominence. Darkly pigmented skin may not have visible blanching; its colour may differ from the surrounding area. The area may be painful, firm, soft, warmer or cooler as compared to adjacent tissue. Category I may be difficult to detect in individuals with dark skin tones. May indicate "at-risk" persons. 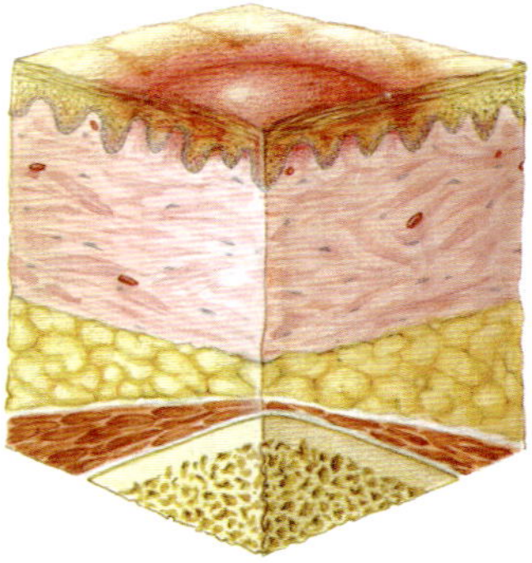 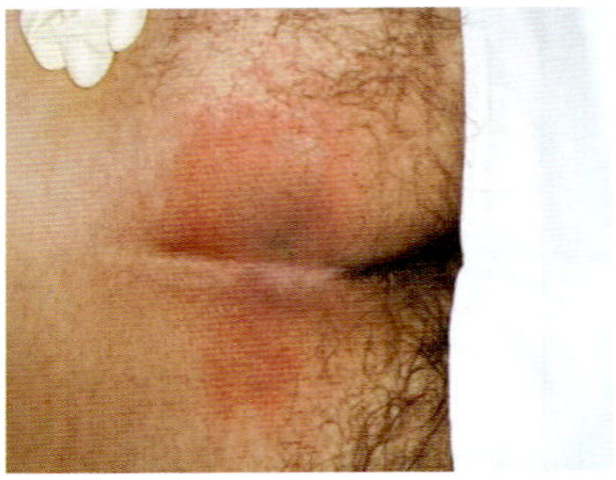
II	**Partial thickness.** Partial thickness loss of dermis presenting as a shallow open ulcer with a red pink wound bed, without slough. May also present as an intact or open/ruptured serum-filled or serosanguinous filled blister. Presents as a shiny or dry shallow ulcer without slough or bruising.* This category should not be used to describe skin tears, tape burns, incontinence associated dermatitis, maceration or excoriation. *Bruising indicates deep tissue injury. 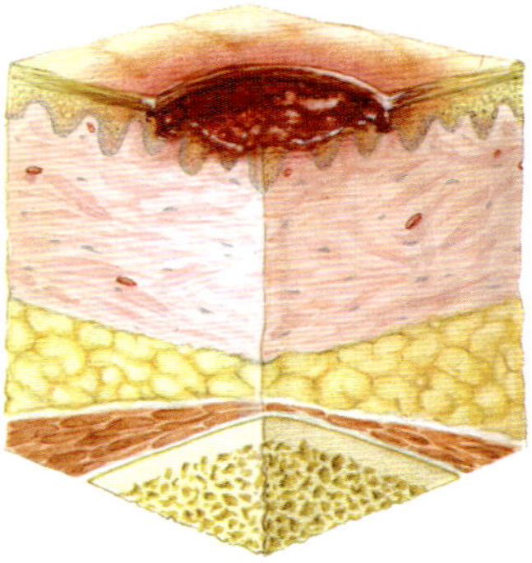 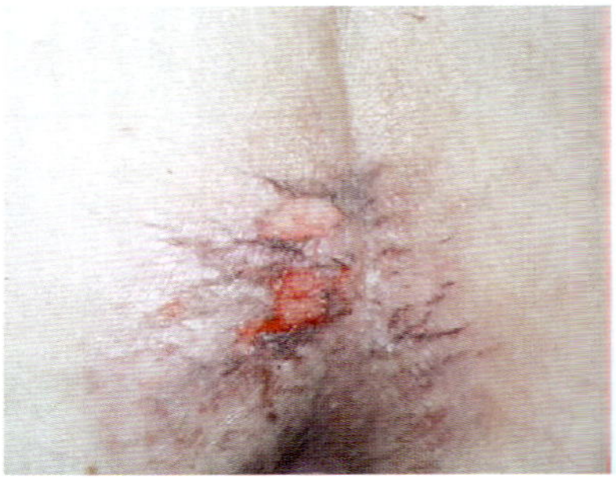
III	**Full-thickness skin loss.** Subcutaneous fat may be visible but bone, tendon or muscle is *not* exposed. Slough may be present but does not obscure the depth of tissue loss. *May* include undermining and tunnelling. The depth of a category/stage III pressure ulcer varies by anatomical location. The bridge of the nose, ear, occiput and malleolus do not have (adipose) subcutaneous tissue and category/stage III ulcers can be shallow. In contrast, areas of significant adiposity can develop extremely deep category/stage III pressure ulcers. Bone/tendon is not visible or directly palpable. 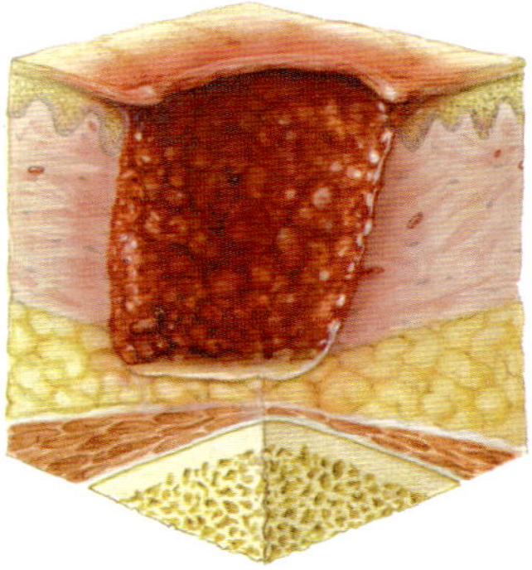 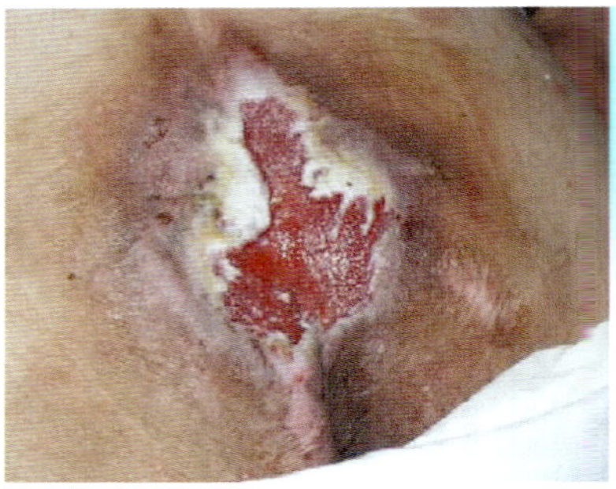

pressure ulcers according to size, exudates and tissue type, with changes in the PUSH score over time indicating the progression or regression of the pressure ulcer.

Although the term "reverse staging" has been used to describe the progression of a later-stage pressure ulcer to a healed stage, the NPUAP has advised against this practice because it does not accurately reflect the pathophysiological processes that occur. The NPUAP provides many educational resources related to the staging classification and the PUSH tool. The tool

TABLE 23-2 Stages of pressure ulcer development (*continued*)

Stage	Description
IV	**Full-thickness tissue loss.** Full-thickness tissue loss with exposed bone, tendon or muscle. Slough or eschar may be present. Often includes undermining and tunnelling. The depth of a category/stage IV pressure ulcer varies by anatomical location. The bridge of the nose, ear, occiput and malleolus do not have (adipose) subcutaneous tissue and these ulcers can be shallow. Category/stage IV ulcers can extend into muscle and/or supporting structures (e.g. fascia, tendon or joint capsule) making osteomyelitis or osteitis likely to occur. Exposed bone/muscle is visible or directly palpable. 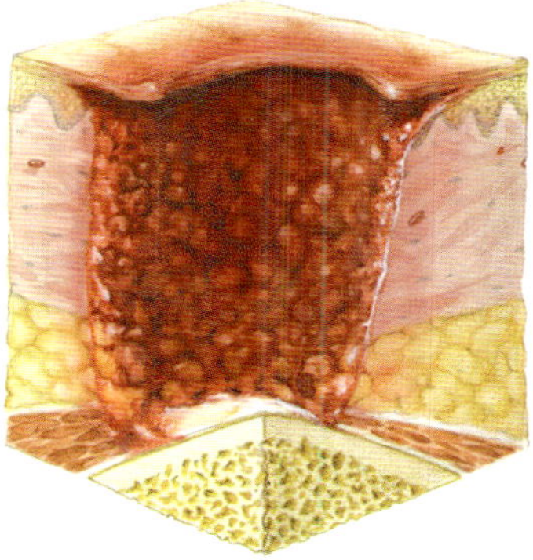 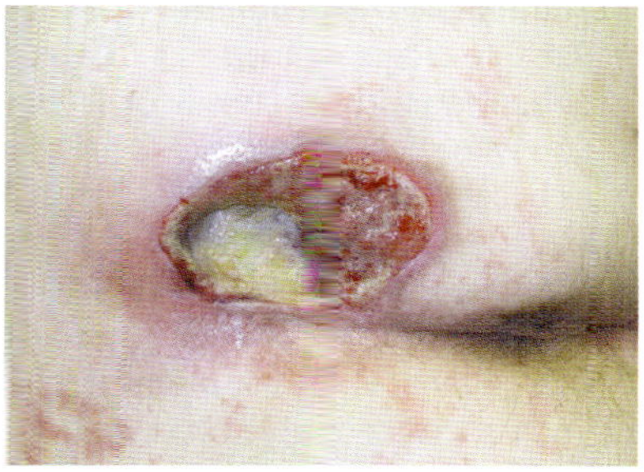
Unstageable	**Full-thickness skin or tissue loss—depth unknown.** Full-thickness tissue loss in which actual depth of the ulcer is completely obscured by slough (yellow, tan, grey, green or brown) and/or eschar (tan, brown or black) in the wound bed. Until enough slough and/or eschar is removed to expose the base of the wound, the true depth cannot be determined, but it will be either category/stage III or IV. Stable (dry, adherent, intact without erythema or fluctuance) eschar on the heels serves as "the body's natural (biological) cover" and should not be removed. 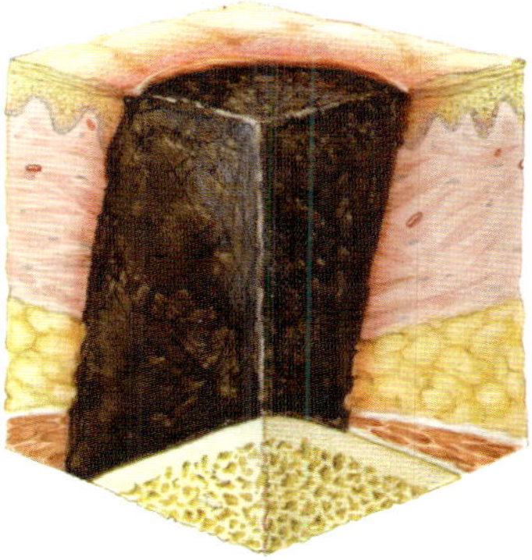
Suspected deep tissue injury	**Depth unknown.** Purple or maroon localised area of discoloured intact skin or blood-filled blister due to damage of underlying soft tissue from pressure and/or *shear*. The area may be preceded by tissue that is painful, firm, mushy, boggy, warmer or cooler as compared to adjacent tissue. Deep tissue injury may be difficult to detect in individuals with dark skin tones. Evolution may include a thin blister over a dark wound bed. The wound may further evolve and become covered by thin eschar. Evolution may be rapid exposing additional layers of tissue even with optimal treatment. 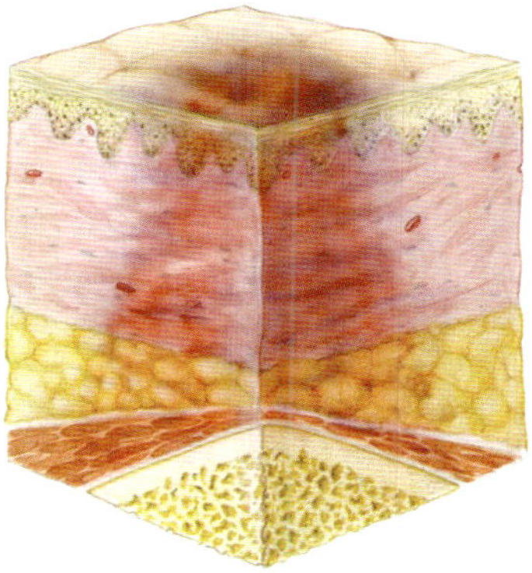

Source: Text reprinted from European Pressure Ulcer Advisory Panel and National Pressure Ulcer Advisory Panel. (2009). Prevention and treatment of pressure ulcers. Available from www.npuap.org. Used with permission of the National Pressure Ulcer Advisory Panel.

includes quick reference guides in English and other languages.

Evidence-based practice for pressure ulcers

Financial and quality of care implications related to pressure ulcers have led to an abundance of information about interventions for preventing and healing pressure ulcers, as summarised in Evidence-based practice 23-1. Although much progress has been made in identifying interventions for preventing and healing pressure ulcers, research is ongoing and recommendations continue to develop. For example, repositioning is consistently identified as an effective measure;

EVIDENCE-BASED PRACTICE 23-1
Pressure ulcers

Statement of the problem

- Pressure ulcers, defined as a localised injury to the skin and/or underlying tissue as a result of pressure or pressure n combination with shear, are a major focus of quality of care initiatives in all healthcare settings.
  - Underlying causative factors are a combination of pressure intensity and duration and tissue tolerance.
- Risk factors include immobility, surgery, frailty, older age, friable skin, incontinence, compromised nutritional status, cognitive impairment, comorbid conditions, and dependence in activities of daily living.
  - The sacrum and heels are the two most common sites for the development of pressure ulcers; other common sites are the ears, elbows, coccyx and ischium.
  - Pressure ulcers differ physiologically from moisture-associated dermatitis or surface injury caused by moisture or friction.
- Pressure ulcer complications include sepsis, cellulitis, osteomyelitis increased length of stay, and financial and emotional cost.
- Detection of stage I pressure ulcers is particularly challenging in people with darkly pigmented skin, and these people are more likely to die from pressure ulcers.

Recommendations for nursing assessment

- Identify risk factors using a valid and reliable tool (e.g. Braden Scale).
- Perform a head-to-toe skin assessment on admission to a facility, on discharge, whenever the person's condition changes, and at appropriate intervals.
  - Additional components of a comprehensive assessment for pressure ulcer risk include a history and physical examination.
- Assess and reassess pressure ulcers according to the most recent NPUAP Pressure Ulcer Staging System.
- During assessments, use natural or halogen lighting rather than fluorescent lighting.
- Because people with darkly pigmented skin may not meet the normal criteria for stage I pressure ulcers, consider additional parameters (e.g. differences in skin over bony prominences compared with surrounding skin, alterations in pain or local sensation, deviations from the usual colour for that person).
- If available, use technological devices to improve the detection of stage I pressure ulcers in people with darkly pigmented skin.

Recommendations for nursing interventions

- Pressure redistribution interventions: individualise repositioning schedules, use pressure redistribution surfaces (e.g. static mattresses and overlays, alternating pressure mattress, gel cushions).
  - Positioning interventions: raise heels to eliminate pressure, keep head of bed in lowest height, maintain 30° tilted side-lying position, avoid positioning directly on the trochanter, avoid doughnut-shaped devices.
  - Use protective methods, such as heel protection boots.
  - Decrease the risk of friction and shear: have the person use trapeze to lift self off bed, staff can use transfer or lifting devices.
- Nutritional interventions: assessment of nutritional status and appropriate referrals for the services of registered dietitians; provision of adequate kilojoules, nutrients and hydration; and appropriate use of supplements.
  - Daily nutrient needs for prevention and treatment of pressure ulcers: 125–150 kilojoules/kg body weight, 1.25 to 1.5 g/kg protein, 1 mL fluid intake per kilocalorie, and vitamin and mineral supplements to compensate for deficiencies. with less than 40 mg elemental zinc.
- Protect skin from moisture: manage incontinence, keep skin clean and dry, use absorbent products, change linens frequently, and use moisture barrier skin protectant.
  - Skin care: individualise bathing frequency; avoid hot water and excessive rubbing; use moisturiser lotion; protect skin from urine, stool and other sources of moisture; and do not massage bony prominences.
- Manage treatment measures, including wound cleansing, moist wound dressings, debridement, pain management, and referral to wound care specialists.
- Education of professionals, older adults and carers.

Cultural considerations for interventions

- Dressings for pressure ulcers may contain animal-derived collagen that conflicts with the person's ideology or cultural background as in the following examples: porcine products for Jewish or Muslim people, bovine products for Hindu people, and honey-based products for people who follow a vegan diet.
- Obtain information about products with animal-based collagen and discuss with people who may have cultural conflicts.

Source: Ayello & Sibbald (2012); Chou, Dana, Bougatsos et al. (2013); Boyer (2013); Institute for Clinical Systems Improvement (2012); Posthauer, Collins, Dorner et al. (2013).

however, the long-standing criterion of turning people every 2 hours has been replaced with the recommendation to individualise repositioning schedules based on the person's condition, care goals, vulnerable skin areas, and type of support surface being used (Chou, Dana, Bougatsos et al., 2013).

Chronic wounds

When a wound heals it usually progresses through 3 phases: the Inflammatory Phase (2–5 days); the Proliferative Phase (2 days to 3 weeks) and finally the Remodelling Phase (3 weeks to 2 years). Wound healing is normally continuous and occurs within an expected time frame. There are usually no complications. However, when a wound remains in the inflammatory phase and does not progress as expected to the proliferative phase or it has not healed within 6 weeks, it is then referred to as a **chronic wound**. Older adults are at an increased risk of developing chronic wounds (Werdin et al., 2009). Ageing skin and delayed wound healing are factors that increase the risk of chronic wound development in older adults. There are other risk factors such as oedema, malnutrition, diabetes and medications, particularly corticosteroids, which also increase the risk. Common chronic wounds that occur in older people are venous, arterial or mixed ulcers, diabetic ulcers; and, as described above, pressure ulcers. Breaks in skin integrity, such as skin tears, also have the potential to develop into a chronic wound if they do not receive optimal wound care.

Billions of dollars are spent annually on treating chronic wounds (Werdin et al., 2009). The consequences of chronic wounds for older adults include pain and a reduction in their quality of life. Many treatments are available and it is beyond the scope of this text to describe these treatments. General wound management principles still apply when treating chronic wounds in older adults. The TIME acronym can also assist with chronic wound management, regardless of the wound type (Schultz & Dowsett, 2012). The letter "T" refers to tissue, where the type of wound tissue is identified. The "I" refers to the presence of inflammation or infection within and surrounding the wound. "M" refers to the state of moisture of the wound bed. Finally, "E" describes the wound edge and re-epithelialisation.

One other distinguishing feature about chronic wounds as opposed to other wounds is that they usually have some level of bacterial contamination. This is referred to as **bacterial burden**. Chronic wounds can be contaminated with bacteria but not be infected or experience a delay in healing (Medical Education Partnership [MEP] 2008). Bacteria in a chronic wound may result in colonisation where the bacteria multiply, but the wound tissues are not damaged. To determine if bacterial contamination is causing infection or delaying healing, assessments are required. A positive wound culture for bacteria can be suggestive of infection. The presence of greater than 10^5 colony-forming units (CFUs) per gram of tissue (as demonstrated by biopsy) is generally accepted as a guideline for diagnosing a clinically infected wound. Also required is an assessment of the wound for infection. Signs and symptoms of infection include purulent discharge, odour, redness, appearance of surrounding skin and pain. Nurses are required to continually monitor the progression of the healing of chronic wounds in older adults. As healing takes longer for older adults, nurses should be very cautious about changing a dressing type because of the appearance of slow healing. It is important to do a thorough wound assessment before this decision is made to ensure that the wound requires an alternative dressing and not a longer period for wound healing.

NURSING ASSESSMENT OF SKIN

Because the skin is the largest and most visible organ of the body it is relatively easy to identify problems that affect it. In addition, the skin may yield clues to other areas of physiological and psychosocial function such as nutrition, hydration and personal care. Nurses collect information about the skin, hair and nails during an assessment interview and through physical examination procedures. Opportunities for direct examination also arise during routine nursing care activities such as assisting with personal care or listening to the lungs and apical heart rate. Noting the characteristics of the skin, hair and nails can also provide information to validate or raise questions about other areas of function. For example, the observation that an older man has a beard of several days' growth, when combined with assessment information about his overall function, may support conclusions about possible depression or the need for assistance with personal care activities.

Identifying opportunities for health promotion

Assessment questions are aimed at identifying the person's perception of any problems, any risk factors that may contribute to skin problems and the person's personal care behaviours that influence hair and skin status. Assessing these aspects of skincare can help identify opportunities for health education about risk factors and healthy skincare practices. Older adults may initiate a discussion about age spots or other noticeable skin changes and they are usually very receptive to information about skin and hair care. Nurses obtain information about medications and other risk factors as part of the overall assessment and they incorporate this information into the skin assessment. Likewise, other pertinent information obtained during a comprehensive assessment, such as information about fluid intake, nutritional status and mobility and safety, is applicable to the assessment of the skin. Box 23-3 summarises assessment questions related to the skin and nails.

Observing skin, hair and nails

Close inspection of the skin in a warm, private and well-lit environment is an essential component of skin assessment.

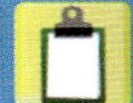

BOX 23-3
Interview questions for assessing the integument

Questions to assess risk factors and skin problems

- Do you have any concerns about or trouble with your skin?
- Do you have any problems with rashes, itching, swelling or dry skin?
- Do you have any sores that will not heal?
- Do you bruise easily?
- Have you been treated for skin cancer or any other skin problems?
- How much time do you spend in the sun?
- Do you spend time in tanning booths?
- Do you do anything to protect yourself from the effects of the sun?

Questions to assess personal care practices

- How do you manage your bathing?
- How often do you take a bath or shower?
- What water temperature do you use?
- Do you use soap every time you bathe?
- What kind of soap do you use?
- Do you use any kind of skin lotion, creams or ointments? What kind do you use and how frequently do you use it? Where do you apply it?
- Do you have any problems with your fingernails or toenails?
- Do you get or need any help with nail care?

Examination of the skin is particularly important because older adults may focus on benign conditions, such as xerosis, but not notice more serious conditions such as skin cancer. Nurses observe skin colour, turgor, dryness, overall condition and any growths or pathological conditions. Nurses also observe and document cultural variations. For example, older adults of Latin, Asian or African ancestry may have faded Mongolian spots (i.e. irregular areas of blue colouration common on the buttocks and lower back and sometimes on the arms, thighs and abdomen) that might be mistaken for bruises. Also, when assessing for erythema or pressure areas, nurses should keep in mind that early skin changes may be difficult to detect in people with darkly pigmented skin.

The common occurrence of various skin lesions complicates the assessment of skin in older adults. Although most of these changes are harmless, except in terms of their cosmetic consequences, some are cancerous or precancerous. An important aspect of health promotion is to reassure the older adult about the harmless changes and to encourage medical evaluation of the questionable ones. In general, the following characteristics of a skin lesion warrant medical evaluation:

- Redness
- Swelling
- Dark pigmentation
- Moisture or drainage
- Pain or discomfort
- Raised or irregular edges around a flat centre.

Also, any lesion that undergoes change or any sore that does not heal within a reasonable time, should be evaluated further. Evaluation is also indicated when, because of its location, a mole or other skin lesion is subject to frequent rubbing or irritation. When nurses observe a questionable skin lesion, they assess and document all the following characteristics: size, shape, colour, location, macular (flat) versus papular (raised), superficial versus penetrating, discrete versus diffuse borders and the presence or absence of inflammation, redness or discharge. Terminology related to various skin lesions in older adults is confusing and many terms are used interchangeably. Table 23-3 describes some of the terms used for skin lesions that are common in older adults; some of these lesions are shown in Figure 23-5.

Nursing assessment of the skin, hair and nails can provide clues to a broad spectrum of physiological functioning, particularly when nursing observations are combined with additional assessment information. For example, brown-stained fingertips are an indication of cigarette use and faeces under the fingernails and around the cuticle may be a clue to constipation. In some circumstances, toenails provide clues to mobility difficulties, particularly when extremely long nails curl under the toes. Observations of the skin may provide the only objective evidence of serious functional problems that the older person might not otherwise acknowledge. For example, multiple bruises, particularly in various stages of healing, may be a significant clue to falls, alcoholism, self-neglect or physical abuse. Observation and documentation of these signs are particularly important when neglect or abuse is suspected but the older adult or carer denies any such problems (see Chapter 10 for a detailed description of elder abuse).

In assessing the skin for clues to the broader aspects of function, keep in mind that some of the usual manifestations may be altered in older adults. For example, nurses often assess skin turgor on the hands or arms as an indication of hydration status. However, because of xerosis and

TABLE 23-3 Common skin lesions in older adults

Common term(s)	Description
Age spots, liver spots, senile lentigines, senile freckles	Pale to dark brown macules, occurring most frequently on exposed areas
Actinic keratosis, solar keratosis	Red, yellow, brown or flesh-coloured papules or plaques; gritty texture; surrounded by erythema; *premalignant*
Senile purpura	Areas of brown or bluish discolouration that look like bruising
Seborrhoeic keratosis	Brown or black papules or plaques with sharp edges and a waxy or wart-like texture; appearing most frequently on trunk and face
Sebaceous hyperplasia	Yellowish, doughnut-shaped elevations; common on face, particularly in men
Senile angiomas, cherry or ruby angiomas, telangiectasia	Bright, ruby-red, pinpoint, superficial elevations of small blood vessels
Spider angiomas	Tiny, red papules with radiating arms; *may indicate a pathological condition*
Venous stars	Bluish, irregular, sometimes spider-shaped lesions, appearing mainly on the legs or the chest
Venous lakes, benign venous angiomas	Bluish papules with sharp borders, appearing mainly on the lips or the ears
Acrochordons, skin tags	Flesh-coloured, pedunculated or stalk-like lesions
Corns, calluses	Hard masses of keratin caused by repeated pressure or irritation
Xanthelasma	Fatty deposits, usually around the eyes; *may be related to a pathological condition*, particularly if large or numerous

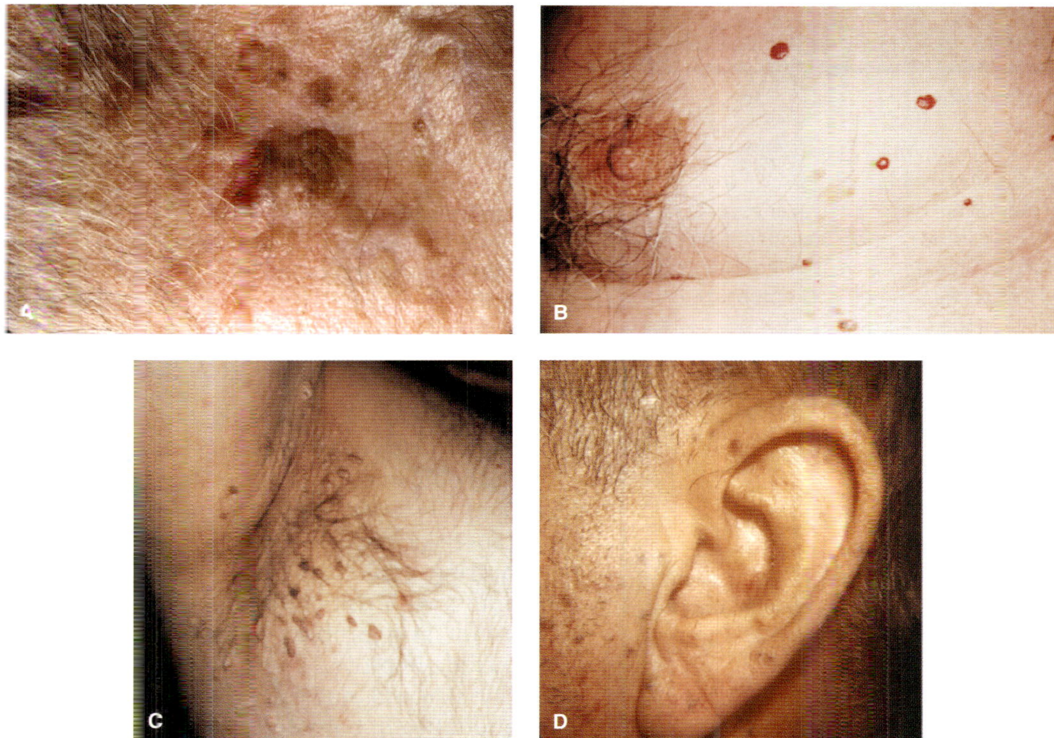

FIGURE 23-5 Common skin lesions in older adults. (**A**) Seborrhoeic keratosis. (**B**) Cherry angioma. (**C**) Skin tag. (**D**) Venous lakes or benign venous angiomas. (A & D, Reprinted with permission from Rosenthal, T. C., Williams, M. E. & Naughton, B. J. [2007]. *Office care geriatrics*. Philadelphia, PA: Lippincott Williams & Wilkins; B, Reprinted with permission from Weber, J. & Kelley, J. [2002]. *Health assessment in nursing* [2nd ed.]. Philadelphia, PA: Lippincott Williams & Wilkins; C, Reprinted with permission from Edwards, L. & Lynch, P. J. [2011]. *Genital dermatology atlas*. Philadelphia, PA: Lippincott Williams & Wilkins.)

decreased elasticity in the skin of older adults, skin turgor is not necessarily a reliable indicator of hydration status. Although the hands or arms may be convenient and socially acceptable sites of inspection, the skin over protected areas, such as the sternum or abdomen, is a more accurate indicator of hydration status in older adults. In non-medicated older adults, the oral mucous membranes are usually reliable indicators of hydration. However, many medications, including over-the-counter preparations containing anticholinergic ingredients, cause dry mouth. Another age-related change that complicates the assessment of the skin is delayed wound healing. This change makes it difficult to assess patterns of wound healing using the same standards that are applied to younger adults.

Observations of the hair, skin and nails provide multiple clues to self-esteem and other aspects of psychosocial function. Physical limitations can interfere with personal grooming, as can psychosocial influences such as lack of motivation or awareness. Thus, evidence of self-neglect in grooming may indicate depression, dementia or social isolation. The use of hair colouring may reflect the person's attitudes about ageing, and unusually deep hues of hair colouring or facial cosmetics may indicate impaired colour perception. Nurses can use Box 23-4 as a guide to assessment observations regarding the integumentary system.

UNFOLDING CASE STUDY

Part A

Ms Swanke is an 84-year-old fair-skinned woman who lives in her own home on the coast of Queensland, Australia. She is quite active and healthy and enjoys golfing and "beach-combing". The local chapter of the Cancer Society is co-sponsoring a skin cancer screening day at an expo for older people, which is held every year in the convention centre. You are a community nurse who has been asked to prepare a health education program titled "Checking Your Skin for Serious Changes". You are also assisting the dermatologist with the screening examinations. Ms Swanke attends the health education part of your program and says she is not sure if she can stay for the screening. She just has one "age spot", and she knows it is not serious because she has "had a couple skin cancers removed, and this one looks different". You look at the questionable spot, and you assess it as a brown, raised plaque with a gritty texture, about 1 cm in diameter.

Thinking points

- What additional assessment information would you want to obtain from Ms Swanke?
- How would you use Table 23-3 and Boxes 23-3 and 23-4 in your assessment?
- What advice would you give to Ms Swanke about her skin?

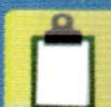

BOX 23-4
Observations regarding the integument

Examination of the skin

- What is the colour?
- Are there any areas of irregular pigmentation?
- Are there any areas of sunburn or tan?
- Are there areas that are discoloured in any way?
- Are there any indications of poor circulation, particularly in the extremities (e.g. varicosities, or areas of red, blue or brown discolouration indicative of chronic stasis problems in the lower extremities)?
- What is the skin temperature?
- Is there a marked difference between the temperature of the extremities and that of the rest of the body?
- How does the skin feel in terms of moisture? Is it dry? Clammy? Oily?
- What is the skin's texture? Is it smooth or rough?
- Does the skin look tissue-paper thin?
- What is the turgor of the abdominal skin?
- Are scars present? (If so, describe their location and appearance.) Are there any signs of falling or physical abuse?
- Are any of the lesions described in Table 23-3 present?

Examination of the hair and nails

- What are the colour, texture and general condition of the hair?
- What is the distribution pattern of the hair?
- Is there any evidence of dandruff, scaling or other problems with the hair?
- What are the colour, length, cleanliness and general condition of the toenails and fingernails?
- What are the colour and general condition of the nail beds of the toes and fingers?

Personal care practices

- What is the person's overall appearance with regard to grooming and attention to personal attractiveness?
- If grooming is poor, does the person express concern about this or provide an explanation?
- Are there any psychosocial factors that influence personal care practices (e.g. is the person socially isolated or overburdened with caregiving responsibilities and, therefore, inattentive to personal care)?
- Are any of the following signs of neglect evident: presence of a body odour; unkempt, uncut or matted hair; unusually long and unkempt fingernails or toenails; patches of brown crust on the skin; bruises; or any pathological skin conditions?

NURSING ISSUES

When older adults have any skin breakdown, nurses can use the nursing issue of *impaired skin integrity*. When older adults have any risk factors for skin tears or pressure ulcers, nurses can use the nursing issue of risk for impaired skin integrity. Related factors that commonly affect older adults include medications, incontinence, dehydration, limited mobility, nutritional deficits or a combination of these factors.

If the older adult has any suspect skin lesion, the nursing issue is of an inability to identify, manage and/or seek out help to maintain health. This nursing issue applies to people who do not use protective measures when they are exposed to ultraviolet radiation (from sunlight or tanning booths).

WELLNESS OPPORTUNITY

Nurses can use the wellness nursing issue of willingness for enhanced skincare knowledge for older adults who are interested in learning how to address risks for conditions such as dry skin and skin cancer.

GOAL PLANNING FOR WELLNESS OUTCOMES

When older adults have conditions that affect skin comfort or integrity, nurses develop goals that achieve wellness outcomes as an essential part of the nursing process. Similarly, when they have risks for conditions that can cause skin problems (e.g. skin cancer or pressure ulcers) nursing goals focus on prevention. For healthy older adults with risk factors (e.g. history of skin cancer) or minor skin problems (e.g. xerosis), applicable goals include improved comfort level; improved tissue integrity: skin and mucous membranes; increased knowledge about health behaviour; development of health-seeking behaviour; improved nutritional status; and prevention of skin cancer.

For older adults with pressure ulcers or other types of wounds or skin breakdown, goals include wound healing by primary intention and wound healing by secondary intention. These goals and wellness outcomes are achieved through interventions discussed in the following section.

WELLNESS OPPORTUNITY

Nurses promote wellness when they plan outcomes to address skin comfort and the prevention of skin cancer.

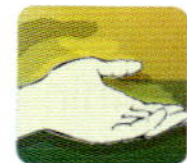

NURSING INTERVENTIONS FOR SKIN WELLNESS

Nurses have many opportunities for promoting wellness with regard to comfort, self-esteem and maintenance of a healthy integumentary system. Nursing interventions for healthy older adults focus on teaching about self-care practices, such as promoting responsibility for identifying and seeking further evaluation for harmful or precancerous lesions. Interventions for physically compromised older adults focus on maintaining intact skin and managing skin tears, pressure ulcers and chronic wounds. Nursing interventions may focus on hair care, health education, health screening, nutrition therapy, positioning, skin tear prevention, pressure management, pressure ulcer prevention, chronic wound prevention, pruritus management, risk identification, self-esteem enhancement, skin surveillance and wound care.

BOX 23-5
Health promotion teaching about skin care for older adults

Maintaining healthy skin

- Include adequate amounts of fluid in the daily diet.
- Use humidifiers to maintain environmental humidity levels of 40% to 60%.
- Apply moisturising lotions twice daily or as needed.
- Use moisturising lotions immediately after bathing, when the skin is still moist.
- Avoid massaging over bony prominences when applying lotions.
- Avoid skincare products that contain perfumes or isopropyl alcohol.
- Avoid multiple-ingredient preparations because unnecessary additives may cause allergic responses.
- Inspect skin monthly for suspicious-looking changes.

Personal care practices

- When bathing or showering, use soap sparingly or use a mild, unscented soap (e.g. Dove).
- Maintain water temperatures for bathing at about 32°C to 37.7°C (90°F to 100°F).
- Rinse well after using soap. Whirlpool baths stimulate circulation, but moderate temperatures should be maintained.
- Apply moisturising products after bathing, rather than using them in the bath water, to minimise the risk for falls on oily surfaces and to maximise the benefits of the emollient.
- Use emollient products containing petroleum or mineral oil (e.g. Vaseline).
- If you use bath oils, take extra safety precautions to prevent slipping.
- If moisturising products are applied to the feet, wear non-skid slippers or socks before walking.
- Dry your skin thoroughly, particularly between your toes and in other areas where your skin rubs together.
- When drying your skin, use gentle, patting motions rather than harsh, rubbing motions.
- Obtain regular podiatric care.

Avoiding sun damage

- Wear wide-brimmed hats, sun visors, sunglasses and long-sleeved garments when exposed to the sun.
- Wear clothing made of cotton, rather than polyester fabrics, because ultraviolet rays can penetrate polyester.
- Apply sunscreen lotions generously and frequently, beginning 1 hour before sun exposure.
- Use sunscreen lotions with an SPF of 30 or higher. Limit exposure to the sun between 10:00 a.m. and 3:00 p.m. to one hour weekly.
- Protect yourself from ultraviolet rays, even on cloudy days and when you are in the water.
- Artificial tanning booths use ultraviolet type-A rays, which are advertised as harmless, but which have been found to cause damage in high doses.

Preventing injury from abrasive forces

- Do not use starch, bleach or strong detergents when laundering clothing or linens.
- Use soft terry or cotton washcloths.
- If waterproof pads are necessary, make sure that an adequate amount of soft, absorbent material is placed near the body.

Promoting healthy skin

Because one's overall health significantly affects the condition of the skin, maintenance of optimal nutrition and hydration is an important intervention in the skin care of older adults. Health promotion interventions also address environmental factors and personal care practices that influence the condition of the skin. Box 23-5 can be used as a guide to teaching older adults, or carers of dependent older adults, about skin health. Although much of the nursing literature advocates limiting baths or showers to one to three times weekly, it is not clear that there is a cause–effect relationship between bathing or showers and dry skin. Other factors, including smoking, dehydration, sun exposure, low environmental humidity, and the use of harsh cleansing products, are likely to contribute to skin problems in older adults.

Currently there is controversy about health promotion recommendations related to exposure to sunlight because sunlight is required for vitamin D synthesis in humans and it is beneficial in treating seasonal affective disorder and many skin conditions, including psoriasis and fungal mycosis (Wilson, Moon & Armstrong, 2012). In contrast, it is a well-recognised cause of wrinkles, photoageing, all types of skin cancer and other skin conditions, as well as increased risk for diseases of other systems (e.g. cataracts, immunosuppression) (Al-Mutairi, Issa & Nair, 2012).

Concerns about vitamin D deficiency from lack of exposure to sunlight include increased incidence of or poor outcome for autoimmune conditions, infectious diseases, cardiovascular disease, and various types of cancers (e.g. skin, breast, and colon) (Mason & Reichrath, 2013). Current recommendations emphasise the importance of a balanced approach that encourages small amounts of sun exposure each day for adequate vitamin D synthesis, but not so much that would lead to increased skin cancer risk (Bonevski, Bryant, Lambert et al., 2013). Although questions have also been raised about the safety and efficacy of sunscreens, recent Food and Drug Administration regulatory guidelines emphasise the following (Jou, Feldman & Tomecki, 2012; Latha, Martis, Shobha et al., 2013):

- All sunscreening agents must be tested and meet requirements for claims about effectiveness.
- Claims for broad-spectrum agents must protect from both ultraviolet A and ultraviolet B rays.
- Claims for reduction of skin cancer and skin ageing can be made only with an SPF between 15 and 50.
- Claims of "waterproof", "sweatproof", or "sunblocks" are not permitted because they overemphasise the product's efficacy.
- Claims of "water resistant" need to be substantiated by tests for 40 or 80 minutes.

- Acceptable forms of sunscreen include oils, gels, sprays, creams, pastes, butters and ointment; forms that are *not* acceptable include wipes, powders, shampoos, towelettes and body washes.

Studies suggest that the use of sunscreens can prevent skin ageing and this is not a contributing factor for vitamin D deficiency (Hughes, Williams, Baker et al., 2013; Lin, Eder, Weinmann et al., 2011). This information can be incorporated in health education about use of sunscreens to protect older adults from skin cancer and other skin changes.

Preventing skin wrinkles

The best methods of preventing skin lesions and wrinkles are avoiding too much exposure to sunlight and using a sunscreen with a sun protection factor (SPF) of 15 or higher when exposure to sunlight is unavoidable. Topical products containing alpha- or beta-hydroxy acids may be beneficial in reversing wrinkles and promoting the regression of solar keratoses. Nurses need to be alert to the possibility that older adults might develop an allergic or sensitivity reaction to some of the ingredients in topical products. Information about the harmful effects of sunlight should be included in health education about the maintenance of healthy skin and prevention of undesirable cosmetic and pathological skin changes. Also, nurses can encourage people who are concerned about wrinkles and dry skin to discuss medical interventions with their primary care provider.

WELLNESS OPPORTUNITY

Nurses promote wellness by teaching that exposure to ultraviolet light—by sunlight or tanning lights—is a major factor in the occurrence of skin wrinkles, skin cancer and other skin changes.

Preventing dry skin

Petrolatum and other emollients are effective in alleviating dry skin discomfort, because they moisturise and lubricate the skin. The effectiveness of an emollient is based on its ability to prevent water evaporation, so the beneficial effects will be enhanced when it is applied to skin that already has some degree of moisture. Thus, an emollient agent is most effective when it is applied to moist skin immediately after bathing. See Box 23-5 for information on the use of emollients and other interventions designed to prevent or care for dry skin in older adults.

Detecting and treating harmful skin lesions

Early detection and treatment of cancerous or precancerous skin lesions are key factors in preventing serious functional consequences, because the cure rate for most skin cancers approaches 100% with early excision. The nurse's role is to detect any suspicious-looking lesions and to encourage or facilitate further evaluation. Nurses can encourage all older adults to use the following guide to identify for themselves any skin changes that require further evaluation:

- **A**symmetric shape: irregular or different-looking sides
- **B**order that is irregular: ragged, notched, blurred, irregular
- **C**olour change: different shades, uneven distribution
- **D**iameter: larger than a quarter of an inch (6 mm) and increasing.

If the older adult or caregiver has avoided medical evaluation because of fears about cancer, the nurse can provide reassurance about the high cure rate and the minimal chance of long-term problems if early treatment is obtained. Similarly, if they have ignored suspicious changes because they attribute them to "normal ageing", nurses can teach about the importance of further evaluation. Box 23-5 includes health promotion information about the prevention and early detection of skin cancer.

WELLNESS OPPORTUNITY

Nurses address the body–mind–spirit interrelationship by allaying unreasonable fears about skin cancer.

EVALUATING THE EFFECTIVENESS OF NURSING INTERVENTIONS

Nursing care for older adults with dry or itching skin is evaluated by determining the degree to which the interventions alleviate the person's complaints. It may take several weeks for older adults to feel the full effects of skincare interventions because of an age-related delay in derma response to external stimuli. Also, there is a great deal of individual variation among older adults in their response to interventions.

Thus, it may be necessary to evaluate the effects of one type of soap or lotion for several weeks before trying a different brand if the problem does not resolve. Because environmental humidity affects skin comfort, environmental conditions may also influence the evaluation of interventions.

The effectiveness of interventions for older adults at risk for skin breakdown is measured by the absence of skin tears, pressure ulcers or chronic wounds. The effectiveness of interventions for skin tears, pressure ulcers and chronic wounds is determined by the rate of healing and prevention of complications such as osteomyelitis. Because significant cost and quality-of-life issues are associated with pressure ulcers and other chronic wounds, preventing skin breakdown can have far-reaching positive consequences for older adults who are at risk for developing pressure ulcers.

UNFOLDING CASE STUDY

Part B

Mrs Swanke is now 92 years old and lives in a long-term residential care facility in Queensland. She ambulates with a walker and needs assistance with meals, medications and personal care. Three months ago, her doctor prescribed hydrochlorothiazide 25 mg every morning for isolated systolic hypertension. She has a history of osteoarthritis but does not take any medication for it. When she comes to see you, she complains of dry skin and discomfort.

Nursing assessment

You interview Ms Swanke about her personal care practices and find out that she soaks in the tub in lukewarm water three times weekly and enjoys using bath salts and perfumed skin lotions. She spends much of her leisure time outdoors on the patio. She does not use sunscreens because she thinks they are unnecessary and too oily. She states that she has not had sunburn for several years, and that she has built up a good tolerance to the sun. She does not wear sunglasses or sun hats. She reports that she has had three skin cancers removed in the past 10 years, one from her cheek, one from her arm and one from her ear lobe. She says she does not worry about recurrent skin cancer because she no longer swims outside or sits by the swimming pool. Also, because she does not get sunburned, she believes she is not at risk for skin cancer.

Inspection of Ms Swanke's skin reveals dry, wrinkled skin on her face and arms and unevenly tanned skin on her face, neck and extremities. She has many age spots over the exposed skin areas but no suspicious-looking lesions. Ms Swanke has blue eyes and fair skin.

Nursing issue

Your nursing issue is ineffective health maintenance related to excessive sunlight exposure and insufficient knowledge of the effects of ultraviolet light. Evidence for this comes from her misconceptions about risk factors for skin cancer and other skin problems. Also, you identify her lack of knowledge about the potential photosensitivity reactions associated with use of hydrochlorothiazide as a factor that contributes to ineffective health maintenance.

Nursing care plan for Ms Swanke

Goals for wellness outcomes	Nursing interventions	Nursing evaluation
Ms Swanke's discomfort from dry skin will be alleviated.	• Discuss and describe age-related skin changes. • Discuss risk factors that contribute to skin discomfort (e.g. bath, bath salts, perfumed lotions, unprotected exposure to sunlight) • Use Box 23-5 to teach Ms Swanke about skincare practices directed towards alleviating dry skin.	• Ms Swanke reports that she no longer experiences skin discomfort and dryness.
Ms Swanke's knowledge about risk factors for skin cancer will be increased.	• Discuss the relationship between skin cancer and exposure to ultraviolet rays. • Explain that any exposure to ultraviolet rays is a risk factor for skin cancer. • Emphasise that a history of skin cancer increases the chance of recurrent skin cancer.	• Ms Swanke verbalises an awareness of the risk factors for skin cancer.
The factors that increase Ms Swanke's risk of skin problems and skin cancer will be eliminated.	• Inform Ms Swanke that hydrochlorothiazide may increase the risk for photosensitivity, making protective measures increasingly important. • Use Box 23-5 as a guide for discussing measures to avoid sun damage. • Emphasise the importance of using sunscreens and wearing wide-brimmed hats when in the solarium or outside.	• Ms Swanke uses measures to reduce the risk for skin cancer and sun damage.

Thinking points

- What risk factors would you address in your care plan?
- How would you promote Ms Swanke's personal responsibility for skincare, including addressing risks for skin cancer?

CHAPTER HIGHLIGHTS

Age-related changes that affect skin wellness

- Decreased rate of epidermal proliferation
- Thinner dermis, flattened dermal–epidermal junction
- Diminished moisture content
- Decreased dermal blood supply
- Fewer sweat and sebaceous glands
- Decreased number of melanocytes and Langerhans cells
- Changes in patterns of hair distribution

Risk factors that affect skin wellness

- Genetic factors (hair colour and distribution, skin cancer)
- Exposure to ultraviolet radiation (sunlight or tanning light)
- Adverse medication effects
- Personal hygiene practices
- Factors that increase the risk for skin breakdown

Functional consequences affecting skin wellness

- Xerosis (dry skin), discomfort
- Irregular pigmentation and other cosmetic changes
- Increased susceptibility to injury, mechanical stress and effects of ultraviolet radiation
- Delayed wound healing, increased susceptibility to infection
- Decreased tactile sensitivity, increased susceptibility to burns
- Diminished sweating and shivering, increased susceptibility to hypothermia and heat-related conditions
- Increased risk for skin cancer
- Increased risk for breaks in skin integrity and pressure ulcers

Pathological conditions affecting skin wellness

- Skin cancer
- Skin tears
- Pressure ulcers
- Chronic wounds

Nursing assessment of skin

- Abnormal skin conditions
- Personal care practices
- Skin lesions common in older adults (Table 23-3, Fig. 23-5)
- Risk of skin tears, pressure ulcers (Figures 23-3 & 23-4) and chronic wounds
- Skin tear classification (Figure 23-2)
- Pressure area staging
- Chronic wound assessment: TIME

Nursing issues

- Willingness for enhanced knowledge: skin
- Impaired skin integrity (or risk for)
- Ineffective health maintenance

Goal planning for wellness outcomes

- Comfort level
- Tissue integrity: skin and mucous membranes
- Improved nutritional status
- Prevention of skin cancer, pressure areas, skin tears, chronic wounds
- Wound healing: primary or secondary

Nursing interventions for skin wellness

- Health promotion teaching about healthy skin
- Preventing skin wrinkles
- Preventing dry skin
- Detecting and treating suspect skin changes
- Preventing and managing skin tears
- Preventing and managing pressure ulcers/preventing and managing chronic wounds

Evaluating effectiveness of nursing interventions

- Alleviation of complaints (e.g. dryness)
- Evaluation of suspect skin changes
- Absence of skin tears
- Absence of pressure ulcers in high risk older adults
- Absence of chronic wounds
- Wound healing

CRITICAL THINKING EXERCISES

1. What changes would a healthy 85-year-old person notice with regard to his or her skin, hair and nails?
2. Describe the questions that you would ask and the observations you would make to assess the skin, hair and nails of an 82-year-old person.
3. Describe at least eight skin lesions that are normal and three skin lesions that require further evaluation.
4. You are asked to give a 20-minute presentation on "Maintaining Healthy Skin" to a group of retirees who belong to a community Probus club. Outline the content of your health education program.
5. What would you teach the family carers of a 74-year-old woman who sits in a wheelchair for 14 hours a day with regard to the prevention of pressure ulcers?

RESOURCES

For an extensive range of additional resources to enhance teaching and learning and to facilitate understanding of this chapter, please see the text's accompanying website located on thePoint at http://thepoint.lww.com.

Clinical tools

Hartford Institute for Geriatric Nursing, ConsultGeriRN.org
http://consultgerirn.org/resources
Try This® assessment series and *How to Try This* resources
General assessment series:
- *Try This*, issue 5: Predicting pressure ulcer risk. Ayello, E. A. (2012). *Best Practices in Nursing Care to Older Adults.*

- *How to Try This* (article): Predicting pressure ulcer risk. Stotts, N. A. & Gunningberg, L. (2007). *American Journal of Nursing, 107*(11), 40–48.
- *How to Try This* (video): *The Braden Scale.*

Evidence-based practice

Ayello, E. A. & Sibbald, R. G. (2012). Preventing pressure ulcers and skin tears. In M. Boltz, E. Capezuti, T. Fulmer & D. Zwicker (Eds), *Evidence-based geriatric nursing protocols for best practice* (4th ed., pp. 298–323). New York: Springer.

Joanna Briggs Institute: http://connect.jbiconnectplus.org

Best practice information sheets:

- Joanna Briggs Institute. (2007). Tropical skin care in aged care facilities. *Evidence-Based Practice Information Sheets for Health Professionals, 11*(3), 1–4.

Evidence summaries:

- Chu, V. (2014). Topical skin care for older people.
- Kunde, L. (2014). Skin tears: Prevention.
- Slade, S. (2014a). Pressure area care: Prevention.
- Slade, S. (2014b). Skin tears: Assessment and management.
- Peters, M. (2013). Skin tears (community setting): Prevention, assessment and initial management.
- Psaltos, S. (2014). Pressure area care: Management.

Recommended practices:

- Campbell, L. (2013). Pressure area care (older adult).
- Pressure area care: Turning an older person in bed (2013).
- Skin tears: Prevention (2013).
- Skin tears: Treatment (2013).

National Guideline Clearinghouse: www.guideline.gov

Search for:

- Early detection of cancers (including skin cancer). In *Guidelines for preventive activities in general practice* (8th ed.). (2012).
- Pressure ulcer prevention and treatment.
- Skin cancer prevention (2013).

Health education

Australian Wound Management Association: www.awma.com.au

American Cancer Society: www.cancer.org

Braden Scale: www.bradenscale.com

National Pressure Ulcer Advisory Panel (NPUAP): www.npuap.org

New Zealand Wound Care Society: www.nzwcs.org.nz

STAR—Skin Tear Classification System: www.silverchain.org.au

REFERENCES

Al-Mutairi, N., Issa, B. I. & Nair, V. (2012). Photoprotection and vitamin D status. *Indian Journal of Dermatology, Venereology and Leprology, 78*(3), 342–349.

Apold, J. & Rydrych, D. (2013). Preventing device-related pressure ulcers. *Journal of Nursing Care Quality, 27*(1), 28–34.

Australian Institute Health and Welfare (AIHW). (2010). *Cancer in Australia 2010: An overview.* Cancer series no. 60. Cat. no. CAN 56. Canberra: AIHW.

Ayello, E. A. & Sibbald, R. G. (2012). Preventing pressure ulcers and skin tears. In M. Boltz, E. Capezuti, T. Fulmer & D. Zwicker (Eds), *Evidence-based practice protocols for best practice* (4th ed., pp. 298–323). New York: Springer.

Bergstrom, N., Braden, B. J., Laguzza, A. & Holman, V. (1987). The Braden Scale for Predicting Pressure Sore Risk. *Nursing Research, 36*(4), 205–210.

Berwick, M. & Erdei, E. (2009). Melanoma epidemiology and public health. *Dermatologic Clinic, 27*(2), 205–214.

Black, J., Berke, C. & Urzendowski, G. (2012). Pressure ulcer incidence and progression in critically ill subjects. *Journal of Wound, Ostomy and Continence Nursing, 39*(3), 267–273.

Bonevski, B., Bryant, J., Lambert, S. et al. (2013). The ABC of vitamin D: A qualitative study of the knowledge and attitudes regarding vitamin D deficiency amongst selected population groups. *Nutrients, 5*, 915–927.

Boyer, D. (2013). Cultural considerations in advanced wound care. *Advances in Skin & Wound Care, 26*(3), 110–111.

Braga, I. A., Pirett, C. C., Ribas, R. M. et al. (2013). Bacterial colonization of pressure ulcers: Assessment of risk for bloodstream infection and impact on patient outcomes. *Journal of Hospital Infections, 83*(4), 314–320.

Briggs, M., Collinson, M., Wilson, L. et al. (2013). The prevalence of pain at pressure areas and pressure ulcers in hospitalized patients. *BMC Nursing, 12*(1), 19.

Bry, K. E., Buescher, D. & Sandrik, M. (2012). Never say never: A descriptive study of hospital-acquired pressure ulcers in a hospital setting. *Journal of Wound, Ostomy, and Continence Nursing, 39*(3), 274–280.

Carville, K. & Smith, J. (2004). A report on the effectiveness of comprehensive wound assessment and documentation in the community. *Primary Intention*, 12(1), 41–49.

Carville, K., Lewin, G., Newall, N., Haslehurst, P., Michael, R., Santamaria, N. & Roberts, P. (2007). STAR: A consensus for skin tear classification. *Primary Intention, 15*(1), 18–28.

Chang, A. L., Wong, J. W., Endo, J. O. et al. (2013). Geriatric dermatology review: Major changes in skin function in older patients and their contribution to common clinical challenges. *Journal of the American Medical Directors Association, 14*(10), 724–730.

Chou, R., Dana, T., Bougatsos, C. et al. (2013). *Pressure ulcer risk assessment and prevention: Comparative effectiveness.* Publication no. 12(13)-EHC148-EF. Rockville, MD: Agency for Healthcare Quality and Research.

Cox, J. (2012). Predictive power of the Braden Scale for Pressure Sore Risk in adult critical care patients. *Journal of Wound, Ostomy, and Continence Nursing, 39*(6), 613–621.

Coyer, F. M., Stotts, N. A. & Blackman, V. S. (2013). A prospective window into medical device-related pressure ulcers in intensive care. *International Wound Journal, 11*(6), 656–664.

Durai, P. C., Thappa, D. M., Kumari, R. et al. (2012). Aging in elderly: Chronological versus photoaging. *Indian Journal of Dermatology, 57*(5), 343–352.

Edwards, L. & Lynch, P. J. (2011). *Genital dermatology atlas*. Philadelphia, PA: Lippincott Williams & Wilkins.

European Pressure Ulcer Advisory Panel and National Pressure Ulcer Advisory Panel. (2009). Prevention and treatment of pressure ulcers. Available from www.npuap.org.

Gadd, M. M. (2012). Preventing hospital-acquired pressure ulcers. *Journal of Wound, Ostomy, and Continence Nursing, 39*(3), 292–294.

Gatherwright, J., Liu, M. T., Amirlak, B. et al. (2013). The contribution of endogenous and exogenous factors to male alopecia: A study of identical twins. *Plastic and Reconstructive Surgery, 131*(5), 794e–801e.

Gatherwright, J., Liu, M. T., Gliniak, C. et al. (2012). The contribution of endogenous and exogenous factors to female alopecia: A study of identical twins. *Plastic and Reconstructive Surgery, 130*(6), 1219–1226.

Geller, A. C. (2009). Educational and screening campaigns to reduce deaths from melanoma. *Hematology/Oncology Clinics of North America, 23*(3), 515–527.

Goodheart, H. P. (2009). *Goodheart's photoguide of common skin disorders*. Philadelphia: Lippincott Williams & Wilkins.

Hughes, M. C., Williams, G. M., Baker, P. et al. (2013). Sunscreen and prevention of skin aging: A randomized trial. *Annals of Internal Medicine, 158*(11), 781–790.

Institute for Clinical Systems Improvement (ICSI). (2012). Pressure ulcer prevention and treatment protocol. Bloomington (MN): Author. Available March 2015 at www.guideline.gov/content.aspx?id=36059.

Jou, P. C., Feldman, R. J. & Tomecki, K. J. (2012). UV protection and sunscreens: What to tell patients. *Cleveland Clinic Journal of Medicine, 79*(6), 427–435.

Kelechi, T. J., Arndt, J. V. & Dove, A. (2013). Review of pressure ulcer risk assessment scales. *Journal of Wound, Ostomy, and Continence Nurses Society, 40*(3), 232–236.

Kelleher, A. D., Moorer, A. & Makic, M. F. (2012). Peer-to-peer nursing rounds and hospital-acquired pressure ulcer prevalence in a surgical intensive care unit. *Journal of Wound, Ostomy, and Continence Nurses Society, 39*(2), 152–157.

Kunde, L. (2014). Skin tears: Prevention. Evidence summary. ID JBI 1659. Joanna Briggs Institute. Available March 2015 via http://joannabriggs.org.

Latha, M. S., Martis, J., Shobha, V. et al. (2013). Sunscreening agents: A review. *Journal of Clinical and Aesthetic Dermatology, 6*(11), 16–24.

Latreille, J., Kesse-Guyot, E., Malvy, D. et al. (2012). Dietary monounsaturated fatty acids intake and risk of skin photoaging. *PLoS One, 7*(9), e44490.

LeBlanc, K. & Baranoski, S. (2009). Prevention and management of skin tears. *Advances in Skin & Wound Care 22*(7), 325–332.

LeBlanc, K., Baranoski, S., Christensen, D. et al. (2013). International Skin Tear Advisory Panel: A tool kit to aid in the prevention, assessment, and treatment of skin tears using a Simplified Classification System©. *Advances in Skin and Wound Care, 26*(1), 459–476.

LeBlanc, K., Baranoski, S., Holloway, S. & Langemo, D. (2013). Validation of a new classification system for skin tears. *Advances in Skin & Wound Care, 26*(6), 263–266.

Lin, J. S., Eder, M., Weinmann, S. et al. (2011). Behavioral counseling to prevent skin cancer: A systematic review for the U.S. Preventive Services Task Force. Evidence syntheses number 82. *Annals of Internal Medicine, 154*(3), 190–201.

Liu, P., He, W. & Chen, H.-L. (2012). Diabetes mellitus as a risk factor for surgery-related pressure ulcers. *Journal of Wound, Ostomy, and Continence Nurses Society, 39*(5), 495–499.

Lyder, C. H., Wang, Y., Metersky, M. et al. (2012). Hospital-acquired pressure ulcers: Results from the national Medicare Patient Safety Monitoring System study. *Journal of the American Geriatrics Society, 60*(9), 1603–1608.

Mason, R. S. & Reichrath, J. (2013). Sunlight vitamin D and skin cancer. *Anticancer Agents in Medicinal Chemistry, 13*(1), 83–97.

Medical Education Partnership (MEP) Ltd. (2008). *Wound infection in clinical practice: A WUWHS international consensus*. Principles of best practice series. London: Wounds International/Schofield Healthcare Media Ltd. Accessed March 2015 via www.woundsinternational.com.

National Pressure Ulcer Advisory Panel (NPUAP). (2009). Prevention and treatment of pressure ulcers: Clinical practice guideline. Washington, DC: National Pressure Ulcer Advisory Panel.

Payne, R. & Martin, M. (1993). Defining and classifying skin tears: Need for a common language … a critique and revision of the Payne-Martin Classification System for Skin Tears. *Ostomy Wound Management, 39*(5), 16–20.

Posthauer, M. E., Collins, N., Dorner, B. et al. (2013). Nutritional strategies for frail older adults. *Advances in Skin & Wound Care, 26*(3), 128–140.

Rosenthal, T. C., Williams, M. E. & Naughton, B. J. (2007). *Office care geriatrics*. Philadelphia, PA: Lippincott Williams & Wilkins.

Schultz. G. & Dowset, C. (2012). Wound bed preparation revisited. *Wounds International, 3*(1), 25–29.

Silver Chain Nursing Association & School of Nursing & Midwifery, Curtin University of Technology. (2010). STAR: Skin Tear Classification System. Viewed March 2015 at www.silverchain.org.au/assets/group/research/STAR-Skin-Tear-tool-04022010.pdf.

Tescher, A., Branca, M., Byrne, T., et al. (2012). All at-risk patients are not created equal. *Journal of Wound, Ostomy, and Continence Nursing, 39*(3), 282–291.

Theisen, S., Drabik, A. & Stock, S. (2012). Pressure ulcers in older hospitalised patients and its impact on length of stay: A retrospective observational study. *Journal of Clinical Nursing, 21*(3/4), 380–387.

Tschannen, D., Bates, O. Talsma, A. et al. (2012). Patient-specific and surgical characteristics in the development of pressure ulcers. *American Journal of Critical Care, 21*, 116–125.

Tucker, M. A. (2009). Melanoma epidemiology. *Hematology/Oncology Clinics of North America, 23*, 383–395.

Turk, B. G., Gunaydin, A., Ertam, I. & Ozturk, G. (2013). Adverse cutaneous drug reactions among hospitalized patients: Five year surveillance. *Cutaneous and Ocular Toxicology, 32*(1), 41–45.

Vierkotter, A. & Kurtmann, J. (2012). Environmental influences on skin aging and ethnic-specific manifestations. *Dermatology & Endocrinology, 4*(3), 227–231.

Weber, J. & Kelley, J. (2002). *Health assessment in nursing* (2nd ed.). Philadelphia, PA: Lippincott Williams & Wilkins.

Werdin, F., Tennenhaus, M., Schaller, H. E. & Rennekampff, H. O. (2009). Evidence-based management strategies for treatment of chronic wounds. *Open Access Journal of Plastic Medicine, 9*, 169–179. Viewed March 2015 at www.ncbi.nlm.nih.gov/pmc/articles/PMC2691645/pdf/eplasty09e19.pdf.

Wilson, B. D., Moon, S. & Armstrong, F. (2012). Comprehensive review of ultraviolet radiation and the current status on sunscreens. *Journal of Clinical and Aesthetic Dermatology, 5*(9), 18–22.

WoundsWest. (2011). Wounds in WA: The facts. Viewed March 2015 at www.health.wa.gov.au/woundswest/facts/index.cfm.

Xu, X., Lau, K., Taira, B. R. & Singer, A. J. (2009). The current management of skin tears. *American Journal of Emergency Medicine, 27*(6), 729–733.

Chapter 24

Sleep and rest

By Carol Miller and Sharyn Hunter

LEARNING OBJECTIVES

After reading this chapter, you should be able to:

1. Delineate age-related changes that affect sleep and rest patterns in older adults.
2. Identify psychosocial, environmental and physiological risk factors that influence sleep and rest in older adults.
3. Discuss sleep changes and problems common in older adults.
4. Assess sleep patterns in older adults to identify opportunities for health promotion to improve sleep.
5. Identify nursing interventions to promote optimal sleep and to address risks that interfere with sleep in older adults.

KEY POINTS

advanced sleep phase
circadian rhythm
Epworth Sleepiness Scale (ESS)
excessive daytime sleepiness (EDS)
obstructive sleep apnoea (OSA)
insomnia
periodic limb movements in sleep (PLMS)
Pittsburgh Sleep Quality Index (PSQI)
restless legs syndrome (RLS)
sleep latency

Approximately one-third of a person's lifetime is spent in sleep and rest activities, yet little attention is paid to the essential physiological and psychosocial functions accomplished through these activities. During periods of sleep and rest, many metabolic processes decelerate, production of growth hormone increases and tissue repair and protein synthesis accelerate. During the deeper stages of sleep, cognitive and emotional information is stored, filtered and organised. Thus, the quantity and quality of sleep affect many aspects of wellness.

Before the 1930s, research on sleep was non-existent, and nocturnal sleep was viewed as the absence of daytime activity, rather than as an activity in its own right. In the 1950s, our understanding of sleep patterns improved significantly based on polygraphic measurements that identified sleep cycles. By the 1960s, scientists had identified rapid eye movement (REM), non-rapid eye movement (NREM) and waking stages as three distinct states of consciousness. In the 1970s, sleep disorder centres were established to conduct research on sleep and offer comprehensive evaluation and treatment programs for people suffering from sleep disorders. In Australia and New Zealand there are sleep research and sleep disorder centres. The sleep disorder centres are usually privately owned, and offer assessment and treatment of a range of sleep disorders.

In the beginning of the 21st century, print and broadcast media focused public attention on the detrimental effects of sleep deprivation and the large numbers of people affected by inadequate sleep. Numerous Internet sites sprang up, and *sleep apnoea syndrome* became part of the common language.

Now, healthcare practitioners are likely to address sleep-related concerns and refer the older adult for comprehensive sleep studies as a health promotion intervention. Because older adults are as likely as younger adults to benefit from newer information and technology, it is important to understand the specific sleep problems of older adults so that they too can take advantage of the most recent approaches to addressing this important health-related quality-of-life concern.

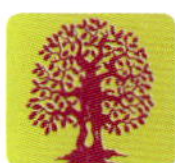

AGE-RELATED CHANGES THAT AFFECT SLEEP AND REST PATTERNS

Half a century of sleep research has provided a strong base of information about age-related changes in sleep patterns, as well as the many sleep disorders that affect older adults. Sleep patterns of older adults are affected by complex relationships among a wide range of physiological, environmental and psychosocial factors. This section describes age-related changes in sleep characteristics according to the quantity of time spent in bed and the depth and quality of sleep.

Sleep quantity

Sleep efficiency, or the percentage of time asleep during the time in bed, influences perceived quality of sleep. Sleep efficiency ranges from 80% to 90% for younger people but diminishes to 50% to 70% for older people (Misra & Malow, 2008). This diminished sleep efficiency is attributed both to prolonged **sleep latency**, which is the time required to fall asleep, and to an increased number of awakenings during the night. Beginning in the fourth

Promoting sleep wellness in older adults

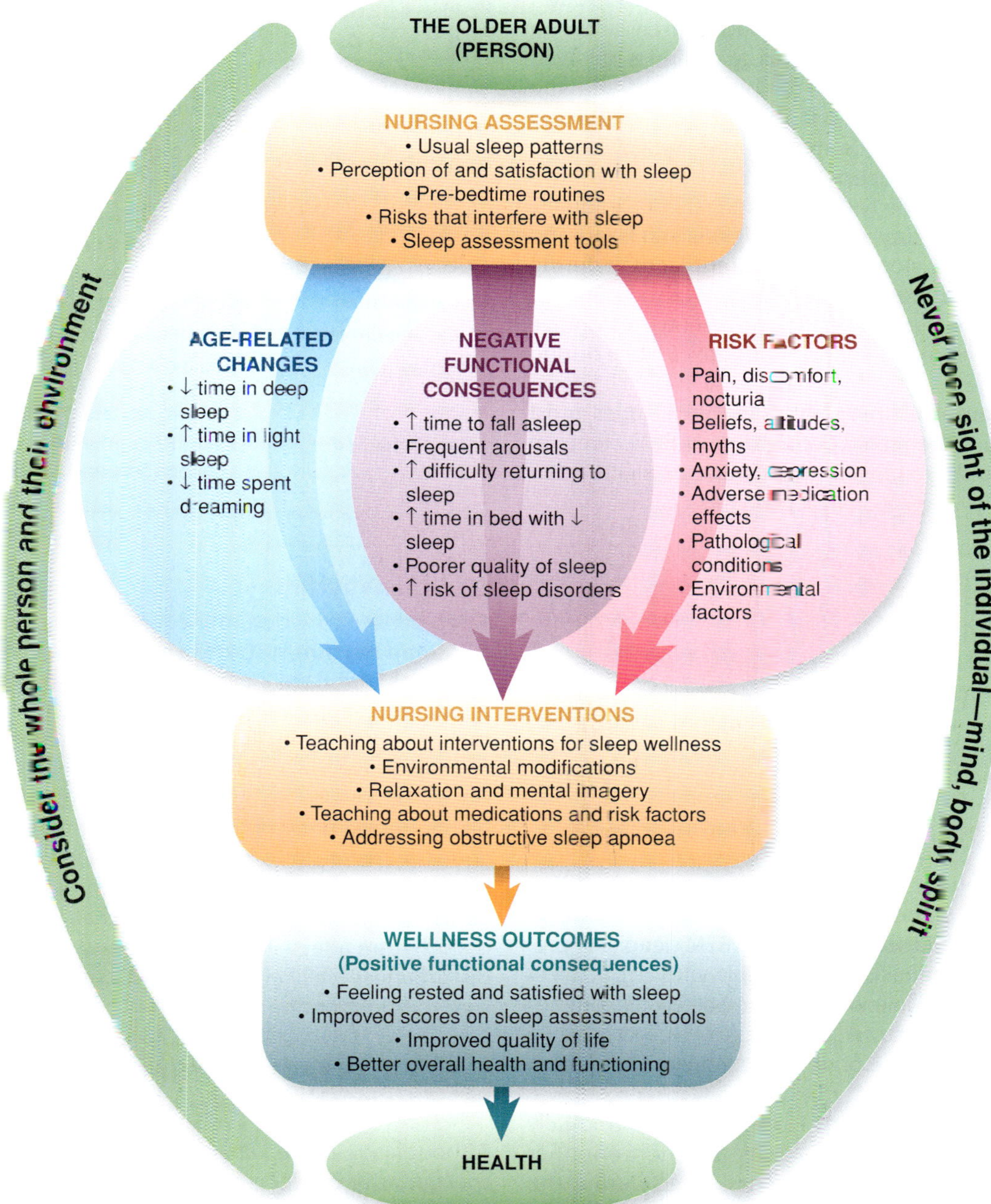

decade, the ability to initiate and maintain sleep gradually declines, with an average loss of 28 minutes per decade of life (Espiritu, 2008).

Older adults spend increasing amounts of time in bed, with a decreasing proportion of time in actual sleep. One study found a 28-minute decrease in sleep duration for each decade between the ages of 16 years and 83 years (Van Cauter et al., 2008). Other studies indicate that healthy older adults take more daytime naps and spend approximately 1 hour per day napping (Espiritu, 2008). Beneficial effects of daytime naps in older adults include compensation for less night time sleep, improved overall functioning and improved alertness and less daytime sleepiness.

Sleep quality

Nocturnal sleep patterns are described in terms of sleep cycles and sleep stages. Each sleep cycle, which lasts between 70 and 120 minutes, is a combination of sleep stages. Sleep stages are classified according to the presence or absence of REMs. A typical cycle consists of four

NREM stages and one REM stage (also called the dream stage). At the beginning of each cycle, the NREM stages occur sequentially from stage I (lightest sleep) through stage IV (deepest sleep). These stages then occur in reverse order until stage I is reached again and is followed by REM sleep. The cycle repeats during the night, with the length of REM increasing and the length of stages III and IV gradually diminishing (i.e. more time is spent in dream stage and less time in deeper NREM stages as the night progresses). During the NREM stages, muscles gradually relax, body systems function at low levels and heart and respiratory rates are slower and more regular than during REM or waking periods. Stages III and IV (also known as delta sleep) are the deepest stages, and essential restorative functions and the release of hormones take place during the fourth stage.

Although some dreaming occurs in NREM stages, most active and vivid dreaming occurs during REM sleep. In addition to rapid eye movement, REM sleep is characterised by the following physiological changes:

- Flaccid muscles
- Fluctuating blood pressure
- Diminished thermoregulatory functions
- Increased gastric acid secretions
- Production of more highly concentrated urine
- An approximately 40% increase in cerebral blood flow
- Irregular and increased rate and rhythm of pulse and respirations
- Clitoral engorgement and increased vaginal blood flow (in women)
- Penile tumescence (in men).

The physiological alterations that occur during REM may exacerbate some medical problems. For example, increased gastric acid secretion during REM sleep may precipitate gastrointestinal pain for people with peptic ulcer disease. Likewise, people with chronic obstructive pulmonary disease (COPD) may experience dyspnoea or even a respiratory crisis because of decreased oxygen saturation during REM periods.

Because the length of stage I sleep increases gradually throughout adulthood, older adults experience longer periods of drowsiness without actual sleep during the early part of the night. In addition, older adults shift more frequently in and out of lighter sleep stages. Between the ages of 20 and 40 years old, the proportion of deep sleep (stages III and IV) decreases gradually until the age of 70 years, when it levels off. In both younger and older adults, stage IV sleep increases significantly during the night after sleep loss. The number of episodes of REM sleep does not change significantly in older adults, but episodes are shorter, resulting in proportionately less time spent in REM. Also, REM sleep stages shift towards the earlier part of the night in older adults. Table 24-1 summarises the usual adult sleep cycle and typical age-related changes in sleep patterns.

TABLE 24-1 Age-related changes in sleep

Sleep characteristics	Healthy older adults (versus healthy younger adults)
NREM	
Stages I and II (light sleep)	Gradual increase in quantity, so it accounts for 70% of total sleep time
Stages III and IV (deep sleep)	Proportionate decrease in quantity
REM (dream stage)	Proportionate decrease in quantity Begins earlier in the night Less intense
Sleep initiation	Longer time to fall asleep
Sleep maintenance	More frequent arousals
Sleep efficiency	Reduced amount of sleep during time in bed, more time in napping to compensate
Sleep schedule	Shift in nocturnal sleep phase to earlier bedtime and wakening

NREM, non-rapid eye movement; REM, rapid eye movement.

Circadian rhythm

Sleep patterns are determined, in part, by an individual's **circadian rhythm**, also known as a *biological clock*. Body functions that have a circadian pattern include thermoregulation, sleep–wake cycles and secretion of many hormones, including cortisol and melatonin. The sleep–wake circadian rhythm generally causes adults to become sleepy between 10 p.m. and midnight, and to awaken feeling rested between 6 a.m. and 8 a.m. With increasing age, **advanced sleep phase** occurs, causing older adults to become sleepy earlier in the evening and to awaken earlier in the morning. Age-related alterations in circadian rhythm affect sleep quantity and quality, and these disturbances are likely to be exacerbated by lack of exposure to bright light.

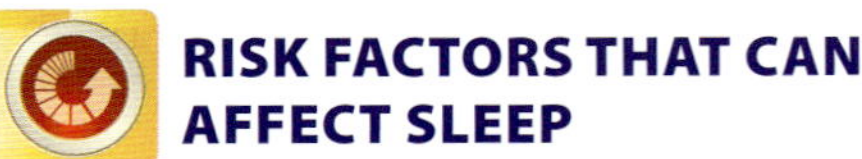

RISK FACTORS THAT CAN AFFECT SLEEP

Although age-related changes affect both the quality and the quantity of sleep, they do not necessarily lead to sleep complaints in healthy older adults. For example, in a study of 180 centenarians, 57.4% reported good quality sleep (Tafaro et al., 2007). Rather, the common complaint of sleep problems among older adults is associated with the many psychosocial or physiological risk factors that frequently affect older adults. In addition, environmental conditions, particularly in institutional settings, can significantly affect the sleep patterns of older adults. Many older adults experience sleep complaints due to several interacting risk factors. One study found that 69% of residents of assisted living facilities reported sleep disturbance, 42% reported primary insomnia and 35% reported daytime sleepiness, with an association between more functional impairment and sleep complaints (Martin et al., 2008).

Psychosocial factors

Beliefs and attitudes about sleep can have a powerful impact, with many beliefs having a detrimental, anxiety-producing effect. For example, older adults who believe that arousals during the night are abnormal and unhealthy may think they have **insomnia** and seek treatment with medications. Rigid beliefs about the amount of sleep required during the night can also lead to false definitions of insomnia and inappropriate treatment. Likewise, excessive worry about the quantity or quality of sleep can have a negative impact on sleep.

Anxiety, dementia and depression are psychosocial disorders associated with disrupted sleep. Anxiety and dementia are associated with difficulty falling asleep, frequent arousals during the night and difficulty returning to sleep. In addition, people with dementia are likely to experience the following sleep alterations: increased time in light sleep stages, very little REM and deep sleep, decreased total sleep time, disrupted sleep–wake cycles and frequent night time arousals and daytime napping. Sleep changes associated with dementia vary according to dementia severity, as discussed in more detail in Chapter 14. Compared with people unaffected by depression, people who are depressed typically take longer to fall asleep, have less deep sleep and more light sleep, awaken more frequently during the night and earlier in the morning and feel less rested in the morning.

Older adults with few or no interesting activities, work demands, social responsibilities or environmental stimuli may find it particularly difficult to establish healthy sleeping patterns. Older adults with dementia or depression who are living alone are particularly susceptible to disturbed sleep patterns because of the tendency to stay in bed during the day out of boredom, lack of motivation, difficulty concentrating on interesting activities or a desire to withdraw from stressful situations. Finally, in any setting, if an older adult spends all of his or her time in the same room, the lack of differentiation between space for waking and sleeping activities may interfere with sleep patterns.

Environmental factors

Environmental circumstances are another factor that can significantly influence sleep patterns. For people who do not live alone, the actions and demands of other people in the setting, particularly those sharing the same sleeping area, influence sleep patterns. For adults at any age, a change in the sleep environment usually requires a period of adjustment before optimal sleep patterns are established. Thus, older adults may have a particularly difficult time sleeping during the first few nights in a new environment.

In institutional settings, a lack of quiet and privacy, the conflicting needs of various people and sleeping in close proximity to others are all factors that can interfere with sleep. Older adults who are accustomed to sleeping alone or with close relations may feel their privacy is being violated in institutional settings where they are required to share a room with people from outside their family.

Difficulty falling asleep may also arise if environmental circumstances do not allow the performance of usual pre-bedtime activities, such as listening to music or reading a book. Schedules of carers/caregivers may also interfere with the sleeping habits of the older adult. For example, in institutional settings, the time for awakening patients/residents is often based on the most efficient use of nursing and dietary time, and patients/residents are expected to adjust their sleep routines accordingly. Likewise, in home settings, dependent older adults may have to adjust their sleep routines to the schedule of their carers, who may have work and other responsibilities.

Uncomfortably low or high temperatures, which are often related to inadequate heating or cooling systems, are another environmental factor that can interfere with sleep. Hot and humid conditions can contribute to sleep disturbances in menopausal women by increasing the number of night time hot flushes. Noise is another environmental factor that can be more problematic for older adults because, around the age of 40 years, people become more sensitive to noise when they are sleeping and can be awakened by less intense auditory stimuli.

Lighting exerts a strong influence on circadian rhythms and can affect sleep patterns in several ways. During the night, excessive light in rooms and hallways, as well as intermittent use of bedside or overhead lighting during care routines, may disrupt sleep. During the day, a lack of sufficient bright light can interfere with night time sleep because exposure to bright light is a strong influence on the circadian rhythm. The strong effect of light on sleep is associated with the fact that the body needs light to produce melatonin, a hormone that regulates many physiological functions, including sleep, body temperature and the setting of the circadian rhythm. Lack of exposure to bright light is especially problematic in long-term care settings because residents are typically exposed to only a few minutes of bright light daily and daytime light levels tend to be quite low (Martin & Ancoli-Israel 2008).

In home settings, environmental factors can interfere with the sleep of older adults. For example, older adults who are carers may have their sleep interrupted by dependent family members who require care during the night. Conditions such as fear, loneliness or neighbourhood noise are environmental factors that can interfere with sleep in home settings. In any of these situations, a move to an institution may provide the supports and security needed for more peaceful sleeping.

Pathophysiological conditions and functional impairments

Pathological conditions interfere with sleep and increase the risk for sleep-related disorders for many different reasons, as delineated in Table 24-2. In addition to these conditions that directly interfere with sleep, many pathological

TABLE 24-2 Pathophysiological factors affecting sleep

Risk factor	Sleep alteration
Arthritis	Chronic pain and discomfort that interfere with sleep
COPD	Awakening as a result of apnoea and respiratory distress
Diabetes mellitus	Awakening secondary to nocturia or poorly controlled blood glucose levels; increased incidence of OSA
Gastrointestinal disorders, ulcers	Nocturnal pain secondary to increased gastric secretions during REM sleep
Hypertension	Early morning awakening
Hyperthyroidism	Increased difficulty falling asleep
Nocturnal angina	Awakening without perception of pain, especially during REM sleep
PLMS, RLS	Awakening caused by recurrent involuntary leg movements
Malignancies	Increased incidence of RLS
Chronic kidney disease	Increase incidence of PLMS, RLS and OSA
Parkinsonism	Increased time awake; decreased amount of sleep
Dementia	Alterations of all sleep stages
Delirium	Increased somnolence *or* inability to sleep

COPD, chronic obstructive pulmonary disease; OSA, obstructive sleep apnoea; PLMS, periodic limb movements in sleep; REM, rapid eye movement; RLS, restless legs syndrome.

conditions are strongly associated with sleep problems, but the cause–effect relationship is unclear. For example, conditions that impair physical or cognitive function (e.g. dementia, Parkinson's disease) have underlying pathophysiological mechanisms that are similar to those involved with sleep disorders (e.g. restless legs syndrome [RLS], circadian rhythm sleep disorders) (Watson & Viola-Saltzman, 2013). There is a strong correlation between lower level of functioning and poor sleep in residents of long-term residential care, but the relationship between these variables is unclear (Fung, Martin, Chung et al., 2012; Valenza et al., 2013). *Nocturia* (discussed in Chapter 19), a common occurrence in older adults, is significantly associated with decreased quantity and quality of sleep (Zeitzer, Bliwise, Hernandez et al., 2013).

WELLNESS OPPORTUNITY

Nurses promote wellness by identifying subtle risk factors, such as chronic pain and discomfort, which are often overlooked and which can be addressed through many types of holistic interventions.

Obstructive sleep apnoea (OSA) is a specific sleep disorder that affects many older adults and is discussed in the section on pathological conditions affecting sleep. In recent years, researchers and clinicians have focused on two sleep-related movement disorders, restless legs syndrome (RLS) and periodic limb movements during sleep (PLMS), which are strongly associated with sleep disturbances. Increased age is a risk factor for both RLS and PLMS, and symptoms may increase over time. Researchers are currently exploring a potential causative relationship between dopamine deficiency and RLS and PLMS (Bliwise, Trotti, Yesavage et al., 2012; Silber, 2013).

Restless legs syndrome, also known as *Willis-Ekbom disease*, is characterised by an almost irresistible urge to move the legs, which is often accompanied by unpleasant leg sensations. Symptoms of RLS occur in a circadian rhythm, with peak severity during the evening and night, which can interfere with both initiating and maintaining sleep. During waking hours, RLS disrupts periods of rest and relaxation. An additional characteristic is that the symptoms are not due to another condition such as leg cramps, fibromyalgia, arthritis or positional discomfort. Risk factors for RLS include genetic predisposition, iron deficiency, chronic renal failure, peripheral neuropathy, and adverse effects of medications (e.g. most antidepressants, antipsychotic agents, and possibly antihistamines) (Silber, 2013). In addition to causing major sleep problems, RLS is associated with increased risk for anxiety, depression and hypertension (Gupta, Lahan & Goel, 2013; Salas & Kwan, 2012).

Periodic limb movements during sleep, also known as *nocturnal myoclonus*, is the occurrence of brief muscle contractions, spaced at intervals of about 20 to 40 seconds, which cause leg jerks or rhythmic movements of muscles in the foot or leg. They may occur several times to more than 200 times nightly, with increased occurrence during the first half of the night. PLMS can contribute to complaints of insomnia, frequent arousals and increased daytime sleepiness. They also are associated with increased risk for cardiovascular disease (Koo et al., 2011). In addition to increased age as a risk factor, PLMS is more common in people with RLS, diabetes, Parkinson's disease, Lewy body dementia, and sleep disorders (Hibi et al., 2012; Roux, 2013; Silber, 2013).

Effects of pharmacological and other substances

Adverse effects of medications and other substances can interfere with sleep in a number of ways. Prescription

TABLE 24-3 The effects of various medications and other chemicals on sleep

Medication or chemical	Sleep alteration
Alcohol	Suppression of REM sleep; early morning awakening
Alcohol or hypnotic withdrawal	Sleep disturbances; nightmares
Anticholinergics	Hyperreflexia; overactivity; muscle twitching
Barbiturates	Suppression of REM sleep; nightmares; hallucinations; paradoxical responses
Benzodiazepines	Awakening secondary to apnoea
Beta-blockers	Nightmares
Corticosteroids	Restlessness; sleep disturbances
Diuretics	Awakening for nocturia; sleep apnoea secondary to alkalosis
Theophylline, levodopa, isoprenaline, phenytoin	Interference with sleep onset and sleep stages
Antidepressants	PLMS; suppression of REM sleep

PLMS, periodic limb movements in sleep; REM, rapid eye movement.

medications that can cause disturbed sleep include steroids, antidepressants, aminophylline preparations, thyroid extracts, antiarrhythmic medications, and centrally acting antihypertensives. These effects are not unique to older adults; however adverse effects of medication are more likely to occur in older adults, as discussed in detail in Chapter 8.

Caffeine is a central nervous system stimulant that lengthens the sleep latency period and causes awakening during the night. Although low doses of nicotine can have relaxing and sedative effects, higher doses interfere with sleep because of nicotine's stimulant effect as well as its effects on respiration. Alcoholic beverages initially induce drowsiness but also suppress REM sleep and cause frequent awakenings, resulting in less total sleep and more daytime sleepiness. People who abstain from alcohol after long-term abuse may experience insomnia for a few years after withdrawing from it. Alcohol and other central nervous system depressants can exacerbate sleep disorders and lead to additional detrimental effects.

Table 24-3 summarises the effects of various medications and other chemicals on sleep in older adults.

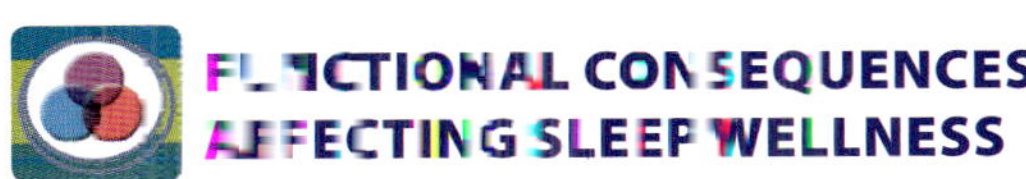

FUNCTIONAL CONSEQUENCES AFFECTING SLEEP WELLNESS

The overall functional consequences of age-related changes in sleep are insufficient, inefficient, and poor quality sleep, as summarised in Table 24-1. In addition, the high prevalence of risk factors that can interfere with sleep increases the vulnerability of older adults to sleep disorders and complaints. Common sleep complaints of older adults include daytime sleepiness, difficulty falling asleep, and frequent arousals during the night. Studies indicate that significant sleep problems affect 25% to 30% of the adult population (National Center on Sleep Disorders Research, 2011). Health consequences of poor sleep include impaired cognitive functions and increased risk for stroke, cancer, obesity, diabetes, depression, metabolic syndrome, substance abuse and all-cause mortality (Harand, Bertran, Doidy et al., 2012; Hung, Yang, Ou et al., 2013; Mander, Rao, Lu et al., 2013; National Center on Sleep Disorders Research, 2011).

Depression is a condition that is strongly associated with sleep problems but it is difficult to determine if it is a risk for or functional consequence (i.e. cause or effect) of sleep problems. People who are depressed take longer to fall asleep, have less deep sleep and more light sleep, awaken more frequently during the night and earlier in the morning, and feel less rested in the morning. Although these sleep problems are commonly viewed as symptoms of depression, recent studies suggest that depression in older adults is a consequence of sleep disorders, particularly insomnia and excessive daytime sleepiness (EDS) (Baglioni & Riemann, 2012; Jaussent, Bouyer, Ancelin et al., 2011).

PATHOLOGICAL CONDITIONS AFFECTING SLEEP: SLEEP DISORDERS

In the late 1970s, sleep disorders were classified systematically and standards were established to diagnose these disorders. **Insomnia** is a chronic or acute sleep disorder characterised by a complaint of poor sleep quality or difficulty initiating or maintaining sleep that causes daytime impairment. Because people with chronic insomnia experience symptoms during the night and day, it is considered a 24-hour condition (Neubauer, 2013). The prevalence of insomnia is 10% to 20% with about half of those having a chronic course (Buysse, 2013).

Excessive daytime sleepiness, defined as the inability to maintain alertness, is characterised by hypersomnolence (i.e. falling asleep at periodic intervals during a 24-hour period). EDS differs from fatigue, which manifests as difficulty sustaining a high level of functioning. An evidence-based geriatric nursing protocol for best practice states that daytime sleepiness should not be dismissed as an insignificant condition; rather, it should be evaluated by healthcare providers because it can have significant health effects (Chasens & Umlauf, 2012). Evidence-based practice 24-1 summarises guidelines for nursing assessment and interventions related to EDS.

Obstructive sleep apnoea is a sleep disorder that has been the focus of much research and clinical attention since 1988, when the U.S. Congress established the National Commission on Sleep Disorders Research. Primary

EVIDENCE-BASED PRACTICE 24-1
Excessive sleepiness

Statement of the problem

- Healthy older adults experience the following changes in sleep: an increase in transient arousals, longer time until sleep onset and stage 1 sleep, and decrease in quantity and quality of restorative slow-wave sleep.
  - Excessive sleepiness—defined as the inability to maintain alertness or vigilance because of hypersomnolence—is common in older adults.
- Primary causes of excessive sleepiness include OSA, insomnia and RLS.
  - Secondary causes include medications, psychiatric illnesses (e.g. depression and anxiety), and medical conditions (e.g. respiratory illness, heart failure, neurological conditions, painful chronic conditions).
  - Lifestyle factors and pre-bedtime behaviours are contributing factors that can be addressed through health promotion.
- Because 22% to 61% of hospitalised in-patients experience sleep disturbances, routine care should include interventions to assess and improve sleep.
- Daytime sleepiness is often viewed falsely as normal or unpreventable in older adults; this misperception reduces the likelihood that this condition will be appropriately evaluated and treated.
- Consequences of sleepiness and decreased alertness are decreased alertness, delayed reaction time, and diminished cognitive performance.

Recommendations for nursing assessment

- Obtain a sleep history from and information from both the older adult and family members, including information about sleep patterns and sleep-related behaviours.
- Use the ESS as a valid and reliable tool for identifying excessive sleepiness.
  - Use the STOP-BANG tool for identifying risks for OSA: Snoring, Tired, Observed gaps in breathing, blood Pressure high, BMI more than 35, Age over 50, Neck circumference greater than 40 cm, and Gender male.
- Assess sleep history and consider primary and secondary causes of excessive sleepiness.
- When possible, observe or snoring, apnoea during sleep, excessive leg movements during sleep, and difficulty staying awake during normal daytime activities.

Recommendations for teaching older adults

Teach older adults and carers about the following sleep-promoting measures:

- Use the bed only for sleeping or sex.
- Develop consistent and rest-promoting bedtime routines and maintain the same schedule daily.
- If awakened during the night, avoid looking at the clock.
- Avoid naps or limit them to 10–15 minutes.
- Sleep in a cool, quiet environment.
- Avoid the following before bedtime: caffeine, nicotine, alcohol, large meals, exercise, emotionally charged activities.
- If you cannot fall asleep after 15 or 20 minutes, go to another room and engage in a quiet activity until you are sleepy again.

Recommendations for care

- Work with medical practitioners to ensure optimal management of medical conditions, psychological disorders and symptoms that interfere with sleep.
- Teach older adults and families about lifestyle measures for improving sleep among all family members.
- Incorporate sleep-hygiene measures and ongoing treatment of existing sleep disorders into the plan of care for older adults in all settings.
- Work with prescribing practitioners to review and, if appropriate, adjust medications that can cause drowsiness or sleep impairment.
- Suggest referral to a sleep specialist for moderate or severe sleepiness or a clinical profile consistent with major sleep disorders.

Source: Chasens, E. R. & Umlauf, M. G. (2012). Excessive sleepiness. In M. Boltz, E. Capezuti, T. Fulmer & D. Zwicker (Eds), *Evidence-based geriatric nursing protocols for best practice* (4th ed., pp. 74–88). New York: Springer; Slater, G. & Steier, J. (2012). Review article: Excessive daytime sleepiness in sleep disorders. *Journal of Thoracic Disease, 4*(6), 608–616.

manifestation of OSA are (1) the involuntary cessation of airflow for 10 seconds or longer (i.e. apnoea) and (2) the occurrence of more than five to eight of these episodes per hour. This condition occurs because the muscles responsible for holding the throat open relax during sleep and block the passage of air. Symptoms of OSA include daytime fatigue, morning headaches, diminished mental acuity, and loud snoring punctuated by brief periods of silence.

OSA is not exclusively a condition of older adults, but the prevalence of apnoea increases with advancing age, beginning around the fifth decade, and is higher in men than in women. Prevalence rates for adults older than 60 years range from 32% to 62% (Sforza & Roche, 2013). Additional factors associated with increased risk for OSA include obesity, diabetes, stroke, Parkinson's disease, congestive heart failure, genetic predisposition, craniofacial anatomical features, and the use of alcohol or medications that depress the respiratory centre (Panossian & Daley, 2013).

OSA is a major focus of researchers and clinicians because of the increasing evidence that it causes serious consequences, and even death, when it is untreated. Studies confirm a strong link between OSA and all the following medical conditions: stroke, hypertension, cerebral ischaemia, and many types of cardiovascular disease (e.g. arrhythmias, coronary heart disease) (Cho, Kim, Seo et al., 2013; Das & Khan, 2012; Levy, Tamisier, Arnaud et al., 2012; Winklewski & Frydrychowski, 2013). Moreover, effective treatment of OSA results in improved cardiac function, reduced cardiovascular disease, and a decrease in mortality rates (Baquet et al., 2012; Kasai, 2012; Vijayan, 2012; Yang, Lin, Lan et al., 2013). In addition, OSA interferes with quality of life because it causes EDS and other cognitive effects. Studies also are investigating a potential causative relationship between OSA and cognitive impairment (Grigg-Damberger & Ralls, 2012; Sforza & Roche, 2013).

DIVERSITY NOTE

Obstructive sleep apnoea affects 24% and 9% of young, middle-aged men and women, respectively, and 70% and 50% of older men and women (Lin, Davidson & Ancoli-Israel, 2008)

NURSING ASSESSMENT OF SLEEP

Identifying opportunities for health promotion

In recent years, nurses and other healthcare professionals have focused on the importance of assessing sleep as an essential aspect of wellness and quality of life. Nurses assess sleep patterns to determine the adequacy of the person's usual sleep and rest pattern and to identify factors that either contribute to or interfere with the quality and quantity of sleep. When the assessment identifies health-promoting behaviours that improve sleep, nurses can support these efforts. When nurses identify dysfunctional sleep patterns or risk factors that interfere with sleep, they plan interventions to address the underlying contributing factors. Nurses can address many of the contributing factors through educational interventions when the assessment identifies that misinformation or a lack of knowledge contributes to sleep complaints. Box 24-1 provides guidelines for interviewing independent older adults and carers of dependent older adults about sleep and rest patterns.

In addition to obtaining information from older adults and their carers, nurses observe behavioural cues of night time and daytime rest and activities. This is especially important when objective observations are contrary to subjective complaints. For example, older adults may complain of not sleeping at all, but when observed by carers, they may appear to be sleeping during the entire night. By contrast, older adults who deny any problems sleeping may nap frequently and readily fall asleep during daytime activities.

WELLNESS OPPORTUNITY

Nurses can help older adults who are dissatisfied with their sleep identify the risk factors that can be addressed through self-care measures to improve sleep quantity and quality, rather than view this as an inevitable consequence of ageing.

Evidence-based assessment tools

Evidence-based sleep assessment tools for self-assessment or for self-reporting to healthcare professionals are two methods of collecting information about sleep. Two easy-to-use and readily available tools that have been tested for validity and reliability are the **Pittsburgh Sleep Quality Index (PSQI)** and the **Epworth Sleepiness Scale (ESS)**. The PSQI assesses sleep quality and patterns over the past month, and the ESS focuses on daytime sleepiness over the past week. The Hartford Institute for Geriatric Nursing recommends the use of both of these tools, and nurses can access the tools and guidelines at http://consultgerirn.org. The *sleep diary* is a useful tool that encourages the collection of comprehensive information about sleep. It is completed daily for at least 2 weeks each morning upon waking (Australian & New Zealand Geriatric Society for Medicine [ANZSM], 2011). The diary includes "... the time the person went to bed, total sleep time, time taken to fall asleep, the number of awakenings per night, use of sleep medications, time getting out of bed in the morning, a rating of subjective sleep quality and daytime symptoms" (p. 9).

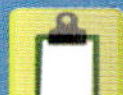

BOX 24-1
Guidelines for assessing sleep and rest

Questions to assess the perception of quality and adequacy of sleep

- On a scale of 1–10, with 10 as the highest, how would you rate your sleep?
- When you awaken in the morning, do you feel like you are rested?
- Do you feel drowsy or sleepy during the day or early evening?
- Does fatigue interfere with your desired daytime activity level?

Questions to identify opportunities for health education

- What is your usual time for getting into bed?
- Describe your usual activities during the daytime and evening.
- What are the factors that help you fall asleep (e.g. food or drink, relaxation strategies, environmental influences)?
- What conditions interfere with good sleep (e.g. pain, discomfort, anxiety, depression)?
- Do you take any medicines to help you sleep?
- Do you take medicines to help you stay awake during the day?
- Do you drink alcohol or caffeinated beverages, or take medicines that contain alcohol or caffeine during the late afternoon or evening? (If yes, how much and what kind?)
- Do you smoke or use nicotine products? (If yes, what kind and how much?)
- Are you aware, or has anyone told you, that you snore or stop breathing during your sleep?
- Do your legs kick or jump involuntarily while you sleep?

Questions to assess night time sleep pattern

- Where do you sleep at night (e.g. bed, couch, recliner chair)?
- How long does it usually take to fall asleep after you get into bed?
- Do you think you lie awake too long before falling asleep?
- After you fall asleep, how many times do you wake up during the night?
- What kinds of things disturb your sleep during the night (e.g. getting up to urinate; activities of roommates or other people in the setting; environmental factors, such as noise or lighting)?
- If changes in living arrangements have occurred in the past few months: Has your sleep pattern changed since ... (e.g. since you came to this facility; since your spouse passed away)?

UNFOLDING CASE STUDY

Part A

Mrs Zilski is 66 years old and recently retired from her job as office manager for a law firm. She considers herself to be in good health, although she has had hypertension for 20 years and osteoarthritis for the past several years. She self-monitors her blood pressure and takes atenolol, 50 mg daily. She occasionally takes an over-the-counter analgesic medication when her osteoarthritis pain bothers her. She attends a local medical clinic. You are the practice nurse at this clinic. During one of her appointments, Mrs Zilski comes to talk with you about her difficulty sleeping. She reports that since she has retired, she often wakes up several times during the night and has difficulty returning to sleep. She used to sleep an average of 7 to 8 hours nightly and could easily return to sleep if she woke up during the night. Now she is lucky if she gets 6 hours of sleep because she lies in bed for several hours. She used to go to bed between 10 and 11 p.m. and get up promptly between 6.30 and 7 a.m. Now that she is retired, she goes to bed around 11 p.m., but stays in bed until 10 a.m. if she wakes up during the night and does not get a full night's sleep.

Thinking points

- What age-related changes may be contributing to Mrs Zilski's dissatisfaction with her sleep?
- What risk factors might be contributing to Mrs Zilski's dissatisfaction with her sleep?
- What further assessment information would you need to obtain, and how would you obtain it?

NURSING ISSUES

Nursing issues pertinent to older adults who have sleep problems include insomnia, disturbed sleep pattern or sleep deprivation. When healthy older adults report dissatisfaction with their sleep and express interest in learning self-care activities to improve their sleep pattern, the nursing issue of willingness for enhanced sleep is applicable.

WELLNESS OPPORTUNITY

Nurses can be alert to opportunities to include the wellness nursing issue of willingness for enhanced sleep for older adults in community or long-term care facilities who are able to explore interventions that improve their sleep patterns.

GOAL PLANNING FOR WELLNESS OUTCOMES

When older adults experience sleep disturbances or have risk factors that affect sleep patterns, nurses create goals that achieve wellness outcomes as an essential part of the nursing process. Wellness outcomes for older adults that are appropriate for sleep disturbance or who are at risk of a sleep pattern disturbance are sleep, rest, comfort level, personal well-being, control of anxiety and knowledge about health behaviour. Goals include: improved sleep or rest; increased comfort level; improved personal well-being; reduction in anxiety; and increased knowledge about health behaviour.

WELLNESS OPPORTUNITY

Quality of life is a wellness outcome that is achieved through nursing interventions directed towards enhancing sleep.

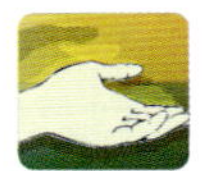

NURSING INTERVENTIONS FOR SLEEP WELLNESS

Nursing interventions to promote sleep wellness for older adults include health education and direct interventions, such as environmental modifications and comfort and relaxation strategies. As with other aspects of nursing care for older adults, it is essential that nurses individualise the care to address each person's identified needs in various settings. For example, community nurses can focus on teaching older adults and their carers about self-care interventions that can improve sleep patterns. In long-term care settings, nurses focus on interventions that can be implemented routinely to improve sleep patterns of residents. In hospital settings, nurses focus primarily on acute medical problems, but sleep disturbances should not be overlooked as an important health concern.

Evidence-based guidelines for interventions to improve sleep and address excessive sleepiness are listed in the resources section at the end of this chapter. All guidelines emphasise initiation of appropriate interventions, including health education about self-care strategies; identification and management of underlying causative conditions; and suitable referrals for further evaluation and treatment. Information in this chapter is based on these guidelines and focuses on interventions that nurses can use in various settings to enhance sleep patterns in older adults. Nursing interventions that may be appropriate include enhancement of sleep strategies, anxiety reduction, exercise promotion, music therapy, environmental changes, pain management, relaxation therapy, and autogenic training.

Health promotion for sleep wellness for older adults

Increasing attention is paid to non-pharmacological interventions for improving sleep and alleviating insomnia with an emphasis on safe and effective alternatives to medications that can have many adverse effects (see the section on educating older adults about medications and sleep). Evidenced-based practice 24-2 summarises current research conclusions about non-pharmacological interventions for improving sleep.

An important aspect of health promotion is to teach older adults about normal age-related changes and help them identify risk factors that can affect their sleep, as described in Tables 24-1, 24-2 and 24-3. When contributing factors are identified, help older adults plan interventions to address risks such as stress and chronic pain or

EVIDENCE-BASED PRACTICE 24-2
Research conclusions about non-pharmacological EBP interventions to improve sleep

- Meditation, mindfulness and mindfulness-based stress reduction are consistently identified as effective interventions for improving sleep (Gross et al., 2011; Nagendra, Maruthai & Kutty, 2012; Ong, Ulmer & Manber, 2012).
- Daily moderate physical activity improves sleep for older adults (Kline, Sui, Hall et al., 2012; Uchida, Shioda, Morita et al., 2012).
- Muscle relaxation techniques (e.g. progressive muscle relaxation, autogenic training) improve sleep, particularly when stress is a contributing condition (Sharma & Andrade, 2012).
- Many studies find strong support for cognitive behavioural treatment for insomnia (e.g. Katofsky, Backhaus, Junghanns et al., 2012; Troxel, Germain & Buysse, 2012; Williams, Roth, Vatthauer et al., 2013).
- Studies find good support for the use of yoga and tai chi (body–mind interventions) in improving sleep (Sarris & Byrne, 2011; Sobana, Parthasarathy, Duraisamy et al., 2013).
- Acupuncture and acupressure may be effective for sleep disorders, based on their effects on serotonin, dopamine and endogenous opioids, with stronger evidence in support of acupressure (Lu, Lin, Chen et al., 2013; Sarris & Byrne, 2011).
- Listening to soothing music is effective for improving sleep quality (Su, Lai, Chang et al., 2012).
- Melatonin, a sleep-regulating hormone produced by the pineal gland, can be effective in managing circadian sleep disorders and jet lag (Kostoglou-Athanassiou, 2013).
- L-tryptophan (an exogenous amino acid that is converted into serotonin) may increase sleepiness and decrease length of time for sleep onset, particularly in healthy adults (Sarris & Byrne, 2011).
- A systematic review of studies found that lavender oil may be helpful for promoting sleep (Fismer & Pilkington, 2012).
- Some, but not all studies, have found that valerian (a herbal product), alone or in combination with hops or kava, may improve sleep (Sarris & Byrne, 2011).
- Earplugs and eye masks can improve sleep in critical care patients (Jones & Dawson, 2012).
- Massage therapy is beneficial for improving sleep, for example, for menopausal symptoms (Oliveira, Hachul, Goto et al., 2012) and for people with dementia in residential care (Harris, Richards & Grando, 2012).

discomfort. In addition, use information in Box 24-2 to teach about self-care actions (sometimes called *sleep hygiene*) for promoting sleep wellness. If older adults are not familiar with relaxation techniques, give them a copy of Box 24-3 and teach them about deep breathing, progressive relaxation, and mental imagery. Encourage older adults to use music players with automatic shutoffs or other devices to listen to soothing music or provide instructions for deep breathing, guided imagery or relaxation exercises.

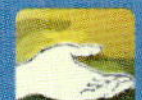

BOX 24-2
Health promotion teaching about sleep

Actions to take

- Establish a bedtime ritual that is effective for you, and try to follow it every night.
- Maintain the same daily schedule for waking, resting and sleeping.
- Take a warm, relaxing bath in the afternoon or early evening.
- After 1.00 p.m. avoid foods, beverages and medications that contain caffeine or stimulants (e.g. tea, cocoa, coffee, chocolate, sugar, refined carbohydrates, and some over-the-counter pain relievers and cold preparations).
- Pre-bedtime foods that promote sleep include milk (warm), chamomile tea, and a light snack of complex carbohydrates (e.g. whole grains).
- Use one or more of the following relaxation methods: imagery, meditation, deep breathing, progressive relaxation, soothing music, body or foot massage, rocking in a chair, reading non-stimulating materials, or watching non-stimulating television.
- Perform daily moderate aerobic exercise, preferably before the late afternoon, but avoid vigorous exercise in the evening.
- Assure adequate intake of the following nutrients: zinc, calcium, magnesium, manganese, vitamin C and vitamin B complex.

Actions to avoid

- Do not drink alcohol before bedtime because it may cause early morning awakening. If you do use alcohol, use it in only small amounts.
- Do not smoke cigarettes in the evening because nicotine is a stimulant.
- If your bedtime is temporarily changed, try to keep your waking time as close to the usual time as possible, and avoid staying in bed beyond your usual waking time.
- Do not use your bed for reading or other activities not associated with sleeping.
- If you awaken during the night and cannot return to sleep, get out of bed after 30 minutes and engage in a non-stimulating activity, such as reading, in another room.
- Arise at your usual time, even if you have not slept well.

Complementary and alternative care practices

- Yoga, tai chi, meditation, imagery, aromatherapy, massage, soothing music, relaxation techniques, and a warm bath or warm footbath may be effective in promoting sleep.
- Melatonin, a sleep-regulating hormone, can be effective in improving sleep, but it can interact with other medications and also can cause daytime sleepiness.

Special precautions

- Although widely promoted as sleep aids, herbs should be used with caution in older adults because of their possible adverse effects.
- Inform your healthcare professionals about any use of herbs, aromatherapy or other complementary and alternative care practices.

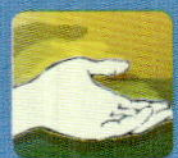

BOX 24-3
Relaxation and mental imagery techniques that promote sleep

Deep breathing

- Focus your attention on your breathing; extend your belly and draw in a deep breath as you count.
- Hold your breath for three or four counts.
- Exhale completely.
- Repeat this pattern, focusing your total attention on breathing.
- Phrases, such as "I am sleepy", or counting may be repeated during each exhalation to help keep your attention focused on breathing.

Progressive relaxation

- Start by focusing your attention on the muscles in your toes.
- Flex or tense these muscles, and then relax them.
- Repeat two or three times.
- Focus your attention on the muscles in your foot.
- Flex or tense, then relax these muscles, two or three times.
- Repeat this process, progressively focusing on different muscle groups and proceeding from your feet to your head.

Mental imagery

- Begin with deep-breathing exercises to relax yourself.
- Focus your attention on a serene and peaceful scene, visualise the setting, and imagine the sounds (e.g. a beach with waves gently washing ashore).
- Imagine yourself in the setting, lying relaxed, enjoying the environment.
- Keep your attention focused on the scene.
- Imagine repetitive motions, such as waves on the beach or sheep jumping over a fence.

Improving sleep for older adults in institutional settings

Older adults in acute and long-term residential care settings have a high prevalence of sleep disturbances, and these disturbances can lead to serious and detrimental health consequences, as already delineated. Nurses who work evening or night shifts have many opportunities to engage in direct care activities that promote good night time sleep, which are in addition to environmental interventions discussed in the next section.

For older adults in any setting, nursing responsibilities include addressing factors that interfere with sleep, ensuring the most comfortable environment possible, and individualising care plans so that they incorporate personal preferences for optimal sleep conditions. The following relatively simple nursing actions can improve sleep in people hospitalised: supporting the person's usual sleeping schedule and routines, providing assistance with personal care and comfortable positioning, providing comfort measures (e.g. warm beverage, a brief massage, maintaining a quiet environment with minimal lighting).

If dementia or depression interferes with sleep onset, a helpful intervention is to simply stay with the older person to provide reassurance until the person is able to fall asleep. In addition, relief of pain, anxiety and physical discomfort are nursing responsibilities that can affect the sleep of older adults. Older adults who are cognitively impaired may not request analgesics but may give non-verbal cues that pain is interfering with sleep, as discussed in Chapter 28. Be alert to this possibility and assess for chronic or acute pain, and recognise that an analgesic taken 30 minutes before bedtime may help induce sleep in people with chronic pain or discomfort.

Because daytime activities influence sleep patterns, care plans in long-term residential care settings should incorporate appropriate types and amounts of activities in each older adult's daily routine. Also, residents should be exposed to adequate bright lights during the day. Evening and night time routines need to be based on a comprehensive assessment of the needs of the older adult and consider any conflicting needs. For example, for some older adults, the need for an uninterrupted night's sleep may outweigh the potential benefits of being awakened for night time care tasks. In many situations, the needs can be addressed during the person's usual waking time, rather than performing the tasks on a rigid schedule designed for the convenience of staff.

WELLNESS OPPORTUNITY

Nurses promote sleep wellness for older adults who experience sleep problems by teaching about the importance of having any sleep disorder evaluated by a knowledgeable professional.

Modifying the environment to promote sleep

Environmental modifications are among the simplest and most effective interventions to improve sleep, especially in institutional settings. Actions such as closing bedroom doors and adjusting bedroom lighting can improve sleep. Elimination of unnecessary staff-initiated noise, especially conversations at the nursing station, is another helpful intervention for in-patients/residents located near the centre of nursing activity. In long-term residential care settings, nurses can document preferences for bedtime routines that promote sleep on each resident's care plan and assure that these measures are carried out by nursing staff. In long-term care settings where residents share rooms, decisions about room assignments should take into consideration the compatibility of individual needs. Once room assignments have been made, roommate behaviours that interfere with sleep can be addressed by a room change, if necessary.

If a noisy environment contributes to sleeping difficulties, and the noise cannot be controlled or eliminated, the older person may wish to use earplugs. However, people who live alone should be cautioned about the danger of blocking out protective noises, such as that of a smoke alarm. If environmental noise cannot be eliminated, it can be masked by white noise (e.g. using a fan, air conditioner, soft music or recordings of white noise). In addition to addressing noise in the environment, interventions address temperature in the sleeping area. The night time room temperature should be comfortable, and is usually slightly lower than during the day. In cooler environments, the older adult should wear a nightcap to prevent loss of heat through the head.

Educating older adults about medications and sleep

Hypnotics may be effective for short-term management of sleep disorders, especially in temporary circumstances, such as in acute care settings; however, the adverse effects of some hypnotics can outweigh their advantages. Guidelines for evidence-based practice emphasise that sedative–hypnotic medications should not be used for treatment of insomnia in older adults, particularly in long-term residential care (Brandt & Piechocki, 2013; ANZGSM, 2011). There is an increased risk of dependence and tolerance with these medications.

Benzodiazepines (e.g. temazepam) was the most commonly prescribed sleep medication for older adults until the early 1990s. However, recent guidelines emphasise that this class of drugs should not be used as hypnotics because they are associated with serious adverse effects, including falls, fractures, cognitive and functional impairments, and increased risk of infections, dementia and coronary artery disease (American Geriatrics Society, 2012; deGage, Bégaud, Bazin et al., 2012; Huang, Mallet, Rochefort et al., 2012).

Non-benzodiazepine agents (e.g. zolpidem and zopiclone) have been available for 20 years, but recent studies indicate that these drugs are associated with serious adverse effects, including increased risk of fractures (Kang, Park, Rhee et al., 2012). Consequently non-benzodiazepines are also only indicated for short-term use (usually less than a month in Australia and New Zealand (ANZGSM, 2011). In addition, older adults often use over-the-counter medications, such as diphenhydramine and other antihistamines, for their sedating effects; however, there is little evidence they are effective for improving sleep when used for more than several days, and they are associated with serious adverse effects because of their strong anticholinergic actions. Box 24-4 summarises pertinent teaching points that nurses can use to educate older adults and their carers about the effects of alcohol, medications and certain chemicals on sleep.

WELLNESS OPPORTUNITY

Nurses have important roles in correcting misperceptions about sleep and teaching older adults about non-pharmacological ways of improving sleep.

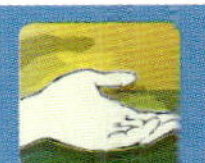

BOX 24-4
Health promotion teaching about medications and sleep

- Older adults are more susceptible than younger adults to the adverse effects of many prescription sleeping medications, including benzodiazepines (e.g. temazepam).
- Over-the-counter sleeping preparations usually contain diphenhydramine and can have adverse effects, such as confusion, constipation or blurred vision, either alone or in combination with other medications.
- Sleeping medications, even over-the-counter ones, are likely to have adverse effects that interfere with daytime function and with the quality of night time sleep.
- Many hypnotic medications are not effective for long-term use because of increasing tolerance, which may develop within the first week and usually develops after a month of regular use.
- Sleep medications can interfere with the dream stage of sleep and cause a rebound effect, characterised by nightmares and excessive dreaming, after they are discontinued.
- Alcohol is likely to cause nightmares and awakenings during the latter part of the night.
- Medications that can interfere with sleep include steroids, diuretics, theophylline, anticonvulsants, decongestants and thyroid hormone.
- Combining a sleeping medication with any other medication can be harmful or even fatal.

Health promotion: Teaching about management of sleep disorders

Evidence-based guidelines emphasise the important role that nurses have in identifying and referring older adults for sleep disorders because they have many opportunities to observe their sleep patterns. Thus, when older adults have sleep disturbances that do not respond to health promotion interventions, it is important to teach them about many safe and effective interventions for addressing sleep problems. Nurses can also emphasise the importance of addressing sleep disorders as a health issue and encourage older adults to talk with their primary care practitioner about a referral for a comprehensive sleep evaluation.

Teaching about interventions for OSA is an important nursing responsibility because of the serious health consequences that develop when the condition is not adequately treated. This is especially important because the disorder affects so many older adults and is associated with serious health consequences, as discussed earlier in this chapter.

Many types of interventions are available for treating OSA, so obtaining a comprehensive evaluation and treatment at a sleep disorders clinic should be considered. The "gold standard" for treating OSA is continuous positive airway pressure (CPAP) therapy, which is effective in improving symptoms and preventing serious complications. Although CPAP adherence is an essential first-line treatment for OSA, there is a high rate of non-adherence, which nurses can address through health education (Carlucci,

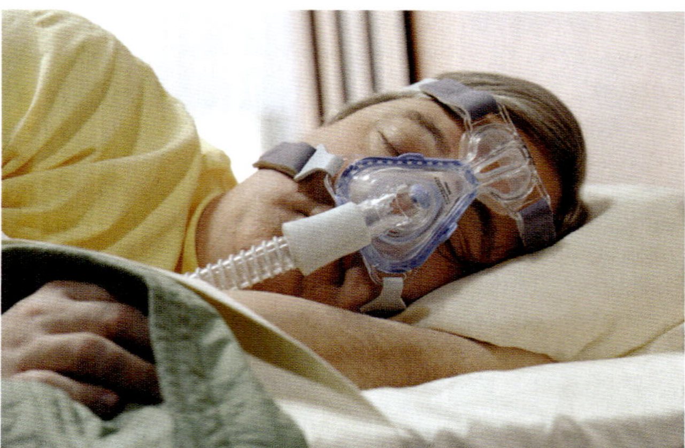

FIGURE 24-1 A continuous positive airway pressure machine. (Used with permission from Philips Respironics.)

Smith & Corbridge, 2013). Although most people who use CPAP equipment do so independently in their homes, older adults in hospitals and long-term residential care settings may need assistance with managing their nightly treatments. Figure 24-1 illustrates an older adult using a CPAP machine.

WELLNESS OPPORTUNITY

Health education about sleep is particularly important in community and long-term care settings because nurses have more opportunities to focus on quality-of-life issues.

UNFOLDING CASE STUDY

Part B

Mrs Zilski returns for further discussion of her sleep problem after filling out the Pittsburgh Sleep Quality Index based on her experiences during the past month. In addition, she has followed your instructions to keep a "sleep log" describing her daily activities, including exercise, and the effect of these activities on her sleep. As per your request, she has documented the types of foods and beverages she consumes regularly. You review the assessment information with her and find out that when she is home, she spends most of her time reading or doing crossword puzzles. She attends the senior centre weekly, plays bridge two evenings a week and goes to lunch with friends a few times every week. She enjoys gardening during the summer but has no other interest in physical activities. She avoids exercise because she is afraid that physical activity "will get the old arthritis all stirred up". On further questioning, she estimates that when she worked, she walked about 800 metres daily. She drinks about "a pot" of coffee daily and has coffee and biscuits at bridge games. She enjoys a glass of wine in the evenings. When she wakes up during the night, she usually gets up and goes to the bathroom, then returns to bed and lies there "thinking" until she returns to sleep. Her sleep log reflects that she often stays awake for as long as 2 hours before returning to sleep. She says she's heard that melatonin is good for insomnia and asks your opinion about trying it.

Thinking points

- What myths and misunderstandings about sleep would you address?
- What risk factors might you address through health education?
- Because you can see Mrs Zilski weekly at the wellness clinic, you can develop a long-term teaching plan. How would you establish priorities for immediate and long-term goals?
- What information from Boxes 24-2, 24-3 and 24-4 would you use for health education with Mrs Zilski?

EVALUATING THE EFFECTIVENESS OF NURSING INTERVENTIONS

The effectiveness of interventions for the nursing issues of disturbed sleep pattern or for the wellness issue of willingness for enhanced sleep can be measured subjectively or objectively. A subjective measurement would be that the older adult reports that he or she feels rested and refreshed upon waking in the morning. If a sleep assessment tool is used during the initial assessment, it can be used again for a reassessment after interventions have been implemented. An example of an objective measurement would be that the older adult is able to sleep for 6 to 8 hours at night with only brief interruptions, and that the person looks and acts rested during the day.

UNFOLDING CASE STUDY

Part C

Mrs Zilski is now 79 years old and is being admitted to a rehabilitation unit for care after a total hip replacement. Her diagnoses include osteoarthritis and osteoporosis. After a few weeks in the facility, she plans to return to her home where she lives with her husband. Before surgery, she was independent in her activities of daily living, and she expects to regain her independence. . The hospital transfer form has orders for Panadol Osteo (paracetamol) 1330 mg every 8 hours and zolpidem tartrate 5 mg at bedtime as needed.

Nursing assessment

During the admission interview, you ask Mrs Zilski about her sleep patterns. She states that for the past few years she has been awakened frequently at night by her hip pain and other arthritic discomforts. In addition, she reports that she would usually get up three or four times during the night to go to the bathroom. When questioned further, she explains that the pain and discomfort would wake her, and so she would go to the bathroom because she wanted to move around, not because she felt an urge to urinate that often. Although her doctor had prescribed medications for pain, she did not take them regularly because she was concerned about adverse effects. During her 1-week hospitalisation, she had taken a sleeping pill several times as well as Panadol with codeine. Mrs Zilski expresses anxiety about sleeping in the long-term care facility because she says that the noise in the hospital was very disruptive to her sleep. She reports that she feels rested in the morning if she gets at least 6 hours of sleep during the 8 hours she spends in bed. During her hospitalisation, she never felt rested in the morning and was unable to sleep for 6 hours except when she took sleeping pills. Mrs Zilski says that listening to relaxing music helps her to fall asleep.

Nursing issues

In addition to nursing issues related to Mrs Zilski's osteoarthritis and hip surgery, you identify a nursing issue of disturbed sleep pattern. Related factors are pain, age-related changes and environmental conditions. You decide that you will not list nocturia as an associated factor because Mrs Zilski does not feel an urge to void during the night. Rather, she wakes up with pain and then goes to the bathroom. You decide to list age-related changes as a related factor because it is important for Mrs Zilski to understand that, even though she may not awaken with pain, she may awaken because of age-related changes.

Nursing care plan for Mrs Zilski

Goals for wellness outcomes	Nursing interventions	Nursing evaluation
Mrs Zilski will identify factors that influence her sleep pattern.	• Describe age-related changes in sleep patterns. • Discuss the important role of pain-relieving measures in promoting good sleep.	• Mrs Zilski describes the age-related changes and other conditions that affect her sleeping pattern.
Mrs Zilski will consistently obtain 6 hours of sleep nightly without the aid of sleeping medications.	• Administer Panadol as ordered and evaluate its effectiveness in controlling Mrs Zilski's pain. • Explain that sleeping medications should be avoided, except for periodic use in short- term situations. • Assign Mrs Zilski to a room that is not close to the nursing station. • Make sure Mrs Zilski's door is closed at night. • Encourage Mrs Zilski to play quiet music at bedtime. • Give Mrs Zilski a copy of Boxes 24-3 and 24-4 and discuss additional non-pharmacological methods for promoting sleep.	• Mrs Zilski reports that she is not awakened by pain. • Mrs Zilski reports that she feels rested upon waking in the morning.

Thinking points

- What additional assessment information pertinent to Mrs Zilski's sleep patterns would you like to have, and how would you obtain this information?
- What additional nursing interventions would you include in the care plan to address Mrs Zilski's disturbed sleep pattern? Would you use any of the information in Box 24-2 or give her a copy of it?
- What concerns specifically related to sleep would you have about Mrs Zilski after she is discharged from the rehabilitation unit to her own home? How would you address these concerns in your health promotion interventions?

CHAPTER HIGHLIGHTS

Age-related changes that affect sleep and rest patterns

- Time in bed and total sleep time
- Diminished sleep efficiency
- Alterations in sleep cycles and stages
- Shifts in circadian rhythm

Risk factors that affect sleep wellness

- Psychosocial factors: beliefs, attitudes, anxiety, depression, boredom
- Environmental factors: noise, light, lack of privacy
- Pathological conditions and functional impairment (e.g. pain and discomfort, medication effects, physiological disorders)
- RLS and PLMS

Functional consequences affecting sleep wellness

- Longer time needed to fall asleep
- Frequent arousals during the night
- More time in bed to achieve same quantity of sleep
- Diminished quality of sleep (less dreaming and deep sleep)
- Increased risk of sleep disorders

Pathological conditions affecting sleep wellness

- Insomnia
- EDS
- OSA

Nursing assessment of sleep patterns

- Perception of quantity and quality of sleep
- Factors that affect sleep

- Usual sleep pattern and behaviours that affect it
- Actual sleep pattern (observed in institutional settings)
- Sleep assessment tools: PSQI, ESS and sleep diary

Nursing issues

- Willingness for enhanced sleep
- Disturbed sleep pattern

Goal planning for wellness outcomes

- Sleep
- Rest
- Comfort level
- Personal well-being

Nursing interventions for sleep wellness

- Teaching about interventions to promote healthy sleep patterns
- Modifying the environment
- Individualising care in institutional settings
- Relaxation and mental imagery techniques
- Teaching about medications that affect sleep
- Addressing obstructive sleep apnoea

Evaluating effectiveness of nursing interventions

- Expressed feelings of being rested upon waking
- Improved score on sleep assessment tool
- Observations that the person is sleeping at night

CRITICAL THINKING EXERCISES

1. What is an older adult likely to experience with regard to sleep and rest patterns? How would you explain these changes to an older adult?
2. Identify three specific factors in each of the following categories that might interfere with sleep: environmental influences, physiological disturbances and psychosocial factors.
3. How would you assess an 82-year-old person who comes to the medical centre where you work as a nurse, and they inform you they feel tired all the time and not getting enough sleep?
4. What would you include in a half-hour presentation on "Tips for Good Sleep" for a group of older adults who are attending a community day care centre for older people?
5. What information about sleep and rest would you include in an in-service program for evening and night shift assistants-in-nursing employed in a long-term residential care centre?

RESOURCES

For an extensive range of additional resources to enhance teaching and learning and to facilitate understanding of this chapter, please see the text's accompanying website located on thePoint at http://thepoint.lww.com.

Clinical tools

Hartford Institute for Geriatric Nursing, ConsultGeriRN.org: http://consultgerirn.org/resources

Assessment tools *Try This*® series and *How to Try This* resources

General assessment series:

- *Try This*, issue 6.1: The Pittsburgh Sleep Quality Index (PSQI). Smyth, C. (2012). *Best Practices in Nursing Care to Older Adults.*
- *How to Try This* (article): Evaluating sleep quality in older adults: Why screen for sleep problems in older patients? *American Journal of Nursing, 108*(5), 44–46.
- *How to Try This* (video). *Evaluating sleep quality in older adults.*
- *Try This*, issue 6.2: The Epworth Sleepiness Scale (ESS). Smyth, C. (2012). *Best Practices in Nursing Care to Older Adults.*

Evidence-based practice

Chasens, E. R. & Umlauf, M. G. (2012). Excessive sleepiness. In M. Boltz, E. Capezuti, T. Fulmer & D. Zwicker (Eds). *Evidence-based geriatric nursing protocols for best practice* (4th ed., pp. 74–88). New York: Springer.

Joanna Briggs Institute: http://connect.jbiconnectplus.org

Evidence summaries:

- Chen, Z. (2014). Residents (high-level aged care): Sleep management.
- Gaikwad, M. (2014). Sleep problems: Cognitive behavioral interventions in adults (age 60+).
- Sayakkara, S. M. L. (2014). Sleep problems (adults 60+): Physical exercise.

National Center for Biotechnology Information (NCBI):

- Martin, J. L. & Ancoli-Israel, S. (2008). Sleep disorders in long-term care settings, *Clinics in Geriatric Medicine, 24*(1), 39-iv. Accessed 19 January 2015 at www.ncbi.nlm.nih.gov/pmc/articles/PMC2215778.

National Guideline Clearinghouse: www.guideline.gov

Search for:

- Clinical guideline for the treatment of primary insomnia in middle-aged and older adults. (2014).
- Excessive sleepiness. Evidence-based geriatric nursing protocols for best practice 2003 (revised 2012).
- Obstructive sleep apnoea.

Health education

American Sleep Apnea Association: www.sleepapnea.org/i-am-a-health-care-professional.html

National Center on Sleep Disorders Research (National Heart, Lung, and Blood Institute [NHLBI]): www.nhlbi.nih.gov/about/org/ncsdr

NIHSenior Health: nihseniorhealth.gov/sleepandaging/toc.html

Sleep Apnoea Association of New Zealand Inc: www.sleepapnoeanz.org.nz

Sleep Disorders Australia: www.sleepoz.org.au

REFERENCES

American Geriatrics Society. (2012). American Geriatrics Society updated Beers Criteria for potentially inappropriate medication use in older adults. *Journal of the American Geriatrics Society, 60*, 616–631.

Australian & New Zealand Society for Geriatric Medicine (ANZGSM). (2011). Sleep and older people. Position statement no. 20, 1–17. Accessed at www.anzsgm.org/documents/PositionStatementNo20SleepandtheOlderPerson.pdf.

Baglioni, C. & Riemann, D. (2012). Is chronic insomnia a precursor to major depression? Epidemiological and biological findings. *Current Psychiatry Reports, 14*(5), 511–518.

Baquet, J. P., Barone-Rochette, G., Tamisier, R. et al. (2012). Mechanisms of cardiac dysfunction in obstructive sleep apnea. *National Review of Cardiology, 9*(12), 679–688.

Bliwise, D. L., Trotti, L. M., Yesavage, J. A. et al. (2012). Periodic leg movements in sleep in elderly patients with Parkinsonism and Alzheimer's disease. *European Journal of Neurology, 19*(6), 18–23.

Brandt, N. J. & Piechocki, J. M. (2013). Treatment of insomnia in older adults. *Journal of Gerontological Nursing, 39*(4), 48–54.

Buysse, D. J. (2013). Insomnia. *Journal of the American Medical Association, 309*(7), 706–716.

Carlucci, M., Smith, M. & Corbridge, S. J. (2013). Poor sleep, hazardous breathing: An overview of obstructive sleep apnea. *Nurse Practitioner, 38*(3), 20–27.

Chasens, E. R. & Umlauf, M. G. (2012). Excessive sleepiness. In M. Boltz, E. Capezuti, T. Fulmer & D. Zwicker (Eds), *Evidence-based geriatric nursing protocols for best practice* (4th ed., pp. 74–88). New York: Springer.

Cho, E. R., Kim, H., Seo, H. S. et al. (2013). Obstructive sleep apnoea as a risk factor for silent cerebral infarction. *Journal of Sleep Research, 22*(4), 452–458.

Das, A. M. & Khan, M. (2012). Obstructive sleep apnea and stroke. *Expert Review of Cardiovascular Therapy, 10*(4), 525–535.

deGage, S. B., Begaud, B., Bazin, F. et al. (2012). Benzodiazepine use and risk of dementia. *British Medical Journal, 345*, e6231.

Desai, A. & Bartlett, D. (2008). Insomnia. *Australian Doctor, April*, 29–36.

Espiritu, J. R. D. (2008). Aging-related sleep changes. *Clinics in GeriatricMedicine, 24*, 1–14.

Fismer, K. L. & Pilkington, K. (2012). Lavender and sleep: A systematic review of the evidence. *European Journal of Integrative Medicine, 4*(4), e436–e447.

Fung, C. H., Martin, J. L., Chung, C. et al. (2012). Sleep durations among older adults in assisted living facilities. *American Journal of Geriatric Psychiatry, 20*(6), 485–493.

Grigg-Damberger, M. & Ralls, F. (2012). Cognitive dysfunction and obstructive sleep apnea: From cradle to tomb. *Current Opinion in Pulmonary Medicine, 18*(6), 580–587.

Gross, C. R., Kreitzer, M. J., Reilly-Spong, M. et al. (2011). Mindfulness-based stress reduction vs pharmacotherapy for primary chronic insomnia. *Explore, 7*(2), 76–87.

Gupta, R., Lahan, V. & Goel, D. (2013). Prevalence of restless legs syndrome in subjects with depressive disorder. *Indian Journal of Psychiatry, 55*(1), 70–73.

Harand, C., Bertran, F., Doidy, F. et al. (2012). How aging affects sleep-dependent memory consolidation? *Frontiers in Neurology, 3*, 8.

Harris, M., Richards, K. C. & Grando, V. T. (2012). The effects of slow-stroke back massage on minutes of nighttime sleep in persons with dementia and sleep disturbances in the nursing home: A pilot study. *Journal of Holistic Nursing, 30*(4), 255–263.

Hibi, S., Yamaguchi, Y., Umeda-Kameyama, Y. et al. (2012). The high frequency of periodic limb movements in patients with Lewy body dementia. *Journal of Psychiatry Research, 46*(12), 1590–1594.

Huang, A. R., Mallet, L., Rochefort, C. M. et al. (2012). Medication-related falls in the elderly. *Drugs & Aging, 29*(5), 359–376.

Hung, H. C., Yang, Y. C., Ou, H. Y. et al. (2013). The association between self-reported sleep quality and metabolic syndrome. *PLoS One, 8*(1), e54304.

Jaussent, I., Bouyer, J., Ancelin, M.-L. et al. (2011). Insomnia and daytime sleepiness are risk factors for depressive symptoms in the elderly. *Sleep, 34*(8), 1103–1110.

Jones, C. & Dawson, D. (2012). Eye masks and earplugs improve patient's perception of sleep. *Nursing in Critical Care, 17*(5), 247–254.

Kang, D. Y., Park, S., Rhee, C. W. et al. (2012). Zolpidem use and risk of fracture in elderly insomnia patients. *Journal of Prevention and Public Health, 45*(4), 219–226.

Kasai, T., (2012). Sleep apnea and heart failure. *Journal of Cardiology, 60*(2), 78–85.

Katofsky, I., Backhaus, J., Junghanns, K. et al. (2012), Effectiveness of a cognitive behavioral self-help program for patients with primary insomnia in general practice. *Sleep Medicine, 13*(5), 463–468.

Kline, C. E., Sui, X., Hall, M. H. et al. (2012). Dose-response effects of exercise training on the subjective sleep quality of postmenopausal women: Exploratory analysis of a randomised control trial. *British Medical Journal, 2*(4), e001044.

Koo, B. B., Blackwell, T., Ancoli-Israel, S. et al. (2011). Association of incident cardiovascular disease with periodic limb movements during sleep in older men. *Circulation, 124*(11), 1223–1231.

Kostoglou-Anthanassiou, I. (2013), Therapeutic applications of melatonin. *Therapeutic Advances in Endocrinology and Metabolism, 4*(1), 13–24.

Levy, P., Tamisier, R., Arnaud, C. et al. (2012). Sleep deprivation, sleep apnea and cardiovascular diseases. *Frontiers in Bioscience, 4*, 2007–2021.

Lin, C. M., Davidson, T. M. & Ancoli-Israel, S. (2008). Gender differences in obstructive sleep apnea and treatment implications. *Sleep Medicine Reviews, 12*, 481–496.

Lu, M.-J., Lin, S.-T., Chen, K.-M. et al. (2013). Acupressure improves sleep quality of psychogeriatric inpatients. *Nursing Research, 62*(2), 130–137.

Mander, B. A., Rao, V., Lu, B. et al. (2013). Prefrontal atrophy, disrupted NREM slow waves and impaired hippocampal-dependent memory in aging. *Nature Neuroscience, 16*(3), 357–364.

Martin, J. L., Alam, T., Harker, J. O., Josephson, K. R. & Alessi, C. A. (2008). Sleep in assisted living facility residents versus home-dwelling older adults. *Journal of Gerontology: Medical Sciences, 63A*, 1407–1409.

Martin, J. L. & Ancoli-Israel, S. (2008). Sleep disturbances in long-term care. *Clinics in Geriatric Medicine, 24*, 39–50.

Misra, S. & Malow, B. A. (2008). Evaluation of sleep disturbances in older adults. *Clinics in Geriatric Medicine, 24*, 15–26.

Nagendra, R. P., Maruthai, N. & Kutty, B. M. (2012). Meditation and its regulatory role on sleep. *Frontiers in Neurology, 3*, 54.

National Center on Sleep Disorders Research. (2011). National Institutes of Health sleep disorders research plan. NIH publication no. 11-7820. Washington, DC: U.S. Department of Health and Human Services.

Neubauer, D. N. (2013). Chronic insomnia. *Continuum, 19*(1), 50–66.

Oliveira, D. S., Hachul, H., Goto, V. et al. (2012). Effect of therapeutic massage on insomnia and climateric symptoms in postmenopausal women. *Climacteric, 15*(1), 21–29.

Ong, J. C., Ulmer, C. S. & Manber, R. (2012). Improving sleep with mindfulness and acceptance. *Behaviour Research and Therapy, 50*, 651–660.

Panossian, L. & Daley, J. (2013). Sleep-disordered breathing. *Continuum, 19*(1), 86–103.

Roehrs, T. & Roth, T. (2008). Caffeine: Sleep and daytime sleepiness. *Sleep Medicine Reviews, 12*, 153–162.

Roux, F. J. (2013). Restless legs syndrome: Impact on sleep-related breathing disorders. *Respirology, 18*(2), 236–245.

Salas, R. E. & Kwan, A. B. (2012). The real burden of restless legs syndrome. *American Journal of Managed Care, 18*(9 Suppl.), S207–S212.

Sarris, J. & Byrne, G. J. (2011). A systematic review of insomnia and complementary medicine. *Sleep Medicine Reviews, 15*, 99–106.

Sforza, E. & Roche, F. (2013). Sleep apnea syndrome and cognition. *Frontiers in Neurology, 4*, 71.

Sharma, M. P. & Andrade, C. (2012). Behavioral interventions for insomnia: Theory and practice. *Indian Journal of Psychiatry, 54*(4), 359–366.

Silber, M. (2013). Sleep-related movement disorders. *Continuum, 19*(1), 170–184.

Slater, G. & Steier, J. (2012). Review article: Excessive daytime sleepiness in sleep disorders. *Journal of Thoracic Disease, 4*(6), 608–616.

Sobana, R., Parthasarathy, S., Duraisamy, K., et al. (2013). The effect of yoga therapy on selected psychological variables among male patients with insomnia. *Journal of Clinical & Diagnostic Research, 7*(1), 55–57.

Su, C. P., Lai, H. L., Chang, E. T. et al. (2012). A randomized controlled trial of the effects of listening to non-commercial music on quality of nocturnal sleep and relaxation indices in patients in medical intensive care unit. *Journal of Advances in Nursing, 69*(6), 1377–1389.

Tafaro, L., Cicconetti, P., Baratta, A., Brukner, N., Ettorre, E., Marigliano, V. & Cacciafesta, M. (2007). Sleep quality of centenarians: Cognitive and survival implications. *Archives of Gerontology and Geriatrics*, 44S, 385–389.

Troxel, W. M., Germain, A. & Buysse, D. J. (2012). Clinical management of insomnia with brief behavioral treatment. *Behavioral Sleep Medicine, 10*(4), 266–279.

Uchida, S., Shioda, K., Morita, Y. et al. (2012). Exercise effects on sleep physiology. *Frontiers in Neurology, 2–3*, 48.

Valenza, M. C., Cabrera-Martos, I., Martin-Martin, L. et al. (2013). Nursing homes: Impact of sleep disturbances on functionality. *Archives of Gerontology and Geriatrics, 56*(3), 432–436.

Van Couter, E., Spiegel, K., Tasali, S. & Leproult, R. (2008). Metabolic consequences of sleep and sleep loss. *Sleep Medicine, 9*(Suppl. 1), S23–S28.

Vijayan, V. K. (2012). Morbidities associated with obstructive sleep apnea. *Expert Review of Respiratory Medicine, 6*(5), 557–566.

Watson, N. F. & Viola-Saltzman, M. (2013). Sleep and comorbid neurologic disorders. *Continuum, 19*(1), 148–169.

Williams, J., Roth, A., Vatthauer, K. et al. (2013). Cognitive behavioral treatment of insomnia. *Chest, 143*(2), 554–565.

Winklewski, P. J. & Frydrychowski, A. F. (2013). Cerebral blood flow, sympathetic nerve activity and stroke risk in obstructive sleep apnoea. *Blood Pressure, 22*(1), 27–33.

Yang, M. C., Lin, C. Y., Huang, C. Y. et al. (2013). Factors affecting positive airway pressure therapy acceptance in elderly patients with obstructive sleep apnea in Taiwan. *Respiratory Care, 58*(9), 1504–1513.

Zeitzer, J. M., Bliwise, D. L., Hernandez, B. et al. (2013). Nocturia compounds nocturnal wakefulness in older individuals with insomnia. *Journal of Clinical Sleep Medicine, 9*(3), 259–262.

Chapter 25

Thermoregulation

By Carol Miller and Sharyn Hunter

LEARNING OBJECTIVES

After reading this chapter, you should be able to:

1. Describe age-related changes that affect an older adult's normal body temperature, febrile response to illness and response to hot and cold environmental temperatures.
2. Identify risk factors that affect thermoregulation in older adults and increase the potential for hypothermia or hyperthermia.
3. Assess the following aspects of thermoregulation: baseline temperature, risks for altered thermoregulation, hypothermia, hyperthermia and febrile response to illness.
4. Discuss the functional consequences of altered temperature regulation in older adults.
5. Implement health promotion interventions for preventing hypothermia and hyperthermia in older adults.

KEY POINTS

accidental hypothermia
acclimatise
heat exhaustion
heat stroke
heat-related illness
hypothermia
hyperthermia
thermoregulation

The primary function of **thermoregulation** is to maintain a stable core body temperature in a wide range of environmental temperatures. In the presence of infections, thermoregulation also assists in maintaining homeostasis. Under normal circumstances, the core body temperature is maintained at 36.1°C to 37.2°C (97°F to 99°F) through complex physiological mechanisms governing heat production and dissipation. Because older adults experience age-related changes and additional risk factors that affect thermoregulation, they are vulnerable to **hypothermia**, an abnormally low body temperature and **hyperthermia**, an abnormally elevated body temperature from, for example, heat stroke, fever or similar conditions. The term **heat-related illness** is used in this chapter when hyperthermia occurs in response to hot environmental temperatures, in contrast to when it is related to pathophysiological causes. This chapter focuses on nursing assessment and interventions related to altered thermoregulation in older adults.

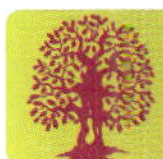

AGE-RELATED CHANGES THAT AFFECT THERMOREGULATION

With increased age, subtle alterations in thermoregulation occur, and these become important considerations in caring for healthy, as well as frail, older adults. Thermoregulation is a complex adaptive process that involves many internal and external influences.

Internal conditions that affect temperature regulation include metabolic rate; pathological processes; muscle activity; peripheral blood flow; amount of subcutaneous fat; function of the cutaneous nerves; ingestion of fluid, nutrients and medications; and the temperature of the blood flowing through the hypothalamus. External influences on thermoregulation include environmental temperature, humidity level, airflow and the type and amount of clothing and covering used. The following sections address these factors in relation to the ability of older adults to respond to environmental temperatures and in relation to normal body temperature.

Response to cold temperatures

In cold environmental temperatures, the body normally initiates physiological mechanisms to prevent loss of body heat and increase heat production. At the same time, individuals usually initiate protective behaviours to warm the body and protect themselves from adversely cold temperatures. Physiological mechanisms that prevent heat loss and increase heat production include shivering, muscle contraction, increased heart rate, peripheral vasoconstriction, dilation of the blood vessels in the muscles, insulation of deeper tissues by subcutaneous fat and release of thyroxine and corticosteroid by the pituitary gland. Protective actions that people commonly initiate in cold temperatures include seeking shelter, ingesting warm fluids, wearing warm clothing or covering and increasing activity to stimulate circulation.

The following age-related changes, which can affect processes involved with heat loss or production, are likely to interfere with an older person's ability to respond to cold temperatures:

- Inefficient vasoconstriction
- Decreased cardiac output
- Decreased muscle mass
- Diminished peripheral circulation
- Decreased subcutaneous tissue
- Delayed and diminished shivering.

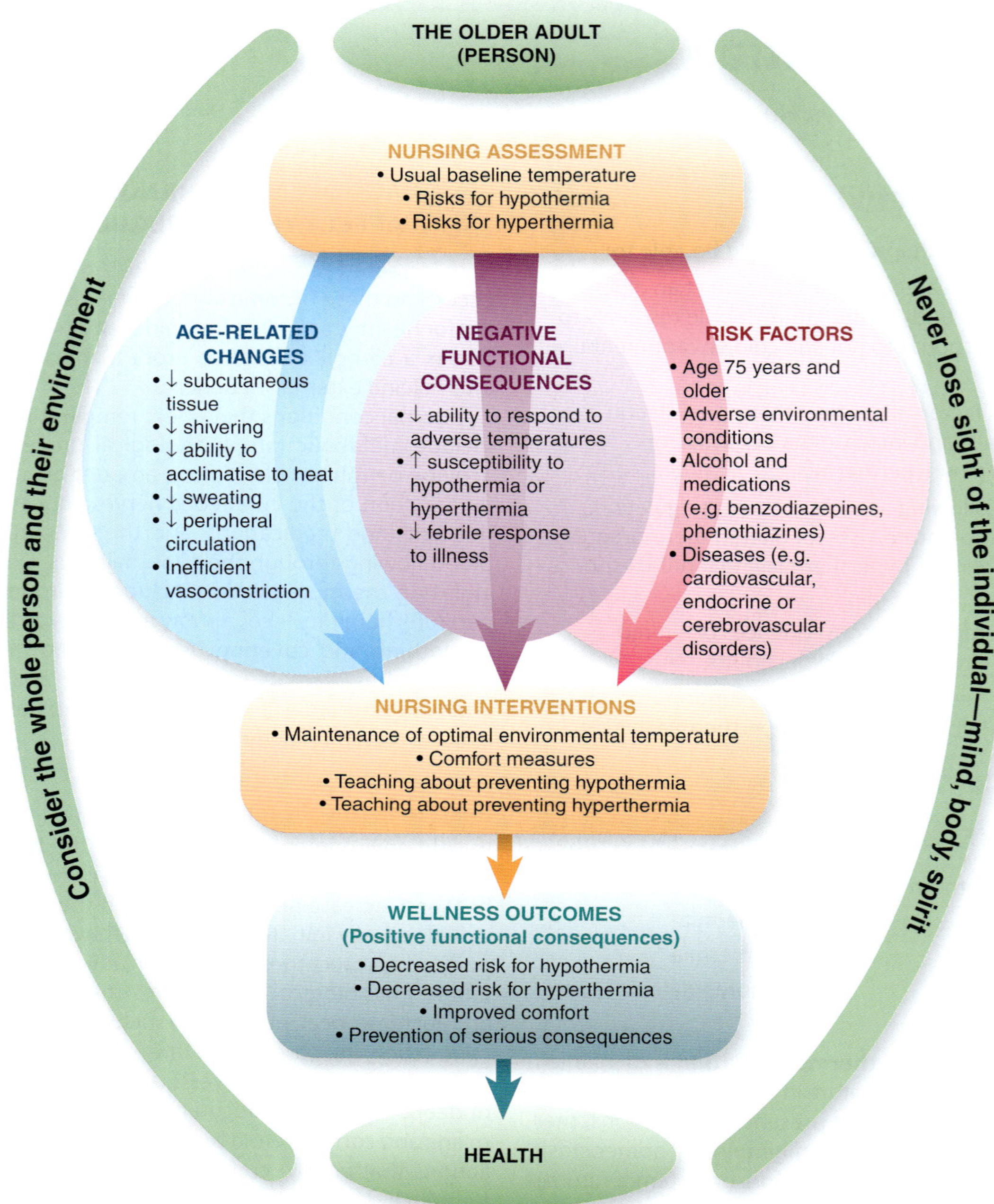

These changes begin during the fifth decade, but their impact is not felt until the seventh or eighth decade. The overall effect of these changes is a dulled perception of cold and a concomitant lack of stimulus to initiate protective actions, such as adding more clothing or raising the environmental temperature.

Response to hot temperatures

In hot environmental temperatures, or when metabolic heat production is high, the normal mechanisms for heat dissipation are the production of sweat to facilitate evaporation and the dilation of peripheral blood vessels to facilitate heat radiation. When exposed to hot climates or engaged in strenuous activity daily for 7 to 14 days, healthy adults are able to **acclimatise** (i.e. gradually increase their metabolic efficiency to adapt to higher temperatures). The older person's ability to acclimatise and respond to heat stress is altered primarily by age-related changes affecting sweating and cardiovascular function. Older adults have an increased threshold for the onset of sweating, a diminished response when sweating occurs and a dulled sensation of warm environments. For example, the sweat response to exercise in healthy adults in their mid-60s is about half of that in adults in their mid-20s. Age-related cardiovascular changes interfere with the ability to acclimatise because cardiac output must be sufficient to produce peripheral vasodilation for heat dissipation. Consequently, even healthy older adults are more susceptible to heat stress because they are less able to adapt to hot environments (Platt & Vicario, 2009).

Normal body temperature and febrile response to illness

The long-standing norm for body temperature has been 37°C (98.6°F); however, a systematic review of studies related to body temperature norms and a study of 18,630 healthy adults concluded that normal body temperature for healthy adults is lower than 37°C, with older adults having an oral temperature range of 36.1°C to 36.3°C (97°F to 97.4°F) (Lu, Leasure & Dai, 2010; Waalen & Buxbaum, 2011).

An elevated temperature, or fever, is the body's protective response to pathological conditions such as cancer, infection, dehydration or connective tissue disease. This protective response is blunted in older adults because of age-related changes involving thermoregulation and the immune system. Implications for nursing care are discussed in the sections on functional consequences and assessment.

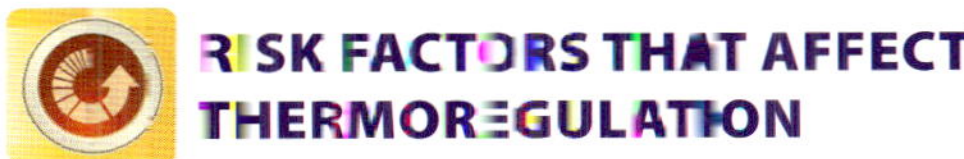

RISK FACTORS THAT AFFECT THERMOREGULATION

Increased age is a risk factor for both hypothermia, defined as a core body temperature of 35°C (95°F) or lower, and heat-related illnesses, which are likely to occur even in moderately cold or hot environments. In addition, pathophysiological disorders, adverse medication reactions and socioeconomic conditions increase the risk for serious consequences related to altered thermoregulation.

Conditions that increase the risk for hypothermia

The risk for hypothermia is increased by conditions that decrease heat production (e.g. inactivity, malnutrition, endocrine disorders, neuromuscular conditions), increase heat loss (e.g. burns, vasodilation), or affect the normal thermoregulatory process (pathological conditions of the central nervous system). Medical disorders that predispose to hypothermia include stroke, sepsis, malnutrition, multiple sclerosis, renal insufficiency, Parkinson's disease, and endocrine disorders (e.g. hypothyroidism, hypoglycaemia, hypoadrenalism) (Davis, 2012)

Medications and alcohol can predispose a person to hypothermia by suppressing shivering, inducing vasodilation, or affecting the central nervous system. Medications most often associated with hypothermia include antipsychotics (including newer atypical ones), benzodiazepines, tricyclic antidepressants, opioids and barbiturates (Davis, 2012; Kreuzer, Landgrebe, Wittmann et al., 2012). Excessive use of alcohol can increase the risk for hypothermia by dulling sensory perceptions and interfering with cognitive skills necessary for initiating protective behaviours.

Conditions that increase the risk for heat-related illness

The risk for heat-related illness is increased by physiological alterations that increase internal heat production (e.g. hyperthyroidism, diabetic ketoacidosis) or interfere with the ability to respond to heat stress (e.g. cardiovascular disease, fluid or electrolyte imbalance). In addition, medical disorders such as cardiovascular disease and Parkinson's disease can worsen the severity of heat-related illness and decrease the chance of full recovery. For example, case studies of heatstroke in people with Parkinson's disease reported multi-organ dysfunction and permanent neurological damage (Yamashita, Uchida, Kojima et al., 2012).

Medications can predispose to heat-related illness by increasing diuresis (e.g. diuretics), increasing heat production (e.g. salicylates intoxication), or interfering with sweating (e.g. anticholinergics) or peripheral vasodilation (e.g. beta-adrenergic blocking agents). A study comparing adverse medication reactions in older adults during heatwaves and normal summers implicated the following medications: diuretics, serotonic antidepressants, angiotensin-converting enzyme inhibitors, and proton pump inhibitors (Sommet et al., 2012). Alcohol increases the risk for heat-related illness by inducing diuresis, and excessive alcohol can increase the risk by increasing heat production.

Environmental and socioeconomic influences

Environmental temperatures can increase the vulnerability of older adults, particularly those older than 75 years, to hypothermia or hyperthermia. Although older adults who live in geographic areas with extreme cold or hot seasonal variations are especially vulnerable, studies have found that hypothermia affects older adults even in temperate climates (Elbaz et al., 2008). Other factors interact with environmental conditions to contribute to an increased risk for altered thermoregulation. For example, heat-related illness can be precipitated by even moderate exercise in hot and humid weather, especially if fluid intake is not adequate. If older adults rely solely on their sensation of thirst to signal the need for fluid intake, they can become underhydrated or dehydrated because of the age-related diminished thirst sensation.

In addition to the obvious influence of hot or cold temperatures, substandard living conditions and diets deficient in protein and kilojoules have been associated with hypothermia and hyperthermia. Heatwaves are especially hazardous for older adults living in environments with poor ventilation. The detrimental effects are magnified when high temperatures combine with high humidity levels and air pollutants. For older adults living in urban areas with high crime rates, keeping windows closed for safety considerations may restrict ventilation. In Great Britain, the

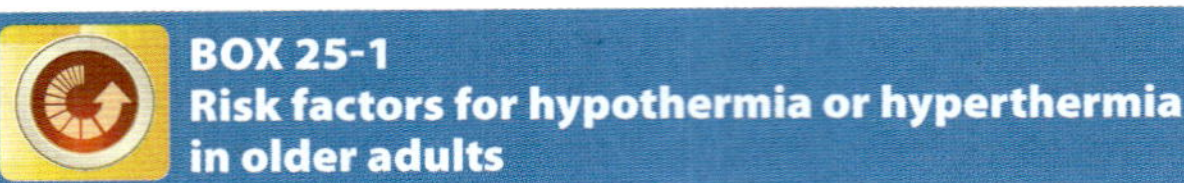
BOX 25-1 Risk factors for hypothermia or hyperthermia in older adults

Risks for hypothermia and hyperthermia
- Age 75+ years
- Adverse environmental temperatures
- Infections or sepsis
- Cardiovascular disorders
- Cerebrovascular disease

Risks for hypothermia
- Alcohol
- Carcinoma
- Diabetes or hypoglycaemia
- Endocrine disorders
- Malnutrition
- Parkinson's disease
- Peripheral neuropathy
- Medications: barbiturates, benzodiazepines, cyclic antidepressants and phenothiazines

Risks for hyperthermia
- Alcohol and alcohol withdrawal
- Dehydration
- Diabetic ketoacidosis
- Hyperthyroidism
- Excessive exercise or even moderate exercise in hot environments
- Medications: alpha-adrenergic blocking agents; anticholinergic agents (including antihistamines, phenothiazines, tricyclic antidepressants); benzodiazepines, beta-adrenergic blocking agents, calcium channel blockers, diuretics and laxatives.

term *urban hypothermia* has been used with reference to older adults living alone in poorly heated dwellings. Likewise, the term *urban hyperthermia* could be applied to older adults living in poorly ventilated houses and apartments, particularly public housing, in cities where heatwaves and air pollution are common.

Social isolation is a factor that increases the risk for progression of hyperthermia or hypothermia because people are rarely able to self-report these conditions. Thus, they may not receive help in a timely manner. Older adults who live alone and have dementia may be at increased risk if they do not have the cognitive skills to adjust the thermostat and wear proper clothing, or the ability to recognise the symptoms and call for help in a timely manner. Homelessness is another socioeconomic factor that increases the risk for both hypothermia and hyperthermia. Additional risk factors are summarised in Box 25-1.

WELLNESS OPPORTUNITY

Although the weather cannot be controlled, it is important to identify the environmental factors that affect thermoregulation and that can be addressed through health education about protective actions.

Behaviours based on lack of knowledge

Lack of knowledge about age-related vulnerability to hypothermia and hyperthermia may create risks secondary to inadequate protective measures. For example, when the use of air conditioning or heating is curtailed as a cost-saving measure, younger adults may be able to adjust to the moderately hot or cool temperature, whereas an older adult might become hypothermic or hyperthermic under the same circumstances. If older adults and their carers, caregivers are not aware of the age-related decrease in the perception of environmental temperatures, they may not take appropriate protective measures, such as removing or adding clothing.

In the presence of infection, lack of knowledge about age-related thermoregulatory changes may result in undetected illnesses. For example, carers and healthcare professionals may falsely assume that no infection is present if there is no fever. Similarly, if they believe that the baseline temperature for all adults is 37°C (98.6°F), they may not recognise an elevated temperature in someone whose baseline temperature is lower than this. In addition, lack of knowledge about diurnal temperature variations and age-related changes may contribute to false expectations and undetected illness.

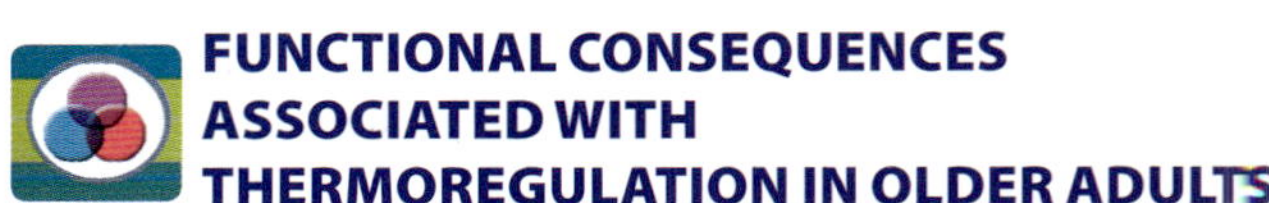
FUNCTIONAL CONSEQUENCES ASSOCIATED WITH THERMOREGULATION IN OLDER ADULTS

A healthy older adult in a comfortable environment will experience few, if any, functional consequences of altered thermoregulation. However, in the presence of any risk factor, hypothermia or hyperthermia may develop in an older adult. Even moderately adverse environmental temperatures can precipitate hypothermia or hyperthermia in an older adult, especially in the presence of additional predisposing factors, such as certain medications or pathological conditions. For older adults in whom hypothermia or hyperthermia develops, the risk of subsequent morbidity or mortality from this condition is greater than that for their younger counterparts. Hyperthermia and hypothermia are usually seasonal hazards that can develop in older adults during heatwaves and cold spells, respectively.

Altered response to cold environments

Increased age is associated with an increased vulnerability to hypothermia because most older adults are less aware of a low core body temperature, less efficient in their physiological response to cold and less apt to take corrective actions when necessary. A low environmental temperature usually contributes to hypothermia, and the term **accidental hypothermia** is used when low environmental temperature is the primary cause of the condition. However, even in normal environmental temperatures, the condition can result from serious alterations in homeostasis, such as can

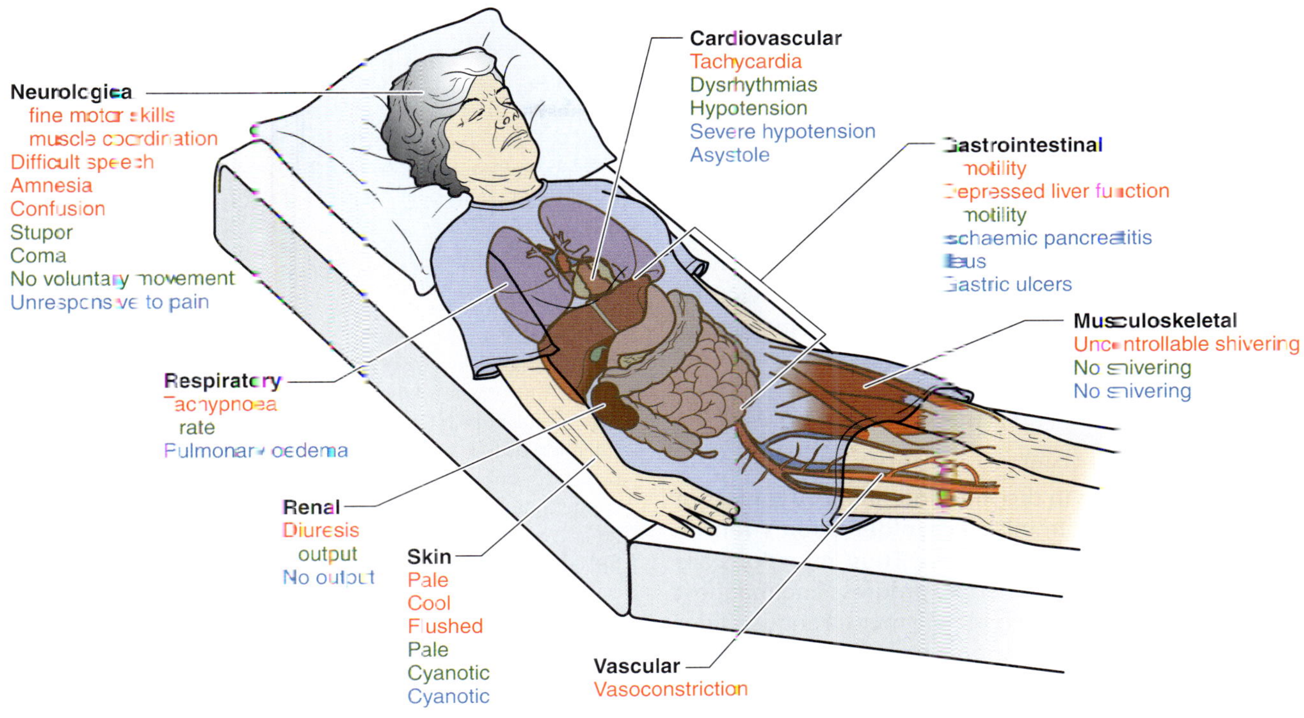

Red = mild (33°C–35°C [91.4°F–95°F]); Green = moderate (29°C–32°C [85.2°F–89.6°F]); Blue = severe (<29°C [<85.2°F]).

FIGURE 25-1 Physiological effects of hypothermia according to stages from mild to severe. (Adapted with permission from Davis, R. A. [2012]. The big chill: Accidental hypothermia. *American Journal of Nursing, 112*[1], 41.)

occur with anaesthesia or endocrine or neurological disorders. Accidental hypothermia can occur in older adults as a consequence of exposure to moderately cool temperatures, and may affect as many as 10% of older adults living in winter climates (e.g. Great Britain, Canada and parts of the U.S.). However, deaths of older adults from hypothermia have also been reported in winter in the temperate climate of Australia (Lim & Duflou, 2008) and New Zealand.

In the early stages of hypothermia, the older adult will probably not shiver or complain of feeling cold. In the absence of any protective measures, hypothermia will progress, clouding mental function. The effects of impaired thermoregulation are cumulative, and hypothermia progresses rapidly after the core body temperature falls to 34°C (93.2°F). The age-related diminished ability of the kidney to conserve water and the common occurrence of inadequate fluid intake in older adults exacerbate the effects of hypothermia (see Chapter 18 for discussion about hydration and ageing and Chapter 19, urinary function and ageing). If the process is not reversed, death from hypothermia will result from the myocardial effects of seriously impaired thermoregulation. Figure 25-1 illustrates the physiological effects of hypothermia according to stages from mild to severe.

Altered response to hot environments

Functional consequences that affect an older adult's ability to respond to hot environments include delayed and diminished sweating and inaccurate perception of environmental temperatures. Because of these functional consequences, the older adult is more likely to have heat-related illnesses such as heat exhaustion and heat stroke.

Heat exhaustion is a condition that develops gradually from depletion of fluid, sodium, or both. It can occur in active or immobilised older people who are dehydrated or underhydrated and exposed to hot environments.

Heat stroke is an even more serious condition that is likely to occur in active older adults because of a combination of age-related thermoregulatory changes and risk factors, such as overexertion and warm environments. Heat stroke can also occur in immobilised older adults in hot environments, either as a progression of untreated heat exhaustion, or as a result of a combination of risk factors. The underlying mechanism in heat stroke is an inability to balance the rates of heat production and dissipation. This balance depends primarily on sweating and cardiac output.

In hot environments, the effects of altered thermoregulation are cumulative, and heat-related illnesses progress rapidly after the body temperature reaches 40.6°C (105.8°F). If fluid volume is not adequate to meet the requirements for effective sweating, then hyperthermia will progress even more rapidly. The age-related decrease in thirst sensation can contribute to inadequate fluid intake and diminished thermoregulation. If hyperthermia is not reversed, death will result from respiratory depression. One study found that heatwaves in Australia were associated with statistically significant increases in cardiovascular and diabetes mortality and higher emergency room admissions for renal disease (Wang, Barnett, Yu et al., 2012). Death rates have been noted to increase during heatwave years in Australia compared with non-heatwave years. In 2009, South Australia and Victoria experienced a most severe heatwave and an increase in sudden deaths was reported (World Socialist Web Site, 2011).

Altered thermoregulatory response to illness

Age-related changes in the thermoregulatory centres of the hypothalamus diminish the older adult's febrile response to illness and infections. Thus, infections are likely to be undetected until they progress and manifest as a functional decline or change in mental status. Older adults with infections commonly have a normal or even lower than normal temperature, but when their temperature is compared with their baseline temperature, at least a slight elevation is evident. An implication of this is that impaired temperature regulation can have deleterious results in older adults and a subtle temperature change may be a significant indicator of an underlying disease that requires medical attention (Chester & Rudolph, 2011).

Altered perception of environmental temperatures

Older adults often report feeling cool or cold, even in very warm environments, and they generally prefer environmental temperatures that are at least 24°C (75°F). Inaccurate perceptions of environmental temperatures are associated with pathophysiological conditions, such as dementia, thyroid disorders or cardiovascular inefficiency, rather than with age-related changes alone.

Psychosocial consequences of altered thermoregulation

Psychosocial consequences are associated with hypothermia, hyperthermia or diminished fever response. If hypothermia or hyperthermia is overlooked, or if interventions are not initiated at an early stage, the condition may progress to the point of impairing cognitive function. Likewise, if a diminished or delayed febrile response to an infection is not recognised, a treatable condition may be overlooked and treatment may unintentionally be delayed or denied. Untreated infections are likely to progress in severity and, in older adults, may manifest primarily as a functional decline, such as impaired cognition.

UNFOLDING CASE STUDY

Part A

Mrs Tully is 76 years old and lives alone on a large farm. She has lived on this farm for 49 years and has been a widow for 2 years. She has four children and eight grandchildren, but they all live in other districts. Mrs Tully has been able to manage her farm with a part-time helper who comes a couple of times a week to help feed the several dozen chickens and collect eggs. When the farm helper doesn't come, she manages by herself. She has hypertension and type 2 diabetes, and manages reasonably well medically. She adheres to her diabetic diet and takes her medications daily. She sends her farm helper to the city once weekly for groceries and drives to the nearby church on Sundays. Once a month she attends the Country Women's Association (CWA). It is the middle of January and summer this year has been unusually hot and humid. A drought and heatwave are predicted. You are planning to present a health education program called "Hot Tips for Surviving the Summer" at the next CWA meeting. You are particularly concerned about Mrs Tully and several other participants who live in isolated areas and have little contact with others.

Thinking points

- What factors increase the risk of Mrs Tully developing a heat-related illness? Which ones would you discuss in your health education program?
- In your health education program, how would you explain heat-related illnesses and the associated signs and symptoms?

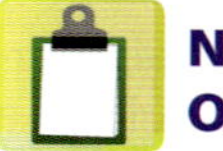

NURSING ASSESSMENT OF THERMOREGULATION

Nursing assessment of thermoregulation addresses the older person's baseline body temperature, any risk factors for altered thermoregulation, manifestations of hypothermia or hyperthermia and febrile response to illness. Nurses use this information for planning health education interventions to prevent hypothermia and hyperthermia. Nurses also use the assessment information to detect hypothermia or heat-related illnesses as quickly as possible so that appropriate interventions can be initiated before serious or irreversible effects occur. Assessment information is also important in detecting infections at an early stage. Nurses obtain much of the pertinent information about risk factors as part of the overall assessment; they also obtain information by observing the environment, measuring the person's body temperature and interviewing the older adult and the carers of dependent older adults.

Assessing baseline temperature

Oral and axillary temperatures are not necessarily an accurate measurement of core temperature in older adults because the difference between their core and skin temperatures is greater and more variable than in younger people. Although rectal temperature has long been viewed as the established standard for measuring body temperature, obtaining it is difficult and very invasive. In recent years, ear thermometry has become the method of choice because it is the least invasive and quickest way of obtaining temperatures, especially in acutely ill patients.

Normal body temperature measurements show a diurnal fluctuation of 1°C (1°F to 2°F) with lower temperatures occurring during sleeping and greater fluctuations during periods of fever-inducing illness. However, because older adults normally have a lower body temperature and may have a diminished febrile response to infection, it is especially important to determine the person's usual temperature, as well as to characterise the usual pattern of diurnal variation. It is important to document the method used for assessing temperature because of the variation in recordings with the different methods of measurement.

Nurses can encourage older adults in home settings to determine their usual temperature by recording their temperature at different times of the day for several days when they are feeling well. Those who live in fluctuating climates should do this seasonally and annually by those who live in stable climates. This recording provides a baseline for comparison when symptoms of illness or functional decline occur. Nurses can follow this procedure in long-term residential care settings and record the results as baseline data on the chart. Box 25-2 summarises the principles underlying nursing assessment of thermoregulation in older adults.

Identifying risk factors for altered thermoregulation

Anyone older than 75 years is at risk for altered thermoregulation, as are older adults who have one or more of the risk factors listed in Box 25-1. Because so many of the risk factors for altered thermoregulation are modifiable, it is important to identify those that can be addressed through health promotion interventions. Nurses usually identify risk factors involving medications and physiological disturbances during the overall assessment, and it is important to consider any conditions predisposing the person to hypothermia or hyperthermia. In addition to assessing for risks for hypothermia or heat-related illnesses, nurses must consider a low baseline body temperature as a risk for undetected fever. It is important to document the person's baseline temperature and note this as a risk factor for both hypothermia and undetected febrile conditions if it is below 36.7°C (98°F).

Most nurses do not have the opportunity to observe and assess the older adult's home environment, but they can ask pertinent questions and listen for clues to detect environmental risk factors. For example, older adults who

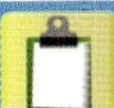

BOX 25-2
Guidelines for assessing thermoregulation

Principles of temperature assessment

- Document the person's baseline body temperature and its diurnal and seasonal variations.
- Assume that even a small elevation above the baseline temperature is a clue to the presence of a pathological process.
- Document actual temperature and deviations from the baseline, rather than using such terminology as "afebrile".
- Carefully follow all the standard procedures for accurate temperature measurement. Use a thermometer that registers temperatures lower than 35°C (95°F).
- Consider the influence of temperature-altering medications when evaluating a temperature reading (e.g. medications that mask a fever).
- Do not assume that an infection will necessarily be accompanied by an elevated temperature.
- Remember that, in the presence of an infection, a decline in function or change in mental status may be an earlier and more accurate indicator of illness than an alteration in temperature.
- Do not assume that an older adult will initiate compensatory behaviours or complain of discomfort when exposed to adverse environmental temperatures.

Questions to assess risk factors for hypothermia or hyperthermia

- Do you have any particular health problems that occur in hot or cold weather?
- Are you able to keep your house or room at a comfortable temperature in both summer and winter months?
- What do you do to cope with hot temperatures in the summer?
- Do you have any difficulty paying your utility bills?
- What forms of protection against the cold do you use in the winter months (e.g. electric blanket, supplemental sources of heat)?
- Have you ever received medical care for exposure to heat or cold?
- Have you ever fallen and not been able to get up or get help?

Observations to assess risk factors for hypothermia or hyperthermia

- Does the older person live in a house where the temperature is kept below 21°C (70°F) during the winter?
- Does the person drink alcohol or take temperature-altering medications (see Box 25-1)?
- Does the person live alone? If so, what is the frequency of outside contacts?
- Does the person have any pathological conditions that predispose him or her to hypothermia (e.g. endocrine, neurological or cardiovascular disorders)?
- Is the person's fluid and nutritional intake adequate?
- Does the person have postural hypotension? (See Chapter 20 for assessment criteria relating to postural hypotension.)
- Is the person immobilised or sedentary? Is the person's judgement impaired because of dementia, depression or other psychosocial disorders?
- Does the person live in a poorly ventilated dwelling without air-conditioning?
- Are atmospheric conditions very hot, humid or polluted?
- Does the person engage in active exercise during hot weather?
- Does the person have any chronic illness that predisposes him or her to hyperthermia?
- Is the person at risk for hyponatraemia or hypokalaemia because of medications or chronic illnesses?

live alone and express concern about keeping the house warm in winter should be considered to be at risk for hypothermia. Likewise, older adults who live in poor housing conditions, or with family members who keep the house at low temperatures during winter months, should be considered to be at risk for hypothermia. Older adults who live in poorly ventilated houses without air conditioning should be considered to be at risk for hyperthermia during heatwaves. Interview questions aimed at identifying risk factors for altered thermoregulation are listed in Box 25-2.

WELLNESS OPPORTUNITY

From a holistic perspective, nurses consider that fears about paying utility bills in the winter or about personal safety when windows are open can increase the risk for hypothermia or heat-related conditions.

Assessing for hypothermia

Hypothermia is best detected by measuring core body temperature with a thermometer that registers below 35°C (95°F). Cool skin in unexposed areas, such as the abdomen and buttocks, is a distinguishing characteristic of hypothermia. The environmental temperature may be only moderately cool and the older person will not necessarily shiver or complain of feeling cold. Even in environmental temperatures of 20°C or 20.6°C (68°F or 69°F), an older person may become hypothermic, especially if other risk factors, such as immobility or hypothermia-inducing medications, are present. When assessing for hypothermia, it is advisable to use several methods and to make sure that the thermometers used are able to detect low body temperatures.

Early signs of hypothermia are subtle, and the most objective assessment tool is a comparison of the person's body temperature with their usual baseline temperature. As untreated hypothermia progresses, additional signs may include lethargy, slurred speech, mental changes, impaired gait, puffiness of the face, slowed or irregular pulse, low blood pressure, slowed tendon reflexes and slow, shallow respirations. Severe stages of hypothermia are characterised by muscular rigidity, diminished urinary function, and a progression of all other manifestations to the point of stupor and coma. The skin will feel very cool, and, contrary to what might be expected, the colour of the skin will be pink. Also contrary to what might be expected, a hypothermic person may not shiver, particularly if the body temperature is below 32.2°C (90°F).

Assessing for heat-related illness

Manifestations of heat-related illnesses range from mild headache to life-threatening respiratory and cardiovascular disturbances. In the early stages of heat-related illness, the person will feel weak and lethargic and may complain of headache, nausea and loss of appetite. The skin will be warm and dry, and the sweating response may be absent, especially if the person's fluid intake is low. As the heat-related condition progresses, these manifestations will be exacerbated and the following signs will become evident: dizziness, dyspnoea, tachycardia, vomiting, diarrhoea, muscle cramps, chest pain, mental impairment and a wide range pulse pressure.

Assessing the older adult's febrile response to illness

Because the manifestations of delayed or diminished febrile response to infections are likely to be very subtle, nurses assess for any temperature changes from the person's baseline as well as for additional signs of illness, such as a decline in function or change in mental status. Nurses should also examine assumptions about temperature regulation that may apply to younger adults but not to older adults. For example, the expectation that pneumonia is accompanied by an elevated temperature is not necessarily applicable to older adults, as discussed in Chapter 21. Thus, nurses in long-term residential care facilities need to be particularly vigilant about subtle temperature changes and other manifestations of fever. A more reliable indicator of elevated temperature in older adults would be an increase of 1.1°C (2°F) above the person's baseline. See Box 25-2 for a summary of some of these considerations.

WELLNESS OPPORTUNITY

A holistic assessment for febrile conditions requires that nurses identify subtle manifestations, such as behaviour changes and slight elevations above the person's baseline temperature, even if the temperature is within the so-called normal range.

NURSING ISSUES

If the nursing assessment identifies risks for impaired thermoregulation in an older adult, pertinent nursing issues include hypothermia, hyperthermia or risk for imbalanced body temperature: hypothermia (and hyperthermia). If conditions increase the risk for hypothermia, hyperthermia and ineffective thermoregulation, the nursing issue of risk for imbalanced body temperature may be appropriate. For example, an 83-year-old woman with diabetes, dementia and hypertension who is taking a diuretic, an antipsychotic and an oral hypoglycaemic would have many risk factors for both hypothermia and hyperthermia. Related factors common in older adults include immobility, advanced age, medication effects, adverse environmental conditions and acute and chronic illnesses. For older adults living alone, social isolation may be a related factor that increases the risk for experiencing more serious consequences if hypothermia or hyperthermia occurs.

WELLNESS OPPORTUNITY

Nurses can use the nursing issue of willingness for enhanced knowledge: prevention of hypothermia (or hyperthermia) for older adults and their carers who are interested in learning to address risks for these conditions.

GOAL PLANNING FOR WELLNESS OUTCOMES

When caring for older adults with risks for hypothermia or hyperthermia, nurses create goals that achieve wellness outcomes as an essential component of the nursing process. Goals that address altered thermoregulation and the risk of altered thermoregulation include: development of health-promoting behaviour, maintaining hydration, increased knowledge about health behaviour, and increased knowledge about personal safety, detection and control of risk factors, a safe home environment and normal body temperature.

Goals will vary depending on the setting. In acute care settings, nurses are more likely to focus on goals that pertain to the person's immediate physical condition (e.g. hydration, thermoregulation and body temperature). The focus of nursing care in long-term residential care settings would be early detection of infections. In home and other community settings, nurses might be able to provide group or individual health education for older adults who are at risk for development of hypothermia or heat-related illness, especially during times of extreme weather conditions. In these situations, nurses focus more on goals about improving self-care and increasing knowledge about environmental modifications to prevent hypothermia or hyperthermia.

WELLNESS OPPORTUNITY

Nurses promote wellness when their care plans include health-promoting behaviours to prevent hypothermia and hyperthermia.

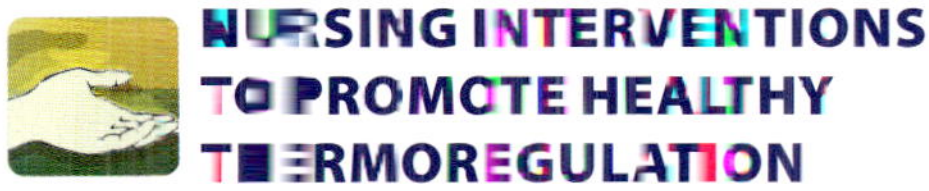

NURSING INTERVENTIONS TO PROMOTE HEALTHY THERMOREGULATION

Health promotion interventions to address altered thermoregulation are directed towards primary prevention of hypothermia and heat-related illness. Health promotion interventions also address early detection of altered thermoregulation and prompt initiation of interventions to restore thermal balance and to prevent detrimental effects. Comfort interventions are initiated to promote well-being in older adults. Other nursing interventions focus on managing the environment, risk protection, health education, risk identification, surveillance of safety, health promotion and temperature regulation.

Addressing risk factors

Maintenance of an environmental temperature of around 24°C (75°F) is the single most important intervention to prevent hypothermia or hyperthermia. In addition, relative humidity can be altered to minimise the discomfort and detrimental effects associated with extremely warm or cool environments.

With comfortable indoor temperatures, the ideal humidity is between 40% and 50%, although an acceptable range is between 20% and 70%. Older adults can be encouraged to humidify the air in their homes during the dry winter months by using humidifiers, either alone or with their heating systems. Simpler measures such as keeping pans of water on heating vents or using a vaporiser near the bed at night may be appropriate if a humidifier is unavailable.

WELLNESS OPPORTUNITY

Nurses promote wellness for socially isolated older adults by identifying ways of developing a system of social contact, such as a friendly phone call program, that ensures daily contact during periods of adversely hot or cold weather.

Promoting healthy thermoregulation

In cool environmental temperatures, interventions to prevent hypothermia include using adequate clothing and covering, especially for the hands, feet and head, because these areas of the body have the heaviest concentration of nerve endings that are sensitive to heat loss. Nurses can encourage older adults to wear caps, thermal socks and several layers of warm clothing when appropriate. Electric blankets used during the night are a relatively inexpensive form of protection in cool environments, but proper safety precautions must be taken. Space heaters are often used to provide intense heat in a small area, but they can create serious fire and safety hazards. In addition to environmental considerations, special attention must be directed towards ensuring adequate nutrition, including fluid intake, and treating any pathological conditions.

During heatwaves hyperthermia can affect older adults living in their own homes or in long-term residential care settings that are not air-conditioned. In long-term residential care facilities without air-conditioning, nurses need to ensure that all residents have adequate fluid intakes. Nurses must also observe for early signs of hyperthermia, especially in residents who are immobile or who have medical problems, such as endocrine or circulatory disorders, that predispose them to hyperthermia. If only parts of the facility are air-conditioned, nurses can encourage residents to spend time in those areas and provide assistance for residents who have mobility limitations.

Nurses can teach older adults living in community settings about measures to cool the environment, such as those summarised in Box 25-3. Older adults may be reluctant to use fans or air-conditioners because of a desire to save money on utility bills; however, if they understand the health risks associated with hyperthermia, they may use these appliances judiciously. If the home setting cannot be cooled adequately during heatwaves, nurses can encourage older adults to spend time in air-conditioned public places. Additional self-care actions to prevent hyperthermia during heatwaves include the provision of adequate fluids and the avoidance of heavy meals and strenuous exercise. Nurses can use Box 25-3, which summarises interventions for the prevention of hyperthermia, as an educational tool for older adults.

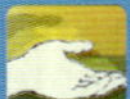

BOX 25-3
Health promotion teaching about hypothermia and heat-related illness

Environmental and personal protection considerations for preventing hypothermia

- Maintain a constant room temperature as close to 24°C (75°F) as possible, with a minimum temperature of 21°C (70°F).
- Use a reliable, clearly marked thermometer to measure room temperature.
- Wear close-knit, but not tight, undergarments to prevent heat loss; wear several layers of clothing.
- Wear a hat and gloves when outdoors; wear a nightcap and socks for sleeping.
- Wear extra clothing in the early morning as this is when your body metabolism is at its lowest point.
- Use flannel bed sheets or blankets.
- Use an electric blanket set on a low temperature.
- Take advantage of programs that offer assistance with utility bills.

Environmental and personal protection action to prevent heat-related illnesses

- Maintain room temperatures below 29°C (85°F).
- If your residence is not air-conditioned, use fans to circulate the air and cool the environment.
- During hot weather, spend time in public air-conditioned settings, such as libraries or shopping malls.
- Drink extra non-caffeinated, non-alcoholic liquids, even if you don't feel thirsty.
- Wear loose-fitting, lightweight, light-coloured, cotton clothing.
- Wear a hat or use an umbrella to protect yourself against sun and heat when you are outside.
- Avoid outdoor activities during the hottest time of the day (i.e. between 10.00 a.m. and 2.00 p.m.); perform them during the cooler hours of the morning or evening.
- Place an ice pack or cold, wet towels on your body, especially on the head, the groin area and armpits. Take cool (about 24°C [75°F]) baths or showers several times daily during heatwaves but do not use soap every time.

Health promotion actions for maintaining optimal body temperature

- Maintain adequate fluid intake by drinking 8 to 10 glasses of non-caffeinated, non-alcoholic liquid daily.
- Do not rely on your thirst sensation as an indicator of the need for fluid.
- Eat small, frequent meals rather than heavy meals.
- Avoid drinking caffeinated beverages, such as cola and coffee.
- Avoid drinking alcohol.
- In cold weather, engage in moderate physical exercise and indoor activities to increase circulation and heat production.

Nutritional considerations

- Maintain good nutrition, especially zinc, selenium and vitamins A, C and E.

Preventive measures and additional approaches

- Know your normal temperature in the morning and in the evening.
- Know the difference in your temperature in the winter and the summer.
- Obtain pneumonia and influenza immunisations (as discussed in Chapter 21).
- Obtain tetanus and diphtheria vaccinations every 10 years.
- Be aware that melatonin and other substances (see Box 25-1) might alter temperature regulation; use these substances only under the advice of a healthcare professional.

WELLNESS OPPORTUNITY

Nurses can use comfort measures to diminish the sensation of being cold, even if the interventions have no effect on core body temperature.

Promoting carer wellness

Carers of older adults who have risks for hypothermia or heat-related illnesses may benefit from the health promotion resources listed at the end of this chapter. For example, carers may be interested in finding out about programs for assistance with utility bills or home repairs for improved energy efficiency and comfort. Use the information in Box 25-3 to teach about strategies for preventing hypothermia and heat-related illnesses. In addition, it is important to encourage carers to establish a plan for at least daily communication with socially isolated older adults, especially during heatwaves or cold spells.

UNFOLDING CASE STUDY

Part B

Recall that Mrs Tully is 76 years old and attends a Country Women's Association where you will be presenting a health education program.

Thinking points

- How would you incorporate assessment information into your health education program?
- How would you use information from Box 25- 3 to teach about preventing heat-related illnesses?
- What specific suggestions would you make about early detection of heat-related illnesses to the participants at this CWA meeting?
- How would you find health education materials to use for your program?

EVALUATING THE EFFECTIVENESS OF NURSING INTERVENTIONS

Nurses evaluate the care of older adults who have been identified with risk for hypothermia/hyperthermia or imbalanced body temperature according to the extent to which the risks are eliminated. It is not always possible to know whether risk factors were eliminated, but nurses can evaluate the effectiveness of their teaching by asking for feedback from older adults and their carers. Nurses also can suggest referrals for resources and ask the older adult about his or her intent to follow through. When nurses teach about preventing hypothermia and heat-related illnesses, its effectiveness is evaluated on the basis of the person's ability to describe ways of decreasing the risk factors for hypothermia or heat-related illnesses.

UNFOLDING CASE STUDY

Part C

Mrs Tully is now 87 years old and continues to live alone in her own home in a rural area. She has a history of hypertension and diabetic retinopathy, and was recently hospitalised for uncontrolled diabetes. Upon discharge from the hospital in May, she was referred to the community nurses for teaching about insulin administration and monitoring of her diabetic care.

Nursing assessment

During your initial visit, you observe that Mrs Tully's house is poorly maintained and has no insulation. Mrs Tully tells you she has lived in this house for 60 years and that, in recent years, she has had difficulty keeping up with maintenance because of her poor eyesight and limited income. She has few social contacts, but her daughter visits her every other week and a neighbour visits weekly and brings her groceries. About once a month, friends pick her up and take her to church. Your assessment reveals that, although Mrs Tully has difficulty preparing meals because of her poor eyesight, she is independent in all other activities of daily living.

During your initial visit you identify several risk factors for hypothermia, so during subsequent visits you follow up with further assessment. You learn that Mrs Tully was taken to the emergency department in July, 2 years ago to be treated for hypothermia. She recalls that her daughter had come for her usual visit and had found her in a very weak and confused state. Her description of the situation is that "they just warmed me up at the hospital and sent me home again. I could have done that myself if my daughter would have just let me be". It is apparent that she did not consider her condition to be of particular concern. In the winter, she keeps her energy bills low by using a small, portable heater in the living room during the day and moving it into the bedroom at night. Mrs Tully keeps her thermostat at 19°C (65°F) during the day and 16°C (60°F) at night.

Nursing issues

In addition to addressing the nursing issues related to Mrs Tully's diabetes, you identify a nursing issue of risk for imbalanced body temperature: hypothermia. Related factors include advanced age, diabetes, social isolation, poor housing conditions, low environmental temperatures and a history of hypothermia.

Nursing care plan for Mrs Tully

Goals for wellness outcomes	Nursing interventions	Nursing evaluation
Mrs Tully's knowledge about risk factors for hypothermia will be increased.	• Discuss risk factors for hypothermia, with emphasis on Mrs Tully's diabetes, social isolation, environmental conditions and history of hypothermia.	• Mrs Tully states at least four factors that place her at risk for hypothermia.
Mrs Tully's knowledge about ways of preventing hypothermia will be increased.	• Use Box 25-3 to discuss interventions to prevent hypothermia and to explore ways of applying these interventions to Mrs Tully's situation.	• Mrs Tully implements strategies aimed at reducing her risk for hypothermia.
The risk factor of low temperatures in Mrs Tully's house will be eliminated.	• Discuss with daughter strategies for improving heating.	• Mrs Tully has her house insulated. • Mrs Tully keeps her thermostat at 21°C (70°F) during the winter.
The risk factor of social isolation will be eliminated.	• Suggest home-delivered meals to Mrs Tully as a means of providing prepared meals and daily contact.	• Mrs Tully accepts home-delivered meals.
	• Emphasise that one of the purposes of such programs is to ensure that socially isolated older adults have daily contact with someone who can monitor their well-being.	• Mrs Tully's daughter phones daily during cold spells.
	• Ask Mrs Tully for permission to contact her daughter to suggest that she call her mother daily during cold spells to make sure she is okay.	

Thinking points

- How would you address Mrs Tully's perception that hypothermia does not have serious health-related implications?
- What additional interventions might you consider to address Mrs Tully's risk for hypothermia?

CHAPTER HIGHLIGHTS

Age-related changes that affect thermoregulation

- Inefficient vasoconstriction
- Decreased cardiac output
- Diminished subcutaneous tissue and muscle mass
- Decreased peripheral circulation
- Delayed and diminished shivering
- Diminished ability to acclimatise to heat

Risk factors that affect thermoregulation

- Environmental factors (e.g. temperatures, humidity)
- Socioeconomic and housing factors (e.g. poor ventilation, inadequate heat, lack of air conditioning)
- Insufficient knowledge about altered thermoregulation
- Medications and alcohol
- Chronic and acute conditions (e.g. infections; cardiovascular, endocrine and neurological conditions)
- Inactivity
- Social isolation

Functional consequences affecting thermoregulation

- Compromised ability to respond to hot or cold environments
- Increased susceptibility to hypothermia and hyperthermia
- Lower baseline temperature
- Diminished febrile response to infections
- Dulled perception of environmental temperatures.

Nursing assessment of thermoregulation

- Establish baseline temperature, including diurnal variations
- Identify risks for hypothermia or hyperthermia
- Observe for additional manifestations of infections

Nursing issues

- Willingness for enhanced knowledge: prevention of hypothermia (or hyperthermia)
- Risk for hypothermia
- Risk for hyperthermia
- Risk for imbalanced body temperature

Goal planning for wellness outcomes

- Health-promoting behaviours
- Knowledge about personal safety
- Risk detection and control
- Safe home environment
- Thermoregulation

Nursing interventions to promote healthy thermoregulation

- Maintaining healthy environmental conditions
- Teaching about measures to protect from hypothermia
- Teaching about measures to prevent hyperthermia
- Instituting comfort measures

Evaluating effectiveness of nursing interventions

- Evidence that risk factors are eliminated
- Feedback about improved knowledge regarding prevention of hypothermia and hyperthermia
- Feedback about referrals for community resources

CRITICAL THINKING EXERCISES

1. Describe four major functional consequences that an older adult is likely to experience with regard to thermoregulation. How would you explain these changes to an older adult?
2. Explain how each of the following factors might affect an older person's thermoregulation: medications, pathological conditions, environmental conditions, socioeconomic factors and lack of knowledge.
3. What would you include in an assessment of thermoregulation in an older adult?
4. What would you teach older adults about hypothermia and its prevention?
5. What would you teach older adults about heat-related illnesses and their prevention?
6. Find appropriate health education materials on the Internet to use in teaching older adults about hypothermia and heat-related illnesses.

RESOURCES

For an extensive range of additional resources to enhance teaching and learning and to facilitate understanding of this chapter, please see the text's accompanying website located on thePoint at http://thepoint.lww.com.

Health education

Age Concern New Zealand Inc., cool tips for winter well-being: www.ageconcern.org.nz

Better Health Channel, heat stress: www.betterhealth.vic.gov.au

Health Direct Australia, seniors' health, hot weather risks: www.healthdirect.gov.au

National Institute on Ageing (U.S.), Hyperthermia: Too hot for your health: www.nia.nih.gov

New Zealand Red Cross, heatwave emergency: www.redcross.org.nz

Victorian Government Health Information, heatwave stress: www.health.vic.gov.au

Search for:

- Heatwave and HACC clients (managing the impact of heatwaves for the elderly).
- Hot Spots Project (directing interventions to vulnerable groups).
- Residential aged care services heatwave-ready resource (revised 2013).

REFERENCES

Chester, J. C. & Rudolph, J. L. (2011). Vital signs in older patients: Age-related changes. *Journal of the American Medical Directors Association, 12*(5), 337–343.

Davis, R. A. (2012). The big chill: Accidental hypothermia. *American Journal of Nursing, 112*(1), 38–46.

Elbaz, G., Etzion, O., Delgado, J., Porath, A., Talmor, D. & Novack, V. (2008). Hypothermia in a desert climate: Severity score and mortality prediction. *American Journal of Emergency Medicine, 26*, 683–688.

Kreuzer, P., Landgrebe, M., Wittmann, M. et al. (2012). Hypothermia associated with antipsychotic drug use: A clinical case series and review of current literature. *Journal of Clinical Pharmacology, 52*(7), 1090–1097.

Lim, C. & Duflou, J. (2008). Hypothermia fatalities in a temperate climate: Sydney, Australia. *Pathology, 40*(1), 46–51.

Lu, S. H., Leasure, A. R. & Dai, Y. T. (2010). A systematic review of body temperature variations in older people. *Journal of Clinical Nursing, 19*(1–2), 4–16.

Platt, M. & Vicario, S. (2009). Heat illness. In J. A. Marx, R. Hockberger & R. Walls (Eds), *Rosen's emergency medicine* (7th ed., pp. 188[illegible]–1892). St Louis, MO: Mosby.

Sommet, A., Durrieu, B., Lapeyre-Mestre, M. et al. (2012). A comparative study of adverse drug reactions during two heat waves that occurred in France in 2003 and 2006. *Pharmacoepidemiology and Drug Safety, 21*(3), 285–288.

Waalen, J. & Buxbaum, J. N. (2011). Is older colder or colder older? The association of age with body temperature in 18,630 individuals. *Journals of Gerontology: Biological Sciences, 66A*(5), 487–492.

Wang, X. Y., Barnett, A. G., Yu, W. et al. (2012). The impact of heatwaves on mortality and emergency hospital admissions from non-external causes in Brisbane, Australia. *Occupational and Environmental Medicine, 69*(3), 163–169.

World Socialist Web Site (2011). Australian heat wave kills 60 people, triggers power and transport chaos. Accessed March 2015 at www.wsws.org/en/articles/2009/02/heat-f02.html

Yamashita, S., Uchida, Y., Kojima, S. et al. (2012). Heatstroke in patients with Parkinson's disease. *Neurological Sciences, 33*(3), 685–687.

Chapter 26

Sexual function

By Carol Miller and Sharyn Hunter

LEARNING OBJECTIVES

After reading this chapter, you should be able to:

1. Describe age-related changes that affect sexual function in older adults.
2. Discuss risk factors that influence older adults' interest in, opportunities for and performance of sexual activities.
3. Discuss the functional consequences affecting sexual wellness in older adults.
4. Assess your own attitudes about sexual function in older adults.
5. Apply assessment guidelines in clinical settings when it is appropriate to address sexual wellness.
6. Teach older adults about interventions to promote sexual wellness.

KEY POINTS

andropause	menopause
erectile dysfunction	perimenopause
female sexual dysfunction	postmenopause
human immunodeficiency virus (HIV)	prostatic hyperplasia
menopausal hormonal therapy (MHT)	urethritis
	vaginitis

Because sexual function in older adults encompasses many physiological and psychosocial aspects of sexuality and intimate relationships, this chapter's perspective is broad. Although sexual function is not a dominant focus of gerontological nursing care in most situations, it is a very important component of quality of life for many older adults. In long-term residential care settings and other situations in which quality of life is a focus of care, nurses need to be prepared to assess sexual function and implement nursing interventions that promote sexual wellness.

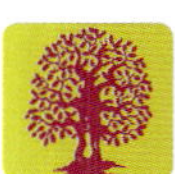

AGE-RELATED CHANGES THAT AFFECT SEXUAL FUNCTION

A loss of reproductive ability at the onset of **menopause** in women is an age-related change in sexual function that is clearly delineated. Additional and more subtle age-related changes in sexual function include diminished reproductive abilities in older men and alterations in both male and female responses to sexual stimulation. Older adults generally can compensate for any age-related changes in their response to sexual stimulation; however, when risk factors are present, they may experience additional changes in sexual function. This section focuses on age-related changes affecting physiological aspects of sexual function. The wide range of commonly occurring risk factors is discussed in the risk factors and pathological conditions sections.

Changes affecting older women

Hormonally regulated cycles, called *menses*, control female reproductive abilities. With the onset of menses during adolescence, the cyclical release of ova marks the beginning of female reproductive abilities. Reproductive abilities decline around the fifth decade, when the frequency of ovulation diminishes and menstrual cycles become shorter and irregular. Menopause (the cessation of menses), which typically occurs around the age of 49 to 51 years, is a clear indicator that reproduction is no longer possible. **Perimenopause** refers to the several years before menopause when women begin experiencing manifestations of approaching menopause (e.g. changes in menstrual cycles, vasomotor symptoms and vaginal dryness). **Postmenopause** begins 12 months after a woman's last menstrual cycle.

In addition to affecting reproductive ability, menopause influences other aspects of sexual function, predominantly because of the accompanying decline in endogenous oestrogen levels. Production of oestradiol by the ovaries is the primary source of oestrogen before menopause. After menopause, the primary source is oestrone, which is converted from androstenedione in skin and fat tissue. Endogenous oestrogen levels decline in all post-menopausal women, but the extent and manifestations of oestrogen deficiency vary. The factors that affect post-menopausal levels of endogenous oestrogen include the interval since the onset of menopause; the production of hormones by the adrenal cortex; changes in the clearance rates of androgens and oestrogens; and body weight, with higher body fat being positively correlated with higher levels of oestrogen.

About 75% to 80% of all menopausal women experience hot flushes (also called hot flashes), with 20% requesting treatment for severe symptoms (Elkins, Fisher,

Promoting sexual wellness in older adults

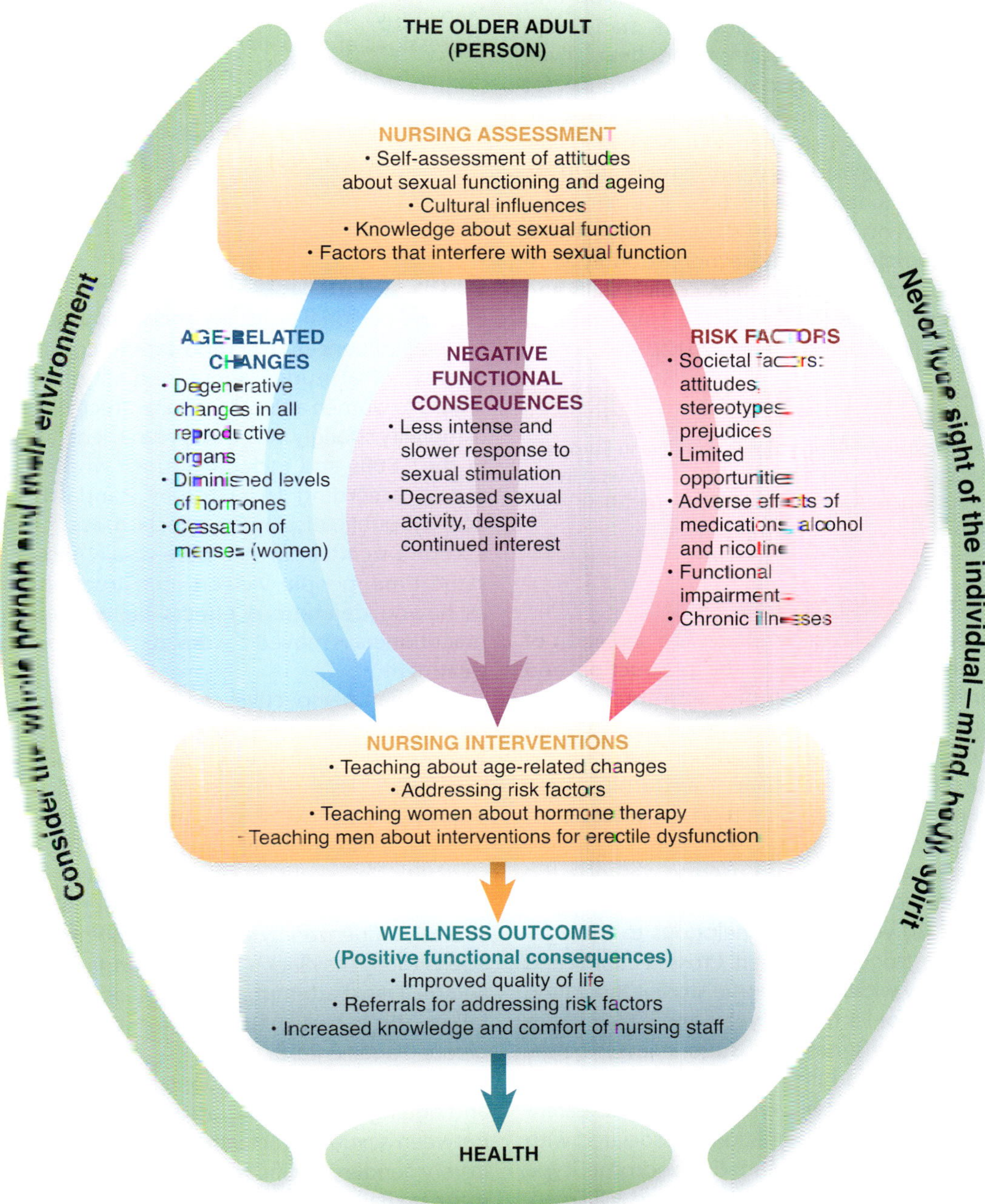

Johnson et al., 2013; Okeke, Ezenyeaku, Ikeako et al., 2013). Hot flushes are a vasomotor symptom characterised by the sudden onset of heat, perspiration and flushing that spreads from the head to trunk. Symptoms last from 1 to 5 minutes and may be accompanied by chills, nausea, anxiety, palpitations and clamminess. Although the severity of symptoms varies significantly, hot flushes can cause embarrassment, sleep disruptions, significant discomfort and interruptions in activities, including sexual activities. Hot flushes gradually subside in most women after 1 to 7 years, but as many as 40% experience them for more than 7 years (Whiteley, Wagner, Bushmakin et al., 2013).

Diminished oestrogen levels can directly affect sexual function for older women in several ways. One of the more obvious effects is that breasts become more pendulous and have more fat and less mammary tissue. Vaginal dryness from diminished secretions is another noticeable effect that can affect sexual pleasure, unless compensatory interventions such as lubricants are used. Less obvious changes include loss of fullness of the labia, diminished quantity of pubic hair and atrophy of sexual organs.

In addition to these effects on sexual function and quality of life, oestrogen deficiency affects many non-reproductive tissues, including brain, bone, heart, liver, muscle tissues, and it is associated with increased risk for osteoporosis, cardiovascular disease, Alzheimer's disease and metabolic dysfunction (Cui, Shen & Li, 2013; Mauvais-Jarvis et al., 2013; Nedergaard, Henriksen, Asser et al., 2013). Menopausal hormonal changes have been identified as a risk factor for depression, but some studies suggest that the relationship is complex and may be more strongly associated with psychosocial factors such as coping skills and social support (Gibbs, Lee & Kulkarni, 2012; Lin, Hsiao, Liu et al., 2013; Pimenta, Leal, Maroco et al., 2012).

DIVERSITY NOTE

Hot flushes are more prevalent in women who live in Europe and North America and are less common in women who live in India, China and Japan (Ayers, Forshaw & Hunter, 2010; Weismiller, 2009).

Changes affecting older men

Male reproductive function depends on the secretion of testosterone and other hormones, the production and release of sperm and the motility of sperm through the urethra. All organs involved in these processes undergo degenerative changes during later adulthood and gradually diminish the production of viable sperm. Despite these age-related changes, however, some men never lose their reproductive abilities.

The term **andropause** has been used to describe the age-related decline in testosterone in men that begins around the age of 30 years and is analogous to the age-related decline in oestrogen in women. Cross-sectional and longitudinal data vary widely, with some studies indicating that up to 20% of men older than 60 years and 50% of those older than 80 years have serum testosterone levels below the lower limits of young adults (Horstman, Dillon, Urban et al., 2012; Surampudi, Wang & Swerdloff, 2012). Researchers emphasise that much of the variation is associated with comorbid conditions such as metabolic syndrome, type 2diabetes and cardiovascular disease (Pantalone & Faiman, 2012). In recent years, the term *androgen deficiency in the older male* (also called *late-onset hypogonadism, testosterone deficiency syndrome*) has been used to describe a condition in which serum testosterone level is abnormally low and is associated with symptoms such as low libido, **erectile dysfunction**, decreased vitality and depressed mood (McGill, Shoskes & Sabanegh, 2012). Recent studies suggest that low serum testosterone levels are associated not only with diminished sexual function but also with increased risk for pathological conditions such as anaemia, diabetes and osteoporosis (Spitzer, Huang, Basaria et al., 2013).

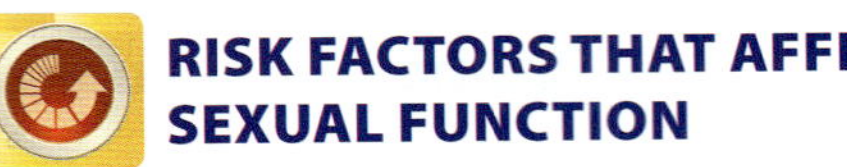

RISK FACTORS THAT AFFECT SEXUAL FUNCTION

Many types of risk factors can affect sexual function and expressions of sexuality, ranging from individual physical functional and psychosocial factors, to broader societal and cultural influences. Although many of these risks affect people at any age, older adults are likely to experience several or more risks and some risks are unique to older adults. This section provides an overview of risk factors that occur most commonly in older adults.

Myths and attitudes in society

Because personal attitudes about sexuality are shaped by societal influences, it is important to consider the societal context of attitudes about sexuality, particularly with regard to women and older adults. Strict Victorian standards of morality strongly influenced many generations, beginning in the 1800s and including those who are older adults today. According to Victorian standards, homosexual activity, public displays of affection, and sex with anyone except a marital partner were totally taboo. During this same time, people viewed menstruation and sexuality as having deleterious effects on women and medical practitioners removed a woman's sexual organs as a usual treatment.

Victorian perspectives were common until 1953 when Kinsey and colleagues published results of their study of *Sexual behaviours in the human female.* This "Kinsey report" brought public attention to previously taboo topics such as orgasm, masturbation, premarital sex and marital infidelity, and was a major turning point in perspectives on female sexuality. In recent decades, attitudes about sexuality changed significantly; however, older adults have been strongly influenced by societal viewpoints of the past. Older adults today may lack accurate information about sexuality, and may resist attempts to discuss topics that they consider taboo. This is particularly true for women born in 1925 or before (Farrell & Belza, 2011).

Another factor that influences perspective on sexuality and ageing is the strong association in Western societies between sexual attractiveness and physical attractiveness in very gender-specific and stereotypical ways. For example, male sexuality is associated with the image of a tanned, muscular and youthful man; female sexuality is associated with the image of a thin, but adequately endowed, young woman. Because these images contrast with typical portrayals of older adults as physically unattractive, they foster a stereotype of "sexless seniors".

These societal influences promote the false perception that older adults have lost the interest in or capacity for sexual activity. This can become a self-fulfilling prophecy if older adults believe this stereotype. Even if older adults do not believe these stereotypes, they may be embarrassed to acknowledge their sexual desires and activities for fear of being considered not normal.

WELLNESS OPPORTUNITY

Nurses need to avoid reinforcing, or even buying into, any pervasive societal attitudes about "sexless seniors".

In addition to being affected by myths and stereotypes, older people who are lesbian, gay, bisexual and transgender (LGBT) usually have long-term experiences of prejudice and misinformation related to their sexual orientation and identity. Even though attitudes have changed in recent years, these diverse groups of sexual minorities have experienced decades of stigma and discrimination and they are more likely than younger generations to be "closeted" and secretive about their sexual orientation. In addition, the disproportionately high death rate among gay men between the ages of 25 and 44 years when the human immunodeficiency virus (HIV)/acquired immunodeficiency syndrome (AIDS) was at its peak (1987–1996) had a strong influence on social networks and personal lives of those who are now reaching older adulthood (Rosenfeld, Bartlam & Smith, 2012). A review of studies identified many health disparities among LGBT older adults; however, studies also identified many areas of strength and resiliency among these groups (Van Wagenen, Driskell & Bradford, 2013).

WELLNESS OPPORTUNITY

Nurses holistically address sexual wellness in older adults by being non-judgemental about with whom they choose to form close relationships.

Social circumstances

Availability of a satisfactory partner is a major factor that influences opportunities for sexual activities during older adulthood and this is especially true for older heterosexual women (Wood, Runciman, Wylie et al., 2012). Although higher levels of sexual interest and activity are reported by men at any age compared with women at a similar age, this gender difference widens during older adulthood. This is partly attributable to the fact that women outnumber men in older age groups. Similarly, the proportion of married women also decreases with increasing age. Another contributing factor for women is the common occurrence of poor health in their male partners (Syme, Klonoff, Macera et al., 2013).

Privacy is generally considered a requisite for sexual activity, and adults who live in their own homes are usually able to arrange for this. However, older adults who live in institutions, group settings or family homes may find it difficult or impossible to arrange for privacy, especially if their sexual needs are ignored or considered not normal. Even if some privacy is possible in institutional settings, additional environmental constraints include the inability to lock doors and ensure total privacy and the unavailability of anything larger than a single bed.

WELLNESS OPPORTUNITY

Nurses in long-term residential care settings need to create opportunities for privacy if a resident desires this.

Adverse effects of medication, alcohol and nicotine

Three decades ago, a study (Slag, Morley, Elson et al., 1983) identified adverse effects of medication as the single largest cause of erectile dysfunction in men. Slag and colleagues found that 34% of 1180 male patients in a medical clinic were impotent, and 25% of the 188 subjects who subsequently underwent further evaluation were found to have medication-induced erectile dysfunction. In recent years, there has been increasing attention to the sexual adverse effects of medications as a major factor that influences quality of life and adherence to prescribed regimens. Although most studies have focused on men, medications are a common cause of sexual dysfunction in both men and women (Wood, Runciman, Wylie et al., 2012).

Medications adversely affect sexual function through a variety of mechanisms, including their influence on the release of hormones and their actions on the autonomic and central nervous systems. Specific adverse medication effects that interfere with sexual function in men include a decreased or absent libido; difficulty obtaining or maintaining an erection; dry, premature or retrograde ejaculation; and an inability to achieve orgasm. Women might experience the following medication-induced limitations in their sexual function: diminished vaginal lubrication, decreased or absent libido, and inability to achieve orgasm. Box 26-1 lists some of the medications commonly associated with sexual dysfunction. These effects usually disappear when the medication is discontinued, and occasionally the effects will disappear if the dose is decreased.

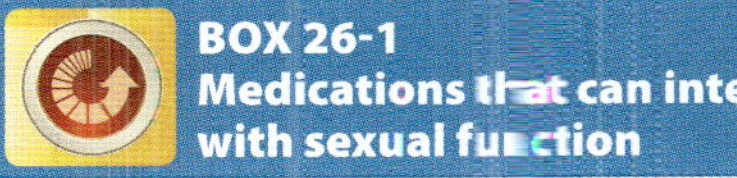

BOX 26-1 Medications that can interfere with sexual function

- ACE inhibitors
- Alpha-adrenergic blockers or agonists
- Antidepressants
- Antihistamines
- Anti-parkinsonism agents
- Antipsychotics
- Benzodiazepines
- Beta-blockers
- Calcium channel blockers
- Diuretics
- Dopamine agonists
- Histamine H_2 antagonists
- Monoamine oxidase inhibitors (MAOIs)
- Non-steroidal anti-inflammatory drugs
- Alcohol, nicotine, recreational drugs

Because alcohol depresses the central nervous system, it can interfere with sexual function. Although alcohol can decrease inhibitions and heighten sensual and sexual interest in social settings, excessive amounts can depress the central nervous system and interfere with sexual performance. Moderate amounts of alcohol normally do not interfere with sexual performance; however, in combination with other risk factors, such as medications or pathological conditions, even small amounts of alcohol may be detrimental to the sexual performance of older adults.

Cigarette smoking was first identified as a cause of erectile dysfunction in the mid-1980s and recent studies have confirmed that smoking increases the risk for sexual dysfunction in both men and women (Glina, Sharlip & Hellstrom, 2013; Harte & Meston, 2012; Kim, Kim, Kim et al., 2011). Nicotine interferes with circulation to the sexual organs and accentuates the effects of other risk factors such as diabetes, hypertension and vascular disease. In addition, cigarette smoking is associated with earlier onset of menopause and increased the intensity and frequency of hot flushes (Hayatbakhsh, Clavarino, Williams et al., 2012; La Marca, Sighinolfi, Papaleo et al., 2013).

Effects of chronic conditions

Chronic conditions that have consistently been identified as having detrimental effects on sexual wellness include pain, cancer, diabetes, cardiovascular disease, and obstructive sleep apnoea (Ryan & Gajraj, 2012; Santos, Drummond & Botelho, 2012; Syme, Klonoff, Macera et al., 2013). Prevalence of erectile dysfunction in men with diabetes is 50% or more, with higher rates being associated with obesity, older age, physical inactivity and taking calcium channel blockers (Shamloul & Ghanem, 2013; Sharifi, Asqhari, Jaberi et al., 2012; Thorve, Kshirsagar, Vyawahare et al., 2011). In addition to erectile dysfunction, men with diabetes are likely to experience retrograde ejaculation (Fedder, Kaspersen, Brandslund et al., 2013). Women with diabetes or metabolic syndrome also have a high prevalence of sexual dysfunction, such as problems with orgasm or lubrication, with increased age being an independent risk factor (Copeland, Brown, Creasman et al., 2012; Martelli, Valisella, Moscatiello et al., 2012; Pontiroli, Contelazzi, Morabito, 2013). Depression is another chronic condition strongly associated with sexual dysfunction in men and women (Pastuszak, Badhiwala, Lipshultz et al., 2013; Wood, Runciman, Wylie et al., 2012).

Cardiovascular disease (e.g. heart failure) is strongly associated with many aspects of sexual dysfunction, including decreased libido, inhibited performance and pleasure, and decreased frequency of sexual activities (Hoekstra, Lesman-Leegle, Luttik et al., 2012). Sexual function is affected not only by the physical manifestations of coronary heart disease (e.g. angina and reduced levels of activity) and adverse effects of medications, but also by psychological factors that commonly occur in people with cardiovascular disease. For example, even when no physiological basis exists for abstaining from sexual intercourse after a myocardial infarction, sexual activity is often limited or absent because of fatigue, depression, diminished sexual desire, and fears and anxiety of the person or the sexual partner.

DIVERSITY NOTE

A review of studies concluded that sexual function in women is significantly affected by coronary artery disease and that nurses play a key role in addressing sexual concerns for women with cardiovascular disease (Steinke, 2010).

Effects of dementia

Gerontologists and clinicians have focused attention on sexual function and intimate relationships in people living with dementia. It has been found that the issues related to sexual expression are often compounded by concerns about competency, decision making, the personal meaning of behaviours, and whether the behaviour arises from dementia. During the later stages of the disease, most people living with dementia are indifferent about sex, but issues related to sexual function and intimate relationships often arise during early and middle stages. Loss of sexual desire is the most common effect of dementia on sexual function; however, some people with dementia experience hypersexuality and demand frequent sexual intercourse, particularly men and especially during the middle stages.

Some people living with dementia exhibit behaviours that are considered sexually inappropriate (e.g. removing clothing or getting into bed with someone); however, these behaviours are caused by cognitive impairments rather than sexual impulses. For example, hypersexual behaviours and increased sexual desire are common manifestations of cognitive impairment due to frontal lobe disorders (e.g. fronto-temporal dementia) (Mendez & Shapira, 2013).

Prevalence of inappropriate sexual behaviours in people with dementia ranges from 2% to 17%, with higher rates reported in men (Lochlainn & Kenny, 2013). It is important to consider that behaviours associated with sexuality may be expressions of unmet needs related to touch, intimacy and interpersonal relationships. Sometimes, the behaviours are normal but they become problematic because of the context or the environment. For example, masturbating or disrobing in public places is considered sexually inappropriate, but these actions may be due to dementia-related disinhibition.

For people living in institutional settings, questions may arise about the ability of the person with dementia to make decisions about intimate relationships and sexual expressions. This is particularly problematic with regard to non-marital relationships and behaviours involving spousal infidelity. These decisions are complex and should consider not only the effect on the spouse but also whether sexual interactions could be beneficial or positive for the person with dementia.

Gender-specific conditions

Prostatic hyperplasia (also called *benign prostatic hypertrophy*) is a pathological condition in which the prostate gland gradually enlarges and affects the urinary tract and sexual function. Estimates of the prevalence of erectile dysfunction in men who have had prostatectomy for prostate cancer range from 25% to 90% (Tutolo, Briganti, Suardi et al., 2012). Prostatic hypertrophy is highly associated with erectile dysfunction and ejaculatory dysfunction and is also a common cause of urinary incontinence, which can interfere with enjoyment of sexual activities (Rosen et al., 2009). Sexual function in older women can be affected by their increased susceptibility to **urethritis** and **vaginitis** because of the thinning of the vaginal tissue and the decreased acidity and quantity of vaginal secretions. These conditions can occur after intercourse and cause urinary urgency and burning that persists for several days. They can also interfere with enjoyment of sexual intercourse.

Functional impairments

Functional impairments associated with chronic conditions can interfere with enjoyment of sexual activity in many ways, as in the following examples:

- Chronic obstructive pulmonary disease may cause hypoxia and severe shortness of breath in response to the high physiological demands of sexual activity
- Arthritis and other musculoskeletal disorders are likely to be associated with pain, stiffness, muscle spasms and limited flexibility
- Urinary incontinence can interfere with satisfying sexual relationships in people of any age, but this condition is more common in older adults
- Medical conditions and adverse medication effects can have physiological effects that interfere with all phases of sexual function
- Dementia, depression and other conditions that affect psychosocial function can also affect sexual function.

Functional limitations increase with advancing age and are likely to combine with other risk factors to interfere with sexual function. In addition to direct effects, disabilities can indirectly affect sexual function because of the common misperception equating disability with lack of sexual function. This cultural bias, along with other effects of disabilities on self-image, can have a negative impact on sexual function. This is particularly relevant to older adults who live in institutional settings because attitudes of the staff members can affect the residents' expressions of sexuality. A study of factors that influence attitudes about late-life sexuality found that young adults expressed less acceptance of sexual expression and more doubt about ability to consent when older women were described as cognitively impaired (Allen, Petro & Phillips, 2009).

Sensory impairments can also interfere with sexual function because sensory stimulation is an important part of sexual pleasure and intimate communication. For example, an older adult with impaired hearing may find it difficult or impossible to carry on the intimate conversations that are often a part of sexual interactions. Similarly, hearing impairments can interfere with professional efforts to assess and counsel older adults on this sensitive topic. Likewise, impairments affecting vision, smell or touch can interfere with some of the usual sensual stimulation associated with sexual activities.

Attitudes and behaviours of families and carers

In addition to societal influences, the attitudes and behaviours of family members and carers/caregivers who are closest to the older adult can negatively affect the older adult's sexual function. Adult children of older people often find it difficult to deal with the sexuality of their parents because they believe the common stereotype that older adults are asexual. In addition, they may discourage intimate relationships if they fear that a serious relationship would jeopardise their inheritance.

In institutional settings, attitudes of staff members can significantly affect the way in which residents express or repress their sexual needs. Staff members in long-term residential care are generally unprepared to address issues related to sexuality and ageing. Moreover, studies have found a notable lack of policies to guide staff responses to residents' sexual expressions or romantic behaviours (Cornelison & Doll, 2012; Elias & Ryan, 2011).

In general, sexual needs of older adults are ignored unless they are expressed in private and not brought to the attention of staff. When staff in long-term residential care observe sexual expressions of residents, they are likely to view these behaviours as a problem rather than an expression of unmet need (Cornelison & Doll, 2012). Another concern in institutional settings is that family members are often involved with decisions about a resident's sexual expressions, even when the person is competent. This occurs either because the staff members initiate the contact with the family or the family requests assistance from the facility in setting boundaries on the resident's expressions of sexuality.

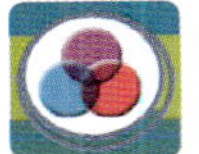

FUNCTIONAL CONSEQUENCES AFFECTING SEXUAL WELLNESS

Sexual function involves reproduction, response to sexual stimulation, and interest and participation in sexual activity. With increased age, reproductive aspects become less significant, but many studies verify that sexual well-being is an important component of overall quality of life throughout older adulthood (Syme, Klonoff, Macera et al., 2013). Although age-related changes directly affect reproduction, other aspects of sexuality are affected more directly by risk factors. In addition, because sexual dysfunctions commonly occur in older men and women as a consequence of risk factors, these are discussed in this section.

Reproductive ability

For women, the loss of reproductive ability is a functional consequence of menopause, caused by the cessation of ova production within 1 year of the last menstrual cycle. Another functional consequence affecting reproduction in women is the increased risk that a fetus will be defective if ova are fertilised during the premenopausal years. On the positive side, older women frequently experience fewer constraints and inhibitions when they no longer are concerned about pregnancy (Gray & Garcia, 2012). The reproductive ability of men, by contrast, gradually declines with age but does not cease completely.

Response to sexual stimulation

The Masters and Johnson (1966) investigation has been widely recognised as the landmark study of human physiological response to sexual stimulation. This study of 694 adults in a laboratory setting identified four phases of physiological response to sexual stimulation in men and women. An analysis of data on older subjects led to the following conclusions:

- Older adults maintain their ability to respond to sexual stimulation, but their response is slower and less intense.
- Regularly engaging in sexual activity helps older adults respond to sexual stimulation.
- Any major changes in response to sexual stimulation are associated with risk factors rather than ageing, per se.

Although older adults were greatly underrepresented in this study, the findings of Masters and Johnson have been widely accepted as the knowledge base about age-related changes in physiological response to sexual stimulation. Normal age-related changes in male and female responses to sexual stimulation and the associated consequences are discussed in the following sections and summarised in Table 26-1.

In recent years, more comprehensive models have been proposed with emphasis on multifactorial factors that influence men and women; however, research on age-related differences is lacking. Current models emphasise the interrelationship between mind and body and conceptualise sexuality in relation to and interaction with such variables as culture, religion and social practices (Wylie & Mimoun, 2009).

Sexual interest and activity

During the 1940s and 1950s, the Kinsey surveys first brought information about sexual behaviours of older adults to public attention by concluding that the frequency of sexual activity gradually declines with increasing age but sexual interest and competence do not necessarily decline. Sexual interest, attitudes, activity and satisfaction are a continuation of lifelong patterns, and they remain stable in older adulthood unless risk factors interfere with sexual function. As discussed in the risk factors section, conditions that commonly affect sexual interest and activity in older adults include social circumstances, poor health, pathological conditions, adverse medication effects, and influences of family and carers. The sexual needs and interests of older adults, including residents of long-term residential care, do not necessarily decrease, but their opportunities for sexual activity are often limited.

In recent decades, studies of sexuality and ageing have focused on broader aspects such as affection, friendships and intimacy. For older adults, these aspects of sexual

TABLE 26-1 Functional consequences for response to sexual stimulation

	Changes in female response	Changes in male response
Excitement phase	Breasts not as engorged Sexual flush diminished Delayed or diminished vaginal lubrication Decreased expansion of vaginal wall Decreased vasocongestion of labia	Longer time required to attain erection Less firm erection Longer maintenance of erection before ejaculation Increased difficulty regaining an erection if lost Reduced scrotal and testicular vasocongestion
Plateau phase	Decreased areolar engorgement Less intense sexual flush Less intense myotonia Decreased vasocongestion of labia Reduced Bartholin's gland secretions Slower/less marked uterine elevation	Diminished nipple turgidity and sexual flush Less intense muscle tension Slower penile erectile response Delayed and diminished testicular elevation Fewer rectal sphincter contractions Diminution of ejaculatory expulsion force by about 50%
Orgasmic phase	Fewer rectal sphincter contractions Decreased number and intensity of orgasmic contractions	Absent or diminished sense of ejaculatory inevitability Fewer and less intense ejaculatory contractions
Resolution phase	Slower loss of nipple erection Quicker return to pre-excitement stage	Slower loss of nipple erection Longer refractory period Rapid penile detumescence and testicular descent

Source: Dementia Collaborative Research Centre (Australia). (2014). Assessment tools. Available at www.dementia-assessment.com.au/cognitive.

function may become more important as the number of opportunities for sexual activities diminishes. For example, one of the first studies addressing sexual behaviours found that the most common sexual activities in a sample of 202 adults aged 80 to 102 years were touching and caressing without sexual intercourse (Bretschneider & McCoy, 1988). More recent studies have confirmed that older men and women who engage in more frequent sexual touching report higher levels of satisfaction (Galinsky, 2012). Additional components of sexuality that are especially important for older adults include kissing, hugging, intimacy, fantasy, masturbation, oral sex, loving words, physical closeness, and expressions of affection (Lochlainn & Kenny, 2013; Muzacz & Akinsulure-Smith, 2013). A study of healthy community-dwelling older women (median age 67 years) found that one-third reported low libido, but half were sexually active and maintained arousal, lubrication and orgasm (Trompeter, Bettencourt & Barrett-Connor, 2012).

In summary, older adults do not lose their interest in or capacity for sexual activity because of age-related changes, but risk factors such as misinformation, social circumstances, pathological conditions, environmental constraints and adverse medication effects commonly interfere with sexual function. Many studies confirm that healthy older adults remain sexually active, particularly if they have positive attitudes, accurate information and access to a healthy partner (DeLamater, 2012; Trompeter et al., 2012; Van Wagenen, Driskell & Bradford, 2013). However, a normal consequence of ageing is that the response of older men and women to sexual stimulation is slower, less intense and of shorter duration. As one 79-year-old man reported, "It's like sparklers, not fireworks."

WELLNESS OPPORTUNITY

Nurses need to recognise that many interacting physical and psychosocial factors affect sexual wellness in a unique way for each older adult.

Sexual dysfunction in men and women

Erectile dysfunction, defined as the inability to achieve or maintain an erection sufficient for satisfactory sexual function, is the term that has been used since the early 1990s to replace the term *impotence*. The U.S. National Institutes of Health proposed this change in terminology to reflect the broader understanding of erectile dysfunction as a complex condition associated with many pathophysiological conditions and other risk factors. Although erectile dysfunction is not the only type of male sexual dysfunction, it is the one that has been studied the most and has received the most public attention since 1998 because of the availability of medications such as sildenafil (Viagra) and the widespread publicity about these medications that continues today. Other types of male sexual dysfunction include problems with ejaculation and diminished desire. Although these problems are associated more strongly with risk factors than with normal ageing, the prevalence increases with increasing age. It is currently viewed as a complex disease associated with multiple interacting factors, as discussed in the risk factors section.

In recent years, healthcare practitioners and pharmaceutical companies have started addressing **female sexual dysfunction**, similar to the way in which erectile dysfunction has been addressed since the early 1990s. Female sexual dysfunction includes disorders that affect sexual desire (including motivation and physical drive), sexual arousal, orgasm or pain during sexual activities (i.e. dyspareunia or vaginismus). Many of the same risk factors associated with erectile dysfunction are also associated with female sexual dysfunction, such as diabetes, cardiovascular disease, cigarette smoking, pelvic surgeries and adverse medication effects. An additional risk factor for women is diminished oestrogen levels.

UNFOLDING CASE STUDY

Part A

You are the nurse at the senior centre where Mr and Mrs Smith come for the meal program and social interaction. Mr Smith is 73 years old and has hypertension and a history of a heart attack. He takes diltiazem, 300 mg daily; frusemide, 20 mg daily; and propranolol, 80 mg three times daily. Mrs Smith, who is 71 years old, describes herself as generally healthy, but with a history of depression and some arthritis. She takes ibuprofen, 400 mg four times daily, and sertraline, 50 mg daily. During your nursing clinics, Mr Smith and several other men have asked you about the drug that is advertised on television for men who have trouble satisfying their partners. The senior centre's director has also noticed an increased interest in this topic and has asked that you plan a group health information session called "Sexuality and Ageing".

Thinking points

- Develop a plan for teaching older adults about the normal changes in sexual function that they are likely to experience.
- What risk factors would you discuss in relation to sexuality and ageing?
- What educational materials would you use?
- What interventions would promote sexual wellness in older adults?

PATHOLOGICAL CONDITION AFFECTING SEXUAL WELLNESS: HUMAN IMMUNODEFICIENCY VIRUS

Nurses who provide care to older adults must also be aware that older adults remain at risk of developing a sexually transmitted infection (STI), including *Chlamydia*, syphilis, gonorrhoea, hepatitis C, and the human immunodeficiency virus (HIV). In Australia and New Zealand, very few older adults become infected with these diseases, but notifications still occur (Australian Government Department of Health [AGDH], 2015; New Zealand Ministry of Health,

2014). In both countries, syphilis has the highest reported incidence of the STIs in older adults.

Older adults remain at risk of infection from the **human immunodeficiency virus (HIV)** and it is becoming more common among older adults. Studies indicate that 11% of new HIV infections occur in adults aged 50 years and older (Brooks, Buchacz, Gebo et al., 2012). The effectiveness of antiretroviral therapy since the late 1980s has enabled many HIV-infected people to live longer with this condition, which is now considered a chronic disease, before it progresses to AIDS. As a result of the use of highly effective antiretroviral treatments during the past two decades, fewer than one-third of the people who have been diagnosed and treated will die from conditions traditionally associated with HIV/AIDS. By 2015, 50% of HIV-infected individuals will be age 50 and older (Adekeye, Heiman, Onyeabor et al., 2012; Cahill & Valadez, 2013). It is estimated that the number of people aged 55 years and over in Australia who are living with HIV/AIDS will almost double, reaching 44% by 2020 (Jansson & Wilson, 2012).

DIVERSITY NOTE

The prevalence of *Chlamydia*, gonorrhoea and hepatitis B in older Indigenous people is much higher than other Australians, while the prevalence of hepatitis C (newly acquired) and HIV/ AIDS is comparable for both groups (AGDH, 2012).

The diagnosis of HIV/AIDS for people at any age is always accompanied by major health-related issues, but some issues are more unique to older adults, as summarised in Box 26-2. Although nurses in are not expected to be experts in all aspects of HIV/AIDS, there is the expectation to holistically assess and address the complex needs of older adults with this condition and, perhaps first and foremost, to communicate a non-judgemental approach in all interactions with people who have risks for or a diagnosis of HIV/AIDS.

An important assessment consideration is that HIV may initially manifest as a non-specific viral illness with signs and symptoms similar to seasonal flu or mononucleosis. These early manifestations may subside after several weeks, and HIV antibodies will appear in the blood between 3 and 6 weeks after the initial infection. If appropriate treatment is initiated in a timely manner, people with HIV can expect to live well into older adulthood, although they are likely to experience additional health issues, as summarised in Box 26-2.

Treatment of HIV generally includes a combination of antiretroviral agents and other types of medications to control disease progression. The pharmacological regimen requires close monitoring for therapeutic and adverse effects. Adherence is a common problem for people with HIV/AIDS for various reasons, including cost of medications and adverse effects, making these issues important aspects of assessing older adults with HIV/AIDS.

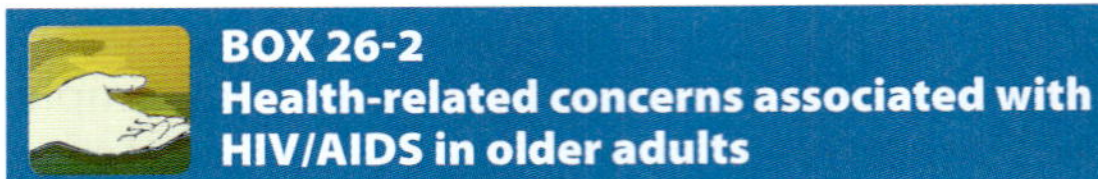

BOX 26-2
Health-related concerns associated with HIV/AIDS in older adults

Issues related to progression of the condition

- Older adults are likely to be diagnosed at a later stage, due to lack of screening, poor awareness of risk factors and failure of healthcare professionals to recognise and treat HIV/AIDS.
- Older adults have a shorter interval before progression to AIDS, particularly if HIV was diagnosed after the age of 60 years.
- Older adults have a shorter time before death.

Associated medical concerns

- HIV/AIDS in older adults increases the risk for diabetes, osteoporosis, parkinsonism, cerebrovascular conditions, cardiovascular conditions, liver disease and some cancers.
- Dementia occurs more frequently in those who are older with HIV.
- Drug regimens for HIV/AIDS increase the risk for interactions, particularly with drugs used for anxiety, depression, hyperlipidaemia and erectile dysfunction.

Additional concerns

- Older adults with HIV/AIDS have higher rates of depression.
- Older adults are more likely to have less social support due to ageism, living alone, perceived stigma and non-disclosure of HIV status.
- Carers of people with HIV/AIDS experience significant levels of stress that is exacerbated by associated factors such as stigma, uncertainty, depression, social isolation and impaired cognitive function.

Nurses have important responsibilities with regard to promoting wellness for older adults with HIV/AIDS including addressing any related psychosocial needs. For example, older gay men with HIV/AIDS are particularly susceptible to depression related to stigma, rejection and social isolation (Jang, Anderson & Mentes, 2011). In addition, nurses can consider cultural needs by suggesting resources specific for people who identify as LGBT or other minority groups.

Teaching about safer sex is a nursing responsibility often overlooked when caring for older adults, but it is particularly important with regard to preventing and managing all STIs. Older adults need to recognise that safer sex practices are imperative for anyone who has sex. Nurses also need to teach about sexually transmitted infections and encourage appropriate testing for anyone with risk factors. Recognise that, even though health professionals are reluctant to initiate discussions with older adults about sexually transmitted infections, older adults themselves are receptive to this information (Slinkard & Kazer, 2011). Nurses can incorporate information about safer sex in their health education about sexual activity for older adults, as discussed in the section on nursing interventions and summarised in Box 26-5 later in this chapter.

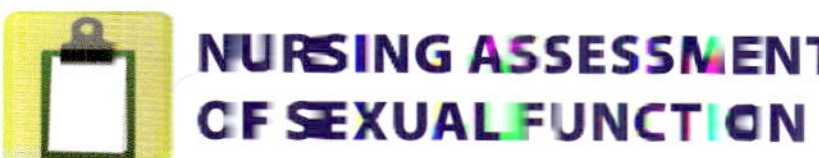

NURSING ASSESSMENT OF SEXUAL FUNCTION

Nurses do not necessarily include sexual function in every assessment, but they should assess it whenever they are addressing quality-of-life issues that affect day-to-day function. Assessment of sexual function is especially important in home care and long-term residential care settings. Sexual function is often neglected in nursing assessments because of the high degree of privacy associated with sexual function and the stereotype of the "sexless senior" that is prevalent in our society. In addition, gender or generational differences between the health professional and the older person may interfere with an assessment of sexual function. Although all of these factors may explain why sexual function in older adults is so often overlooked, they do not justify its exclusion.

Self-assessment of attitudes about sexual function and ageing

Because of the private nature of sexual function and possible associated emotional responses and cultural factors, nurses are often uncomfortable discussing it. Additional discomfort occurs because nurses are not confident in dealing with concerns about human sexuality as an integral part of their nursing practice. They are even less comfortable initiating this topic with older adults or with people who are not in a traditional marital relationship. An assessment of personal attitudes about sexuality and ageing is a prerequisite to addressing sexual wellness. Box 26-3 lists some of the questions nurses can use to examine their own attitudes towards the sexual functioning of older adults. Some questions are specific to adults in long-term residential care facilities because of the dominant role of nurses in addressing sexual function as a quality-of-life issue for residents.

WELLNESS OPPORTUNITY

Nurses should take time for self-assessment to increase their comfort with, openness to and sensitivity about issues related to sexual wellness for older adults.

Significant cultural differences between the nurse and the older adult may increase the difficulty of discussing sexual function. Cultural considerations 26-1 summarises some cultural aspects of sexual function that may be applicable to nursing assessment. Nurses may also be uncomfortable discussing sexual function with older adults who are involved in same-sex or other non-traditional relationships. Thus, an important aspect of self-assessment is to identify attitudes towards non-traditional sexual activities because these attitudes can influence the assessment and care of people who do not conform to the nurse's expectations. When assessing sexual function, it is important that nurses establish a trusting relationship, have an awareness

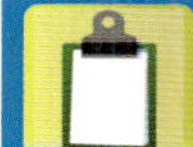

BOX 26-3
Assessing personal attitudes towards sexuality and ageing

What do I believe about sexuality and ageing?

- Do I hold the misconception that older people, especially unmarried ones, are no longer interested in or capable of sexual activities?
- Do I believe the subtle messages that inaccurately associate sexual activities only with youth and attractiveness?
- Do I hold age-specific standards regarding sexual activity and romantic relationships (e.g. Do I think it is okay for young adults to kiss or hold hands, but inappropriate or "cute" for older people to do this?)

What do I believe about the nurse's role with regard to the sexual function of older adults?

- Do I base my nursing practice on the misconception that sexual function is strictly a private matter that health professionals should not address?
- Do I view sexual function as an activity of daily living that should be included in a comprehensive assessment of long-term care needs of older adults?
- Do I feel more comfortable discussing sexual function with people who are of the same gender and age range as myself, but very uncomfortable in discussing this matter with people who are old enough to be my parents or grandparents?
- Do I avoid discussion of sexual function with older adults because I believe they are not interested in sexual activity or are uncomfortable discussing this topic?
- Do I avoid discussing sexual function with older adults who are not in traditional marital relationships?
- What beliefs do I hold about the assessment of sexual function based on the age of the person? For example, do I think sexual function should be assessed in sexually active teenagers who are at risk for unwanted pregnancy, but not older people?
- Am I comfortable incorporating health education about safer sex practices with older adults?

What is my attitude about various expressions of sexual activity?

- How do I view sexual activity and romantic relationships between unmarried people, or between people of the same gender?
- How do I view masturbation?
- Do my views about masturbation or sexual activity between unmarried or same-gender people influence my assessment of and interventions for people who engage in these activities?
- Am I tolerant and non-judgemental towards people whose views and practices are non-traditional or different from mine?

For nurses in settings where long-term needs are addressed

- How do I feel about the rights of residents to engage in sexual activity in private, either with themselves or people of their own choosing?
- Do I try to ensure privacy for those residents who desire it?
- If I am aware of the sexual activities of a resident, do I think that I should inform the administrator, a family member or another "responsible adult?"

CULTURAL CONSIDERATIONS 26-1
Cultural aspects of sexual function

Expressions of sexuality and intimacy

- In some cultures it is taboo for a man to be alone with a woman other than his wife (e.g. Islamic cultures)
- Touching another person (particularly of the opposite sex) is considered taboo in many cultures.
- In some cultures, heterosexual men and women commonly hold hands with another person of the same gender (it is not uncommon for Italian women to do this).
- Only a few cultures value sexual equality between men and women.
- Homosexuality is accepted in some cultures but is considered taboo or is kept secret among family members in others.

Assessment considerations

- In some cultures it is considered taboo for postmenopausal women to have their breasts or vagina examined, even by a healthcare provider.
- Menopausal manifestations may vary in different cultural groups (e.g. most Japanese women do not experience hot flushes).

Terms describing sexual orientation (i.e. one's sexual and romantic attraction)

- *Heterosexual*: sexual attraction to people of the opposite sex
- *Bisexual*: sexual attraction to both men and women
- *Homosexual*: sexual attraction to people of the same sex; the term applies to both men and women and is associated more with biological aspects rather than with lifestyle characteristics
- *Gay*: the term that is associated with lifestyle characteristics of men who feel romantically attracted to other men
- *Lesbian*: the term that is associated with lifestyle characteristics of women who feel romantically attracted to other women

Terms describing sexual orientation (i.e. a combination of biological characteristics and social roles)

- *Transgender*: people whose gender identity, gender expression or behaviour does not conform to that typically associated with the sex to which they were assigned at birth
- *Female-to-male* or *male-to-female transgenders* may be preparing for or recovering from sexual reassignment surgery, or they may be using long-term hormonal therapy as a non-surgical option

of gay and lesbian culture and other non-traditional sexual relationships and communicate a non-judgemental attitude by using gender-neutral terminology. For example, the word *partner* includes a spouse as well as a same-sex relationship and asking about someone who is a *confidant* is broader than asking about marital status. Terminology related to people who identify as LGBT is delineated in Cultural considerations 26-1.

Assessing sexual function in older adults

The goals in assessing sexual function in older adults include providing an opportunity for the older adult to address any issues related to their sexual function and identifying risk factors, including lack of information, which can interfere with the older person's sexual function and quality of life. Although the extent of the assessment varies according to individual circumstances, it should include, at a minimum, questions about the gynaecological aspects of female sexual function and the genitourinary aspects of male sexual function. Nurses can easily incorporate these questions into a routine assessment of overall function. If these questions are followed by an open-ended question about sexual interest and activities, the nurse can then respond to the individual needs of the older adult. If problems or risk factors are identified, the nurse is not expected to conduct an in-depth assessment of all aspects of sexual function but should obtain enough information to suggest appropriate resources for further evaluation. Box 26-4 summarises guidelines for assessing sexual function in older adults.

The Hartford Institute for Geriatric Nursing recommends that nurses use the PLISSIT assessment model as a routine nursing assessment for older adults (Wallace, 2008). The four components of this model are as follows:

- Obtaining ***P****ermission* from the client to initiate sexual discussion
- Providing ***L****imited* ***I****nformation* about sexual function
- Giving ***S****pecific* ***S****uggestions* for the individual to proceed with sexual relations
- Providing ***I****ntensive* ***T****herapy* surrounding the issues of sexuality for the client.

Additional information about the application of this tool in a clinical setting is available through collaboration of the Hartford Institute and the *American Journal of Nursing* at http://consultgerirn.org/resources or at www.nursingcenter.com. Nurses have effectively applied this model to assess and address sexual issues of people who have stomas or cardiovascular disease (Ayaz & Kubily, 2009; Jaarsma, Steinke & Gianottem, 2010).

NURSING ISSUES

When nurses identify the risks that interfere with sexual function or when older adults express an interest in discussing sexual function, the appropriate nursing issue is altered sexuality pattern. Related factors commonly identified in older adults include medication effects; endocrine diseases (e.g. diabetes); cardiovascular diseases; genitourinary conditions; functional impairments secondary to chronic conditions (e.g. limited range of motion as a result of arthritis); psychosocial circumstances (e.g. lack of a partner); and myths and misunderstandings about age-related changes. The case example at the end of this chapter addresses this nursing issue.

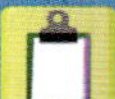

BOX 26-4
Guidelines for assessing sexual function in older adults

Interview atmosphere and communication techniques

- Ensure both privacy and comfort.
- Be non-judgemental and matter-of-fact in verbal and non-verbal communication.
- If feasible, sit face-to-face in chairs, rather than conducting the interview while the person being interviewed is in bed.
- If feasible, allow the person being interviewed to wear usual daytime clothing, rather than a hospital gown.

Initiation and discussion of the topic

- Begin by acknowledging feelings of discomfort and by stating the reason for discussing this topic (e.g. "I know that sexuality is a private matter and people are often uncomfortable discussing this topic. However, as a nurse, I consider sexuality to be an aspect of health and well-being, and it may have a significant bearing on your overall care.").
- Include statements that address stereotypes and require a response from the older adult (e.g. "Our society tends to view older people as being uninterested in sex, but for most older people this is not true. Some older people are less sexually active than when they were younger, but this is not because of age-related changes. Have you experienced any changes in your sexual activities in the past few years?").
- Initiate the topic near the end of a comprehensive assessment interview, and begin with questions about the physiological aspects of male or female function, such as those that follow.
- Incorporate at least one question to assess the appropriateness of including information about safer sex practices in your health teaching (e.g. "If you have sex with partners other than someone who is in a long-term monogamous relationship with you, what precautions do you take?").

Interview questions to assess male sexual function

- Have you ever had prostate problems or related surgery? Have you ever been told that you have or had an enlarged prostate?
- How often do you undergo a complete medical examination? When was your last complete physical examination done?
- Do you ever experience dribbling of urine or have problems holding your water?
- Do you have any trouble initiating the stream of urine?
- After you have urinated (passed water), do you still feel like you haven't emptied your bladder completely?
- Do you have to get up during the night to empty your bladder? If so, how many times?
- Have you ever noticed any blood in your urine?
- Do you ever have any discharge from your penis?
- Do you have any sores, lumps, ulcers, irritations or areas of inflammation on your penis or scrotum?
- Do you have any trouble with erection or ejaculation?

Interview questions to assess female sexual function

- How many children, if any, have you had? How many pregnancies?
- At what ages did your menstrual periods begin and end?
- Have you ever had a Pap (Papanicolaou) test? When were your most recent Pap test and gynaecological examination?
- Have you ever had a mammogram? When was the most recent one?
- Have you ever been taught to examine your breasts for lumps?
- Do you examine your breasts for lumps? How often?
- Have you noticed any changes in your breasts? Do you ever have any discharge from your nipples?
- Do you have any burning, itching or irritation in the vaginal area?
- Do you ever have any vaginal discharge or bleeding?
- Do you have any difficulties with sexual intercourse?

Principles for assessing sexual interest and activities

- If the older adult makes a clear statement that this topic is irrelevant, do not insist on further questions. However, if the older adult responds to questions, do not discontinue the interview because of your own discomfort.
- Do not assume that an assessment of sexual function is irrelevant to unmarried people.
- For both married and unmarried older adults, use open-ended questions to elicit information about intimate relationships (e.g. "Is there anything you would like to ask or discuss about intimate relationships?").
- For a married person, open-ended questions may be asked about the partner's influence on sexual activities (e.g. "Has your husband experienced any changes in his health that have affected your sexual activities?").
- Listen for statements that reflect myths, a negative self-image or self-fulfilling prophecies such as "Of course I stopped being interested in sex after menopause", or "I can't have an erection because I have prostate trouble."
- If risk factors such as certain medications or pathological conditions have been identified earlier in the interview, ask additional questions such as "Have you had any difficulties with sexual activities since your heart attack?" or "Do you have any questions about the possible effects of diabetes on sexual activity?"
- Emphasise the clinical reason for the questions ("Sometimes certain illnesses or medications interfere with sexual function, and we want to identify any problems you might be having in this area.").
- Use open-ended questions that allow for either closure of the topic or a further discussion of issues ("Is there anything you would like to discuss with regard to your sexual relationships?").

WELLNESS OPPORTUNITY

The nursing issue of willingness for enhanced knowledge of sexual functioning would be applicable to older adults who express an interest in learning about the effects of ageing or risk factors on sexual wellness.

GOAL PLANNING FOR WELLNESS OUTCOMES

Increased knowledge about sexual function is a goal for older adults who lack accurate information about age-related changes and risk factors. A goal for residents of long-term residential care would be increased client satisfaction because of the respect of their rights. For a long-term residential care resident who is LGBT, an applicable goal would be increased client satisfaction because their diversity is recognised. Other goals for the promotion of sexual wellness for older adults include improved body image, increased health beliefs, increased knowledge about sexual functioning, improved personal well-being, and improved self-esteem and sexual functioning.

WELLNESS OPPORTUNITY

Quality of life is a wellness outcome for older adults who achieve more satisfying relationships through a variety of expressions of intimacy.

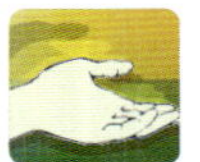

NURSING INTERVENTIONS TO PROMOTE HEALTHY SEXUAL FUNCTION

Nurses have many opportunities to teach older adults about healthy sexual function as an important aspect of quality of life, particularly in home and long-term residential care settings. Nurses have an important teaching role because many older adults, as well as family and carers, hold stereotypes or have little accurate information about sexuality and ageing. Other nursing interventions focus on body image enhancement, health education, rights' protection, risk identification, role enhancement, self-awareness enhancement, self-esteem enhancement and teaching about sexuality.

Health promotion: Teaching older adults about sexual wellness

Although sex therapists provide sex education and direct interventions, nurses are also expected to address sexual function as a quality-of-life concern. Nursing responsibilities also include teaching about safer sex practices for older adults who are sexually active. Health education about sexual wellness for older adults includes the following information:

- Acknowledgment that sexual function is within the usual realm of health promotion for older adults, especially in long-term residential care
- Effects of age-related changes on sexual function
- Risk factors that cause or contribute to problems with sexual function
- Resources for addressing identified problems and risk factors
- Protection from sexually transmitted infections.

In addition, nurses in long-term residential care often need to address attitudes of the staff members, families and residents by providing accurate information and role modelling non-judgemental behaviours.

In some situations, it is appropriate for nurses to teach older adults, as well as their carers, about age-related changes and risk factors that affect sexual function. The privacy of this topic requires that nurses use excellent communication skills when teaching about sexual wellness. It is important to be open, respectful and non-judgemental and to avoid the use of medical terminology when discussing sexuality with older adults. Nurses can use printed information written in non-technical terms, such as the teaching tool in Box 26-5, as the basis of discussion about sexual function for older adults. Nurses can emphasise that any major changes in sexual function are not due to age-related changes alone and they can use Table 26-1, earlier, for further discussion of sexual function in healthy older adults. Many excellent resources for professionals are available. See the resources section at the end of the chapter for some of these.

WELLNESS OPPORTUNITY

Nurses promote personal responsibility for sexual wellness by suggesting sources of accurate information that older adults can use.

Addressing risk factors

If an older adult with significant changes in sexual function also has a pathological condition, takes a medication or uses any substance that might be a contributing factor nurses can teach about the potential influence of these risk factors. This is particularly important when nurses identify pertinent risk factors but the older adult attributes sexual problems to old age. For example, an older man may attribute a problem with attaining an erection to age-related changes when, in fact, he has diabetes and takes an antihypertensive medication that is associated with erectile dysfunction. Nurses can use Box 26-1 to identify some of the medications that can interfere with sexual function. When nurses identify a potential relationship between a risk factor and sexual problems, it is appropriate to suggest that the older adult seek professional advice. A complete medical evaluation by a primary care provider who is knowledgeable about the sexual problems of older adults is usually the best starting point. If medications are causing or contributing to sexual dysfunction, the primary care provider should consider alternative medications or reduced doses if medically feasible. For example, people with hypertension are less likely to have sexual dysfunction when treated with calcium channel blockers, angiotensin-converting enzyme inhibitors or peripheral alpha-adrenergic receptor blockers. After medical problems are addressed, a mental health professional may be an appropriate resource if problems with sexual function persist.

Osteoarthritis is one of the most common pathological conditions affecting older adults and it is often self-managed with little or no medical supervision. Often, the symptoms are not severe enough to motivate the older adult to seek medical evaluation and treatment, but they

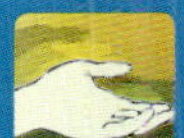

BOX 26-5
Health education about sexual activity for older people

- Older people remain fully capable of enjoying orgasm, but their response to sexual stimulation is usually slower, less intense and of shorter duration. Increasing the amount and diversity of sexual stimulation and experimenting with different positions can compensate for these changes and increase sexual enjoyment.
- Sexual problems in older people occur for the same reasons they occur in younger people. That is, they may be related to illness or disability, medications or alcohol or psychological and relationship factors. A cause of sexual problems that is unique to older people is the self-fulfilling prophecy of the "sexless senior" stereotype.
- The following habits enhance sexual enjoyment: exercising regularly, avoiding or limiting the consumption of alcohol, maintaining optimal health and nutrition, using hearing aids and corrective lenses as needed and engaging in sexual activities when you are relaxed and your energy level is at its peak.
- If you experience problems with sexual function, seek advice from a professional who is skilled in working with older people. Medical help can be obtained from a urologist, gynaecologist or other medical specialist. If there is no medical basis for the problem, a sex therapist or marriage counsellor might be helpful.
- Protect yourself from sexually transmitted infections and talk with your health care practitioner about being tested for them periodically.

Facts specific to older men

- Periodic difficulties with erection and ejaculation do not necessarily indicate that you are impotent.
- After you've reached orgasm, it may be 1 or 2 days before you are able to have full orgasm again.
- Many new treatment options are available for treating erectile dysfunction (impotence). If your health care provider cannot provide up-to-date information about these options, ask for a referral for an appropriate evaluation and discussion of various options.

Facts specific to older women

- Using a water-soluble lubricant will compensate for decreased vaginal lubrication. Do *not* use petroleum jelly because it is not a very effective lubricant for this purpose and can predispose you to infection.
- Oestrogen is beneficial in preventing some problems with sexual function, but the relative risks and benefits of such therapy should be considered and discussed thoroughly with your medical practitioner.
- You may have vaginal irritation or urinary tract infections, especially after sexual intercourse, because of age-related thinning of the vaginal wall. Such problems may be avoided by the following interventions:
  - Drink plenty of fluids.
  - Use an oestrogen cream or vaginal lubricant.
  - Maintain good hygiene in the vaginal area.
  - If you have a male partner, have him thrust his penis downwards towards the back of your vagina.
  - Empty your bladder before and after intercourse.

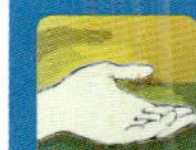

BOX 26-6
Health education about sexual activity for people with arthritis

The pain, fatigue and joint limitations of arthritis may interfere with, but do not have to curtail, your enjoyment of sexual activity. In fact, sexual activity can be beneficial to you because it stimulates the release of cortisone, adrenaline and other chemicals that are natural pain relievers. The following actions may enhance your sexual enjoyment and minimise the effects of arthritis:

- Engage in sexual activity when you feel least fatigued and most relaxed.
- Use analgesic medications and other methods of pain relief before engaging in sexual activity.
- Use relaxation techniques before engaging in sexual activity. Relaxation techniques that may be helpful for arthritis include warm baths or showers and the application of hot packs to the affected joints.
- Maintain optimal health through good nutrition and a proper balance of rest and activity.
- Experiment with different sexual positions and use pillows for comfort and support.
- Increase the time spent in foreplay.
- Use a vibrator if your ability to massage is limited by arthritis.
- Use a water-soluble jelly for vaginal lubrication.

may interfere with sexual activities. In such cases, nurses can use Box 26-6 to teach about self-care interventions that may be effective in improving the quality of sexual activities for the older adult with osteoarthritis. Nurses can also suggest that older adults who have osteoarthritis obtain information from the various arthritis support groups. This information is easily accessed via websites. See Chapter 22 for this information.

Another pathological condition often associated with sexual dysfunction is coronary artery disease, particularly in those who have had myocardial infarctions or who have undergone coronary artery bypass surgery. Nurses have important—but often overlooked—roles in providing information about sexual concerns for males and females and their partners, not only immediately after a myocardial infarction, but also for a prolonged period after initial recovery (Byrne, Doherty, Murphy et al., 2013; Steinke, Mosack, Barnason et al., 2011). Nurses can encourage older adults to discuss these concerns with their medical practitioner and can provide health education using the general guidelines outlined in Box 26-7.

Promoting sexual wellness in long-term residential care

The responsibilities of nurses in long-term residential care to address sexual needs differ from the responsibilities of nurses in acute care or home settings in the following ways:

- Intense medical needs of patients in acute care settings take precedence over sexual needs.

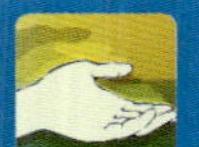

BOX 26-7
Health education about sexual activity for people with cardiovascular disease

- Participation in a medically supervised exercise program can reduce oxygen requirements during sexual activity and improve the quality of your sex life.
- The typical energy expenditure for sexual intercourse is equivalent to that used for climbing two flights of steps.
- Do not engage in sexual activity in extremely hot and humid environments.
- Wait 3 hours after consuming alcohol or a large meal before initiating sexual activity.
- Engage in sexual activity when your energy is at its peak and you are feeling rested and relaxed.
- Avoid sexual activity during times of intense emotional stress.
- Avoid engaging in sexual activity with a partner with whom you are uncomfortable.
- Experiment with different positions to find one that is least demanding of your energy.
- Consider using glyceryl trinitrate, if ordered by your medical practitioner, as needed before sexual activity.
- Know that many types of oral medications for erectile dysfunction can cause serious (even fatal) interactions with nitrates.
- Consult your medical practitioner if you experience chest pain during or after sexual activity, or breathlessness or heart palpitations persisting for 15 minutes after orgasm.

- The short duration of stay in acute care is not conducive to addressing their long-term sexual needs.
- Because of the high degree of privacy and autonomy for people in their own homes, home care nurses are not routinely concerned about sexual needs.

However, older adults in long-term residential care are usually not acutely ill; they stay in the facility for a long time and do depend on the nursing staff to ensure the privacy necessary to meet their personal needs. The nurse in long-term residential care settings must address the sexual needs of residents as an integral part of the overall care plans.

Staff education is an important part of addressing the sexual needs of older adults in long-term residential care because staff members need to understand all aspects of sexuality and ageing, including the lifelong interest in and need for sexual activity and intimate relationships. Audiovisual materials can be used to initiate discussion about the unique aspects of meeting sexual needs in institutional settings and about the responsibilities and limitations of staff. The discussions would utilise a non-judgemental and matter-of-fact approach.

When the ability of a cognitively impaired resident to give informed consent is questionable, a multidisciplinary team can assess competence to participate in an intimate relationship. In Australia, the Charter of Residents' Rights and Responsibilities, as defined by the *Aged Care Act 1997*, can be used to assist with care decisions. The sexual needs of long-term care residents are protected through the rights to:

- Self-determination
- Participation in their own care
- Independence in making personal decisions
- Reasonable accommodation of their needs and their preferences
- Privacy and unrestricted communication with any person of their choice
- Immediate access by their relatives and others, subject to reasonable restriction with the resident's permission.

In addition to educating staff members about the sexual needs and rights of residents, nurses are responsible for ensuring privacy for those residents who desire it. If a resident does not have a private room, staff members try to provide privacy, while still respecting the rights of any roommates. Sometimes, the role of the nurse will be that of a negotiator, assisting residents in reaching mutually acceptable agreements about privacy and shared space.

WELLNESS OPPORTUNITY

Nurses respect autonomy by working with other staff members to assess the ability of someone with dementia to make decisions about expressions of sexuality.

Health promotion: Teaching women about interventions

Hormonal therapy refers to the use of oestrogen alone or with progestogen for symptoms of natural or surgically induced menopause. Use of **menopausal hormonal therapy (MHT)** (also called hormonal replacement therapy) has a long and controversial history, beginning in the 1940s when it was a common medical intervention to alleviate vasomotor symptoms associated with menopause. During the early 2000s, the results of large longitudinal studies such as the Women's Health Initiative raised questions about the safety of MHT, including the increased risk for serious diseases such as cancer and cardiovascular events. As a result of these studies, many women who had been taking MHT for years discontinued these medications and fewer women have initiated this intervention.

Currently researchers continue to investigate the safety and efficacy of MHT and longitudinal data provide information about women who had previously used MHT as well as those who currently or never used MHT. Based on continually evolving evidence, major organisations such as the North American Menopause Society and international consensus groups update their recommendations at least every 2 years. Increasingly, emphasis is placed on the importance of basing decisions about MHT on an individualised assessment of the person's risks and benefits by a knowledgeable healthcare practitioner (deVilliers, Gass, Haines et al., 2013; North American Menopause Society, 2012). These recommendations have been recognised by the Australian Menopause Society. For the latest recommendations regarding MHT, access the website www.menopause.org.au.

Because of the controversy surrounding MHT there is an increasing need for evidence-based recommendations about non prescription therapies for menopausal symptoms. Reviews of well-controlled studies have found little support for phytoestrogens (e.g. red clover and soya extracts) or herbal products (e.g. black cohosh); these reviews also raise concerns about adverse effects (Leach & Moore, 2012; Pitkin, 2012; Villaseca, 2012). Interventions that are highly recommended and without controversy are those that emphasise a healthy lifestyle (e.g. regular exercise, stress management, nutritious food, healthy weight and no smoking). In addition, recent studies indicate that some body–mind interventions (e.g. yoga, hypnosis, relaxation, cognitive behavioural group treatment) have potential for improving quality of life for menopausal women (Cramer, Lauche, Langhorst et al., 2012; Elkins, Fisher, Johnson et al., 2013; Green, Haber, McCabe et al., 2013; Lindh-Astrand & Nedstrand, 2012). Women can be encouraged to use water-soluble lubricants or prescription oestrogen cream for vaginal dryness.

Health promotion: Teaching men about interventions

Interventions for erectile dysfunction have been available for several decades, but until recently, these interventions were not widely used, in part, because men did not seek help for this condition. Since 1998 extensive publicity about oral agents that are safe and easy-to-use interventions has brought much attention to this topic and it is now commonly recognised as a treatable condition. Sildenafil (Viagra) is the most commonly used drug of this type, called oral phosphodiesterase-5 inhibitors, and the two additional drugs in this class are vardenafil and tadalafil. These drugs are widely used as first-line therapies for erectile dysfunction in older adults, with 60% to 80% response rates compared with placebo (Kedia et al., 2013). Common adverse effects of these drugs include nausea, headache, flushing, indigestion and nasal congestion. Some recent studies are finding "emerging evidence" that these drugs are associated with hearing impairments (Thakur, Thakur, Sharma et al., 2013). These drugs are contraindicated for men who are taking nitrate medications because they can cause serious and even fatal adverse effects.

Testosterone replacement therapy has gained increasing attention in recent years, with many questions being raised about the safety and efficacy of this intervention. Current guidelines emphasise that testosterone therapy can improve sexual function in hypogonadal men, but decisions about treatment need to be individualised because information about long-term effects, including adverse effects, is lacking (Baer, 2012). Some herbal preparations (e.g. yohimbine) are promoted for enhancing sexual function in men; however, evidence-based information is unavailable to support these so-called interventions.

In addition to the oral agents that are widely publicised, several types of penile prostheses, such as the vacuum erection device, are used as safe and effective treatments for erectile dysfunction. Some of these devices require a surgical procedure, but some can be self-administered. Another pharmacological approach is the administration of a vasoactive drug such as alprostadil, as either an intracavernosal injection or a transurethral suppository. Nurses do not need to be familiar with the details of these procedures, but they need to know enough about interventions to suggest that men discuss their options with a doctor.

It also is important to discuss interventions to address risk factors that cause or contribute to sexual dysfunction. For example, teach about smoking cessation, healthy lifestyle practices and optimal management of chronic conditions as interventions for sexual wellness. Psychotherapy and behavioural therapy are primary or adjunctive treatment options to address the psychosocial issues that may be contributing to erectile dysfunction. Decisions about appropriate treatment options must be based on a comprehensive evaluation by an urologist or a primary care provider who is knowledgeable about erectile dysfunction. The primary responsibility of nurses is to keep current on the types of interventions that are available and to teach about the importance of seeking help for erectile dysfunction.

EVALUATING THE EFFECTIVENESS OF NURSING INTERVENTIONS

Nursing care for older adults with an issue of altered sexuality patterns is evaluated by the degree to which risk factors are eliminated, particularly through the provision of accurate information. For example, older adults may verbalise an improved understanding of the age-related changes that affect their response to sexual stimulation. In turn, this information can alleviate anxiety about sexual performance and improve quality of life. Interventions to alleviate such risk factors as medical conditions or adverse medication/chemical effects would be considered successful if the older adult follows through with a referral to an appropriate resource. One measure of successful intervention in long-term residential care would be that staff members increase their understanding of the sexual needs of older adults and are comfortable allowing appropriate sexual expressions by the residents.

UNFOLDING CASE STUDY

Part B

Mr and Mrs Smith are now 75 and 73 years old, respectively, and they have moved to a retirement village co-located with a long-term residential care facility. Their health conditions have not changed significantly in the past 2 years, with the exception of Mrs Smith having more difficulty walking because of her osteoarthritis. Mr and Mrs Smith recently moved because they needed help with transportation and wanted to live in a place where they had fewer responsibilities and more time to enjoy life. Since the move Mr and Mrs Smith see their medical practitioner at the residential care facility when he visits. One day, while waiting to see the medical practitioner, in the clinic room Mrs Smith begins to talk to you. Mrs Smith becomes tearful and says she has been disappointed in their move from their own home. She says, "Now we have the time to enjoy our life together, but we seem to be in each other's way all the time. When we lived in our own home, we were so busy with the yard and the housekeeping and all the daily chores, we never had time to think about what we enjoy together. Now I don't have to cook meals and worry about getting to the supermarket, but we aren't enjoying the time we have together."

Nursing assessment

On further discussion, Mrs Smith acknowledges that she has talked with her husband about having more "intimate time and resuming sexual activities that have petered out in the past few years because we were always so tired and never seemed to have much time". In reply, Mr Smith has stated, "We're probably too old to do those things, and old people shouldn't expect to have the fun in bed that we used to have." Mrs Smith says she used to believe that, but recently she's been talking with some of the other women in village who seem to be enjoying sexual activities. Mr and Mrs Smith relate they had a good sexual relationship until Mr Smith's heart attack 5 years ago. After that, he lost interest in sexual activities, even though he was told he could resume all his usual activities except for very strenuous activity. Mrs Smith says she masturbates occasionally, but she doesn't find that very satisfying. Mrs Smith expresses concern about being comfortable in the sexual position they used previously because her arthritis has got worse in the past few years.

Nursing issues

You address ineffective sexuality patterns as your nursing issue for Mr and Mrs Smith. Related factors include myths and lack of information about the age-related changes, and risk factors that influence sexual function. Potential risk factors that you identify are Mr Smith's medications and his lack of information about sexual function after a heart attack.

Nursing care plan for Mr and Mrs Smith

Goals for wellness outcomes	Nursing interventions	Nursing evaluation
Mr and Mrs Smith's knowledge about age-related changes and risk factors that affect sexual function will be increased.	• Use Box 26-5 as a basis for discussion of sexual function in later adulthood.	• Mr and Mrs Smith verbalise correct information about sexual function in later adulthood.
The risk factors associated with Mr Smith's heart attack and medication regimen will be addressed.	• Explain that many medications for heart problems and high blood pressure are associated with problems with sexual function. • Use Box 26-7 as a basis for discussing sexual activity as it relates to people with heart problems. • Encourage Mr Smith to talk with his doctor about his medication regimen and about his heart condition. Suggest that he inquire whether a different medication would effectively treat his high blood pressure without interfering with sexual function.	• Mr Smith agrees to talk with his medical practitioner about the potential relationship between his medications, heart condition and his lack of sexual activity.
The risk factors associated with Mrs Smith's arthritis will be addressed.	• Use Box 26-6 to discuss sexual activity as it relates to people with arthritis.	• Mrs Smith identifies ways to increase her comfort during sexual activities.

Thinking points

- What risk factors are likely to influence Mrs Smith's enjoyment of sexual activity?
- What risk factors are likely to affect Mr Smith's enjoyment of sexual activity?
- What health education would you provide for Mrs Smith, and what would you use for teaching tools?
- What health education would you provide for Mr Smith, and what would you use for teaching tools?

CHAPTER HIGHLIGHTS

Age-related changes that affect sexual wellness

- Diminished levels of hormones and degenerative changes of reproductive organs in both men and women
- Women: cessation of menses, onset of menopause, loss of reproductive ability
- Men: lower testosterone (i.e. andropause), gradual decline but not total loss of reproductive ability

Risk factors that affect sexual wellness

- Societal influences, especially on attitudes, stereotypes and prejudices
- Effects of attitudes and behaviours of families and carers, especially on dependent older adults
- Limited opportunities for sexual activity (lower ratio of men to women, health conditions)
- Adverse effects of medications, alcohol and nicotine
- Chronic conditions
- Gender-specific conditions
- Functional impairments and dementia

Functional consequences affecting sexual wellness

- Reproductive ability: ceases in women, diminishes in men
- Response to sexual stimulation: slower and less intense
- Sexual interest and activity: maintenance of interest and capacity in most older adults, but diminished sexual activity due to risk factors
- Male and female sexual dysfunction

Pathological condition affecting sexual wellness: Human immunodeficiency virus

- Increasing numbers of adults aged 50 years and older have HIV/AIDS
- Health-related concerns associated with HIV/AIDS in older adults
- Risk factors differ for older adults (less likely to be tested or to practise safer sex)
- Nurses have important roles in identifying new cases of HIV, assessing risks for sexually transmitted infections and assessing treatment issues (i.e. adverse effects, drug interactions)
- Nurses need to teach about safer sex practices

Nursing assessment of sexual function

- Self-assessment of attitudes about sexual function and ageing
- Assessment of cultural influences
- General principles of and specific interview questions for nursing assessment
- Using the PLISSIT assessment model

Nursing issues

- Willingness for enhanced knowledge: sexual functioning
- Ineffective sexuality pattern

Goal planning for wellness outcomes

- For older adults in long-term residential care: personal satisfaction; protection of rights; cultural needs' fulfilment
- Body image
- Personal well-being
- Self-esteem
- Sexual functioning

Nursing interventions to promote sexual wellness

- Teaching older adults about sexual wellness: age-related changes and risk factors
- Addressing risk factors: teaching about sexual activity for people with arthritis or cardiovascular disease
- Promoting sexual wellness in long-term residential care: staff education, protection of rights, ensuring privacy
- Teaching women about interventions for menopause and men about interventions for erectile dysfunction

Evaluating effectiveness of nursing interventions

- Verbalisation of accurate information to dispel myths and misconceptions
- Improved quality of life
- Referrals to healthcare professionals for addressing risk factors
- Increased knowledge and comfort of staff in long-term residential care

CRITICAL THINKING EXERCISES

1. Describe the attitudinal risk factors on the parts of society, older adults and healthcare providers that can interfere with healthy sexual function in older adults.
2. Summarise the functional consequences that are likely to affect sexual function in healthy older men and women.
3. What are the responsibilities of nurses in each of the following settings related to assessment of sexual function in older adults: a community setting, an acute care facility and long-term residential care?
4. Describe the assessment and health education approaches you might use for a 73-year old married man who confides that he has difficulty making his wife "happy in bed".
5. Spend a few minutes answering all the questions included in Box 26-3, Assessing personal attitudes towards sexuality and ageing. What did you learn about yourself?

RESOURCES

For an extensive range of additional resources to enhance teaching and learning and to facilitate understanding of this chapter, please see the text's accompanying website located on thePoint at http://thepoint.lww.com.

Clinical tools

Hartford Institute for Geriatric Nursing, ConsultGeriRN.org: http://consultgerirn.org/resources

Assessment tools *Try This*® series and *How to Try This* resources

General assessment series:

- *Try This*, issue 10: Sexuality assessment for older adults. Kazer, M. W. (2012). *Best Practices in Nursing Care to Older Adults*.
- *How to Try This* (article): Assessment of sexual health in older adults. Wallace, M. A. (2008). *American Journal of Nursing, 108*(7), 52–60.
- *How to Try This* (video): *Older adult sexuality: A continuing human need.*

Evidence-based practice

Kazer, M. W. (2008). Issues regarding sexuality. In M. Boltz, E. Capezuti, T. Fulmer & D. Zwicker (Eds), *Evidence-based geriatric nursing protocols for best practice* (4th ed., pp. 500–515). New York: Springer.

National Guideline Clearinghouse: www.guideline.gov

Search: Menopause

- Hormonal therapy in menopausal women.
- The 2012 hormone therapy position statement of The North American Menopause Society.
- Medical care for menopausal and older women with HIV infection.

Health education

Age Concern New Zealand Inc.: www.ageconcern.org.nz/ACNZ_Public/Relationships_in_later_life.aspx

Australian Menopause Society: www.menopause.org.au/health-professionals/information-sheet

Health Direct Australia: www.healthdirect.gov.au/menopause

Impotence Australia: www.impotenceaustralia.com.au/site/default.aspx

NIHSenior Health: www.nia.nih.gov/health/publication/sexuality-later-life

North American Menopause Society: www.menopause.org

NZ Menopause Institute: www.nzmenopause.co.nz/menopause.htm

Relationships Aotearoa (New Zealand): www.relationships.org.nz/intimacy

Relationships Australia: www.relationships.org.au

Senior Action in a Gay Environment (SAGE): www.sageusa.org/index.cfm

Sexual Health Australia: www.sexualhealthaustralia.com.au

Sexual health, HIV/AIDS and viral hepatitis, information for adults: www.qld.gov.au/health/staying-healthy/sexual-health/index.html

REFERENCES

Adekeye, O. A., Heiman, H. J., Onyeabor, O. S. et al. (2012). The new invincibles: HIV screening among older adults in the U.S. *PLoS One, 7*(8), e43618.

Allen, R. S., Petro, K. N. & Phillips, L. L. (2009). Factors influencing young adults' attitudes and knowledge of late life sexuality among older women. *Aging and Mental Health, 13*(2), 238–245.

Anderson, F., Schmedt, N., Weinmann, S., Willich, S. N. & Garbe, E. (2010). Priapism associated with antipsychotics: Role of alpha1 adrenoceptor affinity. *Journal of Clinical Psychopharmacology, 30*(1), 68–71.

Australian Government Department of Health (AGDH). (2012). Aboriginal and Torres Strait Islander Health Performance Framework, 2012 Report. Accessed March 2015 via www.health.gov.au/indigenous-hpf.

Australian Government Department of Health. (2015). National Notifiable Diseases Surveillance System. Available March 2015 at www9.health.gov.au/cda/source/cda-index.cfm.

Ayaz, S. & Kubilay, G. (2009). Effectiveness of the PLISSIT model for solving the sexual problems of patients with stoma. *Journal of Clinical Nursing, 18*(1), 154–156.

Ayers, B., Forshaw, M. & Hunter, M. S. (2010). The impact of attitude towards the menopause on women's symptom experience: A systematic review. *Maturitas, 65*, 28–36.

Baer, J. T. (2012). Testosterone replacement therapy to improve health in older males. *Nurse Practitioner, 37*(8), 39–44.

Bretschneider, J. G. & McCoy, N. L. (1988). Sexual interest and behavior in healthy 80- to 100-year olds. *Archives of Sexual Behavior, 17*, 109–129.

Brooks, J. T., Buchacz, K., Gebo, K. A. & Mermin, J. (2012). HIV infections and older Americans. *American Journal of Public Health, 102*(8), 1516–1526.

Byrne, M., Doherty, S., Murphy, A. W. et al. (2013). The CHARMS Study: Cardiac patients' experiences of sexual problems following cardiac rehabilitation. *European Journal of Cardiovascular Nursing, 12*(6), 558–566.

Cahill, S. & Valadez, M. S. W. (2013). Growing older with HIV/AIDS: New public health challenges. *American Journal of Public Health, 103*(3), e7–e15.

Copeland, K. L., Brown, J. S., Creasman, J. M. et al. (2012). Diabetes mellitus and sexual function in middle-aged and older women. *Obstetrics & Gynecology, 120*(2), 331–340.

Cornelison, L. J. & Doll, G. M. (2012). Management of sexual expression in long-term care: Ombudsmen's perspectives. *Gerontologist, 30*(1), 117–120.

Cramer, H., Lauche, R., Langhorst, J. et al. (2012). Effectiveness of yoga for menopausal symptoms: A systematic review and meta-analysis of randomized controlled trials. *Evidence-Based Complementary and Alternative Medicine*. Article ID 863905. Accessed March 2015 at http://dx.doi.org/10.1155/2012/863905.

Cui, J., Shen, Y. & Li, R. (2013). Estrogen synthesis and signaling pathways during ageing. *Trends in Molecular Medicine, 19*(3), 197–209.

DeLamater, J. (2012). Sexual expression in later life: A review and synthesis. *Journal of Sex Research, 49*(2–3), 125–141.

deVilliers, T. J., Gass, M. L. S., Haines, C. J. et al. (2013). Global consensus statement on menopausal hormone therapy. *Maturitas, 74*, 391–392.

Elias, J. & Ryan, A. (2011). A review and commentary on the factors that influence expressions of sexuality by older people in care homes. *Journal of Clinical Nursing, 20*(11–12), 1668–1676.

Elkins, G. R., Fisher, W. I., Johnson, A. K. et al. (2013). Clinical hypnosis in the treatment of postmenopausal hot flashes. *Menopause, 20*(3), 291–298.

Farrell, J. & Belza, B. (2011). Are older patients comfortable discussing sexual health with nurses? *Nursing Research, 61*(1), 51–57.

Fedder, J., Kaspersen, M. D., Brandslund, I. et al. (2013). Retrograde ejaculation and sexual dysfunction in men with diabetes mellitus. *Andrology, 1*(4), 602–606.

Galinsky, A. M. (2012). Sexual touching and difficulties with sexual arousal and orgasm among U.S. older adults. *Archives of Sexual Behavior, 41*(4), 875–890.

Gibbs, A., Lee, S. & Kulkarni, J. (2012). What factors determine whether a woman becomes depressed during perimenopause? *Archives of Women's Mental Health, 15*(5), 323–332.

Glina, S., Sharlip, I. D. & Hellstrom, W. J. (2013). Modifying risk factors to prevent and treat erectile dysfunction. *Journal of Sex Medicine, 10*(1), 115–119.

Gray, P. B. & Garcia, J. R. (2012). Aging and human sexual behavior. *Gerontology, 58*, 446–452.

Green, S. M., Haber, E., McCabe, R. E. et al. (2013). Cognitive-behavioral group treatment for menopausal symptoms. *Archives of Women's Mental Health, 16*(4), 325–332.

Harte, C. B. & Meston, C. M. (2012). Association between smoking cessation and sexual health in men. *British Journal of Urology International, 109*(6), 888–896.

Hayatbakhsh, M. R., Clavarino, A., Williams, G. M. et al. (2012). Cigarette smoking and age of menopause. *Maturitas, 72*(4), 346–352.

Hoekstra, T., Lesman-Leegte, I., Luttik, M. L. et al. (2012). Sexual problems in elderly male and female patients with heart failure. *Heart, 98*(22), 1647–1652.

Horstman, A. M., Dillon, E. L., Urban, R. J. et al. (2012). The role of androgens and estrogens in healthy aging and longevity. *Journals of Gerontology: Biological Sciences and Medical Sciences, 67*(11), 1140–1152.

Jaarsma, T., Steinke, E. E. & Gianotten, W. L. (2010). Sexual problems in cardiac patients: How to assess, when to refer. *Journal of Cardiovascular Nursing, 25*, 159–164.

Jang, J., Anderson, P. G. & Mentes, J. C. (2011). Aging and living with HIV/AIDS. *Journal of Gerontological Nursing, 37*(12), 4–7.

Jansson, J. & Wilson, D.P. (2012). Projected demographic profile of people living with HIV in Australia: Planning for an older generation. *PLoS ONE, 7*(3), e38334.

Kedia, G. T., Uckert, S., Assadi-Pour, F. et al. (2013). Avanafil for the treatment of erectile dysfunction. *Therapeutic Advances in Urology, 5*(1), 35–41.

Kim, T. H., Kim, S. M., Kim, J. J. et al. (2011). Does metabolic syndrome impair sexual function in middle- to old-aged women? *Journal of Sex Medicine, 8*(4), 1123–1130.

La Marca, A., Sighinolfi, G., Papaleo, E. et al. (2013). Prediction of age at menopause from assessment of ovarian reserve may be improved by using body mass index and smoking status. *PLoS One, 8*(3), e57005.

Leach, M. J. & Moore, V. (2012). Black cohosh for menopausal symptoms. *Cochrane Database of Systematic Reviews, 12*, 9. Art. no. CD007244.

Lin, H. L., Hsiao, M. C., Liu, Y. T. et al. (2013). Perimenopause and incidence of depression in midlife women. *Climacteric, 16*(3), 381–386.

Lindh-Astrand, L. & Nedstrand, E. (2012). Effects of applied relaxation on vasomotor symptoms in postmenopausal women: A randomized controlled trial. *Menopause: Journal of the North American Menopause Society, 20*(4), 401–408.

Lochlainn, M. N. & Kenny, R. A. (2013). Sexual activity and aging. *Journal of the American Medical Directors Association, 14*(8), 565–572.

Martelli, V., Valisella, S., Moscatiello, S. et al. (2012). Prevalence of sexual dysfunction among postmenopausal women with and without metabolic syndrome. *Journal of Sex Medicine, 9*(2), 434–441.

Masters, W. H. & Johnson, V. E. (1966). *Human sexual response*. Boston, MA: Little Brown.

Mauvais-Jarvis, F., Clegg, D. J. & Hevener, A. L. (2013). The role of estrogens in control of energy balance and glucose homeostasis. *Endocrinology Review, 34*(3), 309–338.

McGill, J. J., Shoskes, D. A. & Sabanegh, E. S. (2012). Androgen deficiency in older men. *Cleveland Clinic Journal of Medicine, 79*(11), 797–806.

Mendez, M. F. & Shapira, J. S. (2013). Hypersexual behavior in frontotemporal dementia. *Archives of Sex and Behavior, 42*(3), 501–509.

Muzacz, A. K. & Akinsulure-Smith, A. M. (2013). Older adults and sexuality. *Journal of Mental Health Counseling, 35*(1), 1–14.

Nedergaard, A., Henriksen, K., Asser, K. M. et al. (2013). Menopause, estrogens and frailty. *Gynecology & Endocrinology, 29*(5), 418–423.

New Zealand Ministry of Health. (2014). Sexually Transmitted Infections in New Zealand: Annual Surveillance Report. Viewed March 2015 at https://surv.esr.cri.nz/surveillance/annual_sti.php?we_objectID=3969.

North American Menopause Society. (2012). The 2012 hormone therapy position statement of the North

American Menopause Society. *Menopause: Journal of the North American Menopause Society, 19*(3), 257–271.

Okeke, T. C., Ezenyeaku, C. C., Ikeako, L. C. et al. (2013). An overview of menopause associated vasomotor symptoms and options available in its management. *Nigerian Journal of Medicine, 22*(1), 7–14.

Pantalone, K. M. & Faiman, C. (2012). Male hypogonadism. *Cleveland Clinic Journal of Medicine, 79*(10), 717–725.

Pastuszak, A. W., Badhiwala, N., Lipshultz, L. I. et al. (2013). Depression is correlated with the psychological and physical aspects of sexual dysfunction in men. *International Journal of Impotence Research, 25*(5), 194–199.

Pimenta, F., Leal, I., Maroco, J. et al. (2012). Menopausal symptoms. *Maturitas, 73*(4), 324–331.

Pitkin, J. (2012). Alternative and complementary therapies for menopause. *Menopause International, 18*(1), 20–27.

Pontiroli, A. E., Cortelazzi, D. & Morobito, A. (2013). Female sexual dysfunction and diabetes: A systematic review and meta-analysis. *Journal of Sex Medicine, 10*(4), 1044–1051.

Rosen, R. C., Wei, J. T., Althof, S. E., Seftel, A. D., Miner, M. & Perelman, M. A. (2009). Association of sexual dysfunction with lower urinary tract symptoms of BPH and BPH medical therapies: Results from the BPH registry. *Urology, 73*, 562–566.

Rosenfeld, D., Bartlam, B. & Smith, R. D. (2012). Out of the closet and into the trenches: Gay male baby boomers, aging, and HIV/AIDS. *Gerontologist, 52*(2), 255–264.

Ryan, J. G. & Gajraj, J. (2012). Erectile dysfunction and its association with metabolic syndrome and endothelial function among patients with type 2 diabetes mellitus. *Journal of Diabetes Complications, 26*(2), 141–147.

Santos, T., Drummond, M. & Botelho, F. (2012). Erectile dysfunction in obstructive sleep apnea syndrome. *Review of Portuguese Pneumologica, 18*(2), 64–71.

Shamloul, R. & Ghanem, H. (2013). Erectile dysfunction. *Lancet, 381*(9861), 153–165.

Sharifi, F., Asqhari, M., Jaberi, Y. et al. (2012). Independent predictors of erectile dysfunction in type 2 diabetes mellitus. *ISRN Endocrinology*, Article ID 502353.

Slag, M., Morley, J. E., Elson, M. K. et al. (1983). Impotence in medical clinic patients. *Journal of the American Medical Association, 249*, 1736–1740.

Slinkard, M. S. & Kazer, M. W. (2011). Older adults and HIV and STI screening. *Geriatric Nursing, 32*(5), 341–349.

Spitzer, M., Huang, G., Basaria, S. et al. (2013). Risks and benefits of testosterone therapy in older men. *Nature Reviews Endocrinology, 9*(7), 414–424.

Steinke, E. E. (2010). Sexual dysfunction in women with cardiovascular disease: What do we know? *Journal of Cardiovascular Nursing, 25*(2), 151–158.

Steinke, E. E., Mosack, V., Barnason, S. et al. (2011). Progress in sexual counseling by nurses, 1994 to 2009. *Heart & Lung. 40*(3), e15–e24.

Surampudi, P. N., Wang, C. & Swerdloff, R. (2012). Hypogonadism in the aging male: Diagnosis, potential benefits and risks of testosterone replacement therapy. *International Journal of Endocrinology*. Article ID 625434. Available March 2015 at http://dx.doi.org/10.1155/2012/625434.

Syme, M. L., Klonoff, E. A., Macera, C. A. et al. (2013). Predicting sexual decline and dissatisfaction among older adults. *Journals of Gerontology: Psychological Sciences and Social Sciences, 68*(3), 323–332.

Thakur, J. S., Thakur, S., Sharma, D. R. et al. (2013). Hearing loss with phosphodiesterase-5 inhibitors. *Laryngoscope 123*(6), 1527–1530.

Thorve, V. S., Kshirsagar, A. D., Vyawahare, N. S. et al. (2011). Diabetes-induced erectile dysfunction. *Journal of Diabetes Complications, 25*(2), 129–136.

Trompeter, S. E., Bettencourt, R. & Barrett-Connor, E. (2012). Sexual activity and satisfaction in healthy community-dwelling older women. *The American Journal of Medicine, 125*, 37–43.

Tutolo, M., Briganti, A., Suardi, N. et al. (2012). Optimizing postoperative sexual function after radical prostatectomy. *Therapeutic Advances in Urology, 4*(6), 347–365.

Van Wagenen, A., Driskell, J. & Bradford, J. (2013). "I'm still raring to go": Successful aging among lesbian, gay, bisexual, and transgender older adults. *Journal of Aging Studies, 27*, 1–14.

Villaseca, P. (2012). Non-estrogen conventional and phytochemical treatments for vasomotor symptoms. *Climacteric, 19*(2), 115–124.

Wallace, M. A. (2008) Assessment of sexual health in older adults: Using the PLISSIT model to talk about sex. *How to Try This,* article and video. *American Journal of Nursing, 108*(7), 52–60.

Weismiller, D. G. (2009). Menopause. *Primary Care Clinics in Office Practice, 36*, 199–226.

Whiteley, J., Wagner, J.-S., Bushmakin, A. et al. (2013) Impact of the severity of vasomotor symptoms on health status, resource use, and productivity. *Menopause: The Journal of the North American Menopause Society, 20*(5), 518–524.

Wood, A., Runciman, R., Wylie, K. R. et al. (2012). An update on female sexual function and dysfunction in old age and its relevance to old age psychiatry. *Aging and Disease, 3*(5), 373–384.

Wylie, K. & Mimoun, S. (2009). Sexual response models in women. *Maturitas, 63*, 112–115.

PART 5

PROMOTING WELLNESS IN ALL STAGES OF HEALTH AND ILLNESS

Chapter 27

Caring for older adults who have acute and chronic conditions (includes palliative care)

By Carol Miller and Sharyn Hunter

LEARNING OBJECTIVES

After reading this chapter, you should be able to:

1. Describe characteristics of illness in older adults.
2. Discuss the role of nurses in promoting wellness in older adults who are ill.
3. Describe palliative care as an approach for addressing the needs of older adults during illness.
4. Apply wellness concepts to the nursing care of older adults who have cancer, diabetes and Parkinson's disease
5. Describe the role of nurses in holistically addressing the needs of families and carers.

KEY POINTS

atypical presentation
carer burden
comorbidity
frailty
generalised palliative care
geriatric syndromes
health literacy
palliative care
self-management
specialised palliative care

Several factors differentiate care of older adults from that of other populations and add to the challenge of promoting wellness. Foremost among these is the reality that most older adults—and all of those whom nurses care for in acute and long-term residential care settings—are coping with several or even many pathological conditions that threaten their wellness. Despite pathological conditions, however, nurses can identify numerous opportunities to promote wellness, especially by addressing the whole person instead of focusing only on physiological processes. This chapter describes the characteristics of acute and chronic illness in older adults and discusses the approach to holistic care applicable for older adults. Concepts are applied to nursing care for older adults who have cancer, diabetes and Parkinson's disease. Needs of informal caregivers/carers of older adults also are addressed in this chapter.

CHARACTERISTICS OF ILLNESS IN OLDER ADULTS

Older adults commonly have one or more chronic conditions that gradually accumulate and affect their daily functioning and quality of life. A chronic condition is defined as:

> *A biological or physical condition where the natural evolution of the condition can significantly impact on a person's overall quality of life, including an irreversible inability to perform basic physical and social functions. Serious and persistent chronic conditions are multidimensional, interdependent, complex and ongoing. Chronic and complex conditions are characterised by persistent and recurring health consequences lasting for an extended period of time. (National Health and Medical Research Council [NHMRC], 2011a, p. 21)*

Older adults typically receive health care on a continuing basis for chronic conditions and periodically for acute episodes. Even when acute conditions are the focus of care, interplay between chronic conditions and one or more acute conditions is likely to affect care. Thus, the health of older adults often fluctuates unpredictably and is usually affected by multiple interacting conditions. When nurses care for an older adult who is experiencing illness, it is necessary that they not only address the acute condition but also the interaction between the acute and chronic conditions.

In addition to having more chronic conditions, older adults are more likely than their younger counterparts to have serious pathological conditions (e.g. cancer) and

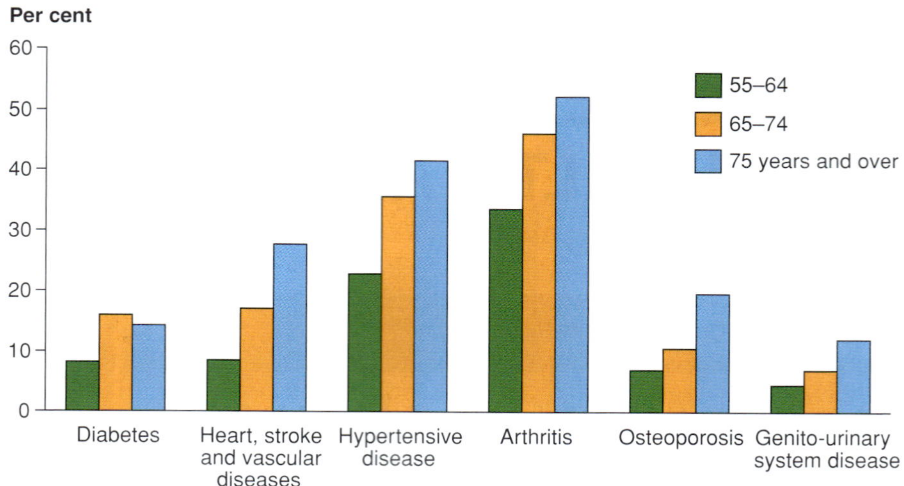

FIGURE 27-1 Prevalence of chronic conditions for older age groups in Australia (2011–12). (Australian Institute of Health and Welfare. [2014]. *Australia's health, 2014.* Australia's health series no. 14. Cat. no. AUS 178. Canberra: Author. Permission granted under a Creative Commons BY 3.0 [CC BY 3.0] licence.)

neurodegenerative conditions (e.g. dementia) that seriously compromise their health and well-being. The conditions most prevalent among older adults are musculoskeletal conditions, stroke, hypertension, cardiovascular disease, cancer, dementia, diabetes, lung conditions, and hearing and vision impairments. They are also more likely to experience adverse effects from the medications they take for these conditions, as discussed in Chapter 8. Prevalence of chronic diseases in older adults in Australia is provided in Figure 27-1 and in New Zealand it is summarised in Box 27-1.

DIVERSITY NOTE

Adult Pacific people have a higher prevalence of chronic diseases such as diabetes, ischaemic heart disease and stroke than for other ethnic groups (Statistics New Zealand and Ministry of Pacific Island Affairs, 2011).

The consequences of illness in older adults may be far reaching and are likely to affect both functioning and quality of life. For example, older adults with heart failure are typically hospitalised when their condition becomes unstable and they are likely to be discharged with some short-term acute care community service. It is possible that this service may encourage increasing levels of dependence if the care delivered does not adequately support or is focused on achieving wellness outcomes. In addition, an illness that threatens the older adult's independence may have serious psychosocial consequences. For example, the fear of being "put away in a nursing home" is a common, although often unfounded, fear among older people. Because of this anxiety, older people may deny symptoms of illness for fear the solution will result in a loss of independence; they also may avoid the healthcare system and experience unnecessary anxiety about minor or treatable illnesses.

The combined and cumulative effects of ageing (which diminish physiological reserves) and disease (which place additional physiological demands on the person) make it more difficult for older adults to adapt to acute and chronic illnesses. The cumulative effects of all these intermittent and interacting forces can lead to a "yo-yoing" effect: the person experiences a cycle of ups and downs in health, with the "yo-yo" failing to return to the height of its previous cycle. With diminishing resiliency during subsequent cycles, the yo-yo eventually loses its ability to bounce back. Promoting wellness involves holistically addressing the changing needs of older adults as they progress through these cycles of ups and downs. Thus, when nurses care for older adults, they typically address several nursing issues simultaneously, reassessing the situation frequently so that they can modify their goals accordingly. When nurses care for older adults holistically, they should be able to identify at least one wellness outcome in every situation.

BOX 27-1
Snapshot of prevalence of chronic diseases in older adults in New Zealand

- Aged 65–74 years: Cancers (29%) and vascular disorders (24%) remain the leading causes of health loss, followed by musculoskeletal conditions (11%)
- Aged 75 years and over: Vascular disorders (35%) overtake cancers (18%) as the leading cause of health loss, with neurological conditions ranked third (10%)

Source: New Zealand Ministry of Health. (2014). New Zealand Burden of Diseases, Injuries and Risk Factors Study, 2006–2016. Wellington: Author.

Comorbidity

In recent years, there has been increasing recognition of the complexity of providing healthcare for older adults who have combinations of chronic conditions and intermittent acute conditions. **Comorbidities** are multiple morbidities associated with higher rates of death, disability, institutionalisation, adverse effects, use of healthcare resources and poorer quality of life. Because there is little evidence-based information about the management of comorbidity and older adults, "guiding principles" of care have been recommended, and these are:

- Elicit and incorporate the person's preferences (i.e. keep the person central) into the medical decision-making process
- Interpret and apply medical literature specifically to older adults with comorbidity, with consideration of the degree to which the evidence base applies to the individual.
- Frame clinical management decisions within the context of risks, burdens, benefits and prognosis (e.g. remaining life expectancy, functional status, quality of life).
- Consider treatment burden, complexity and feasibility when making clinical management decisions.
- Education and assessments must be ongoing, multifaceted, individualised and delivered using a variety of methods, settings and healthcare professionals.
- Choose therapies (including medications) that optimise benefit, minimise harm and enhance quality of life.
- Individualised care plans need to be developed and implemented by interdisciplinary healthcare teams, with coordination of care to include family, friends and paid carers across all sites of care including the home.

Increasingly the roles of nurses when caring for older adults include being advocates, coordinators of care, and communicators with older adults and their families, carers, medical practitioners and other professionals.

Atypical presentation

Atypical presentation (i.e. signs and symptoms of a disease differ from what is expected because they are altered, subtle, absent or non-specific) is common in older adults. For example, falls, changes in behaviour or functioning, and vague physical manifestations (e.g. increased fatigue or loss of appetite) are common atypical presentations of infection (e.g. pneumonia or urinary tract infection). In addition, the expected manifestations of an infection, such as elevated temperature or specific complaints of pain or discomfort, may be absent. Atypical presentation of disease is especially common in those who are cognitively impaired or older than 85 years. Adverse effects of medication also may present atypically, and this can interfere with timely recognition and management (Petrovic, van der Cammen & Onder, 2012). A nursing responsibility is to maintain a heightened awareness of the potential for atypical presentation of disease and to explore all potential underlying causes of signs and symptoms of illness in older adults.

Geriatric syndromes

Geriatric syndromes (GS) is a term that describes a syndrome with a high prevalence in the older adult. GS refers to conditions that do not fit a specific disease category but have a significant negative effect on the older person's level of functioning and quality of life. The most commonly cited geriatric syndromes are falls, frailty, malnutrition, urinary incontinence, functional decline, pressure ulcers and delirium. Although definitions of geriatric syndromes vary, experts agree that these conditions are caused by the interplay among several risk factors and underlying conditions, and the risk is increased when older adults experience an acute illness. GS diminish the person's ability to adapt to stressors and are associated with substantial morbidity and poor outcomes (Kane, Shamliyan, Talley et al., 2012; Wang, Shamliyan, Talley et al., 2013). Current emphasis is on addressing specific risks and causative factors so interventions can be initiated to prevent geriatric syndromes or minimise the serious consequences. For example, much attention focuses on addressing adverse effects of the psychoactive drugs that are strongly associated with falls, delirium and hospitalisation (Wierenga, Buurman, Parlevliet et al., 2012).

Frailty

Since the early 2000s, **frailty** has been discussed in geriatric literature as a syndrome arising from the "physiological triad" of sarcopenia (i.e. loss of muscle mass) and immune and neuroendocrine dysregulation (Fried, Tangen, Walston et al., 2001). Frailty is now widely recognised as a complex geriatric syndrome and people are considered frail when they have three or more of the following conditions: low level of physical activity, slow walking speed, unintentional weight loss (i.e. 4.5 kg or more during the past year), weakness (measured by diminished handgrip strength), and self-reported exhaustion (Koller & Rockwood, 2013).

Experts agree that frailty is multifactorial and that a comprehensive definition should include assessment of six domains: cognition, mental health, nutrition, physical functioning, mobility, and gait speed (Rodriquez-Manas et al., 2013). Many studies find that frailty leads to many serious negative consequences, including increased mortality and admissions to hospitals and long-term care facilities, and decreased functioning and quality of life (e.g. Drubbel et al., 2013; Shamliyan, Talley, Ramakrishnan et al., 2013). Studies also emphasise that identification of frailty in hospitalised older adults should be an important first step in preventing adverse events in this group of people who are at increased risk for serious outcomes (Bagshaw & McDermid, 2013). It is recommended that frailty screening occurs for all people over 70 years and those with significant weight loss related to chronic disease because this condition can potentially be prevented or treated with specific modalities, including exercise, nutritional interventions, vitamin D and reduction of polypharmacy (Morley, Vellas, van Kan et al., 2013). Nurses and other carers are well placed to identify older people who are at risk of becoming frail and can deliver care to prevent the development or to delay the progression of frailty (Heath & Phair, 2009).

WELLNESS OPPORTUNITY

By attending to the body–mind–spirit interconnectedness of older adults, nurses can identify opportunities to provide physical comfort and support emotional and spiritual growth, even in situations involving inevitable physical decline.

A student's perspective

I learned a lot from my interview this past week. The woman I spoke with has gone through a lot of hardships in her life—and is still going through hardships—but she continues to move forward despite setbacks. She is suffering from physical ailments, but her faith in God keeps her head above water. This woman was open to questioning and insightful with her answers. For being a quiet woman, she has a lot of inner strength she pulls on.

For a while after she was diagnosed with multiple sclerosis, she suffered depression and lost five dress sizes unintentionally. She also became fatigued and withdrawn. This was in line with how it has been shown that physical ailments can cause stress in a person, and that this in turn can cause other physical ailments. She was fortunate (if it can be called so) to be able to lose the amount of weight that she did and not have severe consequences. If this were to happen to someone of lesser weight, the results may have been more serious. This is a first-hand experience of how depression can cause more than just sad feelings as effects. Once she accepted her fate, she gained back two dress sizes and is holding there, which she is content with.

Her daughter has also been diagnosed with multiple sclerosis, which is a blessing and burden at the same time. Her daughter has been diagnosed at a much younger age and has more serious problems with it, causing her to be periodically hospitalised. It is difficult for a mother to watch her daughter go through this, but it's a blessing that she has someone to share the experience with.

As stated earlier, her faith in God keeps her head above water. She still has her bouts with frustration, but she believes that God only gives what we can handle and that He is always there for her. Her strength is encouraging to the people around her. I know it has given me strength.

Anita M.

CONNECTING THE CONCEPTS OF WELLNESS, AGEING AND ILLNESS

Although the concepts of wellness and ageing may seem almost contradictory, it is relatively easy to apply wellness to older adults who are healthy, functional and satisfied with their lives. The greater challenge is to apply the concept of wellness to the nursing care of people who are not only in their 80s, 90s or even older but who are seriously ill or dying. It is necessary in these circumstances to emphasise that wellness applies to the broader context of the body–mind–spirit interrelationship as well as one's relationships with self, others and all that is important to the individual. When caring for older adults who are ill, nurses have unique opportunities to promote wellness by addressing needs related not only to physical comfort, health and function but also to emotional comfort and spiritual well-being. For example, nurses can promote wellness during illness through such nursing actions as the following:

- Helping older adults identify personal strengths that are not dependent on their physical health and functioning (e.g. emotional, interpersonal and spiritual qualities), then identifying strategies that build on or improve these personal characteristics
- Supporting and promoting interpersonal relationships, including the development of new relationships and support resources, which can improve the older adult's health, functioning and quality of life
- Helping older adults identify realistic goals for quality of life, which can be identified in any situation when wellness is conceptualised in the context of the body–mind–spirit interrelationship
- Recognising a knowledge deficit, particularly about an aspect of the ageing and/or illness and disease
- Facilitating the access and use of resources and strengthening the support resources that already are in place for older adults, their families and carers
- Identifying ways of supporting wellness for families and carers of dependent older adults.

Health promotion is an essential part of nursing care for *all* older adults, including those who have serious chronic or acute illnesses and even those with life-limiting conditions. Unfortunately, ageist attitudes of health professionals, older adults and family members can create barriers to health promotion. Although healthcare professionals might believe there is little or no benefit from improving health behaviours in later life, this belief is not supported by evidence (Pascucci, Chu & Leasure, 2012). Nurses and other healthcare professionals must be careful not to be influenced by ageist attitudes, suggesting that older adults are too old—or too sick or impaired—to learn or change behaviours and to benefit from improved health behaviours.

Having personal responsibility for health is an important aspect of wellness for older adults because self-care is essential for achieving optimal health in people who have chronic illnesses. Increasingly there are evidence-based **self-management** programs available for many chronic conditions that older adults experience. Nurses have a key role in assisting older adults to undertake the management of their health, despite being dependent on others for care. Self-management involves the older adult

TABLE 27-1 Nursing outcomes and nursing interventions for promoting wellness in older adults during illness

Type of needs	Nursing outcomes	Nursing interventions
Psychosocial needs	Anxiety Level, Coping, Decision Making, Fear Level, Participation in Healthcare Decisions, Personal Autonomy, Personal Well-Being, Self-Direction of Care, Self-Esteem, Social Involvement, Stress Level, Suffering Severity	Anxiety Reduction, Counselling, Coping Enhancement, Decision-Making Support, Emotional Support, Patient Rights Protection, Resiliency Promotion, Support Group, Simple Guided Imagery, Touch
Comfort needs	Comfort Level, Pain Control, Pain: Disruptive Effects, Sleep, Symptom Control, Thermoregulation	Pain Management, Positioning, Simple Massage, Temperature Regulation, Therapeutic Touch
Health promotion needs	Fall Prevention Behaviour; Health Promoting Behaviour; Immunisation Behaviour; Knowledge: Diet, Disease Process, Health Behaviour, Health Resources, Illness Care, Medication; Nutritional Status; Physical Fitness; Risk Control; Risk Detection; Self-Care Status; Safe Home Environment	Anticipatory Guidance, Environmental Management: Comfort/Safety, Exercise Promotion, Fall Prevention, Health Education, Immunisation Management, Nutrition Management, Risk Identification, Self-Responsibility Facilitation, Simple Relaxation Therapy, Skin Surveillance, Sleep Enhancement, Surveillance: Safety
Spiritual needs	Hope, Spiritual Health	Active Listening, Forgiveness Facilitation, Guilt Work Facilitation, Hope Instillation, Presence, Reminiscence Therapy, Religious Ritual Enhancement, Self-Awareness Enhancement, Spiritual Growth Facilitation, Spiritual Support
Quality-of-life needs	Leisure Participation, Personal Well-Being, Quality of Life	Animal-Assisted Therapy, Aromatherapy, Family Involvement Promotion, Humour, Music Therapy

with a chronic illness working in partnership with their carers and health professionals so that they:

- Obtain an understanding of their disease and the treatments available
- Contribute to the development and ongoing review of a documented plan of care
- Engage in lifestyle activities that contribute to their health
- Are able to monitor and manage their disease
- Cope with the impact of the chronic illness has on their physical and psychological functioning and their relationships (Royal College of General Practitioners [RACGP] & Diabetes Australia, 2014)

Health literacy is fundamental to the successful self-management of chronic conditions. It is defined as "the degree to which individuals have the capacity to obtain, process, and understand basic health information and services needed to make appropriate health decisions" (Nielsen-Bohlman et al., 2004). The health literacy of most Australian older adults has been reported as below average (Australian Bureau of Statistics [ABS], 2008). Therefore it is recommended that, before commencing any program, an older adult's health literacy skills are assessed. Once assessed and health literacy identified, nurses and other health professionals can begin working with the older adults. Principles of behaviour change are applied (see Chapter 5) to assist the older adult with the adoption of lifestyle changes.

Self-efficacy is a key aspect of health literacy and health promotion that nurses can influence. This may be particularly important for older adults who live alone and need to self-manage care for one or more chronic conditions (Melchior, Seff, Bastida et al., 2013); for example, by providing positive feedback about the progress older adults are making towards managing a complex medication routine. Another intervention for improving self-efficacy is challenging ageist attitudes and communicating confidence in an older adult's ability to learn and apply new information.

Even when illness compromises the health, functioning and quality of life of older adults, nurses can usually identify wellness-oriented outcomes and interventions if they use a holistic perspective. For example, nurses can suggest that older adults who have difficulty engaging in outdoor walking or exercises requiring good balance and mobility explore other options in group settings, such as aquatic exercise or tai chi programs. Programs such as these are available in most communities and they can provide additional positive outcomes, such as increased socialisation. Table 27-1 lists examples of relevant nursing outcomes and nursing interventions that address psychosocial, comfort, health promotion and spiritual needs of older adults. Nurses can incorporate these outcomes and interventions into care plans, in conjunction with addressing the needs directly related to the primary health conditions.

HOLISTICALLY CARING FOR OLDER ADULTS WHO ARE ILL: FOCUSING ON CARING AND COMFORTING

Care and comfort are core components of all nursing, but they become even more important when a cure is not feasible. Equating ageing with inability to cure is not only inaccurate but is also a great disservice to older adults.

However, it also is a disservice to older adults to focus only on curing disease when they reach the point at which treatments are more detrimental than the underlying conditions. Moreover, because of the complexity of illness in older adults, the "turning point" when the focus changes from cure to care is rarely clearly defined. Clinicians and researchers are increasingly trying to identify ways to improve quality of life for people whose quantity of life is limited.

The emergence of palliative care programs in recent years provides a framework for promoting wellness during serious illness, and this model is increasingly used to address the complex and cumulative effects of conditions for which there is no cure. It is important that palliative care be incorporated in chronic disease management, including Alzheimer's and other dementias, cancer, cardiovascular diseases, cirrhosis of the liver, chronic obstructive pulmonary diseases, diabetes, HIV/AIDS, kidney failure, multiple sclerosis, Parkinson's disease and rheumatoid arthritis (World Health Organization [WHO], 2014). **Palliative care** is defined as:

> *An approach that improves the quality of life of individuals and their families facing the problems associated with life-threatening illness, through the prevention and relief of suffering by means of early identification and impeccable assessment and treatment of pain and other problems, physical, psychosocial and spiritual. (WHO, 2004)*

There are three types of palliative care and it is important to be able to distinguish between them, because each has a different role in caring for a person during the final stages of their life. They are:

1. **Generalised palliative care:** When there is no likelihood of a cure for a person and the symptoms of the disease require management, this approach is appropriate. The person may still be receiving active treatment for their disease alongside palliative care. Health professionals utilise a good basic knowledge of palliative care to improve the person's level of comfort, function and well-being for the remainder of their life.
2. **Specialised palliative care:** This form of palliative care involves referral to a specialised palliative team or healthcare practitioner. The specialised palliative team works with the care team to assist with treating complex symptoms and providing support to the team and families about complex ethical issues.
3. End-of-life (terminal) care: This form of palliative care is provided during the final stage of life (Australian Government Department of Health [AGDH], 2014; New Zealand Ministry of Health [NZMOH], 2001).

Two types, generalised and specialised palliative care, are addressed in this chapter, while end-of-life care is addressed in Chapter 29.

Since the 1980s there has been a quest in Australia and New Zealand for the recognition of the needs of people who are dying and their families, and for services to meet those needs. Since then palliative care has emerged as a specialised area in the healthcare systems of both countries. There has been much growth in the volume and type of palliative care services. Australia and New Zealand have both adopted a national palliative care strategy. Palliative Care Australia has worked with the Australian Government Department of Health to develop policies and strategies that support its National Palliative Care Strategy launched in 2010 and the ongoing National Palliative Care Program (AGDH, 2014). New Zealand also has an organised, informed approach to the provision and funding of palliative care services, which is the New Zealand Palliative Care Strategy (NZMOH, 2001; Palliative Care Subcommittee & New Zealand Cancer Treatment Working Party, 2007; Hospice New Zealand, 2012). The aim of the Australian and New Zealand national palliative care programs is to ensure all people who are dying and their families have access to quality palliative care services that are culturally appropriate and provided in a coordinated way.

Australia and New Zealand's palliative care strategies embrace the three types of palliative care and identify that each type has a role in the care of older adults. Regardless of the type of palliative care received, the goals of palliative care services include:

- Promoting comfort by identifying pain through assessment, initially and ongoing, and the treatment of pain and other distressing symptoms
- Improving the quality of life of the person and their families, and
- Offering psychological, emotional and spiritual support to the person and their families (*whānau*).

Palliative care is based on a multidisciplinary team approach, with nurses assuming essential roles, which support the needs of older adults and emphasise quality of life during chronic illness. Palliative care services are provided at any point during the course of a declining chronic condition and in any setting, including acute care, long-term residential care, and home settings. Palliative care promotes wellness for older adults with chronic conditions by focusing on respect for the individual, sharing caring moments, encouraging older adults to direct their own care, and honouring the intrinsic worth and uniqueness of each person (Mahler, 2010). An example relationship between of the palliative care types as an ongoing approach, recommended for preserving the comfort, dignity, autonomy and quality of life for people living with dementia (Passmore, 2013), is provided in Figure 27-2.

Palliative care is rapidly evolving and it is important to keep up to date on developments. Palliative Care Australia recommends using *ehospice*, which is a global resource that shares hospice and palliative care news, intelligence and best practice. *ehospice* is available at www.palliativecare.org.au/ourwork/ehospice.aspx. Other resources are listed at the end of this chapter.

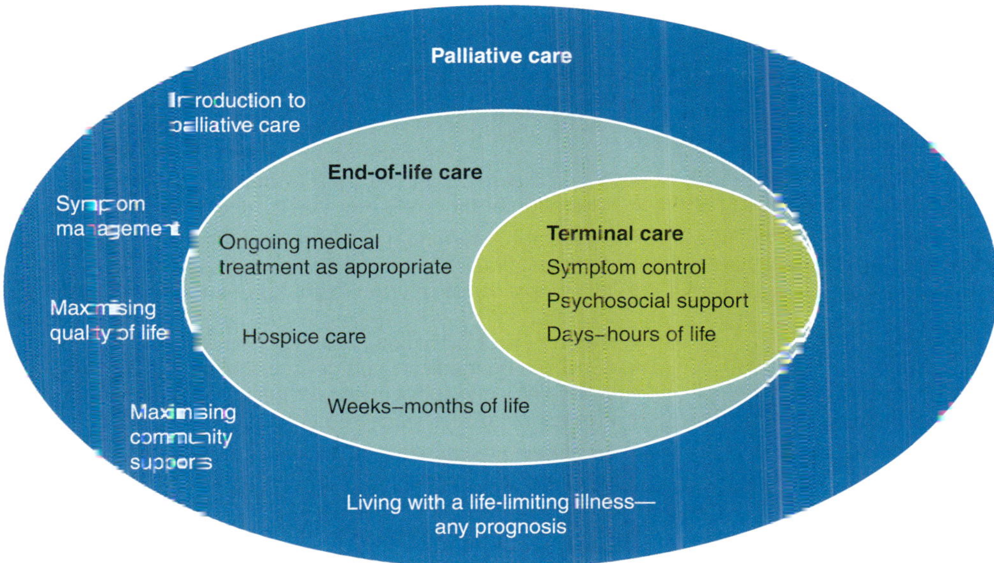

FIGURE 27-2 The palliative care continuum. (© Copyright 2013. Passmore, M. . [2013]. Neuropsychiatric symptoms of dementia: Consent, quality of life, and dignity. *BioMed Research International*. Article ID 230134.)

Generalised palliative care

Older adults with chronic conditions such as diabetes, heart, respiratory and neurological conditions or who are frail all benefit from this generalised form of palliative care. It is the responsibility of all healthcare professionals to provide palliative care. This type of care begins early and is used alongside active ongoing care for the chronic conditions. The World Health Organization (2002) and the Australian and New Zealand Palliative Care organisations describe the following aspects of the generalised palliative care:

- The recipients of care are the person and their families facing problems associated with a broad range of persistent, life-threatening or recurring conditions that adversely affect their daily functioning or will predictably reduce life expectancy.
- Goals are to prevent and relieve suffering, enhance quality of life, optimise function, assist with decision making, and provide opportunities for personal growth.
- It is applicable early in the course of an illness and should be offered as needs develop and before they become unmanageable.
- It is provided concurrently with life-prolonging therapies or as the condition progresses, as a main focus of care.
- It is an organised system for delivering comprehensive care.

When discussing palliative care, nurses can use the term "supportive care" which may be more acceptable (Maciasz, Arnold, Chu et al., 2013). It is recommended that for older adults, especially those living with dementia, that information about the individual's physical, psychological, social and spiritual background be compiled in a *biosketch* (Long, 2009) to facilitate palliative care. Generalised palliative care includes nursing care directed towards optimising function and encouraging physical activity and other healthy lifestyle activities (Resnick, 2012). It also focuses on preparing the person for future care by discussion of the person's understanding of their medical condition and prognosis, values and preferences about their wishes for care as the disease progresses. This planning of care in advance has many benefits for the older adults as it enables them to make decisions while they are still well: it may prevent hospital admissions and unnecessary treatments. Comprehensive discussion about *advance care directives* and *advance care planning* is contained in Chapter 9.

Because of the developing role of nurses in palliative care, nursing organisations in both Australia and New Zealand have developed competencies for nurses. In New Zealand, competencies have been developed for qualified nurses for palliative care, which can be accessed via www.health.govt.nz/publications. These competencies recognise that all nurses work collaboratively with those requiring palliative care and are required to deliver generalist palliative care (Palliative Care Nurses New Zealand, 2014). Specialist competencies have also been developed for palliative nurse specialists. In Australia, despite the expectation that nurses in many care settings will provide palliative care, competencies have only been available for the specialist palliative care nurses (Canning, Yates & Rosenberg, 2005). Also in Australia, a proposed palliative care curriculum for undergraduate nurses has been developed, which can be accessed via www.pcc4u.org.

TABLE 27-2 Examples of conditions and symptoms that indicate a need for palliative care

Conditions	Indicators of the need for palliative care
Cancer	• Pain, dyspnoea, anorexia, and any other symptom that is not well controlled • When condition is likely incurable, even while person is undergoing treatment (e.g. radiation, chemotherapy) • When disease progresses even with treatment • When significant care is required to meet basic needs
Dementia	• Significant behavioural problems that are distressful to the person with dementia or to carers • Nutritional concerns (e.g. weight loss, eating/feeding limitations, risk for choking) • Frequent hospitalisations and/or unstable medical conditions • Concomitant medical conditions (e.g. heart failure, pneumonia) • When decisions about medical care need to be made • Progression to late-stage dementia
Heart failure	• Progression to late-stage heart failure despite optimal medical management • Dyspnoea, pain or other symptoms unresponsive to treatment • The need for frequent medical care or hospitalisations • Significant decline in functioning
Chronic obstructive pulmonary disease	• Orthopnoea, dyspnoea, difficulty managing symptoms related to breathing • Substantial weight loss • Anxiety, fear of death
Parkinson's disease	• Significant decline in functioning • Nutritional concerns, especially involving swallowing difficulties and weight loss

Source: Brown, Sampson, Jones et al. (2013); Miyasaki (2013); Parikh, Kirch, Smith et al. (2013); Passmore (2013); Thoonsen, Engels, Rijswijk et al. (2012).

Specialised palliative care

Nurses have an important responsibility to recognise the appropriateness of a referral for specialised palliative care services and to initiate discussion of this option with older adults and their families. Nurses work with specialised palliative services to help the older adult achieve better symptom management and quality of life. Nurses also access specialised palliative services for advice, education and support. It is not uncommon for a specialist nurse in heart failure to work with a palliative care nurse to manage symptoms and end-of-life care issues for people with heart failure (CareSearch, 2014). A recent study found that a specialised palliative care team provided support in a long-term residential care facility. Positive outcomes of reducing suffering by treating pain and other symptoms, decreasing unnecessary use of emergency and acute care services, and assisting individuals and families address end-of-life issues were obtained (Comart, Mahler, Schreiber et al., 2013).

Nurses can use Table 27-2 as a guide to conditions that may prompt the referral to specialised palliative care service. Many of the indicators, including unintentional weight loss, unstable medical conditions and frequent hospitalisations, are readily identified and can serve as indicators for referral. Information about appropriate referrals and palliative care services is available from Palliative Care Australia (www.palliativecare.org.au) and via Cancer Control New Zealand (www.cancercontrolnz.govt.nz).

APPLYING WELLNESS CONCEPTS IN SPECIFIC CHRONIC CONDITIONS

All clinically oriented chapters in this text identify opportunities for nurses to promote wellness in relation to usual aspects of functioning and some common chronic conditions of older adults. Although it is beyond the scope of this book to address pathophysiological conditions in depth, the next sections highlight some considerations that are more specific to promoting wellness in older adults who have cancer, diabetes or heart failure. These three conditions are selected as examples and are discussed within the framework of the Functional Consequences Theory to illustrate the application of wellness concepts to care of older adults who are ill.

Promoting wellness for older adults with cancer

Because cancer requires the passage of time before it reaches the stage of being a diagnosable disease, the increasing incidence of cancer is associated with increased age. Approximately 60% of cancer incidences and 70% of cancer mortalities occur in individuals older than 65 years (Molina-Garrido et al., 2014). For example, the risk of death from ovarian cancer is twice as high among women age 65 and older, compared with younger women (Freyer, Tew & Moore, 2013). Breast, colon and prostate cancers are the most common diagnoses among older cancer survivors (de Moor et al, 2013). Studies indicate that older adults with cancer are diagnosed at a later stage and are at risk for inadequate treatment (Cataldo, Paul, Cooper et al., 2013; Clough-Gorr et al., 2013).

Decisions about screening and treatment of cancer in older adults can be complicated for several reasons. First, older adults have been underrepresented in clinical trials, so there are fewer evidence-based guidelines about recommendations. Second, they are likely to have coexisting conditions that increase their susceptibility to adverse effects of treatments. Third, decisions about screening and treatment may be influenced by ageism. Current emphasis is on basing decisions not on chronological age alone but on a multidimensional assessment that considers all the following: effects of normal age-related changes, physical and psychosocial health and functioning, effects of accumulated chronic conditions, life expectancy, potential benefits versus harms, and the individual's values and preferences (Eckstrom, Feeny, Walter et al., 2013; Overcash, 2012).

Nursing assessment

From a health promotion perspective, nurses assess older adults to identify their knowledge and attitudes about screening for the types of cancer most likely to develop. For example, skin cancer is one of the most commonly occurring types, and it can be readily detected through self-examination. Thus, nurses can assess whether older adults understand how important it is to check for skin cancer and what they need to look for (as discussed in Chapter 23). Nurses also assess level of knowledge about prevention of cancer because this provides a base for identifying health promotion goals. When caring for an older adult who has cancer, nurses holistically assess such psychosocial aspects as the meaning of cancer for the individual, coping strengths and supports, and the person's ability to participate in decisions about screening and care.

Wellness nursing issues and goal planning for wellness outcomes

Willingness for enhanced knowledge is a wellness nursing issue applicable for older adults who are interested in learning about screening and prevention of cancer. The wellness nursing issue of willingness for enhanced self-care would be applicable for increasing personal responsibility for older adults who have cancer. For example, this would be particularly applicable with regard to complex decision making to do with cancer treatment.

Two goals applicable to prevention and early detection of cancer are the development of health-promoting behaviour and an increase in knowledge about health behaviour. Goals that are pertinent to caring holistically for older adults with cancer include increased comfort and level of coping and improved quality of life.

Nursing interventions

Cancer is an important focus of health promotion efforts because more than half of all cancer deaths could be prevented through healthy lifestyle choices. Health promotion interventions focus on teaching older adults about primary prevention and early detection of cancer through screening, as summarised in Box 27-2. Nurses can encourage older adults and surrogate decision makers to discuss cancer detection and treatment options with their primary care providers with an emphasis on quality of life. Nurses also need to address the need for information about the disease and treatments. Health education for older people with cancer needs be tailored to their identified and individualised needs. Exploring personal treatment goals is important because older people with cancer may be less willing than younger ones to trade increased survival for their quality of life when considering chemotherapy (Posma et al., 2009). Additional wellness-oriented nursing interventions include offering hope, support and encouragement, and considering referrals for hospice and palliative care. Nurses can find additional information about cancer in older adults through the Cancer Council (Australia), and the Cancer Society of New Zealand (see the resources section towards the end of this chapter).

For older adults already diagnosed with cancer, nurses address all aspects of pain and comfort (see Chapter 28). Also, because people with cancer commonly use complementary and alternative therapies, nurses can teach them to obtain information from reliable sources (e.g. CareSearch: Palliative Care Knowledge Network at www.caresearch.com.au).

In addition, nurses can use evidence-based information to teach about self-care practices that may be effective in alleviating some of the symptoms and discomforts associated with cancer and cancer treatments. For example, studies show that guided imagery—one of the most commonly

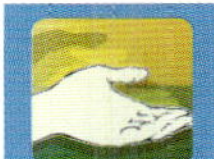

BOX 27-2
Health promotion interventions related to cancer and older adults

Teaching about primary prevention

- Stop smoking (if applicable)
- Avoid second-hand smoke
- Maintain ideal body weight
- Consume at least five servings of fresh fruit and vegetables and 25 g to 30 g of fibre daily
- Limit intake of fats, red meats and fried foods
- Avoid excessive exposure to sunlight
- Avoid excessive alcohol consumption

Screening recommendations for older adults

- Faecal occult blood test every 2 years
- Annual prostate-specific antigen and digital rectal examination for men, as determined by the general practitioner
- Mammogram and Pap test every 2 years for women
- Annual check-up by general practitioner to examine skin, thyroid, oral cavity, breasts, ovaries and testicles
- Bowel screening for people over 50 years every 2 years.

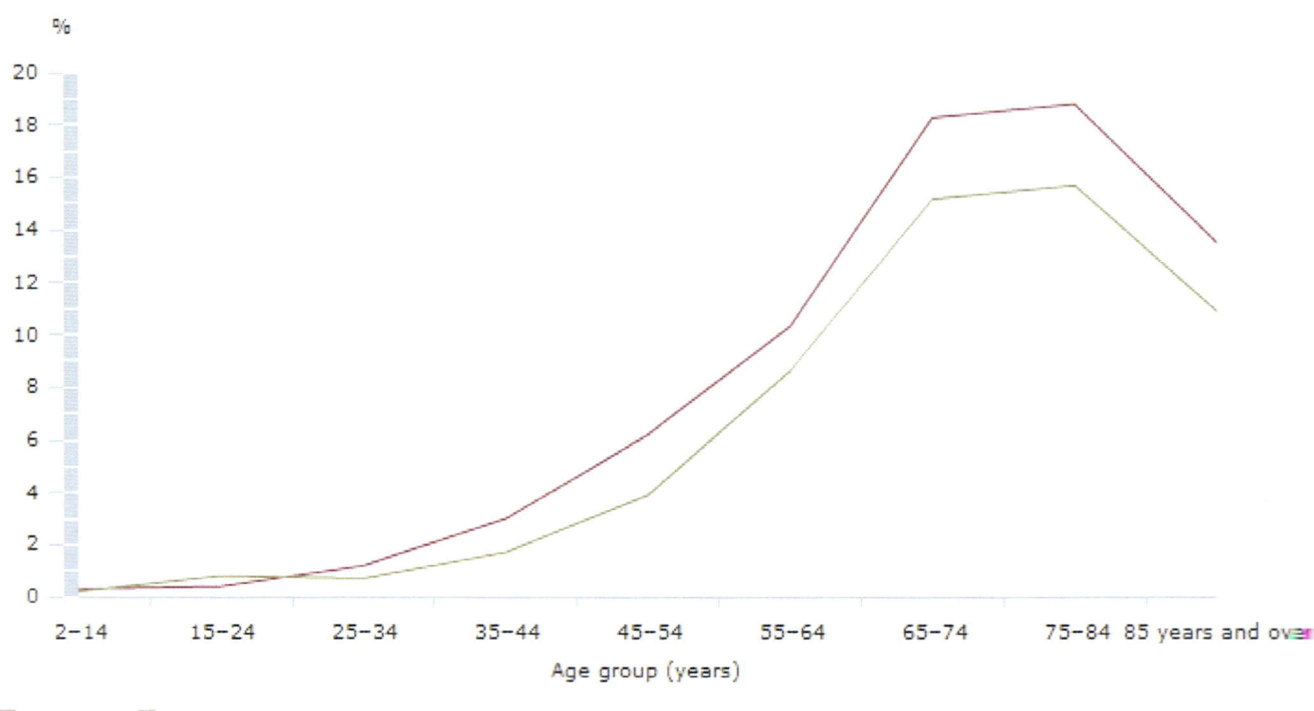

FIGURE 27-3 Percentage of Australians with diabetes by age and gender. (Australian Bureau of Statistics. [2013]. Diabetes. In *Profiles of health, Australia, 2011–13*. Cat. no. 4338.0. Canberra: Author. Permission granted under a Creative Commons BY 3.0 [CC BY 2.5 AU] licence.)

recommended integrative therapies for people with cancer—is most effective for psychosocial and quality-of-life indicators such as anxiety and depression (Fitzgerald & Langevin, 2010). Studies also support the benefits of yoga and meditation for people with cancer (Cameron, 2010; Kreitzer & Reilly-Spong, 2010).

Promoting wellness for older adults with type 2 diabetes

Diabetes is one of the most common chronic conditions in older adults. In Australia, 96% of people with diabetes are over 35 years, and almost half of these are aged 65 years or more (ABS, 2013). Figure 27-3 demonstrates the percentage of people by gender and age with diabetes in Australia. Data about diabetes and New Zealand is contained in Box 27-3.

DIVERSITY NOTE

The proportion of Indigenous Australians verses non-Indigenous Australians who have diabetes has been reported to be 32.1% and 11.6%, respectively (Australian Indigenous Health*InfoNet*, 2007).

Age-related changes that increase the risk for development of type 2 diabetes include declining beta cell function and increased insulin resistance (glucose intolerance). In addition to age-related changes, risk factors for diabetes include obesity, hypertension, family history, physical inactivity, high levels of triglycerides, and low levels of high-density lipoproteins. The serious consequences of diabetes include renal failure, retinopathy, neuropathy, cognitive decline, lower extremity amputations and cardiovascular diseases, including stroke, hypertension, myocardial infarction and coronary artery disease. Additional serious consequences in older adults include higher mortality, decreased functional status, and increased risk of living in long-term residential care (Kirkman, Briscoe, Clark et al., 2012).

BOX 27-3
New Zealand diabetes data snapshot

- 29% of adults who are aged 65 years and over have diabetes
- Pacific people are the population group with the highest prevalence of diabetes
- In 2006–2007, 10% of Pacific people aged over 15 years were diagnosed with diabetes, 90% of whom had type 2. This is approximately three times the rate of the total population
- Diabetes has been reported in Māori to be double that of non-Māori in the 65-years-and-over age group
- It is estimated the number of diabetes cases will increase and the increase will be greater within the Māori, Pacific and Asian populations

Source: New Zealand Ministry of Health. (2013). New Zealand Health Survey: Annual update of key findings 2012/13. Accessed March 2015 via www.health.govt.nz; Statistics New Zealand and Ministry of Pacific Island Affairs. (2011). *Health and Pacific peoples in New Zealand.* Wellington: Statistics New Zealand and Ministry of Pacific Island Affairs. Available March 2015 via www.stats.govt.nz.

Disease management and nursing care related to diabetes are complicated by the common occurrence of concomitant conditions in older adults. For example, infections can trigger hyperglycaemia and the older adult may require additional medication to manage their blood glucose levels (BGL) during this period of illness. Chronic arthritis or periodic flare-ups of gout are likely to affect the older adult's level of activity and can cause a transitory rise in their BGL. Another complicating factor is that older adults are likely to be taking medications that can lead to disease instability. For example, older adults are likely to have acute or chronic conditions that require treatment with prednisone, which, in turn, affects control of glucose in the BGL. Conditions that occur more commonly in older adults such as dementia, depression and functional limitations can interfere with self-management of diabetes, as can dependence on others who interfere with meals or financial constraints that affect the ability to purchase medications and appropriate foods.

WELLNESS OPPORTUNITY

Nurses can teach all older adults about actions they can take to reduce the risk of diabetes by using resources (see the health education resources at the end of the chapter).

Nursing assessment

Although nurses are not expected to diagnose diabetes, they are expected to know about variations in diagnostic indicators that are specific to older adults. For example, the renal threshold for glucose increases in older adults, so glycosuria may not be an accurate indicator. Current recommended diagnostic criteria for type 2 diabetes include:

- Fasting blood glucose ≥7.0 mmol/L (on two separate occasions)
- 2-hour postprandial ≥11.0 mmol/L result from an oral glucose tolerance test (on two separate occasions)
- Glycosylated haemoglobin (HbA1c) ≥6.5% (48 mmol/mol) (on two separate occasions). (RACGP & Diabetes Australia, 2014)

There is also a risk assessment tool that older people can use to assess risk of type 2 diabetes: the Australian Type 2 Diabetes Risk Assessment Tool (AUSDRISK), which is available at www.ausdrisk.au. AUSDRISK calculates the risk of developing diabetes over a 5-year period and scores of 12 or more are considered at high risk. It has also been recognised that the AUSDRISK underestimates the risk in Indigenous people.

Ongoing monitoring of type 2 diabetes-HBA_{1c} is routinely used to monitor glucose control in people with diabetes over the previous 2 to 3 months, with the target goals being recommended to reduce microvascular and neuropathic complications. International guidelines specific for older adults recommend that an HbA_{1c} <7.0% / 53 mmol/L should be used as a warning of possible overtreatment (International Diabetes Federation [IDF], 2013) whereas Australian guidelines recommend that targets for older adults need be individualised and weighted against the person's abilities and the risk of hypoglycaemia (RACGP & Diabetes Australia, 2014). Because older adults have wide ranging disabilities and conditions, the international guideline has categorised older adults into different categories dependent on function. The guideline then recommends targets and care for each category. Table 27-3 contains the recommended targets for HbA_{1c} and functional category.

TABLE 27-3 International guidelines for glycated haemoglobin targets relating to functional category

Functional category	General glycated haemoglobin target
Functionally independent	7.0–7.5% / 53–59 mmol/mol
Functionally dependent	7.0–8.0% / 53–64 mmol/mol
• Frail	• Up to 8.5% / 70 mmol/mol
• Dementia	• Up to 8.5% / 70 mmol/mol
End of life	Avoid symptomatic hyper-glycaemia

Source: International Diabetes Federation. (2013). IDF global guideline for managing older people with type 2 diabetes. Accessed March 2015 at www.idf.org/guidelines.

Older people are at an increased risk of hypoglycaemia because they have reduced sensitivity to its signs and symptoms (Bremer et al., 2009; Kirkman, Briscoe, Clark et al., 2012). Also, since the introduction of generic glycaemia targets there has been an increase in admissions for hypoglycaemia in older adults. One study found that for admissions for hyperglycaemia in older adults has declined by 38.6%, but with a corresponding increase in admissions for hypoglycaemia by 11.7% (Lipska, Ross, Wang et al., 2014). It is recommended that less stringent targets may be safer and more appropriate for older adults who have multiple comorbidities, are hospitalised, or have a reduced life expectancy (Kirkman, Briscoe, Clark et al., 2012). Box 27-4 presents a summary of the IDF recommendations for glucose targets and hypoglycaemia for older adults.

In addition to the usual nursing assessment parameters for diabetes, a holistic nursing approach for older adults addresses such issues as the meaning of the condition to the person, identification of ageist attitudes that may affect management, and socioeconomic and cultural influences. Box 27-5 summarises some questions that are more specific to assessment of diabetes in older adults from a wellness perspective.

Wellness nursing issues and goals for wellness outcomes

Willingness for enhanced knowledge is a wellness nursing issue that is applicable for older adults and their carers, if appropriate, who are interested in learning about diabetes, particularly with regard to improved understanding of how this condition affects their health. Nurses can use the

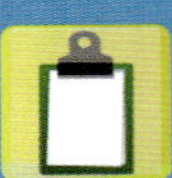

BOX 27-4
Summary of recommendations from the IDF (2013) guidelines about glucose targets and hypoglycaemia

- Healthcare professionals caring for older adults with diabetes should assess each individual's risk of hypoglycaemia and develop an individualised care plan including a blood glucose range to minimise risk
- In routine clinical practice, avoid blood glucose levels below 6.0 mmol/L
- An HbA_{1c} <7.0% / 53 mmol/mol should be used as a warning of possible overtreatment
- Every older adult on insulin and certain sulfonylureas should have a hypoglycaemia management plan that includes blood glucose monitoring
- An episode of severe hypoglycaemia should trigger a detailed diabetes review, including a structured medicine review
- An education strategy should be developed and implemented for healthcare professionals and older adults with diabetes to minimise the risk of hypoglycaemia and its consequences
- A hypoglycaemia management kit should be readily available in hospitals and should be restocked immediately after use
- Every older adult who is self-administering insulin should have an evaluation of their self-administration abilities.

Source: International Diabetes Federation. (2013). IDF global guideline for managing older people with type 2 diabetes. Accessed March 2015 via www.idf.org/guidelines.

BOX 27-5
Assessment guidelines for older adults with diabetes

Considerations about the meaning of diabetes

- What terminology is appropriate for discussing the condition (e.g. older adults may refer to diabetes as "sugar")?
- What is the person's understanding of diabetes?

Considerations for disease management

- What is the person's understanding of personal responsibility for managing diabetes?
- Socioeconomic influences: Who does grocery shopping and meal preparation? What foods are included in the usual meal pattern? What is the usual "budget" for food? Where does the person eat meals?
- What cultural factors affect health beliefs, disease management, food preparation, eating patterns, and health-related behaviours, such as exercise?
- What concomitant conditions affect the older adult's self-care abilities?

Considerations regarding the influence of ageist attitudes

- Do ageist attitudes (of the older adult, carer or healthcare professionals) interfere with setting wellness-oriented goals? (e.g. "I've been eating ice cream all my life, why should I worry about that now at my age?")
- Does the older adult (or do others) inaccurately associate a sense of hopelessness with his or her condition because of advanced age? (e.g. "At my age, I can't do anything about my sugar levels.")

wellness nursing issue of willingness for enhanced self-care when they care for older adults who are interested in improving personal responsibility for management of their condition, including preventing complications. Goals that would be pertinent to promoting wellness in older adults with diabetes include participation in a diabetes self-management program, improved blood glucose level, development of health-promoting behaviour (nutrition, weight and exercise), increased knowledge about diabetes management, and improved self-care status.

Nursing and other health professional interventions

Teaching about self-management is the cornerstone of diabetes care, and group programs are particularly effective for older adults (Tshiananga, Kocher, Weber et al., 2012). Benefits of group interventions for older adults with diabetes include improvements in glycaemic control, self-efficacy, emotional coping and quality of life, and decreased levels of distress and depressive symptoms (Beverly, Fitzgerald, Sitnikov et al., 2013). The aim of a self-management program is to assist skills-based learning and development of a sense of empowerment about diabetes. Thus, in addition to individual teaching about diabetes, a primary nursing responsibility is facilitating referrals for group educational programs. Best practice information about individual teaching about nutrition, activity and diabetes self-management for older adults with type 2 diabetes is contained in Evidence-based practice 27-1.

In addition to teaching about lifestyle interventions, nurses should emphasise the involvement of other health professionals (see below), prevention of injury, and observations of wound healing. Nurses also make referrals when appropriate, for instance:

- A diabetes educator, to assist the older adult with self-management of all aspects of the disease
- A dietitian and exercise physiologist, if the older adult has an issue requiring review or nutrition or exercise
- An ophthalmologist, for surveillance of eyes for diabetic retinopathy
- A podiatrist, for ongoing review of feet
- An oral health professional, especially if oral disease is noted.

Another aspect of care that nurses are involved in with older adults living with diabetes is foot care. Nurses assess feet and promote programs that protect the feet in an endeavour to prevention diabetic complications. Box 27-6 on page 614 lists the key points regarding assessment and protection of diabetic feet.

Older adults with diabetes may also benefit from referrals for community-based services, including home-delivered meals, assistance with grocery shopping or meal preparation, participation in group meal programs, transportation to appointments, and assistance with medication management or glucose monitoring. Providing such services for an older adult with diabetes is often an

EVIDENCE-BASED PRACTICE 27-1
Summary of best practice interventions for nutrition, activity and diabetes self-management for older adults with type 2 diabetes

Nutrition

- All older adults should have a nutritional and biochemical assessment at diagnosis, or admission to long-term residential care, and as part of the annual review.
- The nutrition plan should be individualised and consider the person's food preferences, eating routines, religion and culture, and physical and cognitive health status.
- The meal plan should include a variety of foods to ensure essential vitamins, minerals, protein and fibre are consumed in adequate amounts.
- Medicine administration times must coincide with meal times if the individual is on insulin or sulfonylureas to reduce the risk of hypoglycaemia.
- People with swallowing difficulties should be identified and referred to a speech pathologist if available.

Physical activity

- Older adults with diabetes should be encouraged to be as active as their health and functional status allow.
- A risk assessment should be undertaken before recommending an activity program.
- Timing and type of activity should be considered in relation to the medicine regimen, especially glucose-lowering agents associated with an increased risk of hypoglycaemia.

Education, diabetes self-management and self-monitoring of blood glucose

- Education should be offered to all older adults with diabetes with the teaching strategy and learning environment modified to suit the older person and/or their carer.
- Education should be individualised, include goal setting, and focus on safety, risk management and complication prevention.
- Older adults with newly diagnosed diabetes (and/or their carer) should receive 'survival education' initially and then ongoing education.
- Older adults with established diabetes (and/or their carer) should receive regular education and reviews.
- Provide simple and individualised hypoglycaemia and sick day management plans.
- Appropriate decision aids and cues to action should be developed with the individual and their family carers.
- Consider an individualised blood glucose monitoring plan for people: self-monitoring is usually recommended for those on insulin and oral hypoglycaemic agents (OHAs) that can cause hypoglycaemia or when monitoring hyperglycaemia arising from illness.
- Consider an individualised blood-glucose monitoring plan for people on insulin, as well as some oral glucose-lowering therapy.
- Monitoring of blood glucose could be considered for others as an optional component of self-management where there is an agreed purpose for testing.
- Monitoring of blood glucose should be used only within a care package, accompanied by structured education on how the results can be used to reinforce lifestyle change, adjust therapy or alert healthcare professionals to changes.
- Oral glucose-lowering therapy is commenced when lifestyle interventions alone are unable to maintain target blood glucose levels. Metformin is the first choice unless contraindicated or not tolerated (diarrhoea). Second-line agents, usually sulfonylureas, may be necessary and should be chosen using an individualised approach.
- Maintain support for lifestyle measures throughout the use of these medicines.
- Discuss with the individual and principal carer the goals and medicine dose, regimen and tablet burden before choosing glucose-lowering agents.
- The "start low and go slow" principle is used when initiating and increasing medication. Monitor response to each initiation or dose increase for up to a 3-month trial period.
- Insulin may be commenced if oral hypoglycaemics are not effective. There are a number of delivery options, including insulin pens and insulin syringes, and the selected option will depend on the person's preference and abilities.
- Insulin injectors (pens) assist older adults with self-management, as does the "InnoLet" injecting device (information about which can be found via www.novonordisk.com).
- Discontinuing ineffective and unnecessary therapies should be considered.
- The cost and the risk*-to-benefit ratio should be considered when choosing a medicine.

*Risk includes adverse events, hypoglycaemia, weight gain or weight loss, need for carer involvement, impact of worsening renal or hepatic function, gastrointestinal symptoms.

Source: International Diabetes Federation. (2013). IDF global guideline for managing older people with type 2 diabetes. Accessed March 2015 via www.idf.org/guidelines

essential element in ensuring optimal control and supporting the person's ability to remain in his or her own home.

Nurses may need to address factors that are more common among older adults, such as involving and teaching carers, compensating for memory deficits, and identifying the most cost-effective ways of obtaining medications and glucometer supplies. Health education interventions need to address the needs of specific cultural groups because studies found that culturally relevant lifestyle interventions can improve diabetes-related behaviours and clinical outcomes (Castro et al., 2009). Nurses can use the resources listed in Chapter 5 to find culturally appropriate health education programs pertinent to older adults with diabetes.

Nurses also may need to address fear and anxiety in older adults and carers and to encourage discussion of feelings about diabetes and the impact of this chronic condition on the person's health and lifestyle. Nurses can help older adults identify safe and enjoyable ways of

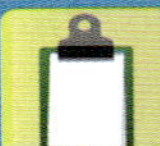

BOX 27-6
Feet assessment and protection program for older adults living with diabetes

Feet assessment

- Observe for calluses, sites of pressure, bony deformities, dry skin, fungal infection, skin discolouration (ischaemia), and breaks in skin integrity
- Palpation of peripheral pulses—dorsalis pedis and posterior tibial
- Test sensation using a monofilament

Feet protection program

- Podiatry
- Hygiene maintenance: advice to inspect and wash feet daily
- Appropriate footwear and hosiery
- Protective shoes: avoid constrictive footwear
- Clinic contact initiated by the person if they are concerned

Source: National Health and Medical Research Council (NHMRC). (2011b). National evidence-based guideline for the prevention, identification and management of foot complications in diabetes. Adelaide: Baker IDI Heart & Diabetes Institute. Available March 2015 via www.nhmrc.gov.au/guidelines-publications/di21.

engaging in physical activity, especially if they have concomitant conditions that affect their ability to exercise. For example, swimming or aqua therapy classes may be more appropriate than walking for an older adult who has arthritis or problems with balance.

Promoting wellness for older adults with Parkinson's disease

Parkinson's disease is a chronic neurodegenerative condition that many older adults develop. Advancing age is the greatest risk factor but genetics and environmental toxins have also been implicated (bestpractice[NZ] Decision Support, 2014). Box 27-7 contains statistics regarding Parkinson's disease in older Australians and New Zealanders. Currently there is no cure for this condition and, as there is no objective test to diagnose Parkinson's disease, misdiagnosis can occur. Diagnosis is usually performed by a specialist medical practitioner. Diagnosis is usually made when the following motor symptoms are present: tremor, muscle rigidity, akinesia/bradykinesia (slowness in the initiation of movement/reduced movement), and postural instability (bestpractice[NZ] Decision Support, 2014). Other symptoms that commonly accompany the disease are called non-motor symptoms and include urinary and bowel changes, pain, sleep disturbance and cognitive changes.

Parkinson's disease is a progressive disease with five different stages. Each older adult will experience these stages differently and it is not uncommon that a stage is missed. Stage 1 and 2 represent early-stage (mild motor symptoms), 2 and 3 mid-stage, and 4 and 5 advanced-stage (immobility, dependence and cognitive decline). Consequently Parkinson's disease, with its all-consuming progressive course, affects all aspects of the person's physical, mental and psychological well-being. Because of these consequences, Parkinson's disease is a major source of chronic disability, increased mortality and impaired quality of life. It is necessary for nurses to work with older adults to promote their health and well-being. It is important for the older adult to maintain a healthy lifestyle in the earlier stages to counter the deterioration they will experience as the disease advances. Older adults with Parkinson's, as the disease progresses, will require increased assistance with all aspects of living. They may be admitted in to long-term residential care, but this will depend on the availability of a carer/s, the carers' abilities and other community care supports.

Nursing assessment

Because of the dynamic nature of parkinsonism symptoms—that is, the fluctuations experienced in the person's motor symptoms—nursing assessment is always challenging. Nurses assess for signs and symptoms of Parkinson's in older adults using the same assessment techniques that apply to adults of any age. However, ongoing management of older adults as the disease progresses requires the inclusion of assessment tools that consider ageing changes.

Wellness nursing issues and goals for wellness outcomes

Nurses can use the wellness nursing issue of willingness for management to promote increased personal responsibility

BOX 27-7
Parkinson's disease statistics regarding older adults in Australia and New Zealand

Currently Australia and New Zealand death rate from Parkinson's disease is located in the high risk zone compared to other global nations. It is estimated that the death rate is 2.5 (New Zealand) and 2.4 (Australia) per 100 people.

Australia

- Parkinson's is the second most-common neurological disease after dementia
- Eighty per cent of sufferers are over 50 years old
- The number of people with Parkinson's has increased by 17% during 2005–2011
- The prevalence of Parkinson's is greater than prostate and bowel cancer

New Zealand

- An estimated 1% of people aged over 65 years have Parkinson's disease
- The median age of onset is 60 years, and the life expectancy following diagnosis is 15 years on average

Source: Deloitte Access Economics. (2011). Living with Parkinson's Disease—Update. Report prepared for Parkinson's Australia. Accessed March 2015 via www.deloitteaccesseconomics.com.au/publications+and+reports/browse+reports; bestpractice[NZ] Decision Support. (2014). The management of Parkinson's disease: Which treatments to start and when? *Best Practice Journal*, 58, 26–39. Accessed March 2015 at www.bpac.org.nz/BPJ/2014/February/parkinsons.aspx.

TABLE 27-4 List of nursing issues and goal planning for wellness outcomes for older adults with Parkinson's disease

Nursing issue	Goal planning for wellness outcomes
Speech difficulties	• Improved voice quality, volume and audibility
Undernutrition and nausea	• Prevention of weight loss and reduction in nausea
Dysphagia	• Improved swallowing, prevention of aspiration
Self-care deficit instrumental activities of daily living and activities of daily living	• Maintenance of independence • Maintenance of safe activity and employment
Difficulties with mobilisation, at risk of falling and increased risk of injury	• Improved gait: improved muscle strength, balance and endurance; prevention of falls; reduction of risk of falls and injury
Altered sleep patterns, nightmares	• Improved sleep pattern
Urinary urgency and frequency	• Prevention of urinary incontinence
Constipation	• Prevention of constipation
Pain: acute and persistent	• Pain is controlled
Psychological disturbances	• Improvement in mood, reduction in anxiety, improved coping, maintenance of resilience, prevention of depression
Altered sexual pattern	• Improvement in sexual function

for the management of Parkinson's motor and non-motor symptoms. Table 27-4 lists the multitude of issues and related goals for wellness outcomes for older adults living with Parkinson's.

Nursing interventions

Wellness-oriented care plans for older adults with Parkinsons disease during the early stages of the disease will focus on teaching about actions the person can take to achieve the best possible level of functioning and quality of life despite the chronic condition. Teaching the older adult about the optimal management and prevention of symptoms that arise from the condition is an important aspect of self-management. There is much that can assist the older adult to maintain their quality of life and well-being as the disease progresses. However, older adults will require ongoing assessment and support from a range of health professionals to achieve these wellness outcomes. Nurses also discuss palliative care with the older adult and their families so they understand the stages of the disease and make plans for future health decline.

Pharmacological interventions

Medications are essential part of the care plan for older adults with Parkinsons. These medications are used to improve the motor symptoms of Parkinson's by increasing the level of dopamine in the brain and thus activate the parts of the brain where dopamine works. As Parkinson's is a very individual condition, medications are prescribed that have been titrated to individual's needs and responses. Not every medication that treats the motor symptoms is suitable for every person. A fundamental guideline that should be followed when Parkinson's medication is being administered is that the older adults receive their medication on time. It is also preferable for those with Parkinson's to self-medicate to optimise drug therapy. Optimisation means achieving the best control of the motor symptoms.

Nurses can assess for optimal medication therapy and, if poor control is detected, then it is recommended that the older adult be referred to their specialist doctor for revision. Common medications prescribed for older adults with Parkinson's disease include:

- Levodopa (dopamine precursor—primary medication used in people over 40 years)
- Carbidopa or benserazide (potentiates levodopa)
- Selegiline (potentiates levodopa)
- Bromocriptine, pergolide, pramipexole, cabergoline and ropinirole (dopamine agonists)
- Benzhexol and benztropine (anticholinergic agents). (Deloitte Access Economics, 2011; bestpractice[NZ] Decision Support, 2014)

While taking these medications a number of other medications must not be administered concurrently. Box 27-8 provides a list of these medications. Of particular importance is that the nurse must be aware the only oral anti-nausea medication that may be prescribed is domperidone.

Non-pharmacological interventions

Many non-pharmacological interventions also are available, which assist with mobility, communication, independence

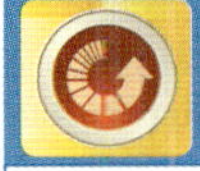

BOX 27-8 Drugs to be avoided when an older adult is prescribed anti-parkinsonism medications

- Haloperidol
- Chlorpromazine
- Metoclopramide
- Flupenthixol
- Trifluoperazine
- Prochlorperazine

TABLE 27-5 Non-pharmacological interventions for symptoms of Parkinson's disease

Nursing issue	Intervention
Increasing difficulty with mobility: shuffling and unsteady gait, stooped posture, freezing (inability to move); increased risk of falls and injury	Nurses can promote exercise to improve mobility. Evidence suggests that people with the Parkinson's disease should aim to complete at least 20 to 30 minutes each day of aerobic exercise such as walking. Referral to a physiotherapist may also be helpful to develop an individualised exercise plan to improve muscle strength, balance and endurance.
Increasing difficulty with communicating: poor articulation, loss of facial expression and body language all contribute	Referral to a speech pathologist for voice training.
Increasing difficulty with activity of daily living (ADLs) and instrumental activities of daily living	Nurses teach the older adults about the importance of receiving the Parkinson's medications on time which reduce the fluctuations in physical function. Also, optimised medication levels will assist with muscle function. Nurses provide education regarding medication optimisation. Referral to an occupational therapist will provide assistive devices and a plan for performance of ADLs (many older adults feel better in the morning).
Postural and postprandial hypotension	Nurses provide information and support to older adults about increasing fluid and salt intake, eating frequent small meals to reduce postprandial hypotension, and wearing compression stockings that extend to above the knee.
Drooling, dysphagia, nausea and undernutrition	Optimised medication levels will assist to minimise these symptoms. Nurses provide education regarding medication optimisation. Thickened fluids reduce the risk of aspiration. Nurses teach older adults about eating slowly and taking smaller mouthfuls of food. Referral to a speech therapist is required depending on the degree of dysphagia. Nurses can advise those older adults with nausea to eat frequent small meals and try to improve posture while eating. See Chapter 18 for wellness management of nutrition.
Constipation	Nurses provide support regarding the development of a bowel management plan and continuous assessment and review of plan. See Chapter 18 for further information about bowel wellness in older adults.
Pain from muscle cramps, spasms and reduced movement	Medication optimisation will assist with musculoskeletal symptoms. Nurses provide education regarding medication optimisation. Physiotherapy has been found to provide relief from pain. See Chapter 28 for further information about pharmacological management of persistent neuropathic pain. Massage, acupuncture and yoga have proved helpful in relieving pain in some people with Parkinson's disease.
Anxiety, depression, hallucinations and at risk of developing dementia	Medication optimisation will assist with cognitive and psychological symptoms. Nurses provide education regarding medication optimisation. See Chapters 12 and 15 for strategies to promote psychosocial wellness in older adults.
Sleep disturbances: excessive daytime sleeping, nightmares	Parkinson's medications can be the cause of nightmares. See Chapter 24 for assessing and managing sleep disorders.
Urinary urgency and frequency and incontinence	See Chapter 19 for wellness management of urinary symptoms.
Sexual difficulties: reduced libido, painful or uncomfortable sex, erectile dysfunction	Reduced libido may be linked to depression and persistent pain. See Chapter 26 for wellness management of sexual difficulties.

Source: bestpractice[NZ] Decision Support. (2014). The management of Parkinson's disease: Which treatments to start and when? *Best Practice Journal,* 58, 26–39. Accessed March 2015 at www.bpac.org.nz/BPJ/2014/February/parkinsons.aspx; Deloitte Access Economics. (2011). Living with Parkinson's Disease—Update. Report prepared for Parkinson's Australia. Accessed March 2015 at www.parkinsons.org.au/ACT/AEReport_2011.pdf.

and the management of other symptoms commonly associated with Parkinson's disease. Table 27-5 provides a summary of some of the key non-pharmacological interventions.

Another consideration is that dementia occurs with Parkinson's disease in 40% of older adults, and it is often the onset of dementia that initiates a transfer from home care to long-term residential care. Dementia symptoms in Parkinson's can be caused by the Parkinson's medication, but a reduction o withdrawal may lead to poor symptom control.

Finally, as Parkinson's disease progresses the olde adult will become increasing reliant on others, usually family, to assist them to complete their daily living activities and maintain their health and well-being. The needs of families and carers are discussed further in the next section.

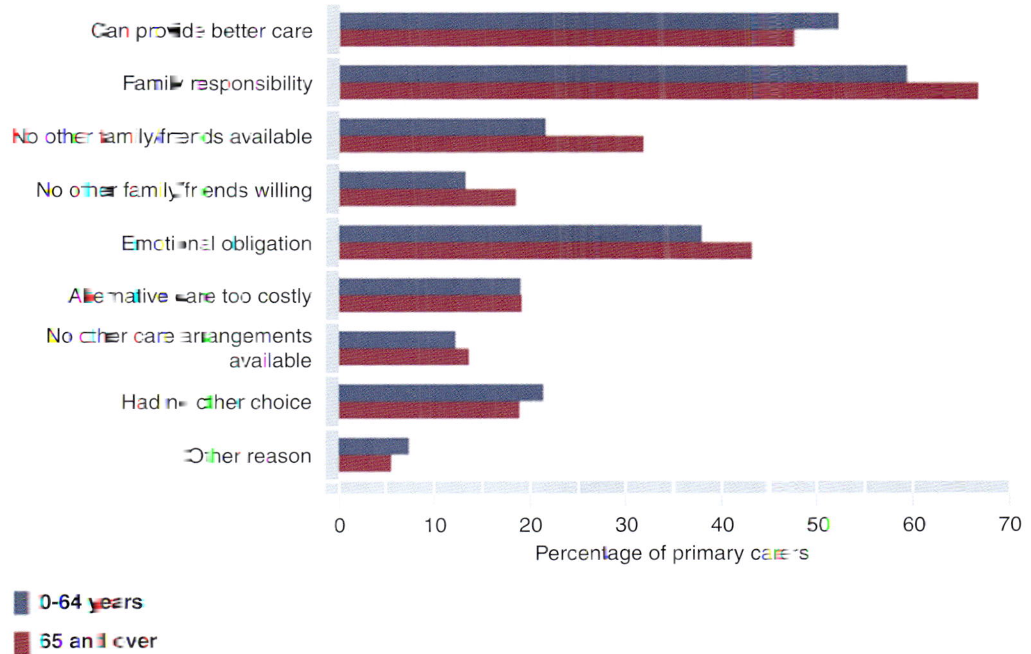

FIGURE 27-4 Reasons for taking on a carer role by age in Australia. (Australian Bureau of Statistics. [2012]. *Disability, ageing and carers, Australia: Summary of findings*. Cat. no. 4430.0. Canberra: Author. Permission granted under a Creative Commons BY 3.0 [CC BY 2.5 AU] licence.)

ADDRESSING NEEDS OF FAMILIES AND CARERS

During periods of illness—whether acute, chronic or declining—the importance of relationships increases in proportion to the need not only for physical care but also for emotional and spiritual care. When nurses care for older adults during illness, families and carers are an integral focus of care. Even with the increasing availability of aged community services for older adults, families and friends continue to provide 80% to 90% of the care given to dependent older adults in the community. In Australia 20% of primary carers were aged 65 years or more and caring for a partner (ABS, 2012). Figure 27-4 presents the reasons that people by age take on a carer role, with the most common reasons being they can provide better care and have a sense of family responsibility.

For older adults who have dementia or other conditions that cause progressive declines in functioning, the role of carer usually evolves gradually and can last for years. Even in situations in which older adults do not have progressively declining conditions, families of older adults frequently deal with intermittent and cumulative conditions that require intense medical care or rehabilitative services. It is not uncommon for the families of older adults to take on the roles of care managers and find themselves negotiating healthcare services for at least one and sometimes several parents, grandparents, aunts, uncles, other relatives and "significant others". It has also been reported that spouses are less likely to seek assistance outside the family network, particularly some ethnic groups, including Pacific people, Māori and Indigenous Australians (Medical Council of New Zealand, 2010).

The term **carer burden** is commonly used to describe the financial, physical and psychosocial problems that family members experience when caring for older adults who are impaired or suffering from illness. Specific functional consequences associated with carer burden include: depression; disturbed sleep; social isolation; family discord; career interruptions; financial difficulties; lack of time for self; poor physical health; psychological/emotional/mental strain; and feelings of anger, guilt, grief, anxiety, hopelessness and helplessness. Some of the stressors that contribute to carer burden are multiple demands on the carer, a lack of control over the situation, lack of social support, impairment of the care recipient, duration and intensity of care, dependency in activities of daily living, unpredictability and recurrence of illness, and problem behaviours of the care recipient (Coon & Evans, 2009; Tamayo et al., 2010). Nurses can use the Modified Caregiver Strain Index (Figure 27-5) to identify families who may benefit from further assessment and follow-up.

Although most studies have focused on the burdens of caregiving, there is increasing recognition that carer well-being can be a positive consequence of caring for a dependent loved one. Positive outcomes identified in

Directions: Here is a list of things that other caregivers have found to be difficult. Please put a checkmark in the columns that apply to you. We have included some examples that are common caregiver experiences to help you think about each item. Your situation may be slightly different, but the item could still apply.

	Yes, On a Regular Basis = 2	Yes, Sometimes = 1	No = 0
My sleep is disturbed (For example: the person I care for is in and out of bed or wanders around at night)			
Caregiving is inconvenient (For example: helping takes so much time or it's a long drive over to help)			
Caregiving is a physical strain (For example: lifting in or out of a chair; effort or concentration is required)			
Caregiving is confining (For example: helping restricts free time or I cannot go visiting)			
There have been family adjustments (For example: helping has disrupted my routine; there is no privacy)			
There have been changes in personal plans (For example: I had to turn down a job; I could not go on a vacation)			
There have been other demands on my time (For example: other family members need me)			
There have been emotional adjustments (For example: severe arguments about caregiving)			
Some behavior is upsetting (For example: incontinence; the person cared for has trouble remembering things; or the person I care for accuses people of taking things)			
It is upsetting to find the person I care for has changed so much from his/her former self (For example: he/she is a different person than he/she used to be)			
There have been work adjustments (For example: I have to take time off for caregiving duties)			
Caregiving is a financial strain			
I feel completely overwhelmed (For example: I worry about the person I care for; I have concerns about how I will manage)			

[Sum responses for "Yes, on a regular basis" (2 pts each) and "yes, sometimes" (1 pt each)] Total Score =

FIGURE 27-5 Modified Caregiver Strain Index. (From Thornton, M. & Travis, S. S. [2003]. Analysis of the reliability of the Modified Caregiver Strain Index. *Journals of Gerontology: Psychological Sciences and Social Sciences, 58*[2], S129. © Copyright The Gerontological Society of America. Reproduced by permission of the publisher.)

EVIDENCE-BASED PRACTICE 27-2
Family caregiving

Statement of the problem

- More than 80% of the care for dependent older adults is provided by family.
- Caregiving activities include assistance with daily activities, illness-related care (medication management, assessing and addressing symptoms, carrying out treatments), and care management activities (advocacy, accessing and coordinating services, navigating healthcare and social service systems).
- Carers typically experience higher levels of stress and depression and lower levels of physical health and subjective well-being.
- Increased carer strain is associated with lack of preparedness for the role, caring for someone with dementia, and poor quality relationships between caregiver and care recipient.

Parameters for nursing assessment

- Caregiving context: roles and responsibilities, duration of caregiving, physical environment, financial status, cultural factors and potential resources
- Carer's perception of health and functional status of care recipient, including functional and cognitive limitations
- Carer preparedness: skills, knowledge
- Quality of relationship between carer and care recipient
- Indicators of problems with care: unhealthy environment, inappropriate financial management
- Carer's health status: self-rated health, physical and mental health, rewards of caregiving

Recommended assessment tool

- Modified Caregiver Strain Index (see Figure 27-5)

Recommendations for interventions

- Form a partnership with carers and use an interdisciplinary approach when working with carers
  - Identify carers' needs, issues and concerns and assist carers in developing a plan to address these
- During hospitalisations, invite family carers to participate in care, based on an assessment of family preference
- Help the carer identify strengths in the caregiving situation
- Assist the carer in finding and using resources

Source: Messecar, D. C. (2012). Family caregiving. In M. Boltz, E. Capezuti, T. Fulmer & D. Zwicker (Eds), *Evidence-based geriatric nursing protocols for best practice* (4th ed., pp. 469–499). New York: Springer.

studies include personal growth, strengthening of relationships, feelings of satisfaction, and increased self-esteem (Winter, Boulton & Andresen, 2010). Carers are more likely to experience positive effects when they have more choice about the situation or when they perceive themselves as interdependent with the care receiver (e.g. as a spouse) (Foulin et al., 2010; Winter et al., 2010).

One study found that a high proportion of carers of family members with dementia or stroke found satisfaction from promoting the care recipient's well-being and from experiencing a sense of fulfilment or personal achievement (Mayor, Ribeiro & Paul, 2009). Cultural factors also significantly affect the experience of being a carer, as discussed in Chapter 1, especially with regard to societal perceptions of family roles and responsibilities (see Cultural considerations 1-1).

Nurses address teaching needs of older adults' families, partners and significant others as an essential nursing responsibility related to continuity of care in all healthcare settings. Consistent with this responsibility, nurses follow standards of care and document the teaching they provide regarding caregiving instructions, but they do not necessarily address the broader needs of carers because of such barriers as time constraints and perception of this as a non-essential aspect of care. However, when nurses care for dependent older adults, it is important to recognise that even the basic needs of the older adult cannot be met without a strong support system. Nurses need to identify outcomes and interventions to prevent carer burnout and enhance the ability of families and other carers to provide the necessary care. For example, studies found that skill-training interventions improved carer health and quality of life (Coon & Evans, 2009; Elliott, Burgio & DeCoster, 2010).

Interventions also need to focus on improving the function and well-being of the care recipient. A study found that the burden experienced by family carers of depressed older adults was alleviated after the care recipient was treated with antidepressants (Martire et al., 2010). As with all aspects of caring for older adults, there is great individual variation among families, carers and care recipients, so there are many varied interventions to address carer issues. Evidence-based practice 27-2 summarises research findings related to interventions for family carers, and Table 27-6 on the next page lists nursing outcomes and interventions that are applicable to promoting wellness for families and carers who are involved with the care of ill or dependent older adults.

Some excellent resources are available for carers in New Zealand. For example, A guide for carers—He Aratohu mā ngā Kaitiaki, provides comprehensive information and is available via the Ministry of Social Development's website www.msd.govt.nz. Another resource at this site is CarersAir, which provides information on well-being and learning assistance for family carers and friends. The Australian Government portal www.myagedcare.gov.au also provides many resources to assist carers.

CHAPTER HIGHLIGHTS

Characteristics of illness in older adults

- Presence of many interacting conditions and factors (e.g. acute illness, chronic conditions, psychosocial factors, environmental conditions, age-related changes, medication effects)

TABLE 27-6 Nursing outcomes and nursing interventions for promoting wellness in carers/caregivers

Type of need	Nursing outcomes	Nursing interventions
Needs related to carer role	Carer Adaptation to the Person's Institutionalisation, Carer Emotional Health, Carer Endurance Potential, Carer Home Care Readiness, Carer Lifestyle Disruption, Carer–Older adult Relationship, Carer Performance: Direct/Indirect Care, Carer Physical Health, Carer Stressors, Carer Well-Being	Carer Support, Case Management, Counselling, Energy Management, Family Support, Family Integrity Promotion, Resiliency Promotion, Role Enhancement, Self-Awareness Enhancement, Support Group
Needs related to using resources and managing care	Information Processing, Knowledge: Health Resources, Participation in Healthcare Decisions, Role Performance	Decision-Making Support, Health Education, Health System Guidance, Referral, Respite Care, Support System Enhancement, Teaching: Individual, Telephone Consultation
Psychosocial needs	Anxiety Level, Coping, Decision Making, Depression Level, Family Coping, Family Resiliency, Fear Level, Grief Resolution, Loneliness Severity, Self-Esteem, Stress Level	Active Listening, Anticipatory Guidance, Anxiety Reduction, Cognitive Restructuring, Coping Enhancement, Emotional Support, Grief Work Facilitation, Mood Management, Presence, Simple Guided Imagery
Spiritual and quality-of-life needs	Hope, Leisure Participation, Quality of Life, Sleep, Social Involvement, Social Support, Spiritual Health	Forgiveness Facilitation, Guilt Work Facilitation, Hope Instillation, Humour, Sleep Enhancement, Spiritual Support

- Complexity of interpreting signs and symptoms (e.g. vague or atypical manifestations)
- Far-reaching consequences (e.g. loss of independence due to fractured hip)
- Cumulative effects of ageing and illness making adaptation difficult
- Older adults possibly experiencing a "yo-yoing" pattern of health, with gradually diminishing resiliency.
- Key concepts: comorbidity, atypical presentation, geriatric syndromes, frailty.

Connecting the concepts of wellness, ageing and illness

- A holistic perspective enables nurses to identify ways of promoting wellness by addressing needs related to physical health and functioning, and emotional and spiritual well-being.
- An important aspect of wellness is promoting personal responsibility for health through self-care measures and management of chronic conditions.
- Nurses can challenge ageist attitudes and provide health education to foster behaviour change when appropriate.
- Nursing interventions and outcomes applicable for older adults when they are ill are listed in Table 27-1.

Holistically caring for older adults who are ill: Focusing on caring and comforting

- Palliative care is a holistic approach to caring for people with advanced progressive illnesses through prevention, assessment and treatment of pain and other physical, psychosocial and spiritual problems.
- Nurses are involved in providing generalist palliative care and assist in obtaining referrals for specialist palliative care. They discuss with older adults and their families about the scope of these services.

Promoting wellness for older adults with cancer

- Older adults are disproportionately affected by cancer, they are less likely to be screened for cancer, and they are diagnosed at a later stage.
- From a health promotion perspective, nurses assess older adults to identify their knowledge and attitudes about screening for the types of cancer they are most likely to develop.
- Nurses holistically address the needs of older adults already diagnosed with cancer.
- Nurses can teach older adults about primary prevention interventions and about screening recommendations.

Promoting wellness for older adults with diabetes

- Diabetes is common among older adults. There is a high prevalence among Indigenous Australians and Māori. Disease management and nursing care related to diabetes are made complex by the common occurrence of concomitant conditions and by the increased vulnerability of older adults to complications.
- Recommended older-adult assessment parameters for diabetes are in Box 27-5.
- Care plans for older adults with diabetes include interventions and additional teaching points that are appropriate for older adults (EBP 27-1; Box 27-6)

Promoting wellness for older adults with Parkinson's disease

- Parkinson's disease is a progressive disease with five different stages.
- Parkinson's disease, with its all-consuming progressive course, affects all aspects of the person's physical, mental and psychological well-being.
- Parkinson's disease is a major source of chronic disability, increased mortality and impaired quality of life.

- Nurses work with older adults to promote their health and well-being throughout all stages of the disease (Boxes 27-7 & 27-8; Tables 27-4 & 27-5).

Addressing needs of families and carers

- Nurses promote carer well-being by identifying and addressing issues related to carer burden (EBP 27-2).
- Nursing interventions and outcomes applicable to carers are listed in Table 27-6.

CRITICAL THINKING EXERCISES

1. Identify an older person (in your personal life or clinical experience) who has recently been hospitalised and address the following in relation to that person:
   - How many different conditions (e.g. acute and chronic illness, functional limitations, support resources, psychosocial factors or environmental factors) affected how the person was able to adapt to the hospitalisation?
   - How did these factors affect the outcome for the person (e.g. longer hospitalisation, increased dependency on others, discharge plans)?
   - Select two nursing outcomes and interventions from Table 27-1 that you could apply to a care plan to promote wellness for this person.
2. Think about your expectations for older adults who are affected by multiple interacting conditions and identify any ageist attitudes or assumptions that are likely to affect your care.
3. Find information about local resources for palliative care and prepare yourself to teach older adults and their families about these services.
4. Identify a situation in your personal life or clinical experience that requires caregiving assistance from a family member at least once weekly and address the following in relation to this situation:
   - What benefits (rewards) and stresses is the carer likely to experience?
   - Select two nursing outcomes and interventions from Table 27-6 that you could apply to a care plan to address the needs of this carer.

RESOURCES

For an extensive range of additional resources to enhance teaching and learning and to facilitate understanding of this chapter, please see the text's accompanying website located on thePoint at http://thepoint.lww.com.

Clinical tools

Hartford Institute for Geriatric Nursing, ConsultGeriRN.org: http://consultgerirn.org/resources

Try This® assessment series and *How to Try This* resources

General assessment series:

- *Try This*, issue 14: The Modified Caregiver Strain Index (CSI). Onega, L. (2013). *Best Practices in Nursing Care to Older Adults*.
- *How to Try This* (article): Helping those who help others: The Modified Caregiver Strain Index. Onega, L. (2008). *American Journal of Nursing, 108*(9), 62–69.
- *How to Try This* (video): *The Modified Caregiver Strain Index*.

Specialty practice series:

- *Try This*, SP2: Informal caregivers of older adults at home: Let's PREPARE! Borneman, T. (2011). *Best Practices in Nursing Care to Older Adults*.
- *Try This*, SP5: Assessment of spirituality in older adults: FICA Spiritual History Tool. Borneman, T. (2011). *Best Practices in Nursing Care to Older Adults*.

Search for:

- Topic-related resources from Visiting Nurse Service of New York (VNSNY).
- Topic-related resources from the Hospice and Palliative Nurses Association.

Evidence-based practice

Balas, M. C., Casey, C. M. & Happ, M. B. (2012). Comprehensive assessment and management of the critically ill. In M. Boltz, E. Capezuti, T. Fulmer & D. Zwicker (Eds), *Evidence-based geriatric nursing protocols for best practice* (4th ed., pp. 600–627). New York: Springer.

Coon, D. W. & Evans, B. E. (2009). Empirically based treatments for family caregiver distress: What works and where do we go from here? *Geriatric Nursing, 30*, 426–436.

Messecar, D. C. (2012). Family caregiving. In M. Boltz, E. Capezuti, T. Fulmer & D. Zwicker (Eds), *Evidence-based geriatric nursing protocols for best practice* (4th ed., pp. 469–499). New York: Springer.

Overcash, J. (2012). Cancer assessment and intervention strategies. In M. Boltz, E. Capezuti, T. Fulmer & D. Zwicker (Eds), *Evidence-based geriatric nursing protocols for best practice* (4th ed., pp. 658–669). New York: Springer.

Schipper, J. E., Coviello, J. & Chyun, D. A. (2012). Fluid overload: Identifying and managing heart failure patients at risk for hospital readmission. In M. Boltz, E. Capezuti, T. Fulmer & D. Zwicker (Eds). *Evidence-based geriatric nursing protocols for best practice* (4th ed., pp. 628–657). New York: Springer.

Health education

Cancer Council: www.cancer.org.au

Cancer Nurses Society of Australia: www.cnsa.org.au

Cancer Society of New Zealand: www.cancernz.org.nz/information/resources

CareSearch: Palliative Care Knowledge Network, multicultural resources: www.caresearch.com.au

Diabetes Australia: www.diabetesaustralia.com.au

Diabetes NSW: http://diabetesnsw.com.au

Diabetes New Zealand: www.diabetes.org.nz

Health Direct Australia, seniors' health: www.healthdirect.gov.au/seniors-health

New Zealand Palliative Care Strategy: www.health.govt.nz/publication/new-zealand-palliative-care-strategy

NZ Guidelines Group: www.nzgg.org.nz/practice-tools/diabetes

Palliative Care Australia: www.palliativecare.org.au
Parkinson's Australia: www.parkinsons.org.au
Parkinson's New Zealand: www.parkinsons.org.nz
Virtual Cancer Centre: www.myvmc.com/?s=cancer

REFERENCES

Australian Bureau of Statistics (ABS). (2008). *Health literacy Australia 2006*. Cat. no. 4233.0. Canberra: Author.

Australian Bureau of Statistics. (2012). *Disability, ageing and carers, Australia: Summary of findings*. Cat. no. 4430.0. Canberra: Author. Accessed March 2015 at www.abs.gov.au/ausstats/abs@.nsf/Lookup/4430.0Chapter4002012.

Australian Bureau of Statistics (ABS). (2013). Diabetes. In *Profiles of health, Australia, 2011–13*. Cat. no. 4338.0. Canberra: Author.

Australian Government Department of Health (AGDH). (2014). Palliative care. Viewed March 2015 at www.health.gov.au/palliativecare.

Australian Indigenous Health*InfoNet*. (2007). Review of diabetes among Indigenous peoples. Accessed March 2015 at www.healthinfonet.ecu.edu.au/chronic-conditions/diabetes/reviews/our-review.

Australian Institute of Health and Welfare. (2014). *Australia's health 2014*. Australia's health series no. 14. Cat. no. AUS 178. Canberra: Author.

Bagshaw, S. M. & McDermid, R. C. (2013). The role of frailty in outcomes from critical illness. *Current Opinions in Critical Care, 19*(5), 496–503.

bestpractice[NZ] Decision Support. (2014). The management of Parkinson's disease: Which treatments to start and when? *Best Practice Journal, 58*, 26–39. Accessed March 2015 at www.bpac.org.nz/BPJ/2014/February/parkinsons.aspx.

Beverly, E. A., Fitzgerald, S., Sitnikov, L. et al. (2013). Do older adults aged 60–75 years benefit from diabetes behavioral interventions? *Diabetes Care, 36*(6), 1501–1506.

Bremer, J. P., Jauch-Chara, K., Hallschmid, M. et al. (2009). Hypoglycemia unawareness in older compared with middle aged patients with type 2 diabetes. *Diabetes Care, 32*(8), 1513–1517.

Brown, M. A., Sampson, E. L., Jones, L., et al. (2013). Prognostic indicators of 6-month mortality in elderly people with advanced dementia: A systematic review. *Palliative Medicine, 27*(5), 389–400.

Cameron, M. E. (2010). Yoga. In M. Snyder & R. Lindquist (Eds), *Complementary & alternative therapies in nursing* (6th ed., pp. 123–133). New York: Springer.

Canning, D., Yates, P. & Rosenberg, J. P. (2005). Competency Standards for Specialist Palliative Care Nursing Practice. Brisbane: Queensland University of Technology.

CareSearch. (2014). Non-malignant/end stage disease. Viewed March 2015 at www.caresearch.com.au/caresearch/tabid/1575/Default.aspx.

Castro, S., O'Toole, M., Brownson, C., Plessel, K. & Schauben, L. (2009). A diabetes self-management program designed for urban American Indians. *Preventing Chronic Disease, 6*(4), 1–5.

Cataldo, J. K., Paul, S., Cooper, C. et al. (2013). Differences in the symptom experience of older versus younger oncology outpatients: A cross-sectional study. *BMC Cancer, 13*(6). Available March 2015 at www.biomedcentral.com/1471-2407/13/6.

Chiu, C.-J. & Wray, L. A. (2010). Factors predicting glycemic control in middle-aged and older adults with type 2 diabetes. *Preventing Chronic Disease, 7*(1), 1–5.

Clough-Gorr, K. M., Noti, L., Brauchli, P. et al. (2013). The SAKK cancer-specific geriatric assessment (C-SGA): A pilot study of a brief tool for clinical decision-making in older cancer patients. *BMC Medical Informatics & Decision Making, 13*, 93.

Comart, J., Mahler, A., Schrieber, R. et al. (2013). Palliative care for long-term care residents: Effect on clinical outcomes. *Gerontologist, 53*(5), 874–880.

Coon, D. W. & Evans, B. (2009). Empirically based treatments for family carer distress: What works and where do we go from here? *Geriatric Nursing, 30*(6), 426–436.

De Moor, J. S., Mariotto, A. B., Parry, C. et al. (2013). Cancer survivors in the United States: Prevalence across survivorship trajectory and implications for care. *Cancer Epidemiology, Biomarkers & Prevention, 22*, 561–570.

Deloitte Access Economics. (2011). Living with Parkinson's Disease—Update. Report prepared for Parkinson's Australia. Accessed March 2015 via www.deloitteaccesseconomics.com.au/publications+and+reports/browse+reports.

Drubbel, I., de Wit, N. J., Bleijenberg, N. et al. (2013). Predictions of adverse health outcomes in older people using a frailty index based on routine primary care data. *Journals of Gerontology: Biological Sciences and Medical Sciences, 68*(5), 301–308.

Eckstrom, E., Feeny, D. H., Walter, L. C. et al. (2013). Individualizing cancer screening in older adults: A narrative review and framework for future research. *Journal of General Internal Medicine, 28*(2), 292–298.

Elliott, A. F., Burgio, L. D. & DeCoster, J. (2010). Enhancing carer health: Findings from the resources for enhancing Alzheimer's Carer Health II Intervention. *Journal of the American Geriatrics Society, 58*(1), 30–37.

Ferraro. K. F. (2006). Health and aging. In R. H. Binstock & L. K. Georde (Eds), *Handbook of aging and the social sciences* (6th ed., pp. 238–256). San Diego, CA: Academic Press

Fitzgerald, M. & Langevin, M. (2010). Imagery. In M. Snyder & R. Lindquist (Eds), *Complementary & alternative therapies in nursing* (6th ed., pp. 663–689) New York: Springer

Freyer, G., Tew, W. P. & Moore, K. N. (2013). Treatment and trials: Ovarian cancer in older women. *American Society of Clinical Oncology Educational Books, 2013*, 227–235. Available March 2015 at http://meetinglibrary.asco.org/content/229-132.

Fried, L. P., Tangen, C. E., Walston, J. et al. (2001). Frailty in older adults: Evidence for a phenotype. *Journals of Gerontology: Biological Sciences and Medical Sciences, 56*(3), M146–M156.

Heath, H. & Phair, L. (2009). The concept of frailty and its significance in the consequences of care or neglect for older people: An analysis. *International Journal of Older People Nursing, 4*(2), 120–131.

Hospice New Zealand. (2012). Standards for palliative care: Quality review programme and guide. Available March 2015 via www.hospice.org.nz.

International Diabetes Federation. (2013). IDF global guideline for managing older people with type 2 diabetes. Accessed March 2015 via www.idf.org/guidelines.

Kane, R. L., Shamliyan, T., Talley, K. et al. (2012). The association between geriatric syndromes and survival. *Journal of the American Geriatrics Society, 60*(5), 896–906.

Kirkman, M. S., Briscoe, V. J., Clark, N., Florez, H. et al. (2012). Diabetes in older adults: A consensus report. *Journal of the American Geriatrics Society, 60*(12), 2342–2356.

Koller, K. & Rockwood, K. (2013). Frailty in older adults: Implications for end-of-life care. *Cleveland Clinic Journal of Medicine, 80*(3), 168–174.

Kreitzer, M. J. & Reilly-Spong, M. (2010). Meditation. In M. Snyder & R. Lindquist (Eds), *Complementary & alternative therapies in nursing* (6th ed., pp. 149–167). New York: Springer.

Lipska, K. J., Ross, J. S., Wang, Y. et al. (2014). National trends in US hospital admissions for hyperglycemia and hypoglycemia among Medicare beneficiaries, 1999 to 2011. *JAMA Internal Medicine, 174*(7), 1116–1124.

Long, C. O. (2009). Palliative care for advanced dementia. *Journal of Gerontological Nursing, 35*(11), 19–25.

Maciasz, R. M., Arnold, R. M., Chu, E. et al. (2013). Does it matter what you call it: A randomized trial of language used to describe palliative care services. *Supportive Care for Cancer, 21*(12), 3411–3419.

Mahler, A. (2010). The clinical nurse specialist role in developing a geropalliative model of care. *Clinical Nurse Specialist, 24*(1), 18–23.

Māori Health. (2011). Diabetes (50+ years). *Health of older Māori chart book*. Accessed March 2015 via www.health.govt.nz/nz-health-statistics.

Martire, L. M., Schultz, R., Reynolds, C. F. III., Karp, J. F., Gildengers, A. G. & Whyte, E. M. (2010). Treatment of late-life depression alleviates carer burden. *Journal of the American Geriatrics Society, 58*(1), 23–29.

Mayor, M. S., Ribeiro, O. & Paul, C. (2009). Satisfaction in dementia and stroke carers: A comparative study. *Rev Latino-Americana de Enfermagem, 17*(5), 620–624.

Medical Council of New Zealand. (2010). Best outcomes for Pacific Peoples: Practice implications. Accessed March 2015 via www.mcnz.org.nz.

Melchior, M. A., Seff, L. R., Bastida, E. et al. (2013). Intermediate outcomes of a Chronic Disease Self-Management Program for Spanish-Speaking Older Adults in South Florida, 2008–2010. *Preventing Chronic Disease, 10*. doi:http://dx.doi.org/10.5888/pcd10.130016.

Messecar, D. C. (2012). Family caregiving. In M. Boltz, E. Capezuti, T. Fulmer & D. Zwicker (Eds), *Evidence-based geriatric nursing protocols for best practice* (4th ed., pp. 469–499). New York: Springer.

Miyasaki, J. M. (2013). Palliative care in Parkinson's disease. *Current Neurology and Neuroscience Reports, 13*(8), 367–372.

Molina-Garrido, M. J., Guillen-Ponce, C., Castellano, C. S. et al. (2014). Tools for decision-making in older cancer patients: Role of the comprehensive geriatric assessment. *Anti-Cancer Agents in Medicinal Chemistry, 14*(5), 651–656.

Morley, J. E., Vellas, B., van Kan, G. A. et al. (2013). Frailty consensus: A call to action. *Journal of the American Medical Directors Association, 14*(6), 392–397.

National Health and Medical Research Council (NHMRC). (2011a). Living well with an advanced chronic or terminal condition: How ethics helps. Viewed March 2015 via www.nhmrc.gov.au/guidelines-publications/rec31.

National Health and Medical Research Council (NHMRC). (2011b). National evidence-based guideline for the prevention, identification and management of foot complications in diabetes. Adelaide: Baker IDI Heart & Diabetes Institute. Available March 2015 via www.nhmrc.gov.au/guidelines-publications/di21.

Nelson, J. E., Puntillo, K. A., Pronovost, P. J., Walker, A. S., McAdam, J. L., Ilaoa, D. & Penrod, J. (2010). In their own words: Patients and families define high-quality palliative care in the intensive care unit. *Critical Care Medicine, 38*(3), 808–816.

New Zealand Ministry of Health (NZMOH). (2001). New Zealand Palliative Care Strategy. Available March 2015 via www.health.govt.nz.

New Zealand Ministry of Health. (2007). Diabetes surveillance: Population-based estimates and projections for New Zealand, 2001–2011. *Public Health Intelligence Occasional Bulletin*, no. 46. Available March 2015 via www.health.govt.nz.

New Zealand Ministry of Health. (2013). New Zealand Health Survey: Annual update of key findings 2012/13. Accessed March 2015 via www.health.govt.nz.

New Zealand Ministry of Health. (2014). New Zealand Burden of Diseases, Injuries and Risk Factors Study, 2006–2016. Accessed March 2015 via www.health.govt.nz.

Nielsen-Bohlman, L., Panzer, A. M., Kindig, D. A. (2004). *Health literacy: A prescription to end confusion*. Washington DC: Institute of Medicine.

Overcash, J. (2012). Cancer assessment and intervention strategies. In M. Boltz, E. Capezuti, T. Fulmer & D. Zwicker (Eds), *Evidence-based practice protocols for best practice* (4th ed., pp. 658–669). New York: Springer.

Palliative Care Nurses New Zealand. (2014). A national professional development framework for palliative care nursing practice in Aotearoa New Zealand. Wellington: Ministry of Health. Accessed March 2015 at www.health.govt.nz/publication/national-professional-development-framework-palliative-care-nursing-aotearoa-new-zealand.

Palliative Care Subcommittee and New Zealand Cancer Treatment Working Party (2007). New Zealand palliative care: A working definition. Accessed March 2015 at www.health.govt.nz/system/files/documents/publications/nz-palliative-care-definition-oct07.pdf.

Parikh, R. B., Kirch, R. A., Smith, T. J. et al. (2013). Early specialty palliative care: Translating data in oncology into practice. *New England Journal of Medicine, 369*(24), 2347–2351.

Pascucci, M. A., Chu, N. & Leasure, A. R. (2012). Health promotion for the oldest of old people. *Nursing Older People, 24*(3), 22–28.

Passmore, M. J. (2013). Neuropsychiatric symptoms of dementia: Consent, quality of life, and dignity. *BioMed Research International*. Article ID 230134. doi: http://dx.doi.org/10.1155/2013/230134.

Pastor, D. K. & Moore, G. (2013). Uncertainties of the heart: Palliative care and adult heart failure. *Home Healthcare Nurse, 31*(1), 29–36.

Petrovic, M., van der Cammen, T. & Onder, G. (2012). Adverse drug reactions in older people: Detection and prevention. *Drugs & Aging, 29*(6), 453–462.

Posma, E. R., van Weert, J. C. M., Jansen, J. & Bensing, J. M. (2009). Older cancer patients' information and support needs surrounding treatment: An evaluation through the eyes of patients, relatives and professionals. *BioMed Central Nursing, 8*(1).

Poulin, M. J., Brown, S. L., Ubel, P. A., Smith, D. M., Jankovic, A. & Langa, K. M. (2010). Does a helping hand mean a heavy heart? Helping behavior and well-being among spouse carers. *Psychology and Aging, 25*(1), 108–117.

Resnick, B. (2012). Differentiating programs versus philosophies of care: Palliative care and hospice care are not equal. *Geriatric Nursing, 33*(6), 427–429.

Ripsin, C. M., Kang, H. & Urban, R. J. (2009). Management of blood glucose in type 2 diabetes mellitus. *American Family Physician, 79*(1), 29–36.

Rodriquez-Manas, L., Feart, C., Mann, G. et al. (2013). Searching for an operational definition of frailty: A Delphi Method based consensus statement. *Journals of Gerontology: Biological Sciences and Medical Sciences, 68*(1), 62–67.

Royal Australian College of General Practitioners (RACGP) and Diabetes Australia. (2014). General practice management of type 2 diabetes, 2014–15. Melbourne: Authors.

Shamliyan, T., Talley, K. M., Ramakrishnan, R. et al. (2013). Association of frailty with survival: A systematic literature review. *Ageing Research Review, 12*(2), 719–736.

Statistics New Zealand and Ministry of Pacific Island Affairs (2011). *Health and Pacific peoples in New Zealand*. Wellington: Statistics New Zealand and Ministry of Pacific Island Affairs. Available March 2015 via www.stats.govt.nz.

Tamayo, G. J., Broxson, A., Munsell, M. & Cohen, M. Z. (2010). Caring for the carer. *Oncology Nursing Forum, 37*(1), E50–E57.

Thoonsen, B., Engels, Y., Rijswijk, E. et al. (2012). Early identification of palliative care patients in general practice. *British Journal of General Practice, 62*(602), e625–e631

Thornton, M. & Travis, S. S. (2003). Analysis of the reliability of the Modified Caregiver Strain Index. *Journals of Gerontology: Psychological Sciences and Social Sciences 58*(2), S129.

Tshiananga, J. K., Kocher, S., Weber, C. et al. (2012). The effect of nurse-led diabetes self-management education on glycosylated hemoglobin and cardiovascular risk factors: A meta-analysis. *Diabetes Education, 38*(1), 108–123.

Wakefield, B. J., Boren, S. A., Groves, P. S. et al. (2013). Heart failure care management programs: A review of study interventions and meta-analysis of outcomes. *Journal of Cardiovascular Nursing, 28*(1), 8–19.

Wang, S.-Y., Shamliyan, T. A., Talley, K. et al. (2013). Not just specific disease: Systematic review of the association of geriatric syndromes with hospitalization or nursing home admission. *Archives of Gerontology and Geriatrics 57*, 16–26.

Wierenga, P. C., Buurman, B. M., Parlevliet, J. L. et al. (2012). Association between acute geriatric syndromes and medication-related hospital admissions. *Drugs & Aging 29*(8), 691–699.

Winter, K. H., Bouldin, E. D. & Andresen, E. M. (2010). Lack of choice in caregiving decision and carer risk of stress, North Carolina, 2005. *Preventing Chronic Disease, 7*(2) 1–5.

World Health Organization (WHO). (2002). *National cancer control programmes: Policies and managerial guidelines* (2nd ed.). New York: World Health Organization.

World Health Organization (WHO). (2004). Better palliative care for older people. Prepared by Davies, E. & Higginson I. J. for the World Health Organization, Geneva. Retrieved March 2015 from www.euro.who.int/document/e82933.pdf.

World Health Organization (WHO). (2014). *Global atlas of palliative care at the end of life*. Geneva: Author. Accessed March at www.thewhpca.org/resources/global-atlas-on-end-of-life-care.

Chapter 28

Caring for older adults experiencing pain

By Carol Miller and Sharyn Hunter

LEARNING OBJECTIVES

After reading this chapter, you should be able to:

1. Differentiate between types of pain: nociceptive, acute, persistent and cancer pain.
2. Discuss unique aspects of pain in older adults, including prevalence, causes and complexities of assessment and management.
3. Examine and dispel commonly held myths and beliefs about pain in older adults.
4. Discuss cultural aspects of pain.
5. Apply evidence-based guidelines for assessment and management of pain in older adults who are cognitively impaired.
6. Describe principles of analgesic medication use in older adults.
7. Discuss evidence-based, non-pharmacological and other additional nursing interventions effective in managing pain in older adults.

KEY POINTS

acute pain
addiction
adjuvant analgesics
cancer pain
dependence
neuropathic pain
nociception
non-opioid analgesics
opioid analgesics
pain
pain intensity
persistent pain
tolerance
WHO pain relief ladder

Pain is a biopsychosocial phenomenon with multiple dimensions, including sensory, cognitive, emotional, developmental, behavioural, spiritual and cultural influences. Pain is very common among older adults, and nursing assessment and management is further complicated by additional factors such as age-related changes, impaired mental status and other concomitant conditions. In addition, the knowledge and attitudes of care providers can enhance or interfere with accurate assessment and effective management of pain, particularly with regard to older adults. This chapter provides an overview of pain and discusses the assessment and management of pain, emphasising aspects that are most pertinent to the care of older adults.

DEFINITIONS AND TYPES OF PAIN

Pain is an unpleasant sensory and subjective experience associated with actual or potential injury. The subjective quality of pain is defined as whatever the experiencing person says it is, existing whenever she or he says it does (McCaffery, 1968). Objectively, pain occurs within the context of a physiological process that is a response to a noxious stimulus. Because pain is a very complex phenomenon, there are many ways of classifying it. The following sections describe commonly used classifications according to underlying mechanisms (i.e. nociceptive and neuropathic) and duration (i.e. acute and persistent). Cancer pain is also described because of its unique characteristics and its common occurrence in older adults.

Nociceptive and neuropathic pain

Nociception, which is the physiological process that leads to the perception of a noxious stimulus as being painful, involves four processes: transduction, transmission, perception and modulation (Figure 28-1). *Transduction* involves the activation of primary nociceptive fibres (i.e. the primary afferent neurons throughout the body) when tissue damage occurs from any of the following sources: mechanical (e.g. surgery, trauma, tumour), thermal (e.g. burn, extreme cold), or chemical (e.g. toxin, chemotherapy). Excitatory compounds are released through local tissues, immune cells or nerve endings and include serotonin, bradykinin, histamine, substance P and prostaglandins. These physiological processes set off an action potential, which is the second phase of nociception, called *transmission*. During transmission, the afferent information passes through the dorsal root ganglia to the spinal cord, where it continues to pass through multiple ascending pathways to the brainstem. The effectiveness of analgesic medications is based on their ability to modify specific aspects of transduction and transmission.

Perception, the third process of nociception, is the point at which pain becomes a conscious experience. Sensory, emotional and cognitive areas of the brain are involved in the perception of pain. The effectiveness of cognitive-behavioural therapies and other body–mind modalities is associated with evidence that brain processes can strongly influence pain perception. The final process of nociception, *modulation*, refers to the body's responses to painful stimuli, which involves both the central and peripheral nervous systems and many neurochemicals, including serotonin, noradrenaline and endogenous opioids. Effectiveness of

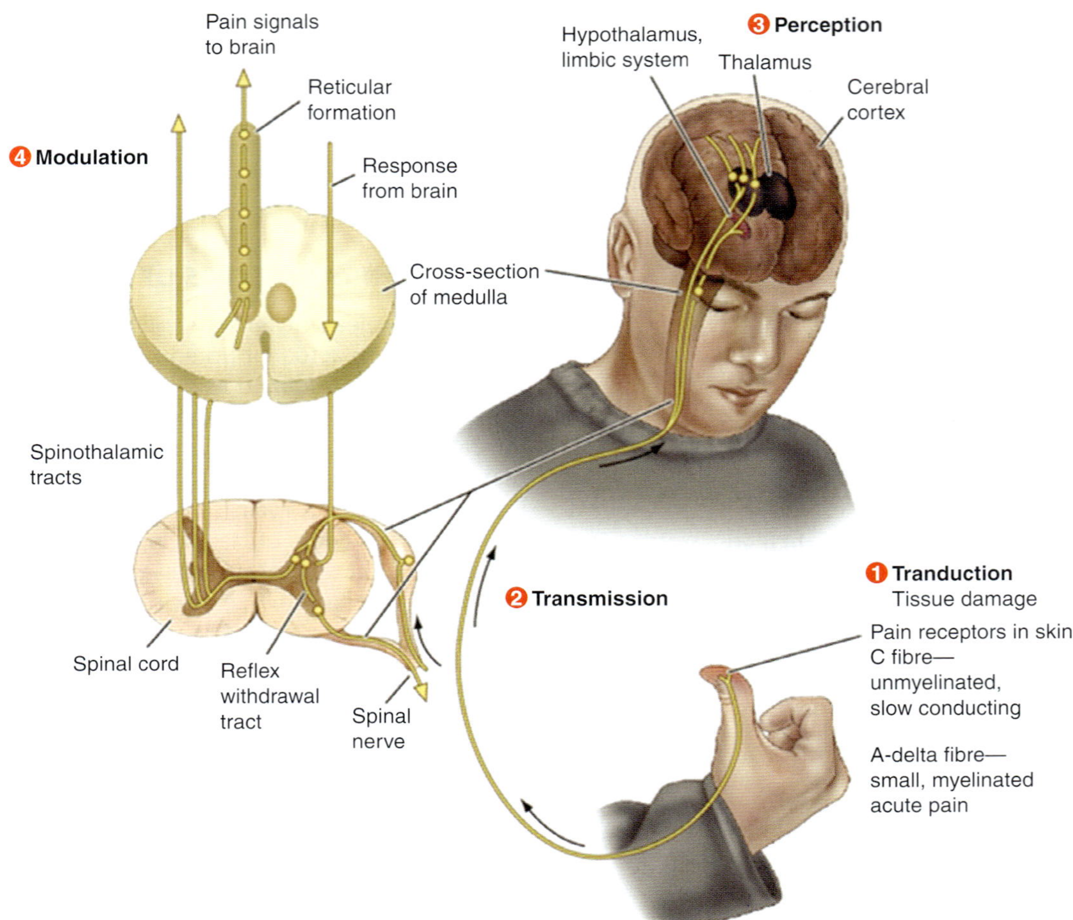

FIGURE 28-1 Processes involved in the physiology of pain. (McKenna, L. & Lim, A. G. [2014]. *McKenna's pharmacology for nursing and health professionals* [2nd ed.]. Sydney: Lippincott, Williams & Wilkins.)

antidepressants for relief of pain is associated with their effects on serotonin and noradrenaline.

Neuropathic pain originates from an abnormal processing of sensory stimuli by the central or peripheral nervous system (i.e. damage to or dysfunction that affects any part of the central or autonomic nervous systems). In contrast to nociceptive pain, which is triggered by an immediate noxious stimulus, neuropathic pain can occur in the absence of immediate tissue damage or inflammation. Also in contrast to nociceptive pain, which serves to warn and protect from further injury, neuropathic pain serves no useful purpose (Pasero & Portenoy, 2011).

Neuropathic pain involves complex responses of many peripheral and central mechanisms. Peripheral mechanisms are activated by actual or potential tissue damage due to mechanical, thermal or chemical stimuli, as described in the section on nociceptive pain. In addition, viruses, infections, ischaemia, metabolic disease (e.g. diabetes), nutritional deficiencies and neurological diseases can activate peripheral pain mechanisms. Abnormalities in processing information during transduction and transmission combine with dysfunctions in central mechanisms to cause sensitisation, which leads to increasingly stronger responses in the pain transmission pathway. When this occurs, pain is experienced with little or no stimulus. Table 28-1 compares characteristics of nociceptive and neuropathic pain and lists examples of types.

Acute and persistent pain

Although the term *persistent pain* (also called *chronic pain*) describes the length of time the pain is experienced, there is increasing evidence that this type of pain has additional unique characteristics. Whereas acute pain has a sudden onset and is linked to a specific event, injury or illness, persistent pain develops when the central nervous system continues to process pain signals as though new injuries were occurring. Researchers are focusing on identifying the many factors that affect the transition from acute to persistent pain, which is sometimes referred to as "pain chronification". Risk factors currently under investigation include genetic predisposition, enhanced pain perception, presence of pre-existing pain, and psychological factors (e.g. distress, catastrophising) (Pergolizzi, Raffa & Taylor, 2012).

TABLE 28.1 Comparison of nociceptive and neuropathic pain

Characteristic	Nociceptive pain	Neuropathic pain
Underlying mechanism	*Normal* processing of noxious stimuli in response to actual or potential tissue injury or inflammation	*Abnormal* processing of sensory input sustained by damage to or dysfunction of the nervous system
Physiological processes	Transduction, transmission, perception, modulation	Sensitisation due to abnormal peripheral and central processing of noxious stimuli
Subtypes and examples according to origin	Somatic: skin, bone, joint, connective tissue, mucous membranes, subcutaneous tissue (e.g. burn, bruise, arthritis, tendonitis, fibromyalgia, myofascial pain) Visceral: gastrointestinal, urinary tract or other internal organs due to blockage, pressure or infection (e.g. tumours, cholecystitis, kidney stones)	Central pain from injury to or dysfunction of the central nervous system (e.g. post-stroke pain, multiple sclerosis, spinal cord injury) Peripheral mononeuropathy results in pain along nerve pathway (e.g. nerve root compression or trigeminal neuralgia) Peripheral polyneuropathy results in pain along the distribution of many peripheral nerves (e.g. trigeminal neuropathy, postherpetic neuralgia, phantom limb, diabetic neuropathy, chronic postsurgical pain)
Common descriptors	Somatic: aching, deep, throbbing, dull, sharp, tender, gnawing, pressure Visceral: cramping, squeezing, shooting, pressure	Burning, shooting, knife-like, tingling, pins and needles
Sensory symptoms	Not common except hypersensitivity in immediate area of injury	Numbness, tingling, pricking, hypersensitive to touch
Distribution	Proximal radiation common	Distal radiation common
Motor symptoms	Weakness due to pain experience	Neurologically associated weakness if motor nerves are involved

Acute pain is sharp, immediate pain from an injury to tissue, and it also can be triggered by physiological malfunction or severe illness. It is the normal, predictable physiological response to an adverse chemical, thermal or mechanical stimulus and its purpose is to lead to resolution of the causative agent or event. Common causes of acute pain include burns, trauma, medical or surgical procedures, or chronic medical problems such as cancer or postherpetic neuralgia. Acute pain is generally time limited and responds effectively to anti-inflammatory and opioid medications as well as other approaches.

Persistent pain lasts longer than 3 to 6 months or beyond the expected time of healing from the initial causative event. National data indicate that prevalence of persistent pain has been steadily increasing among all demographic groups, with people age 65 and over consistently reporting the highest rates (Institute of Medicine [IOM], 2011). Physiologically, the perception of persistent pain involves many neurotransmitters and receptors involved with peripheral sensitisation, central sensitisation and modulation at many sites of the autonomic and central nervous system. Although the phenomenon is not well understood, there is increasing evidence that the pathophysiology of persistent pain begins with an acute nociceptive process that at some point combines with neuropathic characteristics (Taverner, Closs & Briggs, 2014). Because this is a complex pathophysiological process, effective management includes a pharmacological approach with drugs that target several pain pathways in combination with non-pharmacological interventions.

Research has led to the following conclusions about persistent pain, which have been summarised by the Institute of Medicine (2011):

- Persistent pain represents a pathological transition from acute pain.
- Causes of persistent pain include underlying pathological process, injury, medical treatment, surgical interventions, inflammation, and neuropathic pain.
- The cause of persistent pain is not always identifiable.
- In most cases, persistent pain should be considered a disease in its own right.
- Persistent pain can affect every aspect of a person's life.
- The management of persistent pain requires biopsychosocial approach that addresses physiological, psychological, social, emotional and spiritual aspects of the person.

Recent studies have focused on the complex mechanisms involved with the development of persistent postsurgical pain, finding that its incidence can be reduced with the use of aggressive and early analgesic therapy (Deumens, Steyaert, Forget et al. 2013; Van de Ven & John Hsai, 2012). This is particularly pertinent to care of older adults recovering from surgical procedures in acute care settings, nursing facilities, and independent settings. Similarly, studies of postherpetic neuralgia emphasise early treatment with antiviral medication (McGreevy, Bottros & Raja, 2011).

Cancer pain

Cancer pain is a complex phenomenon caused by the cancer itself, concomitant disease or adverse effects of treatments.

Cancer pain can be acute, persistent, nociceptive, neuropathic or—as is most often the case—a combination of these types. Pain is caused directly by the cancer and indirectly by effects of the cancer, such as compression due to tumour infiltration and neuropathy from chemotherapy. Studies have documented high prevalence rates of cancer pain as in the following examples (IOM, 2011):

- Multiple myeloma (100%)
- Metastatic or advanced-stage disease (64%)
- During anticancer treatment (59%)
- Breast cancer (58%)
- Lung cancer (56%), colorectal cancer (41%).

Because half of all cancers occur in people age 65 or older, addressing cancer pain is particularly pertinent when caring for older adults.

UNIQUE ASPECTS OF PAIN IN OLDER ADULTS

Although many aspects of pain differ in older adults, research on pain in older adults lags behind other areas of pain research. There is widespread agreement, however, that pain is underdetected and poorly managed among older adults (Horgas, Yoon & Grall, 2012). Nursing assessment and management of pain is challenging not only because of age-related changes but also because of coexisting conditions, such as dementia, delirium, surgery, or acute or chronic illness, that affect many—if not most—older adults. Additional complicating factors include lack of evidence-based information, misconceptions and misinformation, and the presence of several types of pain (e.g. neuropathic pain plus acute pain, pain at more than one site, acute pain superimposed on persistent pain, cancer pain combined with persistent pain). This section provides an overview of unique aspects of pain in older adults, and the assessment and interventions sections address specific aspects of pain in older adults who are cognitively impaired as a result of delirium or dementia.

Age-related changes

Although many processes involved with pain perception can be altered by age-related changes in neurochemical, neuroanatomical, and neurophysiological mechanisms, little is known about the functional consequences of these changes in older adults. Whereas some studies indicate that older adults have a diminished response to noxious stimuli, numerous studies also find that they are more vulnerable to experiencing severe or persistent pain, and have a diminished ability to tolerate severe pain (IOM, 2011).

Age-related changes in pharmacokinetics and pharmacodynamics, as discussed in Chapter 8, can affect analgesic medications in older adults and increase the risk for adverse effects. Even this aspect, however, is variable, because studies have found no age-related difference in appropriate doses of postoperative morphine, particularly when doses were normalised according to body weight (Pasero & McCaffery, 2011a). A guiding principle with regard to pain in older adults is to consider the person's age as one of the many variables that can influence assessment and management.

Prevalence and causes

Pain is a widespread problem for older adults. Some studies have reported that 25% to 50% of community-dwelling older adults and 50% to 80% of adults in long-term residential care facilities experience pain (Dumas & Ramadurai, 2009; Planton & Edlund, 2010; National Pain Summit Initiative, 2010). In addition, is has been reported 80% to 85% older adults experience at some point in time a significant health problem that predisposes them to pain (Rustoen et al., 2005; Tsai & Means, 2005). Older adults have higher rates of hospital admissions and medical procedures, many of which cause acute pain (National Pain Summit Initiative, 2010). Although acute pain is a predictable consequence of surgical procedures, approximately 50% of surgical inpatients report inadequate pain relief, resulting in unnecessary moderate-to-severe pain (Polomano et al., 2008). People older than 65 years have an increased rate of chronic conditions that are associated with persistent pain and pain-associated declining physical function. Common causes of persistent pain in older adults include arthritis, osteoporosis, post-herpetic neuralgia and diabetic peripheral neuropathy. Further information about pain and older adults from Australia and New Zealand is contained in Box 28-1.

Barriers to pain management

Despite the progress in understanding the physiology of pain and the advances in its assessment and treatment

BOX 28-1
Snapshot of pain in older adults in Australia and New Zealand

Australia

- Prevalence of pain rises to one in three people over the age of 65
- Persistent pain is Australia's third most-costly health condition after cardiovascular diseases and musculoskeletal conditions (also associated with persistent pain)
- In long-term residential care, 92% of people are taking at least one analgesic medication daily, and 80% of people list pain as a problem

New Zealand

- About 25% to 30% of older adults experience persistent pain
- About 50% of older women and 35% older men have arthritis

Source: Pain Australia. (2014). Why we need the National Pain Strategy. Accessed March 2015 via www.painaustralia.org.au; New Zealand Ministry of Health. (2012). *The health of New Zealand adults 2011/12: Key findings of the New Zealand Health Survey*. Wellington: Author.

TABLE 28-2 Barriers to effective pain management

Source of the barrier	Problems contributing to the barrier	Possible solutions to overcoming the barrier
Patients and families	• Attitude that pain cannot be effectively managed and is a normal part of ageing • Family burnout (families are often involved in educating, goal setting and primary caregiving) • Belief that pain is an atonement for past actions that must be endured • Belief that pain is inevitable • Belief that "complaining" equals "burden", or results in retribution • Belief that healthcare providers are "always right"; self-advocacy is not appropriate • Belief that morphine is used only at the end of life • Fear of addiction to medication • Stigma of opiate use • Side effects, which may be difficult to manage or impossible to treat • Fear of the underlying meaning of the pain (e.g. that it indicates worsening of the disease process)	• Provide education about the treatments for side effects • Explain the mechanism of action of morphine and its appropriate use for pain management • Explain the differences between "addiction" and "tolerance" • Present nonpharmacological alternatives: • Physical therapy • Massage • Body/energy work • Acupuncture • Chiropractic or naturopathic care • Behavioural or mental health therapies • Biofeedback • Pilates, yoga
Healthcare providers	• Belief that older adults have a higher pain tolerance • Belief that patients with dementia do not experience pain • Belief that older adults cannot tolerate potent opioid analgesic medication • Fear of being investigated for excessive prescribing of opioids • Fear of the consequences of hospital policies for aggressive pain treatment • Lack of resources in rural/outlying areas • Insufficient communication between members of the healthcare team • Inadequate knowledge about pain and how best to manage it	• Complete continuing education in pain management • Attend educational seminars provided to healthcare workers by hospitals on prescription regulations with strategies for providing safe, structured pain management • Participate in a pain management clinic or team for referral of complex pain management cases
Healthcare system/institution	• Cultural and political climate resistant to change in the standards of care • Systems do not encourage a multidisciplinary approach to pain management • Lack of a shared language among disciplines for communicating about pain • Lack of motivation to improve pain management standards (belief that the problem is already being adequately addressed) • Lack of healthcare provider accountability for effective pain relief	• Encourage institutions to: • Identify key players among upper management and clinicians to include in discussions for change to standards of care • Select a system-wide pain rating system, using clear, concise terminology for routine pain assessment and documentation • Offer education from a policy perspective on the implications of unrelieved pain (e.g. increased length of stay and healthcare costs) • Implement measures to hold individual providers responsible for appropriate pain assessment and treatment

Source: Shillam, C. (2005). Caring for older adults who are experiencing pain. In Miller, C. (Ed.), *Nursing for wellness in older adults* (6th ed.). Philadelphia, PA: Lippincott Williams & Wilkins. Copyright. Used with permission; National Pain Summit Initiative. (2010). National Pain Strategy: Pain management for all Australians. Accessed March 2015 via www.painaustralia.org.au.

there are many barriers nationwide to the appropriate recognition and management of pain (National Pain Summit Initiative 2010). These obstacles exist at many levels, from healthcare systems and providers, to older adults and family members. Nurses need to recognise these barriers so they can not only assess and manage pain but also advocate for the needs of the older person. Table 28-2 lists some of the barriers to pain management, along with problems and possible solutions.

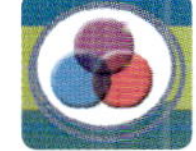

FUNCTIONAL CONSEQUENCES OF PAIN IN OLDER ADULTS

Pain is associated with numerous immediate and long-term consequences, and older adults are particularly vulnerable because pain is often superimposed on other undesirable conditions. An important functional consequence of acute pain, especially if it is undertreated, is the increased risk of developing persistent pain. Additional functional consequences commonly experienced by older adults include the following:

- Diminished physical function to the point of disability
- Psychosocial effects: fatigue, anxiety, depression
- Increased risk for falls
- Sleep disturbances
- Weight loss
- Increased dependency
- Decreased quality of life
- Social isolation and negative effects on relationships.

One study of community-living older adults identified the following functional consequences associated with pain: walking (38%), general activity (23%), mood (19%), enjoyment of life (16%), sleeping (15%), concentration (10%), and relationships (8%) (Brown, Kirkpatrick, Swanson et al., 2011). Similarly, studies of long-term care residents found that pain had significant negative effects on both physical and psychological health, including mobility, activities of daily living, depression and life satisfaction (Tse, Wan & Vong, 2013). Studies also found that chronic pain is an independent risk factor for falls (Eggermont, Penninx, Jones et al., 2012). Overall, any degree of pain diminishes one's quality of life and causes suffering not only for the person who experiences pain but also for all those who live with and care about that person.

An essential aspect of optimal pain management is recognising the unique way in which each individual experiences pain. Pain is interpreted differently by each person and is influenced by many factors. Past pain experiences can influence one's current perception of pain by triggering "memories" in the pain pathways. In addition, age, sex, beliefs, values and culture can influence the meaning and interpretation of pain for each individual. Moreover, expectations of what the pain means and attitudes about the pain can affect the degree of tolerance. Box 28-2 lists specific factors that can worsen or improve pain for older adults.

BOX 28-2
Factors affecting the experience of pain

Factors that worsen pain

- Insomnia/fatigue
- Anxiety
- Fear
- Isolation
- Boredom
- Anger
- Sadness
- Depression

Factors that improve pain

- Non-pharmacological approaches
- Medications
- Sleep/rest
- Understanding/validation
- Companionship
- Diversional activity
- Reduction in anxiety
- Elevation of mood

Source: Shillam, C. (2005). Caring for older adults who are experiencing pain. In Miller, C. (Ed.), *Nursing for wellness in older adults* (6th ed.). Philadelphia, PA: Lippincott Williams & Wilkins. Copyright. Used with permission.

CULTURAL ASPECTS OF PAIN

Cultural factors can significantly influence the way people experience, express and manage their pain, as illustrated by the examples and associated nursing implications in Cultural considerations 28-1. As with all aspects of culturally appropriate care, it is imperative to be aware of different expressions of pain commonly used by cultural groups, while at the same time avoiding stereotypes and basing care on the characteristics of each person as an individual.

It also is important to recognise disparities and diversities in pain prevalence and management, as in the following examples, which are particularly relevant to care of older adults:

- People age 65 or older receive inadequate doses—or even no doses—of analgesic medications for cancer or postoperative pain
- Racial and ethnic minorities are at high risk for receiving inadequate pain relief
- Women are more likely than men to be undertreated for pain
- People with low health literacy or low English proficiency, particularly recent immigrants, report greater pain
- Higher pain rates are strongly associated with lower income and level of education
- Across all groups, women consistently report a higher prevalence of persistent pain than men
- Fears, concerns and misconceptions about analgesic types and doses affect prescribing behaviours and therapeutic adherence by older adults and their carer/caregivers
- Older adults commonly fear negative consequences of analgesics. A common, but misconceived, fear is that of addiction. (IOM, 2011; Pasero & McCaffery, 2011b; Reid, Bennett, Chen et al., 2011)

A first step in assessing and managing pain in older adults is to recognise the actual and potential influences of personal biases, attitudes, experiences, misconceptions, and lack of information with regard to assessing and managing pain. For example, studies using vignettes found that assessment and management of pain by nurses is influenced by their personal experiences of pain and also by their perceived acceptability of the person's lifestyle (Pasero & McCaffery, 2011b). These factors can be addressed by self-assessment and by keeping up-to-date on evidence-based guidelines, as reviewed in the following sections.

CULTURAL CONSIDERATIONS 28-1
Expressions of pain associated with selected cultural groups

Group	Pain expression	Nursing implications
Asians	Pain is accepted as part of suffering and is to be endured. They are less likely to complain. Pain medication may be refused when initially offered and they may not want to bother the nurse for medication.	Nurses should ask about the pain levels and offer pain treatment again even if it has been initially refused. Asians require education about how to use a pain scale and the benefits of relieving pain and the contribution of pain relief to recovery.
Indigenous Australians	Might have a higher threshold for pain, especially the men. They are less likely to complain. There may be a fear of Western pain medicines (McGrath, 2006). They may not be able to communicate pain via standard pain tools (Palmer n.d.).	VAS may not be appropriate (Palmer n.d.). Consider using non-verbal pain assessment tools to assess pain. Indigenous Australians require support and information about pain medicines to minimise their fears (McGrath 2006).
Italians (Cores IT 2006)	Italians generally respond emotionally to pain. They express pain by groaning, moaning and crying. They also require sympathy and prefer not to be alone when in pain.	Nurses will acknowledge the person's pain and provide them with comfort and reassurance. If the person is very distressed about the pain and cannot be consoled by the nurse then it is appropriate to ask the person if they want their family to be present to provide support.
Japanese	Bearing pain is considered a virtue and a matter of family honor. *Itami* is the word for pain. Because addiction is a strong taboo, patients may be reluctant to accept pain medication.	Encourage the expression of pain as an important component of accurate assessment. Consider the use of regularly scheduled medications rather than a patient-controlled approach.
Jews	Verbalisation of pain is acceptable and common. Individuals want to know the cause of the pain which is just as important as obtaining relief.	Talk with patients about causes of pain.
Māori (Fennell, 2005)	Pain is perceived as a multidimensional experience and impacts physiological, psychological and spiritual dimensions.	Assessing and treating pain from a multidimensional perspective is appropriate.
Pacific people	They may not be confident to speak about their pain. They might answer health professional's questions with a simple yes or no. They may be reluctant to ask for analgesia, even when they desire it.	Initiate discussion about pain. Use open-ended questions as well as specific questions.
Somalians	May express pain as being one half of the body. Pain may be an expression of sadness or social and psychological discomfort.	Assess whether pain is an expression of physical or emotional symptoms.
Turks	Pain may be expressed through emotional outbursts or verbal complaints.	Recognise a wide range of pain expressions.

Source: Purnell, L. D. (2014) *Guide to culturally competent health care*. Philadelphia, PA: F.A. Davis.

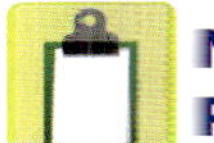

NURSING ASSESSMENT OF PAIN IN OLDER ADULTS

An accurate assessment of pain is based on recognising the unique way in which each individual experiences and expresses pain, as described in the classic definition of pain being whatever the person experiencing it says it is (McCaffery, 1968). Despite the simplicity of this classic definition, assessment of pain is very complex, even when people can describe their pain. When a person's level of cognition is altered—for example, by delirium or dementia—or when other communication barriers exist, assessment of pain is even more challenging (as discussed in the next section). Additional complications are associated with the common occurrence of concomitant conditions in older adults. For example, studies indicate that nurses in acute care settings often overlook issues related to pre-existing chronic pain (Siedlecki, Modic, Bernhofer et al., 2014).

Identifying common misconceptions

Despite the common occurrence of pain in older adults, it is a major mistake to view pain as a "normal part of ageing". This false belief is one of many misconceptions that can affect assessment and management of pain in older adults. Although the study of pain is an evolving and inexact

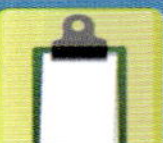

BOX 28-3
Misconceptions that can affect assessment and management of pain

Misconceptions commonly held by healthcare professionals

- Older adults have a high pain tolerance
- People with dementia do not experience pain
- People who are sleeping are not experiencing pain
- Chronic pain is not as painful as cancer pain or acute pain
- Changes in vital signs are an important indicator of pain
- Behavioural manifestations are more reliable than a persons' self-report
- Anxiety and depression directly cause pain
- Opioids should not be used for chronic pain

Misconceptions commonly held by older adults

- Desire to avoid a diagnosis that is serious, untreatable or life-threatening
- Fears related to addiction to or adverse effects of analgesics
- Concern about being perceived as a complainer
- Desire to maintain stoicism or avoid expression of feelings that may be perceived as a weakness
- Perceptions about pain being an atonement or punishment that should not be addressed by analgesics or other medical interventions
- Belief that morphine and strong analgesics are used only for terminal situations
- Stigma associated with prescription analgesics

science—with many unanswered questions—evidence-based information is available to dispel many of the long-held beliefs that can affect pain assessment and management (Pasero & McCaffery, 2011b). For example, a misconception that is commonly incorporated in pain assessments is that changes in vital signs are a good indicator of pain in people who cannot vocalise pain. Evidence-based guidelines emphasise that although changes in vital signs may occur concomitantly with acute pain, these indicators are not necessarily related to the presence or absence of pain (Wysong, 2014). Thus, an initial step in assessing pain is to identify misconceptions, such as the ones delineated in Box 28-3. An associated step is to keep up-to-date on evidence-based guidelines related to pain in older adults.

Collecting information about pain

An important guiding principle is to assess for pain during initial contact with the person, at frequent intervals, whenever the person's condition changes, and as an essential component of pain management interventions. During an initial contact and whenever pain is of recent onset, a comprehensive assessment, as described in this section, is imperative. A less comprehensive but comparative assessment needs to be conducted at appropriate intervals after analgesics and other pain management interventions have been administered, and whenever pain management interventions are changed. For example, in acute care settings, effectiveness of analgesics should be assessed 30 to 60 minutes after administration. A comparative reassessment typically includes questions about pain intensity and length of time the intervention was effective.

Self-report

Because a person's self-report about pain is considered the "gold standard" for pain assessment, begin by asking about the person's experience of pain. Allow older adults enough time to process the information and respond, and recognise that they may refer to pain by words such as *burning*, *discomfort*, *aching*, *soreness* or *hurting*. Another good communication strategy is to "contextualise the older adult's pain experience" by asking older adults to describe how chronic pain affects their daily life (Clarke, Anthony, Gray et al., 2012).

Assessment of pain components

Nurses assess the following components of the pain experience: intensity, person's responses, impact on ADLs, quality, location, physical findings, temporal characteristics, aggravating and alleviating factors, analgesic history, the person's goals, expectations, meaning of pain and attitudes and, finally, the effectiveness of analgesia. Box 28-4 can be used as a guide to assessing components of pain. Mnemonics can be useful when performing a baseline assessment of pain (see Box 28-5).

Intensity

Pain intensity is the state of being unpleasant, or the subjective determination of the strength, concentration or force of the symptom of pain. The subjective report of the intensity is the component most often addressed in pain assessment because it is the most easily identified indicator of improvement or worsening. Intensity is the component that is often considered the "fifth vital sign" and it is assessed by using a rating scale, such as the Numerical Rating Scale (NRS), to document the person's report on a scale of 0 to 10. The Verbal Descriptor Scale (VDS) rates pain on a continuum with verbal cues ranging from no pain to mild pain, moderate pain, severe pain, very severe pain, to the worst pain possible. Often this scale is used in conjunction with the NRS. Figure 28-2 illustrates three commonly used pain intensity scales. It is important to document the person's self-report of his or her pain rating, not your personal impression of what you think the rating "should" be. In addition to consistently using the same tool each time, nurses should document additional assessment comments in the chart when appropriate.

Person's responses

Essential assessment information also is obtained by observing for non-verbal indicators of pain such as grimacing, muscle tension, rubbing or protecting body parts, rapid or

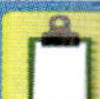

BOX 28-4
Questions to assess pain in older adults

Initial questions to ascertain need for further assessment:

- Are you experiencing pain, discomfort, aching, right now?
- Do you have more than one type of pain?
- Have you had this before or is this new? (If pain has been present before, ask about how it differs, what makes it better or worse and other questions.)
- Describe the pain in your own words. If the person acknowledges having pain, use a pain rating scale and document location(s) on this figure.

Ask about the following characteristics for each type of pain reported:

- Frequency
- Duration
- Precipitating factors
- Alleviating factors
- Variations, such as changes in intensity
- Previous medical evaluation
- Usual management strategies (pharmacological and non-pharmacological)

Ask about effects of pain on functioning and quality of life:

- Daily activities (sleep, eating, appetite, ability to get around, level of independence, driving and so forth)
- Level of physical activity for functioning or enjoyment
- Relationships with others (e.g. social interactions, family activities)
- Emotions (e.g. anger, happiness, irritability, mood)
- Cognitive abilities (e.g. concentration, thinking)
- Participation in enjoyable activities (e.g. hobbies, travel)

Assess the following aspects of analgesic history:

- Current and past use of analgesics
- Names, doses and effectiveness of prescription and non-prescription analgesics
- Experiences with adverse effects
- Analgesics taken on set schedule or as needed
- Use of analgesics during previous 24 hours and influence of these on pain rating scale and other assessment information

Assess concerns about, or fear of, adverse effects, including addiction.

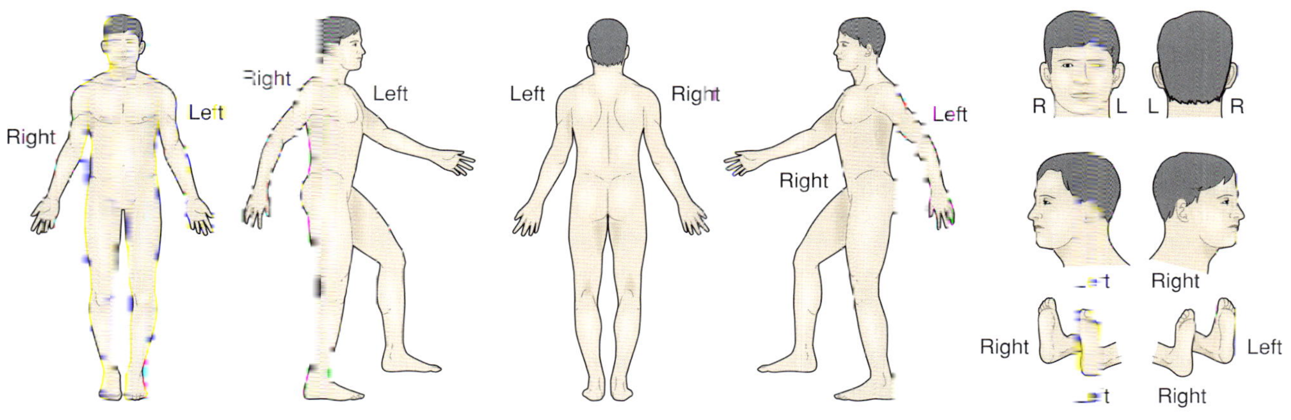

excessive eye blinking, or a sad or frightened facial expression. Information also can be elicited from family members and carers when additional input would be helpful, particularly if the older adult is not a reliable reporter for any reason. If the person's level of functioning has changed recently, find out if pain or discomfort is a contributing factor.

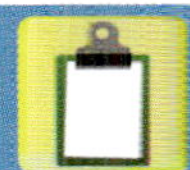

BOX 28-5
The OPQRSTU mnemonic that assists with pain assessment

OPQRSTU

O—Onset of pain
P—Provoking or precipitating factors
Q—Quality of pain (person's description—sharp, achy, etc.)
R—Radiation of pain (does the pain extend from the site?)
S—Severity of the pain (intensity 1 to 10)
T—Timing (occasional versus constant)
U—The person's understanding of pain

Source: Registered Nurses Association of Ontario (RNAO). (2013). *Assessment and management of pain in the elderly* (3rd ed.). Toronto: Author. Available March 2015 via http://rnao.ca.

Effects on ADLs

Assessing the effects of pain on ADLs not only provides additional information for the nurse but also may help older adults recognise subtle ways in which pain interferes with their lives. Thus, nurses should ask how often in the past week the pain or discomfort has interfered with self-care or the usual ability to perform activities such as bathing, eating, dressing and going to the toilet. Limiting the timeframe to the past week helps the person to focus attention on the present, rather than recalling how pain has fluctuated over the course of months or years. Nurses should also ask about the effects of pain states on complex activities such as driving, paying bills, preparing meals, shopping for groceries and taking care of home-related chores.

Quality

Assessing the quality of the pain based on specific descriptors used by older adults is helpful in determining the underlying pain mechanism as somatic, visceral or neuropathic, as discussed in the section on types of pain. Nurses should document the location of the pain on a figure

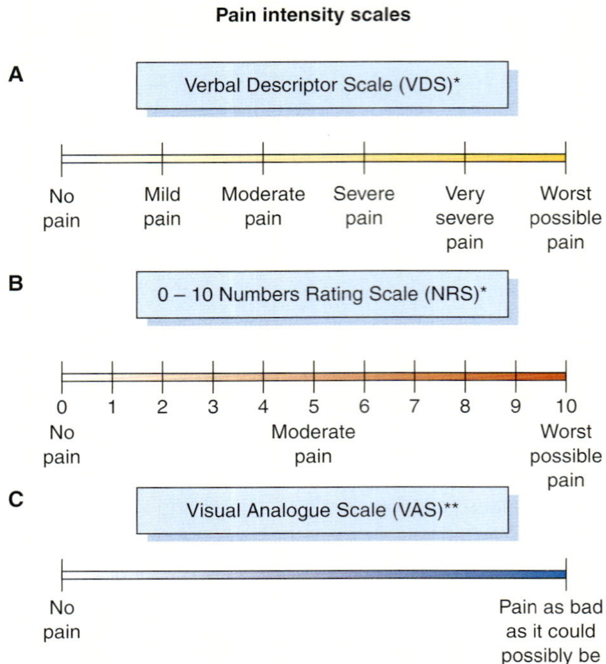

FIGURE 28-2 Examples of pain rating scales: (**A**) Verbal Descriptor Scale, (**B**) Numerical Rating Scale, and (**C**) Visual Analogue Scale.

drawing in the person's chart. Location can be identified simply by asking the person to mark the location on a figure drawing, or by having the person point to the location on his or her own body. If there is more than one site, letters may be used for distinguishing the different sites for documentation (e.g. A, B, C and so forth). This step of assessment is critical for delineating different areas of pain because they may be different types of pain. Each location may require an individual approach to management.

Physical findings

Physical findings may also aid in assessing the location of the pain. Although pain assessment cannot rely only on physical findings, the nurse must observe the site of pain; note any changes in skin colour, warmth, irritation or integrity; and review any pertinent physical assessment data.

Temporal characteristics

Temporal characteristics describe the course of the pain experience using the following parameters: onset, duration of episodes, frequency (i.e. constant or intermittent) and variations with time of day or certain activities. It is logical to assess aggravating and alleviating factors in conjunction with temporal characteristics. This goal is accomplished by inquiring about what makes the pain better or worse, if the pain is affected by movement or changing position, and if any non-pharmacological methods help to alleviate the pain.

Analgesic history

Analgesic history can also be taken at this time and should include information on the older adult's current medication use, the onset and duration of maximal analgesia with medication use, and the number of medications being taken on a set schedule versus those taken only as needed (*prn*). The nurse must also thoroughly assess and document analgesic use within the previous 24 hours because a person can have very different pain ratings, depending on whether analgesics have been taken on the day of the assessment. This is also the time to inquire about problems the older adult has had with side effects of medications as well as any fears of potential side effects or addiction to pain medication.

Goals, expectations and understanding

When assessing pain, nurses must evaluate the person's goals and expectations, as well as the meaning he or she associates with the pain. Some older adults may fear the onset of pain as an indicator of a progressive terminal illness or disease process, and others may view pain as a positive sign that they are still alive for another day. Nurses assess the meaning and context of the pain in relation to actual and potential effects on functional and psychosocial activities such as sleep, physical activities, recreational activities, personal relationships and work. These areas can influence older adults' perception of the severity of the pain and their willingness to participate in a pain management regimen.

This time is also the point at which to gain an understanding of the person's short- and long-term goals of treatment. Does the person expect to return to baseline functioning, or is he or she expecting to continue to experience some pain? Another important issue to determine is the person's acceptable level of pain and to incorporate this acceptable level as a goal of the pain management regimen. Is a pain level of 5 on the 0-to-10 NRS acceptable to the person, or is 3 the target pain level?

Effectiveness of analgesia

A crucial step that is often overlooked is the reassessment of pain frequently and regularly. In acute care settings, nurses should assess the effectiveness of the treatment shortly after the administration of pain medication (30 to 60 minutes) and whenever pain management interventions are changed. Nurses also need to reassess whenever older people experience changes in any of the critical components of pain. This reassessment includes questions regarding pain severity and length of time the pain was relieved with the previous intervention.

Assessing persistent pain

There are tools that have been developed to assist with the assessment of persistent pain. Pain diaries are useful for the assessment of pain. An older adult who is experiencing pain is encouraged to record their perceptions of pain using their own words. The diary enables the person to better understand their pain, the effectiveness of pain interventions and thereby facilitating self-management of persistent pain. The diary also enables the person to share their experience of pain with health professionals and this has been found to be very useful when there has been a change in treatment (Palliative Care, 2014).

Another assessment tool useful to assess persistent pain is the Brief Pain Inventory. It assesses the severity of pain and the impact of pain on daily functions, location of pain, pain medications and amount of pain relief in the past 24 hours or the past week. See Figure 28-3 for an example of a Brief Pain Inventory.

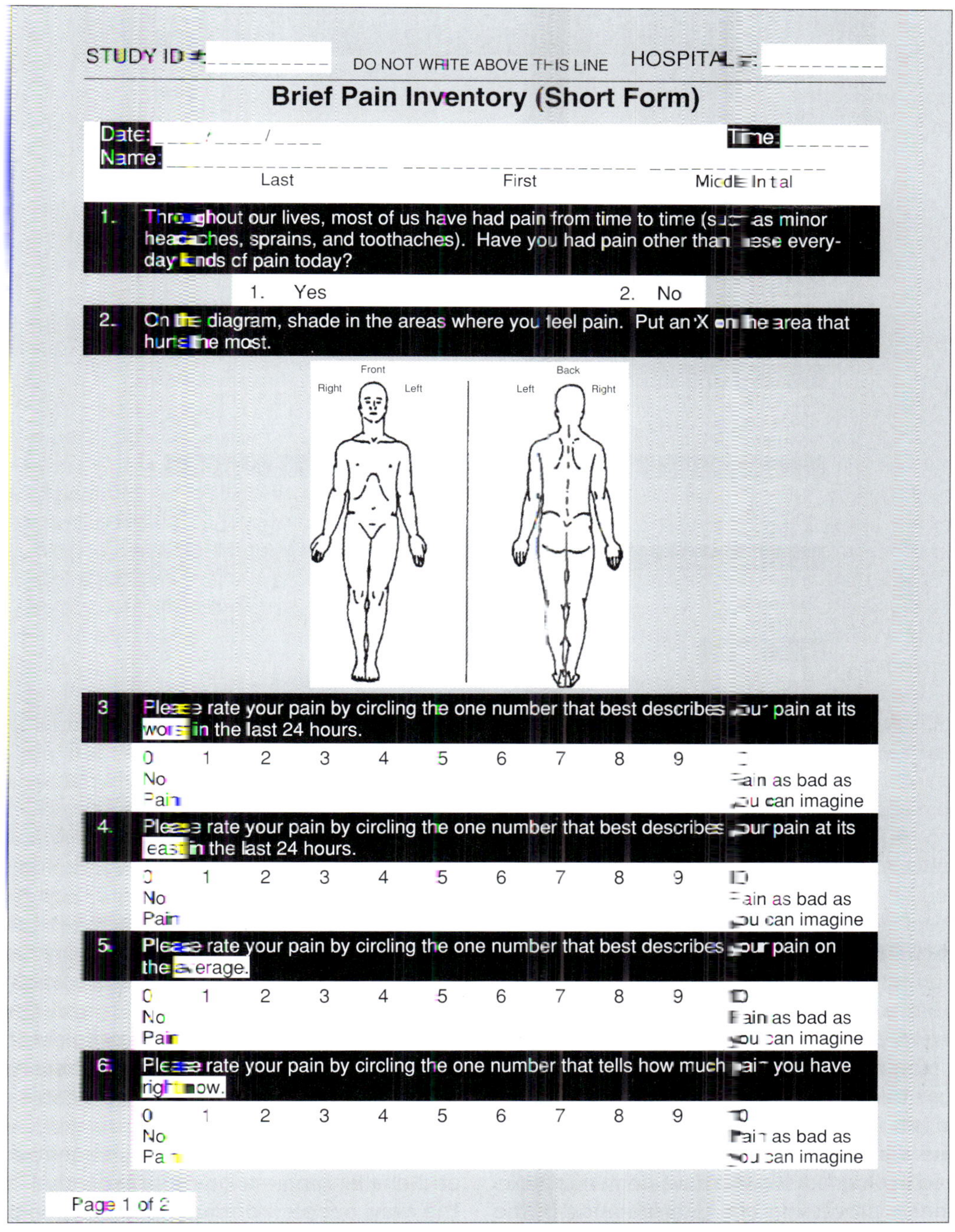

STUDY ID#: __________ DO NOT WRITE ABOVE THIS LINE HOSPITAL#: __________

Brief Pain Inventory (Short Form)

Date: ___/___/___ Time: _______

Name: ____________ ____________ ____________
Last First Middle Initial

1. Throughout our lives, most of us have had pain from time to time (such as minor headaches, sprains, and toothaches). Have you had pain other than these everyday kinds of pain today?

1. Yes 2. No

2. On the diagram, shade in the areas where you feel pain. Put an X on the area that hurts the most.

3. Please rate your pain by circling the one number that best describes your pain at its worst in the last 24 hours.

0 1 2 3 4 5 6 7 8 9 10
No Pain — Pain as bad as you can imagine

4. Please rate your pain by circling the one number that best describes your pain at its least in the last 24 hours.

0 1 2 3 4 5 6 7 8 9 10
No Pain — Pain as bad as you can imagine

5. Please rate your pain by circling the one number that best describes your pain on the average.

0 1 2 3 4 5 6 7 8 9 10
No Pain — Pain as bad as you can imagine

6. Please rate your pain by circling the one number that tells how much pain you have right now.

0 1 2 3 4 5 6 7 8 9 10
No Pain — Pain as bad as you can imagine

Page 1 of 2

FIGURE 28-3 Brief Pain Inventory—Short Form (page 1 of 2). (Copyright Charles Cleeland [1991]. Permission granted from the Department of Symptom Research, MD Anderson Cancer Centre, University of Texas, Houston.) *(continued)*

STUDY ID #:__________ DO NOT WRITE ABOVE THIS LINE HOSPITAL #:__________

Date: ____/____/____ Time: ________

Name: ____________________ ____________________ ______________

Last First Middle Initial

7. What treatments or medications are you receiving for your pain?

____

8. In the last 24 hours, how much relief have pain treatments or medications provided? Please circle the one percentage that most shows how much relief you have received.

0% No Relief	10%	20%	30%	40%	50%	60%	70%	80%	90%	100% Complete Relief

9. Circle the one number that describes how, during the past 24 hours, pain has interfered with your:

A. General Activity

0 Does not Interfere	1	2	3	4	5	6	7	8	9	10 Completely Interferes

B. Mood

0 Does not Interfere	1	2	3	4	5	6	7	8	9	10 Completely Interferes

C. Walking Ability

0 Does not Interfere	1	2	3	4	5	6	7	8	9	10 Completely Interferes

D. Normal Work (includes both work outside the home and housework)

0 Does not Interfere	1	2	3	4	5	6	7	8	9	10 Completely Interferes

E. Relations with other people

0 Does not Interfere	1	2	3	4	5	6	7	8	9	10 Completely Interferes

F. Sleep

0 Does not Interfere	1	2	3	4	5	6	7	8	9	10 Completely Interferes

G. Enjoyment of life

0 Does not Interfere	1	2	3	4	5	6	7	8	9	10 Completely Interferes

Page 2 of 2

FIGURE 28-3 Brief Pain Inventory—Short Form (*continued*) (page 2 of 2).

Assessment in cognitively impaired older adults

Another tool, the Abbey Pain Scale, has been recommended for use (APS, 2005) for non-verbal older adults with dementia (see Figure 28-4).

Many studies confirm that the pain transmission process is unaltered in older adults who have dementia; however, the cognitive processing and interpretation of the pain stimulus may be impaired (Pasero & McCaffery, 2011c). Despite this evidence, many carers and healthcare professionals falsely believe that people with dementia do not experience pain. Consequently, there is a high prevalence of unrecognised and undertreated pain in older adults with dementia.

As with all aspects of pain assessment, it is essential—and challenging—to identify individual differences in the way people communicate their experience. This becomes even more challenging when assessing older adults who are cognitively impaired because dementia

Abbey Pain Scale

For measurement of pain in people with dementia who cannot verbalise.

How to use scale: While observing the resident, score questions 1 to 6

Name of resident: ....

Name and designation of person completing the scale: ....

Date: ....**Time:** ....

Latest pain relief given was..**at** ....**hours.**

Q1	**Vocalisation** **e.g.: whimpering, groaning, crying** *Absent 0 Mild 1 Moderate 2 Severe 3*	**Q1**	☐
Q2	**Facial expression** **e.g.: looking tense, frowning grimacing, looking frightened** *Absent 0 Mild 1 Moderate 2 Severe 3*	**Q2**	☐
Q3	**Change in body language** **e.g.: fidgeting, rocking, guarding part of body, withdrawn** *Absent 0 Mild 1 Moderate 2 Severe 3*	**Q3**	☐
Q4	**Behavioural change** **e.g.: increased confusion, refusing to eat, alteration in usual patterns** *Absent 0 Mild 1 Moderate 2 Severe 3*	**Q4**	☐
Q5	**Physiological change** **e.g.: temperature, pulse or blood pressure outside normal limits, perspiring, flushing or pallor** *Absent 0 Mild 1 Moderate 2 Severe 3*	**Q5**	☐
Q6	**Physical changes** **e.g.: skin tears, pressure areas, arthritis, contractures, previous injuries.** *Absent 0 Mild 1 Moderate 2 Severe 3*	**Q6**	☐

Add scores for 1 – 6 and record here ⇨ **Total pain score** ☐

Now tick the box that matches the total pain score ⇨

0 – 2 No pain	3 – 7 Mild	8 – 13 Moderate	14+ Severe

Finally, tick the box which matches the type of pain ⇨

Chronic	Acute	Acute on chronic

FIGURE 23-4 Abbey Pain Scale. (Abbey, J., De Bellis, A., Piller, N., Esterman, A., Giles, L., Parker, D. & Lowcay, E. [2004]. Funded by the JH & JD Gunn Medical Research Foundation 1998–2002.)

affects communication abilities to varying degrees. It is imperative to recognise that many older adults with mild to moderate dementia can verbally communicate about pain and, in these situations it is appropriate to use the nursing assessment guidelines already discussed. It also is imperative to supplement the information with input from family and all carers, including nursing assistance staff in long-term care facilities.

In people with moderate or advanced dementia, disruptive behaviours may be the key indicator of pain and assessment focuses on non-verbal indicators and reports from reliable observers (e.g. family and carers). A recent analysis of assessment data for nursing home residents found that disruptive behaviours (e.g. aggression and agitation) that do not involve locomotion were more strongly correlated with pain in comparison to behaviours (e.g. wandering) that involved locomotion (Ahn & Horgas, 2013). In all situations when caring for older adults who are cognitively impaired keep in mind that dementia does not directly affect one's experience of pain but it does alter the ability to express pain, as well as other needs.

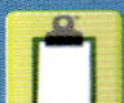

BOX 28-6
Assessing pain in older adults who have dementia

General principles

- Know the person and recognise that the person's ability to communicate may fluctuate.
- For people with mild to moderate dementia, use numerical rating scales as appropriate.
- Base assessment conclusions on multiple sources of information.
- Assess the person under several types of conditions: for example, resting, active, different times of day, during activities of daily living.

Identify verbal indicators of pain

- Vocalisations such as sighing, moaning, chanting
- Repeated calling out "Help"
- Response to touching: "Ow", "Ouch", swearing or cursing
- Response to care-related activities: "Stop" or "Don't do that"
- Facial expressions, such as grimacing or furrowed brows
- Rubbing or protecting an extremity

Observe for non-verbal indicators

- Changes in behaviour
- Increased confusion, disorientation
- Diminished appetite
- Resistance to or combativeness during care activities
- Withdrawal from social activities
- Decreased participation in physical activities
- Spending more time in bed (with or without sleep)

Look for clues to potential causes of pain (as in the following examples)

- Skin infection: swelling, inflammation, breakdown
- Arthritis: joint swelling, guarding, limited use, diminished mobility
- Gout: joint inflammations
- Oral problems: check mouth for sores, redness, open areas
- Low back pain: gait changes, diminished level of activity, abnormal posture
- Urinary tract infection: changes in behaviour, urinary frequency or incontinence

Obtain pertinent information from family, carers and reliable sources

- Identify history of chronic conditions associated with pain (e.g. gout, arthritis, peripheral or postherpetic neuropathy)
- Observe for exacerbations of previously controlled chronic conditions
- Ask about usual manifestations of pain (e.g. wandering, agitation, withdrawal from activities)
- Find out about previous use of analgesics and non-pharmacological interventions
- Ask about recent falls or acute problems that could cause pain (e.g. urinary tract infections, skin tears or injuries or bacterial infections such as pneumonia), as well as chronic conditions.

Pain assessment in older adults who are cognitively impaired involves all the following actions:

- Elicit as much verbal and non-verbal information directly from the person as possible.
- Assess for indicators of underlying causes of pain, such as chronic conditions (e.g. arthritis, gout, neuralgia) or recent falls or surgical procedures.
- Use astute observations to identify behavioural indicators of pain, such as aggression, agitation, verbalisations or resistance to care activities.
- Obtain information from family members, carers and other reliable sources who are familiar with the person.
- Compare current assessment findings with the person's baseline function, but recognise that the person's usual level of functioning may be affected by undiagnosed and undertreated pain.

Box 28-6 summarises specific actions nurses can take to assess pain in older adults who are cognitively impaired.

Many pain assessment tools have been developed specifically for older adults with dementia. The Pain Assessment in Advanced Dementia (PAINAD) and the Pain Assessment Checklist for Seniors with Limited Ability to Communicate (PACSLAC) are two commonly used tools. Both of these tools provide a checklist of observations that may be indicative of pain in people who cannot self-report, with each tool having different characteristics, as summarised in Table 28-3. The PACSLAC is more detailed, with 60 specific indicators listed (see Figure 28-5). Any

TABLE 28-3 Characteristics of PAINAD and PACSLAC

Tool characteristic	PAINAD	PACSLAC
Indicators	Breathing independent of vocalisation Negative vocalisation Facial expression Body language Consolability	Activity/body movement Negative vocalisations Facial expression Social/personality/mood Physiological changes (e.g. sleeping, appetite)
Scoring	0 to 2 for each of five indicators (total 0 to 10), with higher score related to degree of pain	Checkmarks for 60 specific indicators in four subscale groups, with more checkmarks indicating pain
Recommended use	Best for daily use in acute care or frequent intervals	Best for comparisons at longer intervals for persistent pain or in long-term care settings
Validity and reliability	Supported by research	Supported by research
Original reference	Warden, V., Hurley, A. C. & Volicer, L. (2003)	Fuchs-Lacelle, S. & Hadjistavropoulos, T. (2004)
Recent reference	Monroe, T. B. & Mion, L. C. (2012)	Lints-Martindale, Hadjistavropoulos, T., Lix, L. & Thorpe, L. (2012)

PACSLAC: Pain Assessment Checklist for Seniors with Limited Ability to Communicate; PAINAD: Pain Assessment in Advanced Dementia.

Pain Assessment Checklist for Seniors with Limited Ability to Communicate (PACSLAC)

Indicate with a checkmark, which of the items on the PACSLAC occurred during the period of interest. Scoring the subscales is derived by counting the checkmarks in each column. To generate a total pain, sum all subscale totals.

Facial Expression	Present
Grimacing	
Sad Look	
Tighter Face	
Dirty Look	
Change in Eyes (Squinting, dull, bright, increased eye movements)	
Frowning	
Pain Expression	
Grim Face	
Clenching Teeth	
Wincing	
Open Mouth	
Creasing Forehead	
Screwing Up Nose	

Activity/Body Movement	Present
Fidgeting	
Pulling Away	
Flinching	
Restless	
Pacing	
Wandering	
Trying to Leave	
Refusing to Move	
Thrashing	
Decreased Activity	
Refusing Medications	
Moving Slow	
Impulsive Behaviors (Repeat movements)	
Uncooperative/Resistance to Care	
Gaurding Sore Area	
Touching/Holding Sore Area	
Limping	
Clenching Fist	
Going into Fetal Position	
Stiff/Rigid	

Social/Personality/Mood	Present
Physical Aggression (e.g., pushing people and/or objects, scratching others, hitting others, striking, kicking).	
Verbal Aggression	
Not Wanting to Be Touched	
Not Allowing People Near	
Angry/Mad	
Throwing Things	
Increased Confusion	
Anxious	
Upset	
Agitated	
Cranky/Irritable	
Frustrated	

Other (Physiological Changes/Eating Sleeping Changes/Vocal Behaviors)	Present
Pale Face	
Flushed, Red Face	
Teary Eyed	
Sweating	
Shaking/Trembling	
Cold Clammy	
Changes in Sleep Routine (Please circle 1 or 2) 1) Decreased Sleep 2) Increased Sleep During the Day	
Changes in Appetite (Please circle 1 or 2) 1) Decreased Appetite 2) Increased Appetite	
Screaming/Yelling	
Calling Out (i.e., for help)	
Crying	
A Specific Sound of Vocalization for Pain ("ow," "ouch")	
Moaning and groaning	
Mumbling	
Grunting	
Total Checklist Score	

FIGURE 28.5 Pain assessment checklist for seniors with limited ability to communicate. [Reprinted with permission from Fuchs-Lacelle, S. & Hadjistavropoulos, T. (2004). Development and preliminary validation of the pain assessment checklist for seniors with limited ability to communicate (PACSLAC). *Pain Management Nursing*, 5(1), 37–49. © Copyright Shannon Fuchs-Lacelle and Thomas Hadjistavropoulos.]

positive score on these tools should trigger further assessment and plans for interventions, for example, consideration of using an analgesic medication on a trial basis (Monroe & Mion, 2012; Zwakhalen, van der Steen & Najim, 2012).

All tools for assessing pain in people with dementia focus on observation and documentation of behaviours that are indicative of pain, but false-positive results on assessment tools may be associated with psychosocial distress or delirium (Jordan, Hughes, Pakresi et al., 2011;

Lints-Martindale, Hadjistavropoulos, Lix et al., 2012). A review of six tools concluded that the measurements most strongly associated with pain were facial expression, vocalisations and body movements (Lints-Martindale, Hadjistavropoulos, Lix et al., 2012). Keep in mind that the numerical value of any tool is not correlated with NRSs and that pain severity (i.e. the characteristic measured by NRSs) can be assessed only when the person is able to self-report (Monroe & Mion, 2012).

If assessment findings indicate that the person with dementia is likely to be experiencing pain, it is important to do all the following: assume pain is present, initiate a trial of analgesic medication, and observe changes in the person's behaviour in response to the analgesic (Pasero & McCaffery, 2011c). An analgesic trial is an integral part of the assessment, and it also can be an intervention for promoting comfort and for addressing dementia-related behaviours. In recent years, pain management is increasingly viewed as an evidence-based but underused strategy that can be incorporated with other behavioural interventions for older adults with dementia who are at risk for developing aggressive behaviour (Bradford, Shrestha, Snow et al., 2012). Recommended doses of acetaminophen for an analgesic trial are 325 to 500 mg every 4 hours, or 500 to 1000 mg every 6 hours initially, with titration to stronger analgesics if pain continues to be suspected and there is no change in behaviour (Herr, Coyne, McCaffery et al., 2011). In addition, non-pharmacological comfort interventions (e.g. touch, communication, music, massage, reflexology and environmental modifications) are essential components of assessment and management of pain in people with dementia (Lu & Herr, 2012).

In addition to considering an analgesic trial, consider initiating appropriate non-pharmacological interventions, as described in the section on non-pharmacological nursing interventions for managing pain. Because many of these interventions require active participation by the person experiencing pain, assess the individual's ability to engage in the intervention. For people with advanced dementia, consider non-pharmacological interventions, such as music therapy, that are safe and can be used in almost any situation. Case study one provides an opportunity to apply knowledge about pain assessment.

CASE STUDY ONE

John Rolff is a 79-year-old man who has been transferred to long-term residential care after being in hospital for 6 days recovering from the surgical repair of a left fractured neck of femur. John has a diagnosis of Alzheimer's dementia. Prior to his hospital admission he was mobile but did receive care for some activities of daily living from a community service. John also lived with his wife, Vera.

When John arrives in the facility he is moaning quietly and his eyes are closed. When you go to transfer him into the bed, he stiffens and becomes resistive. You and the ambulance officers take some time moving him. Once the transfer is complete, John begins to pull at the sheets. Vera arrives and asks you what is happening to John?

Thinking points

- Could John be in pain?
- Is so, what screening tools/information would you use to assess/monitor John's pain, and what is the rationale for their use?
- Would Vera participate in the assessment process?

DEVELOPING A WELLNESS-FOCUSED PAIN MANAGEMENT PLAN

Although the management of pain in older adults is complex, principles of wellness focus on developing a comprehensive and individualised pain management care plan based on the assessment. Nursing interventions for managing pain depend on the nature of the pain (acute versus persistent) as well as on the person's own experiences and preferences. Incorporating wellness approaches to the care of this population includes the older adult as a partner in decision making and planning.

Pharmacological interventions for managing pain

Analgesic medications are the foundation of effective pain management and are the first intervention for acute and serious pain. Selection of type and dose of analgesic is based on careful evaluation of the person's many variables, including age, weight, concomitant conditions and medications, and concerns about actual and potential adverse effects (including drug interactions). Keep in mind that with careful analgesic selection and monitoring there is less risk of adverse effects from medications as compared with the serious risks associated with undertreatment of pain in older adults. Nurses have major responsibilities in preventing the undertreatment of pain and, at the same time, providing astute assessment and management of both therapeutic and adverse effects. This is particularly important when caring for older adults who are in long-term residential care facilities and those who have dementia.

Principles of analgesic medication

The principles of medication management specific to older adults, is presented in Box 28-7.

Classifications and administration of analgesics

Analgesics are divided into three different groups: non-opioids, opioids and adjuvants.

Non-opioid analgesics include paracetamol; non-steroidal anti-inflammatory drugs (NSAIDs); and aspirin. Non-opioids act at the site of the injury to decrease pain. **Opioid analgesics** are natural, semisynthetic or synthetic drugs that relieve pain by binding to multiple types of opioid

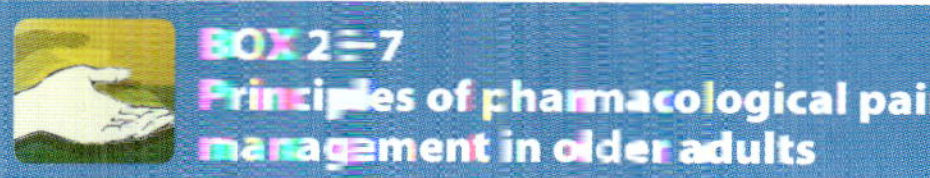

BOX 28-7
Principles of pharmacological pain management in older adults

1. Use a combination of pharmacological and non-pharmacological pain management strategies
2. Give adequate amounts of medication at the appropriate frequency to control pain based on regular assessment
3. Use round-the-clock dosing; avoid PRN dosing
4. Use a combination of drugs that potentiate each other
5. The prescription of analgesics should use a step-wise approach (WHO pain relief ladder)
6. With narcotic analgesic drugs, start low and increase dose slowly
7. Anticipate and prevent side effects common in the older adult
8. Consult an equianalgesic potency table when changing medications
9. Pethidine is not recommended because of the build-up of a toxic metabolite, which can cause seizures. Pethidine is not reversible by naloxone
10. The intramuscular route should be used cautiously because of possible muscle atrophy in older adults varies the medication's effectiveness

Source: Registered Nurses Association of Ontario (RNAO). (2013). *Assessment and management of pain in the elderly* (3rd ed.). Accessed March 2015 via http://rnao.ca; Australian Pain Society (APS). (2005). Pain in residential aged care facilities: Management strategies. Sydney: APS. Accessed March 2015 via www.apsoc.org.au

receptors in the central nervous system. As a result of this action, the release of neurotransmitters is blocked and the pain impulse cannot cross the synapse into the dorsal horn during the transmission phase of the pain pathway. See examples of opioids in Table 28-4. **Adjuvant analgesics** are medications that have a primary indication other than the treatment of pain, such as an antidepressants or anticonvulsants, but relieve pain in some conditions. Adjuvants most often act on the modulation phase of the pain pathway by interfering with the reuptake of serotonin and noradrenaline, which inhibit the transmission of nociceptive impulses. See examples of non-opioid and adjuvant analgesics in Table 28-5. All three groups are effective in the perception phase, acting in different ways to decrease the conscious experience of pain perception.

There are many different forms of analgesics that enable different routes of administration and delivery systems. Box 28-8 lists the routes and the analgesics that may be administered via that route.

Tolerance and dependence: Misconceptions and realities about analgesics

The many misconceptions about different analgesics may affect selection of medications for pain management. Table 28-6 identifies misconceptions and realities about analgesics that are most relevant to pain management for older adults.

Because misconceptions and lack of information can lead to fears and reluctance to take appropriate medications, it is important to teach older adults and their families about tolerance, dependence and addiction. Medication **tolerance** is a physiological protective mechanism that helps the body become accustomed to the medication so that adverse effects (except for constipation) gradually diminish. Tolerance is characterised by a decrease in one or more therapeutic effects of the medication (e.g. less analgesia) or its adverse effects (e.g. nausea, sedation or respiratory depression). Tolerance to analgesia usually occurs during the first several days to 2 weeks of therapy.

Dependence is a normal physiological response manifested by the development of withdrawal symptoms when an opioid is suddenly discontinued after being administered repeatedly for more than 2 weeks. Tapering (i.e. gradually reducing) the dose of an opioid as pain resolves usually prevents withdrawal symptoms. Dependence is not necessarily an indicator of addiction; rather, it indicates that the medication is medically necessary for managing symptoms.

In contrast to dependence and tolerance, **addiction** is a chronic disease with biological, neurological and psychological characteristics, including one or more of the following in relation to a drug: craving, compulsive use inability to control its use, and continued use even when harm occurs. In reality, addiction rarely occurs in relation to analgesic medications, whereas tolerance and dependence are normal responses that should be expected when opioids are taken for 2 to 4 weeks or longer (Pasero & McCaffery, 2011b).

World Health Organization three-step pain relief ladder for pain management

The World Health Organization (WHO) pain relief ladder is used as a guide for the treatment of persistent pain in older adults (Australian Pain Society [APS], 2005). The three steps of the **WHO pain relief ladder** (Figure 28-6) address different

TABLE 28-4 Different forms of opioids used to alleviate pain

Oral forms		Other forms	
Immediate release	**Slow release**	**Injectables**	**Transdermal (patches)**
Morphine liquid	MS Contin	Morphine	Fentanyl
Oxycodone	MS Contin Suspension	Hydromorphone	Buprenorphine
Hydromorphone	OxyContin	Fentanyl	
Methadone	Kapanol		

TABLE 28-5 Non-opioid and adjuvant analgesics used to manage common pain types

Medication group	Mechanism of action	Indications
Non-opioid analgesics		
Paracetamol	Not completely understood Inhibits prostaglandin release in tissues but limited effect on inflammation	Mild aches and pains, bone pain
Aspirin	Inhibits prostaglandin release in tissues and decreases inflammation	Bone pain and pain caused by inflammation
NSAID (celecoxib, ibuprofen)	Inhibits prostaglandin release in tissues and decreases inflammation	Bone pain and pain caused by inflammation
Adjuvant analgesics		
Tricyclic antidepressants (amitriptyline)	Blocks the descending pain pathway by inhibiting the actions of serotonin and noradrenaline. Despite lower doses being used to treat pain than depression, older adults are at increased risk of adverse effects	Neuropathic pain
Steroids (dexamethasone)	Inhibit prostaglandin release. Decreases swelling and inflammation in tumour mass	Pain associated with compression from a cancerous growth, neuropathic pain, and bone pain
Anticonvulsants (phenytoin, sodium valproate, gabapentin)	Suppression of neuronal hyperexcitability	Neuropathic pain
Antispasmodics (hyoscine)	Decrease myotonic activity in smooth muscle (hyoscine is an anticholinergic and older adults at increased risk of adverse side effects)	Bladder spasm and renal colic

levels of pain intensity, and also allow people who experience pain differently to be managed consistently. Additionally WHO recommends four other key principles of pain management. See Box 28-9 for WHO's key principles of pain management.

Step 1 of the WHO pain relief ladder addresses mild pain (i.e. ranging from 1 to 3 out of 10 on an NRS) by recommending the use of non-opioid analgesics initially, with the addition of an adjuvant if it is deemed appropriate. Although non-opioids are generally viewed as having fewer risks of side effects than

BOX 28-8
Administration routes of different forms of analgesics and delivery systems

Oral route
1 Opioids and tramadol
2 Non-selective non-steroidal anti-inflammatory drugs and coxibs
3 Paracetamol

Intravenous route
1 Opioids and tramadol
2 Non-selective non-steroidal anti-inflammatory drugs and coxibs
3 Paracetamol

Intramuscular and subcutaneous routes
1 Opioids and tramadol
2 Non-selective non-steroidal anti-inflammatory drugs and coxibs

Rectal route
1 Opioids
2 Non-selective non-steroidal anti-inflammatory drugs
3 Paracetamol

Transdermal route
1 Opioids
2 Other drugs

Epidural
1 Anaesthetic drugs

Intrathecal
1 Opioids
2 Antispasmodic—baclofen

Transmucosal routes
1 Intranasal route
2 Sublingual and buccal routes
3 Inhaled

Delivery systems
1 Patient-controlled analgesia
2 Pain pumps
3 Syringe drivers

TABLE 28-6 Misconceptions and realities about analgesics

Misconception	Evidence-based reality
Daily use of non-opioids is safer than long-term use of opioids	Long-term use of NSAIDs is associated with more severe and life-threatening adverse effects, whereas the most common adverse effect of opioids is constipation, which can be addressed
Non-opioids are not effective for severe pain	Non-opioids alone rarely relieve severe pain, but they have an important role as adjuvants
Polypharmacy with different types of analgesics is unacceptable	Because different types of analgesics have unique mechanisms, it is acceptable and often recommended to use different types for specific purposes
Rectal or parenteral administration of NSAIDs reduces the risks of GI adverse effects	NSAIDs administered by any route inhibit prostaglandins, which are necessary to maintain the protective barrier in the GI tract
Administering NSAIDs with an antacid reduces the risk of GI adverse effects	Antacids may decrease the risk of GI effects, but they also decrease effectiveness of NSAIDs because they cause the drug to be released in the stomach instead of the small intestine
Taking opioids for pain relief leads to addiction	Addiction as a result of taking opioids for analgesia occurs less than 1% of the time
Opioids are not effective for all types of pain	All pain responds to opioids, but they are more effective in relieving visceral and somatic pain and less effective for neuropathic pain
Opioids should be avoided during early stages of progressive conditions to prevent the development of tolerance	Tolerance to opioids does not necessarily develop and the dose usually stabilises if the pain is stable. There is no ceiling to opioid doses and patients develop tolerance to respiratory depression
Opioids commonly cause clinically significant respiratory depression	If opioid doses are titrated slowly and decreased when sedation occurs, respiratory depression is rare. Tolerance to respiratory effects develops within 72 hours of regular daily doses

GI, gastrointestinal; NSAID, non-steroidal anti-inflammatory drug.
Source: Pasero, Portenoy & McCaffery (2011); Pasero, Quinn, Portenoy et al. (2011).

opioids, this misconception is a dangerous one. The use of NSAIDs poses many serious side effects for older adults because they can cause significant end-organ toxicity. Excessive use of NSAIDs can also result in renal insufficiency, decreased platelet aggregations and even death.

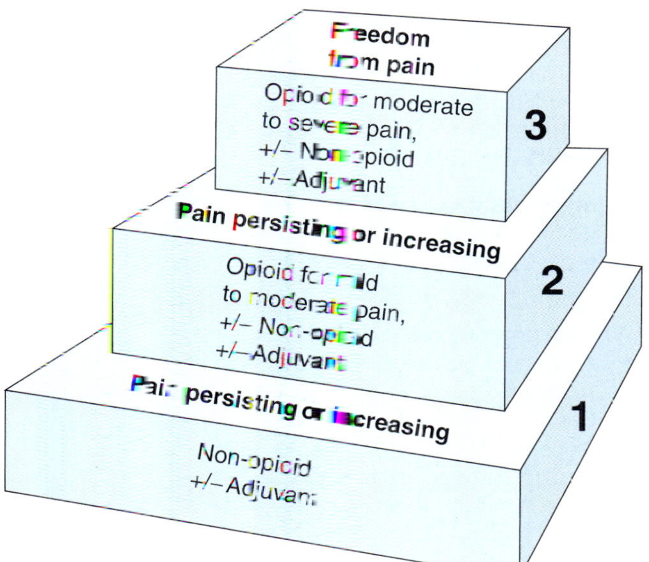

FIGURE 28-6 World Health Organization's pain relief ladder. (Copyright 2005 World Health Organization. Redrawn with permission.)

BOX 28-9
Summary of the World Health Organization's five principles for managing pain

1. **By the mouth**—the oral route for analgesia should always be used, unless the individual has a pre-existing condition that makes this route unpractical, such as ongoing nausea and vomiting, a bowel obstruction or swallowing problems.
2. **By the clock**—analgesia should be given regularly to prevent the pain from coming back. PRN medications should be reserved for breakthrough doses of analgesia or if the pain is intermittent.
3. **By the ladder**—refers to the three-step WHO ladder:
   - Step 1 refers to non-opioid medication such as paracetamol.
   - Step two refers to opioids for mild to moderate pain such as Panadeine Forte, codeine or tramadol. It is important to remember that analgesics such as tramadol and Panadeine Forte have a ceiling effect on their action. Therefore, once that dose is reached, step-three opioids need to be commenced.
   - Step three refers to opioids used for moderate to severe pain such as morphine, oxycodone and fentanyl.
4. **For the individual**—because an opioid's effect varies tremendously from person to person, one cannot prescribe standard dosages.
5. **Attention to detail should be given.**

Source: World Health Organization. (2015). Essential medicines and health products: Impact of impaired access to controlled medications. Accessed March 2015 at www.who.int/medicines/areas/quality_safety/Impaired_Access/en.

Paracetamol is often considered a "safe" alternative to NSAIDs because it is a very effective analgesic with few side effects and does not cause problems with the stomach, kidneys or platelets. However, the most common side effect associated with the overuse of paracetamol is a deadly one: hepatotoxicity. It is important to recognise that the recommended ceiling dose for paracetamol (i.e. 4 g daily) is for *healthy individuals* with no previous liver or metabolic complications. Additional factors that increase the risk of hepatotoxicity include the following:

- Malnutrition or fasting
- Daily consumption of more than two standard alcohol drinks
- Liver disease or hepatic insufficiency
- Use of other potentially hepatotoxic mediations.

Extreme caution must be taken with older adults using any non-opioid medication. Levels of paracetamol must also be carefully monitored if an older adult is using a combination medication (an opioid, e.g. codeine, plus paracetamol) for breakthrough pain because levels greater than the safe maximum can easily be reached. This principle is critically important for teaching because older adults may not realise that many over-the-counter products contain paracetamol that must be factored into the daily maximum dose.

If the pain progresses to the mild-to-moderate range (e.g. it worsens from a 3 to a 5 of 10 on an NRS), and is not adequately relieved by the use of a non-opioid, then Step 2 suggests adding a weak opioid, or opioid combination, to the regimen. This step *builds on* the previous one; it does not replace the use of the Step 1 non-opioid analgesics. Step 2 should also include a method of providing around-the-clock analgesia by using a breakthrough medication.

If the pain persists or worsens (i.e. ranging from 7 to 10 on an NRS) the interventions in Step 3 should be considered. Although both Steps 2 and 3 include the use of an opioid, different types of opioids are used in each step. The use of stronger opioids is appropriate in Step 3. Step 3 builds on Steps 1 and 2, with the continued use of non-opioids and adjuvants. Opioid use in Step 3 must be scheduled around the clock and still include some type of breakthrough pain medication. Opioids prescribed for breakthrough pain should also have a short half-life so that they can be rapidly titrated for severe pain episodes. Opioids for around-the-clock administration should be delivered in a controlled-release formula, ensuring that the administration rate remains constant. One final point to make about the pain relief ladders: pain treatment does not necessarily begin at Step 1 and progress sequentially. For example, it may be appropriate to begin at Step 3 or titrate more rapidly for an older adult who is experiencing excruciating pain.

When adding analgesic medication into the wellness approach to pain management, nurses need to communicate with other members of the healthcare team to formulate a plan that clearly establishes and addresses the person's pain goals, anticipated side effects, and proposed interventions for those side effects. The person and their designated family members are included as members of the decision-making team. Also, proposed interventions should be based on evidence-based guidelines (i.e. the WHO pain relief ladder) and should include non-pharmacological interventions, when appropriate. Although nurses cannot be expected to know all the implications of all analgesics, they can become experts on frequently used drugs and keep references handy for more detailed information about additional interventions.

Other considerations when using opioid analgesics

Nurses are required to have an understanding of the management of side effects of opioids because of there are many adverse effects, and these effects are usually dose-dependent. Many of these side effects will subside as the person develops tolerance. Constipation is the most common adverse effect, however, it is the one that does not subside. Conditions that increase the risk of developing constipation include increased age, diminished mobility, gastrointestinal conditions and medication interactions. Additional adverse effects of opioids include nausea, vomiting, sedation, dry mouth and altered mental status (i.e. delirium, confusion). Less common side effects included urinary retention, pruritus, agitation and respiratory depression. Interventions for preventing and addressing constipation and altered mental state are discussed in Chapters 18 and 14, respectively. Additionally, Box 28-10 summarises a recommended

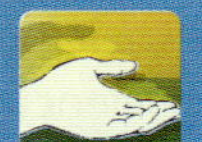

BOX 28-10
Recommendations for maintaining bowel function in people taking opioid medications

Points to remember

- *Tolerance* is your ally with regard to all side effects except constipation
- The hand that writes the opioid order should also write an aperient order, usually coloxyl and senna
- Constipation is an expected adverse effect that should be dealt with from the start

Before requesting a laxative

- Rule out other causes of constipation
- Do not give laxatives if abdominal pain is present
- Reassess daily for responses

A bowel program can include

- Senna and docusate tablets (Senokot)
- Lactulose
- Bisacodyl (Dulcolax)
- Magnesium hydroxide
- Macrogol plus electrolytes (Movicol)
- Non-pharmalogical remedy: daily administration of a fruit paste (including such ingredients as senna tea leaves, prunes, raisins, figs, Nu-lax)

Source: Shillam, C. (2005). Caring for older adults who are experiencing pain. In Miller, C. (Ed.), *Nursing for wellness in older adults* (6th ed.). Philadelphia, PA: Lippincott Williams & Wilkins. Copyright. Used with permission.

BOX 28-11
Commonly used oral analgesics and their approximate equivalence to oral morphine

Panadeine (codeine 8 mg)	=	Oral morphine 1 mg
Panadeine Forte (codeine 30 mg)	=	Oral morphine 3.75 mg
Codeine phosphate 30 mg	=	Oral morphine 3.75 mg
Tramadol 50 mg	=	Oral morphine 10 mg
Endone 5 mg	=	Oral morphine 7.5 mg

regimen for maintaining bowel function in people taking opioid analgesics.

When older adults receive opioid analgesia over long periods the dose, formulation or route of the opioid may be changed. Nurses must have an understanding of the dosage equivalence of the different opioids. Box 28-11 lists common oral opioid doses and their approximate equivalence to oral morphine, while Table 28-7 describes the dose equivalence of transdermal fentanyl patches to morphine.

Pain is a common symptom that requires management when an older adult is receiving palliative care. The principles of analgesic medications are also applicable during palliative care; however, during the end-of-life phase, particularly when the older adult is actively dying, oral administration of analgesia may not be suitable. In the next chapter analgesic considerations is described during the last days and hours of an older adult's life.

A student's perspective

My ageing client complains periodically about pain in her shoulder. She has stated that she does not want to take anything besides Panadol when she has pain and that Panadol seems to take care of her pain. She does not take the Panadol every day. She's afraid of taking pain medications because she does not want to rely on strong medications and she is afraid of becoming addicted. I explained to her the consequences of untreated pain and also tried to ease her fears of pain medication. She assured me that she will see her doctor if the pain becomes severe when Panadol does not help her.

Thelma M.

Non-pharmacological interventions for managing pain

Although analgesics are the mainstay of pain management, non-pharmacological interventions are an essential component of a comprehensive approach for all types of pain. A wellness-oriented approach to pain management for older adults involves the use of a wide variety of interventions to supplement, enhance or diminish the need for pharmacological interventions. One major advantage of non-pharmacological interventions is that they rarely have adverse effects. In addition, non-pharmacological approaches often have broader benefits, such as improved comfort, reduced anxiety and improved quality of life. Lu and Herr (2012) suggest that nurses consider the following non-pharmacological interventions as an integral part of pain management:

- Physical strategies: massage, reflexology, heat and cold, mild exercise, physical therapy, transcutaneous electrical nerve stimulation (TENS units)
- Cognitive-behavioural approaches: relaxation, distraction, hypnosis, biofeedback, guided imagery, music therapy, and spiritual and religious coping strategies (e.g. prayer)
- Biofield therapies and energy medicine techniques: reiki, healing touch therapeutic touch, acupressure, qi therapy
- Education for the person and family: addressing fears and misbeliefs by teaching about nature of pain, signs of its presence, and management goals related to comfort and function, use of pharmacological and non-pharmacological approaches. Evidence-based practice 28-1 summarises recent research related to non-pharmacological approaches to pain management.

Another major role of nurses in pain management is making referrals for specialised services when pain does not respond to usual analgesic approaches, or when people experience persistent pain. For example, palliative care professionals are available in most hospitals and through hospice programs. These programs, which include nurses, doctors, psychologists and other practitioners, use a multidisciplinary approach to assess and manage pain.

Teaching about rehabilitation and self-management strategies is another important aspect of wellness-oriented care for older adults with persistent pain. For example, rehabilitation programs, which include exercise, physical modalities, manual techniques and assistive devices, have been found to provide pain relief, reduce disability and improve function in people with osteoarthritis of the knee and hip (Iversen, 2012). The following case study is about an older adult with osteoarthritis and it provides the opportunity to

TABLE 28-7 Dose equivalence of transdermal fentanyl patches to morphine

Patch strength (mg)	Delivery rate (mcg/hour)	Parenteral morphine dose equivalent (mg/day)	Oral morphine dose equivalent (mg/day)
25	25	30–40	60–100
50	50	60–80	120–200
75	75	90–120	180–300
100	100	120–160	240–400

EVIDENCE-BASED PRACTICE 28-1
Non-pharmacological interventions for persistent pain

Systematic reviews

- Low back pain: evidence in support of yoga, massage, acupuncture, spinal manipulation, progressive relaxation (Cramer, Lauche, Haller et al., 2013; National Center on Complementary and Integrative Health, 2011).
- Acupressure is effective for relieving persistent pain of various types, including chronic headache and low back pain (Chen & Hsiu-Hung, 2013).
- Acupuncture is effective for many types of chronic pain, including osteoarthritis and back, neck and shoulder pain (Vickers, Cronin, Maschino et al., 2012).
- Music is a safe, inexpensive and an independent nursing function that can be used as an adjuvant approach to pain control in hospitalised people (Cole & LoBiondo-Wood, 2014).

Individual studies

- Healing touch may be beneficial for some older adults in long-term care settings as an adjunct for chronic pain (Wardell, Decker & Engebretson, 2012).
- Listening to personal choice of music may be a simple, safe and effective method of reducing pain in people after open heart surgery (Ozer, Karaman, Arslan et al., 2013).
- Using music as a routine part of nursing care is an effective practice for reducing pain intensity in people with neuropathic pain (Korhan, Buyer, Eyigor et al., 2014).
- Relaxation exercises are effective in reducing postoperative pain following upper abdominal surgery (Topcu & Findik, 2012).

Osteoarthritis

(National Center on Complementary and Integrative Health, 2012; Shengelia, Parker, Ballin et al., 2013)

- Acupuncture is the CAM with the most promising evidence of potential benefit in reducing pain and improving joint mobility.
- Some research supports the use of massage and tai chi for reducing pain and improving mobility.
- Yoga may be beneficial for symptoms associated with osteoarthritis (e.g. stress and anxiety), but people with osteoarthritis need to be cautious about overstretching of affected joints and ligaments.
- A few, but not all, studies have found that a combination of glucosamine and chondroitin has potentially beneficial effects for knee osteoarthritis.
- A few, but not all, studies have found that S-Adenosyl-Methionine (SAMe) was effective for small improvements in pain and function.
- There is some evidence to support the use of dietary supplements of devil's claw and avocado–soybean unsaponifiables (ASUs).
- Modalities with little or no evidence of benefits: homeopathy, magnets, topical dimethyl sulfoxide (DMSO), oral methylsulfonylmethane (MSM).

apply knowledge about pharmacological and non-pharmacological interventions.

CASE STUDY TWO

Mrs Vivian Bellagora suffers from osteoarthritis in both knees. She takes two Panadol four times a day (waking, lunch, dinner and bedtime) and whenever the pain gets intolerable.

A brief pain inventory was completed and found that her pain is a "constant aching", especially in her knees. The pain is worse when she is doing the housework and gardening, and moderate in severity (5 to 7 out of 10). However, she further manages her pain by doing short stints of house work or gardening then resting.

Thinking points

- Using the WHO pain ladder, what is the next step in treating Mrs Bellagora's pain from a pharmacological perspective?
- Are there any non-pharmacological interventions recommended that will assist with the management of Mrs Bellagora's pain?

CHAPTER HIGHLIGHTS

Definitions and types of pain

- Nociceptive and neuropathic pain (Figure 28-1; Table 28-1)
- Acute and persistent pain
- Cancer pain

Unique aspects of pain in older adults

- Age-related changes: Aged related changes can affect pain perception and pain management, and pain symptoms may present differently in older and younger adults.
- Prevalence and causes (Box 28-1)
- Barriers to pain: nurses need to identify and address problems that create barriers to effective pain management in older adults (Table 28-2)

Functional consequences of pain in older adults

- The functional consequences of pain in older adults include diminished physical function, loss of mobility, higher levels of disability and decreased quality of life.
- Untreated pain can lead to anxiety, depression or even suicide.

Cultural aspects of pain

- Cultural consideration 28-1

Nursing assessment of pain in older adults

- Identifying common misconceptions (Box 28-3)
- Obtaining information about pain (Figure 28-2; Boxes 28-4 & 28-5)
- Assessing persistent pain (Figure 28-3)
- Assessment in older adults who are cognitively impaired (Table 28-3; Box 28-6; Figures 28-4 & 28-5)

Pharmacological interventions for managing pain

- Principles of analgesia management (Box 28-7)
- Classification of analgesics (Tables 28-4 & 28-5; Box 28-8)
- Misconceptions and realities about analgesics (Table 28-6)
- The WHO three-step pain relief ladder (Figure 28-6; Box 28-9)
- Other considerations when using opioid analgesics (Tables 28-6 & 28-7; Box 28-10; Evidence-based practice 28-1).

Non-pharmacological interventions for managing pain

- Non-pharmacological interventions (Evidence-based practice 28-1)
- Referrals for specialised services
- Teaching about self-management strategies

CRITICAL THINKING EXERCISES

1. Identify an older person in your recent clinical experience who has talked with you about persistent pain and address the following in relation to that person:
   - What factors listed in Box 28-3 affect the person's experience of pain?
   - What characteristics from Box 28-4 are applicable to assessment of pain in that person?
2. Review the barriers to effective pain management related to older adults and families (Table 28-2) and identify ways in which you could overcome these barriers when you care for older adults in clinical practice.
3. Review the information about tolerance, dependence and addiction and write a sentence for each of these concepts in terms that you would use for teaching older adults and their carers.

RESOURCES

For an extensive range of additional resources to enhance teaching and learning and to facilitate understanding of this chapter please see the text's accompanying website located on thePoint at http://thepoint.lww.com.

Clinical tools

City of Hope, Pain & Palliative Care Resource Center: http://prc.coh.org

Hartford Institute for Geriatric Nursing, ConsultGeriRN.org: http://consultgerirn.org/resources

Assessment tools *Try This®* series and *How to Try This* resources

General assessment series

- *Try This* issue 7: Pain assessment for older adults. Flaherty, E. (2012). *Best Practices in Nursing Care to Older Adults.*
- *How to Try This* (article): Using pain-rating scales with older adults. Flaherty, E. (2008). *American Journal of Nursing 108*(6), 40–47.
- *How to Try This* (video): *Pain assessment in older adults.*

Specialty practice series:

- *Try This*, issue SP1: Assessment of nociceptive versus neuropathic pain in older adults. Arnstein, P. (2010). *Best Practices in Nursing Care to Older Adults.*
- View topic-related resources from American Society for Pain Management Nursing (ASPMN).

Dementia series:

- *Try This*, issue D2: Assessing pain in older adults with dementia. Horgas, A. (2012). *Best Practices in Nursing Care to Older Adults.*
- *How to Try This* (article): Pain assessment in people with dementia. Horgas, A. & Miller, L. (2008). *American Journal of Nursing, 108*(7), 62–70.
- *How to Try This* (video): *Pain assessment in people with dementia.*

Evidence-based practice

Australian and New Zealand College of Anaesthetists and Faculty of Pain Medicine. (2010). Acute pain management: Scientific evidence. Available via www.anzca.edu.au.

Australian and New Zealand Society for Geriatric Medicine. Pain in older people. Position statement 21.

Australian Pain Society. (2005). Pain in residential aged care facilities management strategies. Available via www.apsoc.org.au.

Joanna Briggs Institute: http://connect.jbiconnectplus.org

Evidence summary:

- Rathnayake, T. (2014). Pain: Assessment tools.

Systematic review

- Ng, S. Q., Brammer, J. D. & Creedy, D. K. (2012). The psychometric properties, feasibility and utility of behavioural observation methods in pain assessment of cognitively impaired elderly people in acute and long-term care: A systematic review. *Joanna Briggs Institute Library of Systematic Reviews, 10*(17), 977–1085.

National Health and Medical Research Council (NHMRC). Clinical practice guidelines (portal). Available at www.clinicalguidelines.gov.au.

Health education

Australian Pain Society: www.apsoc.org.au

International Association for the Study of Pain: www.iasp-pain.org

National Pain Strategy. Australia: www.chronicpainaustralia.org.au/files/PainStrategy2010Final.pdf

New Zealand Pain Society: www.nzps.org.nz

Pain Australia: www.painaustralia.org.au/healthcare-professionals/research.html

REFERENCES

Abbey, J., De Bellis, A., Piller, N., Esterman, A., Giles, L., Parker, D. & Lowcay, B. (2004). The Abbey Pain Scale: A 1-minute numerical indicator for people with end-stage dementia. *International Journal of Palliative Nursing, 10*(1), 6–13. Accessible March 2015 via www.apsoc.org.au.

Ahn, D. & Horgas, A. (2013). The relationship between pain and disruptive behaviors in nursing home residents with dementia. *BMC Geriatrics, 13*(14). Available March 2015 at www.biomedcentral.com/1471-2318/13/14.

Australian Pain Society (APS). (2005). *Pain in residential aged care facilities: Management strategies*. Sydney: Author. Accessed March 2015 via www.apsoc.org.au.

Bradford, A., Shrestha, S., Snow, A. L., Stanley, M. A., Wilson, N., Hersch, G. & Kunik, M. E. (2012). Managing pain to prevent aggression in people with dementia: A nonpharmacologic intervention. *American Journal of Alzheimer's Disease and Other Dementias, 27*(1), 41–47.

Brown, S. T., Kirkpatrick, M. K., Swanson, M. S. et al. (2011). Pain experience of the elderly. *Pain Management Nursing, 12*(4), 190–196.

Chen, Y.-W. & Hsiu-Hung, W. (2013). The effectiveness of acupressure on relieving pain: A systematic review. *Pain Management Nursing, 15*(2), 539–550.

Clarke, A., Anthony, C., Gray, D. et al. (2012). "I feel so stupid because I can't give a proper answer ..." How older adults describe chronic pain: A qualitative study. *BMC Geriatrics, 12*(78). Available at www.biomedcentral.com/1471-2318/12/78.

Cleeland, C. (1991). Brief Pain Inventory. Houston: Department of Symptom Research, MD Anderson Cancer Centre, University of Texas. Available March 2015 at www.mdanderson.org/education-and-research/departments-programs-and-labs/departments-and-divisions/symptom-research/symptom-assessment-tools/brief-pain-inventory.html.

Co.As.It. (Italian Association of Assistance). (2008). *A profile of Italian Australian culture for aged care service providers*. Sydney: Author.

Cole, L. C. & LoBiondo-Wood, G. (2014). Music as an adjuvant therapy in control of pain and symptoms in hospitalized older adults: A systematic review. *Pain Management Nursing, 15*(1), 406–425.

Cramer, H., Lauche, R., Haller, H. et al. (2013). A systematic review and meta-analysis of yoga for low back pain. *Clinical Journal of Pain, 29*(5), 450–460.

Deumens, P., Steyaert, A., Forget, P. et al. (2013). Prevention of chronic postoperative pain. *Progress in Neurobiology, 104*, 1–37.

Dumas, L. G. & Ramadurai, M. (2009). Pain management in the nursing home. *Nurse Clinicians of North America, 44*, 197–208.

Eggermont, L., Penninx, B., Jones, R. et al. (2012). Depressive symptoms, chronic pain, and falls in older community-dwelling adults: The MOBILIZE Boston Study. *Journal of the American Geriatrics Society, 60*, 230–237.

Fennell, J. A. (2005). Understanding the experience of pain from a Māori perspective. Unpublished Master's Thesis. University of Auckland.

Fuchs-Lacelle, S. & Hadjistavropoulos, T. (2004). Development and preliminary validation of the Pain Assessment Checklist for Seniors with Limited Ability to Communicate (PACSLAC). *Pain Management Nursing, 5*(1), 37–49.

Herr, K., Coyne, P., McCaffery, M. et al. (2011). Pain assessment in the patients unable to self-report. Position statement with clinical practice recommendations. *Pain Management Nursing, 12*(4), 230–250.

Horgas, A. L. Yoon, S. L. & Grall, M. (2012). Pain management. In M. Boltz, E. Capezuti, T. Fulmer & D. Zwicker (Eds), *Evidence-based practice protocols for best practice* (4th ed., pp. 246–267). New York: Springer.

Institute of Medicine (IOM). (2011). *Relieving pain in America: A blueprint for transforming prevention, care, education, and research*. Washington, DC: National Academies Press.

Iversen, M. D. (2012). Rehabilitation interventions for pain and disability in osteoarthritis. *American Journal of Nursing, 112*(3 Suppl. 1), S32–S37.

Jordan, A., Hughes, J., Pakresi, M. et al. (2011). The utility of PAINAD in assessing pain in a UK population with severe dementia. *International Journal of Geriatric Psychiatry, 26*(2), 118–126.

Korhan, E. A., Uyar, M., Eyigor, C. et al. (2014). The effects of music therapy on pain in patients with neuropathic pain. *Pain Management Nursing, 15*(1), 306–314.

Lints-Martindale, A. C., Hadjistavropoulos, T., Lix, L. M. et al. (2012). A comparative investigation of observational pain assessment tools for older adults with dementia. *Clinical Journal of Pain, 28*(3), 226–237.

Lu, D. F. & Herr, K. (2012). Pain in dementia: Recognition and treatment. *Journal of Gerontological Nursing, 38*(2), 8–13.

McCaffery, M. (1968). *Nursing practice theories related to cognition, bodily pain and man-environmental interactions*. Los Angeles, CA: UCLA Students Store.

McGrath, P. (2006). The biggest worry ... Research findings on pain management in Aboriginal peoples in Northern Territory, Australia. *Rural and Remote Health, 6(3)*, 549.

McGreevy, K., Bottros, M. M. & Raja, S. N. (2011). Preventing chronic pain following acute pain. *European Journal of Pain, 5*(2), 365–372.

McKenna, L. & Lim, A. G. (2014). *McKenna's pharmacology for nursing and health professionals* (2nd ed.). Sydney: Lippincott, Williams & Wilkins.

Monroe, T. B. & Mion, L. C. (2012). Patients with advanced dementia: How do we know if they are in pain? *Geriatric Nursing, 33*(3), 226–228.

National Center on Complementary and Integrative Health. (2011). Get the facts: Chronic pain and CAM—At a glance. Available March 2015 at https://nccih.nih.gov/health/pain/chronic.htm.

National Center on Complementary and Integrative Health. (2012). Get the facts: Osteoarthritis and complementary health approaches. Available March 2015 at https://nccih.nih.gov/health/arthritis/osteoarthritis.

National Pain Summit Initiative (2010). National pain strategy: Pain management for all Australians. Accessed March 2015 at www.painaustralia.org.au/the-national-pain-strategy/national-pain-strategy.htm .

New Zealand Ministry of Health (2012). *The health of New Zealand adults 2011/12: Key findings of the New Zealand Health Survey*. Wellington: Author. Accessed March 2015 at www.health.govt.nz/publication/health-new-zealand-adults-2011-12.

Ozer, N., Karaman, O., Arslan, S. et al. (2013). Effect of music on postoperative pain and physiologic parameters of patients after open heart surgery. *Pain Management Nursing, 14*(1), 20–28.

Pain Australia (2014). Why we need the National Pain Strategy. Accessed March 2015 at www.painaustralia.org.au/the-national-pain-strategy/why-we-need-the-nps.html.

Palliative Care (2014). Facts about morphine and other opioid medicines in palliative care. Accessed March 2015 at www.palliativecare.org.au/portals/46/resources/FactsAboutMorphine.pdf.

Palmer, D. (n.d.). Pain relief. In Central Australian Rural Practitioners Association (CARPA). (2003). *Reference book for the remote primary health care manuals* to accompany *CARPA standard treatment manual* (4th ed.). Alice Springs: Centre for Remote Health. Accessed March 2015 at www.carpa.org.au/drupal/node/35 and www.carpa.org.au/Ref%20Manual%204th%20Ed/Emergency%20&%20assessment/Pain_relief.pdf.

Pasero, C. & McCaffery, M. (2011a). Initiating opioid therapy. In C. Pasero & M. McCaffery (Eds), *Pain assessment and pharmacologic management* (pp. 442–461). St Louis, MO: Mosby Elsevier.

Pasero, C. & McCaffery, M. (2011b). Misconceptions that hamper assessment and treatment of patients who report pain. In C. Pasero & M. McCaffery (Eds), *Pain assessment and pharmacologic management* (pp. 20–48). St Louis, MO: Mosby Elsevier.

Pasero, C. & McCaffery, M. (2011c). Assessment tools. In C. Pasero & M. McCaffery (Eds), *Pain assessment and pharmacologic management* (pp. 49–142). St Louis, MO: Mosby Elsevier.

Pasero, C. & Portenoy, R. K. (2011). Neurophysiology of pain and analgesia and the pathophysiology of neuropathic pain. In C. Pasero & M. McCaffery (Eds), *Pain assessment and pharmacologic management* (pp. 1–12). St Louis, MO: Mosby Elsevier.

Pasero, C., Portenoy, R. K. & McCaffery, M. (2011). Nonopioid analgesics. In C. Pasero & M. McCaffery (Eds), *Pain assessment and pharmacologic management* (pp. 177–180). St Louis, MO: Mosby Elsevier.

Pasero, C., Quinn, T. W., Portenoy, R. K., McCaffery, M. & Rizos, A. (2011). Opioid analgesics. In C. Pasero & M. McCaffery (Eds), *Pain assessment and pharmacologic management* (pp. 277–282). St Louis, MO: Mosby Elsevier.

Pergolizzi, J. V., Raffa, R. B. & Taylor, R. (2012). Treating acute pain in light of the chronification of pain. *Pain Management Nursing, 15*(1), 380–390.

Planton, J. & Edlund, B. J. (2010). Regulatory components for treating persistent pain in long-term care. *Journal of Gerontological Nursing, 36*(4), 49–56.

Polomano, R. C., Rathmell, J. P., Krenzischek, D. A. & Dunwoody, C. J. (2008). Emerging trends and new approaches to acute pain management. *Pain Management Nursing, 9*(1), S33–S41.

Purnell, L. D. (2014). *Guide to culturally competent health care* (6th ed.). Philadelphia, PA: F. A. Davis.

Registered Nurses Association of Ontario (RNAO). (2013). *Assessment and management of pain in the elderly* (3rd ed.). Accessed March 2015 via http://rnao.ca.

Reid, M. C., Bennett, D. A., Chen, W. G., Eldadah, B. A., Farrar, J. T., Ferrell, B. et al. (2011). Improving the pharmacologic management of pain in older adults. *Pain Medicine, 12*(9), 1336–1357.

Rustoen, T., Wahl, A. K., Hanestad, B. R., Lerdal, A., Paul, S. & Miaskowski, C. (2005). Age and the experience of chronic pain: Differences in health and quality of life among younger, middle-aged, and older adults. *Clinical Journal of Pain, 21*(6), 513–523.

Shengelia, R., Parker, S. J., Ballin, M. et al. (2013). Complementary therapies for osteoarthritis: Are they effective? *Pain Management Nursing, 14*(4), e274–e288.

Shillam, C. (2005). Caring for older adults who are experiencing pain. In Miller, C. (Ed.), *Nursing for wellness in older adults* (6th ed.). Philadelphia, PA: Lippincott Williams & Wilkins.

Siedlecki, S. L., Modic, M. B., Bernhofer, E. et al. (2014). Exploring how bedside nurses care for patients with chronic pain: A grounded theory study. *Pain Management Nursing, 15*(3), 565–573.

Taverner, T., Closs, S. J. & Briggs, M. (2014). The journey to chronic pain: A grounded theory of older adults' experiences of pain associated with leg ulceration. *Pain Management Nursing, 15*(1), 186–198.

Topcu, S. Y. & Findik, U. Y. (2012). Effect of relaxation exercises on controlling postoperative pain. *Pain Management Nursing, 13*(1), 11–17.

Tsai, P. & Means, K. M. (2005). Osteoarthritic knee or hip pain: Possible indicators in elderly adults with cognitive impairment. *Journal of Gerontological Nursing, 31*(8), 39–45.

Tse, M., Wan, V. & Vong, S. (2013). Health-related profile and quality of life among nursing home residents: Does pain matter? *Pain Management Nursing, 14*(4), e173–e184.

Van de Ven, T. J. & John Hsia, H. L. (2012). Causes and prevention of chronic postsurgical pain. *Current Opinion in Critical Care, 18*(4), 366–371.

Vickers, A. J., Cronin, A. M., Maschino, A. C. et al. (2012). Acupuncture may be helpful for chronic pain: A meta-analysis. *Archives of Internal Medicine, 172*(19), 1444–1453.

Wardell, D., Decker, S. A. & Engebretson, J. C. (2012). Healing touch for older adults with persistent pain. *Holistic Nursing Practice, 26*(4), 194–202.

Warden, V., Hurley, A. C. & Volicer, L. (2003). Development and psychometric evaluation of the Pain Assessment in Advanced Dementia (PAINAD) scale. *Journal of the American Medical Directors Association, 4*, 9–15.

World Health Organization (WHO). (2005). Pain Relief Ladder. Accessed March 2015 at www.who.int/cancer/palliative/painladder/en.

World Health Organization (WHO). (2015). Essential medicines and health products: Impact of impaired access to controlled medications. Accessed March 2015 at www.who.int/medicines/areas/quality_safety/Impaired_Access/en.

Wysong, P. (2014). Nurses' beliefs and self-reported practices related to pain assessment in nonverbal patients. *Pain Management Nursing, 15*(1), 176–185.

Zwakhalen, S. M., van der Steen, J. T. & Najim, M. D. (2012). Which score most likely represents pain on the observational PAINAD pain scale for patients with dementia? *Journal of the American Medical Directors Association, 13*(4), 384–389.

Chapter 29

Caring for older adults at the end of life

By Carol Miller and Sharyn Hunter

LEARNING OBJECTIVES

After reading this chapter, you should be able to:

1. Define end of life, the terminal phase and the actively dying process.
2. Describe how perspectives on end-of-life care have changed in response to demographic and healthcare trends.
3. Identify cultural factors that influence end-of-life care.
4. Describe palliative care and hospice services.
5. Explain components of a dignified death.
6. Describe nursing interventions to address physical symptoms commonly experienced by older adults during the end of life and during the terminal phases
7. Discuss ways of meeting emotional needs of patients and families and self-care needs of nurses.

KEY TERMS

active dying
death
dignified death
end of life
hospice care
medicalisation of end-of-life care
palliative care

Because of the dramatic increases in both life expectancy and the length of time living with chronic conditions, there has been increasing emphasis on providing supportive care during chronic and life-limiting illness and at the end of life. Because many illnesses that once were fatal have become chronic conditions, much of the healthcare focus is on helping older adults achieve quality of life while living with disabilities and chronic conditions and at some point experience a dignified death. Major emphasis also is on addressing the complex and diverse needs of family and all those people who assume caregiving roles for older adults during times of illness and at the end of life. Chapter 27 discusses care of older adults during progressive chronic conditions, and this chapter addresses care at the end of life.

PERSPECTIVES ON END-OF-LIFE CARE

Concepts related to death, dying and end of life have changed since the 1900s when the average life expectancy at birth was much lower than it is today (see Chapter 1). In the early 1990s people usually died at home with their family, friends and community caring for them. Dying was usually after a short, acute illness from either an infection or injury. Today most people die in healthcare institutions, and they are older and dying as a consequence of a chronic illness. Many factors have contributed to major shifts in the perceptions of death and dying and the ways in which end-of-life care is provided.

When does end-of-life care begin?

Death has traditionally been defined as the cessation of all biological functions. In many situations, however, major medical and technological developments have changed the perception of death from a clearly defined event, to an evolving process. This is especially common in acute care settings, where, for example, a person can be considered legally dead resulting from the absence of brain function, but not be clinically dead if medical technology has sustained heart and lung functioning. For many older adults, the **end of life** (EOL) may be a gradual process that is associated with the cumulative effects of chronic illness and many interacting conditions, rather than a single cause. In many cases, a major medical event, such as sepsis or a fractured hip, becomes the "tipping point" that causes the older adult to transition from a state of chronic illness to an end-of-life state in which death occurs. Consequently, end-of-life is not clearly defined, that is, "… what is the interval referred to as end of life or what is end-of-life care" (Izumi et al., 2012, p. 608). In the literature there are a range of definitions, from the last 2 years of life to the final 3 days. In Australia it is defined as the last 12 months or so of a person's life (National Health and Medical Research Council [NHMRC], 2011, p. 21). New Zealand's definition is "The end of life phase begins when a judgement is made that death is imminent. It may be the judgement of the health/social care professional or team responsible for the care of the patient, but it is often the patient or family who first recognises its beginning (Palliative Care Council of New Zealand, Hospice New Zealand & the Ministry of Health, 2012, p. 5).

In this chapter EOL refers to the phase of life when care is focused on comfort and supports a dignified death. Within EOL there is another phase of care when the person is actively dying, and this is referred to as the *terminal phase* or the *actively dying process*. However, recognising when an older adult enters the terminal phase is not easy and is complicated by disease and ageing changes. The different progressions of end-of-life have been described as:

1. Expected death trajectory: steep progressive decline, with prolonged terminal phase
2. Mixed death trajectory: initial successful treatment and period of stability, followed by steep decline and short terminal phase
3. Unexpected death trajectory: slow decline (i.e. periodic exacerbations with recovery never reaching former level of health), followed by extremely short terminal phase. (Penrod, Hupcey, Baney et al., 2011)

Irrespective of the phase of EOL, the goal of care is to prepare the person for death and promote comfort by managing the symptoms that are commonly experienced by those who are dying. Providing practical, psychological and spiritual support to the carer/caregivers while the person is dying and into bereavement period is also a key role of nurses during EOL care (Palliative Care Council of New Zealand, Hospice New Zealand & the Ministry of Health, 2012). Some researchers suggest that carers need to be encouraged to "seek normal" during each phase of the different EOL trajectories (Penrod, Hupcey, Shipley et al., 2012). This is illustrated in Figure 29-1. However, the early phase of these trajectories is not always definitive and may be subtle and recognised only in retrospect, as is often the case with older adults living with dementia.

Views of death and dying in Western culture

Western culture tends to deny or ignore the universality of death and this influences the type of healthcare services provided to people who are dying. Social gerontology studies have identified the following four contemporary values or beliefs that shape perceptions about ageing and death in Western societies (Markson, 2003):

1. Work and activity are intertwined with a person's self-worth, and chronic illness or disability is associated with the end of productivity and loss of purpose. Consequently, people may not acknowledge illness and ageing because they are viewed as predecessors to death.
2. Through self-determination and individual responsibility, anyone can do anything if he or she tries hard enough. Because human life has inherent limitations, this false mentality is a major underpinning to the denial of ageing and death in the 21st century.
3. Medical advances of the last several decades foster the belief that ageing, illness and even death can be manipulated, managed and controlled.
4. Authority over and responsibility for death has subtly transferred from religious leaders to physicians. Consequently, the ability to cure illness and prolong life has imbued life and death with qualities that are more humanistic and less spiritual.

Despite these prevalent attitudes and beliefs, the acknowledgement and acceptance of death has been increasing, along with a focus on a more holistic view of end-of-life care. This change is due largely to the baby boom generation facing its own ageing process while simultaneously dealing with their parents' ageing and health issues. In addition, people living with serious and progressive conditions that significantly limit quality of life are increasingly expressing a desire to control their destiny.

Older adults' perspectives on death and dying

Although younger generations may feel they are invincible and immune to disease or death, older adults tend to be more aware and accepting of the inevitability of death, in part because they have experienced the deaths of family and friends, often including those who are younger than they are. Even though illness and functional limitations are common during older adulthood older adults who develop a holistic perspective recognise that old age can present opportunities for fulfilment and self-actualisation. As such, a "good death" is viewed as part of the process of "ageing well", and both processes are individualised. Defining a "good death" for older adults is extremely personal and strongly influenced by one's level of function, independence and quality of life. Also, although older adults may have an increased awareness of the inevitability of death, true acceptance of death is not a clearly defined process and, even at the end of life, humans "rhythmically oscillate between acceptance and non-acceptance of death" (McLeod-Sordjan, 2013, p. 391).

Culturally diverse perspectives on death and dying

Because cultural perspectives exert a strong influence on end-of-life experiences, all healthcare professionals need to be aware of their own culturally based perceptions as well as those that influence older adults. Cultural influences can affect all of the following aspects of end-of-life care:

- Perceptions of a good death
- Acceptance of hospice and palliative care services
- The role of family, carers and others
- Lines of communication about pending death and end-of-life decisions
- Expectations about medical interventions (e.g. decisions about resuscitation)
- Place where death occurs
- Practices and rituals near the end of death and immediately following death
- Decisions about autopsy or organ donations.

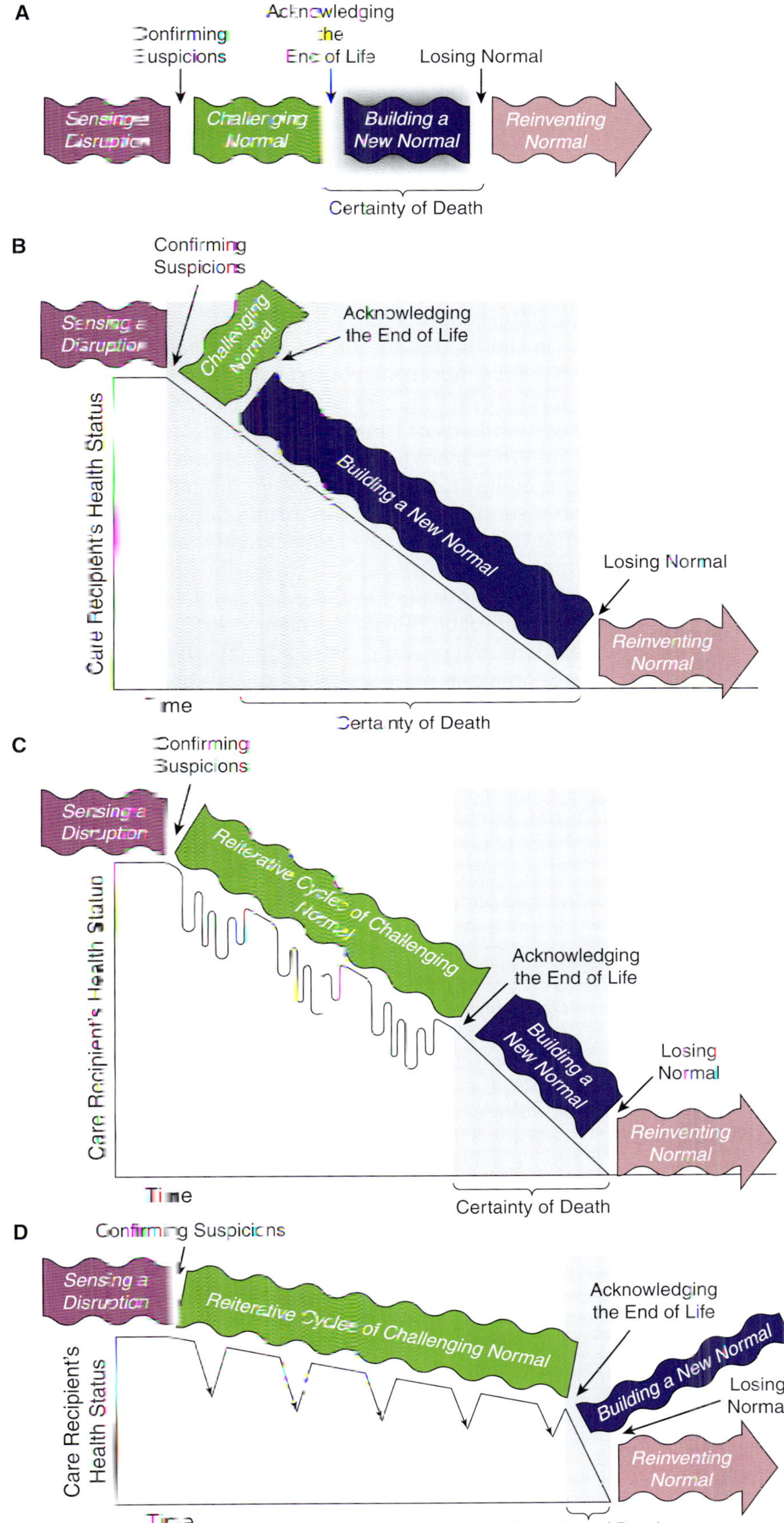

FIGURE 29-1 A model of caregiving through the end of life that illustrates variations in the course and duration of phases. (**A**) Basic model, (**B**) caregiving across the expected death trajectory, (**C**) caregiving across the mixed death trajectory, (**D**) caregiving across the unexpected death trajectory. (Adapted with permission from Sage Publications: Penrod, J., Hupcey, J. E., Shipley, P. Z. et al. [2012]. A model of caregiving through the end of life: Seeking normal. *Western Journal of Nursing Research, 34*[2], 175–193.)

A student's perspective

This week, I learned that it is okay to accept that an older patient is ready to die and that is his/her wish. I had a patient who requested that we not perform any measures—just give him his beer with lunch, wine with dinner, and some pain medicine to make him comfortable. He stated that he has led a good life and is ready to go see God. That is really hard for me because it's my job to help people and save lives. The other aspect of that is helping people die a dignified death—it's just a really TOUGH aspect!!!

Sarah E.

Because the experience of death and dying is very personal, nurses should incorporate cultural considerations into individualised assessments and be aware of diverse beliefs and attitudes associated with the experience of death and dying. (See Chapter 2 for more information about culture and provision of healthcare for the major cultural groups in Australia and New Zealand.) Both the National Palliative Care Strategy and the New Zealand Palliative Care Strategy utilise a coordinated approach that respectively addresses cultural considerations appropriate for Australia and New Zealand. More information about caring for Indigenous Australians who are dying is provided through the Aboriginal and Torres Strait Islander Health Branch of Queensland Health. Its guide, Sad news, sorry business: Guidelines for caring for Aboriginal and Torres Strait Islander people through death and dying, can be accessed via www.health.qld.gov.au and via the Australian Indigenous Health*InfoNet*'s palliative care section at www.healthinfonet.ecu.edu.au.

Booklets are available from the Medical Council of New Zealand that contain information about death and dying in Māori and Pacific cultures via www.mcnz.org.nz. Another worthwhile resource is a presentation by Warihi Campbell, titled, A Māori approach to ageing, spirituality and palliative care, accessible via www.familycentre.org.nz/About/ICPCC/index.html.

An important step in providing culturally safe nursing care is to explore one's own beliefs about death, dying and end of life. Some questions to ponder for self-awareness and insight include the following:

- When you hear the word "death", what comes to your mind? What do you personally fear the most? What are you most curious about?
- How old were you the first time someone close to you died? How was grief handled in your family? What do you believe happens to you when you die?
- Have you ever seen anyone die? What was that like for you?
- How do your own attitudes and previous experiences affect the way you work with dying patients now? (Ohio State University Health Sciences Center, 2003)

In addition to being aware of one's own culturally-based beliefs and attitudes, nurses need to identify those held by each person for whom they provide care. Religion and spirituality are two aspects of culture that are particularly powerful in relation to beliefs about death, dying and end-of-life decisions. Although it may be easy to ask about a person's religious affiliation as part of a nursing assessment, the more challenging aspect of providing culturally appropriate care is identifying the person's beliefs and values that affect their care. Nurses accomplish this by asking exploratory questions with a non-judgemental approach about customs, beliefs and concerns about death, dying, afterlife and end of life, as described in the section on communication.

In clinical settings, nurses are integrally involved with one of the most concrete aspects of end-of-life care: post-mortem care. This care is directed by institutional policies and standards of care and is a routine aspect of nursing care. What is not routine, however, is the incorporation of end-of-life rituals, which are often culturally based and are an essential aspect of supporting families and carers. A study of long-term care nurses found that those who were foreign born stressed the need for end-of-life rituals, whereas those born in the U.S. did not see this as important (Periyakoil, Stevens & Kraemer, 2013). Cultural considerations 29-1 provides information about death rituals that are commonly associated with specific groups. It also suggests interventions that nurses can apply in different situations. As with other aspects of culturally appropriate care, it is important to be aware of different practices associated with particular groups and at the same time avoid stereotypes. An effective way of addressing this issue is to inquire ahead of time about the preferences of older adults, families and carers, and incorporate pertinent information in the care plan.

A student's perspective

I found myself in a situation today in which I quickly recognised the importance of the lesson on cultural sensitivity in nursing. An ageing client unfortunately had a significant change over the weekend, and her husband requested for her to be transported to the hospice. As she and I sat on her bed, she verbalised her acceptance that her disease is terminal. She wept as she voiced her heartache in telling her family of her "disappointment". Even though she is Catholic, because of her Chinese heritage and her family's Buddhist belief in "saving face", she worries that she has let her family down. While she expressed her thoughts, I listened and provided emotional support, which seemed to ease some of her grief. We transported her to the hospice, and I assisted in making her comfortable with the new environment.

When I went out to the nurses' station to give my report, the receiving nurse's first comment to me was, "I see she is Asian and you have her religious preference documented as Catholic. Are you sure that is correct?" Because of our recent discussions and reading on cultural sensitivity, I quickly realised how we as nurses can make incorrect assumptions in categorising individuals based on their ethnicity. I reported about my client's childhood history, her parents' belief in Buddhism, the Catholic

CULTURAL CONSIDERATIONS 29-1
Death rituals commonly associated with specific groups

Group	Death ritual	Intervention
Chinese (Buddhists)[*]	Funeral details are discussed only by family; Monk to be in attendance.	Do not discuss funeral details openly with family. Summon Monk.
Europeans	Believe that the dying person should not be left alone.	Make accommodations for family members to be present at all times.
Filipinos	A large gathering of relatives and friends may attend the dying person and place religious artifacts around the person; candles are lit after death to illuminate the path of the spirit to the afterlife.	Arrange for a gathering place close to the dying person, find electric candles if open flames are not allowed; summon clergy for religious rituals; do not move religious items.
Greek—Greek Orthodox	Priest to be in attendance. The deceased's body is considered highly sacred. The body is placed eastward. Family may be highly emotional.	Summon clergy. Facilitate positioning of bed. Offer understanding of grief behaviours.
Hindus, Indians	Priest and eldest son may perform death rites, with all male relatives assisting; women may respond with loud wailing.	Provide a supportive and private environment; offer understanding of death rituals and grief behaviours.
Indigenous Australians[†]	Where death is expected there is usually a gathering of many family and friends. It is taboo for Aboriginals to mention the name of the deceased person.	Provide a larger private room for the person to accommodate the large number of visitors. Ask the family for the appropriate word to use instead of their name following death.
Italian Catholics	Last rites must be performed. A large gathering of family and relatives may gather at the bedside. Emotions can be openly displayed. Emotional support is usually by family and not nurses.	Summon clergy. Arrange privacy for family and relatives during this time. Organise an area for family and relatives to express their emotions in private. Offer understanding of grief behaviours.
Japanese	Family members gather at the bedside at the time of death, with the eldest son having particular responsibilities at the time.	Notify eldest son of pending death; identify lines of communication if eldest son is not available.
Jews	Dying person should not be left alone; death rituals vary and some are not performed on the Sabbath or holy days.	Ask the closest relative specifically about postmortem practices.
Khmer (Buddhist)	The deceased's body to be handled by family.	Provide a supportive private environment for family to wash and dress the deceased person.
Koreans	Family members are expected to stay with the person who is dying and assist with care.	Support family in caring for the person.
Māori[‡]	Death is an occasion for family. When the person dies the Māori believe the body is not vacated immediately by the spirit. The deceased will be visited at all times and the visitors will be talking and recalling the deceased's life. The family may wish to handle the deceased's body.	Provide a supportive private environment for family to wash and dress the deceased person.
Pacific people[§]	Funeral rites are very important complex and vary depending on the Pacific culture. It is not uncommon for the families to want to remain with the deceased and they may wish to wash and dress the body.	Is it important that this information is accessed preferably well before the death.
Muslim groups	The bed should be turned to face the holy city of Mecca; family recites prayers from the Qur'an.	Facilitate positioning of the bed whenever possible; provide privacy for prayers.
Vietnamese	Flowers are avoided during illness because they are usually reserved for rites of the dead.	Ask permission from the patient or family before placing flowers in a room.

Purnell, L. D. (2014). *Guide to culturally competent health care*. Philadelphia, PA: F. A. Davis.
*Palliative Care Australia. (1999). Multicultural palliative care guidelines. Available March 2015 via www.palliativecare.org.au.
†Australian Government Department of Health and Ageing (DoHA). (2004). Providing culturally appropriate palliative care to Aboriginal and Torres Strait Islander peoples: Resource kit. Accessible March 2015 via http://webarchive.nla.gov.au.
‡bpac[nz] (2006). Providing palliative care to Māori. Accessed March 2015 at www.bpac.org.nz/resources/campaign/palliative/palliative_maori.asp.
§Medical Council of New Zealand. (2010). Best health outcomes for Pacific peoples: Practice implications. Accessed March 2015 via www.mcnz.org.nz.

she was taught in school, and her long and strong Catholic faith. I found myself really understanding the importance of educating ourselves as nurses about different cultures and the effect of cultural belief systems on individualised healthcare. As difficult as it was for me to leave my client in a strange environment, I felt that the information I had learned and shared would enable the staff to be respectful of her beliefs, which in turn would be a positive experience for my client during her stay.

Deborah L.

Trends in providing end-of-life care

Just as medical and technological advances have changed perspectives on death (such as control of communicable diseases and medical and surgical treatments for serious illnesses), major medical advances that began during the 20th century have shifted approaches to end-of-life care. By the middle of the 20th century, healthcare facilities had become centres for curing disease, and healthcare professionals viewed death as something to be avoided because it symbolised failure. Prolonging life, even at the expense of quality, was viewed as the ultimate accomplishment: a symbol of success for patients, families and the healthcare teams involved. The term **medicalisation of end-of-life care** describes care that focuses on prolonging life through the use of medical technology rather than on interventions for comfort and quality of life.

Despite the move away from this type of care, studies confirm that patients continue to experience pain, indignity, social isolation and uncomfortable symptoms related to ineffective and unwanted life-sustaining treatments, particularly in intensive care units (Seaman, 2013). Much of this concern is associated with poor communication between professionals and families about end-of-life decision making (Wiegand, Grant & Cheon, 2013). An expected outcome of the inclusion of palliative care is that many of these issues will be resolved.

Hospitals remain one of the most common sites of death for people living in Australia and New Zealand. In Australia in 2008, people aged 65 years and over accounted for about 80% of all deaths, of which 50% were aged 80 and over (Palliative Care Australia, 2010). Approximately 51% of these deaths occurred in hospital (Australian Institute of Health and Welfare [AIHW], 2014). Three-quarters of these deaths were due to a chronic disease and could have been anticipated. In New Zealand, approximately 80% of the deaths in 2014 were for people aged 65 and over (Palliative Care Council, 2014). Most deaths in New Zealand occurred in long-term residential care, 38%, then 34% in hospitals, 18% in private households, and 5% in a hospice. New Zealand has a higher level of deaths in long-term residential care than Australia, at 32%.

In Australia and New Zealand, **palliative care** can be provided in a person's own home, a specialist inpatient hospice, a hospital, long-term residential care or other healthcare facility. Where the person receives palliative care is now increasingly dependent on their needs and wishes. It has been reported in Australia that 36.8% of patients living with dementia and 58% of patients with motor neuron disease were referred to palliative care services while in hospital (AIHW, 2011). However, people with other chronic diseases such as COPD and heart failure were less so.

It is expected that older adults in Australia and New Zealand will increasingly access palliative care services. The national palliative care programs that exist in both Australia and New Zealand have facilitated this trend. Also in Australia, the implementation of the palliative approach for older adults in long-term residential care and in the community has reduced the incidence of transfer of older adults during the final stage of their life to hospitals (AIHW, 2014).

As the various types of palliative care—including end-of-life care—are becoming a more integral part of the medical mainstream, the issue of quality of life versus quantity of life at all costs has broadened the professional perspective. Nurses and other healthcare professionals increasingly realise they can find meaning, rewards and satisfaction in caring for people at the end of life and for families and others who are an integral part of the dying person's support network. Palliative care professionals play a key role in promoting awareness and understanding of holistic end-of-life care, both as direct providers of care and as consultants for those who are less skilled in this area, as discussed in the section on hospice and palliative care.

HOSPICE AND PALLIATIVE CARE

Both hospice and palliative care refer to an interdisciplinary approach to care that holistically addresses the needs of people with life-limiting conditions as well as their families and others who care for and care about them. All hospice programs include palliative care, but palliative care is also provided outside hospice programs. Palliative care is discussed in Chapter 27 and, in this chapter, it is presented as an integral part of hospice and end-of-life care.

Hospice care

Hospice care refers to a philosophy of care that seeks to support dignified dying or a good death experience for people with terminal illnesses and for their families and carers. The term *hospice* (from the same linguistic root as "hospitality") was first applied to specialised care for dying patients in the 1960s by physician and nurse Dame Cicely Saunders, who founded the first modern hospice—St Christopher's—in a residential suburb of London.

Another influencing factor was the publication of the book *On death and dying* by psychiatrist Elisabeth Kübler-Ross in 1969. This book, based on interviews with dying patients, identified five stages through which many terminally ill patients progress: denial, anger, bargaining, depression and acceptance (Kübler-Ross, 1969). Since the 1980s the growth of hospice programs has increased the percentage of deaths at home and studies confirm that this has led to better symptom management and overall satisfaction with care (Lysaght & Ersek, 2013). Hospice services usually include the following:

- Hospice treats the person, not the disease; focuses on the family, not the individual; and emphasises the quality of life, not the duration
- Hospice care relies on the combined knowledge and skill of an interdisciplinary team of professionals, including medical practitioners, nurses, home care assistants, social workers, counsellors and volunteers
- Hospice care is a cost-effective alternative to the high costs associated with hospitals and traditional institutional care. (World Health Organization [WHO], 2014, p. 5)

Hospice services are provided by interdisciplinary teams and include the following services: doctors; nurses; home care workers; social workers; spiritual counsellors; volunteers; bereavement counsellors; and speech therapists, physiotherapists and occupational therapists. Some programs offer additional services such as music, art, Reiki and pet therapy. These services are provided by public and private agencies in any setting, including homes, hospitals, long-term residential facilities, or free-standing hospice centres.

In New Zealand hospice services are provided differently than in Australia. There are 29 hospice services operating throughout the country—each an independent not for profit organisation whose services are specifically designed to meet the needs of the community in which they work. Box 29-1 contains an overview of Hospice New Zealand, the national organisation representing all the hospice services in New Zealand. Hospice care is provided free of charge and is funded primarily from contracts with central government, but also from community contributions via fundraising.

In Australia the national government, through Medicare, funds hospice services. To access hospice services, a referral from a medical practitioner is required. Hospice programs offer the following services:

- Medical and nursing care
- Home/outreach services
- Therapies such as music, art and other supportive services
- Social work and counselling services
- Spiritual care
- Bereavement counselling, including support programs for 1 year after death
- Inpatient care for pain and symptom management
- Carer respite
- Advisory services to other professionals in the field of palliative care
- Education and training, including university students; for example nurses, social workers and medical students.

BOX 29-1
Overview of Hospice New Zealand

Hospice New Zealand

Our purpose is to ensure all New Zealanders have access to the best possible hospice care at the end of their lives.

Our mission is to be recognised leaders of the hospice movement and support our members:

1. To enhance quality and consistency in the delivery of hospice care
2. To support a high performing hospice/palliative care workforce
3. By advocating for the provision of hospice-palliative care for all New Zealanders and providing central leadership and direction
4. By increasing awareness of hospice in New Zealand
5. By being a highly effective, well resourced and well managed national organisation.

All hospices throughout the country share the same vision that anyone who is dying has the opportunity to celebrate their life with the help of hospice

Our organisational values are a cornerstone of our work:

Patients always come first—every decision we make is based on this belief

Caring—we genuinely care about our people, patients and their families' needs

Respect—we demonstrate respect in all our dealings with patients and their families' needs, recognising diversity

Professionalism—in all instances we will act professionally and with compassion

Determined—we are driven to work in partnership with our communities

Source: Hospice New Zealand. Accessed March 2015 at www.hospice.org.nz.

An important role for nurses in all settings is to encourage older adults and their families to find information about hospice, even in the absence of a clearly defined "terminal" phase. Hospice programs usually arrange for exploratory meetings to discuss services and they can suggest alternative programs (e.g. palliative care) if the person is not immediately eligible.

PROMOTING WELLNESS AT THE END OF LIFE

Wellness at the end of life is closely connected to the concept of a "good death". Terms such as **dignified death** or dignified care are more appropriate for describing a good death. The degree to which hospital care is perceived as dignified is influenced by many variables, such as the following ones that are directly related to nurses: attitude and behaviours, promotion of patient independence, professional commitment and competency, and verbal and non-verbal communication, including compassionate behaviour and taking enough time (Lin, Watson & Tsai, 2013; Manookian, Cheraghi & Nasrabadi, 2014).

Some characteristics of dignified care identified in studies (Cairns, Williams, Victor et al., 2013; van Gennip et al.,

2013) that are most pertinent to promoting wellness for older adults at the end of life are as follows:

- Being treated as an individual and with respect
- Maintaining independence, while having basic care needs met
- Being involved in decision making
- Having privacy and a safe environment
- Being listened to and having needs and wishes respected
- Experiencing good communication
- Feeling peaceful and ready to die
- Absence of anxiety and depressive mood.

These characteristics are in accord with the "Dying Patient's Bill of Rights" (Austin ,1975), to identify concretely the dignified care that dying people deserve (Box 29-2). This document continues to be helpful as a guide for defining goals and interventions for individualised end-of-life care.

Nurses can use the terms "dignified death" and "dignified life closure" to describe issues related to EOL. Dignified life closure is defined as "personal actions to maintain control when approaching end of life". The following goals that achieve wellness outcomes are related to the issue of dignified life closure: maintenance of physical independence, participation in decisions related to care, sharing feelings about dying, maintenance of sense of control of remaining time, completion of meaningful goals, sharing of feelings about dying, discussion of spiritual concerns and experiences, the exchange of affection with others, and involvement in treatment choices, including food and drink intake (Moorhead, Johnson, Maas et al., 2013, p. 201). Nursing interventions to achieve these outcomes are discussed in the next section.

BOX 29-2
The Dying Patient's Bill of Rights

I have the right to be treated as a living human being until I die.
I have the right to maintain a sense of hopefulness, however changing its focus may be.
I have the right to express my feelings and emotions about my approaching death in my own way.
I have the right to participate in decisions concerning my care.
I have the right to expect continuing medical and nursing attention even though cure goals must be changed to comfort goals.
I have the right not to die alone.
I have the right to be free from pain.
I have the right to have my questions answered honestly.
I have the right not to be deceived.
I have the right to have help from and for my family in accepting my death.
I have the right to die in peace and with dignity.
I have the right to retain my individuality and not be judged for my decisions, which may be contrary to the beliefs of others.
I have the right to be cared for by caring, sensitive, knowledgeable people who will attempt to understand my needs and will be able to gain some satisfaction in helping me face my death.
I have the right to be cared for by those who can maintain a sense of hopefulness, however changing this might be.
I have the right to expect that the sanctity of the human body will be respected after death.
I have the right to discuss and enlarge my religious and/or spiritual experiences, whatever these may mean to others.

Source: Austin, L. (1975). Dying Patient's Bill of Rights. Created at The Terminally Ill Patient and the Helping Person Workshops. Sponsored by the Southwest Michigan Inservice Education Council in Lansing, MI.

DIVERSITY NOTE

Perceptions of dignity at the end of life are influenced by religious teachings. For example, the dignity of life in the Catholic faith is rooted around Jesus, who was human and gave respect to all human life. In the Jewish faith, dignity of life is based in the belief that life and death are in God's hands, and humans have the responsibility to live life to the fullest and have life last as long as possible (Zamer & Volker, 2013).

A student's perspective

When I left the nursing home today I felt better about working with people facing the certain end of their lives. Mr F. had a really positive attitude about his inoperable brain tumour and it made me understand that I am the one who feels uncomfortable with death. He expressed that his life has meaning and that he is here for a reason. He told me about some of his goals in life: he plans to get out of the nursing home so that he can travel around the country in an RV with his wife. He seemed to imply that even if that goal never occurred, it was okay, that it was mostly something to look forward to. All of the communication with Mr F. had a huge impact on me. It gave me a whole new perspective on how people view their lives. This man is suffering from this terrible disease, yet he still finds hope and has goals in life.

Erin H.

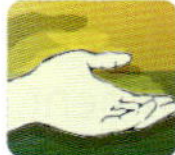

NURSING SKILLS AND INTERVENTIONS FOR END-OF-LIFE CARE

Caring for people at the end of life is one of the most challenging aspects of nursing and, when it is done well, it can be rewarding for all involved. The following nursing skills as essential for quality end-of-life care:

- Aggressive and comprehensive symptom management
- Open and honest communication about prognosis, treatment and the dying process
- Ongoing discussion about patients' goals of care
- Psychological and spiritual support for patients and their families
- Bereavement services. (Hospice & Palliative Nurses Association, 2011)

The next sections discuss nursing skills in relation to communication and management of symptoms. It is beyond the scope of this text to offer comprehensive information about this topic, but resources located at the end of this chapter provide for more in-depth information.

Communication

A number of transitions are experienced by people at the end of their life. These include physical, emotional, spiritual and financial transitions. *Advance care directives* (ACD) and *advance care planning* (ACP) are considered essential aspects of end-of-life care. ACD and ACP provide the basis for communication about care and decision making as older adults experience these transitions. A detailed discussion about ACD and ACP is contained in Chapter 9.

Communication is the cornerstone of building interpersonal relationships when caring for people who are dying. Communication is critically important to all involved, and its importance is magnified by the unpredictability of the situation. Nurses can help dying people express their needs by using open honest, direct and empathetic communication, even when they may be uncertain about what to say. (See Box 29-3 for examples of appropriate communication.) Dying people value the ability to express themselves; in particular, older adults value the opportunity to achieve closure and say goodbye. Additionally, nurses have many opportunities to intervene in each of these realms by using particular communication strategies and interpersonal skills. These interventions include presence, compassion, touch, recognition of an individual's autonomy and honesty (Box 29-4).

DIVERSITY NOTE

For good communication it is recommended that health professionals listen to the Indigenous person's story and then let the story guide the care that is delivered (Palliative Care Australia, 2014).

BOX 29-3
Communicating with dying patients and their families

What to say

Tell me more about ...
What questions do you have about your condition?
What are you most concerned about right now?
How are you feeling right now?
I hear your concern (worry, frustration).
How can I be helpful?
I'm here to listen and I'll do my best to help (support, alleviate discomfort).
Take your time.
Is there someone I can call to help with this (e.g. family, religious person, medical professional)?
It's okay to cry. I know this is very sad for you.
Would you prefer to be left alone?
Would you like to share some memories?

Non-verbal communication

Maintain active presence.
Use touch purposefully.
Communicate patience and respectful waiting.
Learn to be comfortable with silence.
Allow yourself to cry and express emotions in an appropriate and supportive way.

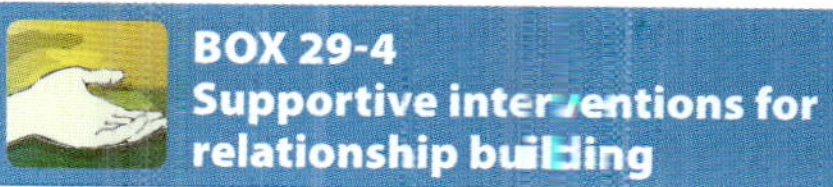

BOX 29-4
Supportive interventions for relationship building

Presence

- A core nursing intervention, presence can be described as a "gift of self" in which the nurse is available and open to the situation.
- Presence can be demonstrated through verbal communication, valuing what the person says, accepting the person's meaning for things and remembering or reflecting.

Compassion

- The nurse strives to be totally and compassionately with the person and family, allowing the most positive experience.

Touch

- A powerful therapeutic intervention, touch communicates an offer of unconditional acceptance. It can be both healing and life affirming, a means of communicating genuine care and compassion.

Recognition of autonomy

- The nurse realises and respects the individual's right to make all end-of-life decisions.

Honesty

- The nurse is often in a front-line position to communicate/explain what can be expected. Compassionate honesty builds trust with the older adult facing death and his or her family.

Expert communication

- At any given moment, nurses need to be able to assess the person and family, implement a plan to comfort them and communicate clearly and supportively throughout.

Assisting in transcendence

- At the highest level of care, nurses provide emotional support that facilitates the experience of self-transcendence and a sense of triumph over death.

Source: Saunderson, C. A. & Brener, T. H. (Eds). (2007). *End of life: A nurse's guide to compassionate care* (p. 78). Philadelphia, PA: Lippincott Williams & Wilkins.

Offering spiritual support

Spiritual care is an essential aspect of nursing care at all times and it becomes even more important at the end of life. Specific ways in which nurses can address spiritual needs at the end of life include:

- Listening reflectively to the person's and family's story with a compassionate presence
- Demonstrating empathy and the ability to journey with others in their suffering
- Recognising and responding to spiritual distress and facilitating the discovery of meaning in the experience of illness, suffering, grief and loss
- Eliciting key concerns with respect, including feelings of hopelessness, loss, brokenness, and other unmet spiritual and religious needs

- Identifying and responding to ethical issues and conflicts, and assisting and supporting others in the application of their own values in decision making
- Willingness to create therapeutic and healing spaces in which spiritual expression can occur
- Facilitating the use of symbolism and rituals according to the needs and values of the person and family
- Offering sensitivity, prayer, music, scripture or other readings that are meaningful to the person and family
- Supporting spiritual strengths of the person and family
- Seeking additional resources as needed by the person and family, including chaplaincy or other spiritual providers.

Chapters 12 and 13 in this text provide additional information about nursing assessment and intervention related to spiritual care for older adults. A tool has been developed, the FICA Spiritual History Tool, so that older adults' spirituality during end-of-life can be supported by nurses (Borneman, 2011) (see Box 29-5).

Nursing issues pertinent to spiritual care during the end of life are risk for spiritual distress, spiritual distress, and readiness for enhanced spiritual well-being. The nursing interventions relevant to spiritual care at the end of life are active listening, coping enhancement, emotional support, guilt-work facilitation, hope instillation, presence, religious-ritual enhancement, spiritual support, and touch. Nurses also make referrals for pastoral care, hospital chaplains or other spiritual support resources when appropriate.

BOX 29-5
Taking a spiritual history using FICA

F—Faith and belief

"Do you consider yourself spiritual or religious?" or "Do you have spiritual beliefs that help you cope with stress?" If the patient responds "No", the clinician might ask, "What gives your life meaning?" Sometimes people respond with answers such as family, career or nature.

I—Importance

"What importance does your faith or belief have in your life? Have your beliefs influenced how you take care of yourself in this illness? What role do your beliefs play in regaining your health?"

C—Community

"Are you part of a spiritual or religious community? Is this of support to you and how? Is there a group of people you really love or who are important to you?" Communities such as churches, temples and mosques, or a group of like-minded friends can serve as strong support systems for some patients.

A—Address in care

"How would you like me, your healthcare provider, to address these issues in your healthcare?"

Source: Puchalski, C. (2001). The role of spirituality in health care. Table 1: The FICA method of taking a spiritual history. *Baylor University Medical Center Proceedings, 14*(4), 352–357.

Hospice programs (New Zealand) provide spiritual support and can provide resources to assist nurses in addressing the spiritual needs of patients and families.

Managing physical symptoms

Although the end-of-life process is individualised and unpredictable, some symptoms occur commonly and require expert and timely nursing care. A systematic review of the prevalence of symptoms during the last 2 weeks of life identified the following symptoms as the most commonly occurring ones: dyspnoea (56.7%), pain (52.4%), respiratory secretions (51.4%) and confusion (50.1%) (Kehl & Kowalkowski, 2013). Additional symptoms that are often addressed at the end of life include fatigue and weakness, constipation, nausea and vomiting, dehydration and decreased appetite. Because these symptoms usually occur in combination, management is challenging and it is not always possible to control every symptom completely.

Nurses can use a symptom assessment scale, the Edmonton Symptom Assessment Scale, to identify and determine the severity of common symptoms that older adults experience during the end of life (see Figure 29-2). Table 29-1 and the following sections provide guides for nurses in the assessment and interventions for some of the commonly occurring symptoms.

In addition, nurses can use information in Chapter 28 to further assess for pain, which is a symptom that occurs frequently at the end of life and is one of the most feared symptoms associated with death. This chapter addresses the symptoms only in relation to end of life; other pertinent topics are discussed more comprehensively in other chapters: confusion or delirium (Chapter 14), depression (Chapter 15), constipation (Chapter 18) and sleep problems (Chapter 24).

A student's perspective

I had a special experience with a man at the nursing and rehab centre. "Mort" and I had great conversations, and he quickly became a friend. Mort was suffering from cardiovascular failure, and I knew he did not have long to live. I interviewed Mort and then wrote a paper about his life. I wrote the paper early so that I could read it to Mort before his health declined any more.

I read my paper to Mort one morning, and he listened with a seeming sense of sacredness about the words being read. This was his life, and I could tell that it meant a lot to him that I wrote it all down. When I finished, Mort simply said, "I thank you … I thank you." He asked me to put the paper in a safe place so it would not get ruined. Mort and I had a special connection; he was a hero to me. The following week, I went to the clinic and found out that Mort had passed away. I am grateful that I had the opportunity to know Mort and to grow and learn from his good life. I am glad that I could serve him at this final time and help him reflect on his life.

Amy C.

Alberta Health Services | Covenant Health

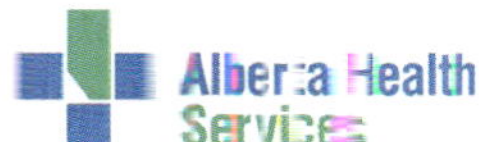

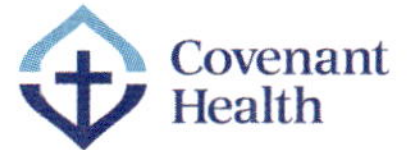

Edmonton Symptom Assessment System:
(revised version) (ESAS-R)

Please circle the number that best describes how you feel NOW:

No Pain	0	1	2	3	4	5	6	7	8	9	10	Worst Possible Pain
No Tiredness *(Tiredness = lack of energy)*	0	1	2	3	4	5	6	7	8	9	10	Worst Possible Tiredness
No Drowsiness *(Drowsiness = feeling sleepy)*	0	1	2	3	4	5	6	7	8	9	10	Worst Possible Drowsiness
No Nausea	0	1	2	3	4	5	6	7	8	9	10	Worst Possible Nausea
No Lack of Appetite	0	1	2	3	4	5	6	7	8	9	10	Worst Possible Lack of Appetite
No Shortness of Breath	0	1	2	3	4	5	6	7	8	9	10	Worst Possible Shortness of Breath
No Depression *(Depression = feeling sad)*	0	1	2	3	4	5	6	7	8	9	10	Worst Possible Depression
No Anxiety *(Anxiety = feeling nervous)*	0	1	2	3	4	5	6	7	8	9	10	Worst Possible Anxiety
Best Wellbeing *(Wellbeing = how you feel overall)*	0	1	2	3	4	5	6	7	8	9	10	Worst Possible Wellbeing
No ________ Other Problem *(for example constipation)*	0	1	2	3	4	5	6	7	8	9	10	Worst Possible ________

Patient's Name ______________________

Date ____________ Time ____________

Completed by (check one):
- ☐ Patient
- ☐ Family caregiver
- ☐ Health care professional caregiver
- ☐ Caregiver-assisted

BODY DIAGRAM ON REVERSE SIDE

ESAS-r
Revised: November 2010

FIGURE 29-2 The Edmonton Symptom Assessment Scale. (Watanabe et al. [2011]. A multi-centre comparison of two numerical versions of the Edmonton Symptom Assessment System in palliative care patients. *Journal of Pain Symptom Management, 41*, 456–468; Bruera, E. et al. [1991]. The Edmonton Symptom Assessment System [ESAS]: A simple method for the assessment of palliative care patients. *Journal of Palliative Care, 7*, 6–9.)

Pain

Pain is a frequent symptom experienced by older adults during EOL. Pain that is not well managed is a significant cause of distress and is not associated with a dignified death. Effective management of pain is an essential component of EOL care. With the increasing complexity of medical treatments and longer periods that older adults are living with life-limiting illnesses, approaches to pain management must be holistic, multimodal and begin at diagnosis, with ongoing assessment for effectiveness. These approaches are addressed in Chapter 28, where the principles of pain management have been discussed.

Fatigue (asthenia)

Fatigue is one of the most commonly reported symptoms at the end of life. Fatigue is often described as tiredness, or

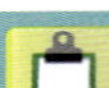

TABLE 29-1 Guide to nursing assessment and interventions for common symptoms during palliation

Symptom	Nursing assessment	Nursing interventions	Pharmacological interventions
Fatigue (asthenia)	Assess for associated conditions, including infection, fever, pain, depression, insomnia, anxiety, dehydration, hypoxaemia, medication effects.	Inform older adult and family of the normality of fatigue at end of life. Pace activities and care according to tolerance. Exercise if tolerated. Promote optimal sleep, with regular times of rest, sleep and waking.	Corticosteroids, although generally contraindicated in older adults, may decrease fatigue in patients with cancer. Treat associated conditions (e.g. with antibiotics, antidepressants).
Constipation	Identify risks (e.g. chronic laxative users, medications). Perform abdominal assessment, including palpation for distension, tenderness or masses and auscultation of bowel sounds and pitch. Assess patients taking pain medications daily. Monitor the character of the bowel movements. Check the rectum if the older adult has not had a bowel movement in more than 3 days or is leaking liquid stool (which can occur with an impaction).	Anticipate and prevent constipation with emphasis on fibre, fluid intake and activity, but recognise that patients may have difficulty tolerating the optimal interventions. Promote regular routine. Strongest propulsive contractions occur after breakfast; provide patient privacy at this time.	Individualise laxative regimen based on the cause(s) of constipation, history and preferences. Use bulk-forming and stool-softening agents for patients with normal peristalsis. A laxative regimen (with stimulant laxative) may be ordered for patients taking a pain medication known to cause constipation. Stimulant laxatives are the most appropriate for opioid-induced constipation.
Dyspnoea	*Respiratory:* Assess vital signs, including oxygen saturation, breathing pattern and use of accessory muscles. Auscultate breath sounds. Assess cough (type, if present). Check for tachypnoea and cyanosis. *General:* Assess for restlessness, anxiety and activity tolerance.	Pace activities and rest. Provide oxygen, usually at 2–4 L per cannula (avoid using face mask because of discomfort and sensation of smothering). Provide calm reassurance. Use a fan to circulate air and help reduce the feeling of breathlessness. Position for optimal respiratory function (e.g. leaning forward over a table with a pillow on top is helpful for COPD; on the side with head slightly elevated for unresponsive patient). Teach patient to use pursed-lip breathing, and encourage relaxation techniques to reduce muscle tightness and associated sensation of breathlessness.	Treat causes. Treat symptoms with morphine or hydromorphone, which relieves the breathless sensation in almost all cases. Use antianxiety agents or antidepressants if appropriate (and if perception of breathlessness is exaggerated because of anxiety or depression). Corticosteroids can be used for their anti-inflammatory effects in certain conditions (e.g. COPD, radiation pneumonitis).
Nausea and vomiting	Assess for potential cause (e.g. constipation, bowel obstruction). Palpate abdomen and check for distension. Assess vomitus for faecal odour. Assess heartburn and nausea, which may occur after meals in squashed stomach syndrome. Assess pain (e.g. pain on swallowing may indicate oral thrush; pain on standing may be caused by mesenteric traction). Hiccups occur with uraemia.	Offer frequent, small meals; serve foods cold or at room temperature. Apply damp, cool cloth to face when nauseated. Provide oral care after vomiting.	Medications need to be specific to the cause: • Squashed stomach syndrome, gastritis and functional bowel obstruction: metoclopramide (contraindicated in full bowel obstruction) • Chemical causes, such as morphine, hypercalcaemia or renal failure: haloperidol • If caused by dysfunction of vomiting centre (e.g. associated with mechanical bowel obstruction, increased intracranial pressure, motion sickness): diphenhydramine

TABLE 29-1 Guide to nursing assessment and interventions for common symptoms during palliation (*continued*)

Symptom	Nursing assessment	Nursing interventions	Pharmacological interventions
Dehydration	Assess for clinical signs of hydration (e.g. skin turgor over the upper chest or forehead). Assess buccal membranes for moistness. Assess vital signs: pulse, orthostatic blood pressure.	Encourage fluids as tolerated; offer ice chips and popsicles if swallowing. Provide frequent oral care; use swabs or moistened toothettes.	Give intravenous fluids if medically appropriate. Discuss continued diuretic use with doctor.
Anorexia and cachexia	Assess for weight loss. Assess for levels of weakness and fatigue. Conduct physical examination for decreased fat, muscle wasting, strength. Assess mental status, including depression.	Remove unpleasant odours. Provide frequent oral care. Treat pain optimally. Provide frequent, small meals. Provide companionship. Serve meals in a place that is separate from the bed area. Involve patient with meal planning. Collaborate with dietitian for nutritional analysis and meal planning. Encourage culturally appropriate foods. Consider using an alcoholic beverage before meals.	Medications that are used to stimulate appetite, promote weight gain and provide a sense of well-being: megestrol acetate, corticosteroids and mertazapine. Metoclopramide is used to improve gastric motility and appetite.
Pain	Use the appropriate assessment tools, depending on the level of cognitive impairment and the pain type (see Chapter 28)	As discussed in Chapter 28, apply the principles of pain management in older adults	See discussion about pharmacological management in Chapter 28

COPD, chronic obstructive pulmonary disease.

lack of physical strength and endurance, or decreased mental concentration. Older adults may have reduced energy or activity tolerance caused by chronic conditions, so it is important for the nurse to establish a baseline for comparison and meaningful interpretation. Fatigue is generally a symptom with underlying causes related to disease processes or conditions such as anaemia, malnutrition, infection, drug therapy or depression. Other concurrent end-of-life symptoms such as pain and dyspnoea may exacerbate fatigue.

Constipation

Constipation, a reduced frequency of bowel movements, can include passing hard stools, straining to pass a stool or impaction (hard stool that is blocked). Constipation may be accompanied by pain, abdominal fullness and reduced bowel sounds. In general, older adults are at increased risk for constipation because of medications, dietary patterns and decreased physical activity. Factors that increase the risk for constipation at the end of life include pain medications (discussed in Chapter 28), dehydration, kidney failure, elevated calcium levels and disease effects (e.g. ascites, spinal cord damage, colon or pelvic cancers).

Dyspnoea

Dyspnoea occurs commonly in conditions involving cardiorespiratory function (e.g. heart failure, lung cancer and chronic obstructive lung disease), and it also occurs during advanced stages of other conditions. Studies have identified dyspnoea as the most distressing symptom experienced by many people with advanced progressive diseases and it often evokes feelings of fear, anxiety and panic (Campbell, 2012; Yates & Zhao, 2012). Descriptive terms include shortness of breath, breathlessness, suffocation, and being smothered. A recent nursing review of literature by Lowey, Powers and Xue (2013) recommended the following framework, called the ADRA (Assess, Document, Reassess, Advocate), as an integral part of care for people with end-stage illnesses:

- Assess all patients for dyspnoea intensity and severity, using a standardised and validated tool.
- Document comprehensive information about assessment, pharmacological and non-pharmacological interventions, and the person's responses.
- Reassess dyspnoea and response to interventions.
- Advocate for the person by discussing wishes and preferences for care.

Nausea and vomiting

Nausea and vomiting are common symptoms associated with terminal illness. Causes of nausea and vomiting at the end of life include the following:

- Irritation/obstruction of gastrointestinal tract (bowel obstruction, constipation, cancer, tumour, delayed emptying of stomach from ascites, tumour pressure [often called *squashed stomach syndrome*])

- Medication side effect (particularly opioids such as morphine)
- Ear infection or labyrinthitis
- Electrolyte imbalance, sepsis
- Kidney failure, liver failure
- Increased intracranial pressure (brain tumour, cerebral oedema, intracranial bleeding, metastasis)
- Foul odours
- Anxiety, fear.

Dehydration

Because older adults normally have an age-related decrease in body water, they become dehydrated more easily. Causes of dehydration at the end of life include reduced or inadequate oral intake, medications such as diuretics, vomiting, diarrhoea and fever. Symptoms of dehydration can interfere with comfort by causing dry mouth, constipation, confusion and skin impairment.

Anorexia and cachexia

Additional symptoms include anorexia, a lack of appetite that progresses to the inability to eat and cachexia, which is a general state of malnutrition in which there is loss of fat, muscle and bone mineral content. Even before the terminal illness, older adults often have less lean tissue, so there is less reserve and malnutrition can progress quickly. Factors that contribute to anorexia and cachexia include nausea and vomiting, constipation, dehydration, weakness, depression, pain, oral candidiasis or dry mouth, gastritis and medication side effects.

Symptoms during the actively dying process

When it becomes apparent that a dying person has only a few days to live, it is especially important that the nurse work closely with the individual and his or her family to help them understand the dying process and anticipate changes. Guidance about what to expect helps reduce fear and anxiety. Characteristic physical signs indicate the **active dying** process (see Table 29-2). In most situations, the individual has become totally dependent on others for all aspects of care, with less wakeful or alert time. Levels of consciousness may change or fluctuate. The person has little or no interest in the oral intake of food or fluids. Physiological changes occur in breathing patterns, circulation slows down, sensory awareness decreases, and muscle weakness occurs as a result of decreased tone.

The overall focus of nursing care during the terminal phase of EOL is to continue to promote physiological and psychological comfort, while assisting the older adult in achieving a dignified death. There are five symptoms associated with this phase that require particular management (Hudson, Remedios, Zordan et al., 2010). These include dyspnoea, nausea and vomiting, pain, respiratory tract secretions and terminal restlessness/agitation. Evidenced-based guidelines from the WA Cancer and Palliative Care Network

TABLE 29-2 Signs and symptoms of death within days

Physiological change	Signs and symptoms
Altered breathing patterns	• Breathing initially becomes more shallow • Cheyne-Stokes respirations • Noisy breathing (death rattle)
Changing circulation	• Limbs, ears and nose become cold to touch or mottled in appearance • Decreased blood pressure • Pulse may weaken and become irregular • Diaphoresis • Possible increase in dependent oedema • No urine output or small amount of very dark urine (anuria or oliguria)
Decreased muscle tone	• Relaxed facial muscles, lower jaw drops, mouth open • Decreased/loss of gag reflex • Difficulty swallowing • Abdominal distension due to decreased gastrointestinal activity • Possible urinary and faecal incontinence due to relaxation of sphincter muscles
Decreased senses	• Reduced level of consciousness • Blurred or distorted vision • Decreased taste and smell (probable continued sense of hearing)

Source: Saunderson, C. A. & Brener, T. H. (Eds). (2007). *End of life: A nurse's guide to compassionate care*. Philadelphia, PA: Lippincott Williams & Wilkins.

(2011) are available that provide protocols for each symptom and support a dignified death.

The management of the symptoms of dyspnoea, nausea and vomiting, and pain have been discussed already in the chapter, but there are some other interventions unique to the terminal phase that require description of these symptoms. During this phase opioids have been found to be effective in improving the sensation of dyspnoea. Air flowing over the face may also help. Promethazine may be appropriate to administer if metoclopramide has not been effective for nausea and vomiting. Morphine is the opioid recommended to control pain during the phase. Most older adults will not be able to swallow and the morphine is administered subcutaneously (see the next section on medication administration during the actively dying process for further discussion about morphine administration).

The remaining two symptoms, respiratory tract secretions and terminal restlessness, also require management. Respiratory tract secretions can be caused by a number of factors, including aspiration, or by pooling of normal oral secretions in an older adult who is not swallowing or coughing effectively (Hudson, Remedios, Zordan et al.,

2010). This is referred to as the *death rattles*. Death rattles occur in many older adults who are dying. Studies report its incidence between 23% and 92%. If death rattles are not managed they can cause significant levels of distress to families. Nurses can prepare families for the development of this symptom and inform them of the care required when or if this symptom occurs. Changes in position and use of medications have been found to be effective. Medications such as hyoscine or atropine can be used if the older adult has developed death rattles, and also to prevent the development of the death rattles if they have been assessed as being at risk. Routine suctioning is not recommended but may be useful if the secretions are thick and positioning is not effective.

Terminal restlessness's incidence has been reported, from 62% to 88%, suggesting many older adults will experience this symptom (Hudson, Remedios, Zordan et al., 2010). Again, family members can find this symptom distressful. Terminal restlessness has been described as '… an agitated delirium that occurs … during the last days of life" (p. 17). Despite there being limited evidence about the use of drugs to treat terminal restlessness, a low dose of haloperidol is recommended. Benzodiazepines may be added to haloperidol if sedation is required.

Care pathways during the actively dying process

Care pathways during the terminal phase have been developed to promote comfort, assist the older adult with a dignified death and provide support to families. The Liverpool Care Pathway for the Dying Patient (LCP) is one pathway that is used in both Australia and New Zealand. In New Zealand the LCP's use is encouraged by the New Zealand Ministry of Health (bpac[NZ], 2011). There are five categories with the pathway: comfort, psychological insight, spiritual support, communication with family and with the primary healthcare team and summary. There are 11 goals within these five categories and these direct the care delivered during the actively dying phase.

Medication administration during the actively dying process

When other administration routes become inappropriate or ineffective (that is, when the person can no longer swallow), the subcutaneous route is recommended to administer medications to control the symptoms that are experienced during the terminal phase. Medications that are administered subcutaneously treat unrelieved pain and other distressing symptoms, including agitation and terminal restlessness (Palliative Care Australia, 2014). Subcutaneous infusion devices are commonly referred to as *syringe drivers*. The most commonly used syringe driver used during EOL in Australia is the Niki T34® (Queensland Government, 2010), while the AC ambulatory syringe driver is recommended for use in New Zealand (New Zealand Ministry of Health, 2009).

BOX 29-6
Nine medications commonly used in subcutaneous infusions during the actively dying process

- Morphine sulfate/tartrate (opioid)
- Hydromorphone (opioid)
- Haloperidol (antipsychotic/antiemetic)
- Midazolam (short-acting benzodiazepine)
- Metoclopramide (antiemetic)
- Hyoscine hydrobromide (antimuscarinic/antiemetic)
- Clonazepam (benzodiazepine)
- Hyoscine butylbromide (antimuscarinic)
- Fentanyl (narcotic)

Source: Queensland Government. (2014). *Guidelines for subcutaneous infusion device management in palliative care* (2nd ed.). Accessed via www.health.qld.gov.au.

In Australia and New Zealand pharmacological agents commonly used in subcutaneous infusions to address the symptoms commonly experienced during the actively dying phase are listed in Box 29-6.

Excellent guidelines that assist with the development of policy and procedures and provide education for subcutaneous infusion management during EOL care are:

- In Australia, the *Guidelines for subcutaneous infusion device management in palliative care*, available via www.health.qld.gov.au
- In New Zealand, the *Guidelines for syringe driver management in palliative care in New Zealand*, available via www.health.govt.nz.

Use of complementary and alternative medicine during the actively dying process

Complementary and alternative medicines (CAM) therapies have been shown to benefit some people during the terminal phase. There is evidence to support the use of some CAM therapies for symptom management and to improve well-being. The understanding of the role of complementary therapies in is still in its infancy during terminal care, as many studies have methodological problems that make their findings unreliable (CareSearch, 2012). However, aromatherapy, massage and music therapy all have evidence to support their use and are particularly effective in the reduction of agitation and the support of the person's well-being. The Australian Pain Society (2005) has developed guidelines to assist with using CAM therapies and they are as follows:

- For safety reasons, members of the care team must always be informed before a CAM therapy is used (e.g. St John's wort interacts with numerous prescription medications). This principle also facilitates a comprehensive care plan to be developed, based on the needs of each person. Current information on using herbs safely is available from the Memorial Sloan Kettering's Integrative Medicine Department's About Herbs section at www.mskcc.org.

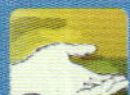

BOX 29-7
Providing emotional support and self-care

The CARES tool addresses Comfort, Airway, Restlessness and delirium, Emotional and spiritual support, and Self-care for dying patients and their carers. CARES was developed by Bonnie Freeman, RN, DNP, ANP, Department of Supportive Care Medicine, City of Hope National Medical Center, in Duarte, California.

Emotional, spiritual, psychosocial and cultural support

Providing emotional, spiritual, psychosocial and cultural support to the patient and family allows nurses to provide spiritual care. This is the very foundation of caring for the dying. It is important to implement various resources. For example:

- Notify supportive care team members for assistance and specify whether the resources are for patient, staff or both.
- Always work to retain the patient's dignity and feelings of value.
- Remember every family is unique and grieves differently.

Good communication is essential

- Make sure that communication exists with the family and all disciplines.
- Take your cues from family members. Do not assume you know what they are thinking or feeling.
- Clarify how much the family wants to know.
- Clarify goals of care.
- Clarify privacy needs.
- Just be with the patient and family and sit in silence.
- Work with family to provide favourite activities, smells, sounds, etc.
- Support rituals and assist with obtaining desired clergy or equipment.

Other activities and methods of support

- Your humanity is needed the most now. Always be available. Your very presence is reassuring to the family.
- The family is an important part of your patient care and becomes your focus as the patient becomes more unresponsive:
  - Be sure families are getting rest and breaks.
  - Provide coffee, water, etc.
  - Continue to be available to answer questions.
  - You cannot take away their pain. Acknowledge their emotions and be present.
- Play patient's favourite music.
- Position bed so patient can see out through a window.
- Encourage family to provide patient's favourite hat, clothing, etc.
- Lower or mute lighting in the patient's room.
- Consider bringing in a favourite pet.

Self-care

Healthcare providers must allow themselves to be human and expect some personal emotional response to the death of their patient and for the grieving family. Care providers may need supportive services. Often a review and debriefing can assist with professional grieving and promote emotional health by:

- Recognising the stressful event and thanking the supportive team members.
- Reviewing what went well and what challenges need to be addressed.
- Sharing bereaved family comments.
- Addressing moral distress issues.
- Expressing issues of death anxiety and obtaining support.
- Exploring challenges and privileges of assisting a fellow human being through the dying process.
- Acknowledging the spiritual impact of witnessing death.
- Exploring how your care made a difference to the grieving family.
- Reviewing effective communication techniques, available resources and support.

Adapted with permission from Freeman, B. (2013). CARES: An acronym organized tool for the care of the dying. *Journal of Hospice & Palliative Nursing*, [illegible], 147–153. Used with permission from B. Freeman, RN, DNP, ANP and *Journal of Hospice & Palliative Nursing*.

- To reduce the risk of possible assault claims, clear approval from the person, whether cognitively or communication impaired, bedridden or fully capable, is essential before a CAM therapy is used on the recommendation of family, friends, staff or doctors.
- Residents who are interested in any CAM therapy should be fully informed about its safety and effectiveness.
- CAM therapists should be carefully selected so that the resident has confidence in their credentials and qualifications.
- It is advisable to check with private health insurers to determine whether a CAM therapy is covered. (NHMRC, 2006, p. 114)

Providing emotional support and caring for oneself

Two aspects of end-of-life care that are particularly challenging are providing emotional support for the older adult and family, and caring for self. Box 29-7 contains a guide for providing emotional support and self-care.

In Australia, a clinical practice guideline has been developed for the psychological and bereavement support of carers of palliative care recipients. There are 20 guidelines that health professionals are encouraged to follow to provide for the psychological, social, financial, spiritual and physical well-being of the carers. Table 29-3 contains the guidelines.

UNFOLDING CASE STUDY

Part A

Mr Bauer is a 91-year-old man with medical diagnoses that include hypertension, type 2 diabetes mellitus, history of cerebrovascular accident, and benign prostatic hyperplasia. He was taking the following medications: lisinopril 20 mg daily; aspirin, 81 mg daily; frusemide 40 mg daily; potassium, 20 mEq daily; and paracetamol as needed for arthritis pain. He has lived at home by himself for the last 15 years since the death of his wife. He has three adult children, all living interstate, who visit on average once a month. He is very well known in his neighbourhood as the older man who helps everyone. He loves his home and

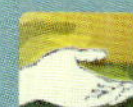

TABLE 29-3 Guidelines for the psychological and bereavement support of carers of palliative care recipients

Guideline 1	Confirm the person who has agreed to receive palliative care that the palliative care also supports their carer/s. This will be the individual's most important support and might be a partner or a friend rather than their next of kin.
Guideline 2	Ensure the person's preferences for their carer's involvement in health and lifestyle decision making are recorded. Identify another carer if only one is involved.
Guideline 3	Ensure the caregiver understand the role and responsibilities they have undertaken.
Guideline 4	Ensure the person and their carer/s understand/s advance care planning and its legal implications.
Guideline 5	The carer/s is/are the key informants for about the person receiving palliative care.
Guideline 6	Provide an explanation of available services and resources that are provided by palliative care services, which enables informed decision making.
Guideline 7	Regularly conduct a case conference with the person and their carers.
Guideline 8	Assess the needs of the carer/s holistically.
Guideline 9	As a result of the assessment, develop a plan of care involving the carer/s.
Guideline 10	Conduct appropriate interventions to assist the carer/s with their psychological health and grief.
Guideline 11	Assist carer/s to understand the signs of imminent death of the person.
Guideline 12	Ensure the carer/s are prepared for the death of the person.
Guideline 13	Ensure that an understanding has been obtained of the carers' support requirements during the terminal phase and immediately after death.
Guideline 14	Identify a communication strategy between the interdisciplinary team and the carer/s and, if required, provide information about external supports.
Guideline 15	Inform the interdisciplinary team of the person's death.
Guideline 16	One of the interdisciplinary team is required to contact the carer/s after the person's death to offer support.
Guideline 17	If appropriate, plan a follow-up assessment with the caregivers for approximately 3 to 6 weeks after the death of the person.
Guideline 18	As a result of the assessment, develop a bereavement plan of care based on the identified caregivers' needs.
Guideline 19	If appropriate, complete the follow-up assessment of caregivers approximately 6 months after the death of the person.
Guideline 20	An interdisciplinary team discussion is advised to occur after the death of the person about the care provided.

Source: Adapted from Hudson, P., Remedios, C., Zordan, R. et al. (2012). Clinical practice guidelines for the psychosocial and bereavement support of family caregivers of palliative care patients. *Journal of Palliative Medicine*, 15(6), 696–702.

spends his day "keeping house". His favourite chores include mowing the grass and blowing the leaves in autumn. He owns and drives a car to the local supermarket and barber and to the cemetery to visit his wife's grave. In late summer, he had an accident with his lawn mower that drew his family's attention to the fact that he was losing his strength. While mowing his grass, he fell over the lawn mower, scraping his face on the cement. He required emergency department (ED) evaluation and treatment, including stitches for facial lacerations. He later admitted that, before his fall, he had been experiencing dizziness, especially when getting out of his easy chair.

Three weeks after his ED evaluation, Mr Bauer's daughter came to visit. She was shocked to see her father looking so "thin and gaunt". Mr Bauer admitted that he had lost a few kilograms over the summer and still didn't have much energy. He stated that he wasn't sleeping well at night, with his sleep disrupted every 30 to 45 minutes because of the need to urinate. To control his urination, he had decided to limit his drinking of fluids to less than three glasses. Mr Bauer's daughter noticed that, in spite of his weight loss, his abdomen was very large and distended. "Do you have any aches?" she asked her father. He nodded yes, and grabbed his lower abdomen.

Thinking points

- Based on symptoms and history, what points would you address in your nursing assessment?
- What nursing problems would you address in Mr Bauer's nursing care plan?
- What are some probable causes of Mr Bauer's abdominal discomfort?
- What would the appropriate nursing interventions be?
- What health teaching would you provide?

UNFOLDING CASE STUDY

Part B

Mr Bauer and his daughter have a follow-up office visit with his general medical practitioner. On arrival, his vital signs are as follows: temperature, 35°C; apical pulse, 82 beats per minute and irregularly irregular; respirations, 24 per minute; and blood pressure sitting, 98/50. When standing to walk to the scale for his weight measurement, he swayed a bit, grabbed the wall, and then steadied himself. "I just got a little dizzy," he admitted. As the office nurse, you immediately grabbed the blood pressure cuff and took his blood pressure in the standing position. It was 70/40. Mr Bauer's pulse at that time was 90 and irregular. Noting the vital sign changes, the doctor ordered some laboratory tests. Blood samples for testing were drawn in the office. With results pending, no changes were made in his medical care at that time.

Thinking points

- What are your immediate nursing concerns for Mr Bauer based on information about his decline during the past 6 months?
- What risk factors are likely to be contributing to Mr Bauer's dizziness?
- What teaching is indicated at this time?

UNFOLDING CASE STUDY

Part C

Mr Bauer's blood test results come back the next day, confirming dehydration and malnutrition:

- Sodium: 150
- Potassium: 3.7
- Serum albumin: 3.0
- Prealbumin: 14
- Blood urea nitrogen: 35
- Serum creatinine: 1.7

The doctor discontinued Mr Bauer's frusemide and lisinopril and suggested a follow-up visit in 2 weeks. Two days before his next appointment, Mr Bauer's daughter called the office to relay that her father had fallen and was taken to the hospital for evaluation. A work-up revealed that he had a transient ischaemic attack and was now too weak to eat and he was experiencing difficulty swallowing.

Thinking points

- Identify two priority nursing issues appropriate for Mr Bauer at this time.
- For each issue, list two to three nursing interventions.
- Mr Bauer died in the hospital 1 week after his fall, on the day he was scheduled for discharge.

CHAPTER HIGHLIGHTS

Perspectives on end-of-life care (Figure 29-1; Box 29-1)

- EOL refers to the phase of life when care is focused on comfort and supports a dignified death.
- Within EOL there is another phase of care when the person is actively dying, and this is referred to as the terminal phase or the actively dying process. The end-of-life time for older adults is often a gradual process associated with the cumulative effects of chronic illness and many interacting conditions, making it difficult to recognise when an older adult enters the terminal phase.
- Views of death and dying in Western societies have shifted as a result of demographic and healthcare trends (e.g. increased life expectancy, medical and technical advances).
- Cultural perspectives—of society, patients and health-care providers—exert a strong influence on all aspects of end-of-life care.

Hospice and palliative care

- Hospice and palliative care services are an interdisciplinary approach to care that holistically addresses the needs of people with life-limiting conditions as well as their families and carers.
- To qualify for hospice services, patients usually have a short life expectancy of months.
- Palliative care services can be provided throughout a continuum of illness for people with serious illnesses.

Promoting wellness at the end of life

- Wellness at the end of life is achieved through a dignified death, as described in the Dying Patient's Bill of Rights (Box 29-2).
- The nursing issues of dignified death and dignified life closure are applicable to promoting wellness for patients at the end of life.

Nursing skills and interventions for end-of-life care (Boxes 29-3 through 29-5; Tables 29-1 & 29-2)

- Nurses use verbal and non-verbal communication skills that are appropriate for addressing the complexity of end-of-life situations.
- Nurses have numerous opportunities to provide spiritual care for patients and families as an integral part of end-of-life care.
- Nurses are responsible for managing physical symptoms that occur during the end of life: pain, fatigue, constipation, dyspnoea, nausea and vomiting, dehydration and anorexia.
- Nurses holistically address needs of patients and families during the actively dying process.
- Five symptoms associated with the actively dying phase include dyspnoea, nausea and vomiting, pain, respiratory tract secretions and terminal restlessness/agitation.
- The Liverpool Care Pathway for the Dying Patient (LCP) is one pathway used during the actively dying phase to assist with the delivery of quality end-of-life care.
- Medication administration during the actively dying phase is usually via subcutaneous infusion.
- Complementary and alternative medicine can be administered by nurses during the actively dying phase.
- Interventions for emotional support for patients and families and self-care for nurses are essential aspects of end-of-life care.

CRITICAL THINKING EXERCISES

1. Review the section on healthcare professionals' perspective on death and dying, and spend a few minutes answering the list of questions for self-reflection.

2. Review Cultural considerations 29-1 and think about how each of the points listed applies to your personal perspectives on death and dying.
3. From a nursing perspective, identify the ways in which caring for people at the end of life differs from caring for people with acute care needs.
4. From a nursing perspective, identify the ways in which caring for people at the end of life differs from caring for people who have chronic illnesses.

RESOURCES

For an extensive range of additional resources to enhance teaching and learning and to facilitate understanding of this chapter please see the text's accompanying website located on thePoint at http://thepoint.lww.com.

Clinical tools

Center to Advance Palliative Care: www.capc.org
Promoting Excellence in End-of-Life Care, palliative care tools: www.promotingexcellence.org/tools
TIME: Toolkit of Instruments for Measuring End-of-life Care: www.chcr.brown.edu/pcoc/toolkit.htm
Hartford Institute for Geriatric Nursing, ConsultGeriRN.org: http://consultgerirn.org/resources

- *Try This* Issue 5: Assessment of spirituality in older adults: FICA spiritual history tool. Borneman, T. (2011). *Best Practices in Nursing Care to Older Adults.*

Evidence-based practice

Australian Government Department of Health. (2014). Guidelines for a palliative approach in residential aged care (enhanced version). Available via www.health.gov.au.
Australian Government Department of Health. (2011). Guidelines for a palliative approach for aged care in the community setting. Available via www.health.gov.au.
Government of Western Australia Department of Health. (2010). WA Cancer and Palliative Care Network: Evidence based clinical guidelines for adults in the terminal phase. Accessible via www.healthnetworks.health.wa.gov.au.
Hudson, P., Remedios, C., Zordan, R. et al. (2010). Clinical practice guidelines for the psychosocial and bereavement support of family caregivers of palliative care patients. Melbourne: Centre for Palliative Care, St Vincent's Hospital. Available at http://centreforpallcare.org/assets/uploads/CP-Guidelines_web.pdf.
Joanna Briggs Institute: http://connect.jbiconnectplus.org
Evidence summary:

- Chen, Z. (2014). Palliative care: Dementia.

National Guideline Clearinghouse: www.guideline.gov
Search for: Palliative care

- End of-life care
- Quality palliative care
- Interventions to improve palliative care of pain, dyspnoea and depression at the end of life
- Family preparedness and end-of-life support before death of a nursing home resident.

World Health Organization. (2011). Palliative care for older people: Better practices. Available at www.euro.who.int/__data/assets/pdf_file/0017/143153/e95052.pdf.

Health education

Australian Government Department of Health, National Palliative Care Strategy: www.health.gov.au
Australian Indigenous Health*InfoNet*, Sad news, sorry business; palliative care: www.healthinfonet.ecu.edu.au
Cancer Control New Zealand, palliative care: www.cancercontrolnz.govt.nz/palliative-care
Cancer Council: www.cancer.org.au
Cancer Nurses Society of Australia: www.cnsa.org.au
Cancer Society of New Zealand: www.cancernz.org.nz
CareSearch, Palliative Care Knowledge Network: www.caresearch.com.au
Grattan Institute, Dying Well Report: http://grattan.edu.au/report/dying-well
Growth House, guides to death, dying, grief, bereavement and end of life resources: www.growthhouse.org
Health Direct Australia, end-of-life health: www.healthdirect.gov.au/end-of-life-health
Medical Council of New Zealand, Māori and Pacific people palliative care: www.mcnz.org.nz
New Zealand Palliative Care Strategy: www.health.govt.nz/publication/new-zealand-palliative-care-strategy
Palliative Care Australia: www.palliativecare.org.au
Virtual Cancer Centre: www.myvmc.com/?s=palliative+care
World Health Organization: www.who.int/cancer/palliative/links/en

REFERENCES

Austin, L. (1975). Dying Patient's Bill of Rights. Created at the Terminally Ill Patient and the Helping Person Workshops. Sponsored by the Southwest Michigan Inservice Education Council in Lansing, MI.
Australian Government Department of Health and Ageing (DoHA). (2004). Providing culturally appropriate palliative care to Aboriginal and Torres Strait Islander peoples: Resource kit. Accessible March 2015 via http://webarchive.nla.gov.au.
Australian Institute of Health and Welfare (AIHW). (2011). *Trends in palliative care in hospital.* Cat. no. HWI 112. Canberra: Author.
Australian Institute of Health and Welfare (AIHW). (2014). *Palliative care services in Australia 2014.* Cat. no. HWI 128. Canberra: Author.
Australian Pain Society. (2005). *Pain in residential aged care facilities: Management strategies.* North Sydney: Author. Available March 2015 via www.apsoc.org.au.

Borneman, T. (2011). Assessment of spirituality in older adults. *Try This* series, issue SP5, 1–2. *Best Practice for Hospitalized Older Adults.* Accessed March 2015 at http://consultgerirn.org/uploads/File/trythis/try_this_sp5.pdf.

bpac^{NZ}. (2006). Providing palliative care to Māori. Accessed March 2015 at www.bpac.org.nz/resources/campaign/palliative/palliative_maori.asp.

bpac^{NZ}. (2011). End-of-life care, and training to the people providing it. Treatment for the dying patient: Liverpool Care Pathway. *Best Practice Journal, 36*, 6–13.

Bruera, E., Kuehn, N., Miller, M., Selmser, P. & Macmillan, K. (1991). The Edmonton Symptom Assessment System (ESAS): A simple method for the assessment of palliative care patients. *Journal of Palliative Care, 7*, 6–9.

Cairns, D., Williams, V., Victor, C. et al. (2013). The meaning and importance of dignified care: Findings from a survey of health and social care professionals. *BMC Geriatrics, 13*, 28. Accessed at www.biomedcentral.com/1471-2318/13/28.

Campbell, M. L. (2012). Dyspnea prevalence, trajectories, and measurement in critical care and at life's end. *Current Opinion in Supportive and Palliative Care, 6*(2), 168–171.

Campbell, W. (2011). A Māori approach to ageing, spirituality and palliative care. Presentation at 9th World Congress of International Council on Pastoral Care and Counselling, Rotorua, August 2011. Wellington: The Family Centre. Viewed March 2015 via www.familycentre.org.nz/About/ICPCC/index.html.

CareSearch. (2012). Clinical evidence: Complementary therapies. Accessed at www.caresearch.com.au/caresearch/tabid/1258/Default.aspx.

Freeman, B. (2013). CARES: An acronym organized tool for the care of the dying. *Journal of Hospice & Palliative Nursing, 15*(3), 147–153.

Hospice and Palliative Nurses Association. (2011). HPNA position statement: Legalization of assisted suicide. Available October 2013 via www.hpna.org.

Hudson, P., Remedios, C., Zordan, R., Thomas, K., Clifton, D., Crewdson, M., Hall, C., Trauer T., Bolleter, A., Clarke, D. M. & Bauld, C. (2012). Guidelines for the psychosocial and bereavement support of family caregivers of palliative care patients. *Journal of Palliative Medicine, 15*(6), 696–702.

Izumi S., Nagae, H., Sakurai, C. & Imamura, E. (2012). Defining end-of-life care from perspectives of nursing ethics. *Nursing Ethics, 19*(5), 608–618.

Kehl, K. A. & Kowalkowski, J. A. (2013). A systematic review of the prevalence of signs of impending death and symptoms in the last 2 weeks of life. *American Journal of Hospice & Palliative Care, 30*(6), 601–616.

Kübler-Ross, E. (1969). *On death and dying*. New York: Macmillan.

Lin, Y. P., Watson, R. & Tsai, Y. F. (2013). Dignity in care in the clinical setting: A narrative review. *Nursing Ethics, 20*(2), 168–177.

Lowey, S. E., Powers, B. A. & Xue, Y. (2013). Short of breath and dying: State of science on opioid agents for the palliation of refractory dyspnea in older adults. *Journal of Gerontological Nursing, 39*(2), 43–52.

Lysaght, S. & Ersek, M. (2013). Settings of care within hospice: New options and questions about dying "at home". *Journal of Hospice & Palliative Nursing, 15*(3), 171–175.

Manookian, A., Cheraghi, M. A. & Nasrabadi, A. N. (2014). Factors influencing patients' dignity: A qualitative study. *Nursing Ethics, 21*(3), 323–334.

Markson, E. (2003). *Social gerontology today*. Los Angeles, CA: Roxbury.

McLeod-Sordjan, R. (2013). Human becoming: Death acceptance. Facilitated communication with low-English proficiency patients at end of life. *Journal of Hospice & Palliative Nursing, 15*(7), 390–395.

Medical Council of New Zealand. (2010). Best health outcomes for Pacific peoples: Practice implications. Accessed March 2015 via at www.mcnz.org.nz.

Moorhead, S., Johnson, M., Maas, M. L. & Swanson, E. (Eds). (2013). *Nursing outcomes classification (NOC).* Philadelphia, PA: Elsevier.

National Health and Medical Research Council (NHMRC). (2006). Guidelines for a palliative approach in residential aged care: A systematic review. Canberra: Author. Accessible March 2015 at www.nhmrc.gov.au/guidelines-publications/ac15.

National Health and Medical Research Council (NHMRC). (2011). Living well with an advanced chronic or terminal condition: How ethics helps. Accessed March 2015 at www.nhmrc.gov.au/_files_nhmrc/publications/attachments/rec31a_advanced_chronic_terminal_ethics_guide_110908.pdf.

New Zealand Ministry of Health. (2009). *Guidelines for syringe driver management in palliative care in New Zealand*. Accessed at www.health.govt.nz/publication/guidelines-syringe-driver-management-palliative-care-new-zealand.

Ohio State University Health Sciences Center, Office of Geriatrics & Gerontology. (2003). Series to understand, nurture and support end-of-life transitions (SUNSET). Retrieved via http://sunset.osu.edu.

Palliative Care Australia. (1999). Multicultural palliative care guidelines. Available March 2015 at www.palliativecare.org.au/Portals/9/docs/publications/guidelines.pdf.

Palliative Care Australia. (2010). Health system reform and care at the end of life: A guidance document. Accessed at www.palliativecare.org.au/Portals/46/Policy/Health%20system%20reform%20-%20guidance%20document%20-%20web%20version.pdf.

Palliative Care Australia. (2014). Improving access to quality care at the end of life for Aboriginal and Torres Strait Islander Australians. Position statement. Accessed at www.palliativecare.org.au/Policy/PositionStatements.aspx.

Palliative Care Council, Hospice New Zealand and the Ministry of Health. (2012). New Zealand palliative care glossary. Accessed at www.palliativecarecouncil.govt.nz.

Palliative Care Council. (2014). Deaths in New Zealand: Regional and ethnic projections 2014–2026. Accessed March 2015 via palliativecare.hirc.org.nz.

Penrod, J., Hupcey, J. E., Baney, B. et al. (2011). End-of-life caregiving trajectories. *Clinical Nursing Research, 20*(1), 7–24.

Penrod, J., Hupcey, J. E., Shipley, P. Z. et al. (2012). A model of caregiving through the end of life: Seeking normal. *Western Journal of Nursing Research, 34*(2), 174–193.

Periyakoil, V. S., Stevens, M. & Kraemer, H. (2013). Multicultural long-term care nurses' perceptions of factors influencing patient dignity at the end of life. *Journal of the American Geriatrics Society, 61*(3), 440–446.

Puchalski, C. (2001). The role of spirituality in health care. Table 1: The FICA method of taking a spiritual history. *Baylor University Medical Center Proceedings, 14*(4), 352–357.

Purnell, L. D. (2014). *Guide to culturally competent health care* (3th ed.). Philadelphia, PA: F.A. Davis.

Queensland Government. (2010). *Guidelines for subcutaneous infusion device management in palliative care* (2nd ed.). Brisbane: Author. Accessed March 2015 via www.health.qld.gov.au/cpcre/subcutaneous/guidelines.asp.

Saunderson, C. A. & Brener, T. H. (Eds). (2007). *End of life: A nurse's guide to compassionate care*. Philadelphia, PA: Lippincott Williams & Wilkins.

Seaman, J. B. (2013). Improving care at end of life in the ICU. *Journal of Gerontological Nursing, 39*(3), 52–58.

van Gennip, I. E., Pasman, H. R., Kaspers, P. J. et al. (2013). Death with dignity from the perspective of the surviving family: A survey study among family caregivers of deceased older adults. *Palliative Medicine, 27*(7), 616–624.

Wiegand, D. L., Grant, M. S. & Cheon, J. (2013). Family-centered end-of-life care in the ICU. *Journal of Gerontological Nursing, 39*(8), 60–68.

Watanabe, S. M., Nekolaichuk, C., Beaumont, C., Johnson, L., Myers, J. & Strasser, F. (2011). A multi-centre comparison of two numerical versions of the Edmonton Symptom Assessment System in palliative care patients. *Journal of Pain Symptom Management, 41*, 456–468.

WA Cancer and Palliative Care Network. (2011). *Evidence based clinical guidelines for adults in the terminal phase* (2nd ed.). Perth: Government of Western Australia Department of Health. Available via www.healthnetworks.health.wa.gov.au.

World Health Organization (WHO). (2014). Global atlas of palliative care at the end of life. Accessed at www.thewhpca.org/resources/global-atlas-on-end-of-life-care.

Yates, P. & Zhao, I. (2012). Update on complex nonpharmacological interventions for breathlessness. *Current Opinion in Supportive and Palliative Care, 6*(2), 144–151.

Zamer, J. A. & Volker, D. L. (2013). Religious leaders' perspectives of ethical concerns at the end of life. *Journal of Hospice & Palliative Nursing, 15*(7), 396–402.

Index

Note: Page numbers followed by f, t, and b indicate figures, tables, and boxes respectively.

E

R

S

LUSTER

Concrete Homes

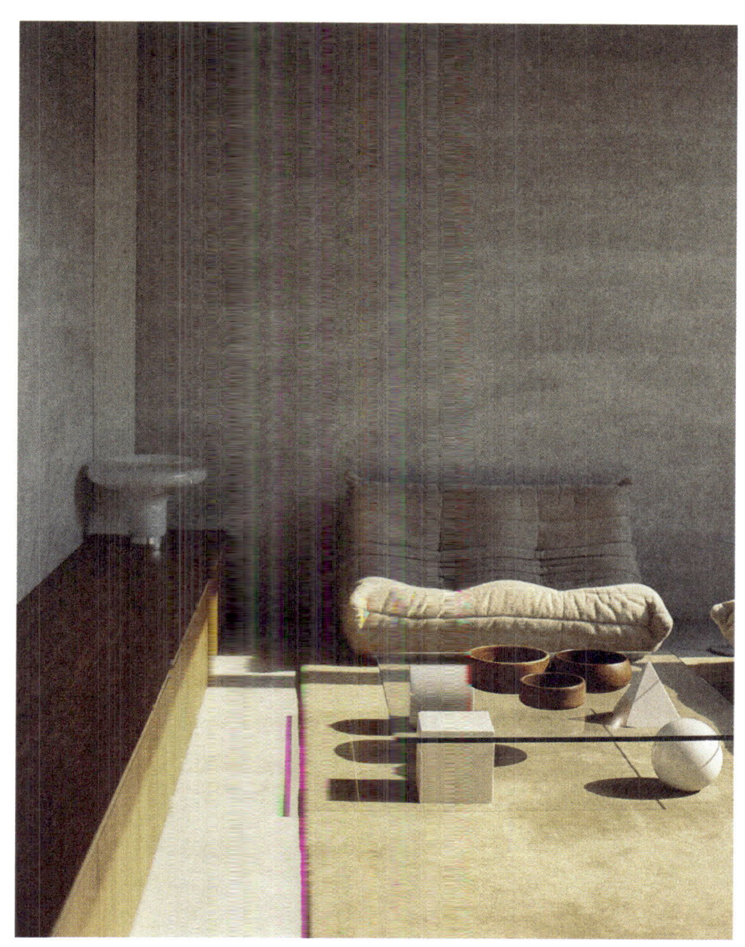

LUSTER

Concrete Homes

Pieter Peulen

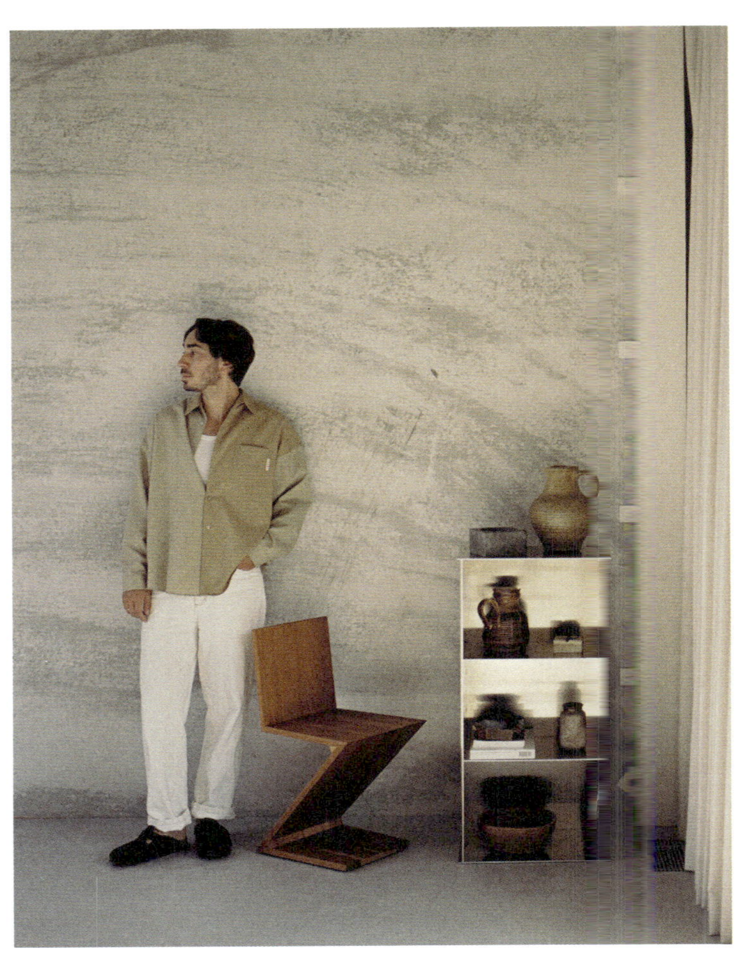

In a quiet corner of Belgium, I live in a house made of concrete. It's not large or loud, but it's carefully designed with clean lines, natural light, and honest materials. For me, concrete has always had a certain appeal. Since I was sixteen, studying at art school, my projects have consistently had a connection to concrete and brutalism. It's not decorative, it doesn't try to impress, it just is. And in that simplicity, there's a kind of beauty that feels grounding.

I'm Pieter Peulen. I studied interior architecture and now work mostly with images: capturing spaces and sharing them online. Over the past few years, my home has become part of that story. I began documenting it, and people started following along. Not because it's perfect, but perhaps because it's different, quiet, and clear. A space that speaks for itself.

In this book, I don't just want to tell the stories of these homes, I want to show them. The images you'll see were captured with my own eyes, through the lens of a 35 mm film camera. The analogue format allows me to stay connected to the rawness and authenticity of concrete and brutalism. There's a kind of respect in using film that echoes the process behind the architecture itself. It's about slowing down, paying attention, and capturing the moment in its most genuine form.

This book started with a simple idea: to look inside homes where concrete plays a central role as structure, texture, atmosphere. I visited thirteen houses across Belgium and Europe: some urban, some remote, some new, and others adapted over time. Each one reflects the mindset of the people who live there and how they relate to space, light, and material.

These stories are shaped by conversations, by walking through rooms, and by paying close attention to details. I wanted to understand how people make choices when they build – what they keep, what they let go of – and what it's like to live with concrete, not just as a design feature, but in daily life.

All of the homes in this book are different, but they share certain values: simplicity, clarity, and a strong sense of intention. They're not about trends or luxury in the usual sense. They're about depth, about creating space that feels calm and lasting.

Concrete Homes is not about showcasing, but about sharing. I hope it offers new ways of thinking about how we live and how architecture can shape that, quietly and powerfully.

Pieter Peulen

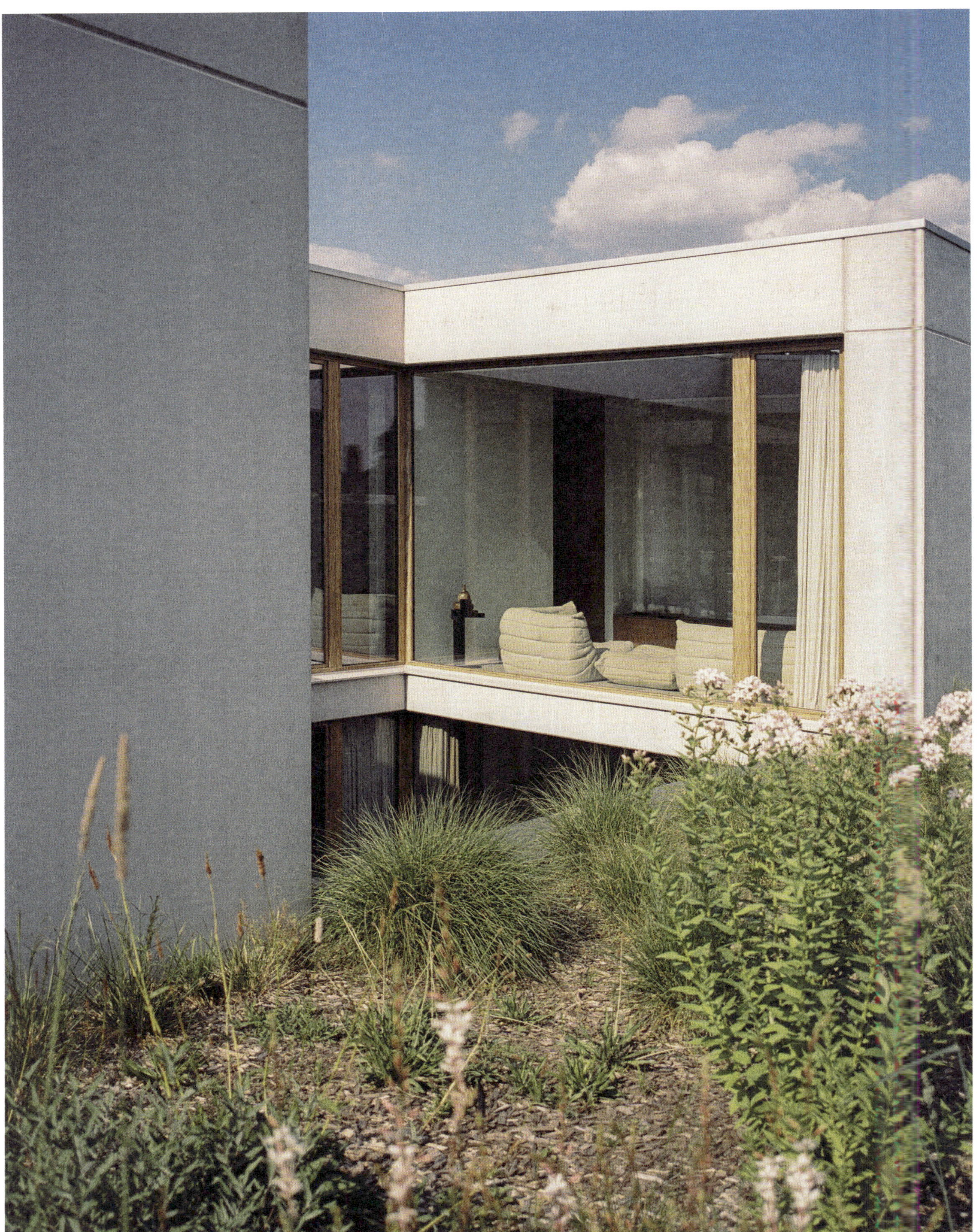

7

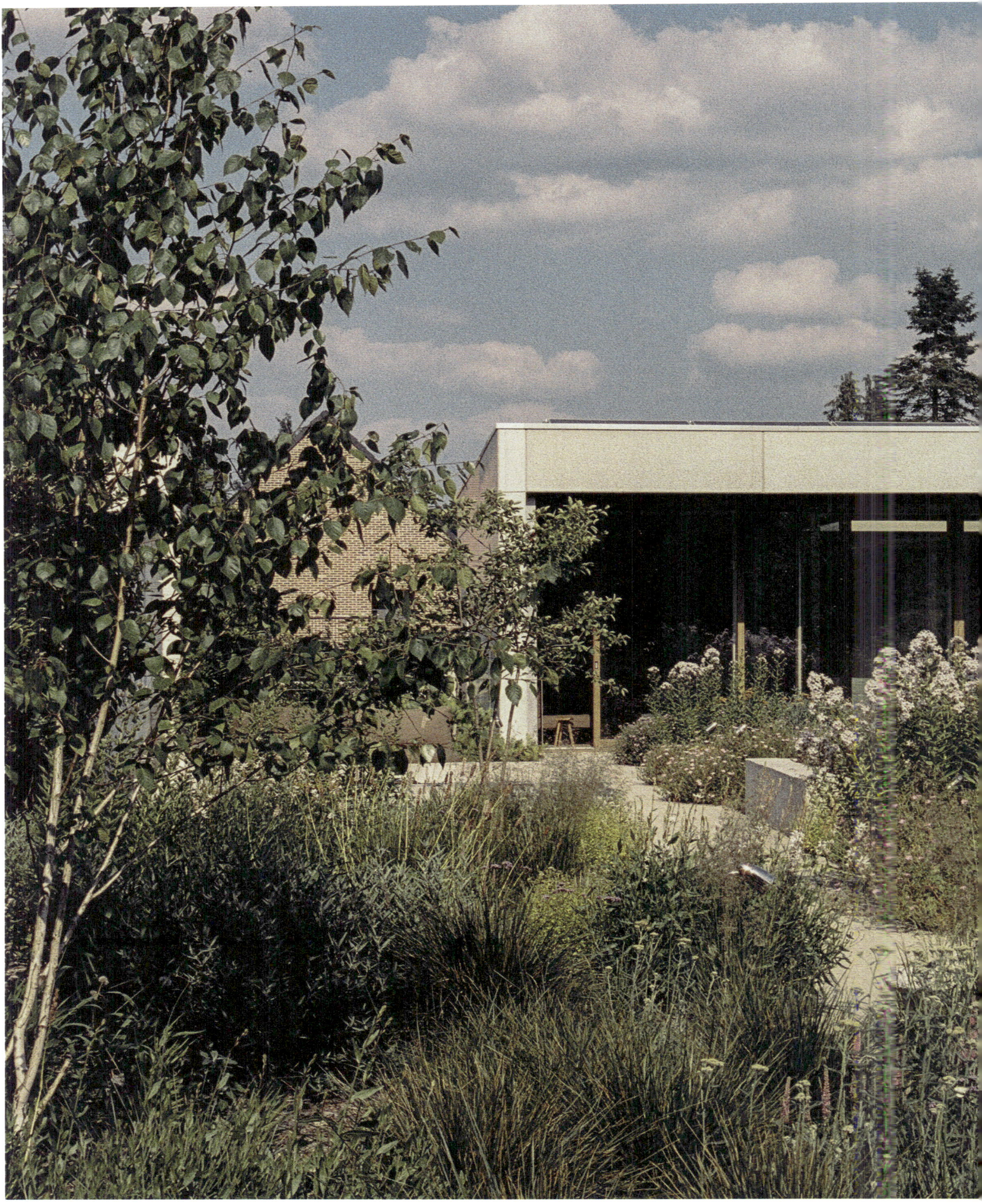

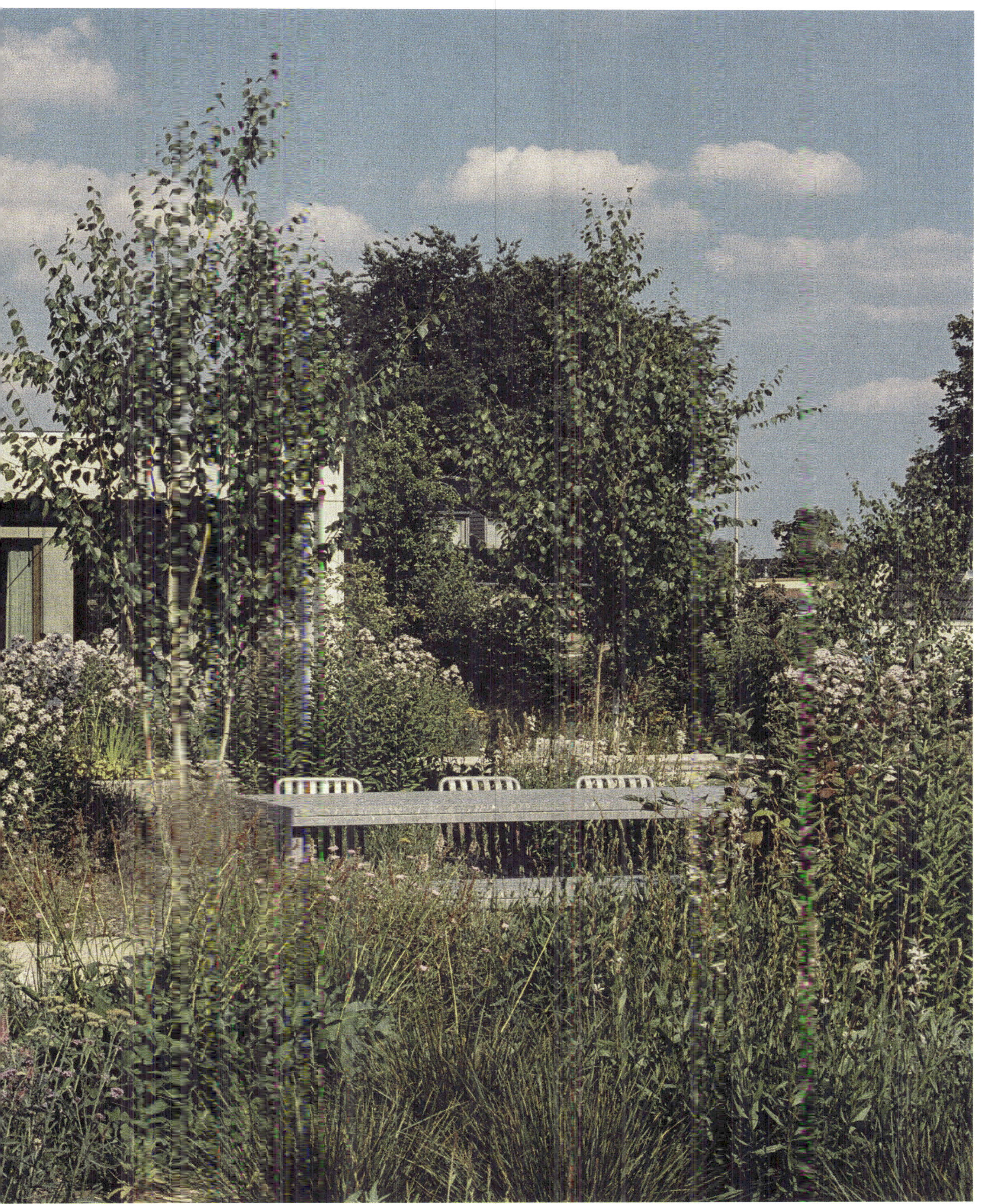

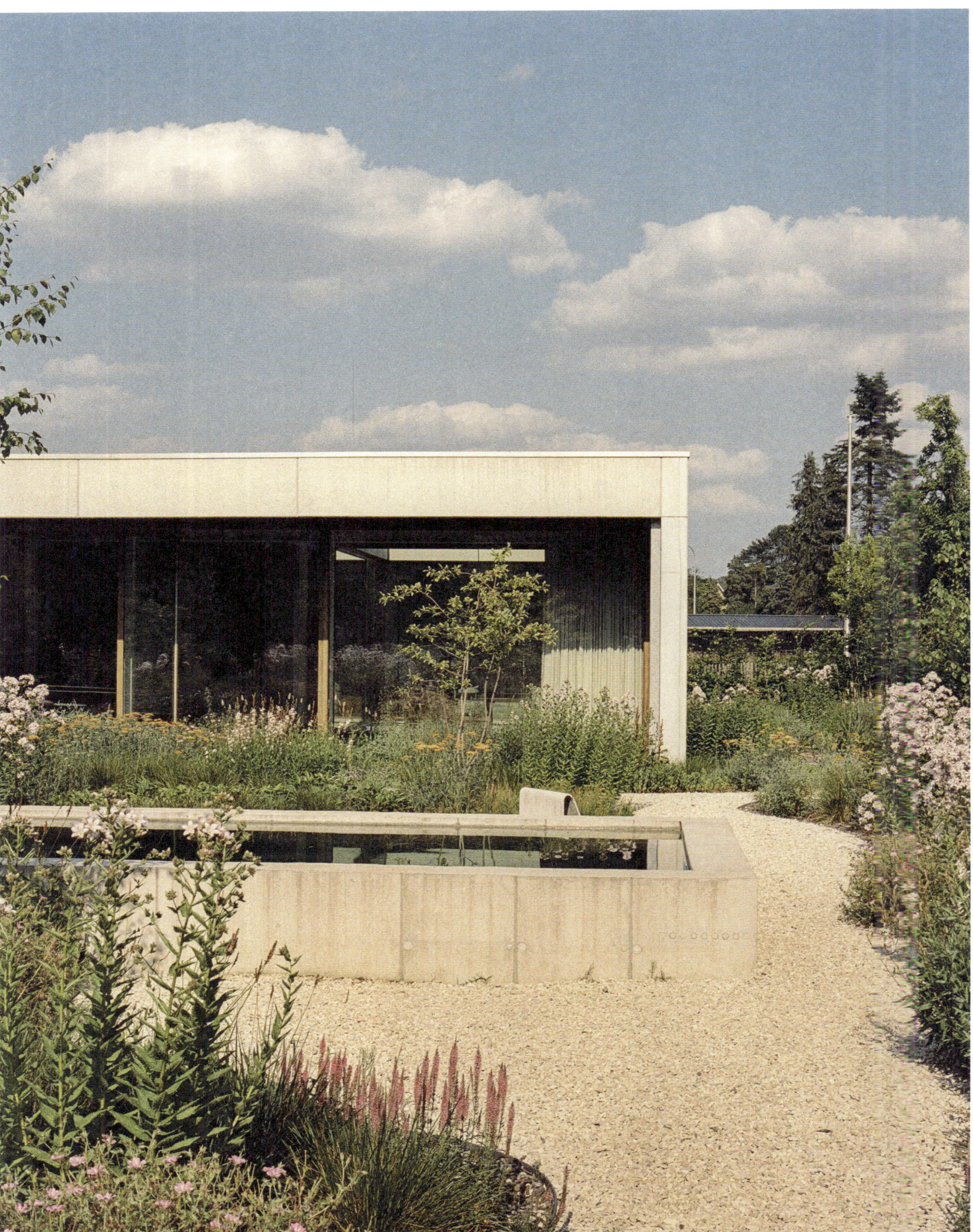

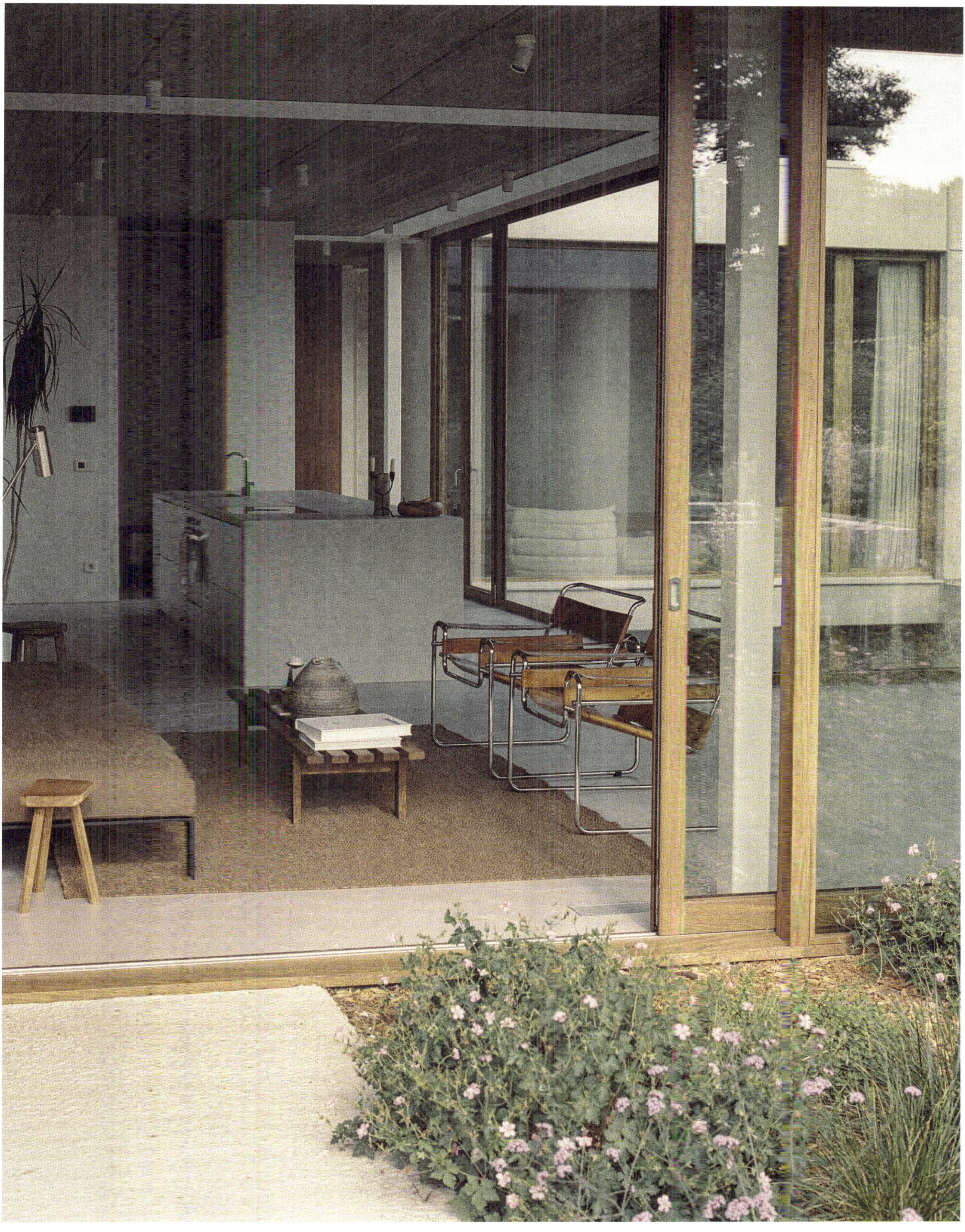

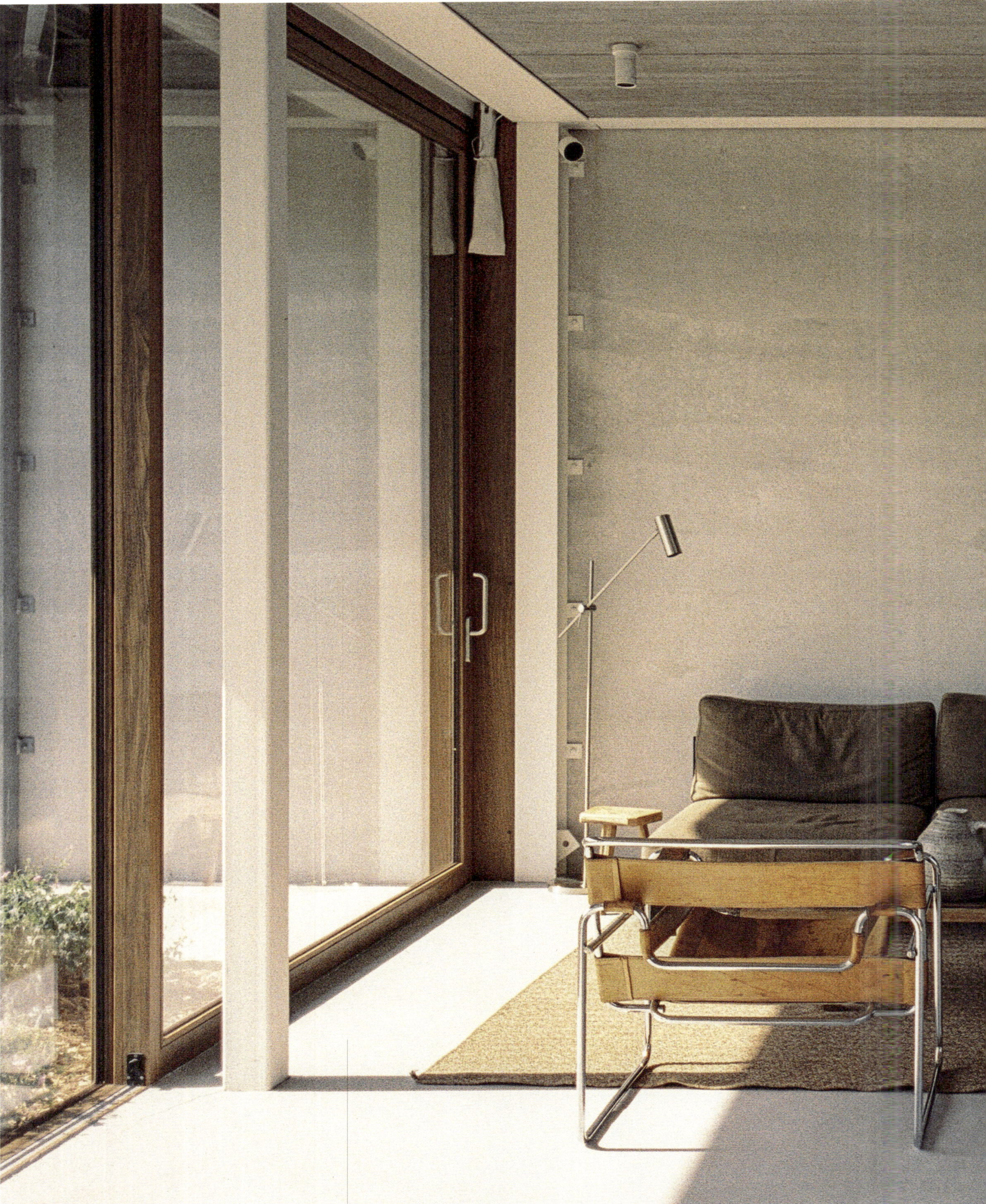

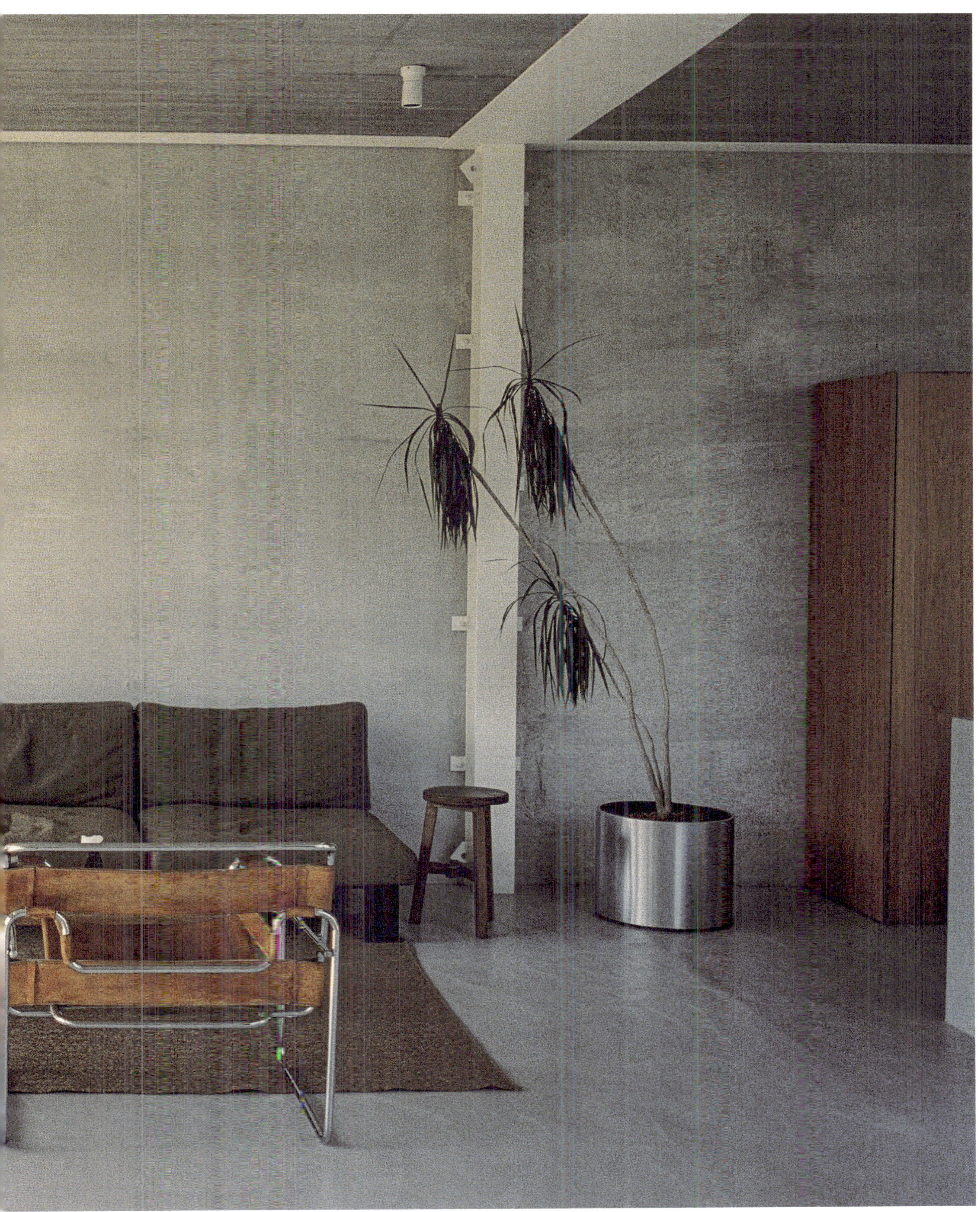

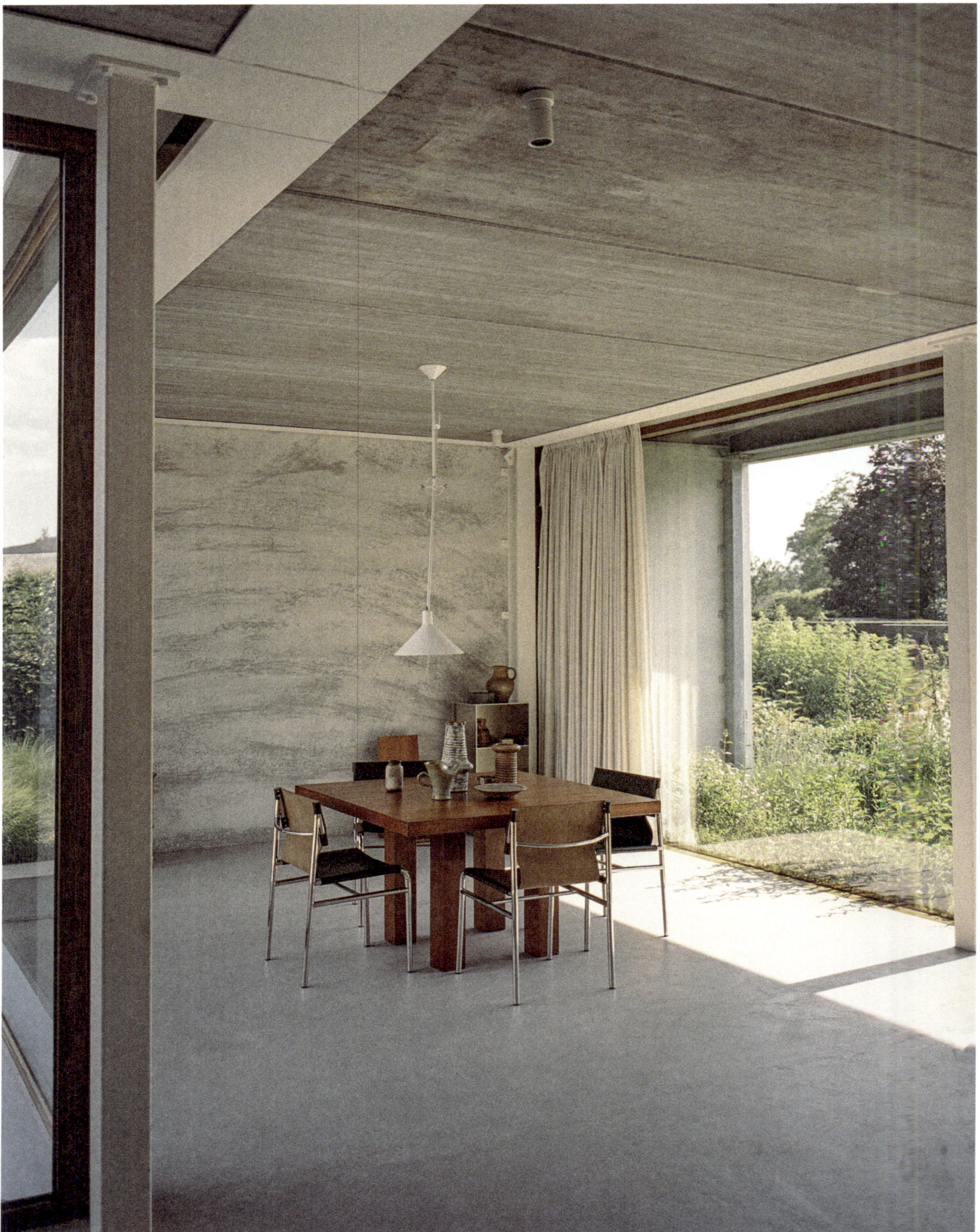

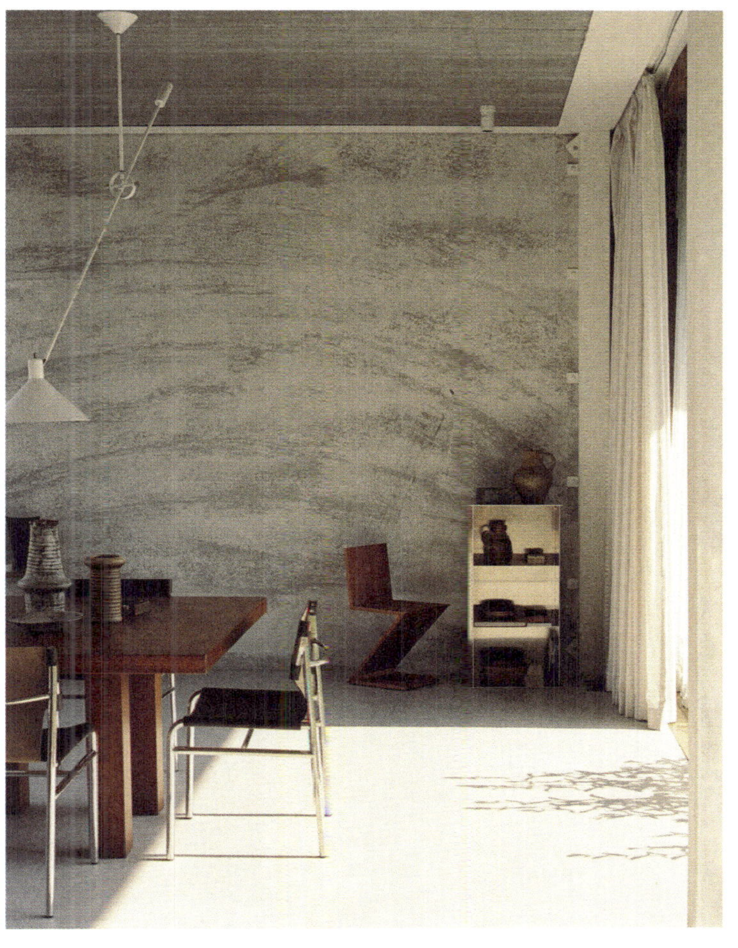

Intro

Villa Stuyven

Atelier Rosa

Missionsstrasse House

Casa D'Estate

Solo Pezo von Ellrichshausen

SpronkenHouse

La Maison H

Project STU

destroyers / builders

Schuppen

Casa Riera

House SS

House WESP

Outro

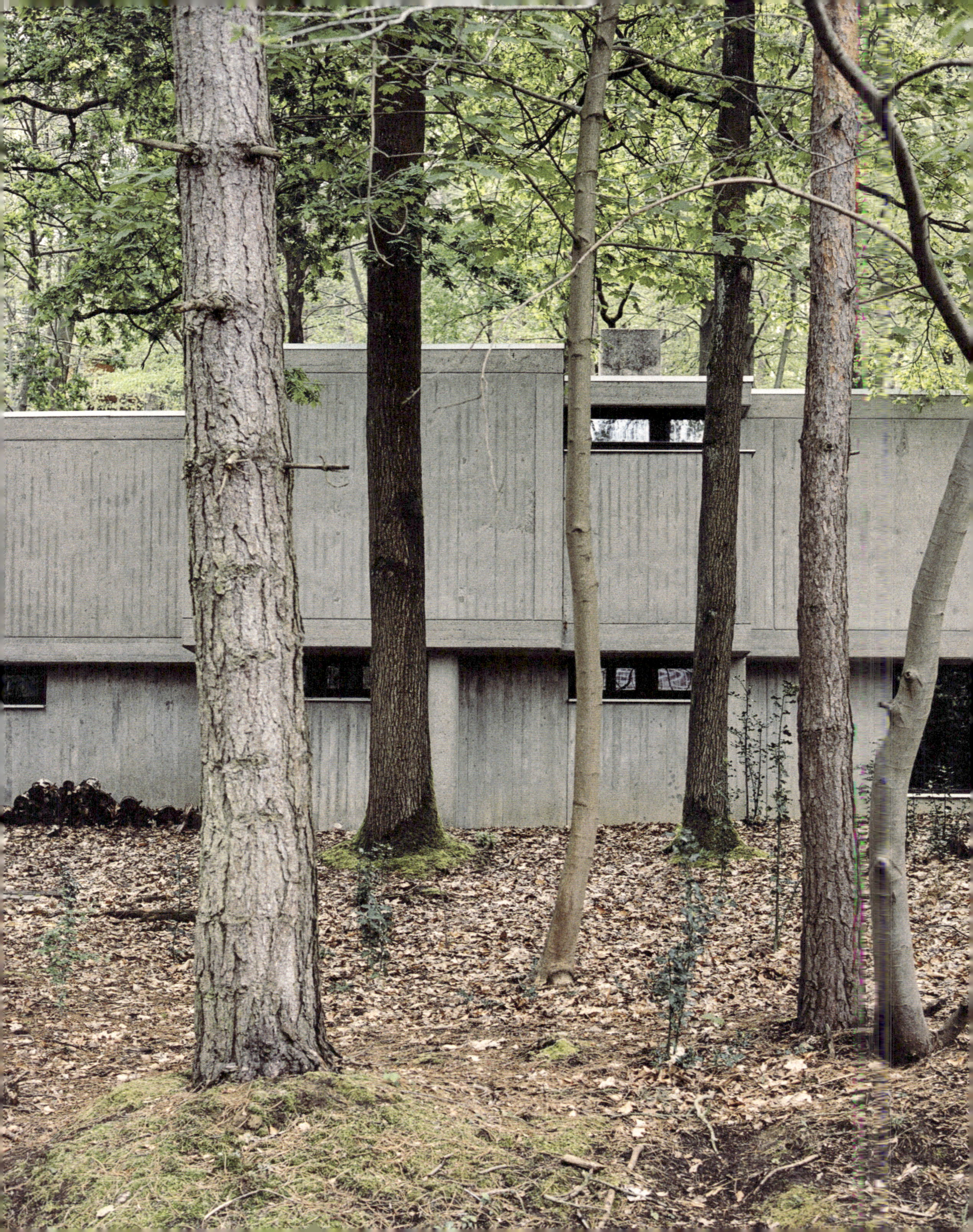

Villa Stuyven
Belgium

In the village of Holsbeek, near Leuven, sits a house that has remained largely unchanged since its construction. Villa Stuyven was built in 1977 for artist and philosopher Jef Stuyven and designed by Belgian architects Vanderbiest & Reynaert. It's a clear expression of Belgian brutalism where exposed concrete, structural honesty, and a deeply human scale come together with remarkable clarity.

Today, it is home to designer Bram Kerkhofs and network architect Lore Baeyens, together with their three children. When they purchased the house, their intention was not to rework it but to preserve it. They chose to live within the logic of the original design, maintaining the wooden ceilings, tiled floors, built-in storage, and even the original green tiled bathroom. The choices reflect respect, not nostalgia.

From the outside, the house is simple and direct. A flat roofline, rectangular forms, and visible board-formed concrete give it a low-key but confident presence. The structure is modest but intentional, sitting low in the landscape, with large glazed openings facing the garden and more closed surfaces facing the street. The contrast between openness and privacy is stark, but never forced.

Inside, the layout has remained almost entirely intact. The family made only a few technical upgrades, such as improved insulation and a new heating system, but otherwise left the structure and flow of the house untouched. Narrow corridors, closed rooms, and modest dimensions are not seen as flaws to fix, but as original decisions worth adapting to. Rather than modernising, they chose to understand.

The materials have aged visibly, but not poorly. Floors are worn, doors creak, finishes are matt and raw. These signs of use are not corrected; they're accepted. The house doesn't feel frozen, it feels lived-in, with light entering selectively through carefully positioned openings, creating contrast and calm. Each space serves its purpose without overreaching.

This respect for the original extends beyond everyday life. The house is part of a quiet but active cultural context. Through collaboration with the Leuven-based arts platform Cas-co, Villa Stuyven occasionally hosts artist residencies. These aren't exhibitions or events, but working stays where guests live and create in the rhythm of the house. The programme connects contemporary makers with a piece of architectural heritage, without spectacle.

The presence of children brings a sense of informality to the space. Toys, books, and drawings integrate effortlessly into the house's quiet aesthetic. And the robust materials seem suited for daily family life. Nothing feels fragile, yet everything is handled with care.

What stands out most is the restraint. Villa Stuyven isn't a showpiece; it's not trying to impress. But it is a rare example of a home from its era that has been preserved without compromise. Not by turning it into a museum, but by living in it attentively. By accepting the architecture on its own terms, the family has found a form of calm that feels grounded and clear.

This is not a nostalgic restoration, it's a lived philosophy. The house invites a different pace, a different attitude. It asks for understanding and in return, it offers clarity.

Project: Villa Stuyven
Location: Belgium
Architect: Vanderbiest & Reynaert
Year of construction: 1977
Year of purchase: 2022
Floor area: 462 m²
Resident: Bram Kerkhofs
Resident's profession: designer, teacher

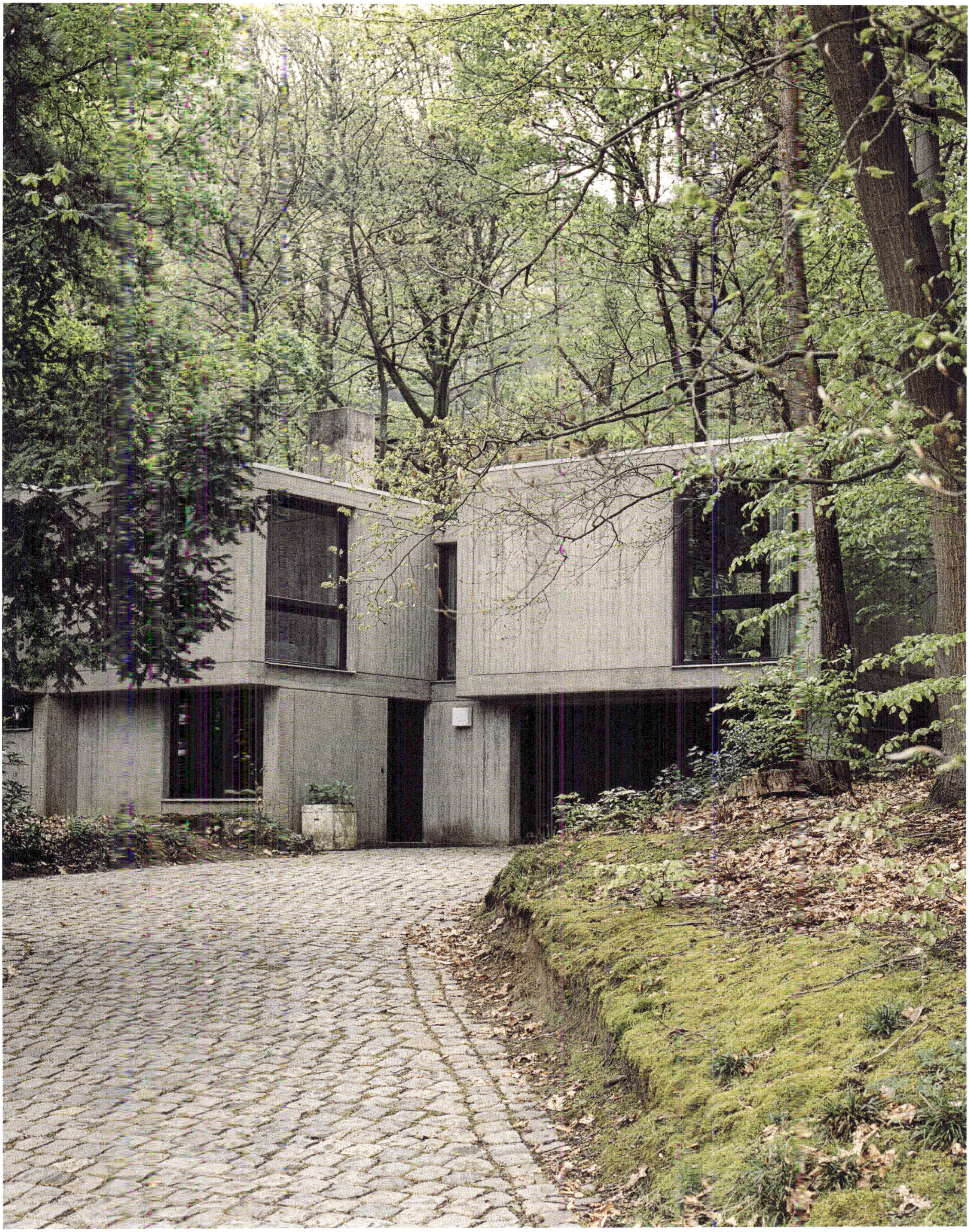

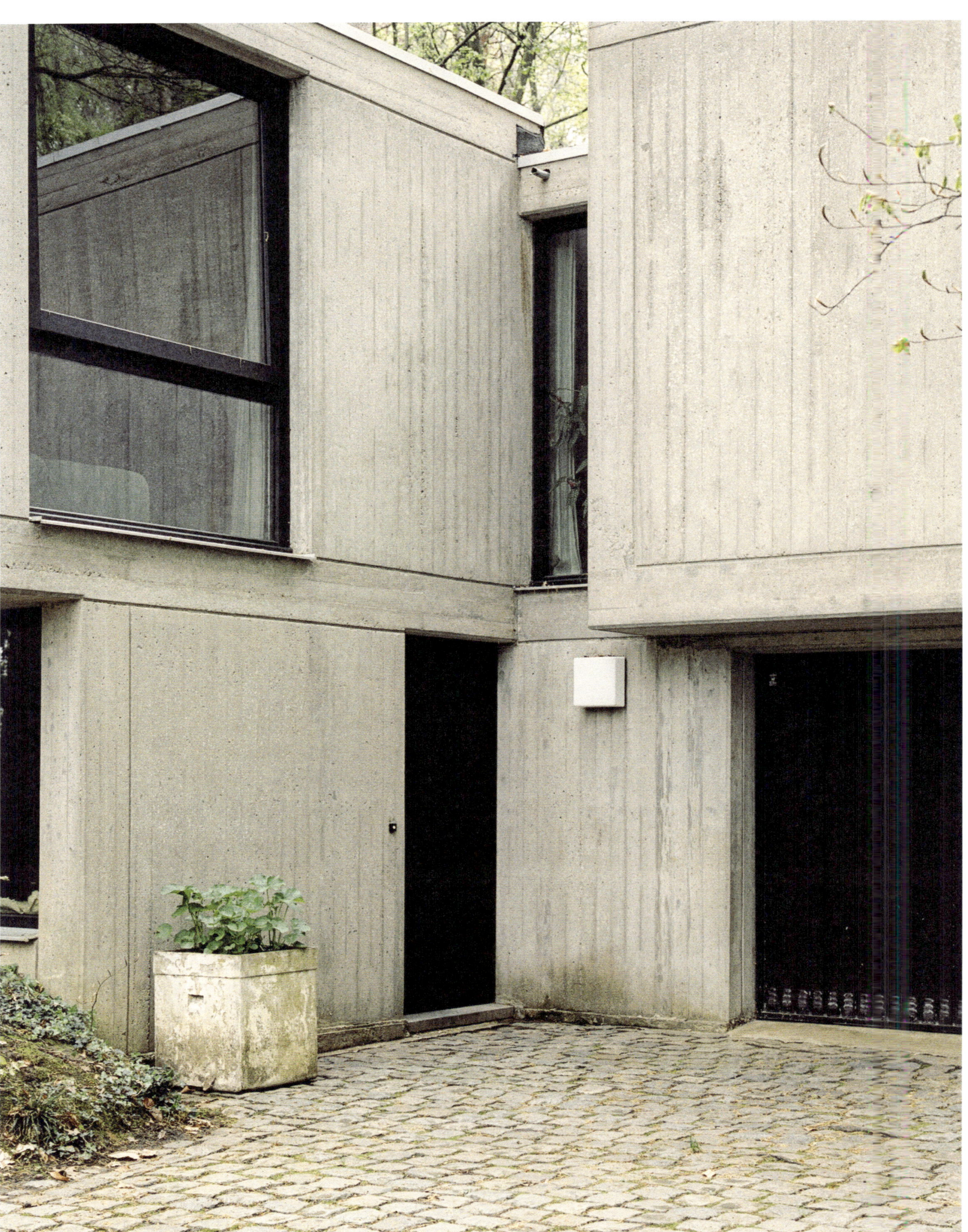

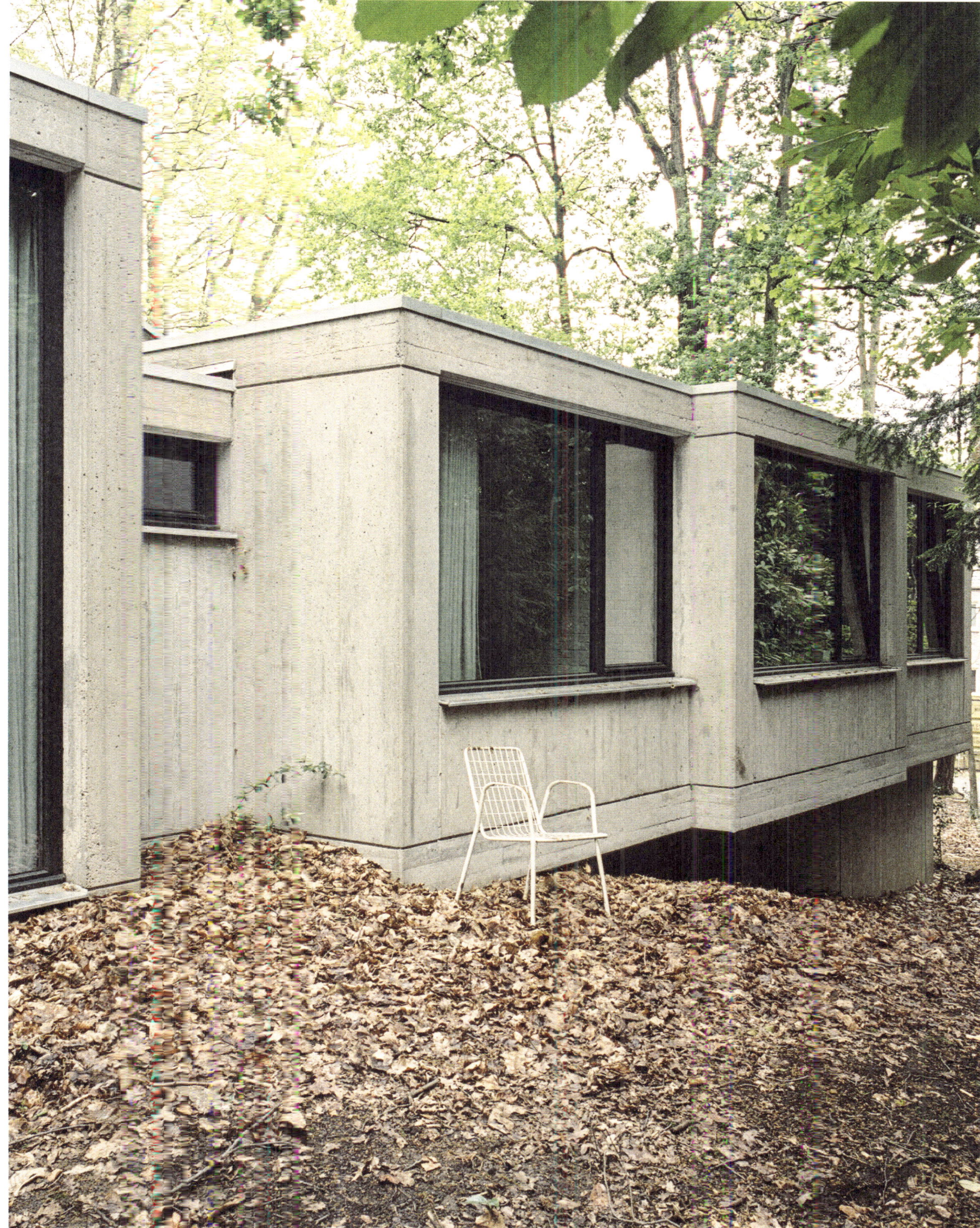

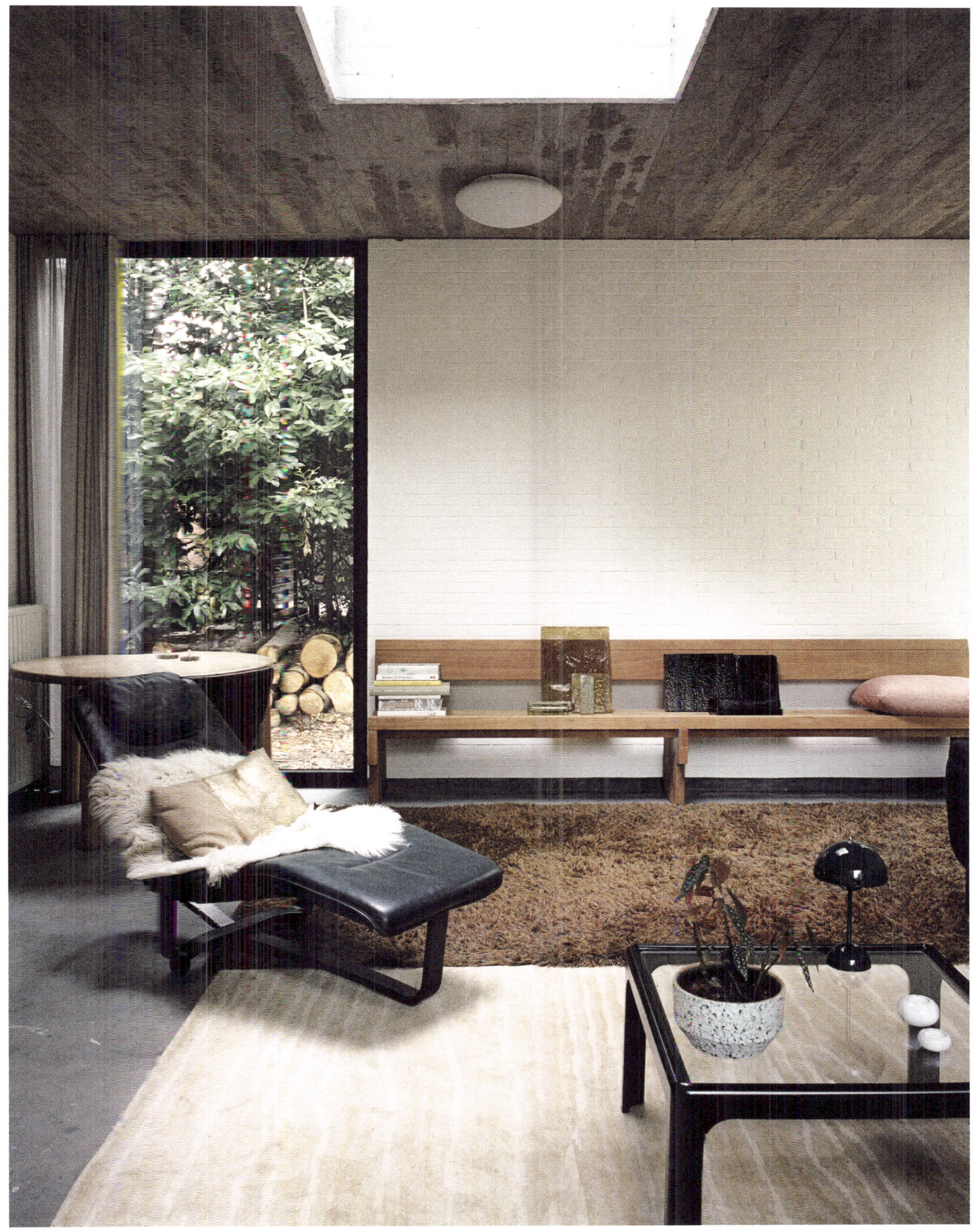

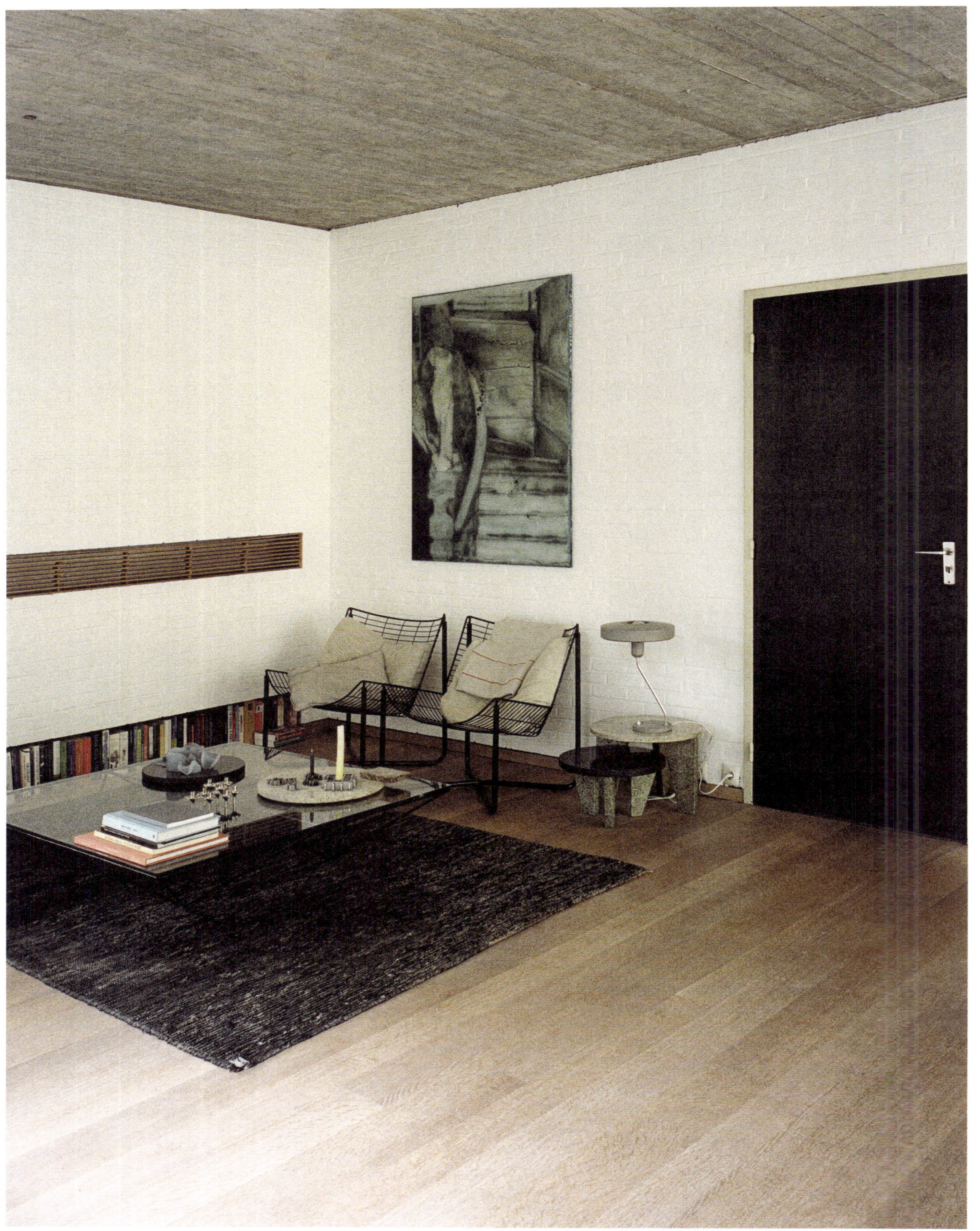

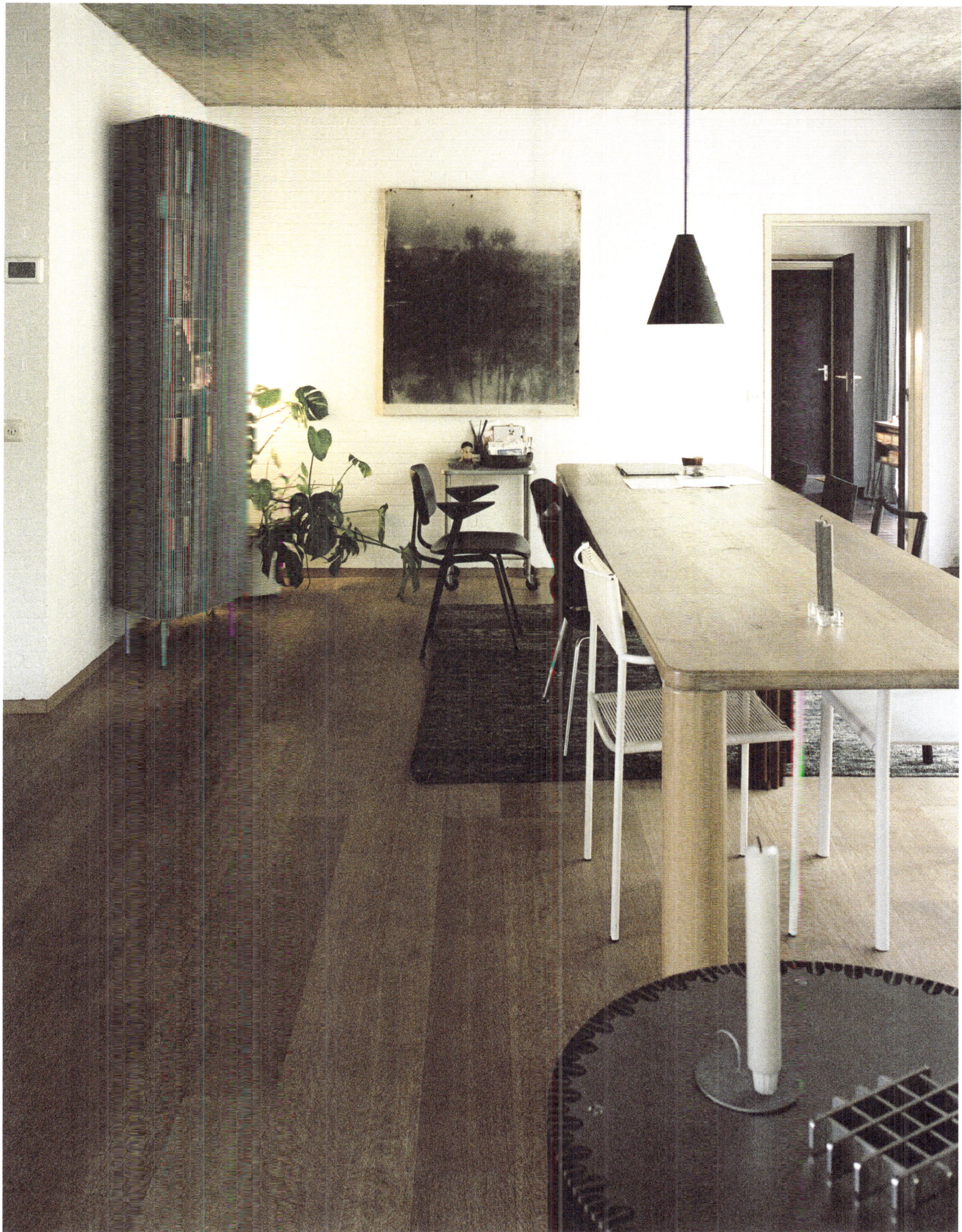

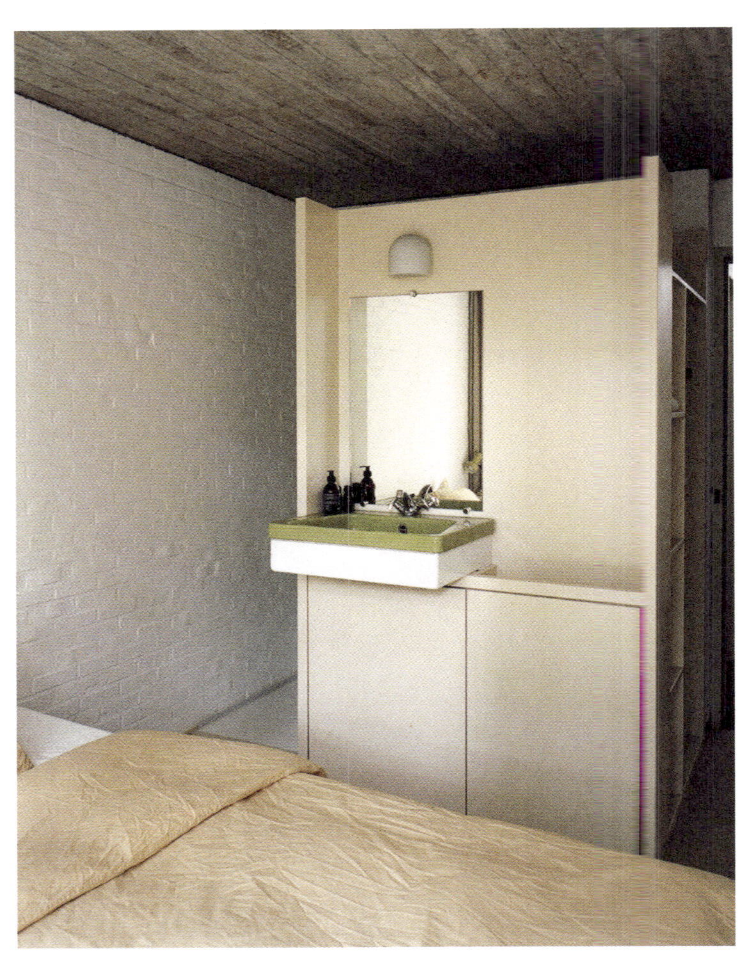

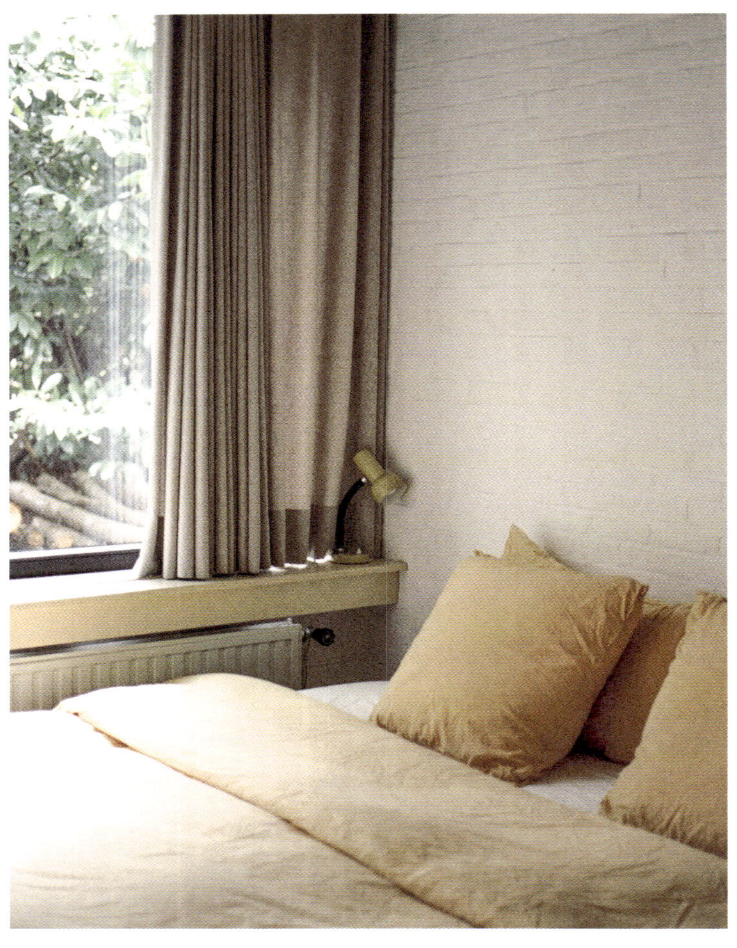

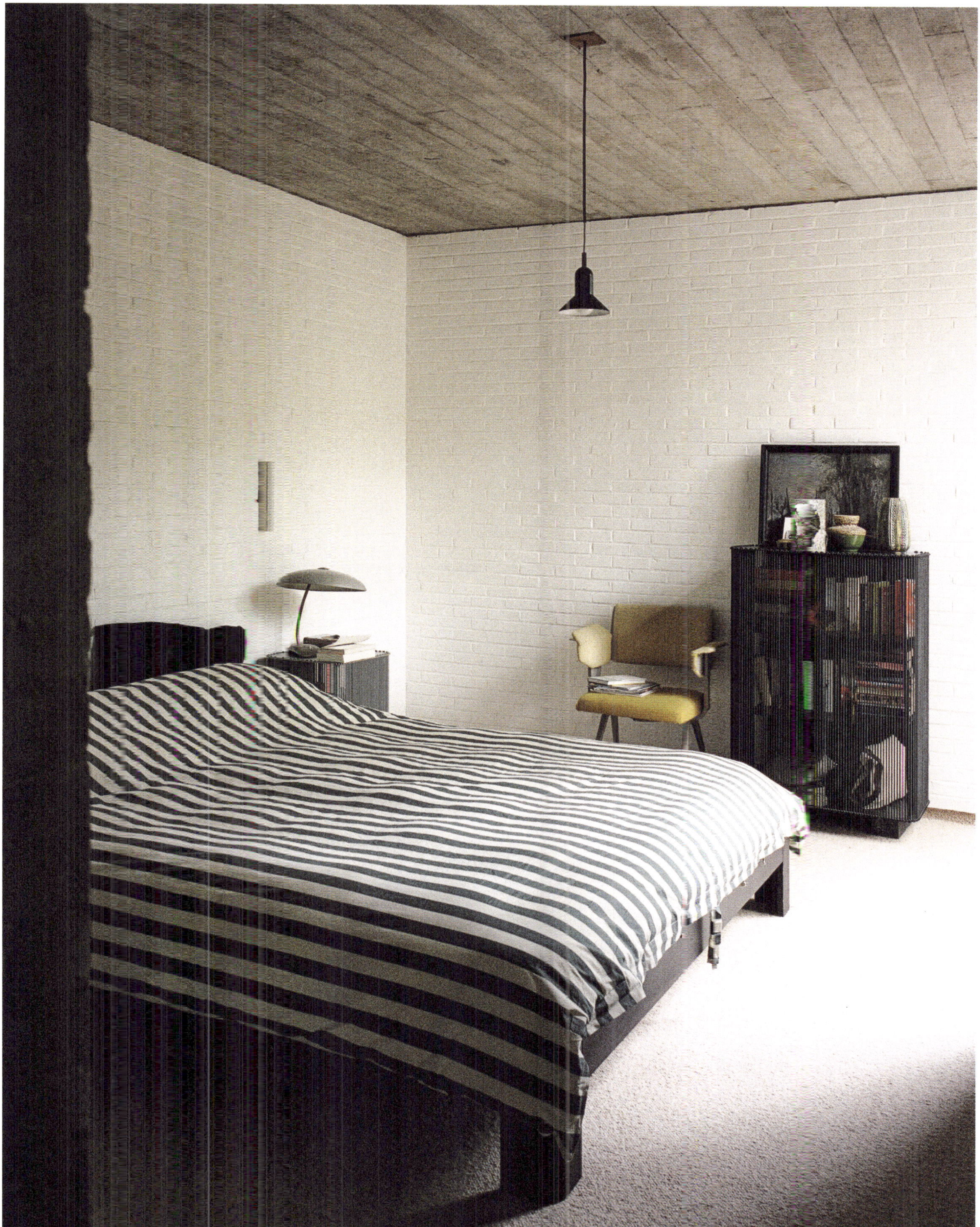

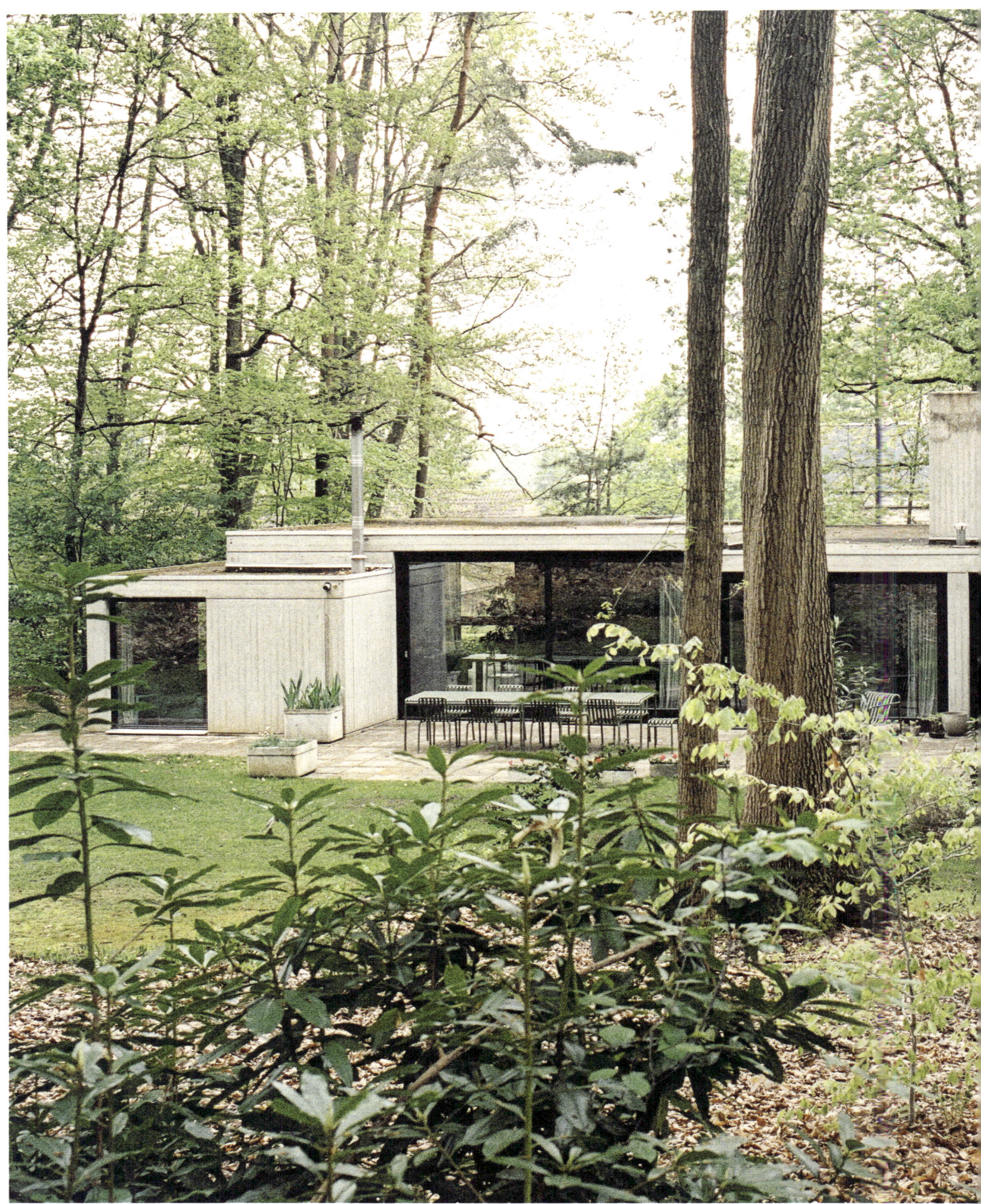

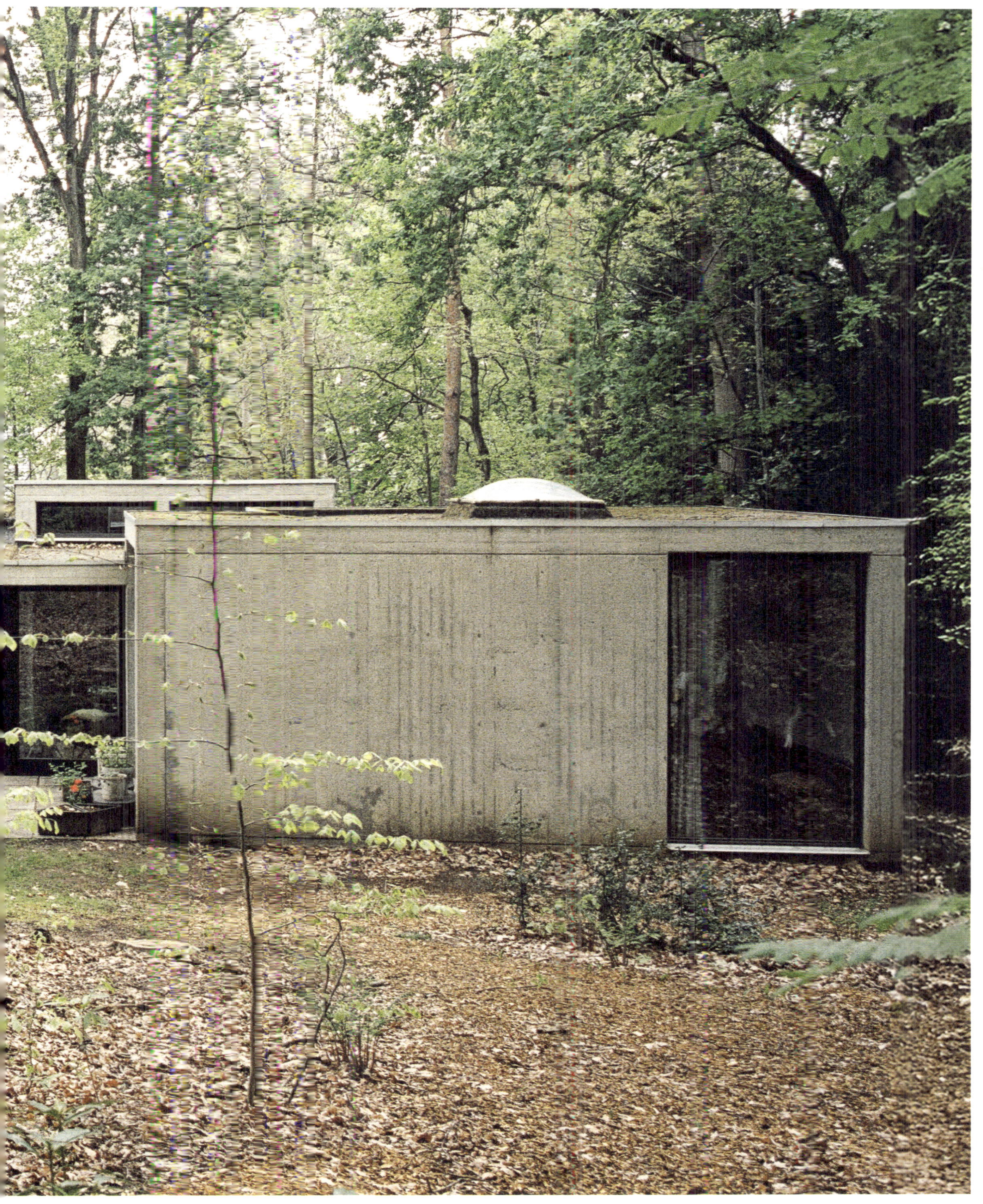

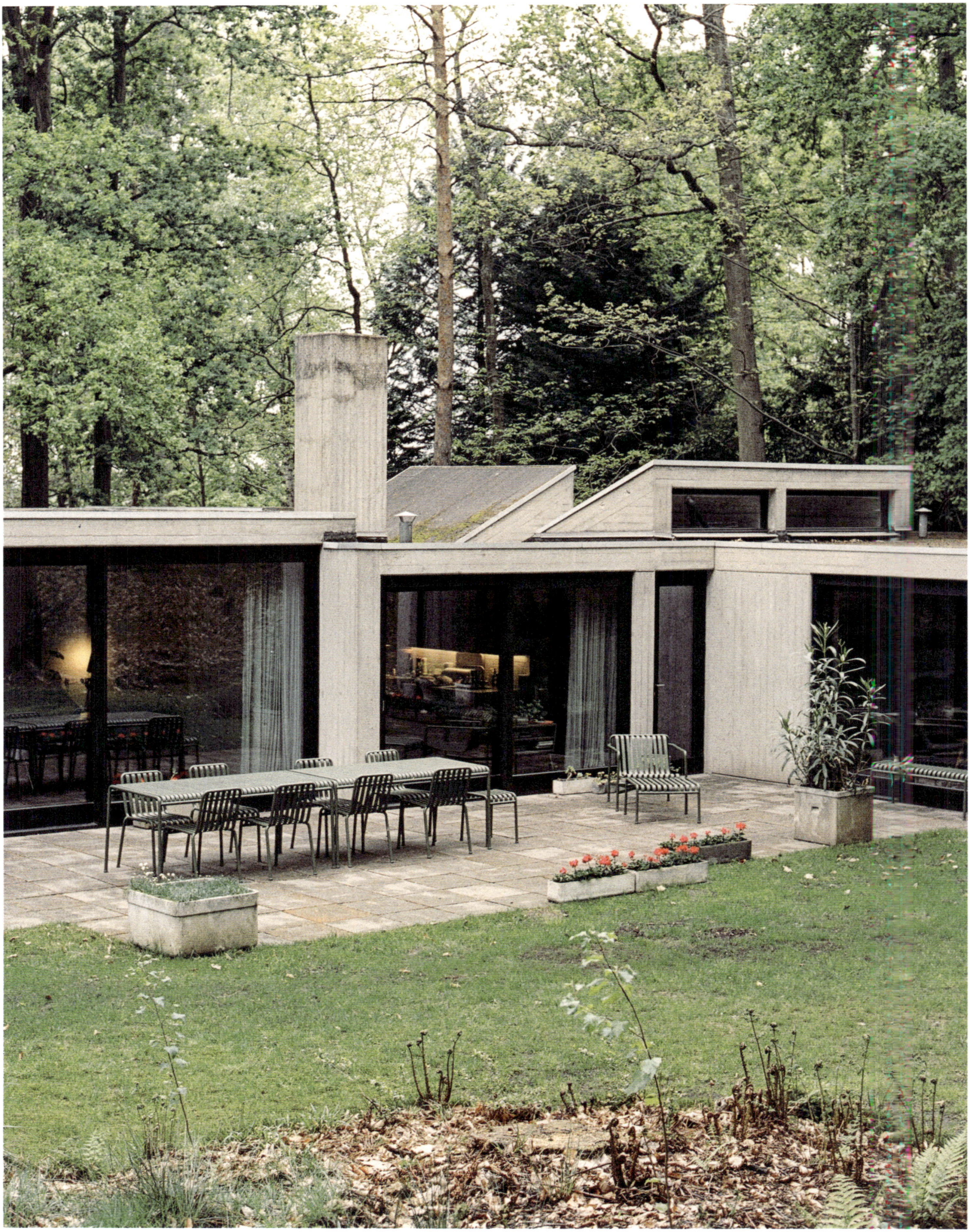

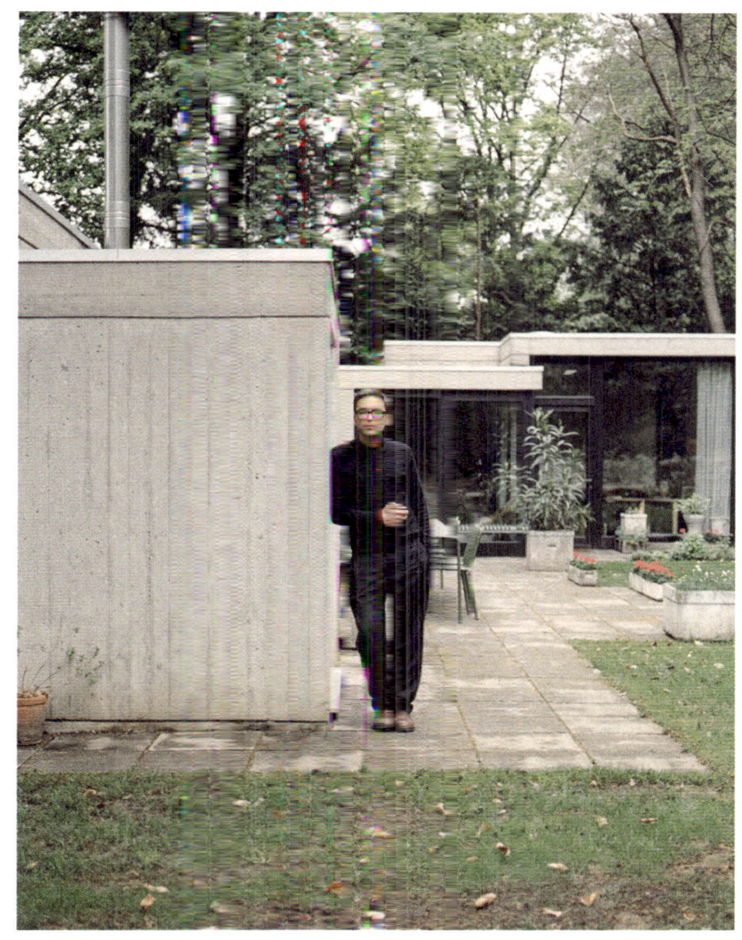

"Living in a brutalist house surrounded by old trees and pure nature, reveals the importance of both details and light in experiencing beauty."

– Bram Kerkhofs

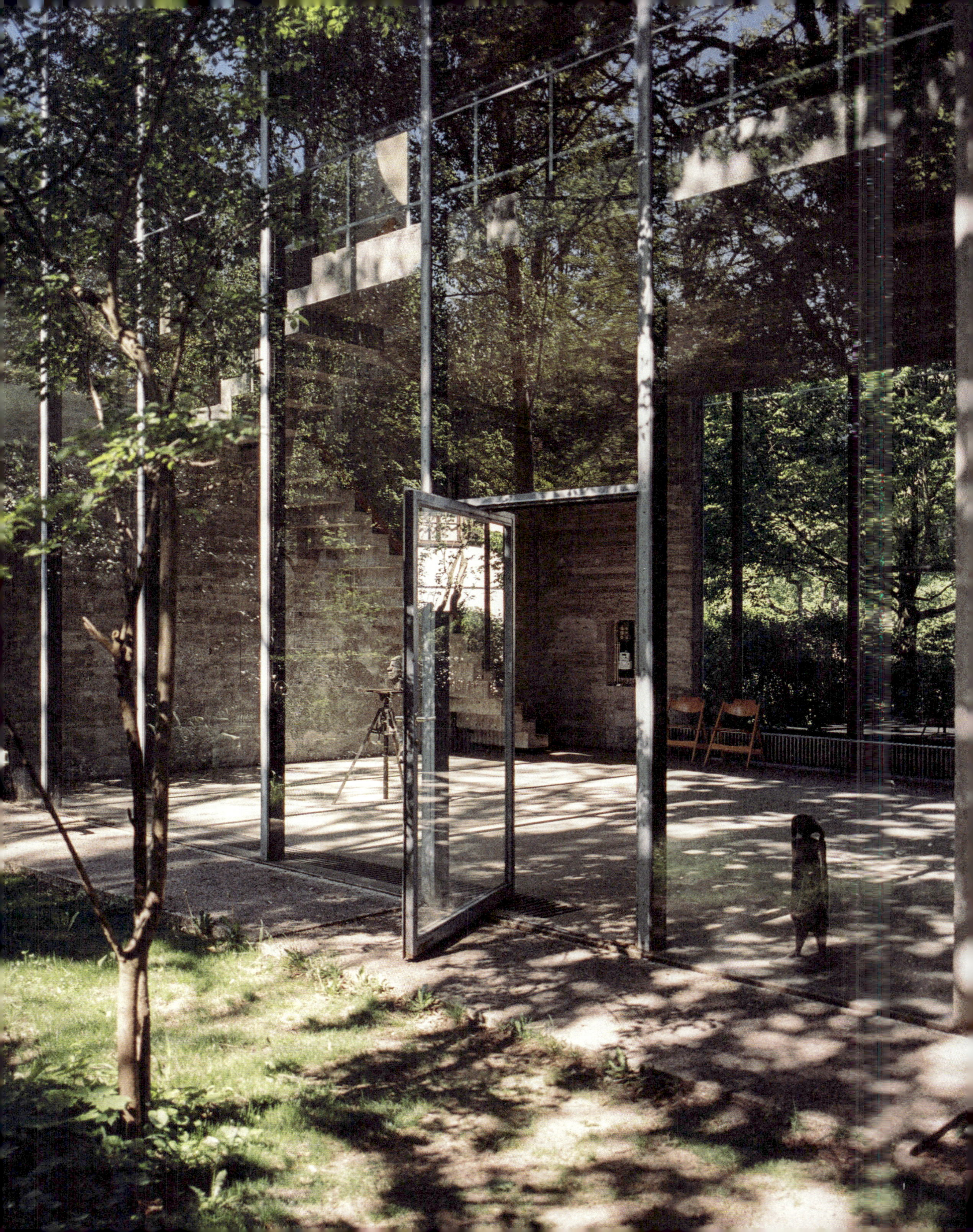

Atelier Rosa
Germany

This place was built slowly, over eight years, by just two people. One of them was Hermann Rosa, a sculptor. The other was a friend, also a sculptor, who came from Schönau to help. They mixed concrete by hand, using two machines, and worked without a construction company. Everything you see here was made this way: careful, physical, and precise.

Rosa had already built other houses before this one, but he had to sell them. This one he kept. It wasn't his home, but his studio. A space for thinking and making. It's strong and quiet, built almost entirely from raw concrete. But it's more than a building; it feels like a sculpture you can walk into. The atelier sits just behind Munich's Englischer Garten, hidden in a quiet residential street.

From the outside, the shape is compact. There are no overhangs or decorations. The walls are simple and straight. But nothing is quite symmetrical. The drainpipe, for example, is not in the middle. The front door isn't centred either. Rosa chose this on purpose. "Normally, you would end the form here", his son explains. "But he ended it there." It's slightly off, and that's the point.

Rosa didn't like traditional architecture. He didn't like buildings that followed the same rules or tried to look pretty. He wanted his work to feel solid and honest. That is why he used concrete. It allowed him to shape the structure like a sculptor. He had also trained in stone and glass work, so he trusted his hands. "You're not always allowed by regulation", his son says. "But you are allowed by the material."

The inside is arranged over three levels. There is a main workspace, a raised area in the corner, and a lower part near the back. A round skylight in the roof brings daylight into the centre of the space. You can see the staircases, the pipes, and the joints. None of it is hidden. Everything is part of the building's story.

Some wood was added later, not as decoration but to finish certain parts. A stair tread, a handrail. Always practical; never too polished. The details are simple but carefully considered.

Today, the building is still used as a studio. It is also open to visitors, but only by appointment. Exhibitions are held here from time to time and, occasionally, a film crew or a photographer may ask to use the space. But the family decides what feels right. "It happens", his son says, "when it fits."

There are other buildings by Rosa in Munich, some he built for others, some he had to leave behind. But this one was his – it holds his ideas and his way of working. He believed that art and architecture should be direct, physical, and real. Not soft, not showy, just honest.

Even though the city around it has grown, the atelier still feels calm and grounded. It doesn't try to stand out, but it doesn't disappear either. It is simply there – clear, careful, and built by hand.

Project: Atelier Rosa
Location: Germany
Architect: Hermann Rosa
Year of construction: 1960
Floor area: 150 m²
Caretaker: Veit Rosa
Caretaker's profession: retired lawyer

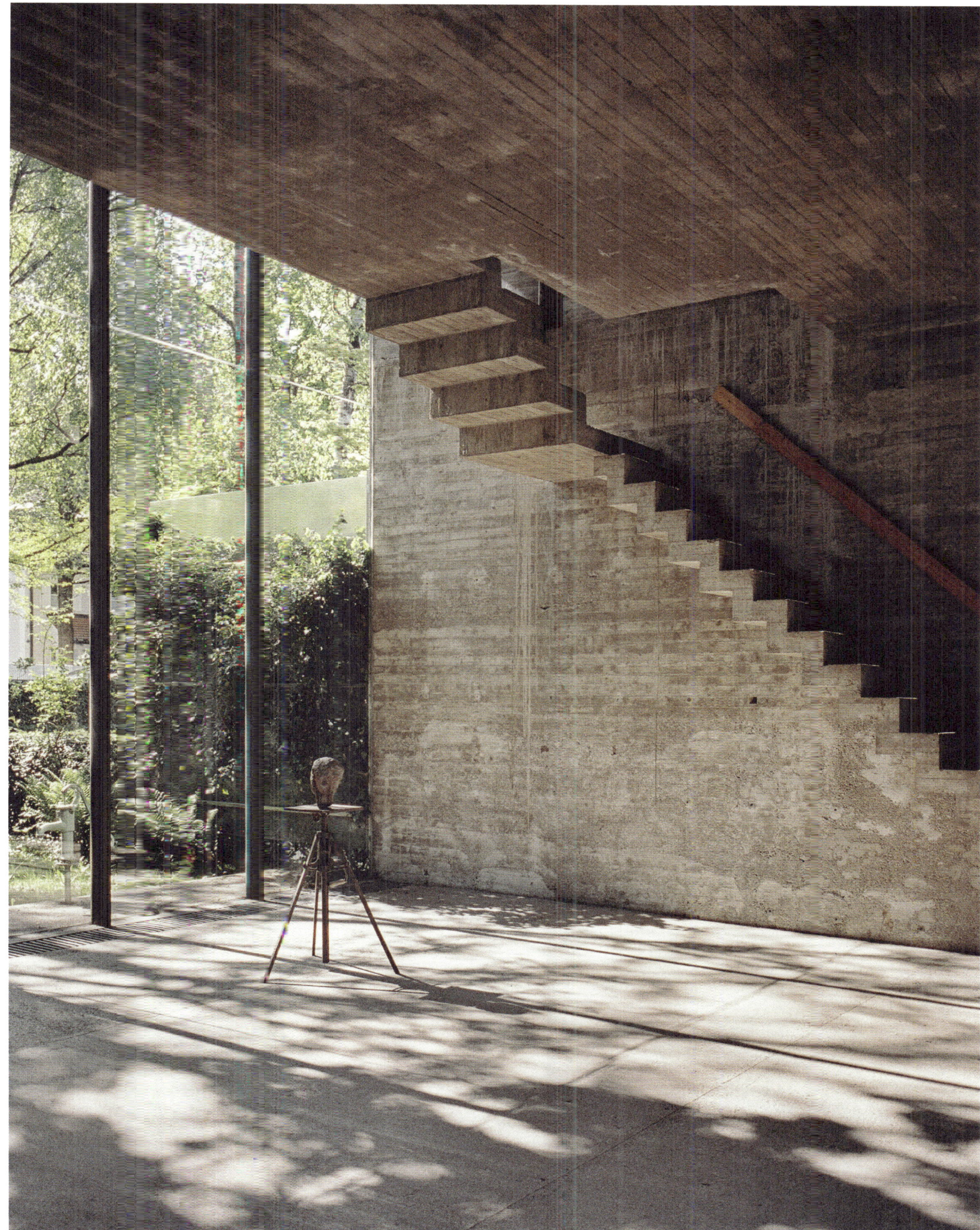

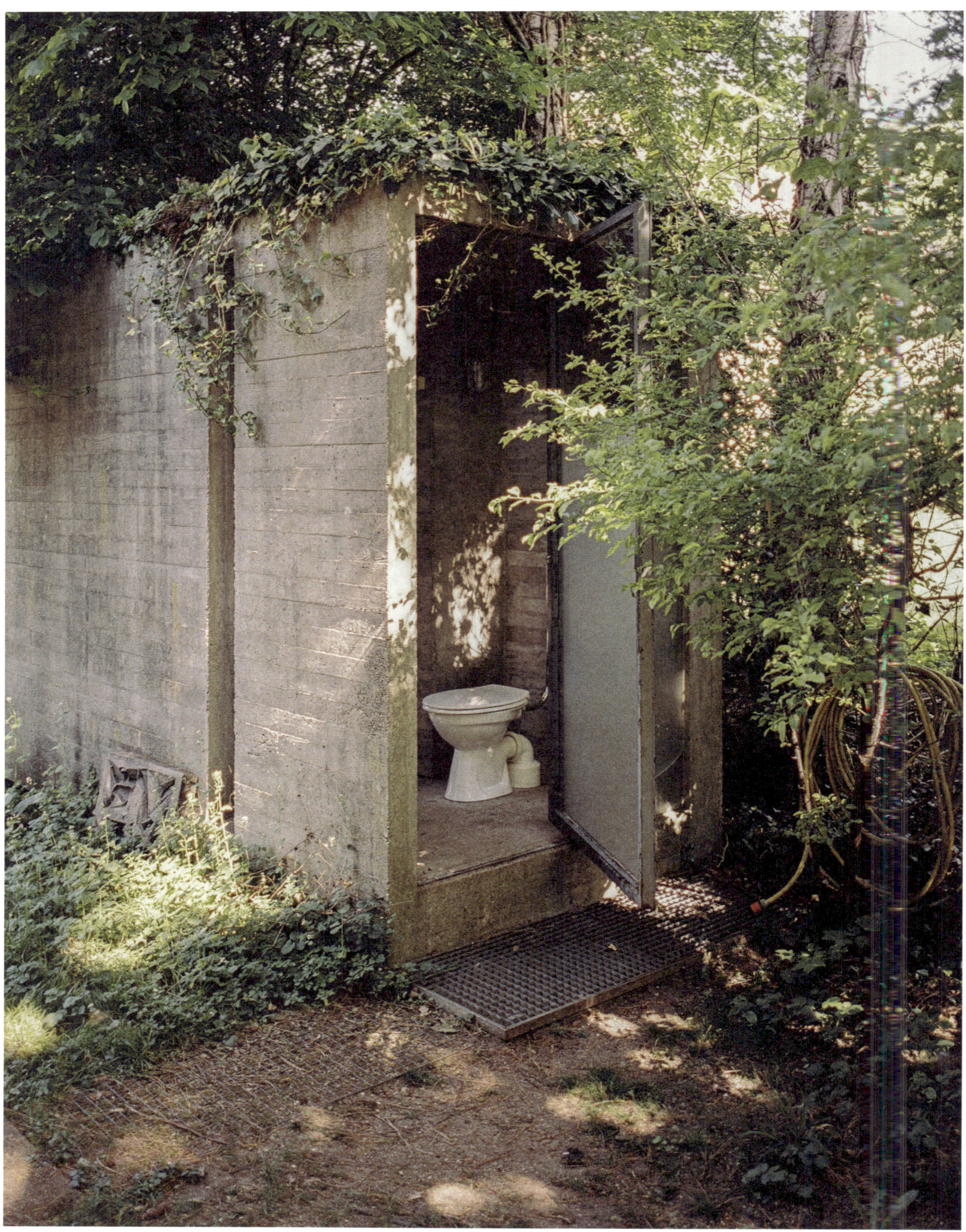

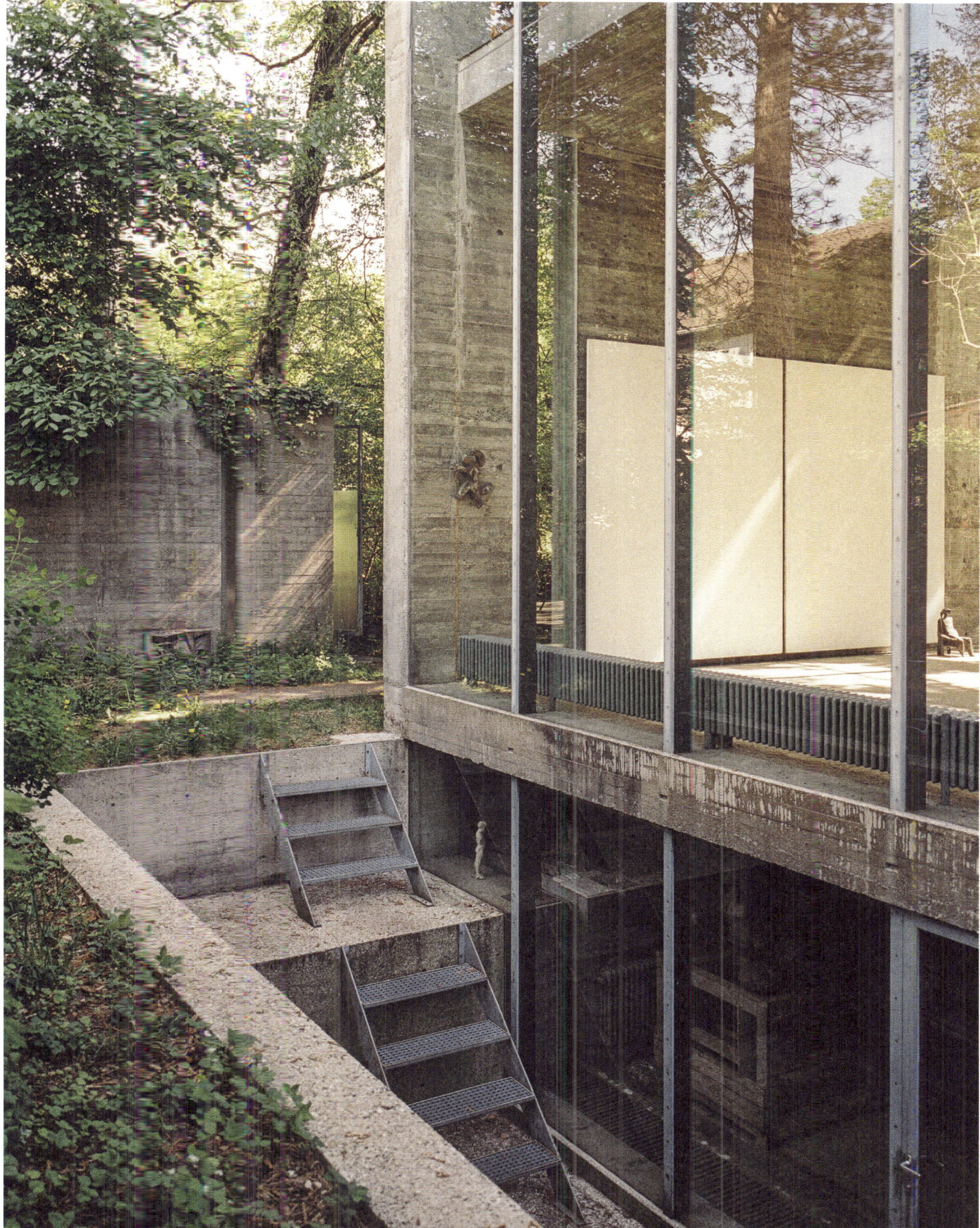

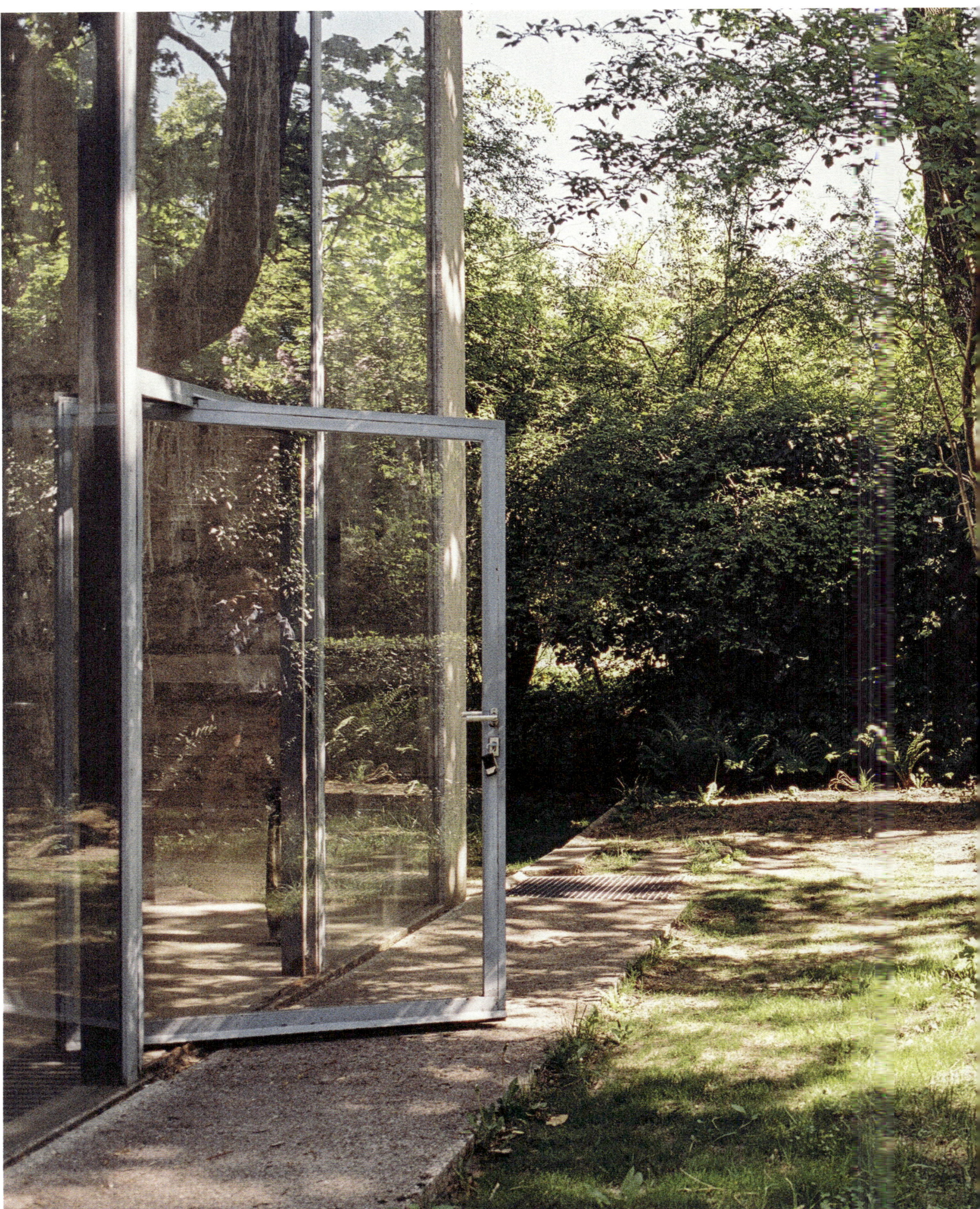

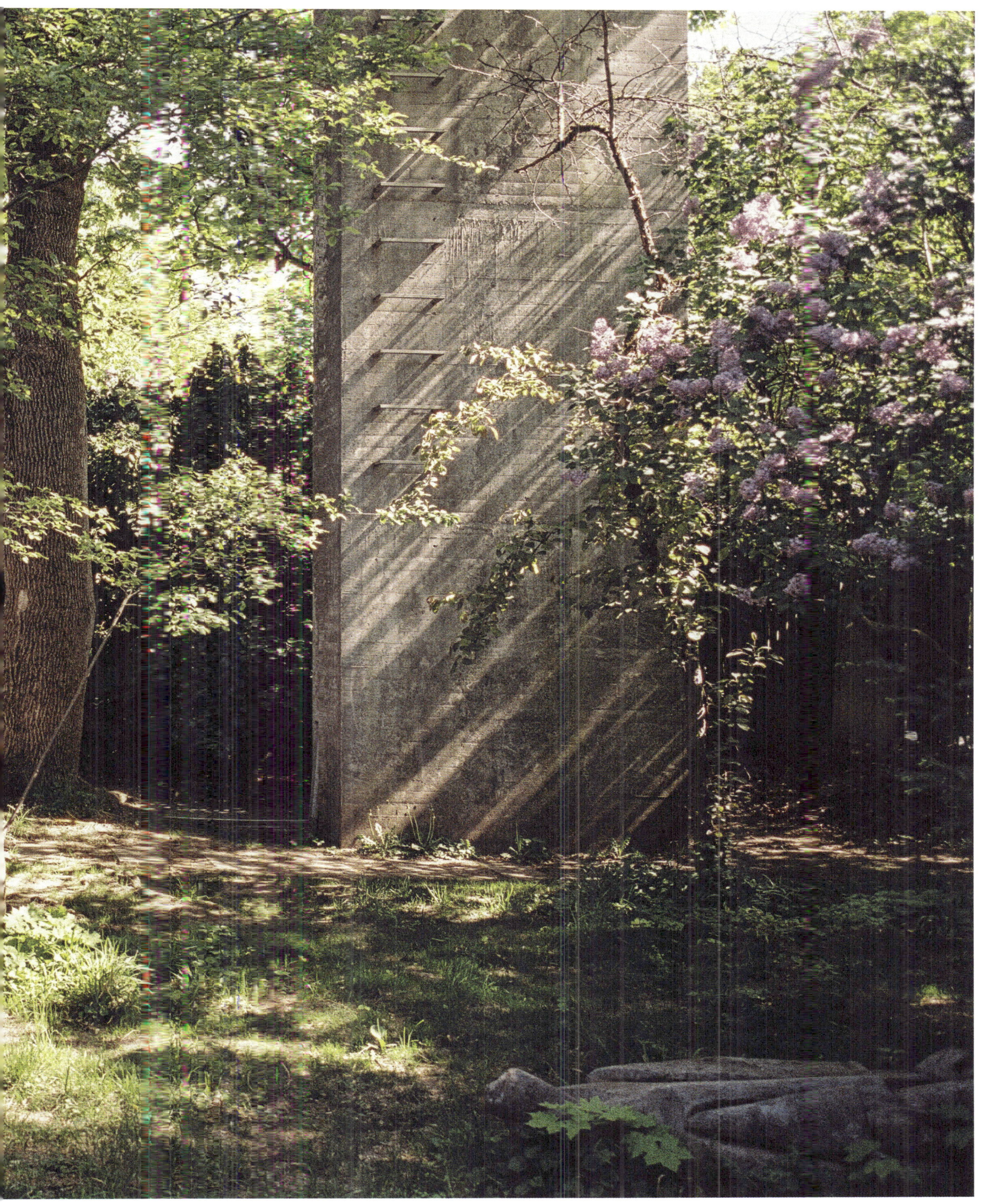

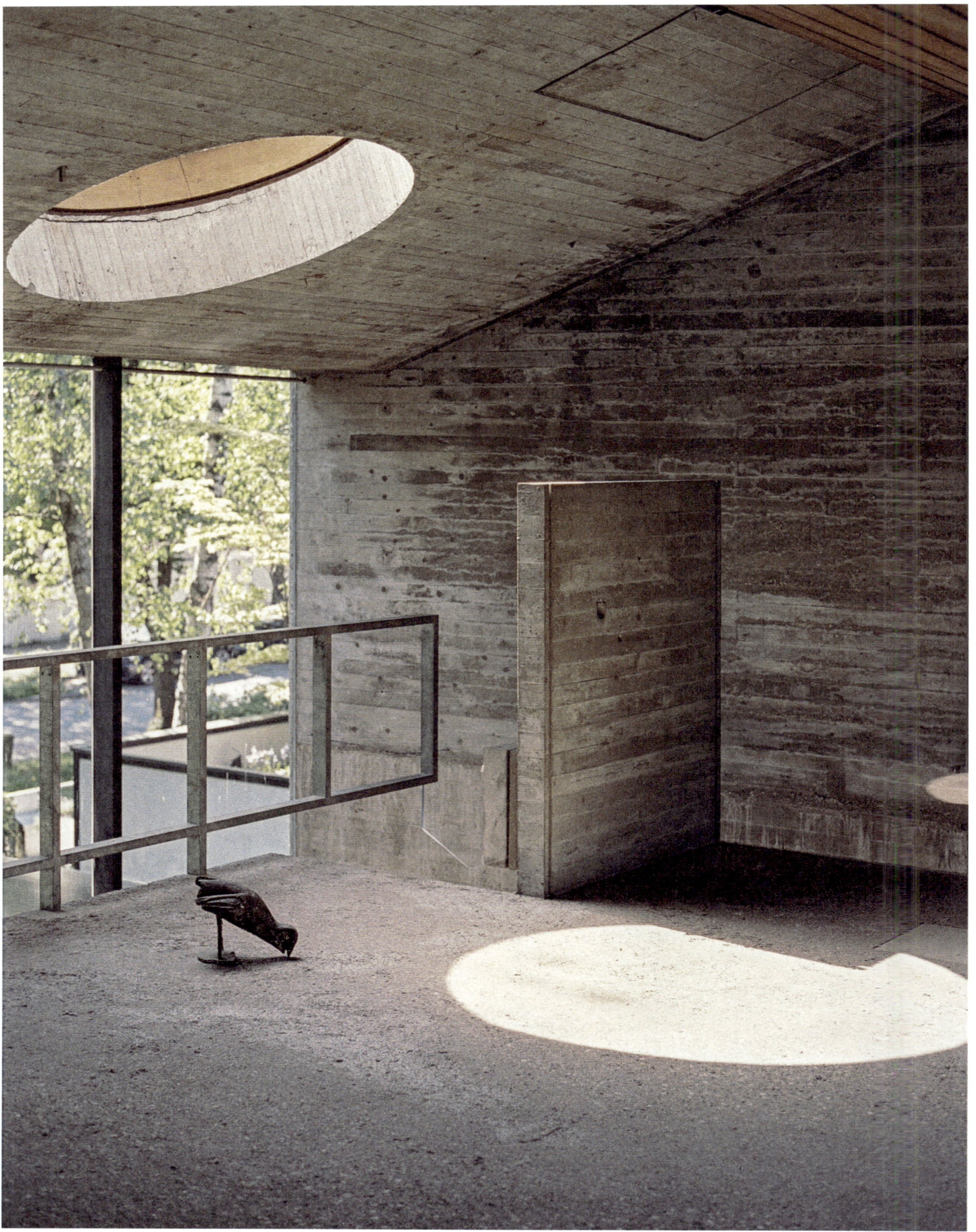

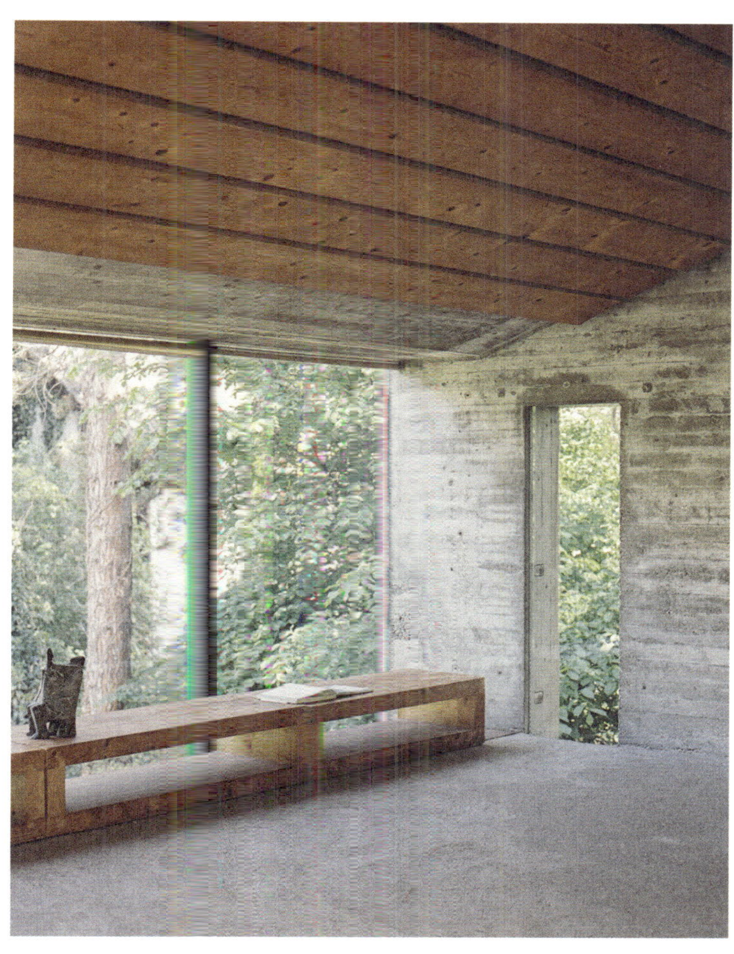

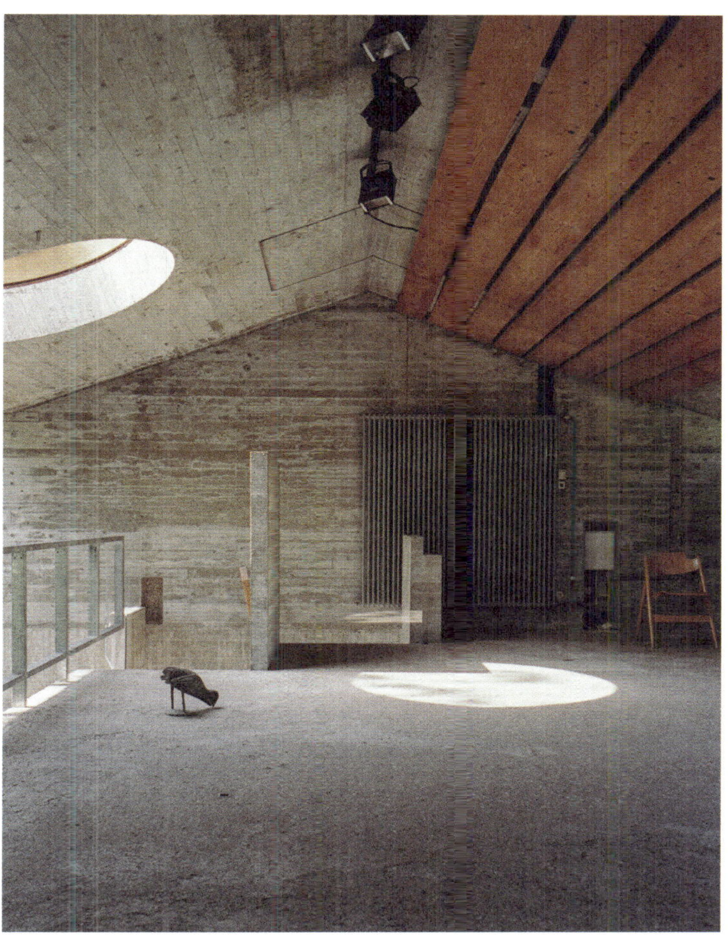

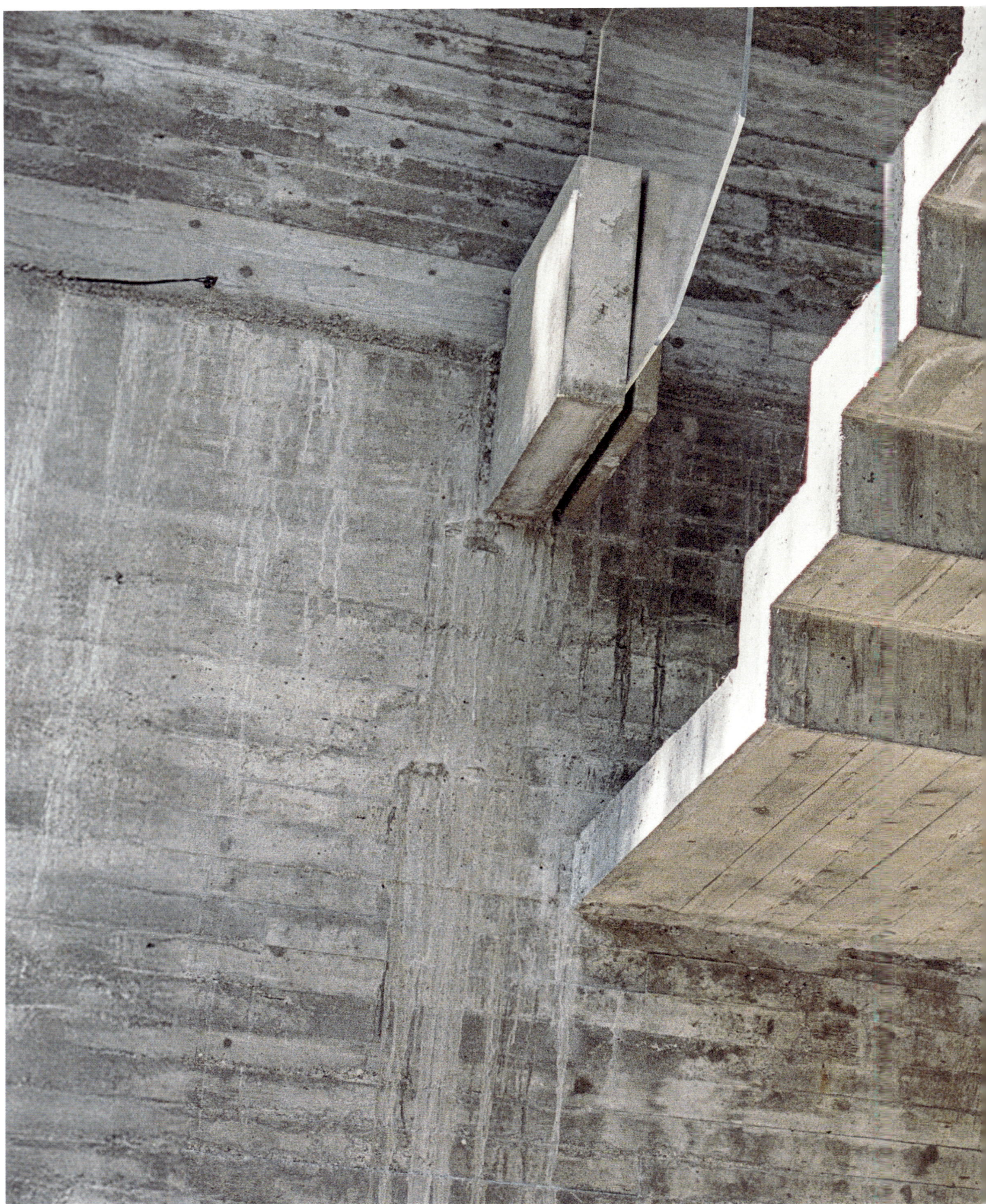

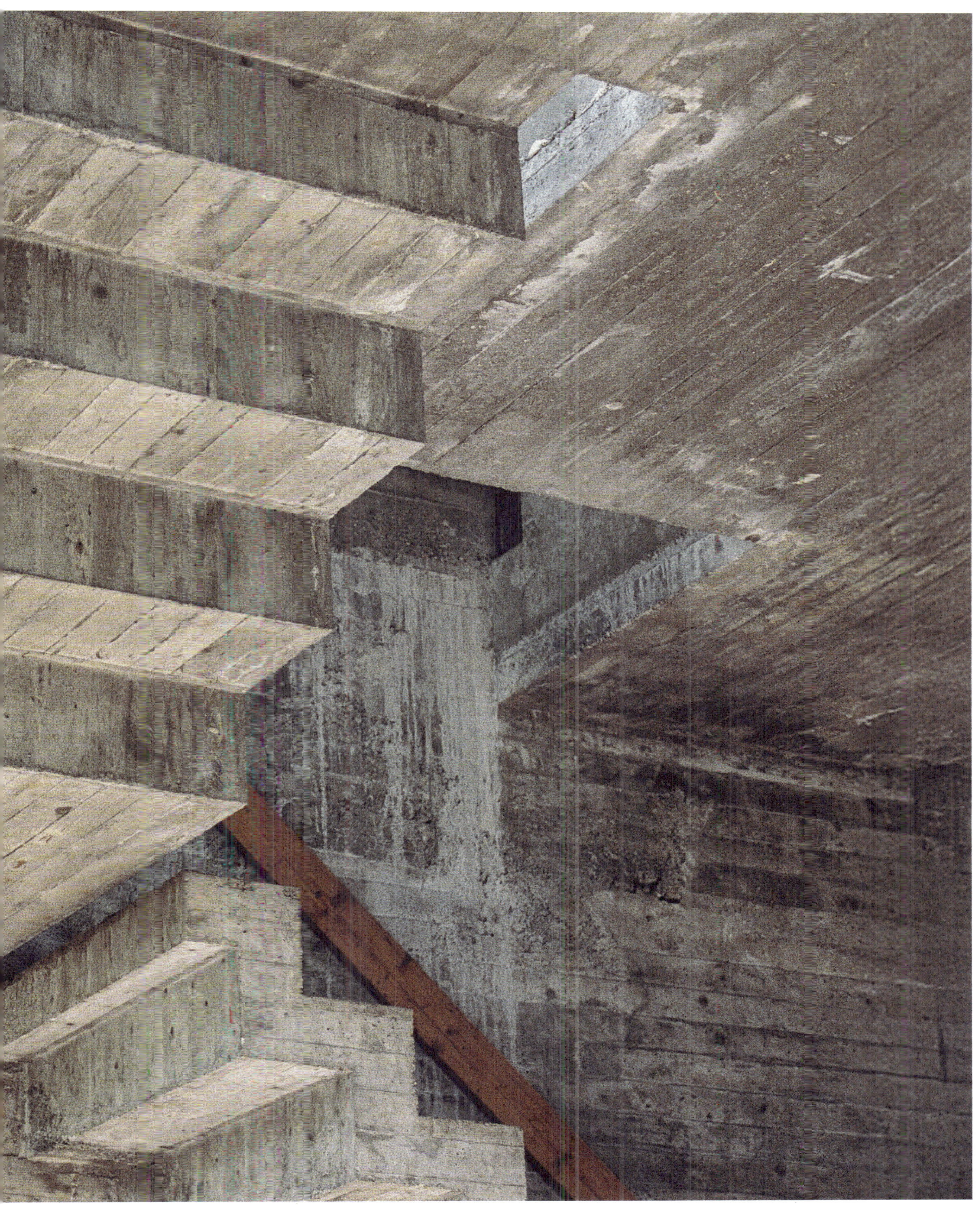

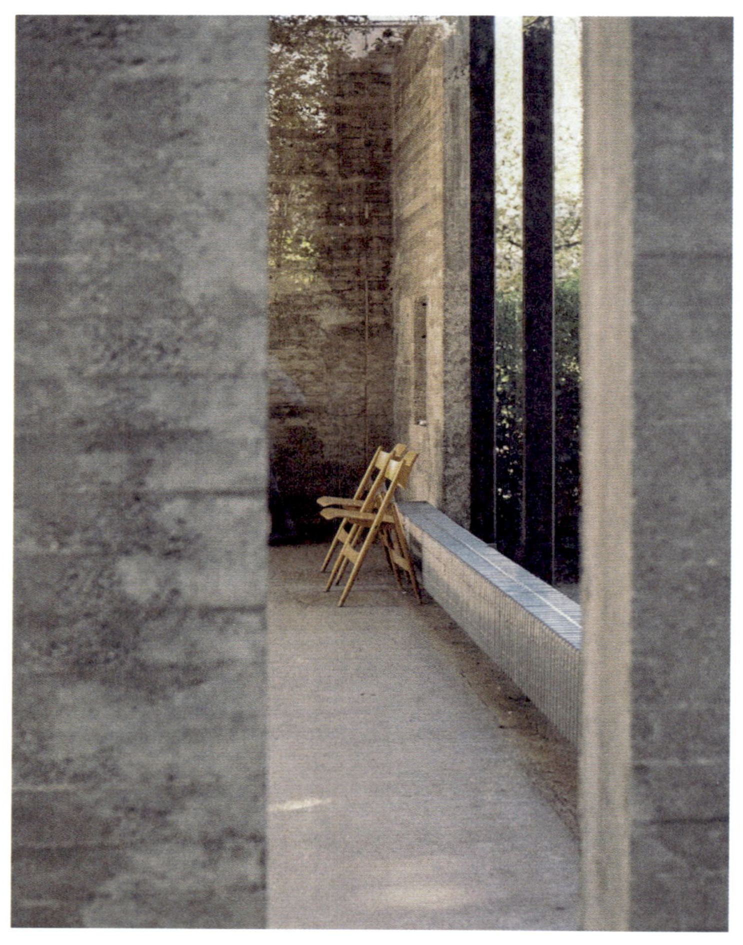

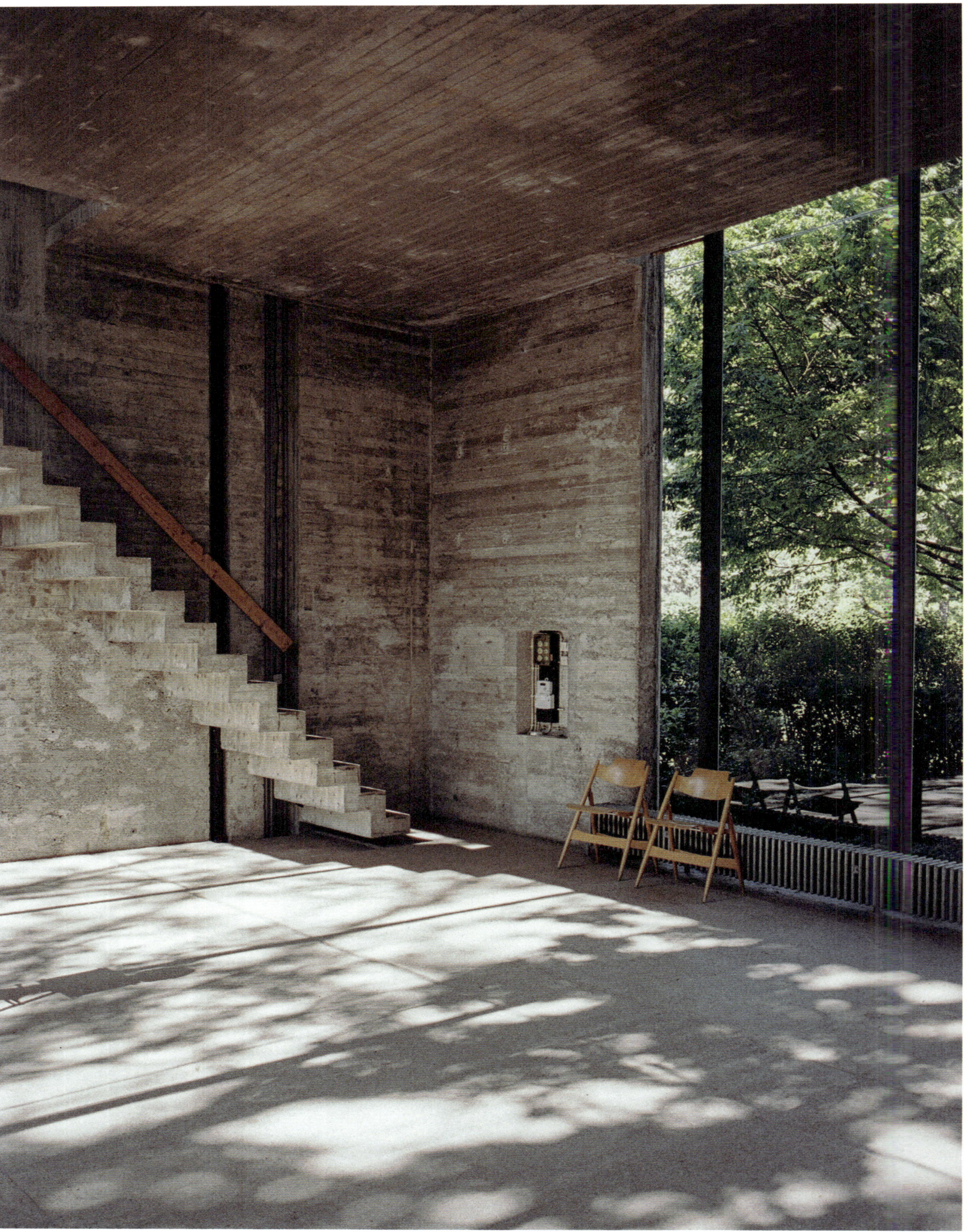

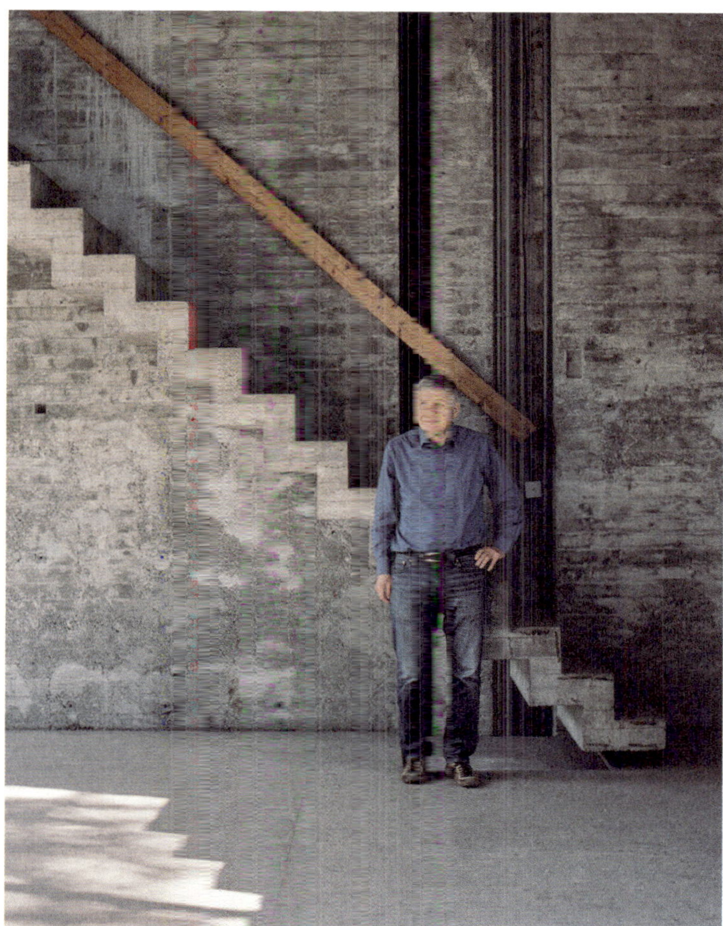

"The studio is a house of light and silence, a place where architecture itself becomes part of the portrait."

– Veit Rosa

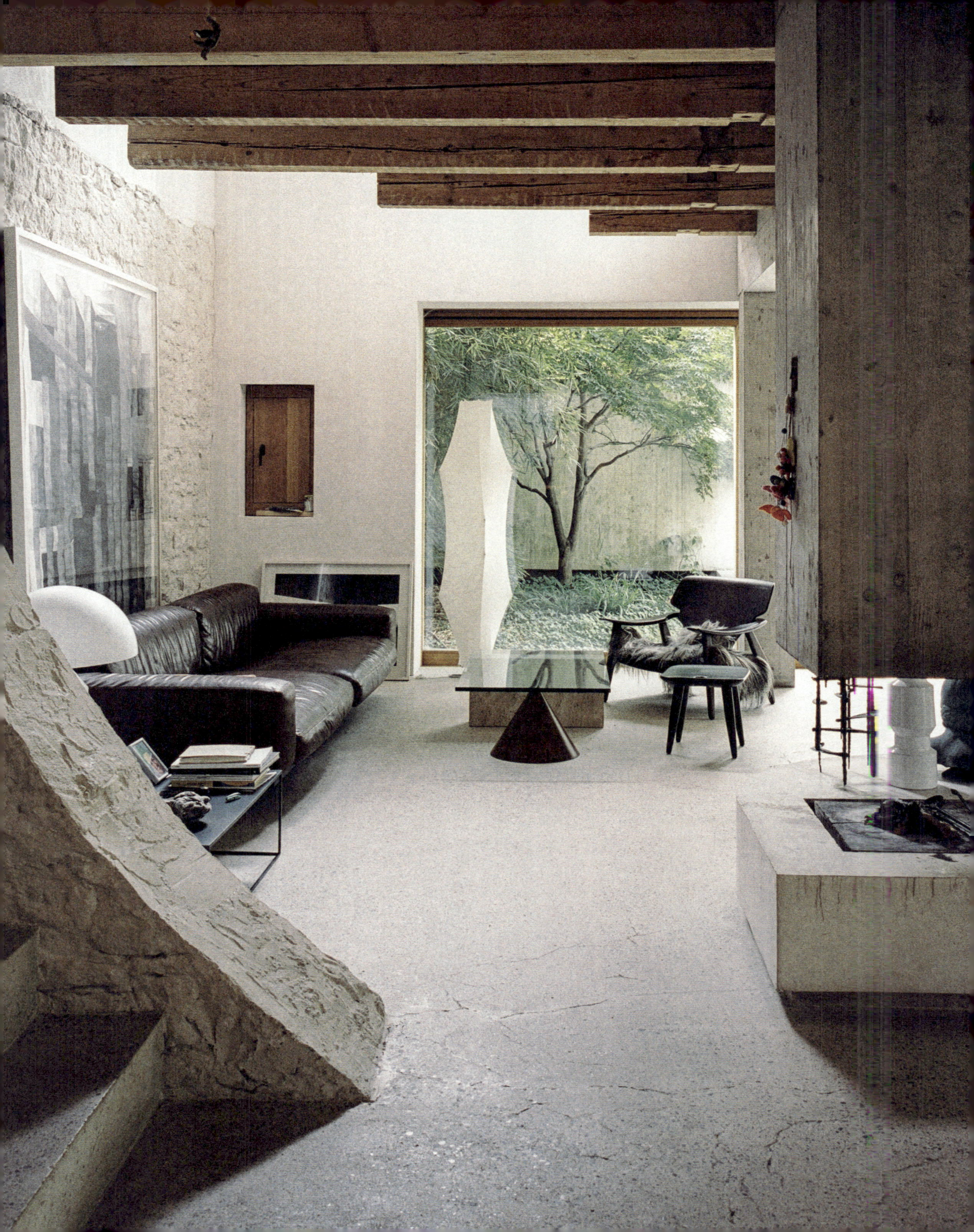

Missionsstrasse House

Switzerland

You can't see the house from the street. It sits behind another building, hidden in a leafy courtyard near Basel's Spalentor. From the public side, there's no trace of what's behind. That sense of seclusion – green, quiet, inward-looking – defines how the house feels. You're in the city, but it doesn't feel like it.

The structure dates back to around 1880. Over the years, it served many purposes: a stable, a coach house, a hayloft, and an artist studio. But it was never properly renovated. When the current owner, also the architect, took over, the building was rundown and fragmented. Still, the idea was never to erase the past. The project became about reframing what was there, structurally and spatially.

Much of the existing envelope was kept, but the interior was rebuilt almost entirely. A new concrete core was inserted, like a house within a house. This gave the structure stability, but also opened up new possibilities: taller rooms, larger spans, and more natural light.

Two vertical voids, triangular in shape, were carved into the plan to bring daylight deep into the building. Light now enters from above, tracing the rough walls and casting shadows across the surfaces. These openings are not just practical, they break up the geometry and add a sense of stillness and space.

The most dramatic gesture is a large circular cut-out across two floors – a softened void that connects levels and rooms, making the building feel lighter and more open.

One of the biggest changes was made to the right-hand façade. Previously closed off and heavy, it now opens to the garden with large pivoting doors and sliding glass. From inside, this transforms the experience entirely: light floods the ground floor, the concrete feels warmer, and the outside becomes part of the daily rhythm of the house.

The material palette is minimal but expressive: concrete, natural stone, oiled oak, and pine. Every surface feels tactile. You see formwork lines and subtle imperfections. The house doesn't hide its process, it shows how it was made.

There are no fixed separations between functions. The kitchen merges into the living space. And built-in cabinetry and careful openings define parts without enclosing them. Nothing dominates, nothing shouts. The atmosphere remains focused, but soft.

Upstairs are bedrooms, bathrooms, and study rooms. Spaces shift in ceiling height and proportion, guided by the geometry of the old structure. And skylights draw in daylight where side windows aren't feasible. Even the most internal spaces don't feel cut off.

Outside, the small garden plays a central role. Trees along the edges offer privacy, while the glazed side wall allows for a constant view to the outside. When the doors are open, the boundary between house and garden disappears. "It's not big", the architect says, "but it's enough. You can breathe here."

This house doesn't chase contrast or nostalgia. It doesn't restore the past or reject it. It uses what was found, holds on to what belongs, and builds with intention. Not to impress, but to clarify, to create space that feels both grounded and new.

Project: Missionsstrasse House
Location: Switzerland
Architect: Buchner Bründler Architekten
Year of construction: 1880
Year of purchase: 2018
Floor area: 405 m^2
Resident: Andreas Bründler
Resident's profession: architect

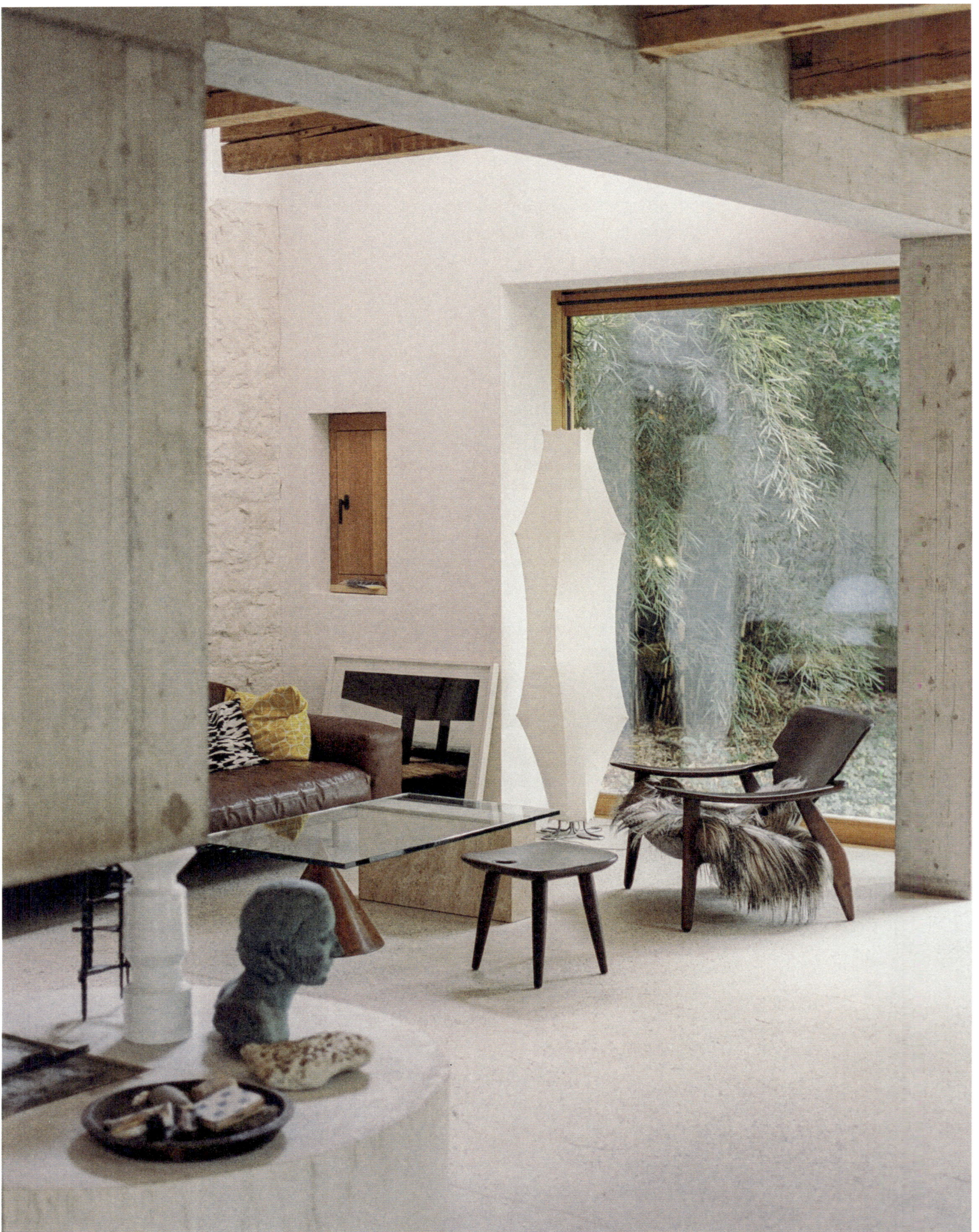

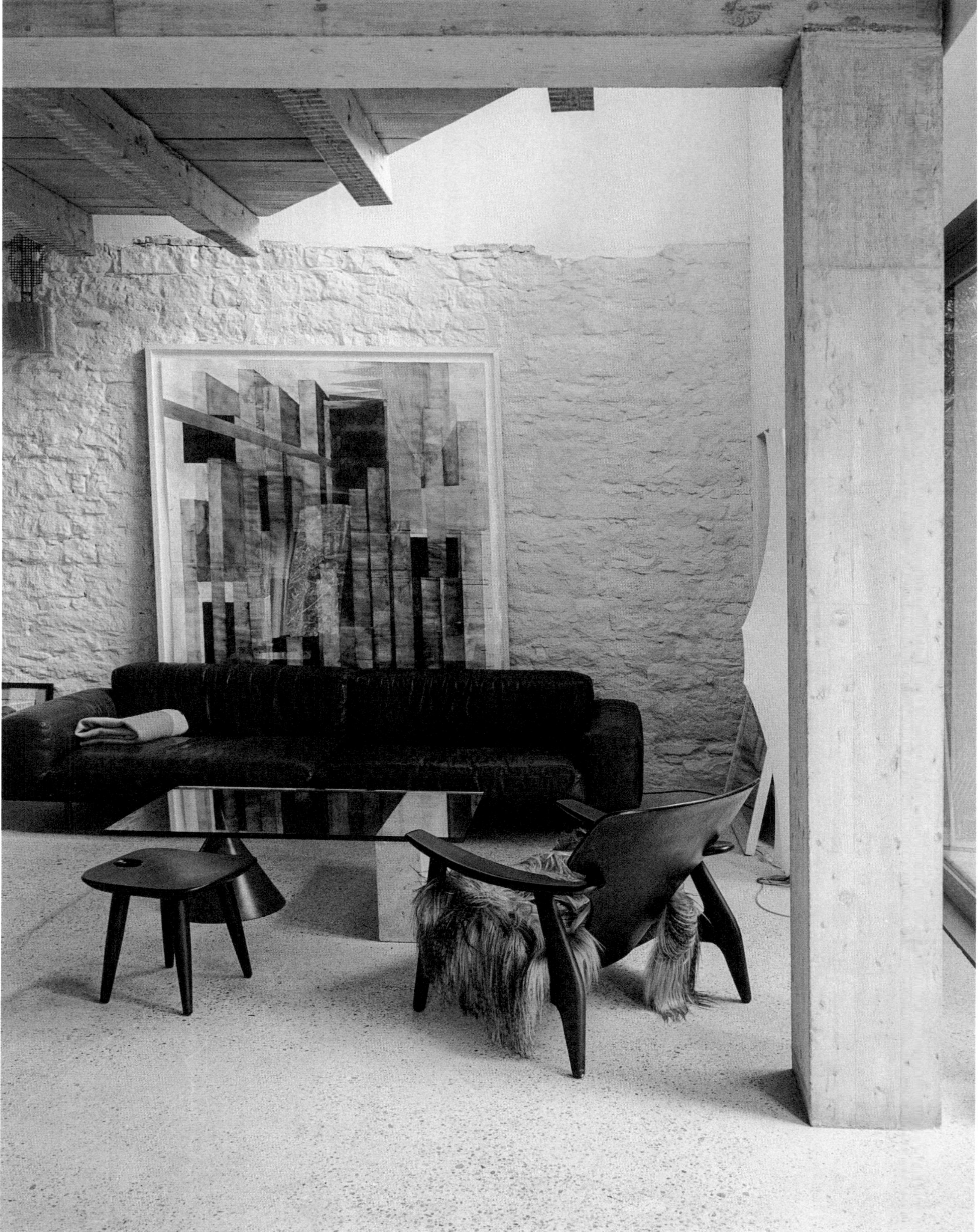

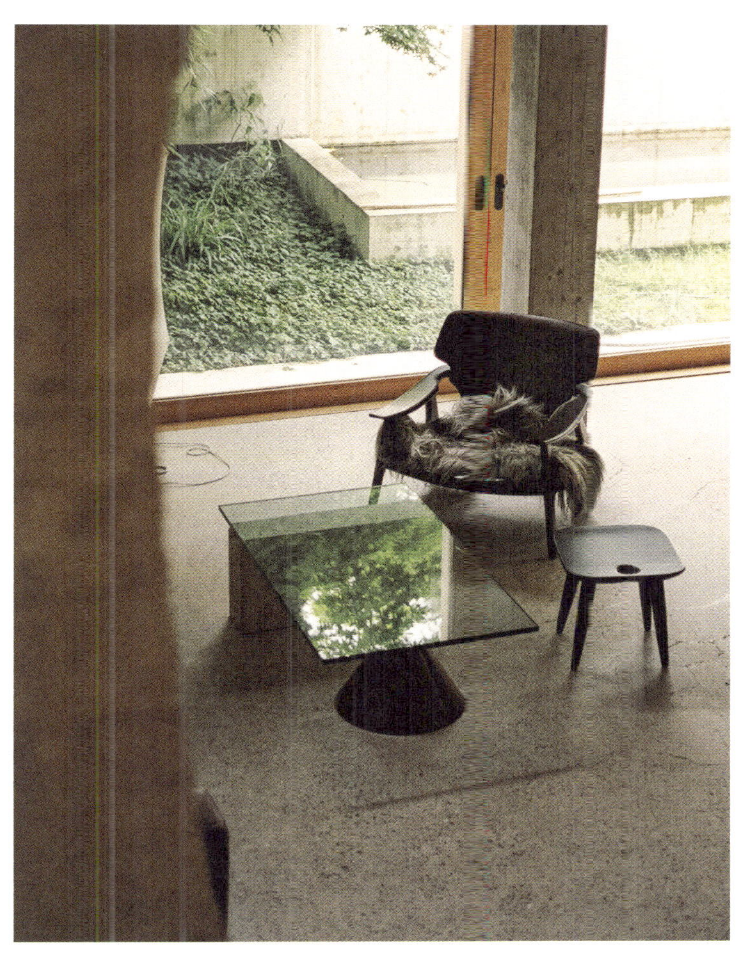

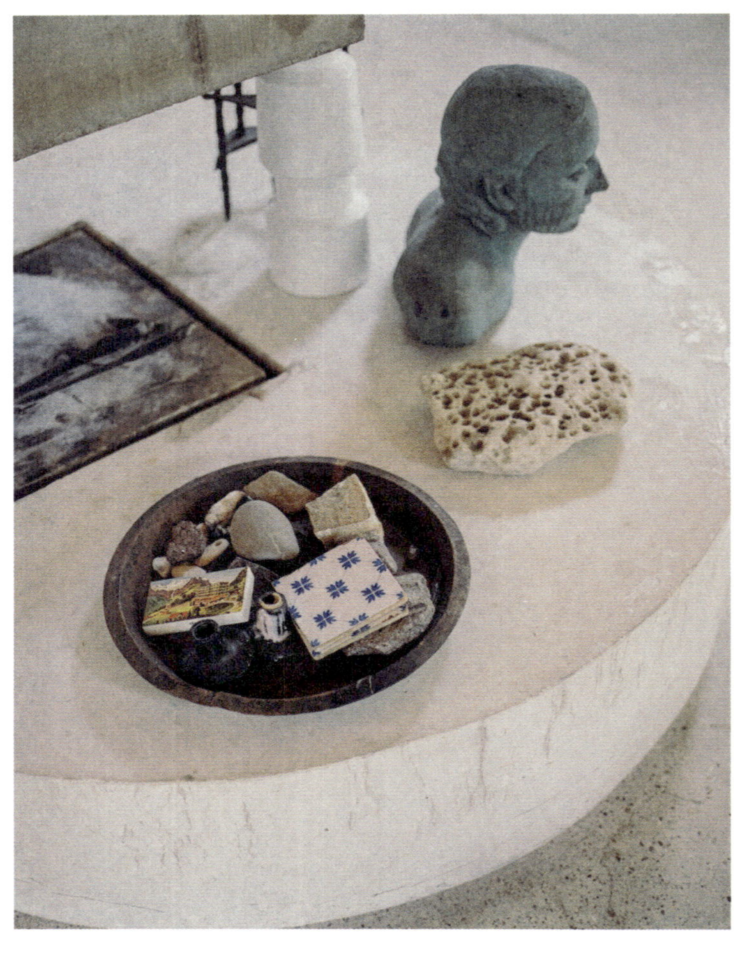

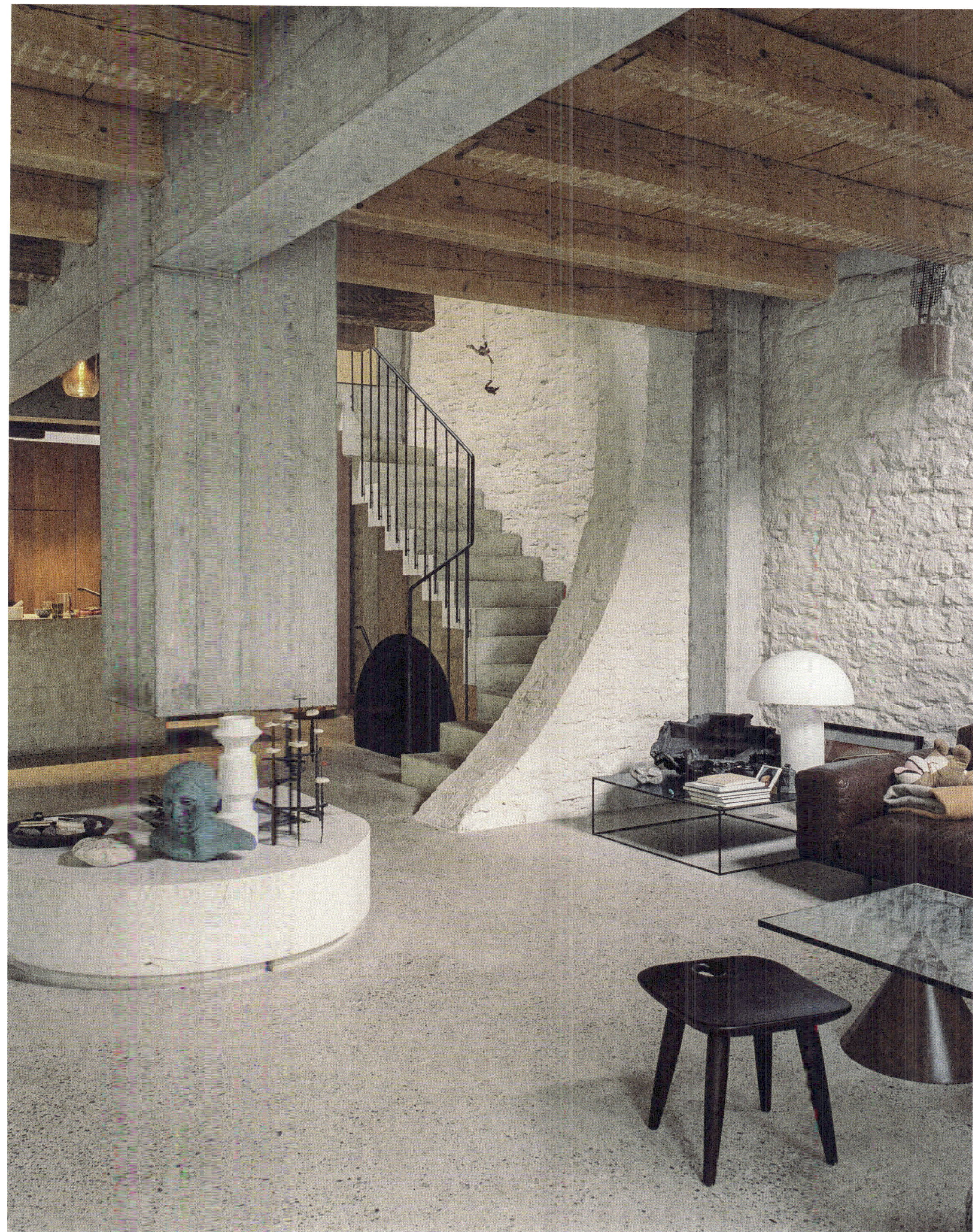

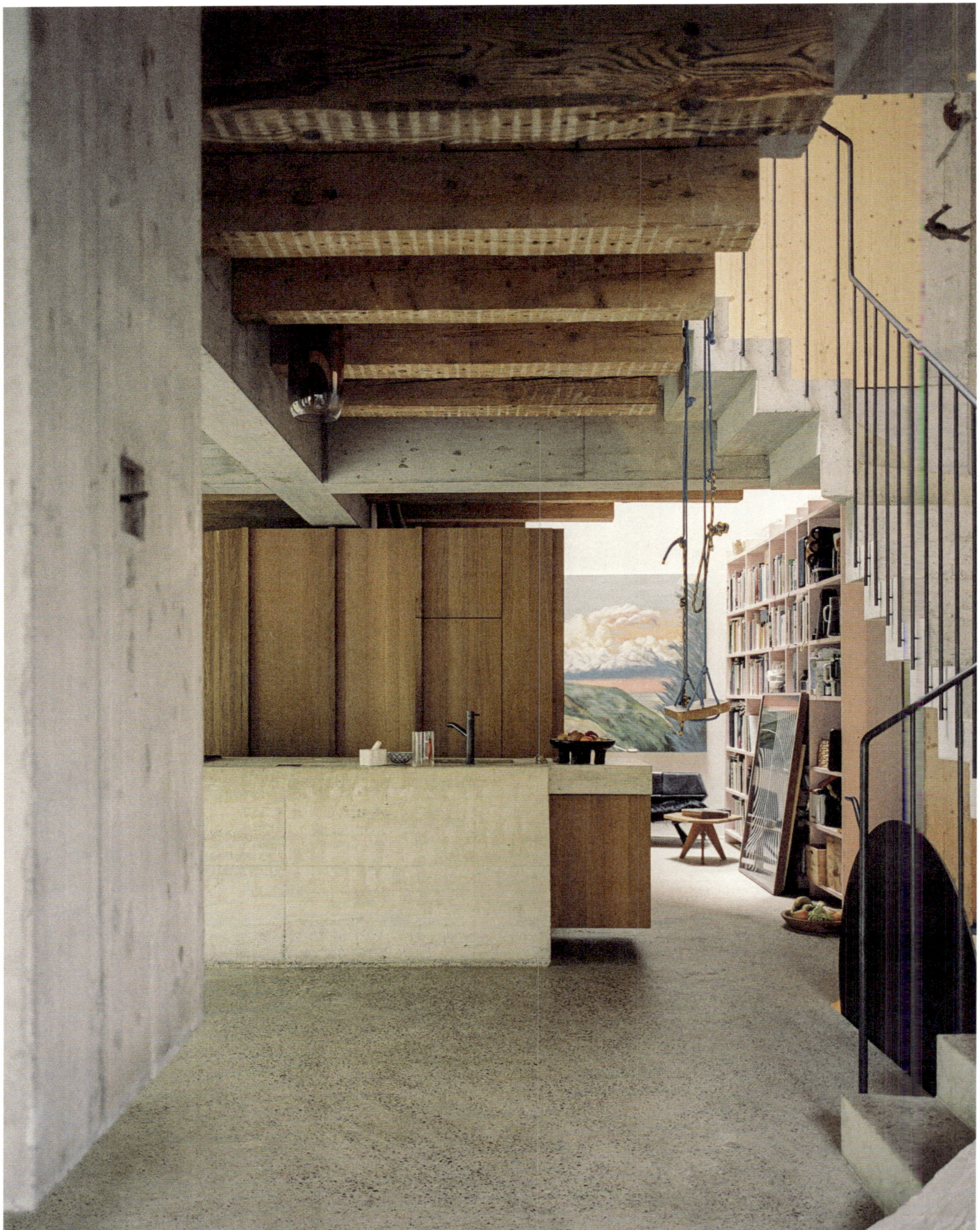

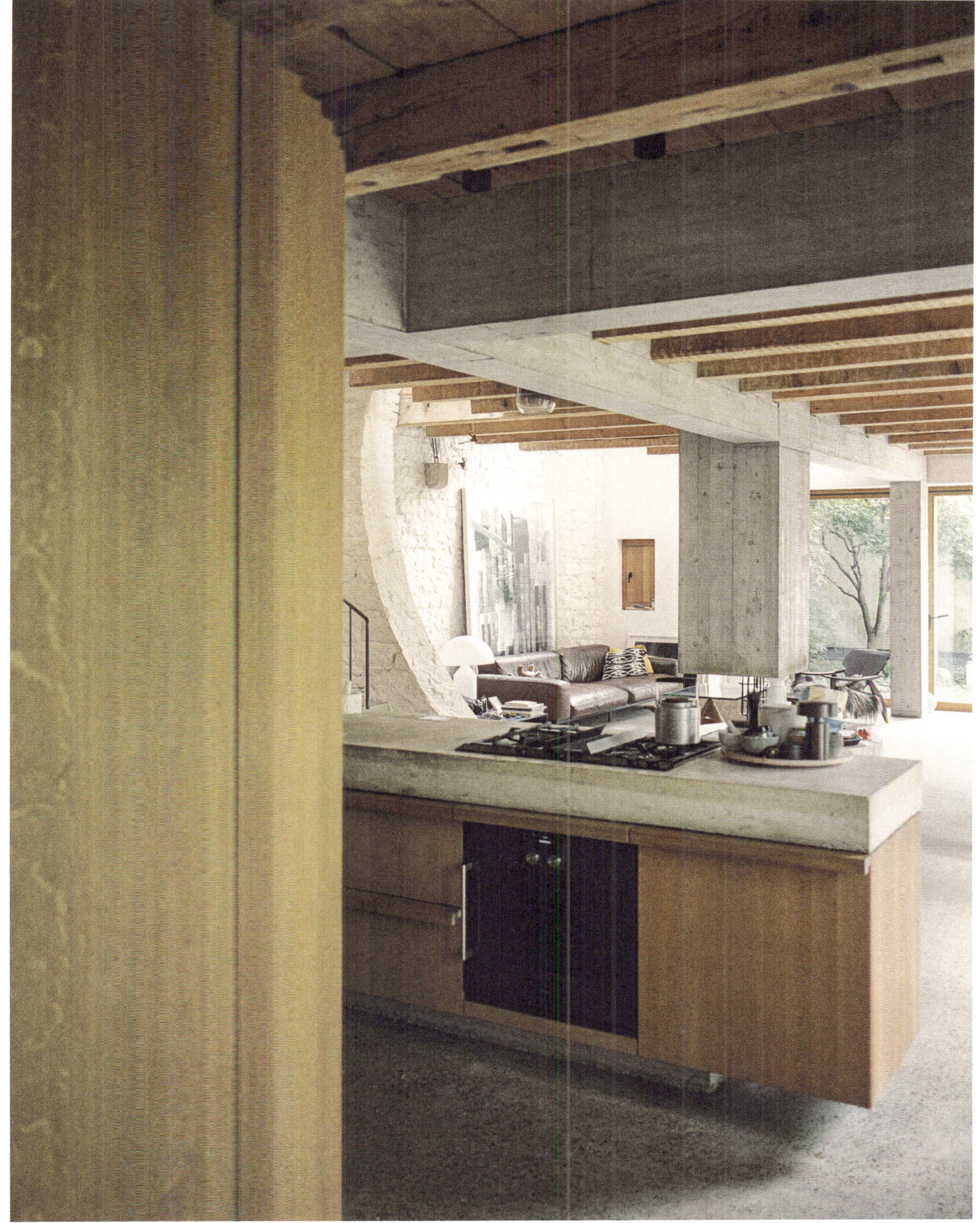

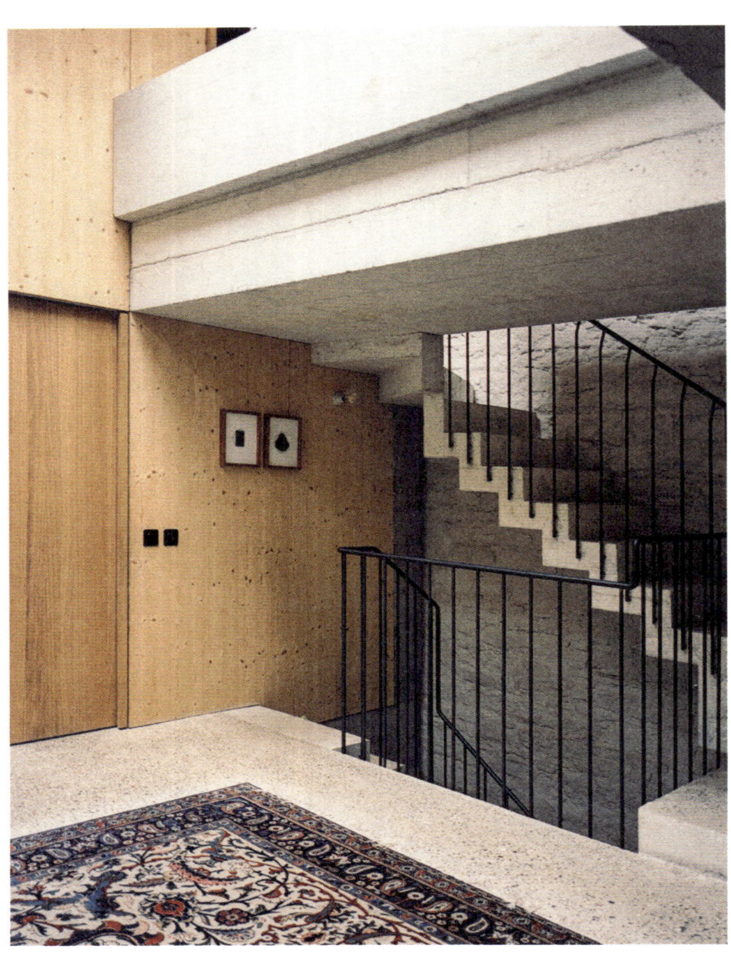

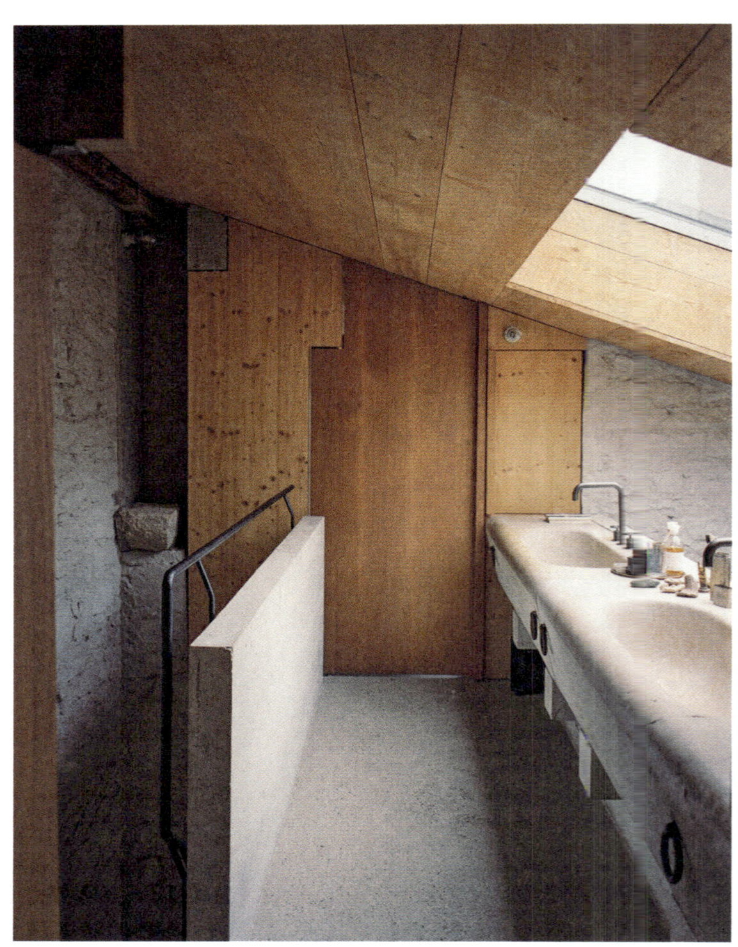

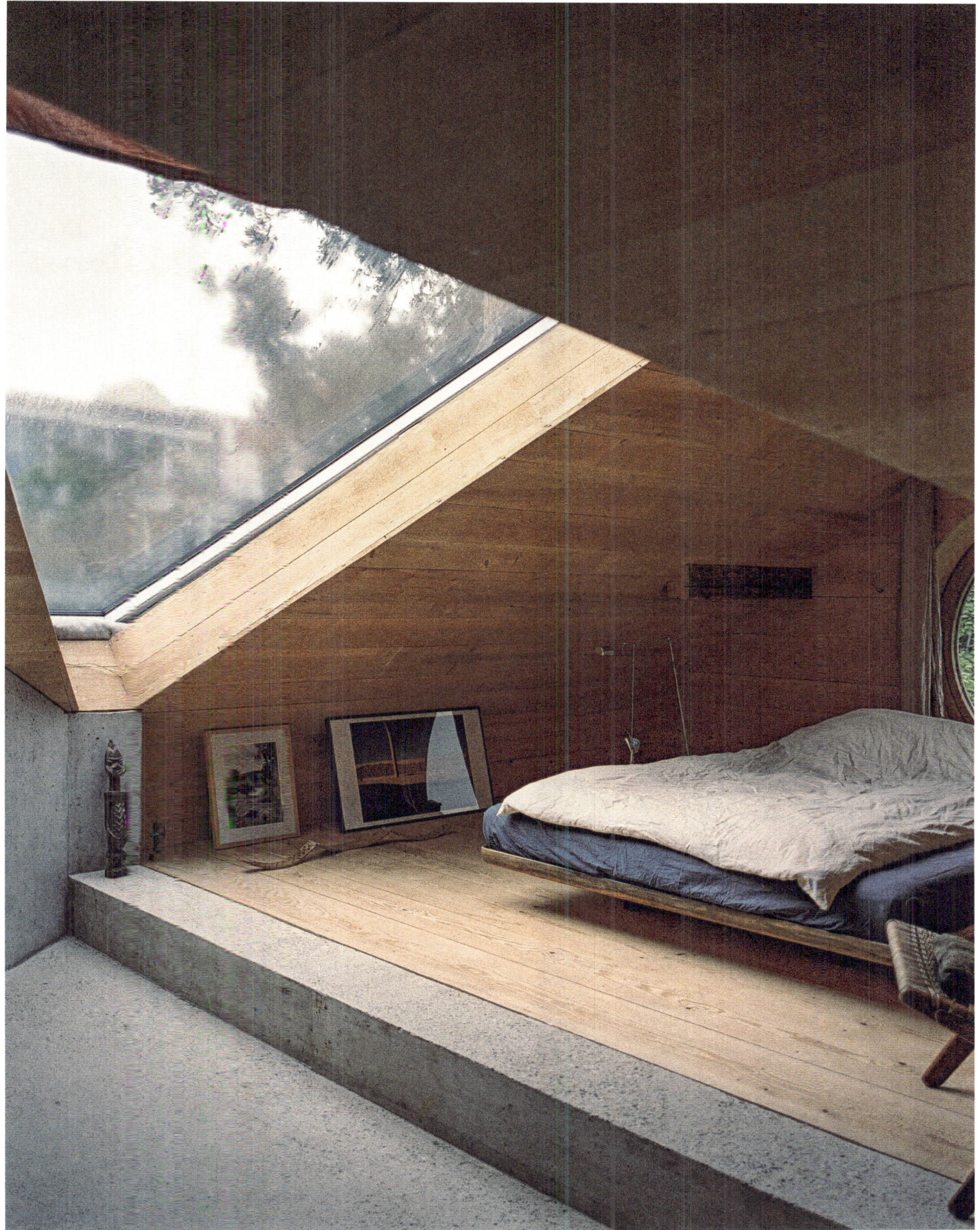

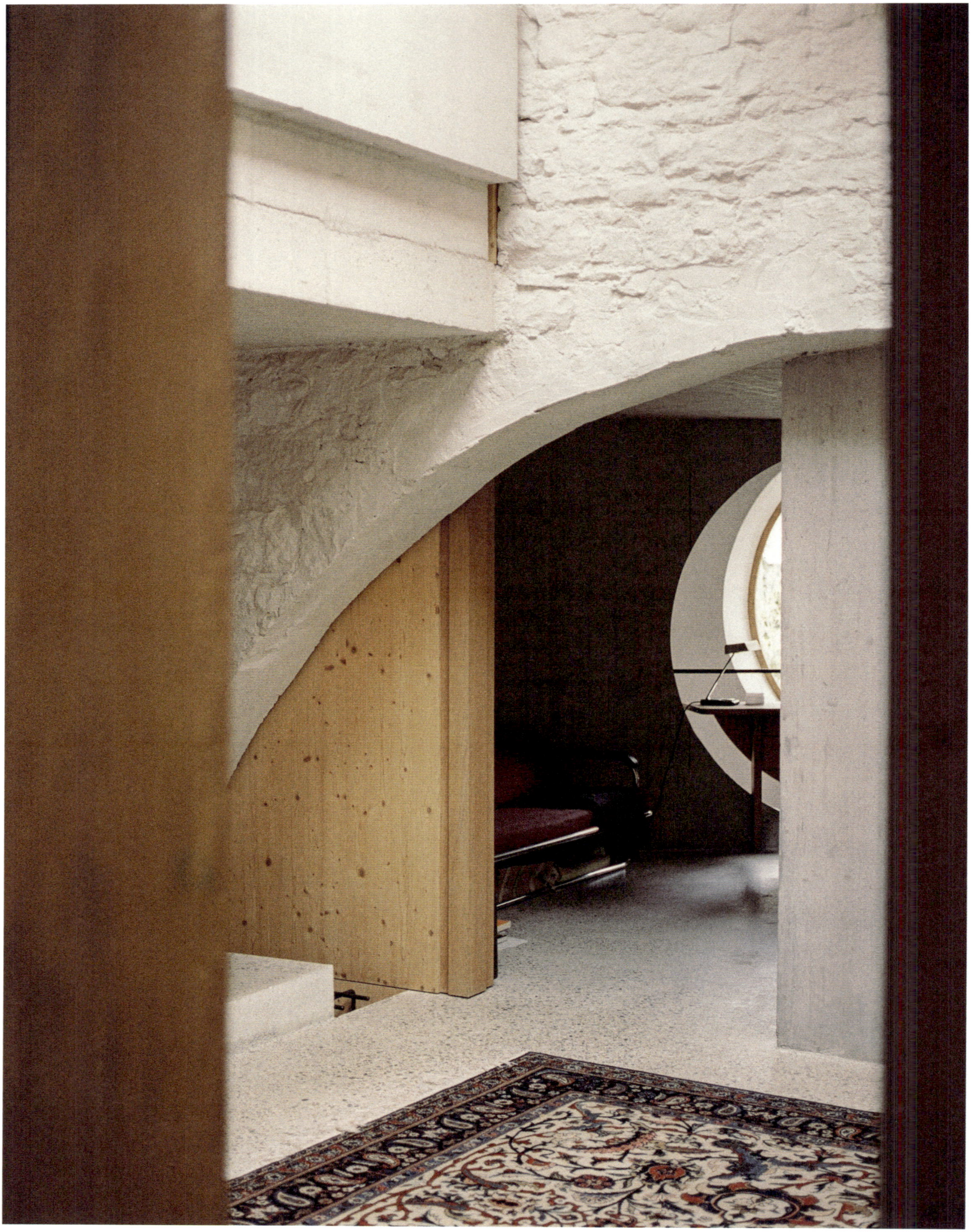

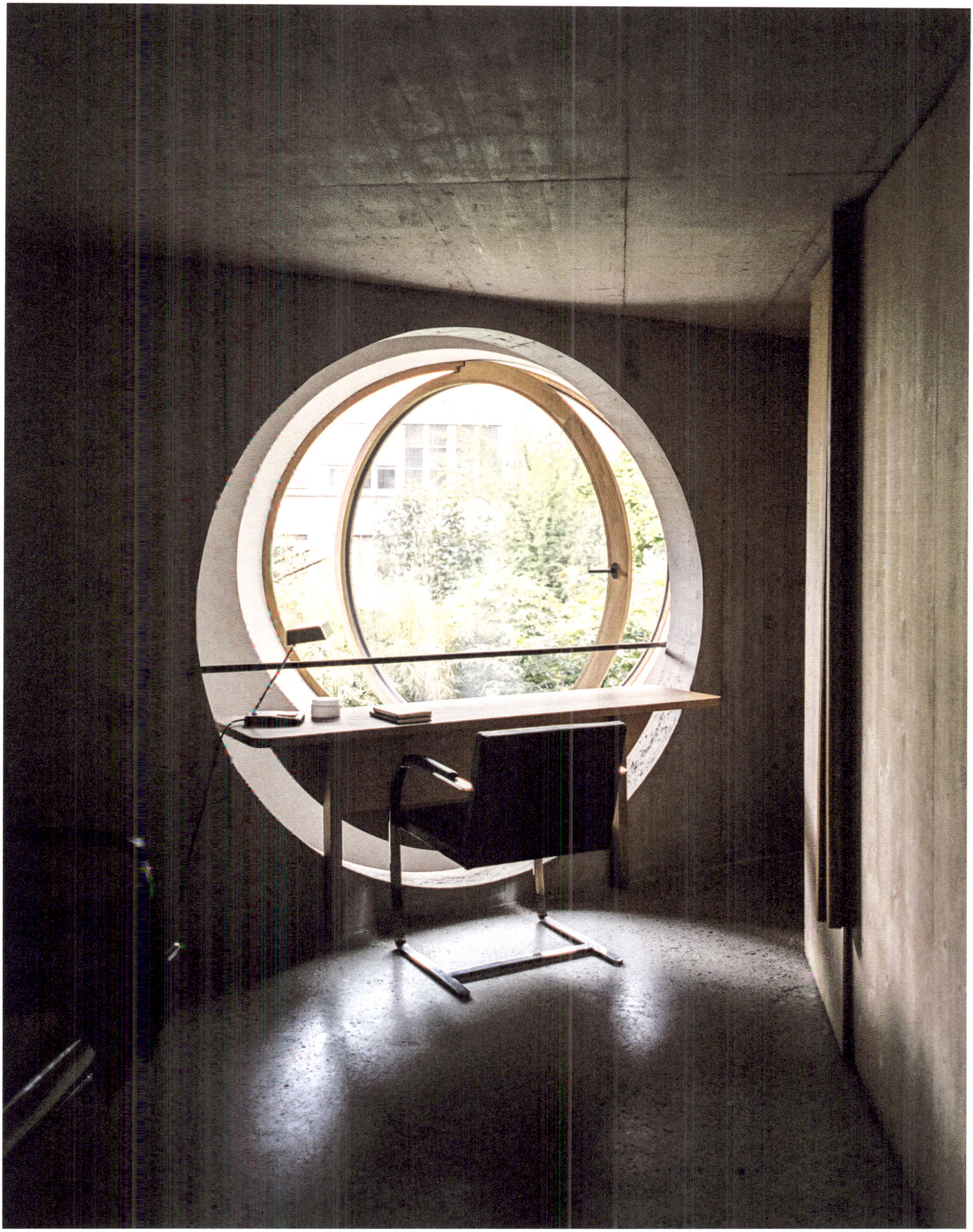

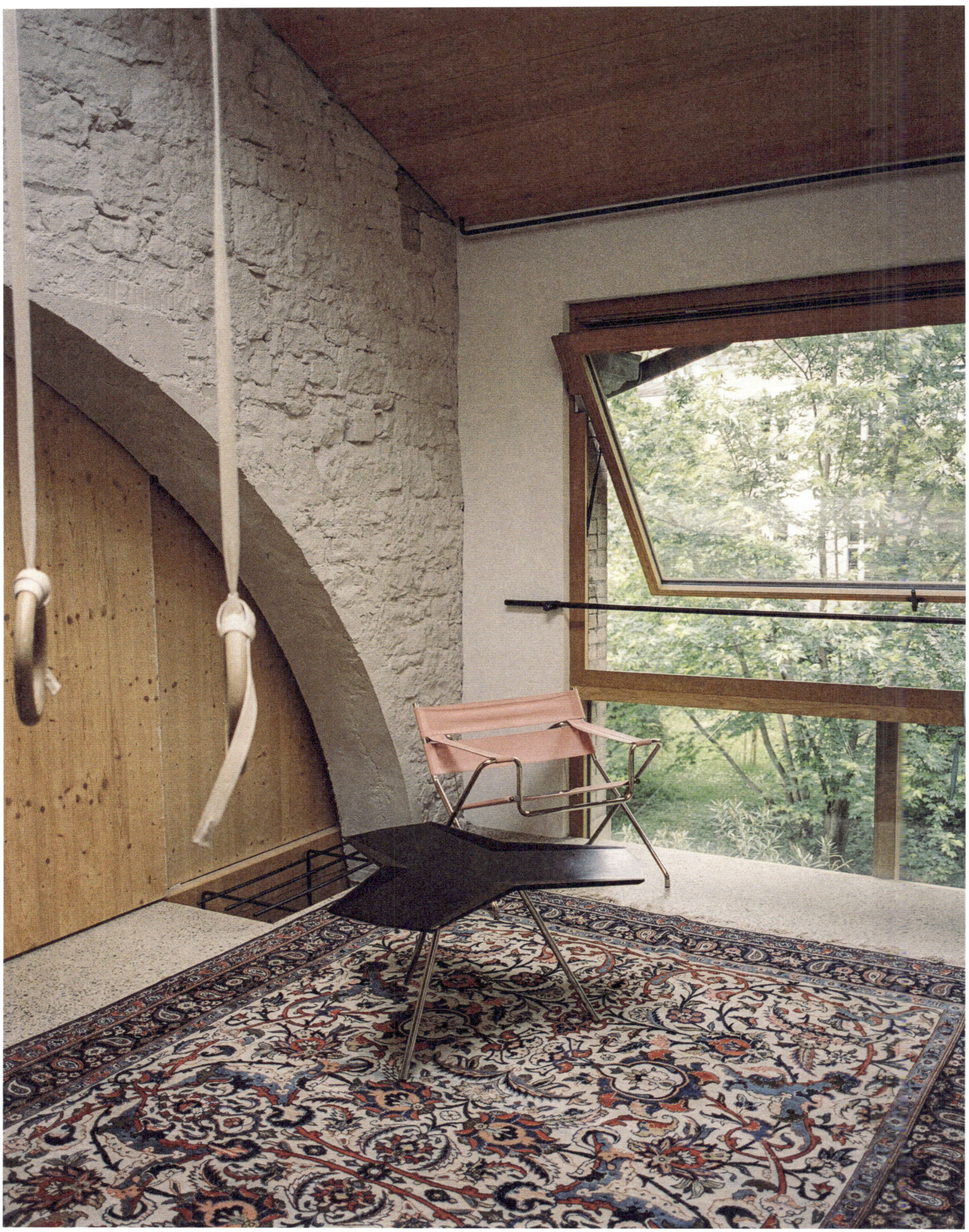

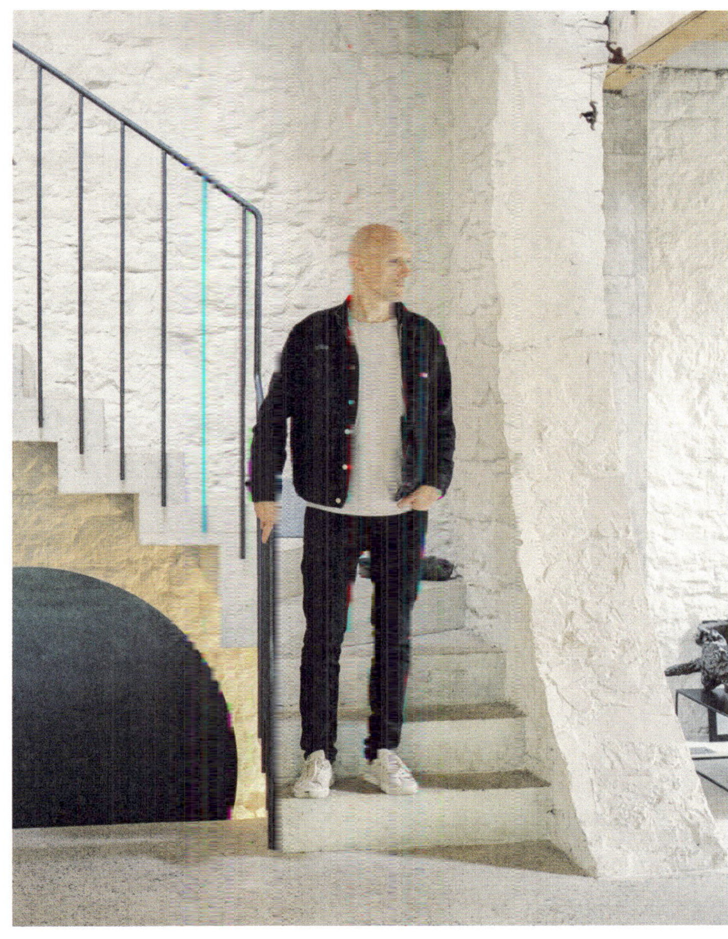

"The versatile use of concrete in different colours and forms complements and continues the historical material canon of the house."

– Andreas Bründler

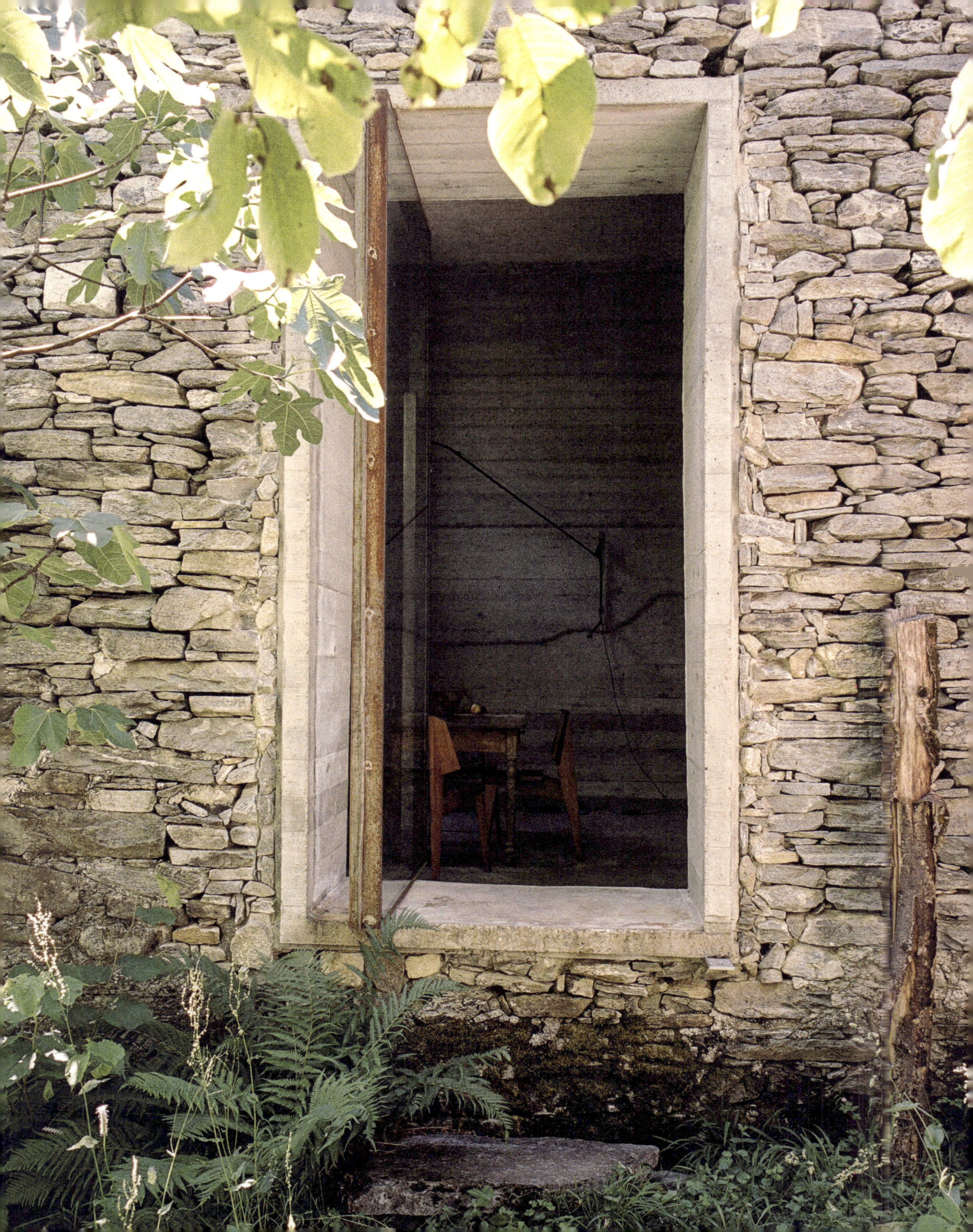

Casa D'Estate
Switzerland

At the far end of the Valle di Campo, in the Italian-speaking part of Switzerland, the village of Linescio rests quietly on the slope. It's a place shaped by stone, shadow, and centuries of seasonal rhythm. For decades, many of the small stone houses here stood empty, slowly abandoned, as agriculture retreated and the younger generations moved away.

This one, compact and strong, was built in the early 1800s. It served different purposes over time: a stable for animals, a place to dry chestnuts, a storage space for hay and winter fuel. For more than fifty years, it stood unused. Not damaged, but forgotten. Then, in the early 2000s, someone saw its potential. And work began.

The approach wasn't to restore the house, or to imitate the past. Instead, a new structure was inserted into the existing one: a concrete volume, carefully poured, that now sits inside the old stone walls. It doesn't pretend to be traditional; it respects the outer shell but brings in a new kind of clarity. The result is something between memory and reimagining.

You still enter through the original doorway. From the outside, almost nothing has changed. The proportions remain the same; the roofline is untouched. But once you're inside, the contrast is clear: smooth concrete floors, light bouncing off mineral surfaces, sharp edges set against the roughness of the stone, and windows placed behind existing openings. The house doesn't shout, it simply reorients itself from within.

The space is simple: one large room on the ground floor, stairs tucked to the side, and a bathroom underneath the sleeping area. Everything is compact, but generous in feeling, with light coming in from both sides. The roof is steep, the ceiling high. You feel the volume of the house all at once.

The house is used as a summer home. There's no central heating, and no insulation beyond the mass of stone and concrete. It doesn't aim to be comfortable in all seasons. "You live with the weather", the owner says. "You wake up with the sun. You adapt."

It was built slowly, by hand, by a single local builder. No machines, no cranes. The concrete was mixed on-site and the wooden formwork was set piece by piece. Every corner of the interior was cast with intention. Nothing here is decorative, every gesture has weight.

Outside, nature presses close. The house is surrounded by stone paths, dry grass, and chestnut trees. You hear water running in the valley below. You feel time differently. There's no signal here, no passing traffic, just wind, light, and structure.

This is not a house of convenience, it's a place for pause. It invites stillness, without requiring silence. It allows you to see the structure of things – how they hold, how they shift, how they remain.

Project: Casa D'Estate
Location: Switzerland
Architect: Buchner Bründler Architekten
Year of construction: early 1800s
Year of purchase: 2008
Floor area: 57 m²
Resident: Daniel Buchner
Resident's profession: architect

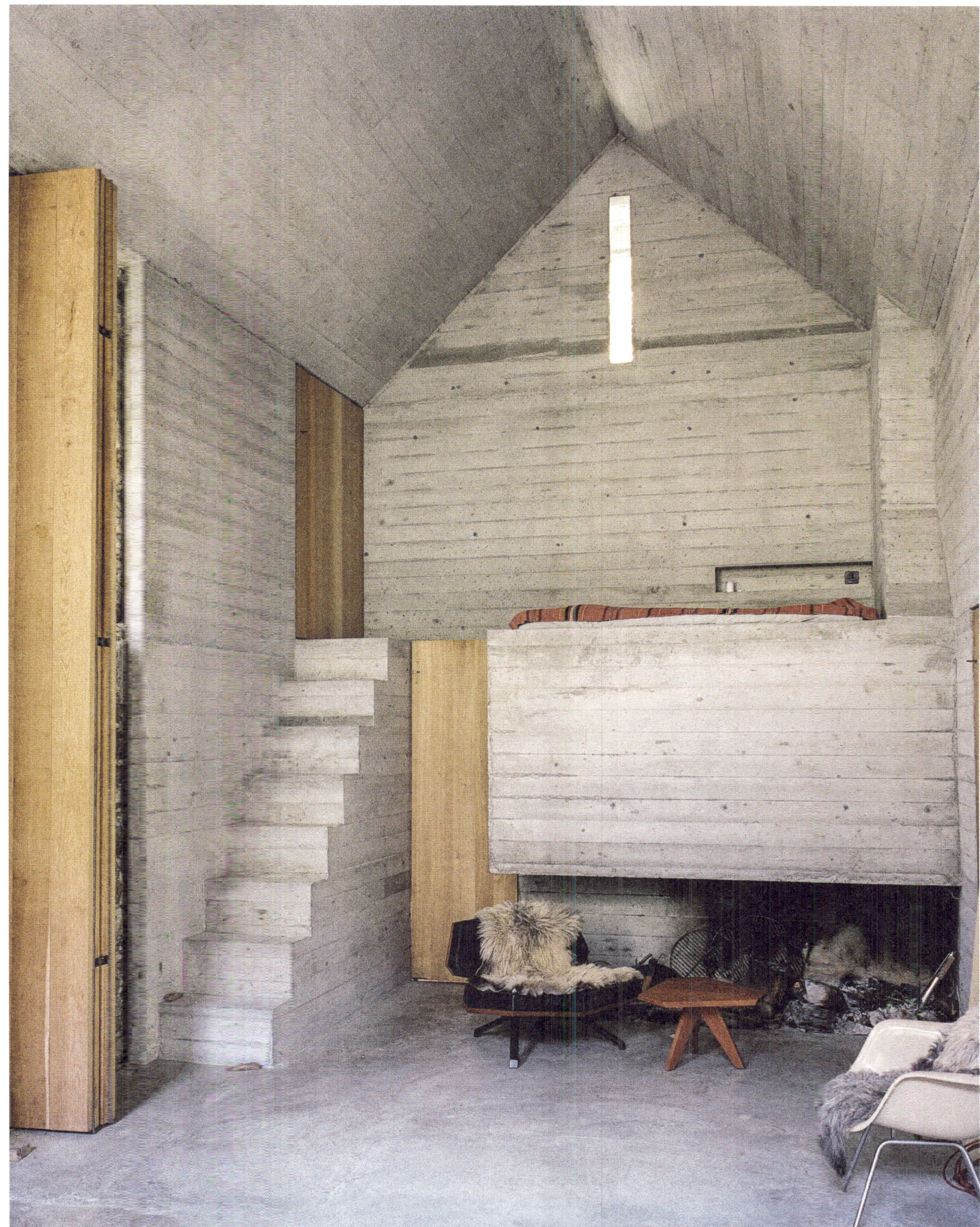

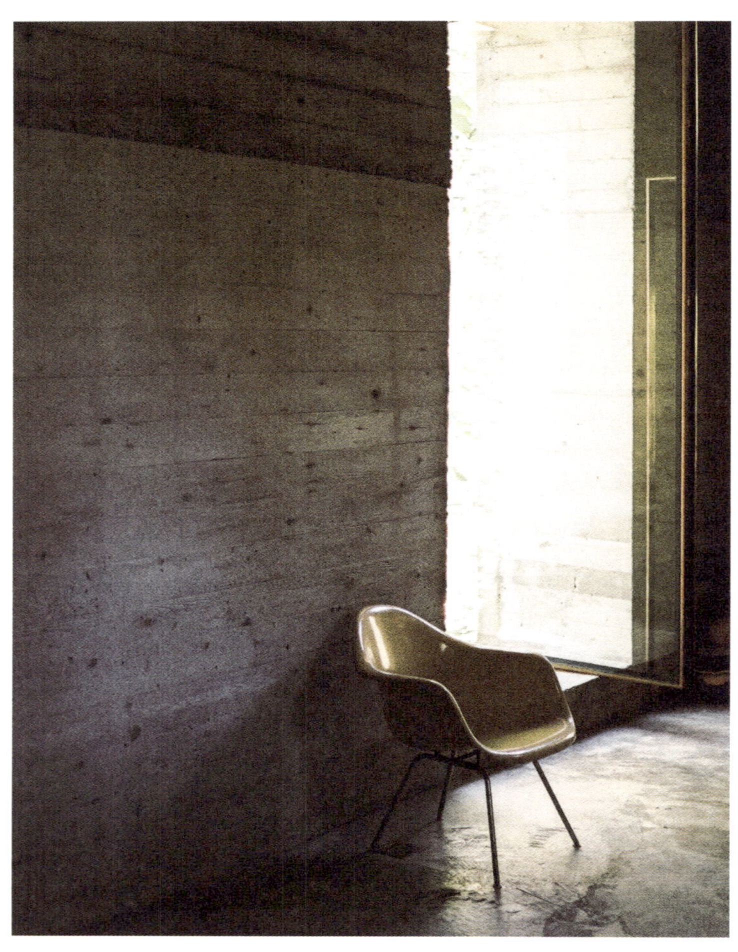

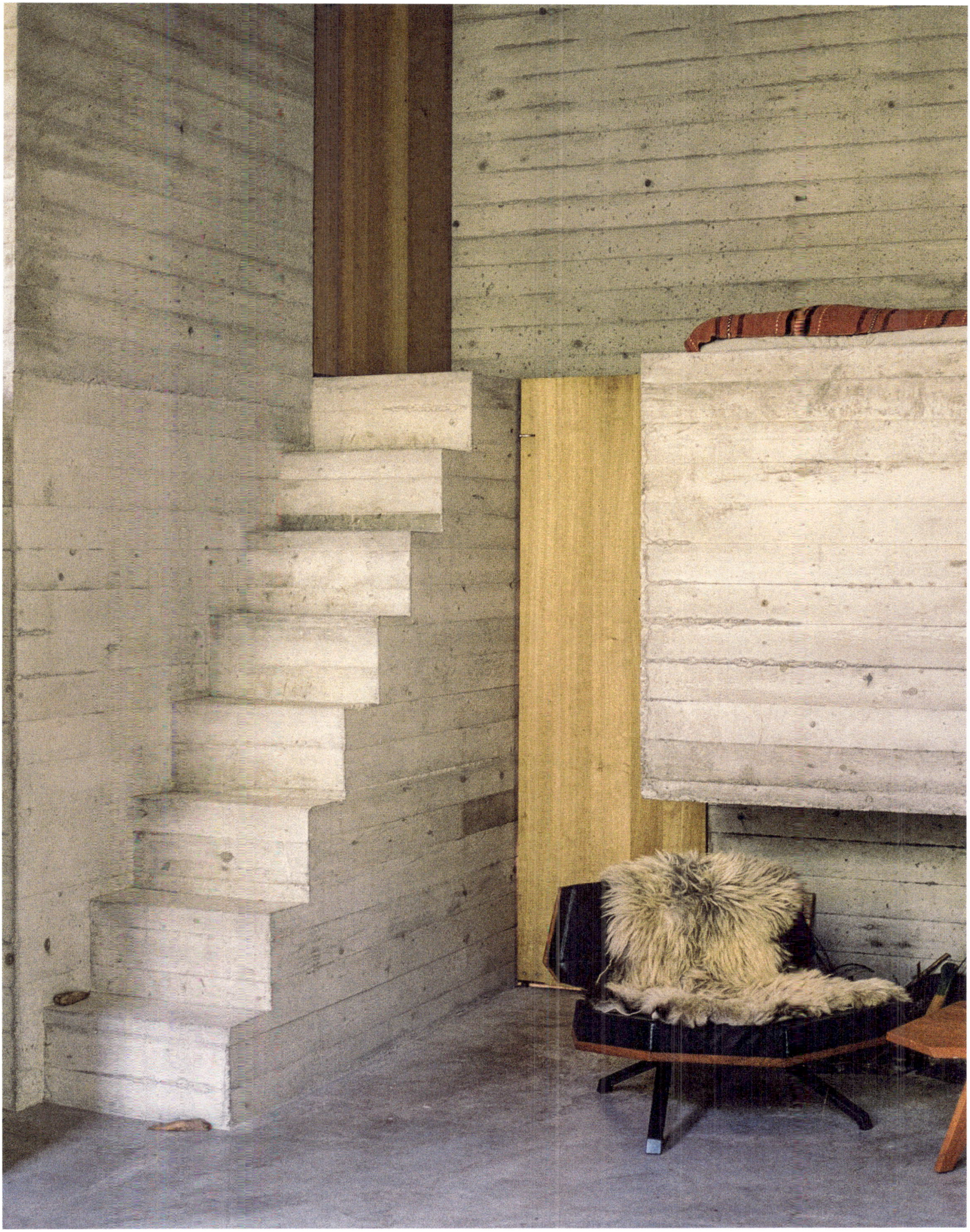

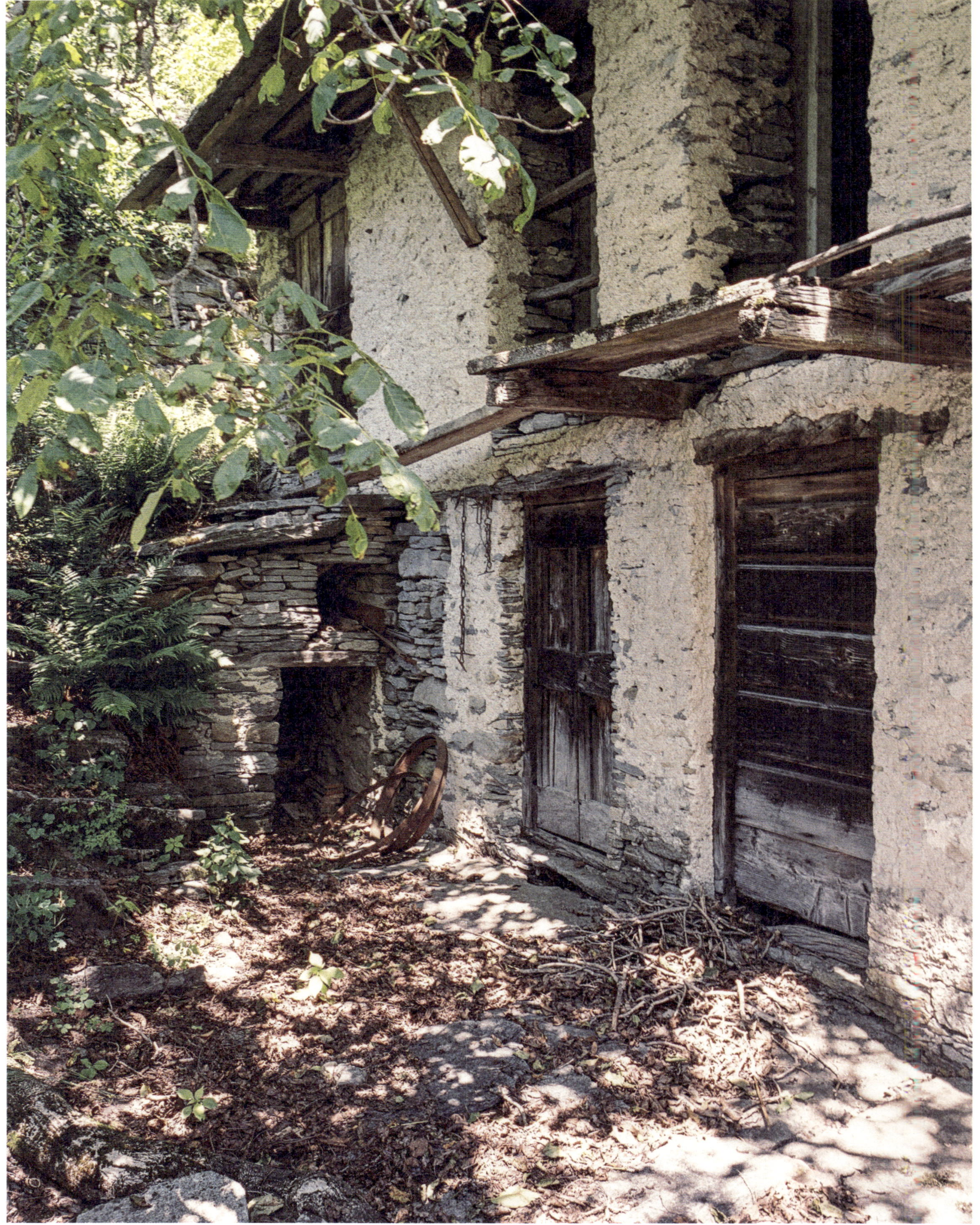

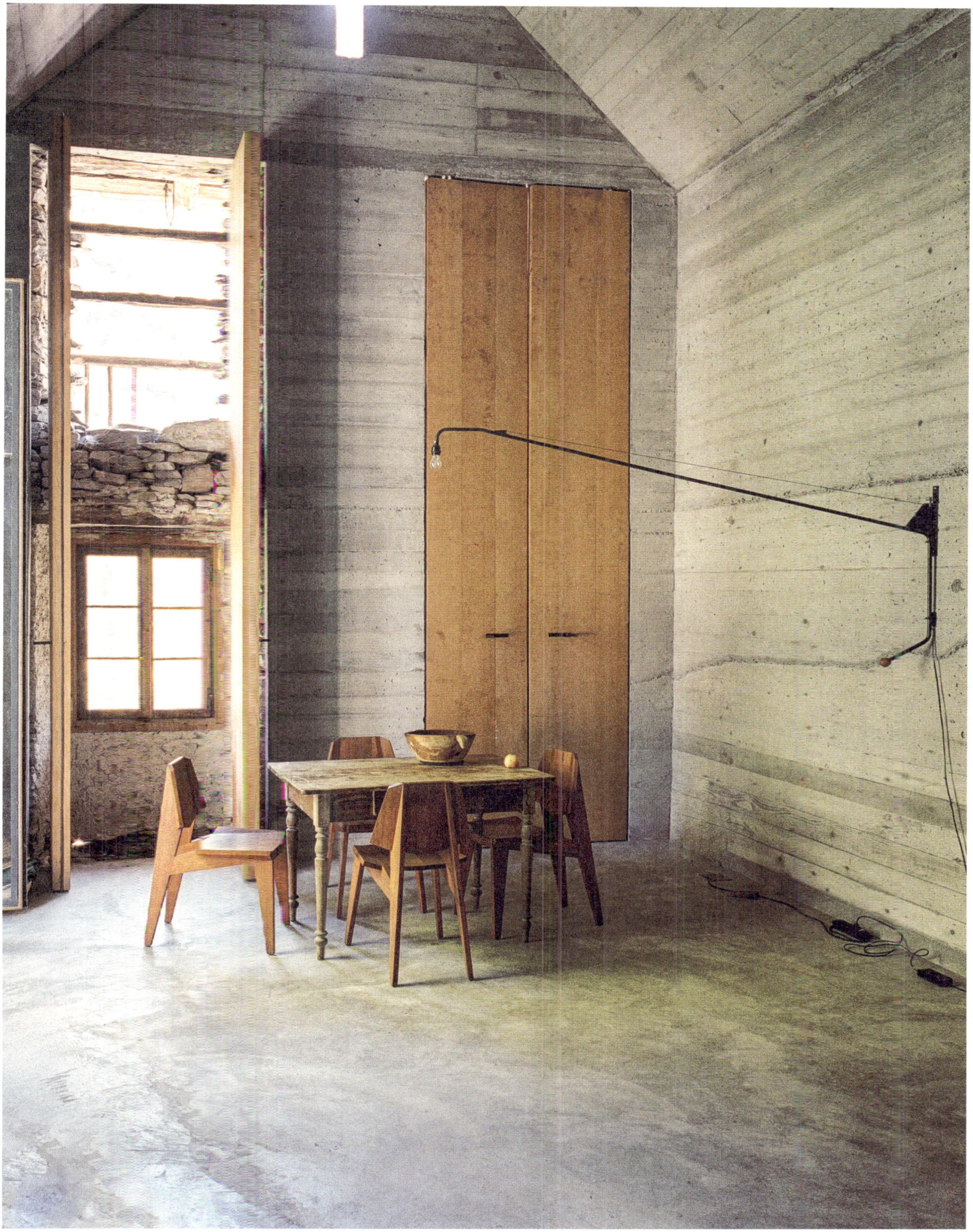

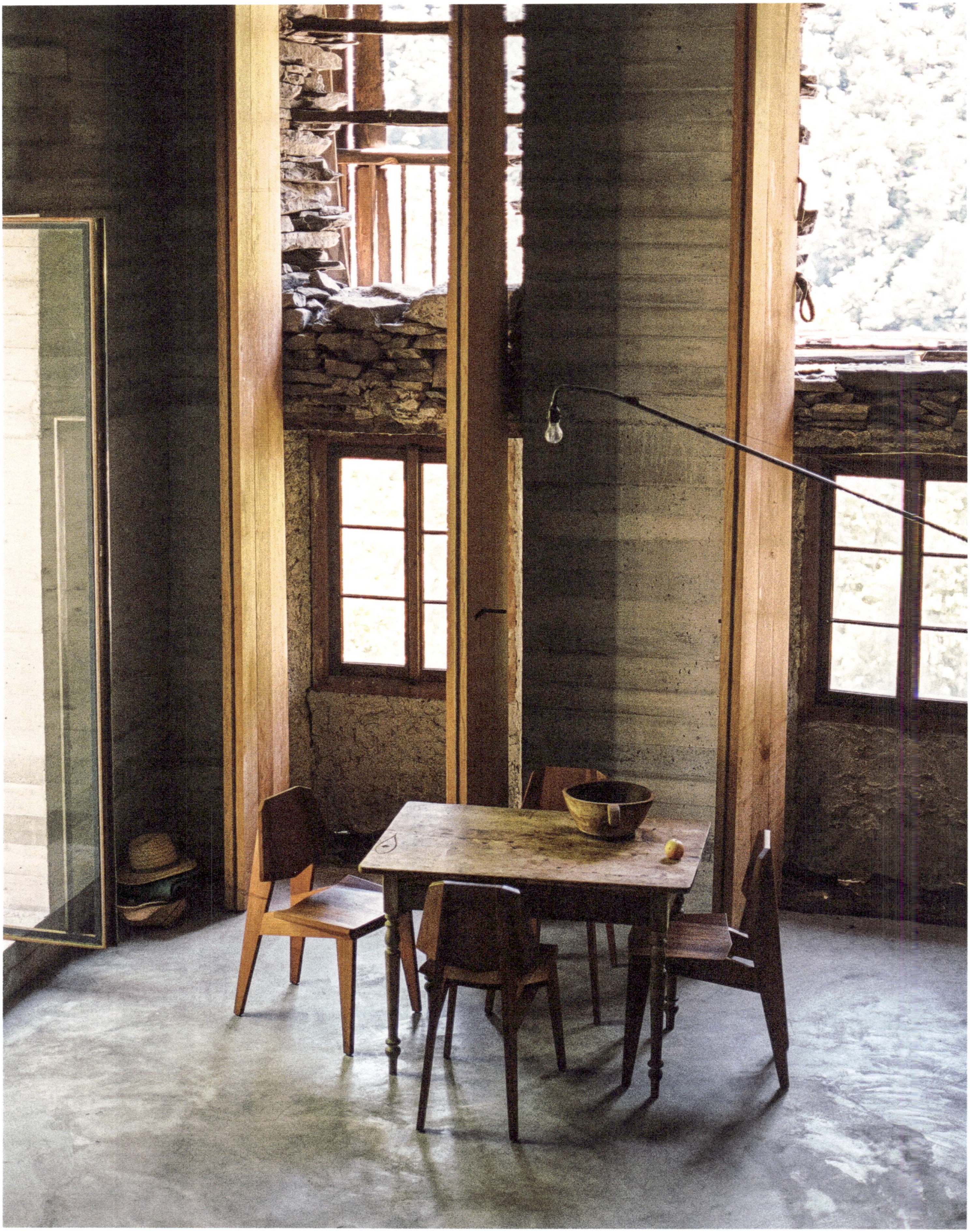

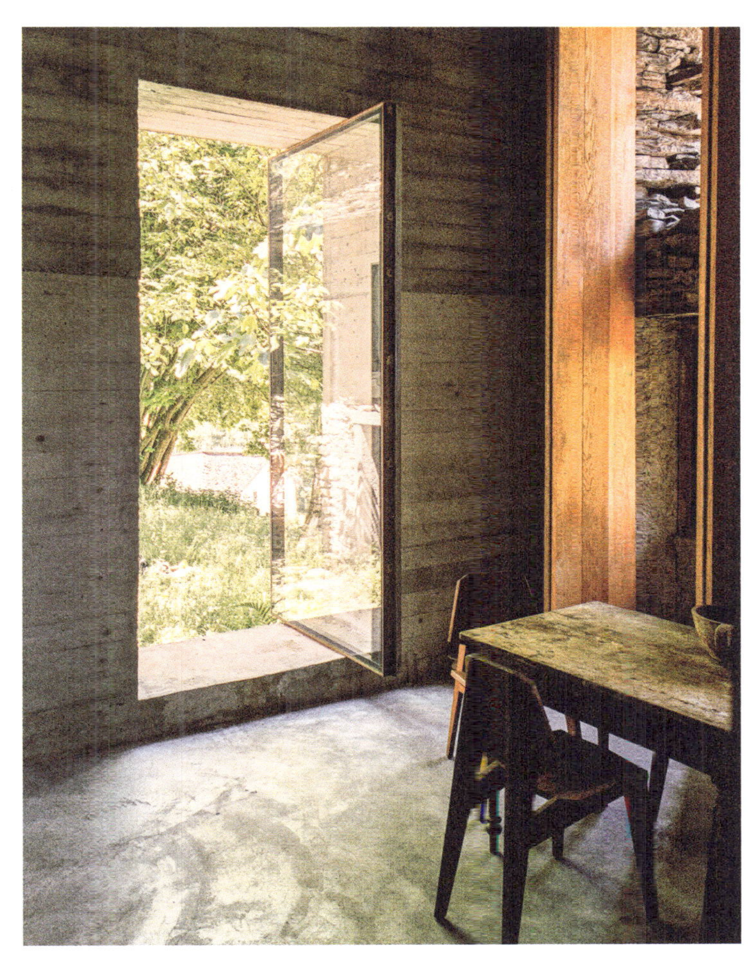

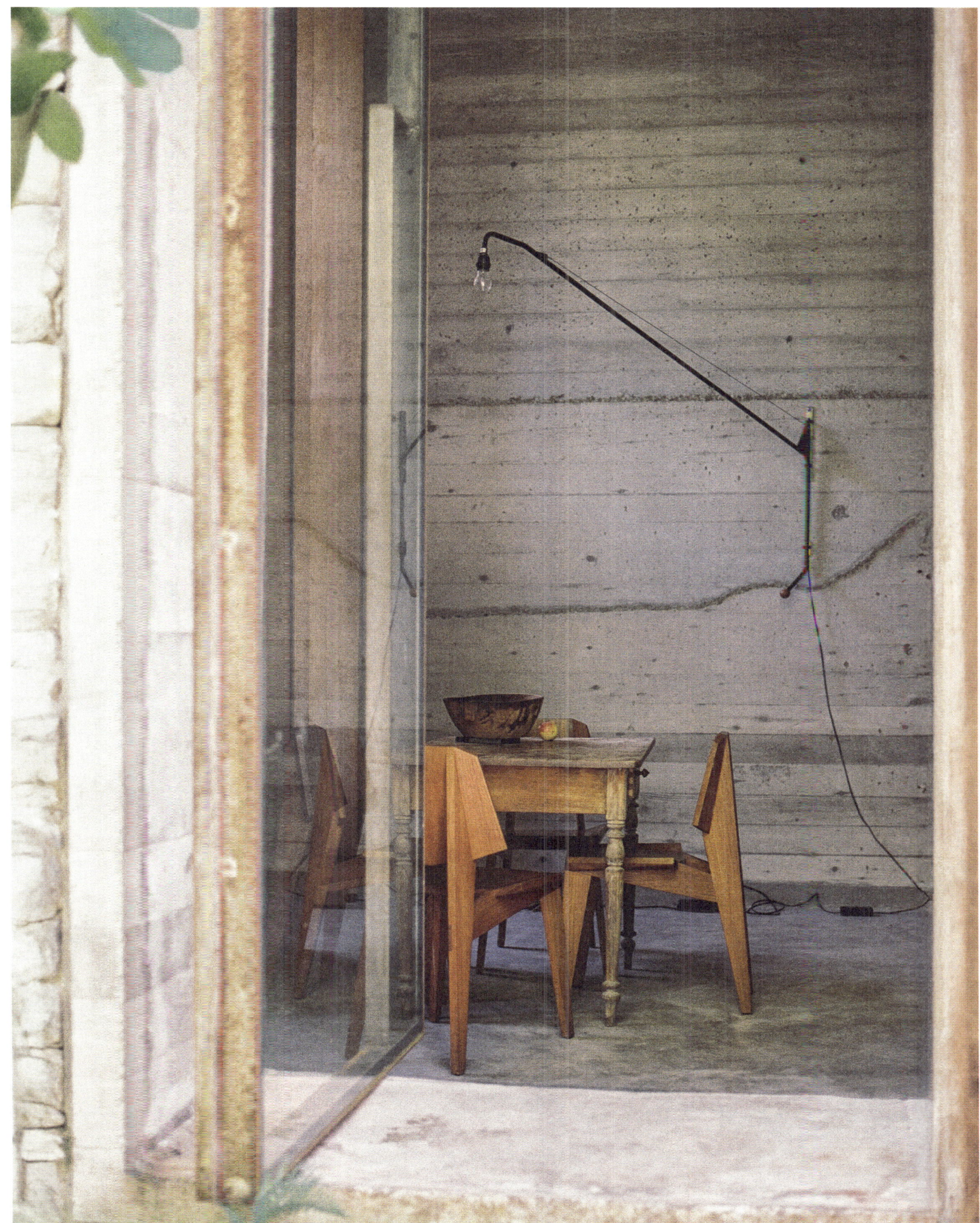

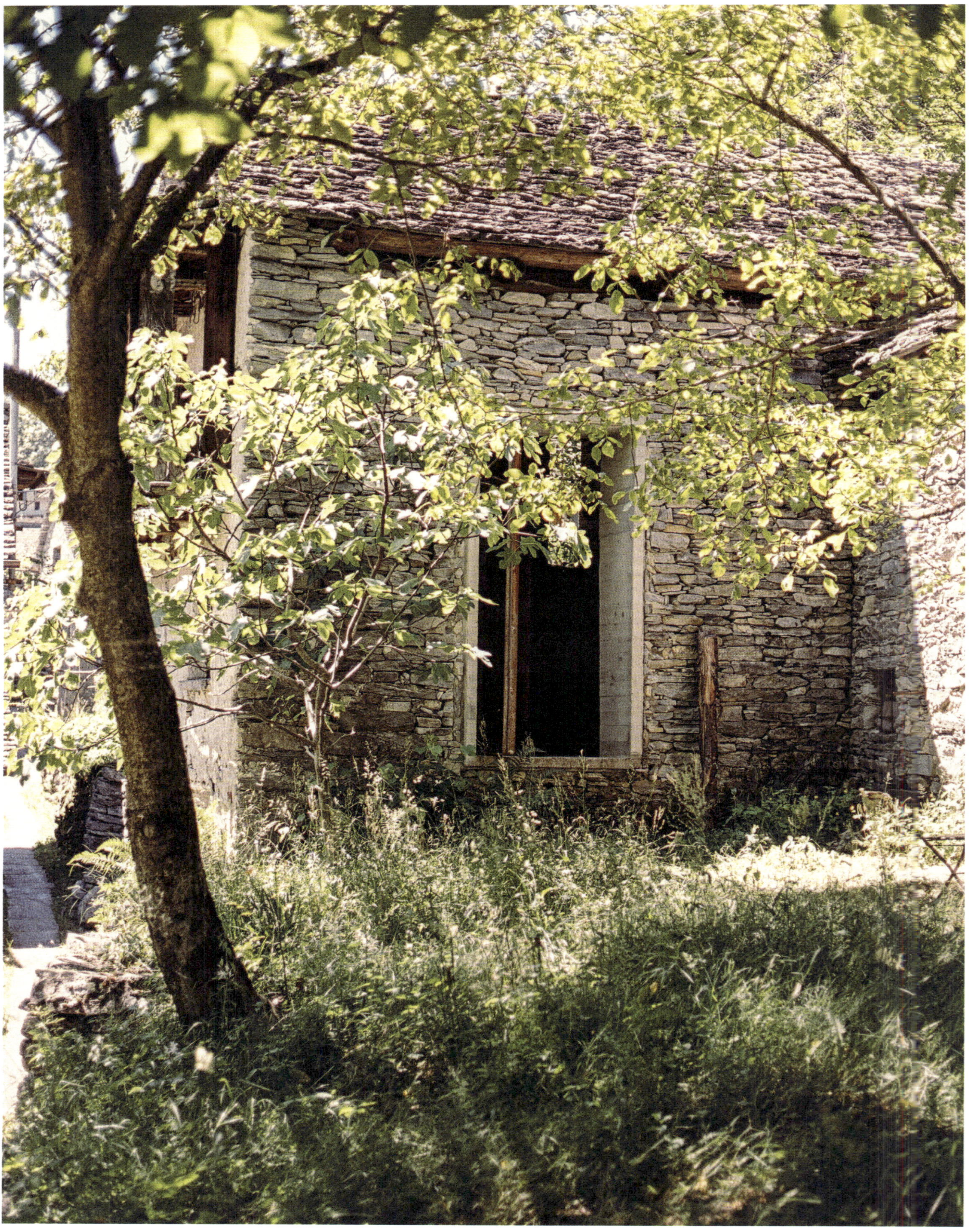

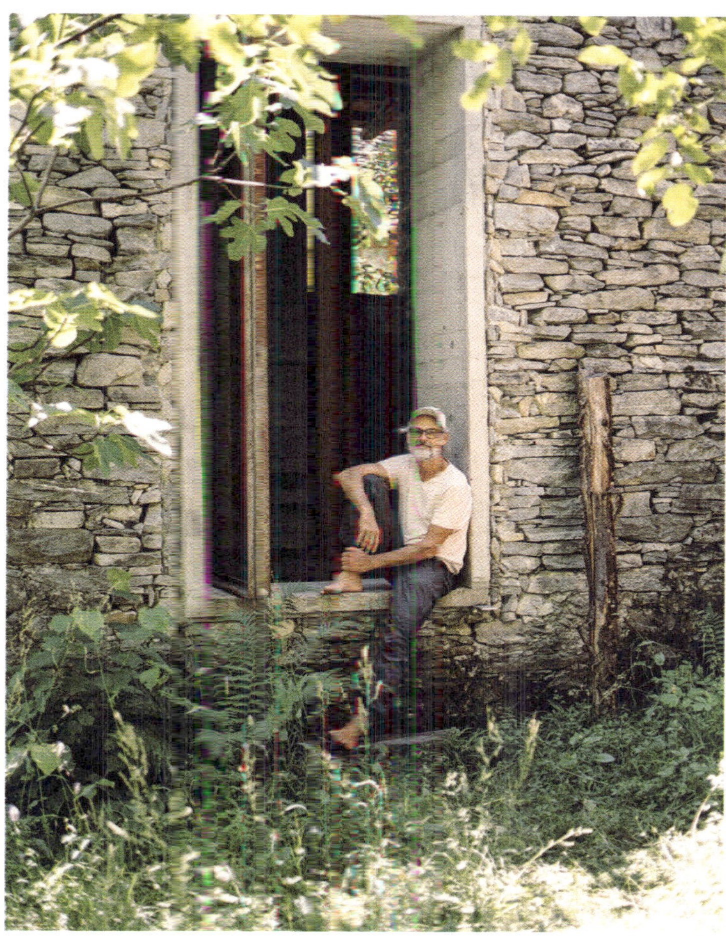

"In this home, the concrete is a reference to the tranquillity and grandeur of the surrounding mountain landscape. An expression of protection and security."

– Daniel Buchner

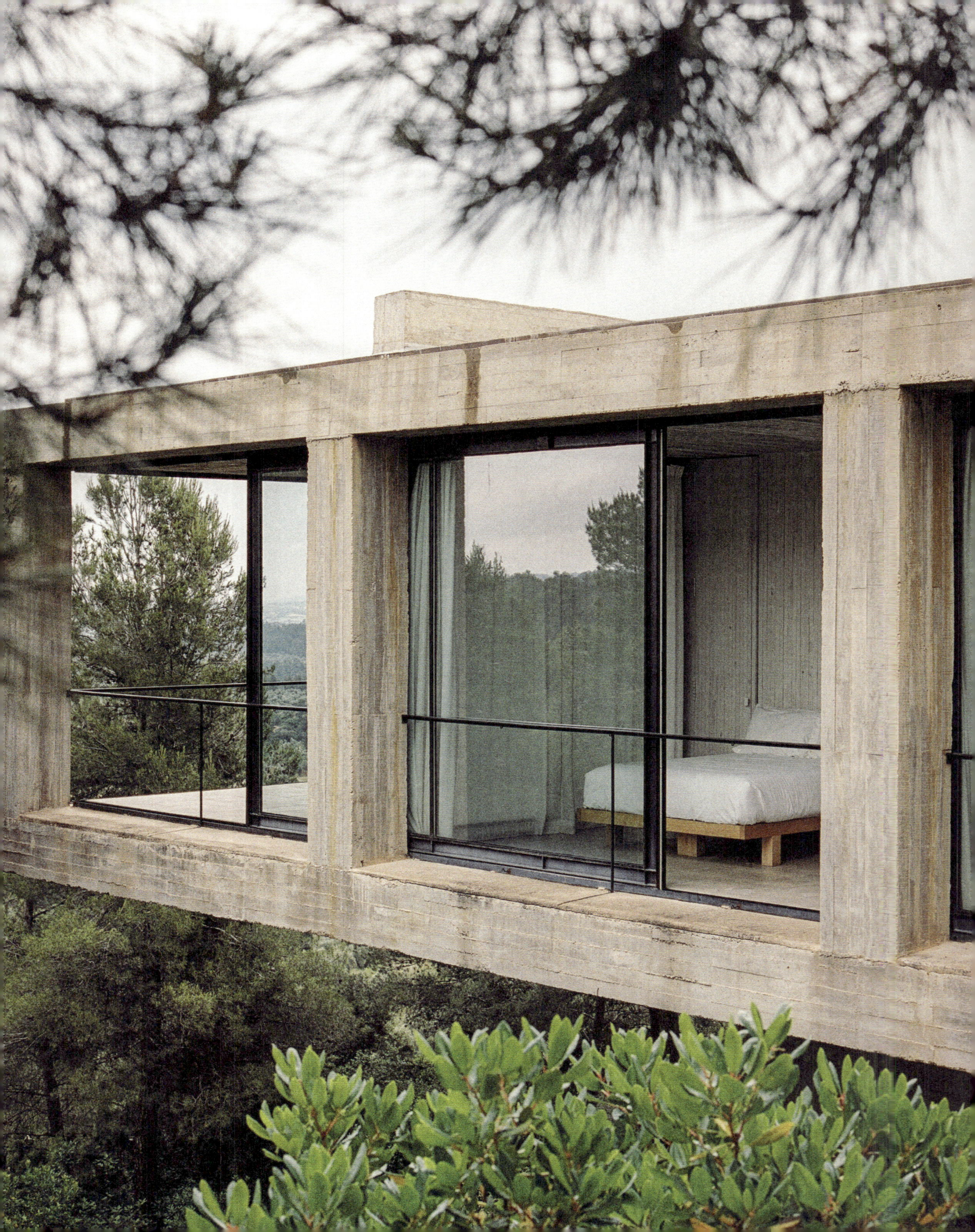

Solo Pezo von Ellrichshausen
Spain

Solo Pezo von Ellrichshausen doesn't reveal itself gradually, it arrives all at once – a concrete square on a plateau in eastern Spain, surrounded by wild hills and silence. The shape is strict, the material is raw, but the experience is open. You feel the wind from all sides, and you see the horizon in every direction.

The house is the work of Pezo von Ellrichshausen, a Chilean architecture studio known for radical clarity. It was built as part of the Solo Houses project, an initiative by gallery owners Eva Albarrán and Christian Bourdais which started in 2010: a collection of experimental retreats, each by a different architect, set in the rural Matarranya region. The goal was simple: allow for total freedom, no brief, no programme, just the landscape.

Solo Pezo von Ellrichshausen is a raised concrete ring, a perfect square, each side measuring twenty metres. In the middle: a patio open to the sky. Around it: four rooms, one in each corner, all of them different in size and proportion, and all facing both inwards and outwards. Every wall facing the landscape can slide open, turning every room into a terrace.

The materials are reduced to the essentials: concrete for structure and floors, glass for openings, wood for detail. There's no insulation, no air conditioning. The temperature is controlled with air and shade. At night, the temperature drops. In the morning, the light returns. It sets the rhythm.

From inside, the landscape feels infinite. There are no fences, no neighbours, no background noise, just hills, trees, and distant light. The house doesn't point in any direction; it's equally open on all sides. You're inside, but always aware of what's outside.

The central patio acts as both anchor and void. In summer, it holds shade; in winter, it collects light; and rainwater flows towards its centre. Sometimes it's used for a table, sometimes just left empty. It's not designed to be useful, it's there to slow things down.

The rooms are sparing but generous. There's a kitchen with no upper cabinets, a bedroom with nothing on the walls, and a long room that sometimes serves as a living space, sometimes as a passage. The furnishings are minimal. There's no screen, no system. You adapt to the house, not the other way around.

The house was poured in place, monolithic. It doesn't hide its material: formwork lines run across the surface, and edges are sharp but never polished. Over time, the concrete has taken on tones from the red soil and dry wind. It's not cold, it's honest.

Solo Pezo von Ellrichshausen is not a home in the usual sense, it's a structure to live inside for a brief time – a place to slow down, observe, and realign. You come here to be with the architecture, with the air, with the distance. There's no distraction, no comfort layered over functionality, just structure, shadow, and sky.

It doesn't try to blend into the land, nor to rise above it. It sits there, clear, silent, definite. And in that stillness, something opens.

Project: Solo Pezo von Ellrichshausen
Location: Spain
Architect: Pezo von Ellrichshausen
Year of construction: 2013
Floor area: 320 m²
Caretaker: Julia Cajaraville
Caretaker's profession: director of Solo Houses

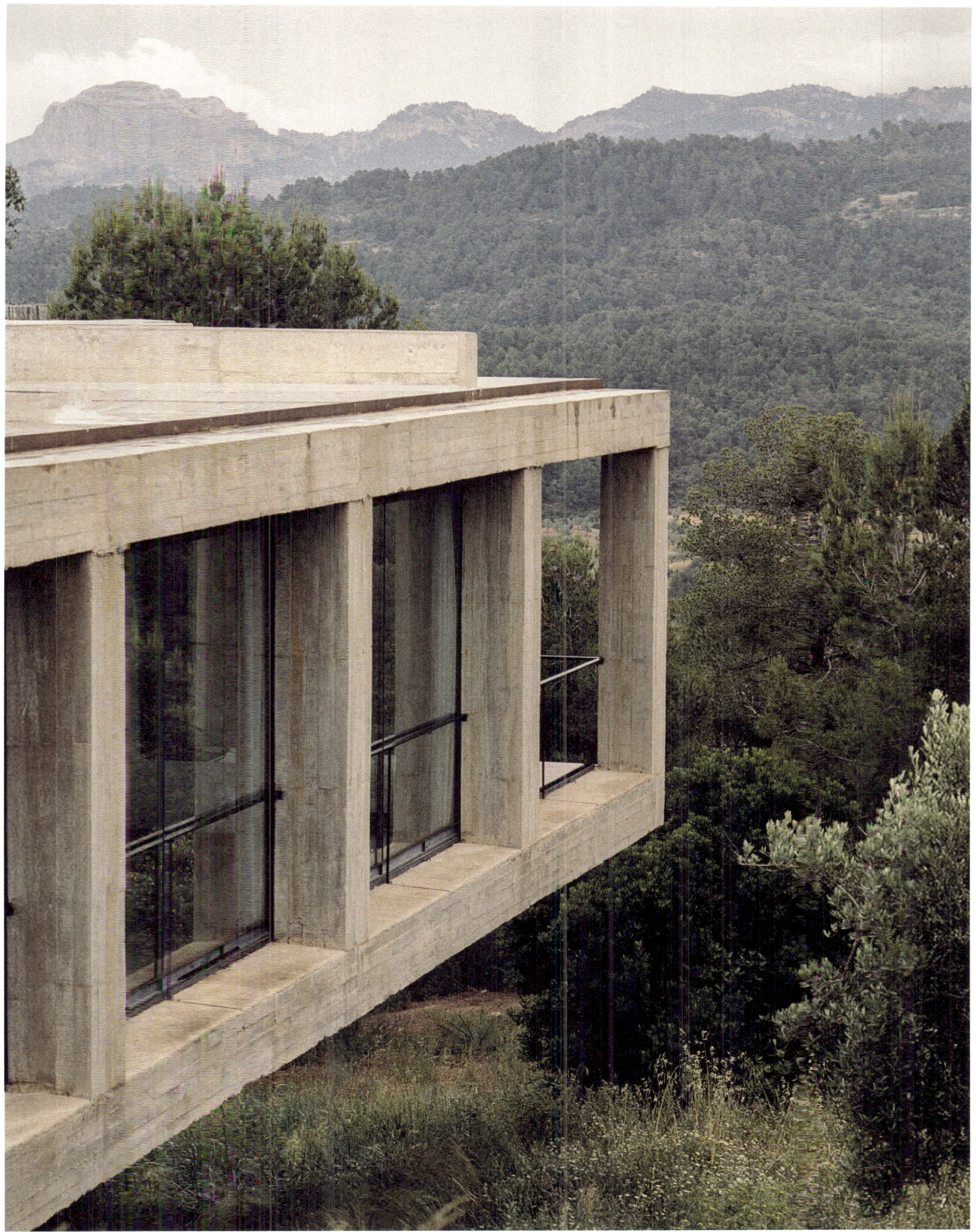

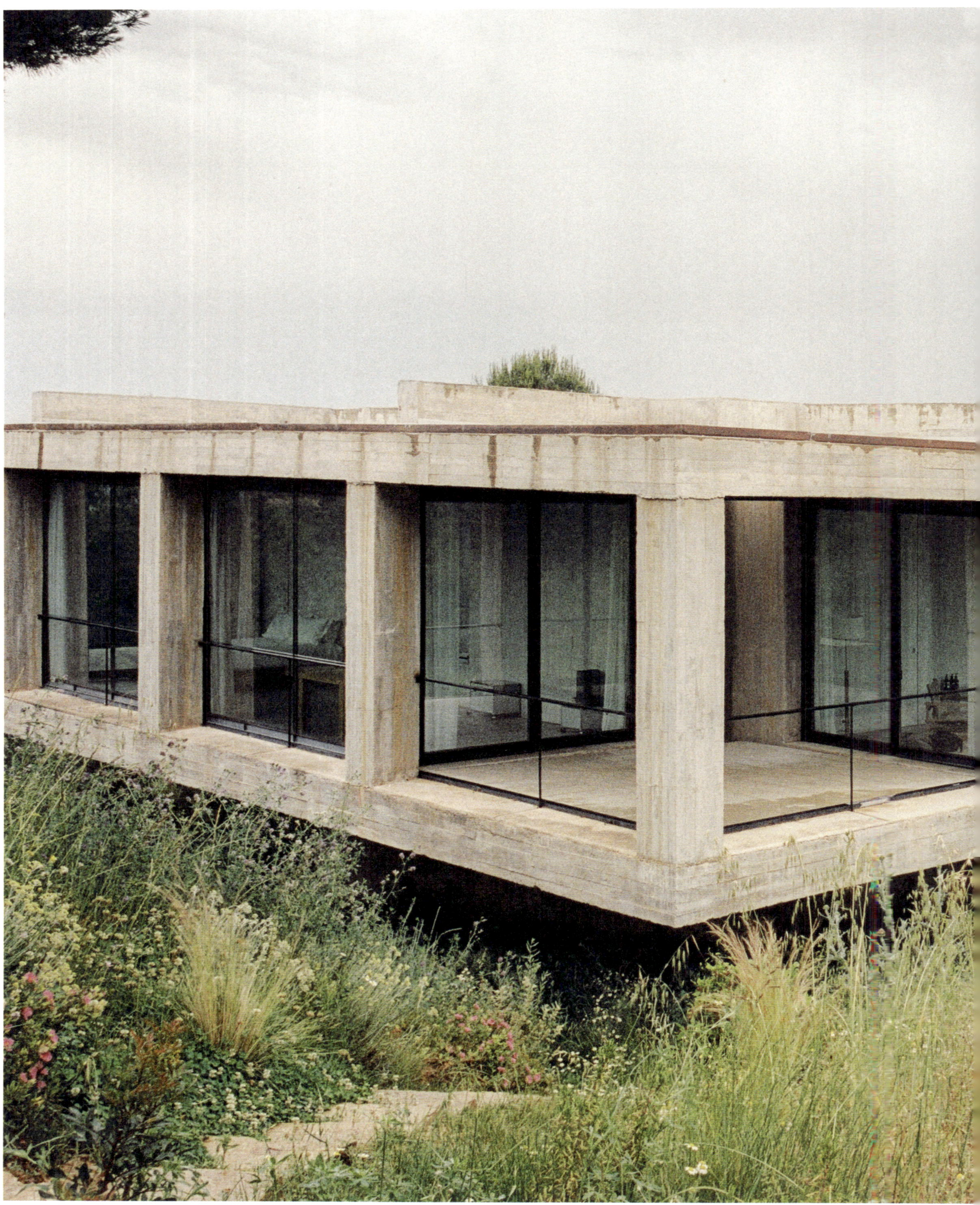

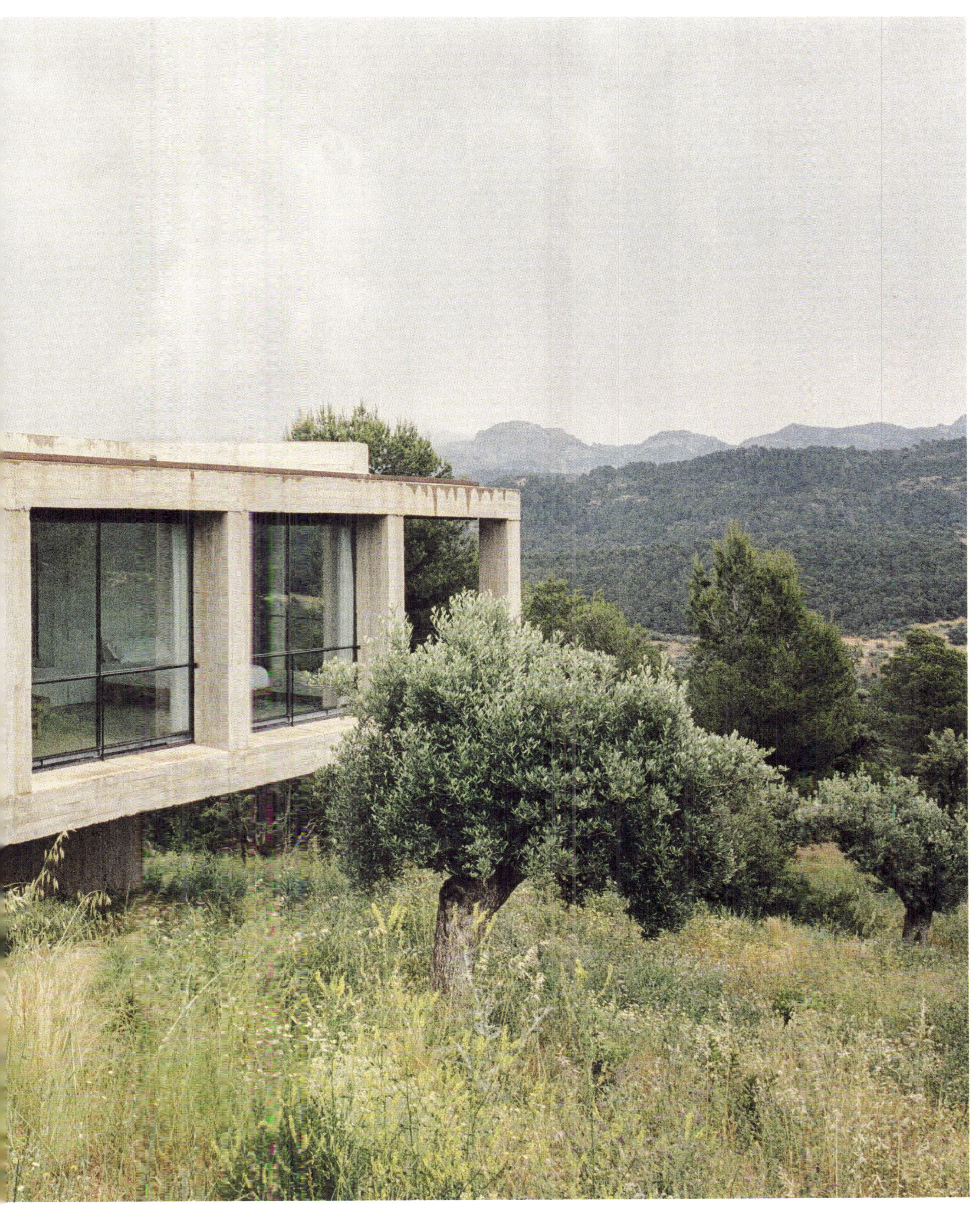

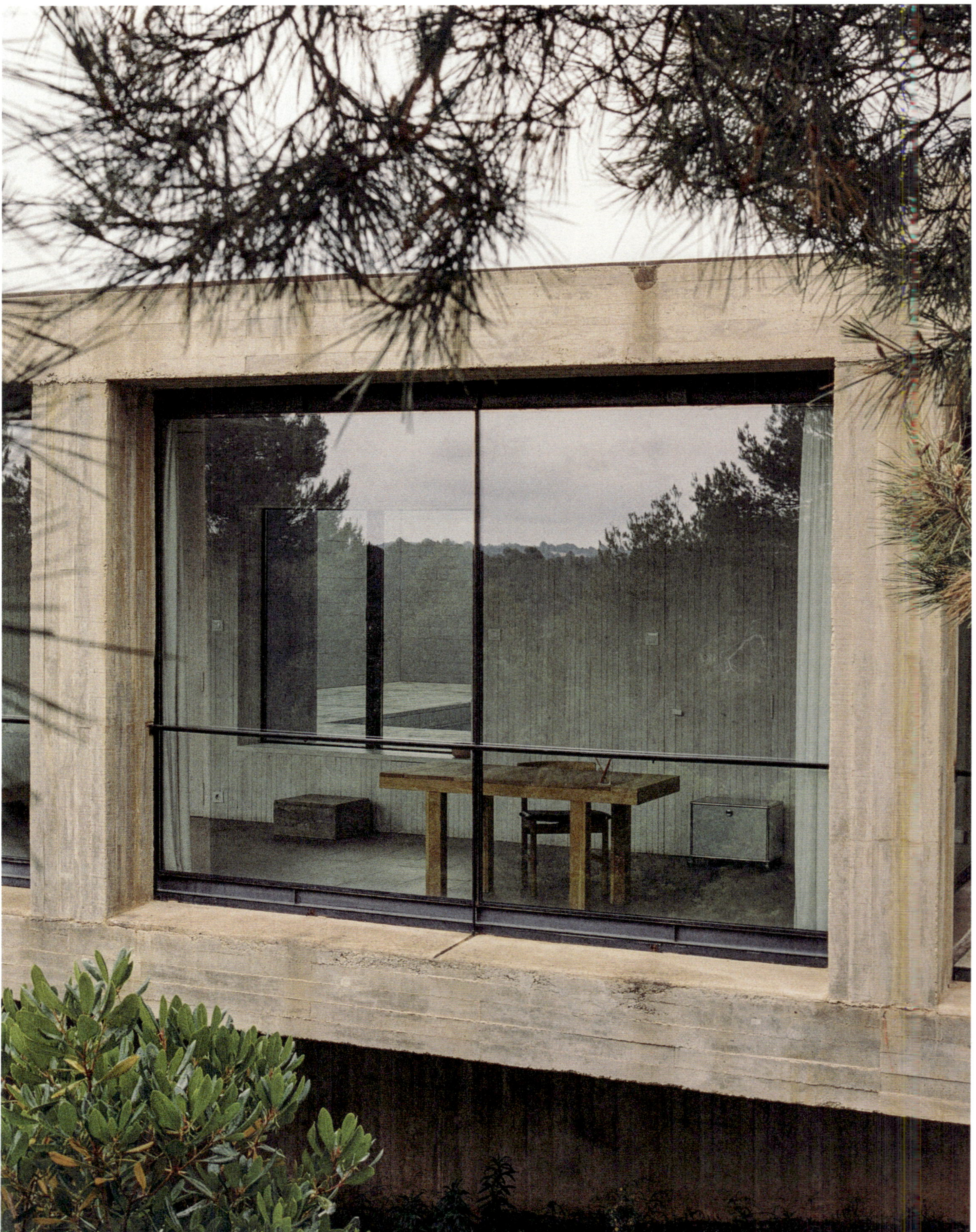

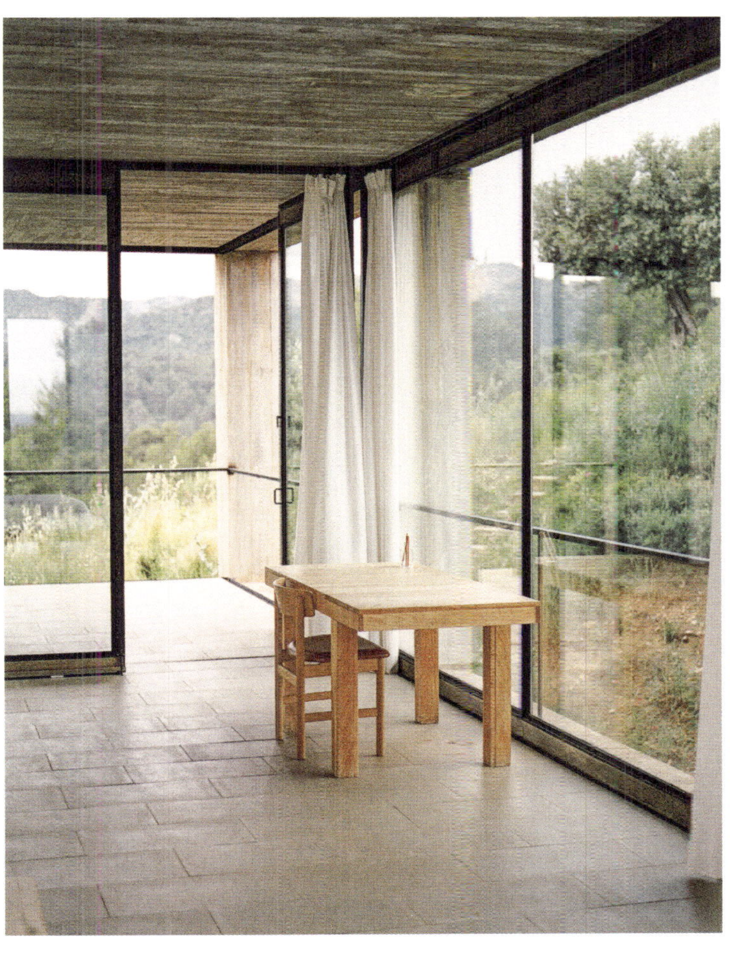

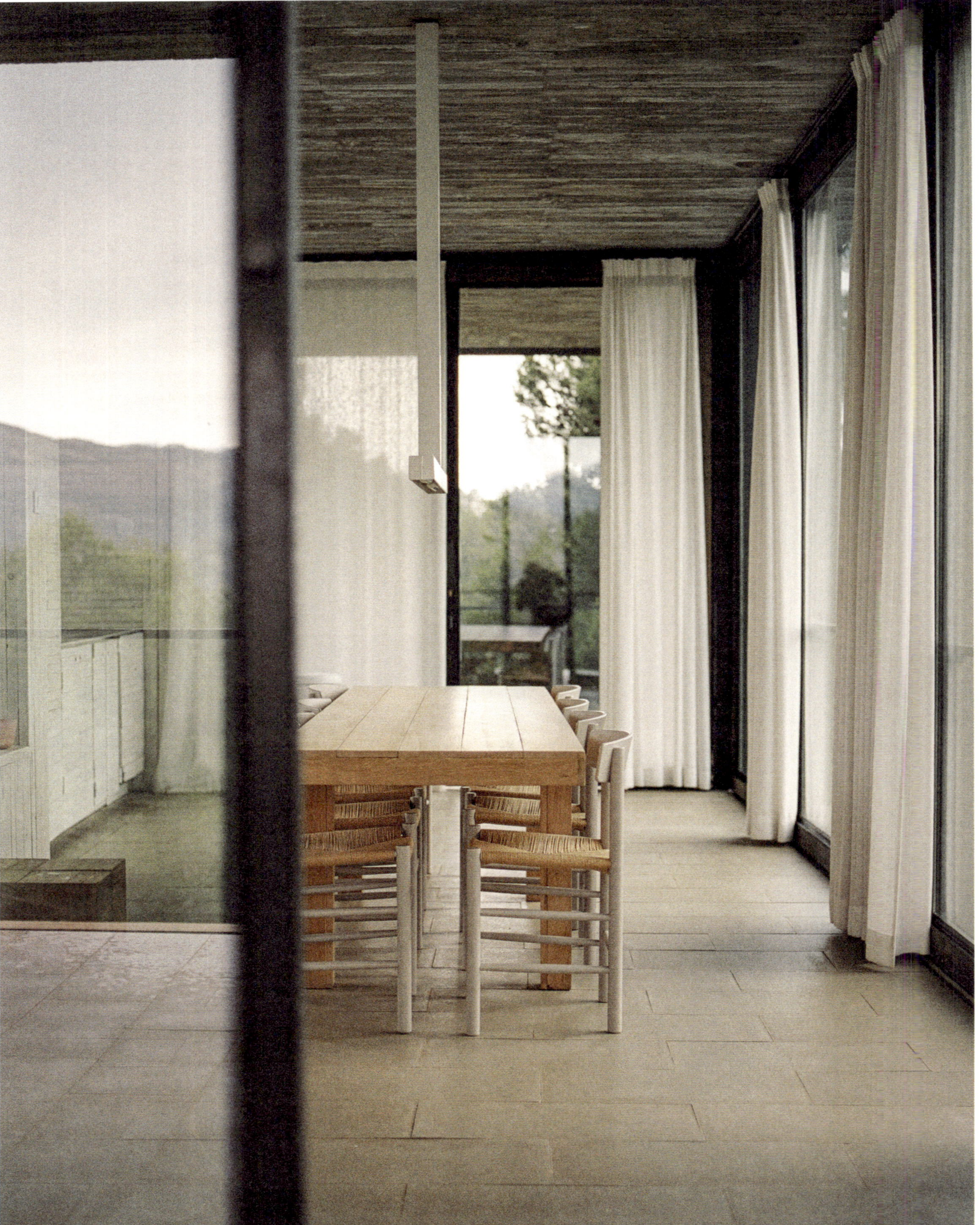

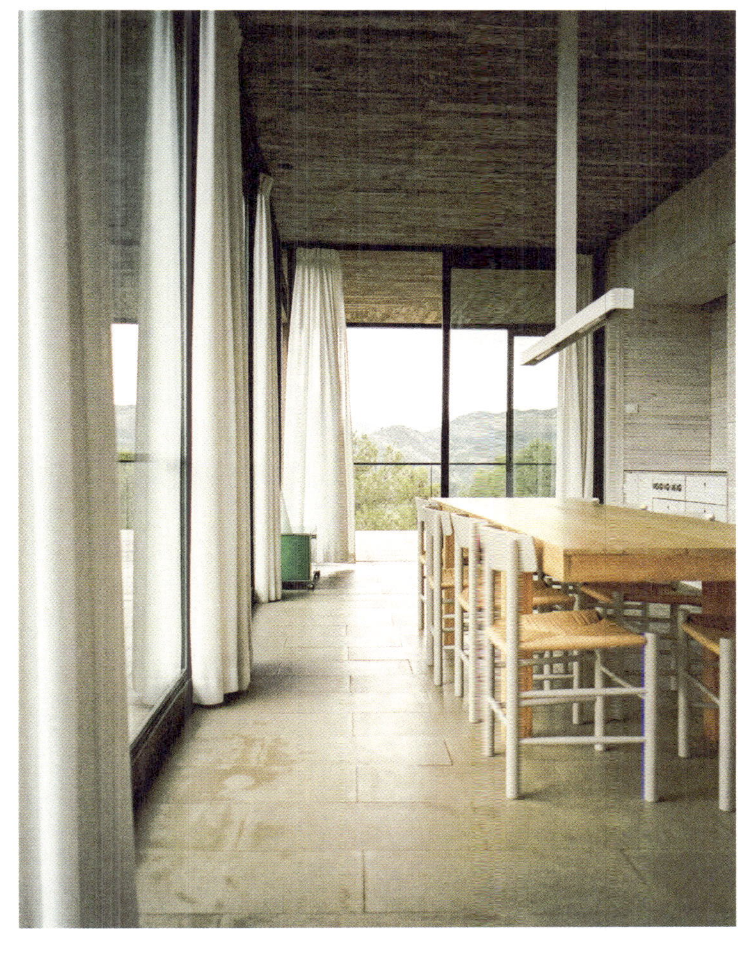

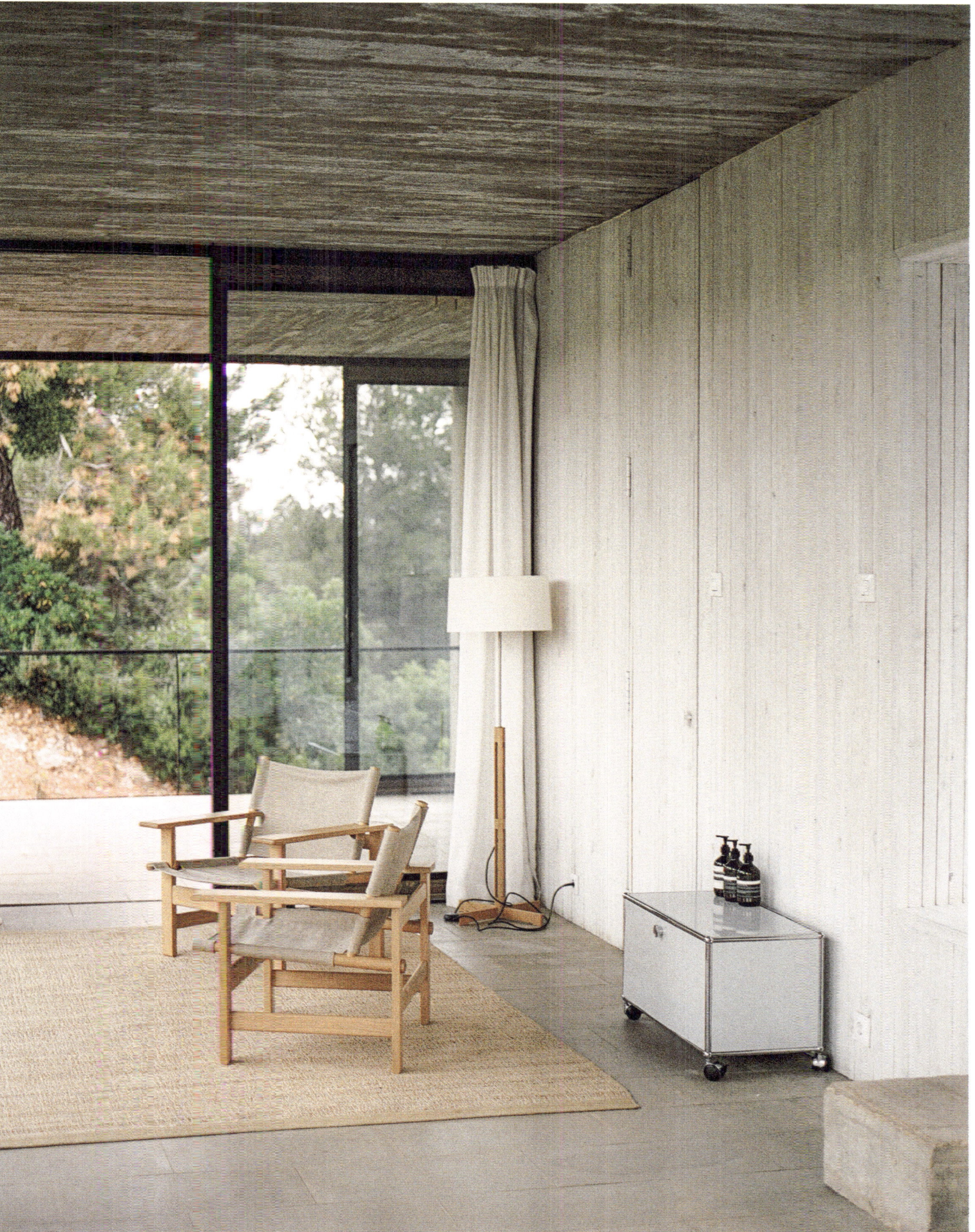

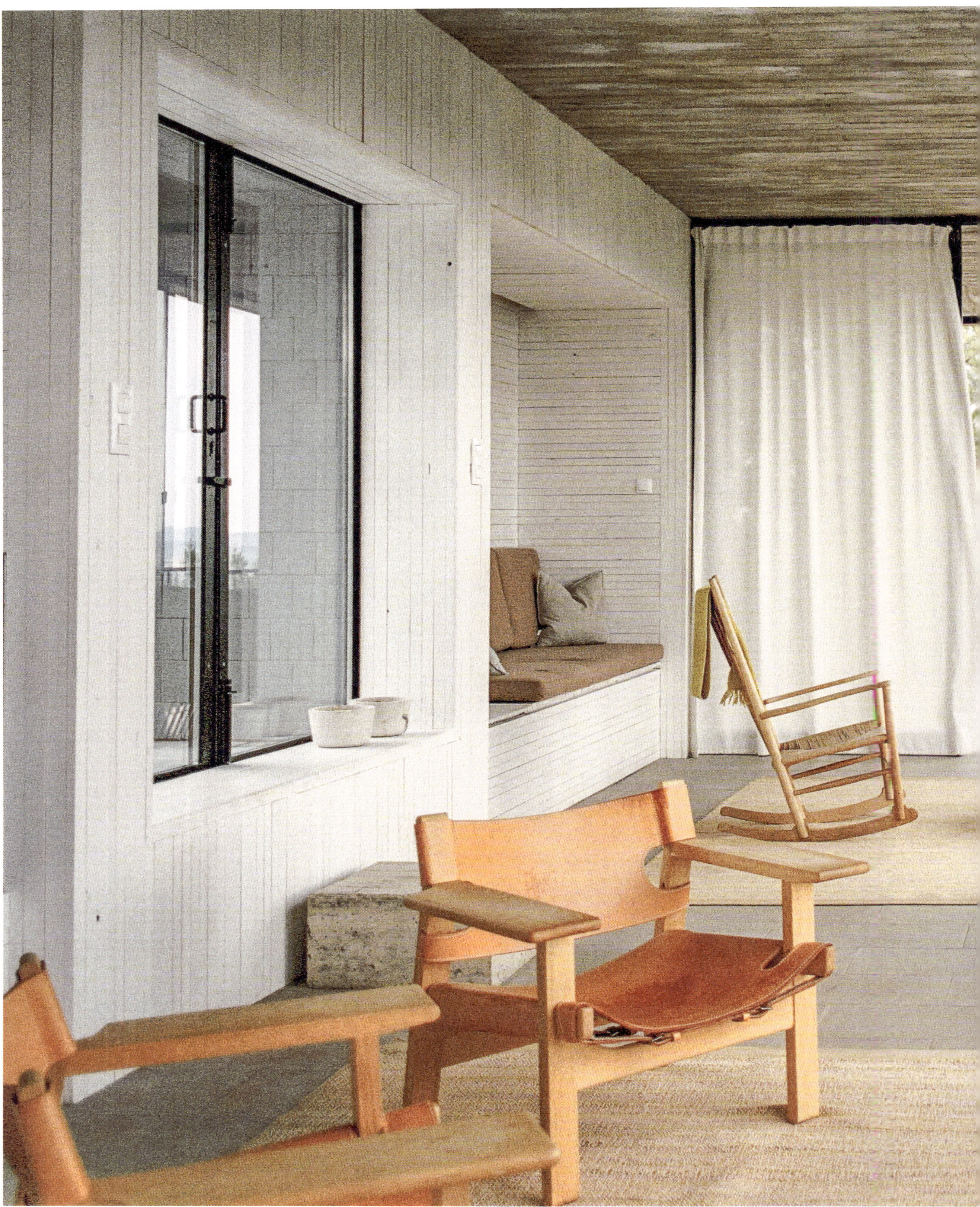

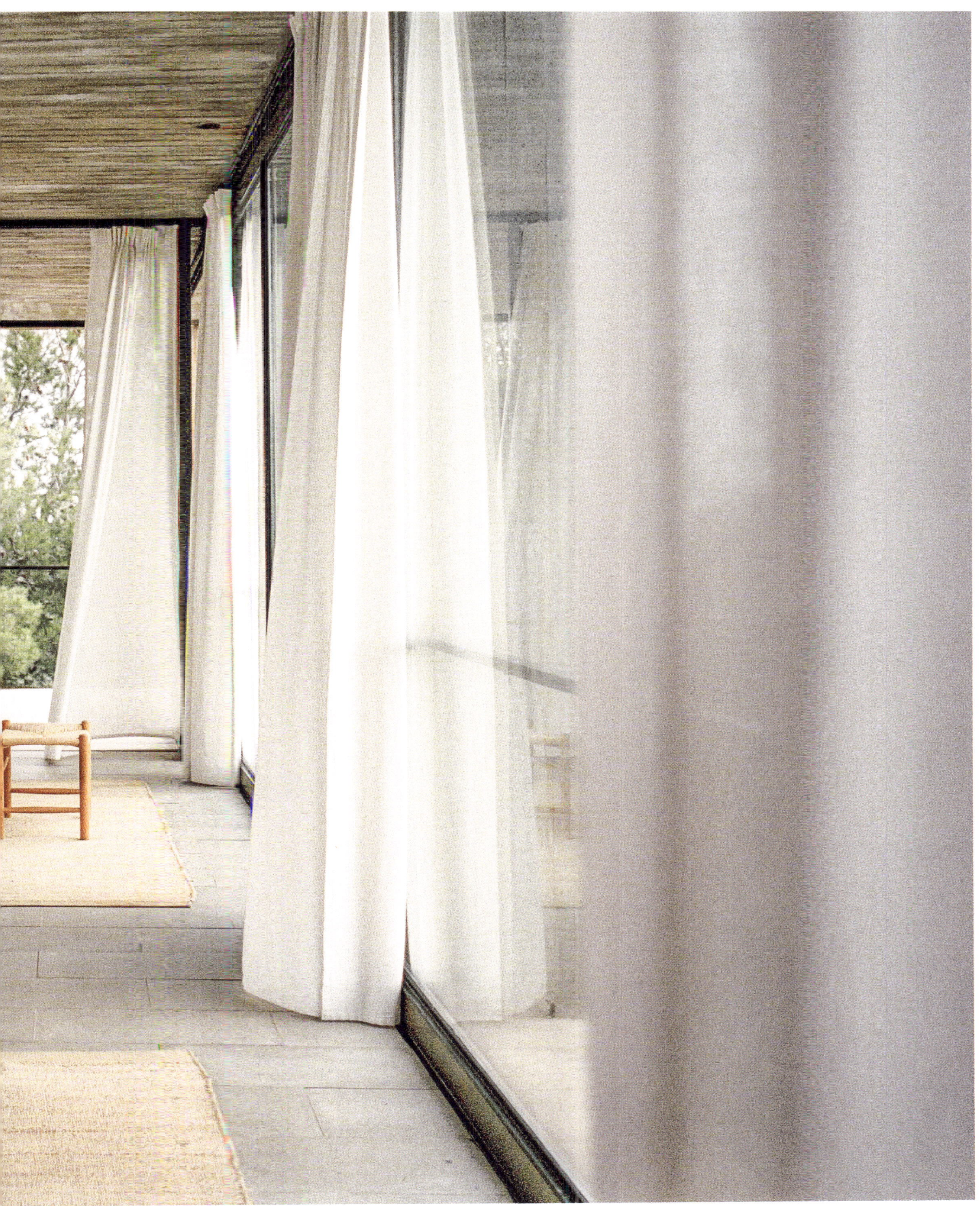

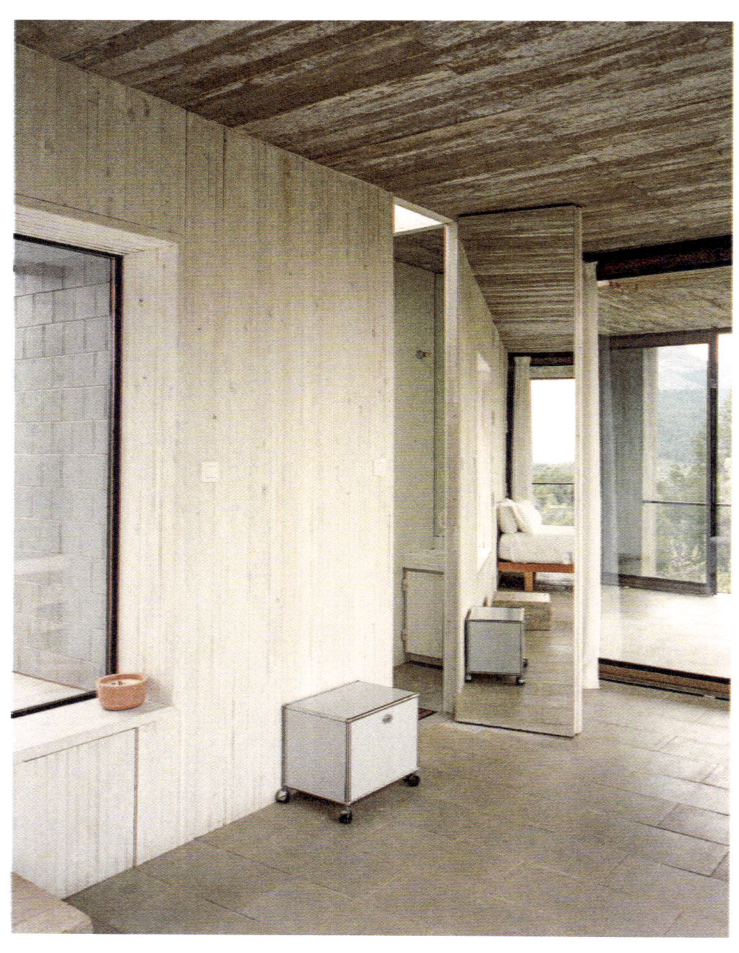

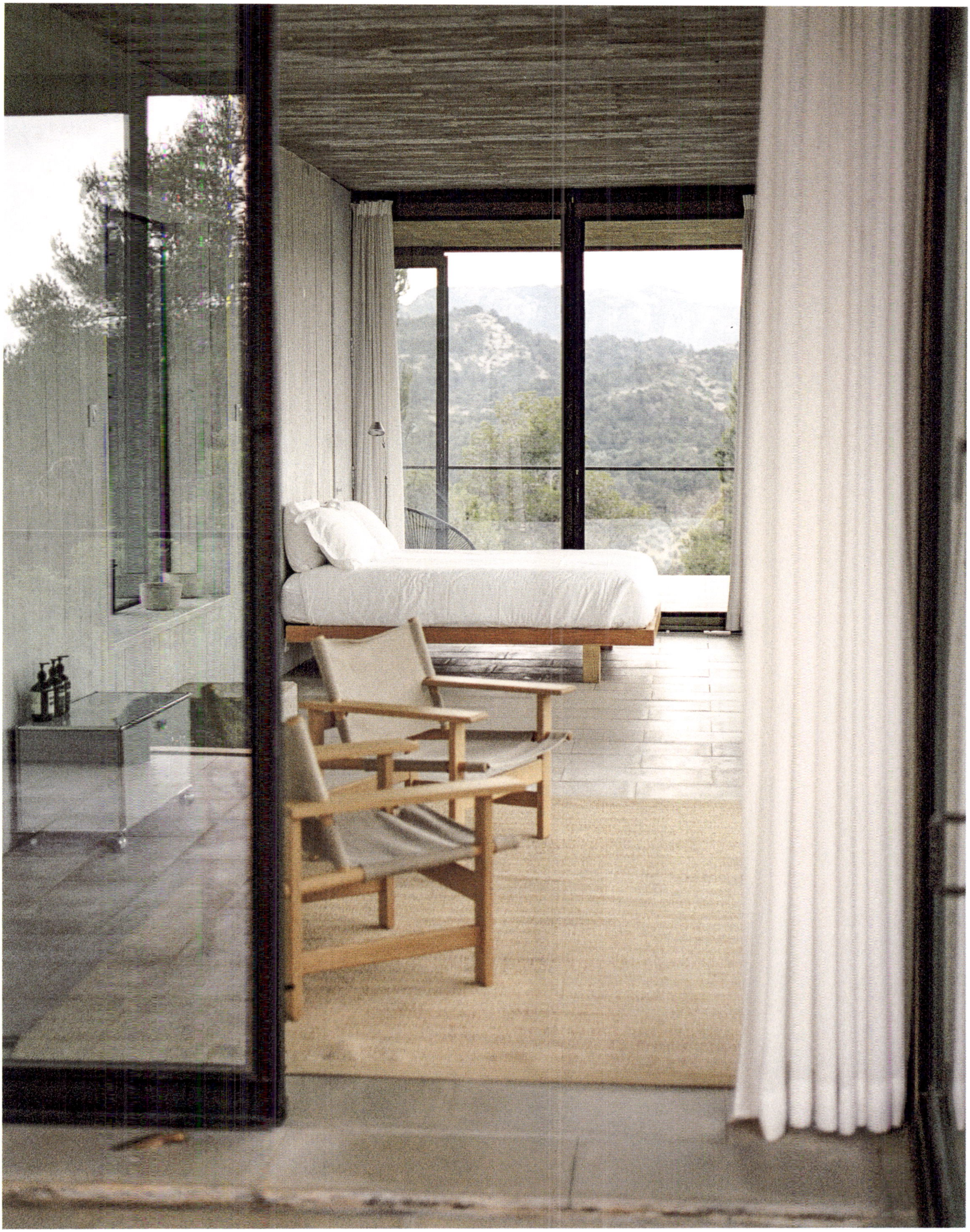

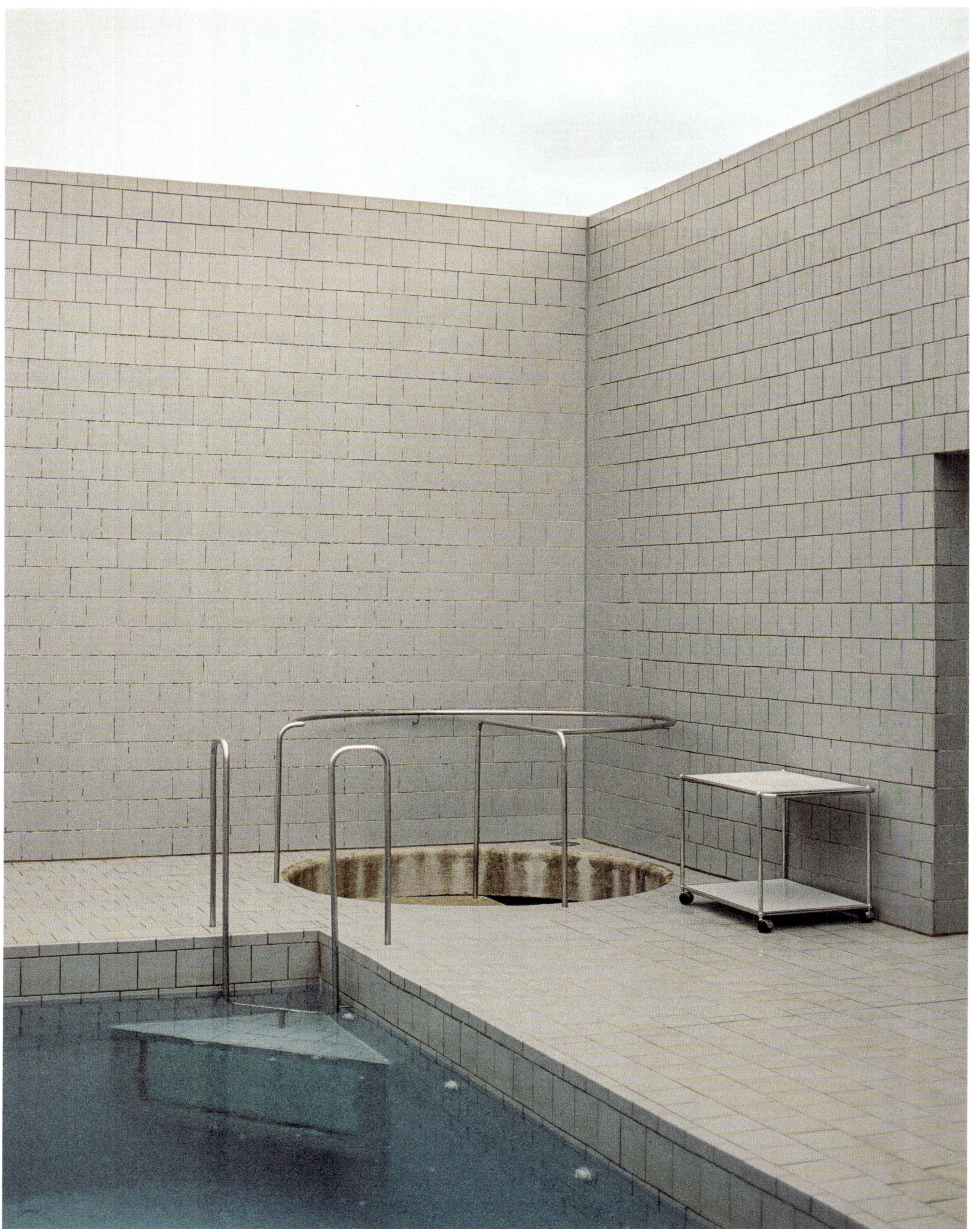

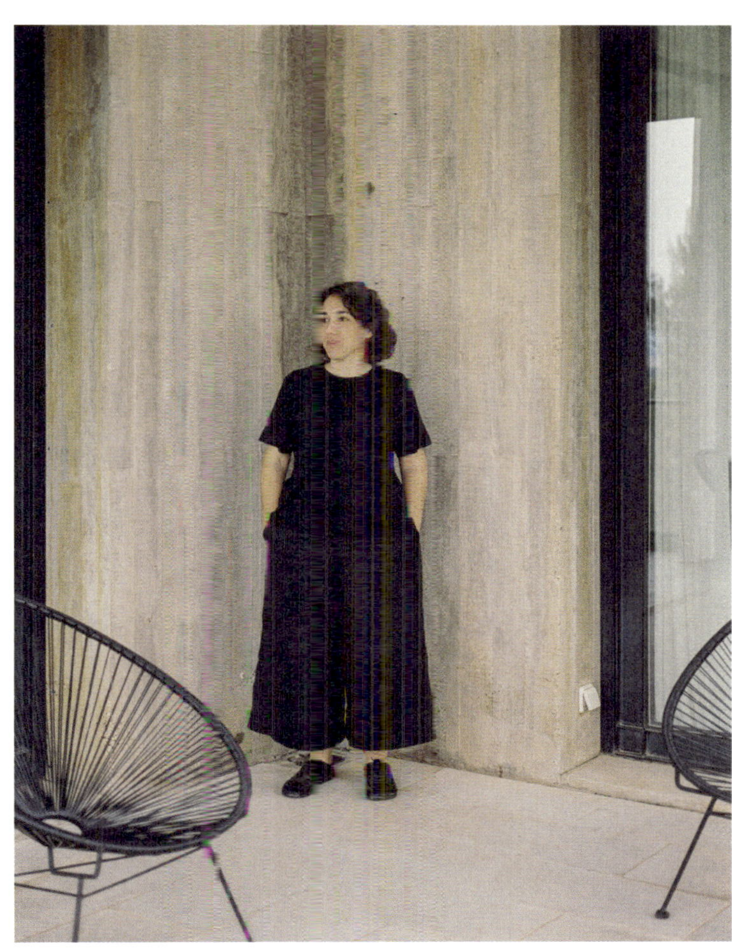

"Throughout the day, as shifting light animates the concrete surfaces and reveals new dialogues between material and nature, the house becomes a place of continual rediscovery."

– Julia Cajaraville

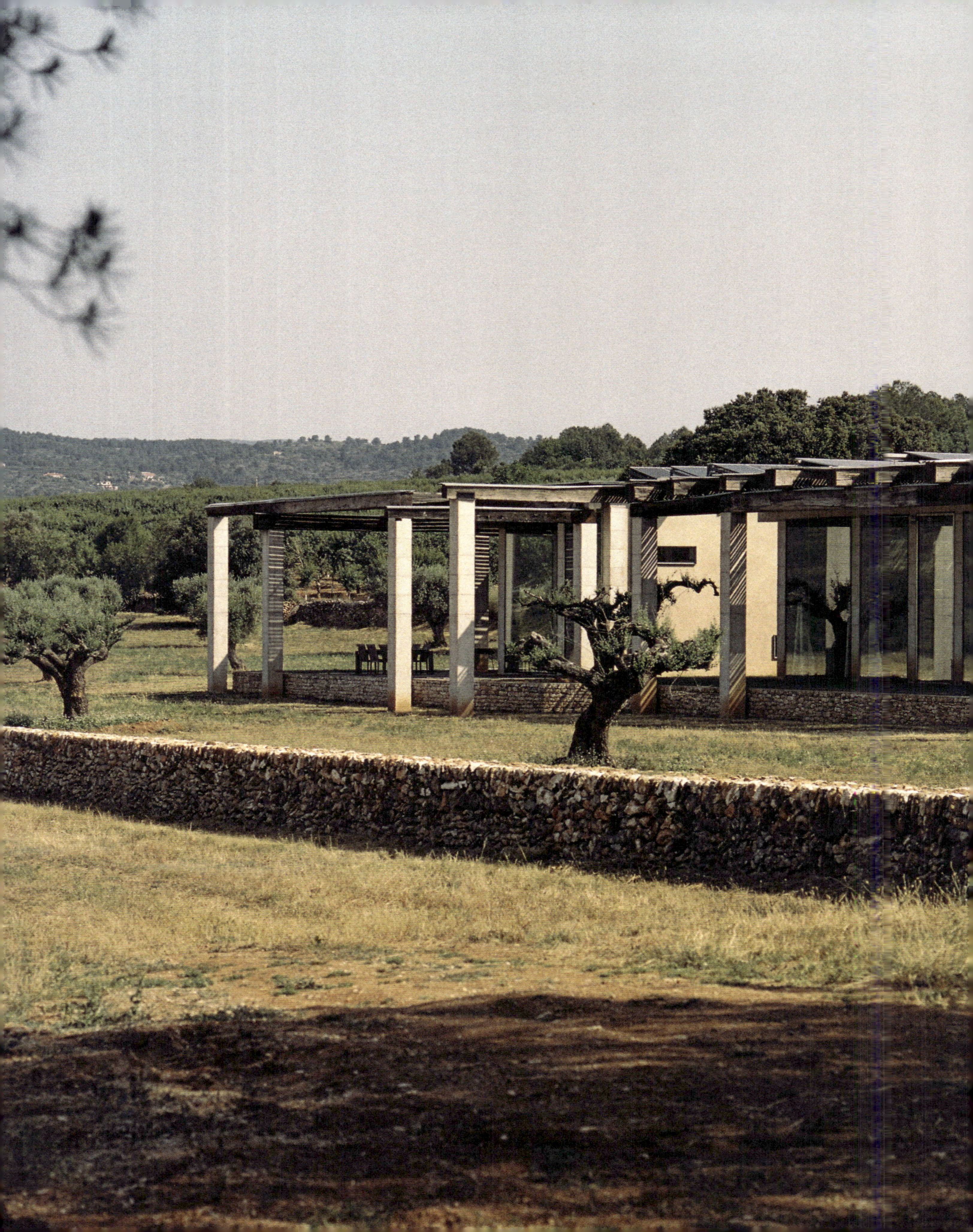

SpronkenHouse
Spain

In the hills of Les Useres, between olive trees and dry stone walls, stands a structure that feels more like a sculpture than a house. SpronkenHouse is the life's work of Dutch artist Xander Spronken. It is a vast, open composition of raw steel and concrete, designed not just to be lived in, but to be experienced.

It is made of 56 vertical columns, each one hand-welded and individually placed. The grid is strict and almost temple-like, with a rhythm based on the golden ratio giving it its proportions. The house is monumental in size but never heavy. It sits lightly in the landscape, wide and low, open to sun and wind.

Spronken built it as his final project. He wanted to create something permanent – a sculpture you could walk through – something that would last. He found the land by chance and pointed to the spot where it should be built. Once built, he left. The house remained.

Years later, it was taken over by a member of his extended family. Someone who understood its intention and wanted to live within it, not change it. And it was carefully adapted over time. The volumes were refined. The landscape was cleaned, repaired, and extended. The interior was furnished slowly and deliberately, without decoration.

The house consists of two residential units, each just over one hundred and thirty square metres. They sit inside the grid, tucked between columns. The materials are minimal: concrete, steel, leather, and glass. Nothing distracts. Inside, a few pieces of custom furniture and vintage design create balance. There are benches by American artist Stephen Kenn, made from repurposed parachute fabric; a kitchen that blends into the wall; a sofa that becomes part of the space. Everything speaks softly.

The rear of the site is being cultivated. Old olive trees have been relocated, dry stone walls rebuilt, and an old winery restored. The long-term vision is not one of expansion, but of completion. The goal is to allow the place to mature without losing its strength and to extend the work with care.

SpronkenHouse was never meant to be finished. It is an open structure, both physically and conceptually. It frames the sky, it holds the wind, and invites people to stop and listen. It is a house, but also something else, a place that stays with you.

Project: SpronkenHouse
Location: Spain
Architect: Xander Spronken
Year of construction: 2017
Floor area: 310 m²
Resident: Joris Dassen
Resident's profession: retired, in real estate

03

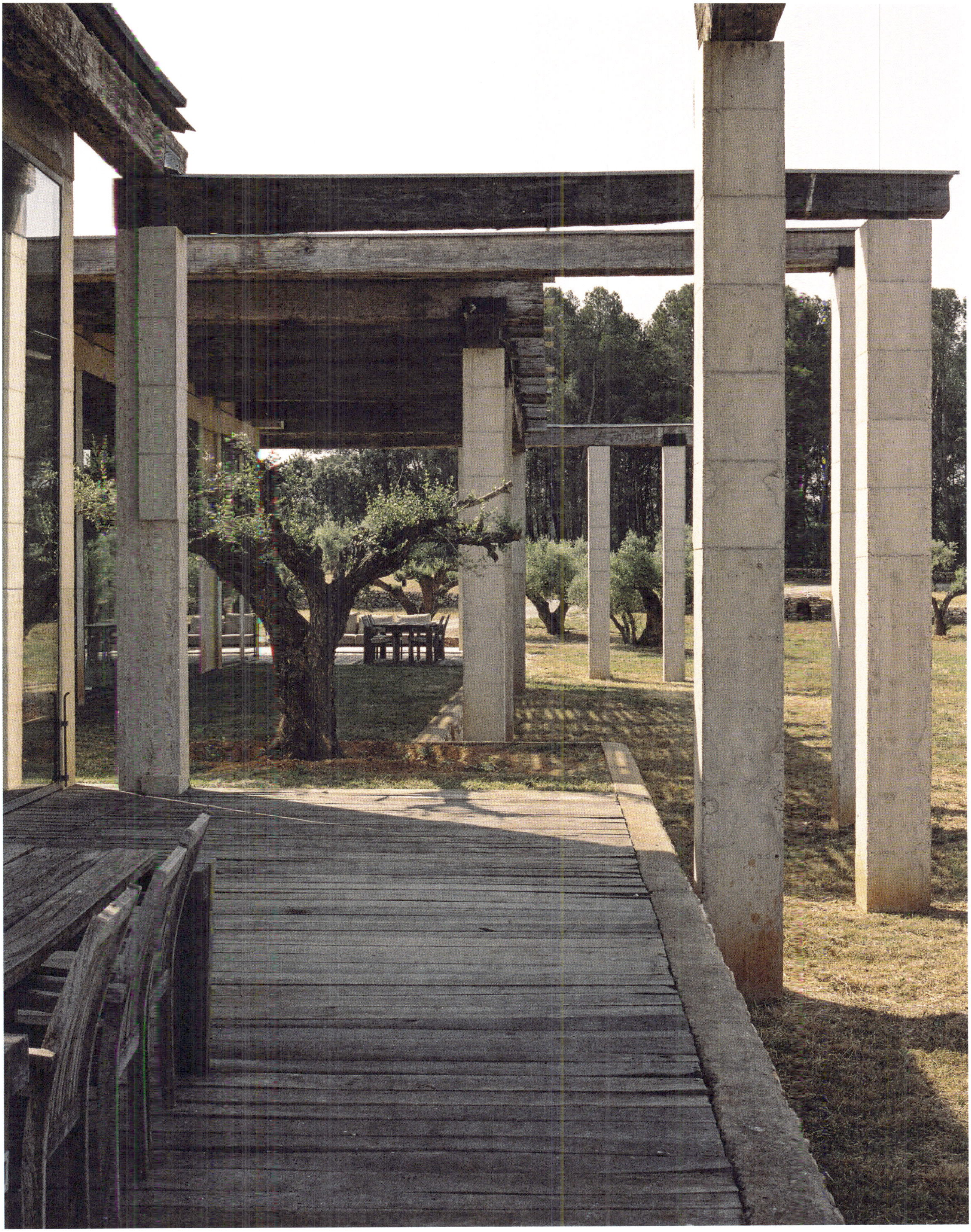

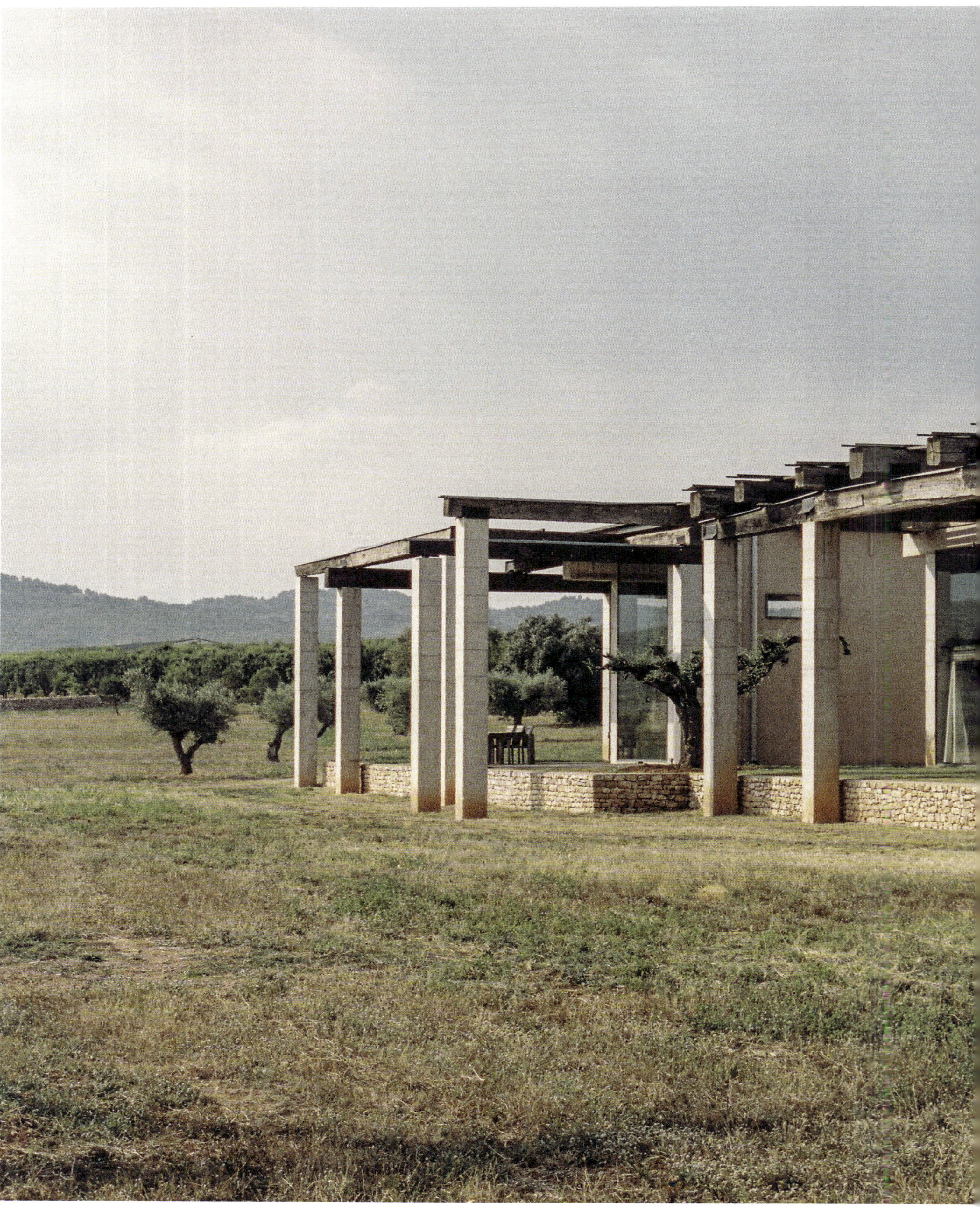

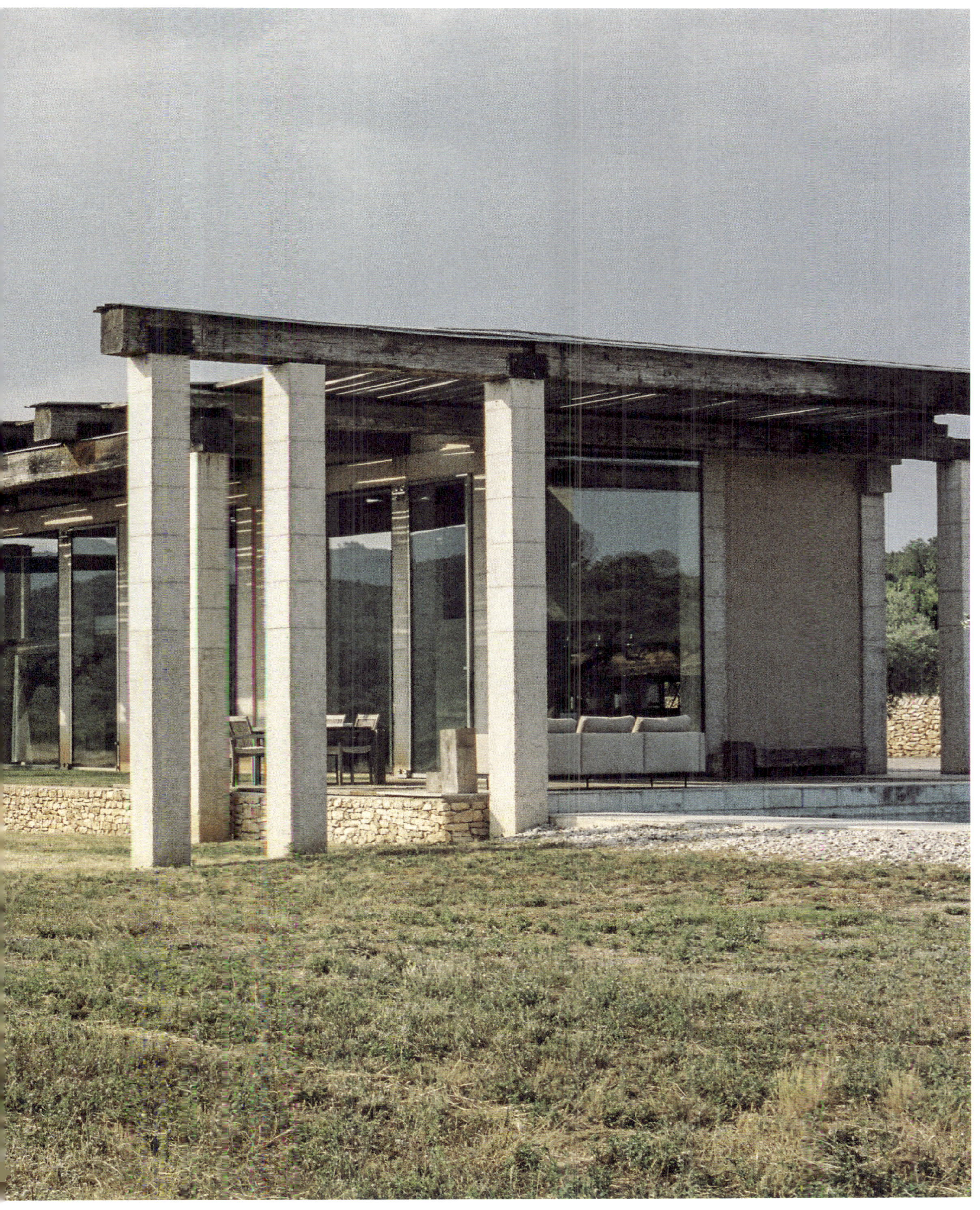

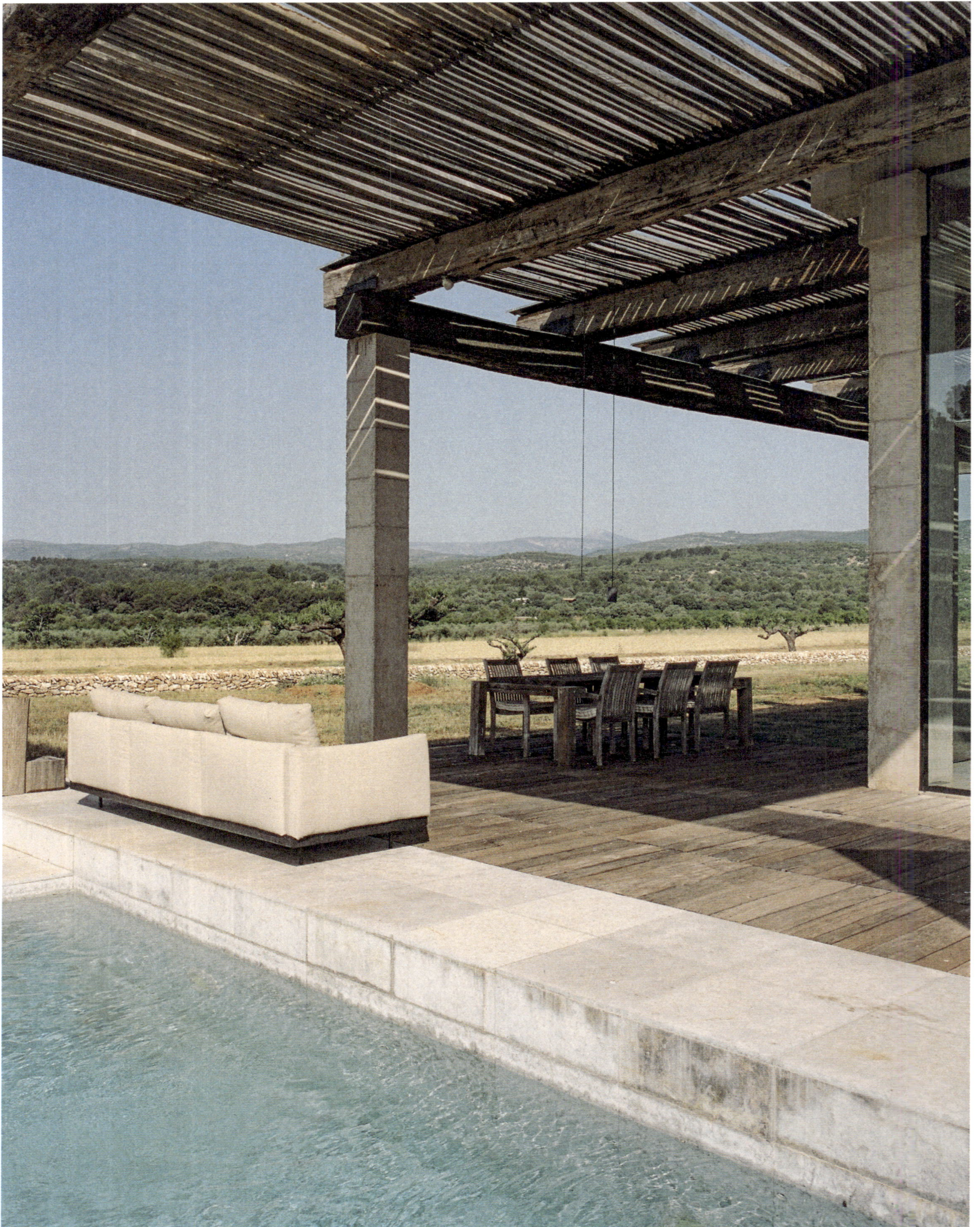

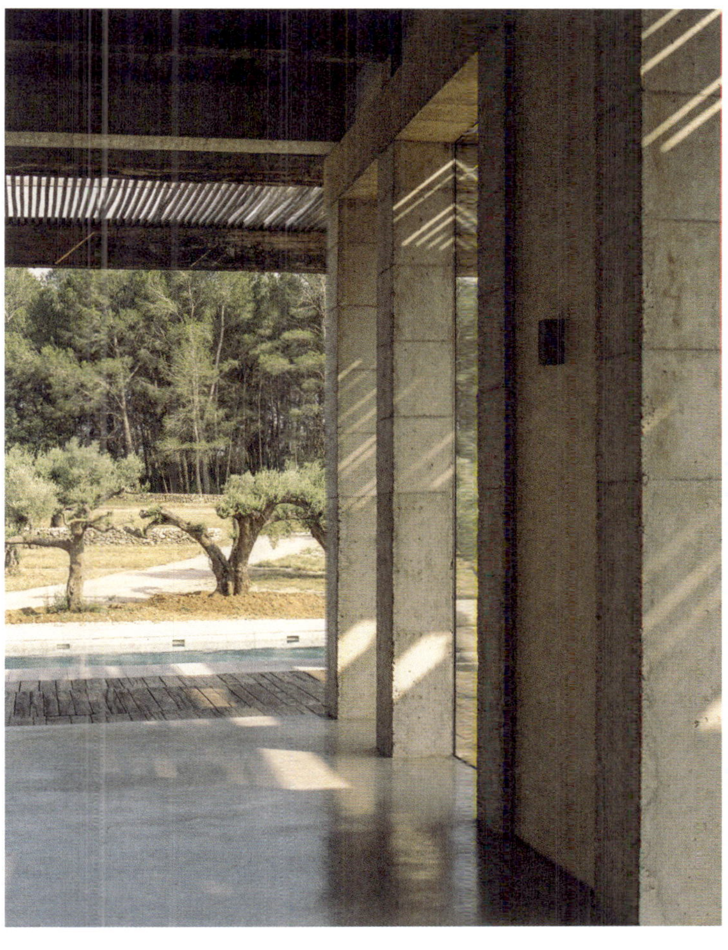

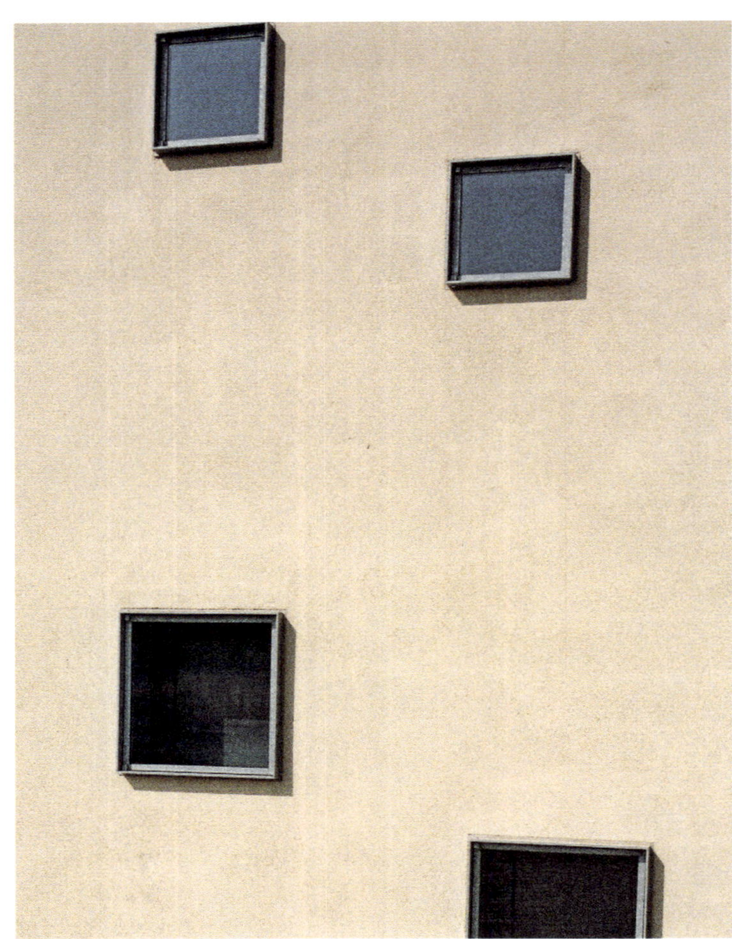

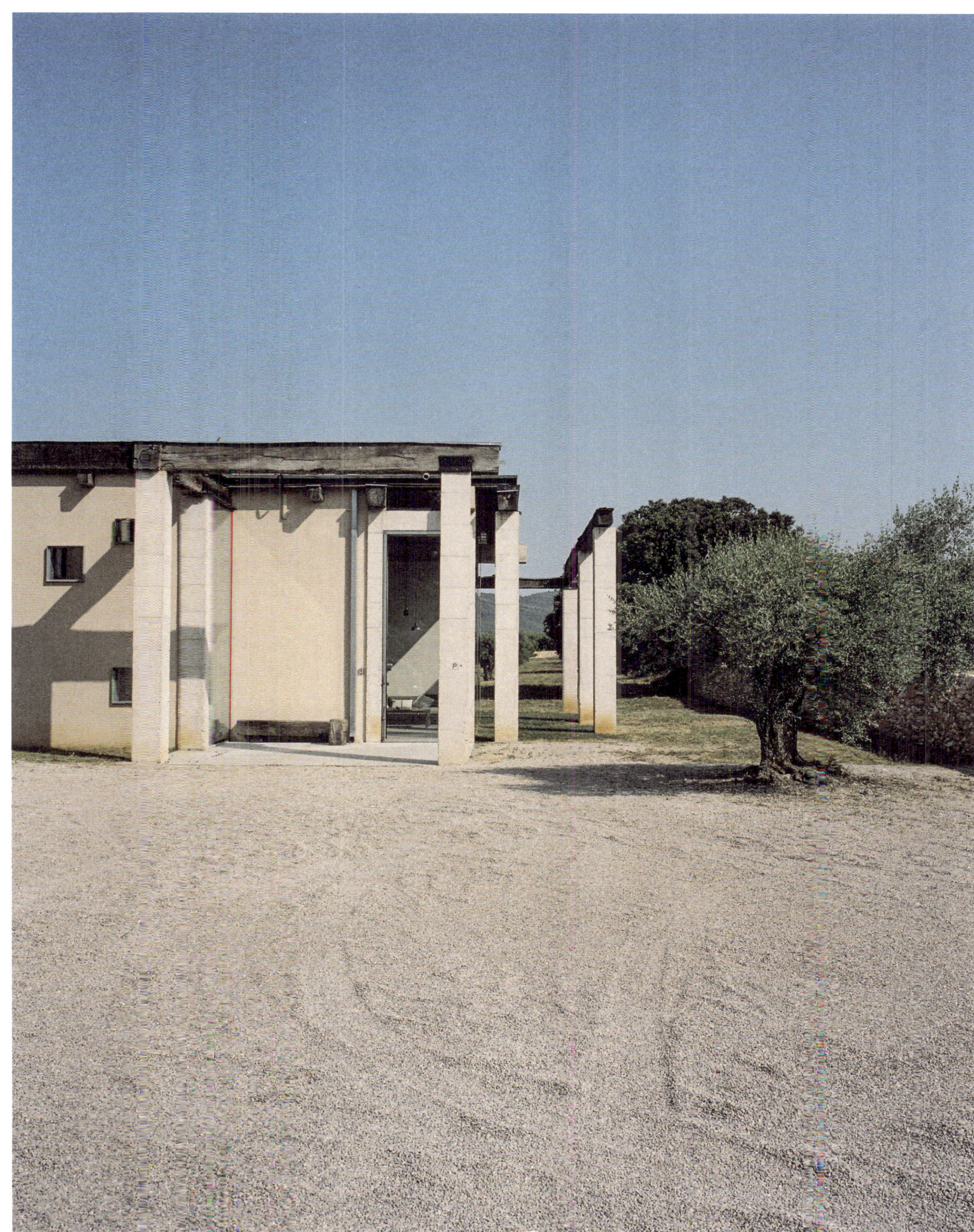

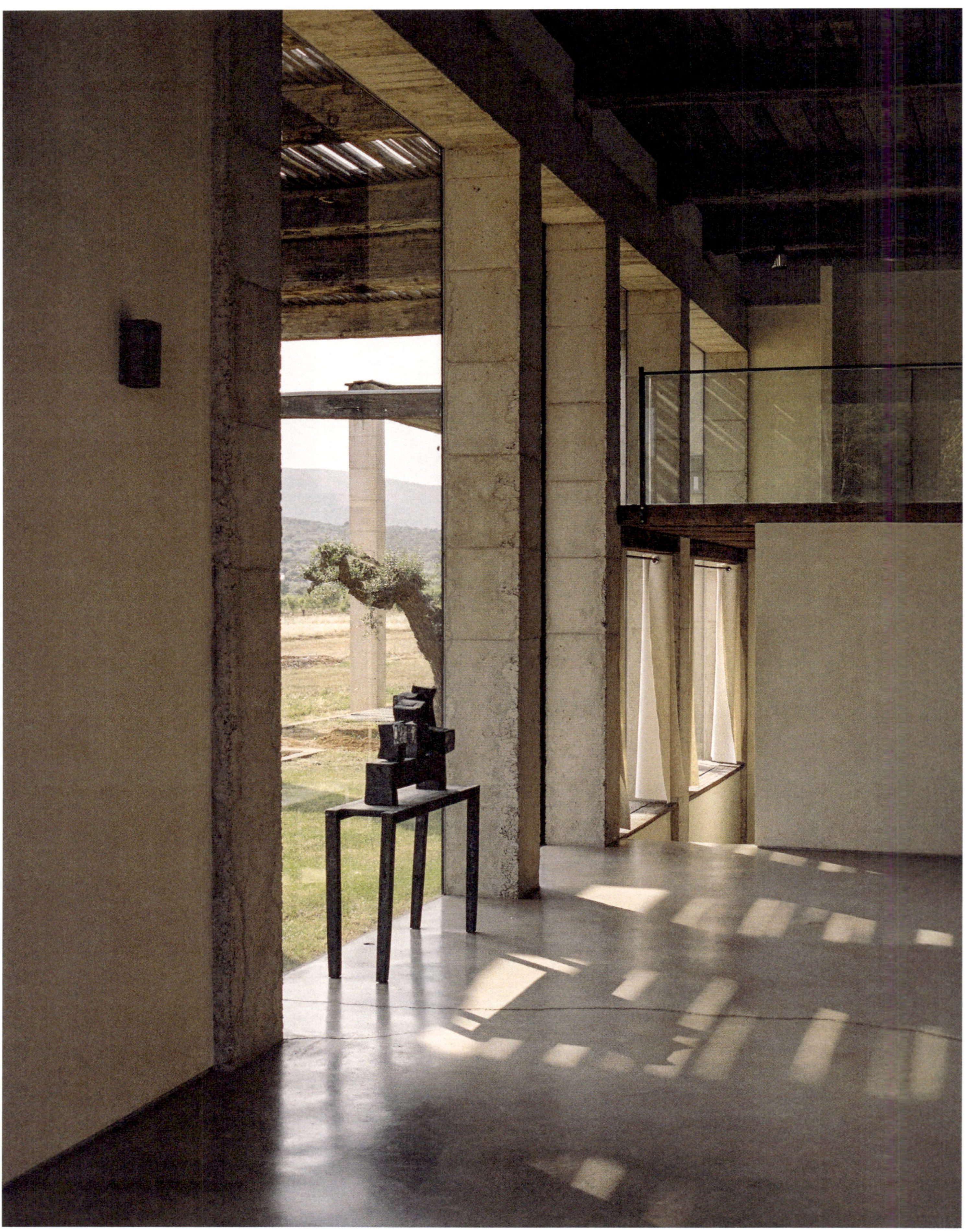

1

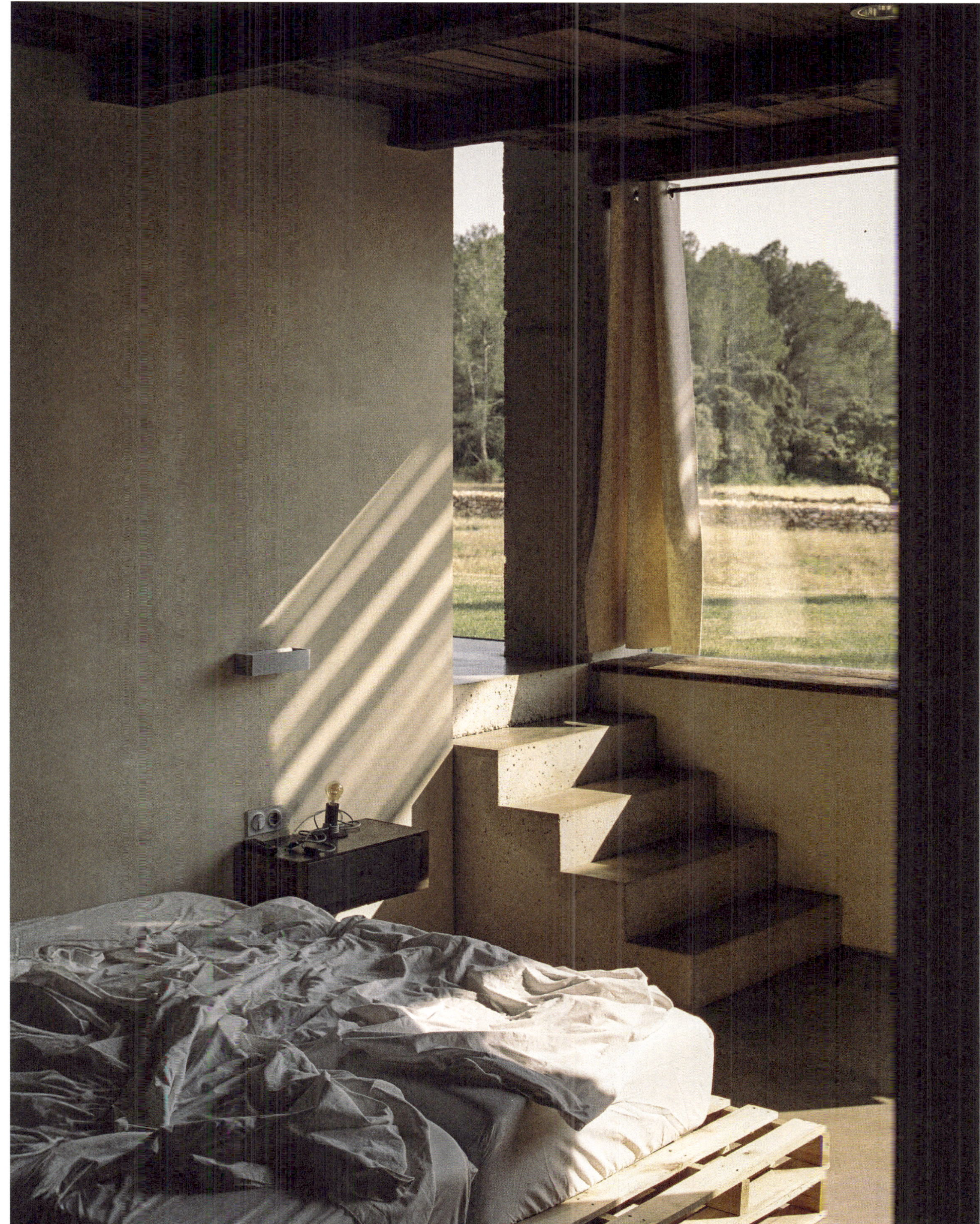

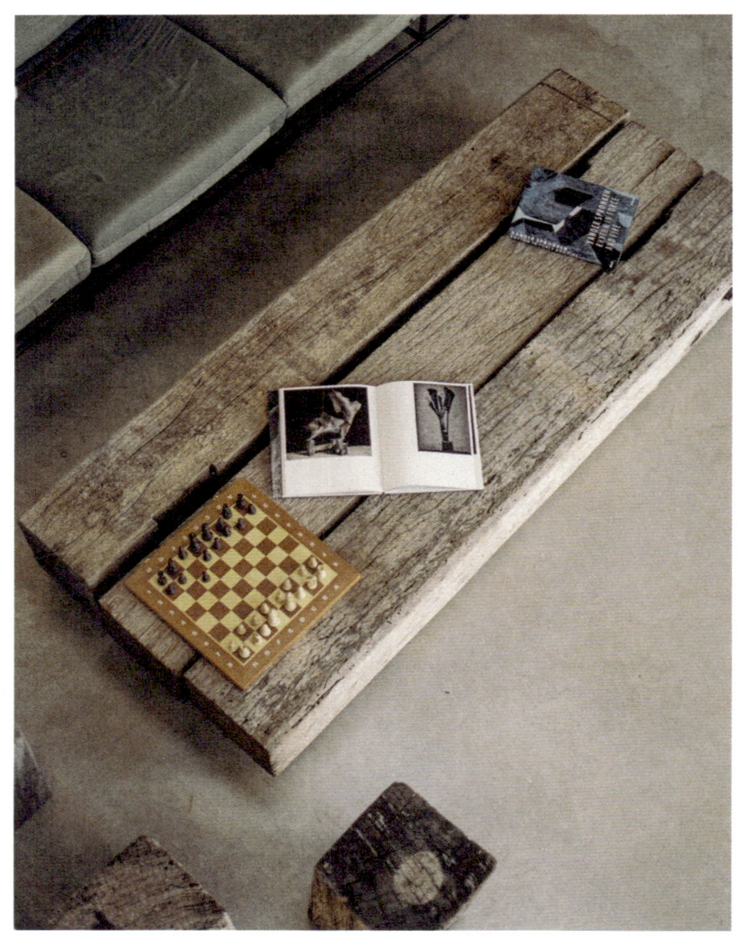

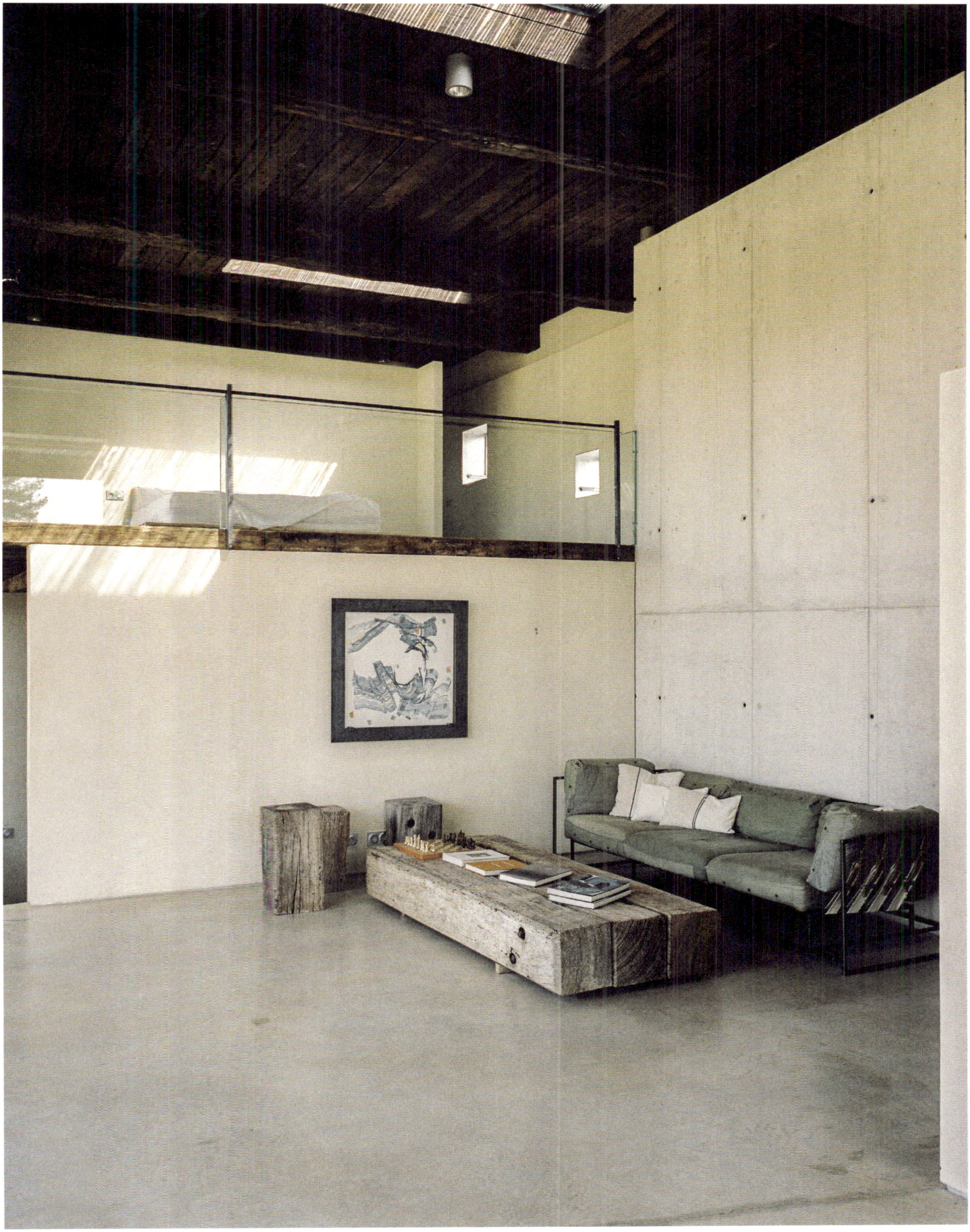

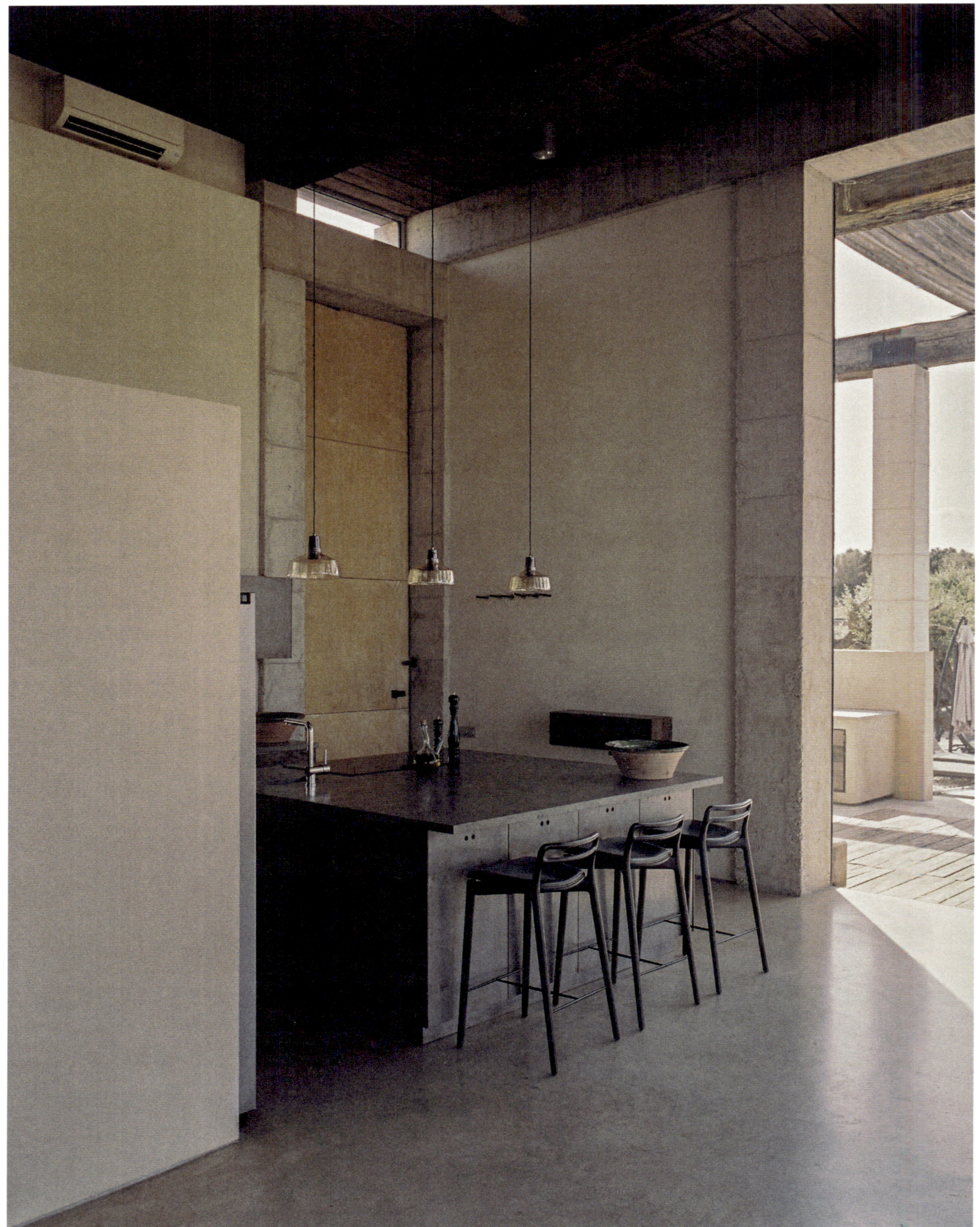

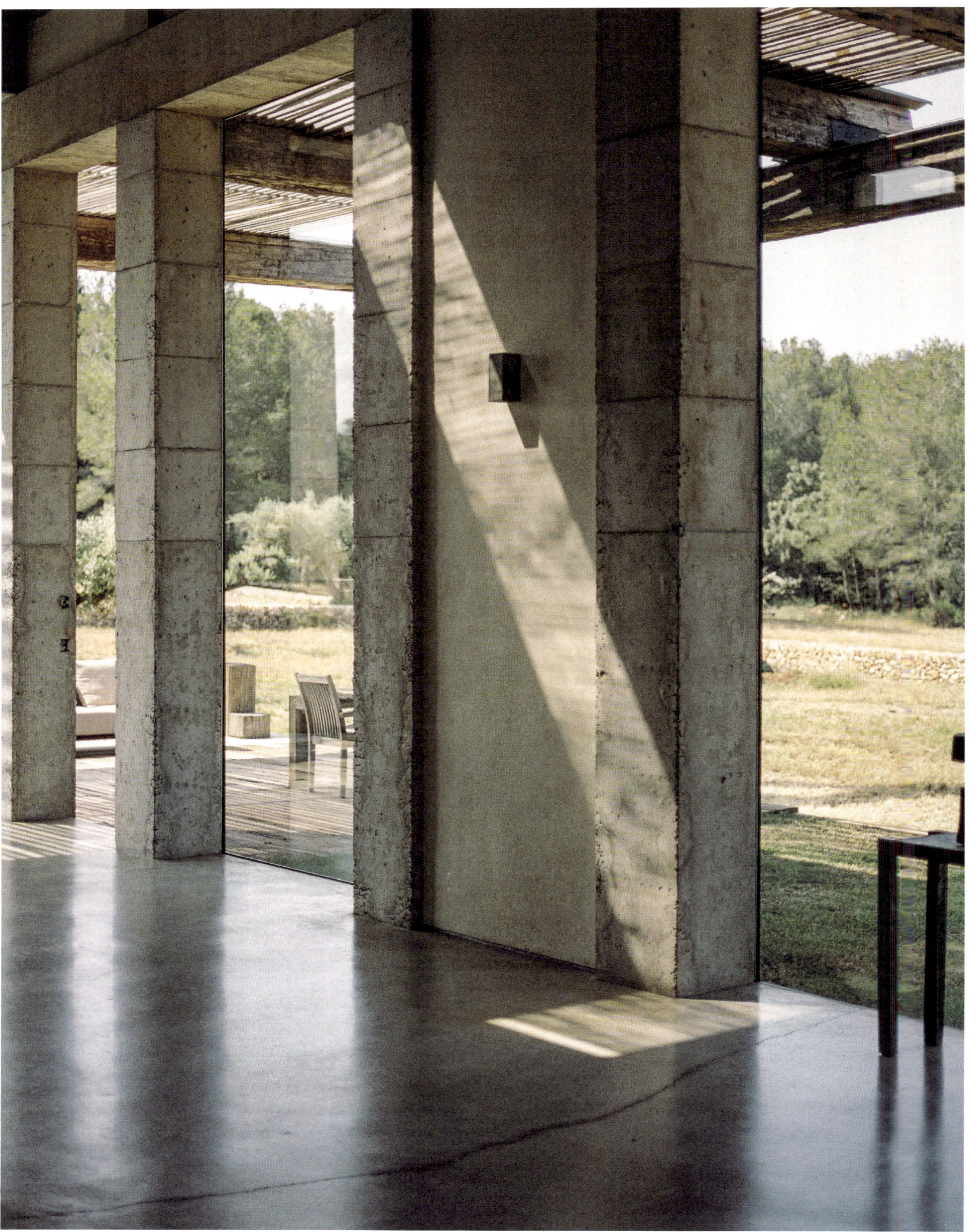

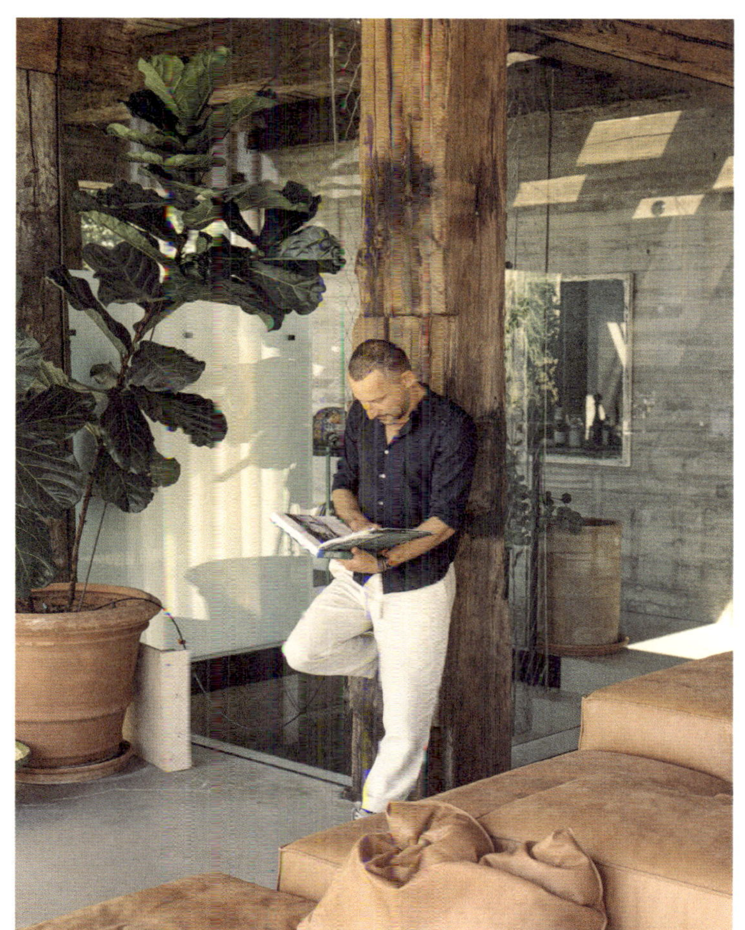

"The concrete and its warm colour make me feel humble and at peace."

– Joris Dassen

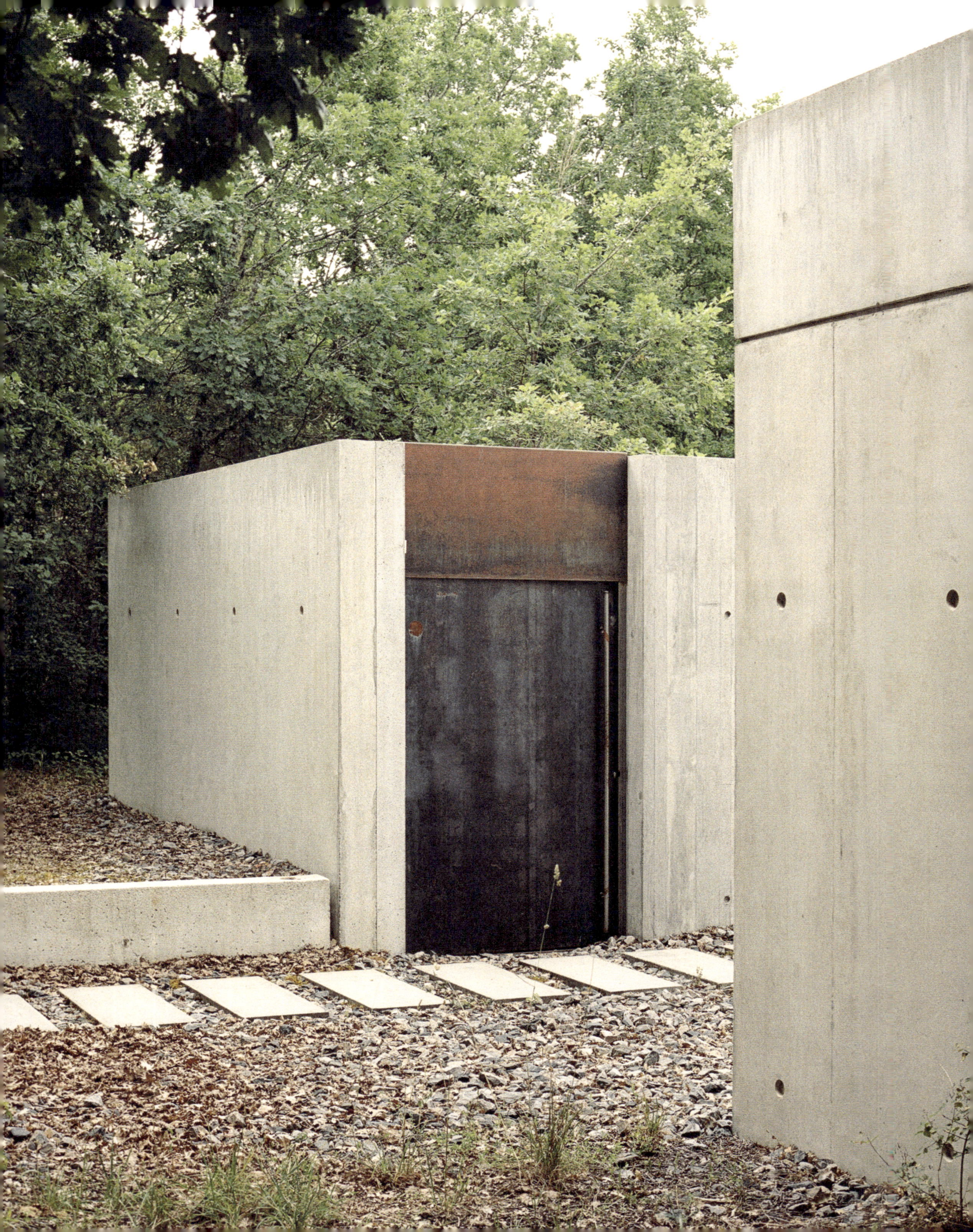

La Maison H
France

In the hills near Cahors, in the southwest of France, there's a house that seems to rest rather than stand. It doesn't sit on the land, it lies in it. Low, horizontal, and silent, La Maison H doesn't draw attention, it absorbs it.

The house was designed by architect Franck Martinez as a home for himself and his family. Built in 2015, it has the clarity of a sketch turned into a structure. The plan is shaped like a large H: two wings joined by a central axis. From above, it reads like a diagram. From the ground, it's harder to define. Concrete walls lead your eye, then stop. Spaces shift from open to enclosed. Nothing announces itself; everything unfolds.

From the road, you don't really see it. The terrain drops slightly, the roofline is flat, and wild grass grows right up to the façade. There's no clear boundary between building and land. No fence, no front garden, no path. You arrive without ceremony.

Inside, the house is structured but not strict, with long corridors leading to wide rooms. Each wing holds different functions – sleeping on one side, living and working on the other – but everything feels connected. Light moves across surfaces through large openings, with views framing the forest. The rooms are not large, but they feel generous in proportion and restraint.

There's no ornamentation, just form. The concrete is left bare – a soft grey with grains from the formwork. Ceilings are wooden, floors are polished, matt, and continuous, and the palette is limited but rich in texture. There are no tricks, no decoration, just a quiet confidence in what things are.

One of the most striking choices is what's missing: there are no baseboards, no handles, no visible lighting fixtures. Doors slide into pockets and windows open without fuss. It feels complete, but never over designed.

The house is now in new hands. A music producer from Paris uses it to work and host other creatives. It's not a performance space, but a backdrop for focus. A place to create and listen.

From inside, the landscape is always present. Trees line the horizon; birds move through the sky. The house doesn't frame nature as a scene, it opens up to it, calmly, without control.

La Maison H doesn't aim to surprise, it doesn't try to impress. It offers something rarer: consistency. A house that doesn't shift with mood or season; a house that holds.

Project: La Maison H
Location: France
Architect: Franck Martinez
Year of construction: 2015
Year of purchase: 2021
Floor area: 200 m²
Resident: Matthieu Tessier
Resident's profession: music producer

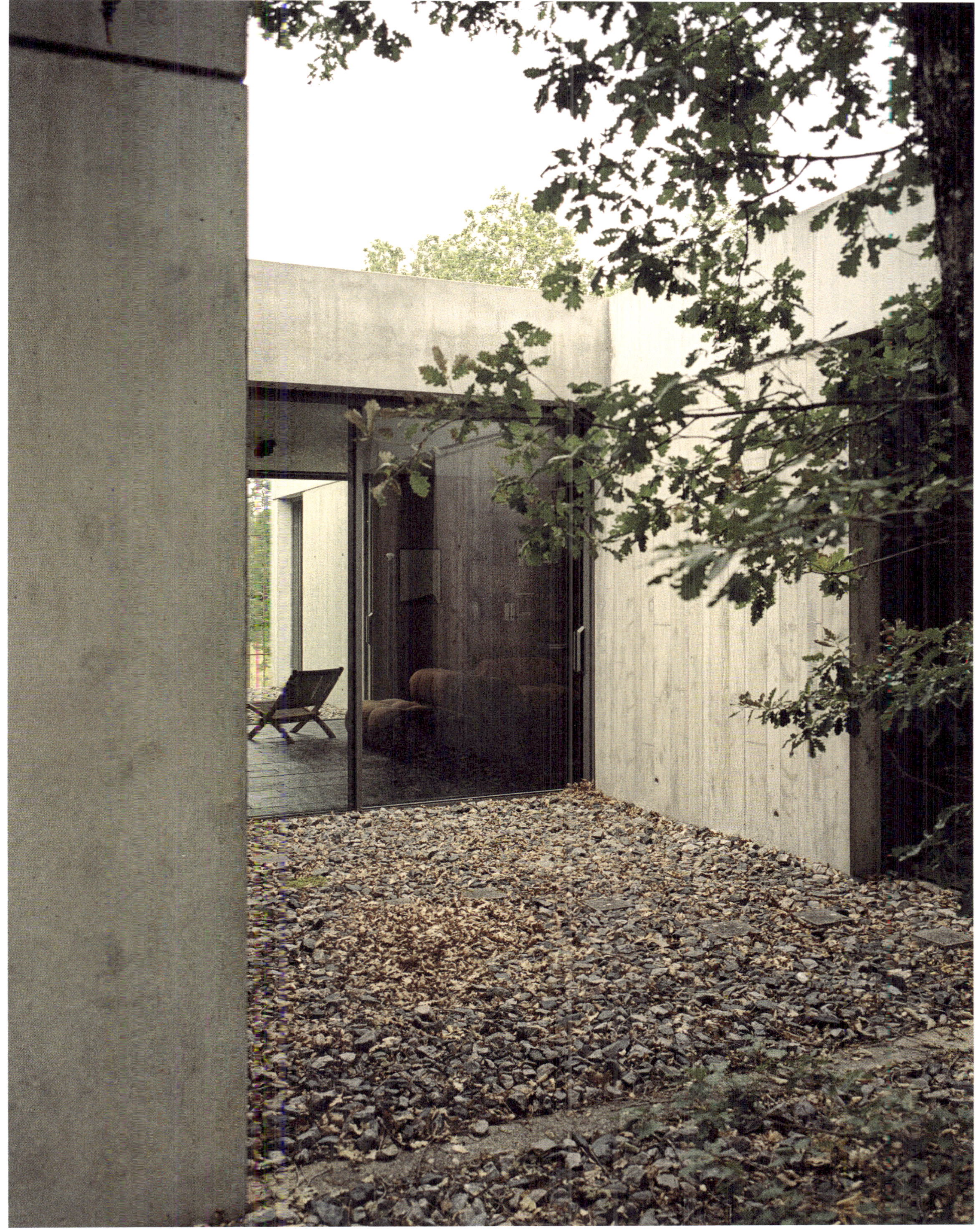

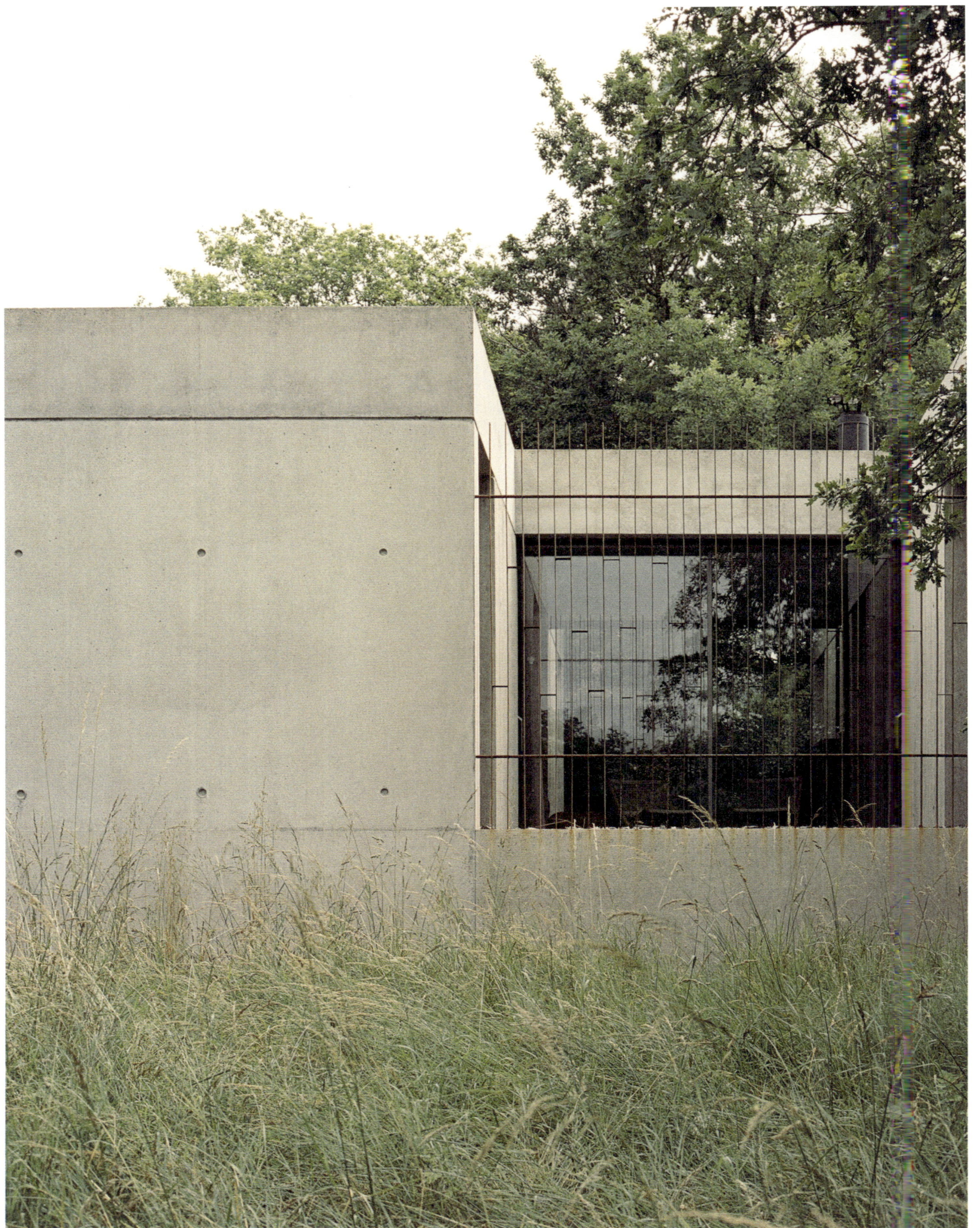

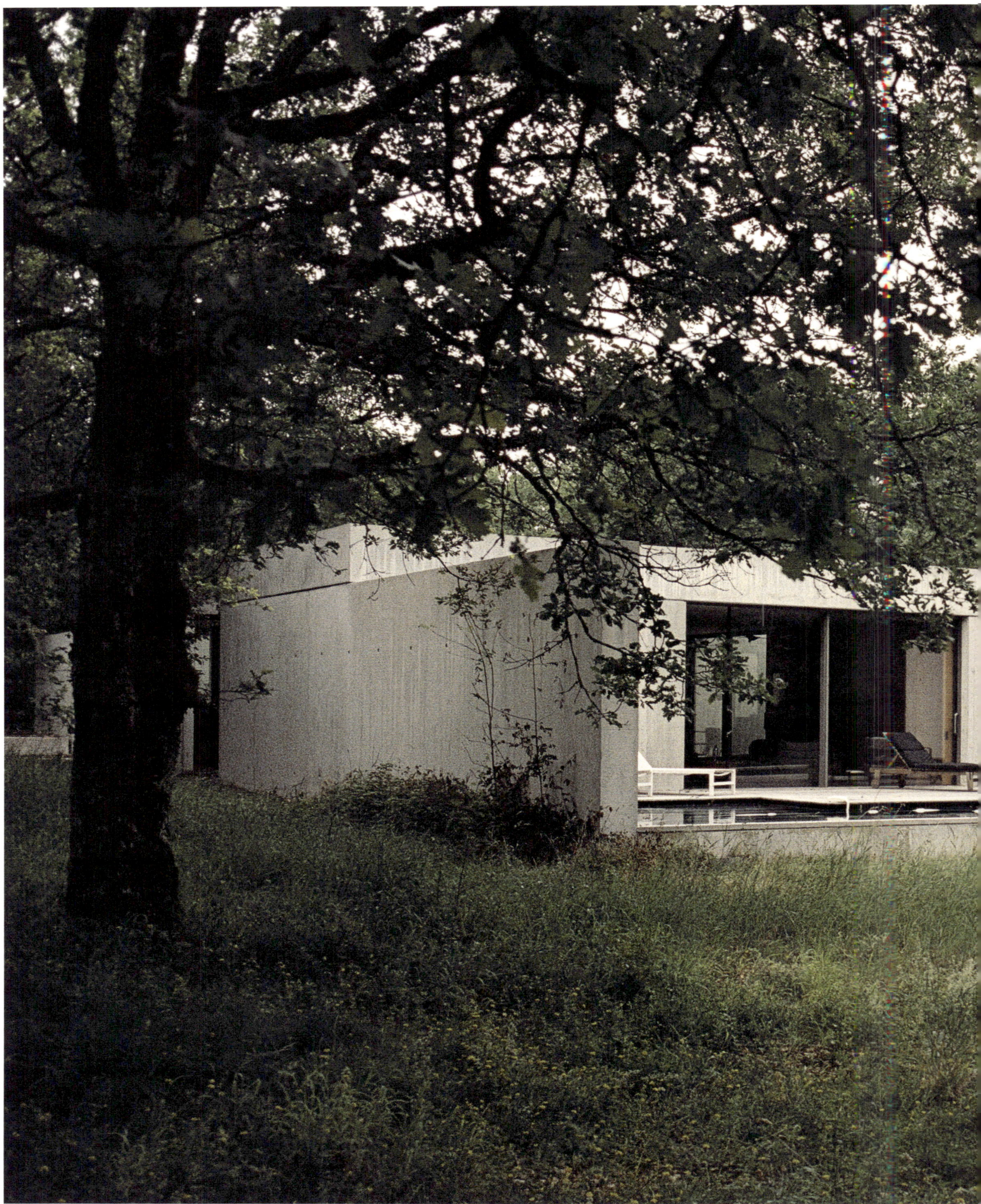

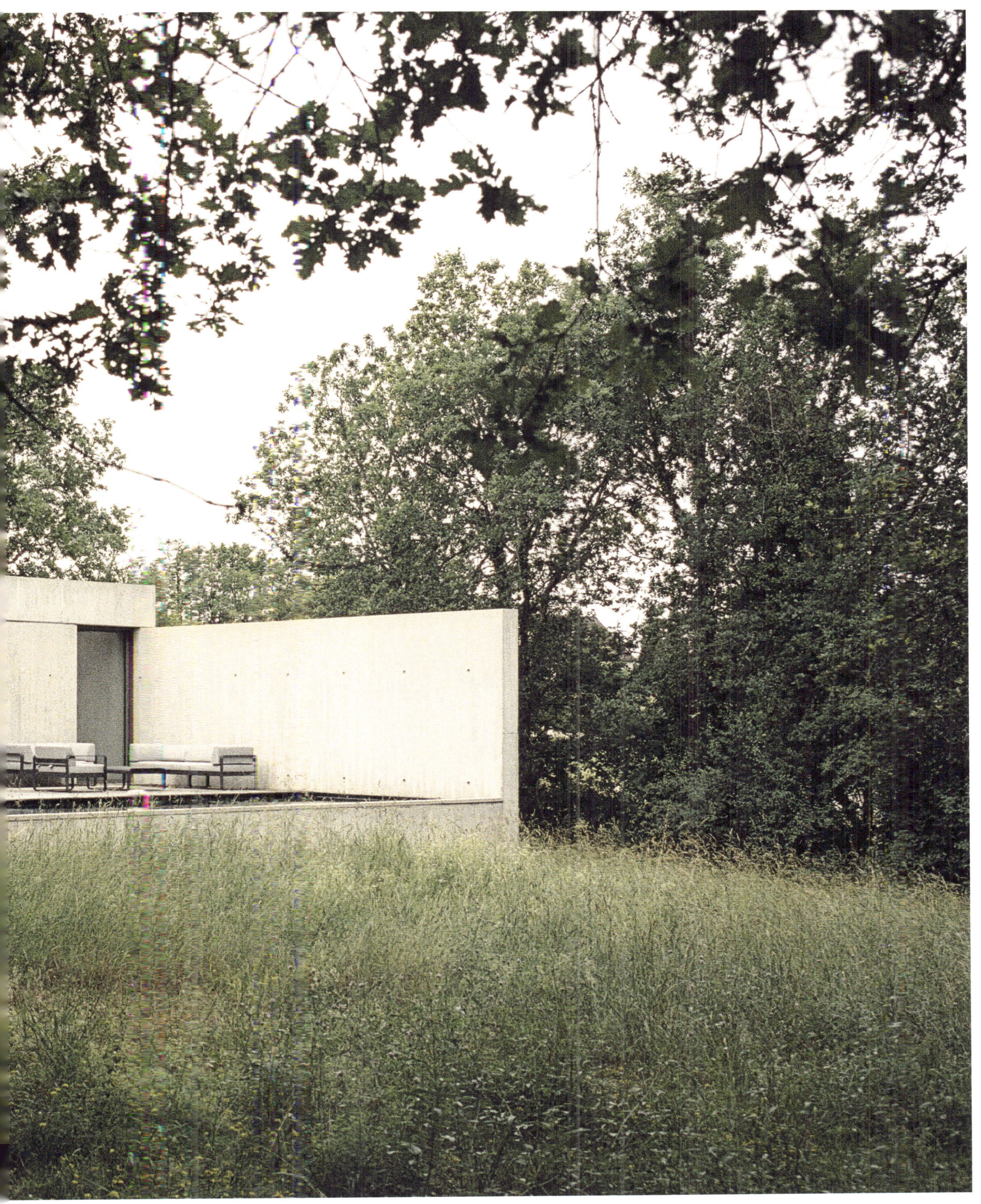

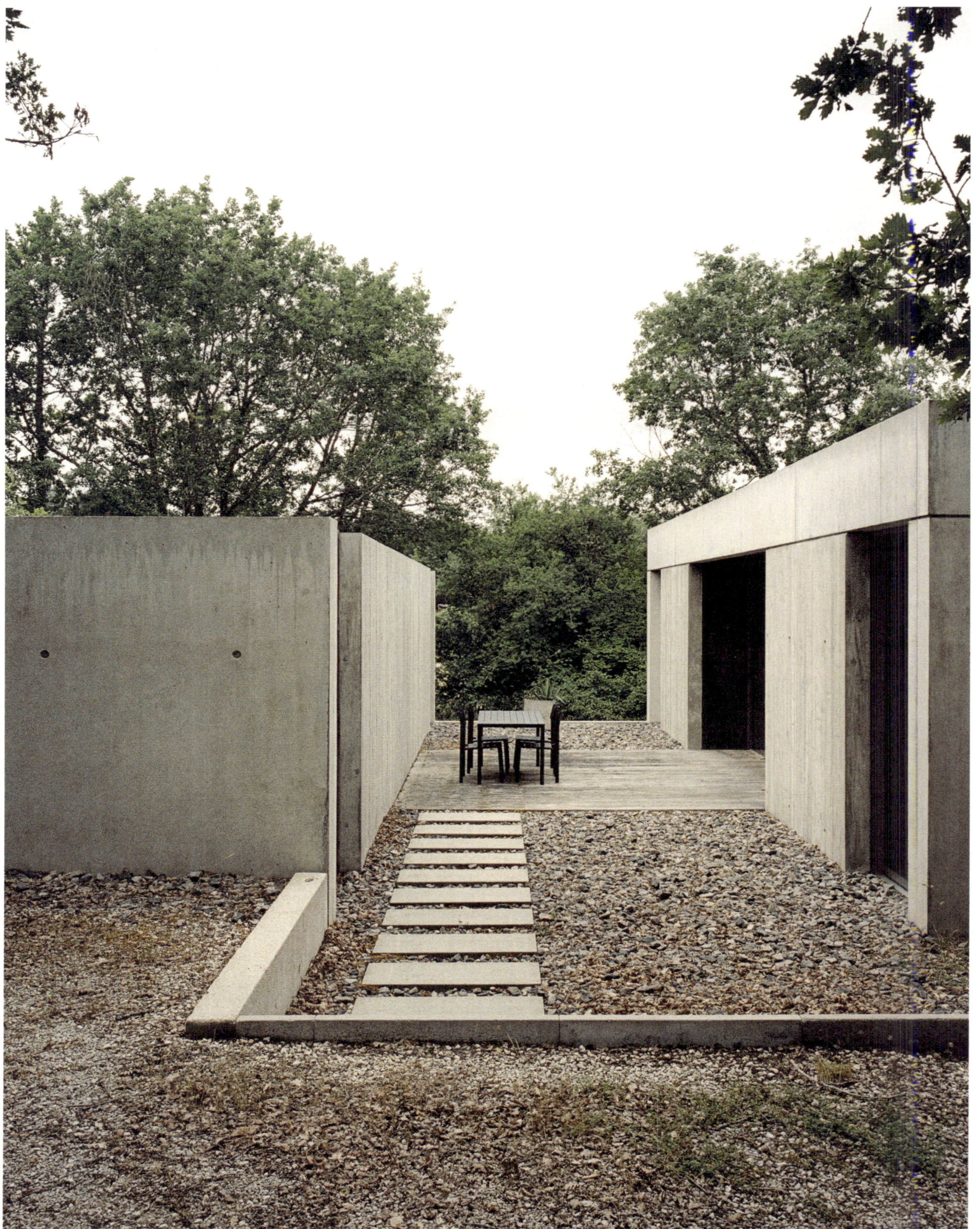

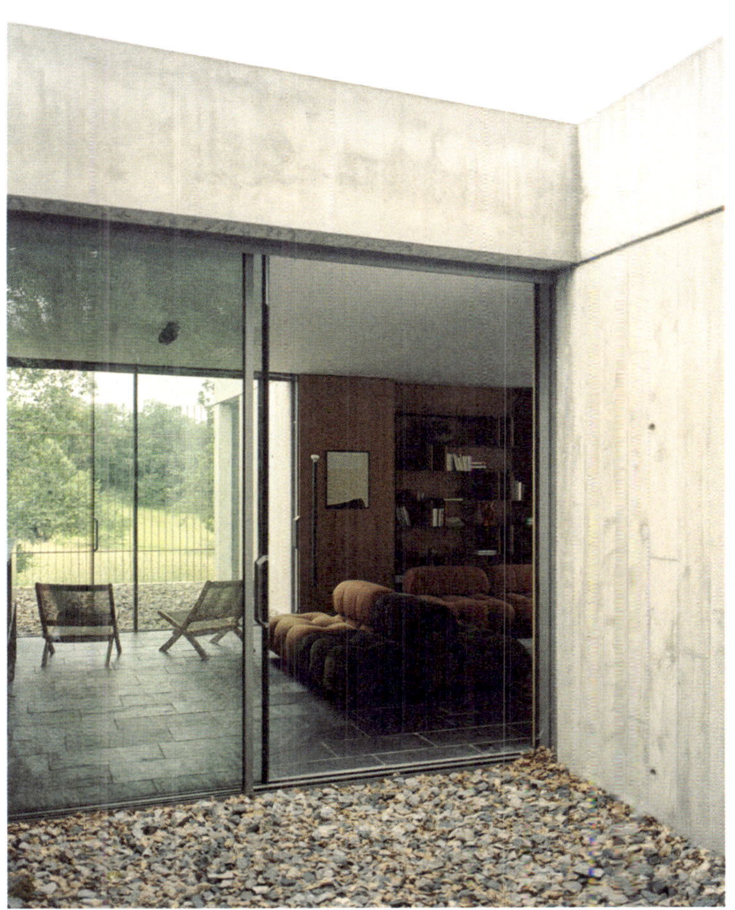

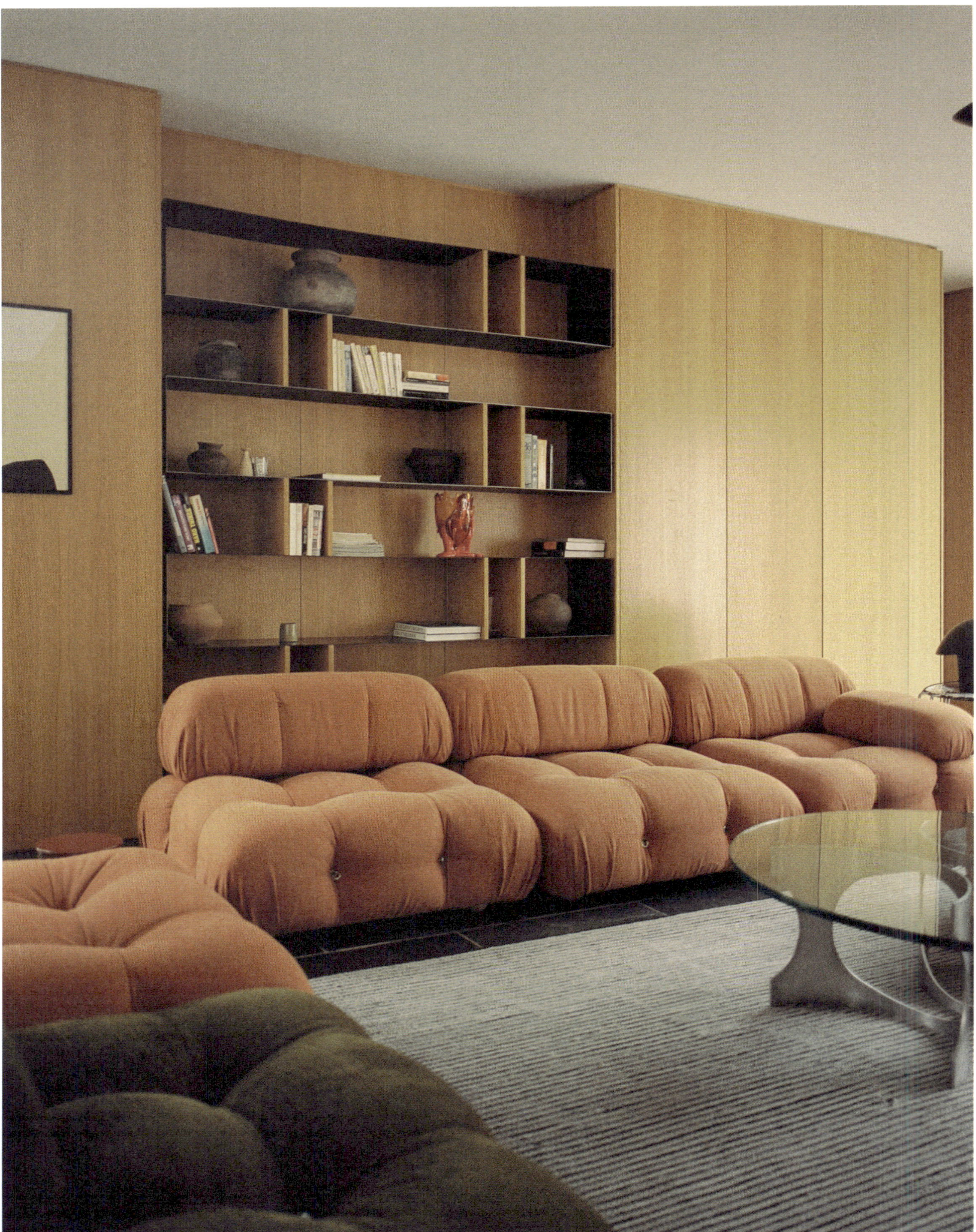

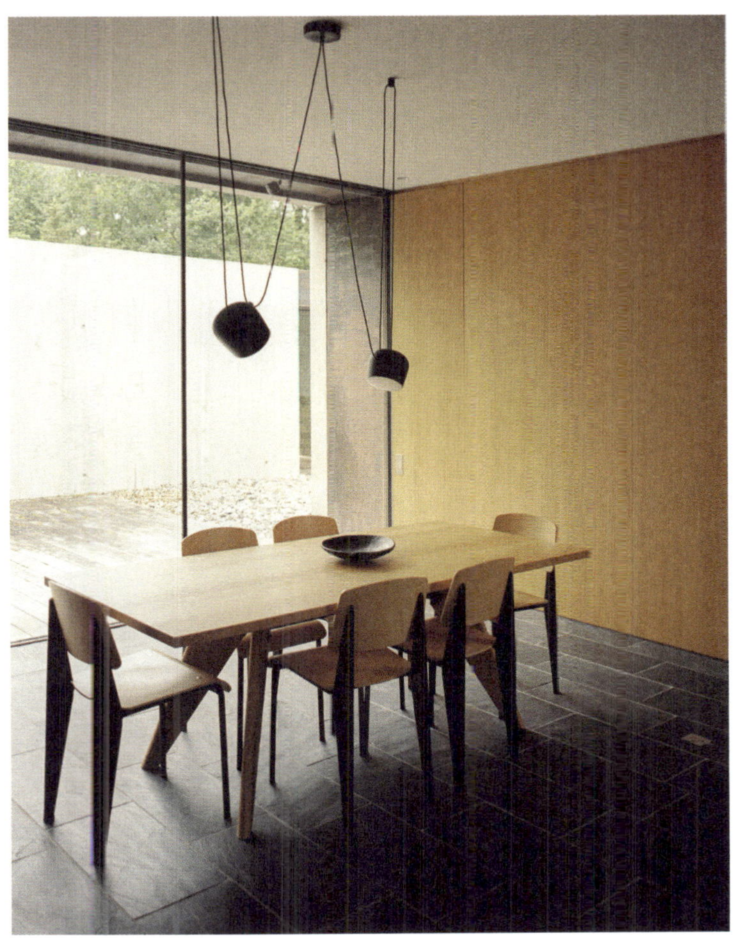

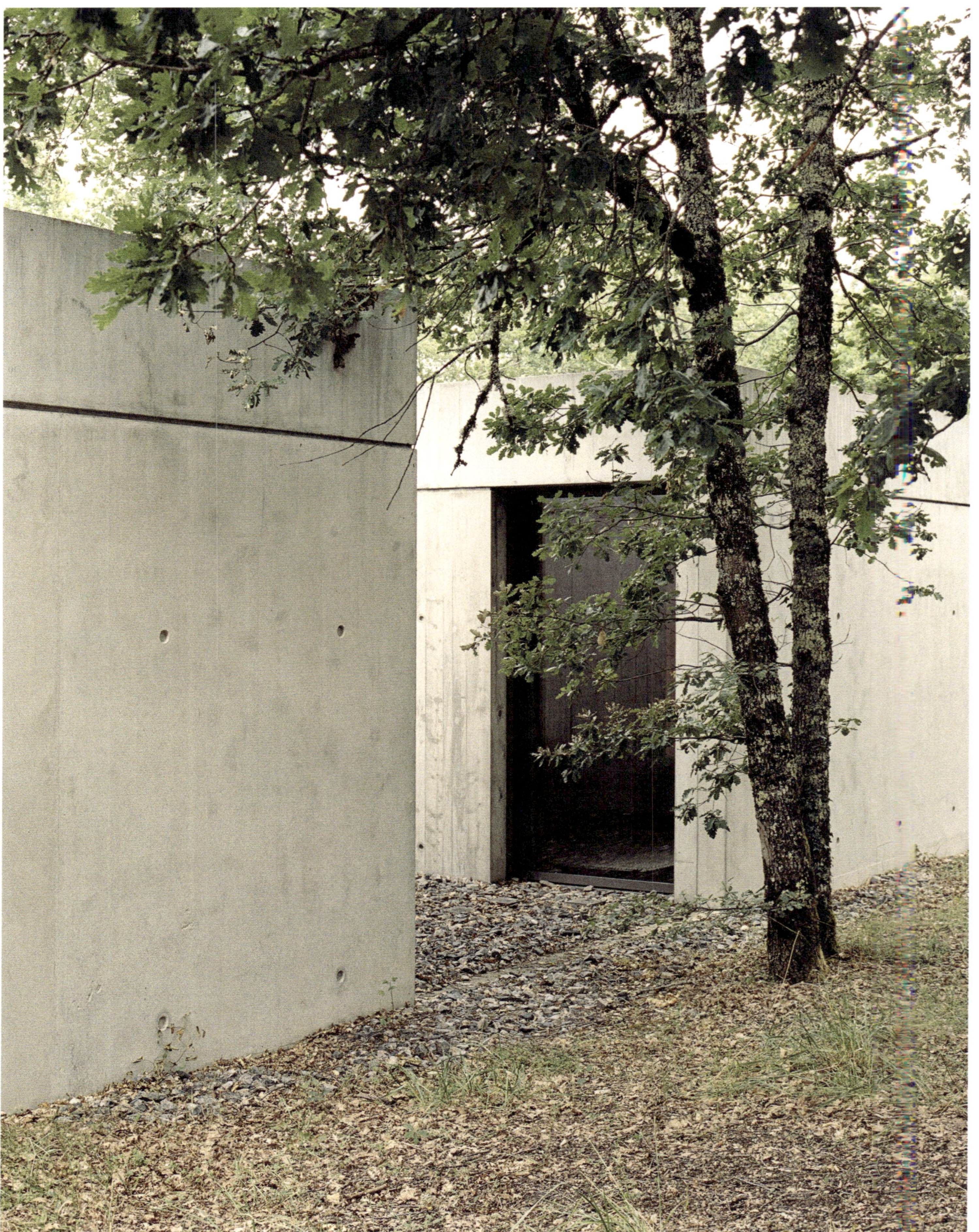

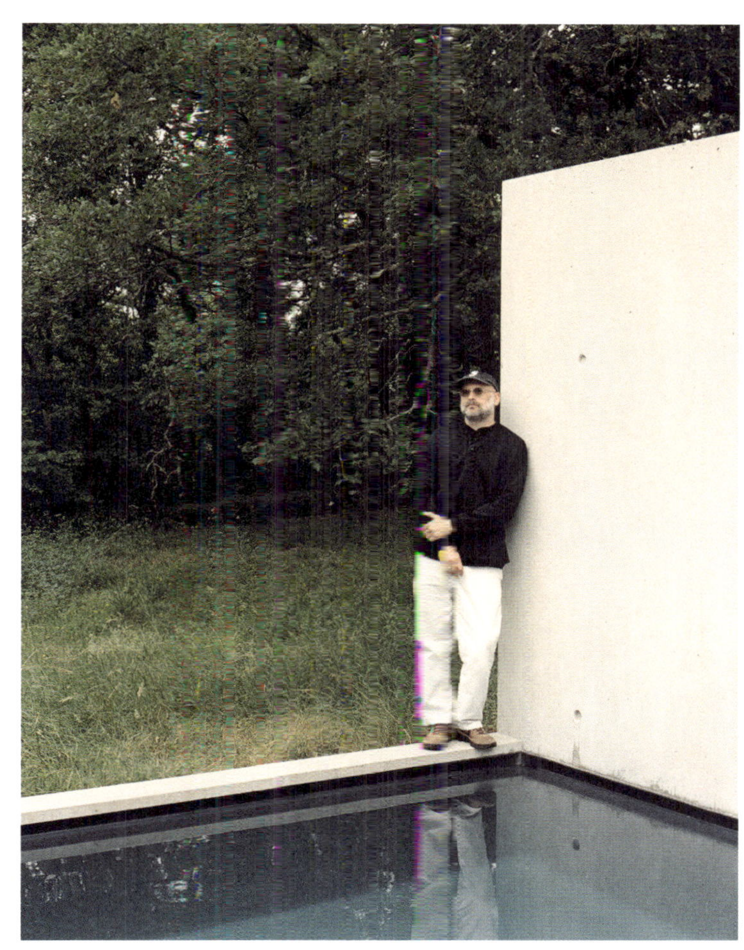

"To me, concrete is the perfect shell, as its raw aspect balances perfectly with nature and frames its surroundings. I love the idea that the material used to build the house isn't hidden behind some other decorative element."

– Matthieu Tessier

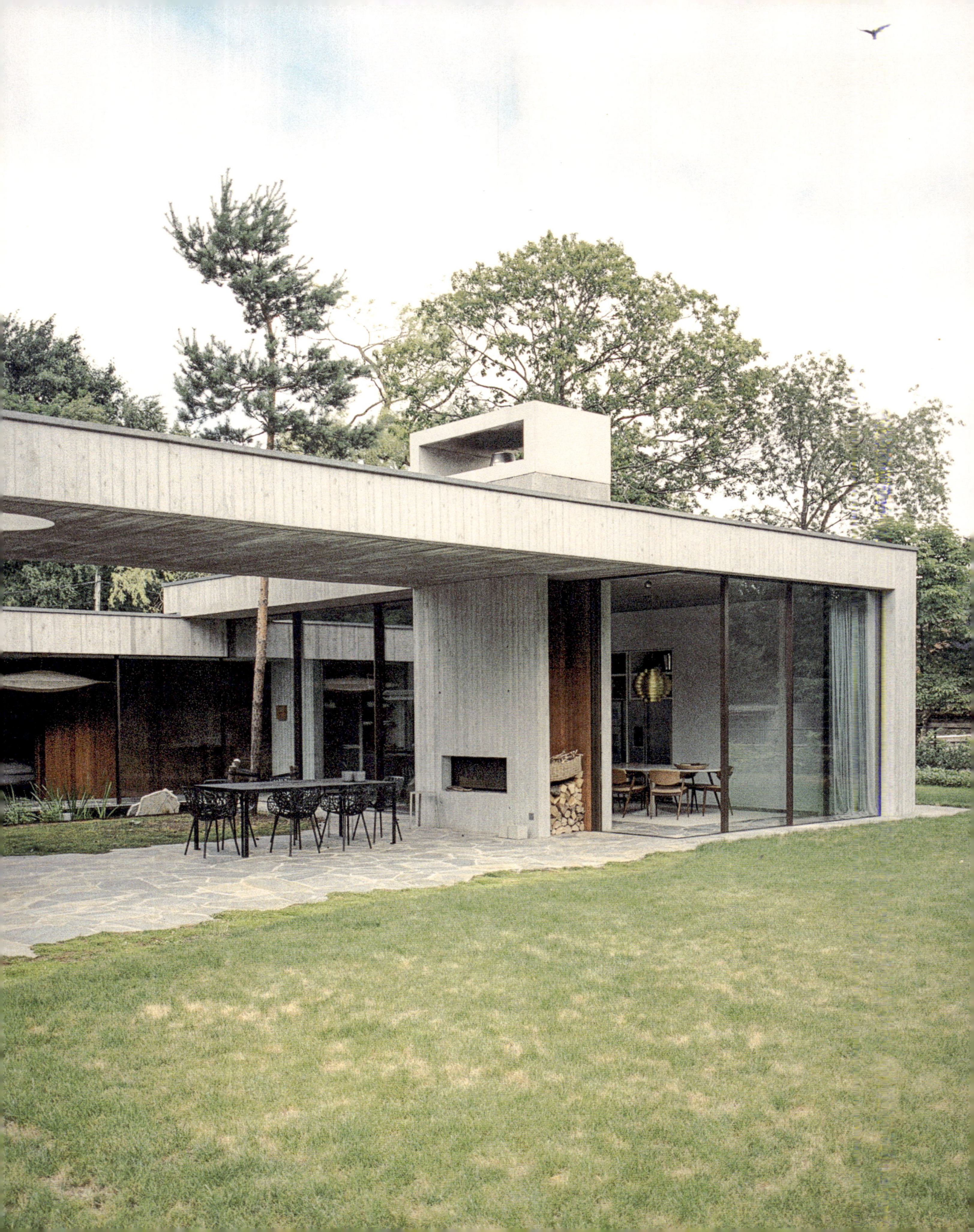

Set just outside a Flemish town, this home sits quietly among tall trees and shaped terrain. It is low, horizontal, and understated. A row of pine trees offers some privacy, though the house never feels closed off. On first approach, it feels grounded, as if it belongs to the land rather than being placed on top of it.

The couple who live here were closely involved in its design. They had collaborated with the same architect before, including on a renovation project in a nearby village. Their brief was straightforward: a house that felt open yet private, spacious but not showy. A place to cook, host, and be outside. The building had to support daily living, without fuss or excess.

The plot once held a modernist home, locally known for its expressive lines and sculptural details. But its internal layout proved difficult to rework. Instead of imitating its style, the architect proposed something new. A design that emphasised clarity, material honesty, and long-term ease of use. The result is contemporary but restrained, formal yet welcoming.

The house is composed of three areas: one accommodates the bedrooms and bathrooms, the second forms the heart of the kitchen and pantry areas, and the third is dedicated to the living room, generous in proportion with long views across the garden. These volumes are positioned around a central outdoor space. They connect via wide openings and sheltered transitions, creating a rhythm of movement through the house and into the landscape.

Though large, the house never feels excessive, and everything is scaled to human usage. Sliding glass doors allow for openness when desired, but the structure also offers protection and stillness. The central patio provides shade and softness, and the house follows the sun across the day without chasing it.

Every element in the house feels intentional. Materials were chosen to age well. And surfaces are left exposed, not as a statement, but to allow for time to leave its mark. The concrete is smooth, but not polished, and timber is left untreated where possible.

The surrounding garden is evolving slowly, shaped by the seasons and the owners' preferences. In one corner of the site, they grow their own vegetables, and nearby, animals are kept behind a simple enclosure, framed in corten steel like the carport and other structures. Nothing feels ornamental. Even the smallest decisions reflect a way of living that is deliberate, grounded, and slow.

The architects behind the project have long worked with concrete. In this case, it is not used to impress, but to anchor. It gives the house a kind of permanence, not heavy but assured. The beauty of the design lies in its balance: the way spaces relate to one another, the softness of one material against another, and the quiet confidence of a home that doesn't need to explain itself.

This is a house made for long days and slow use. You notice the warmth of the timber, the filtered light through the canopy, the rhythm of ordinary routines. It does not ask for attention, but it rewards it.

Project: Project STU
Location: Belgium
Architect: ANTE Architecten
Year of construction: 2023
Floor area: 230 m^2

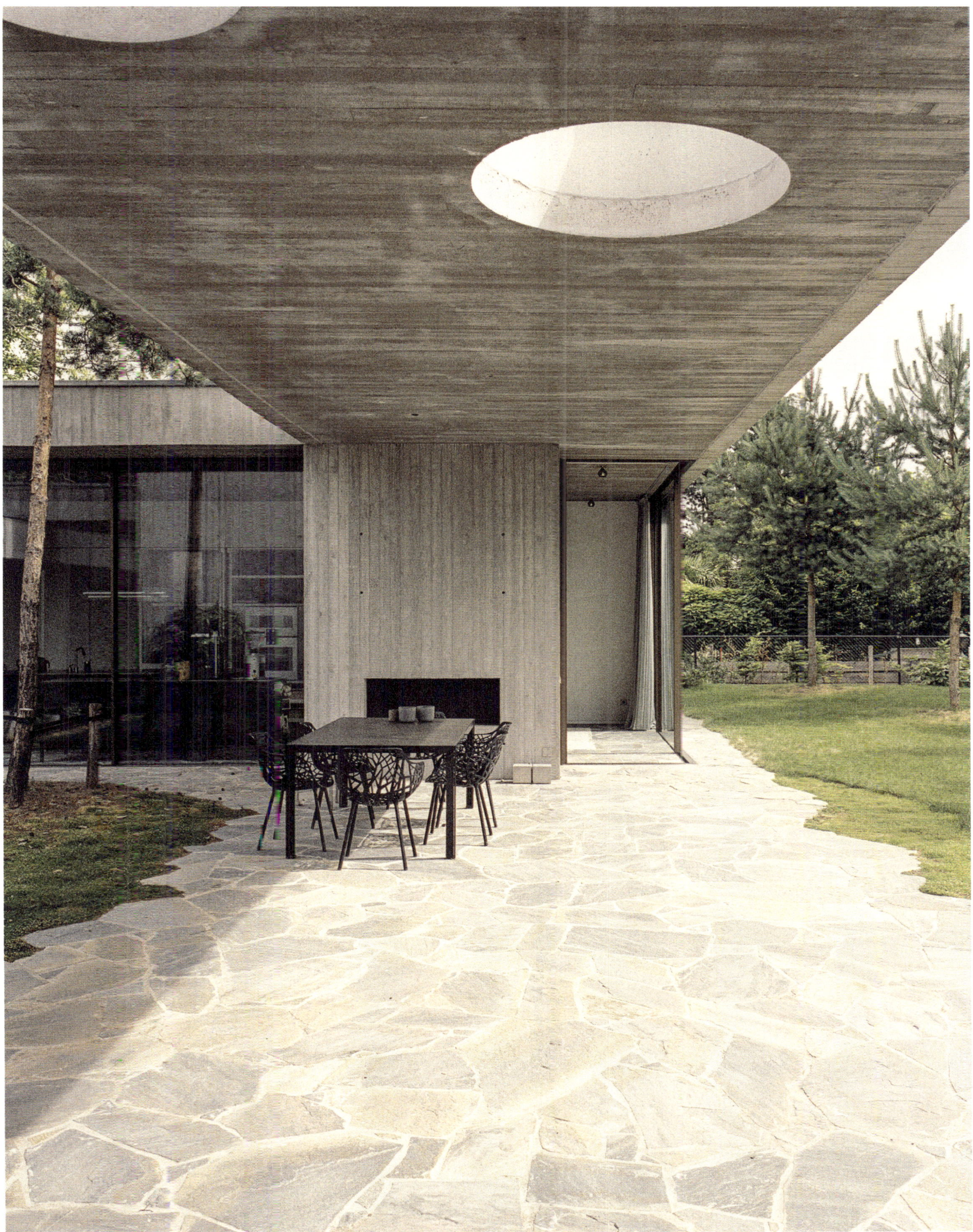

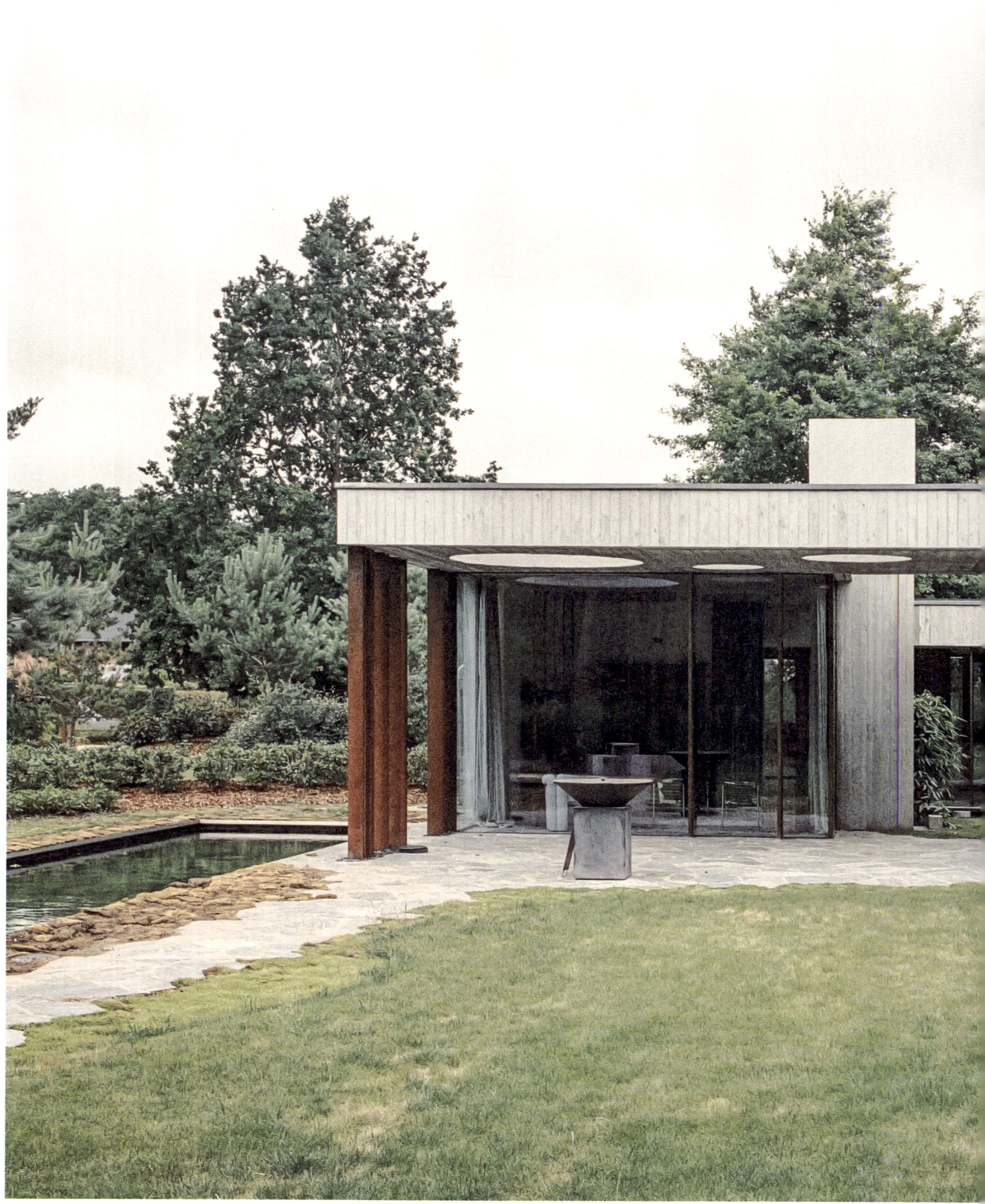

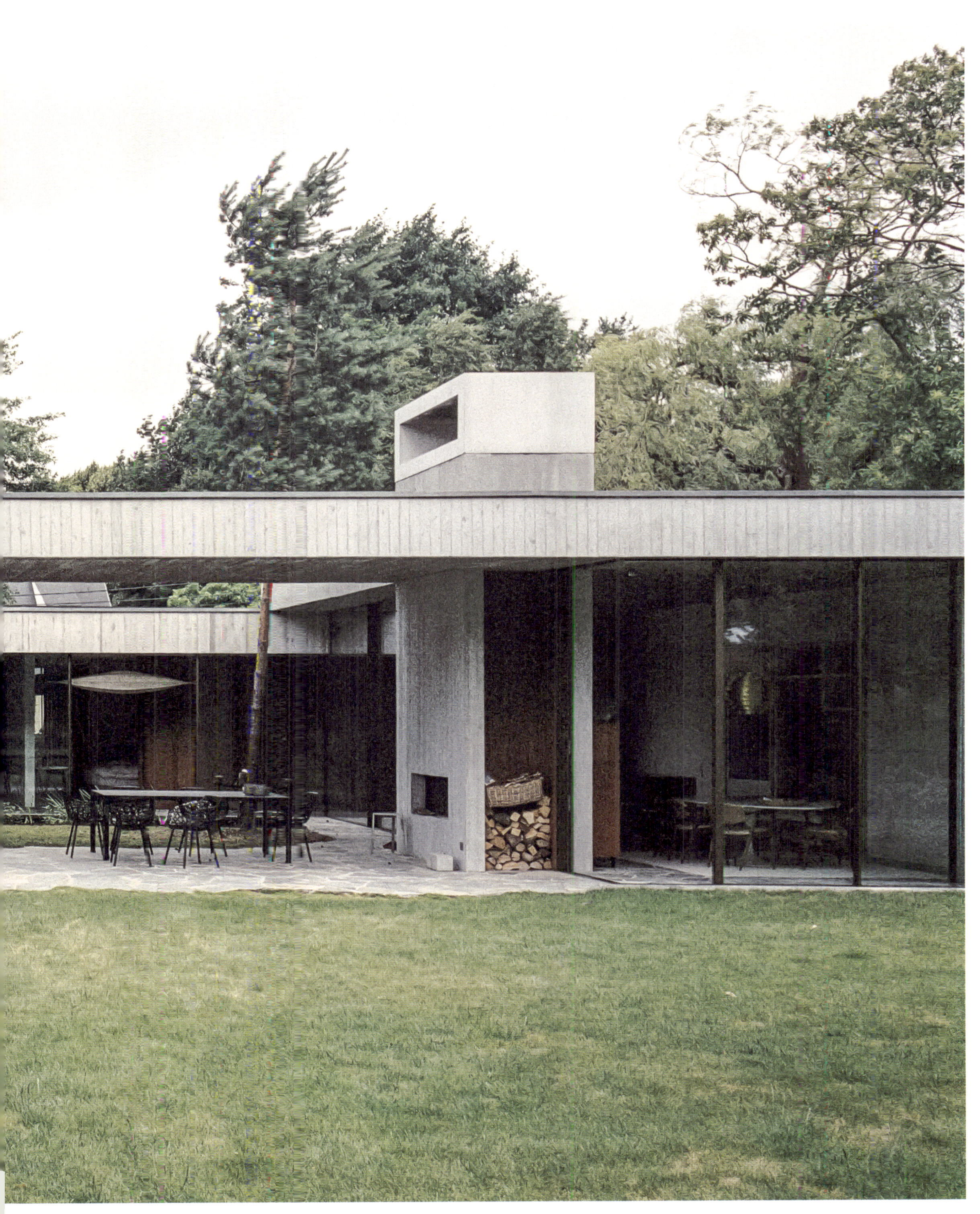

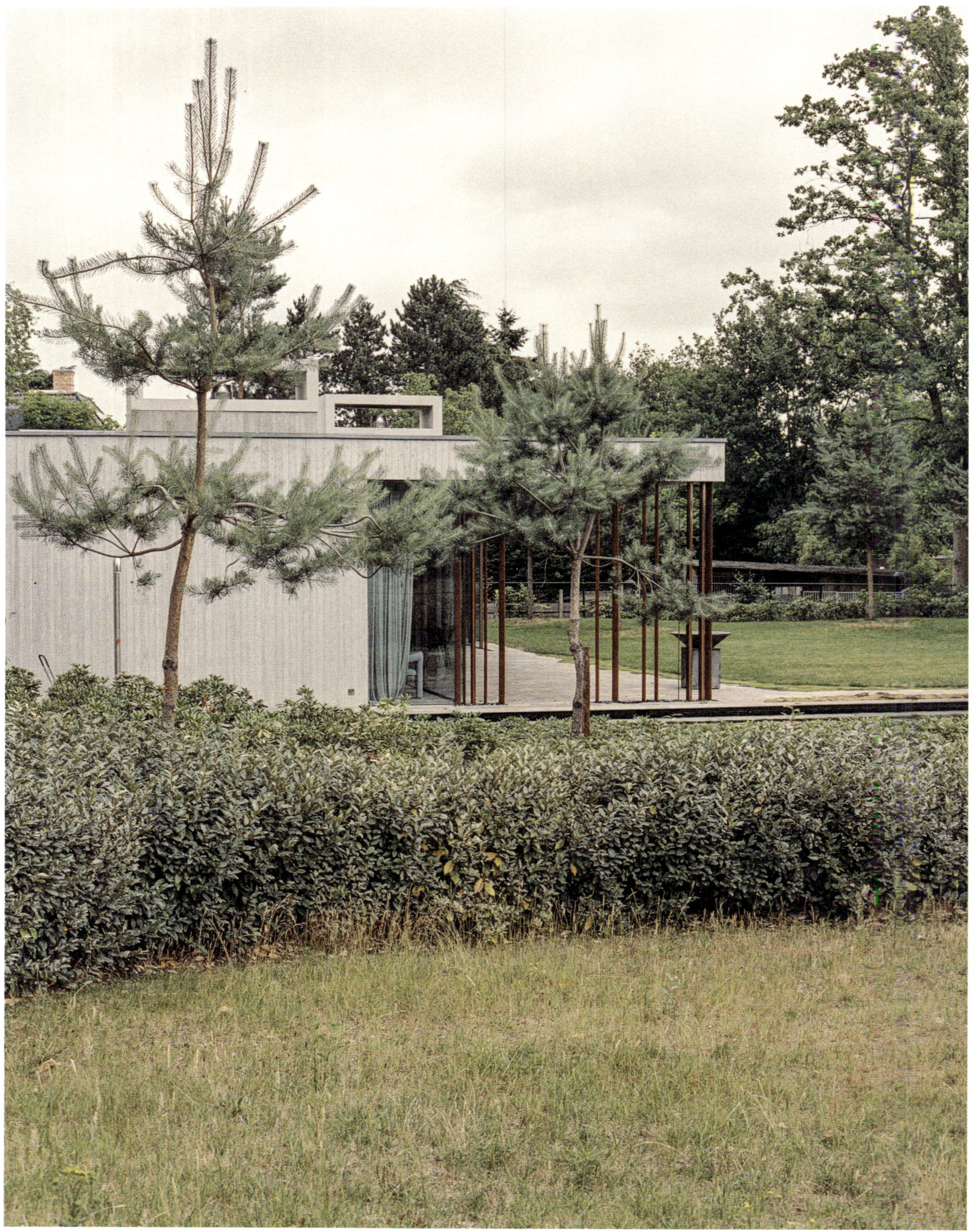

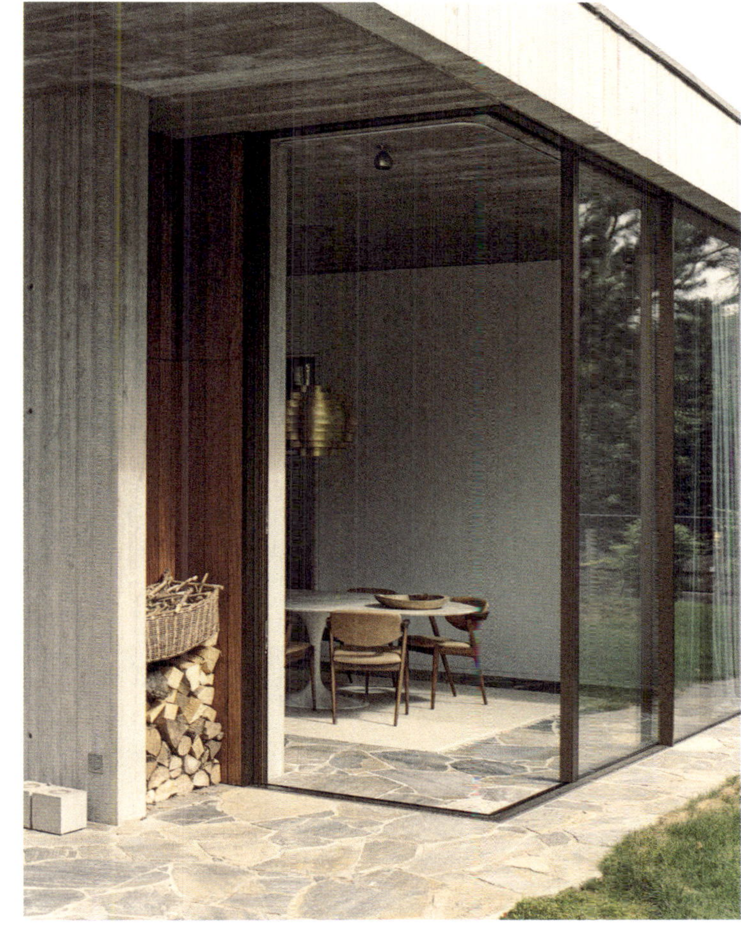

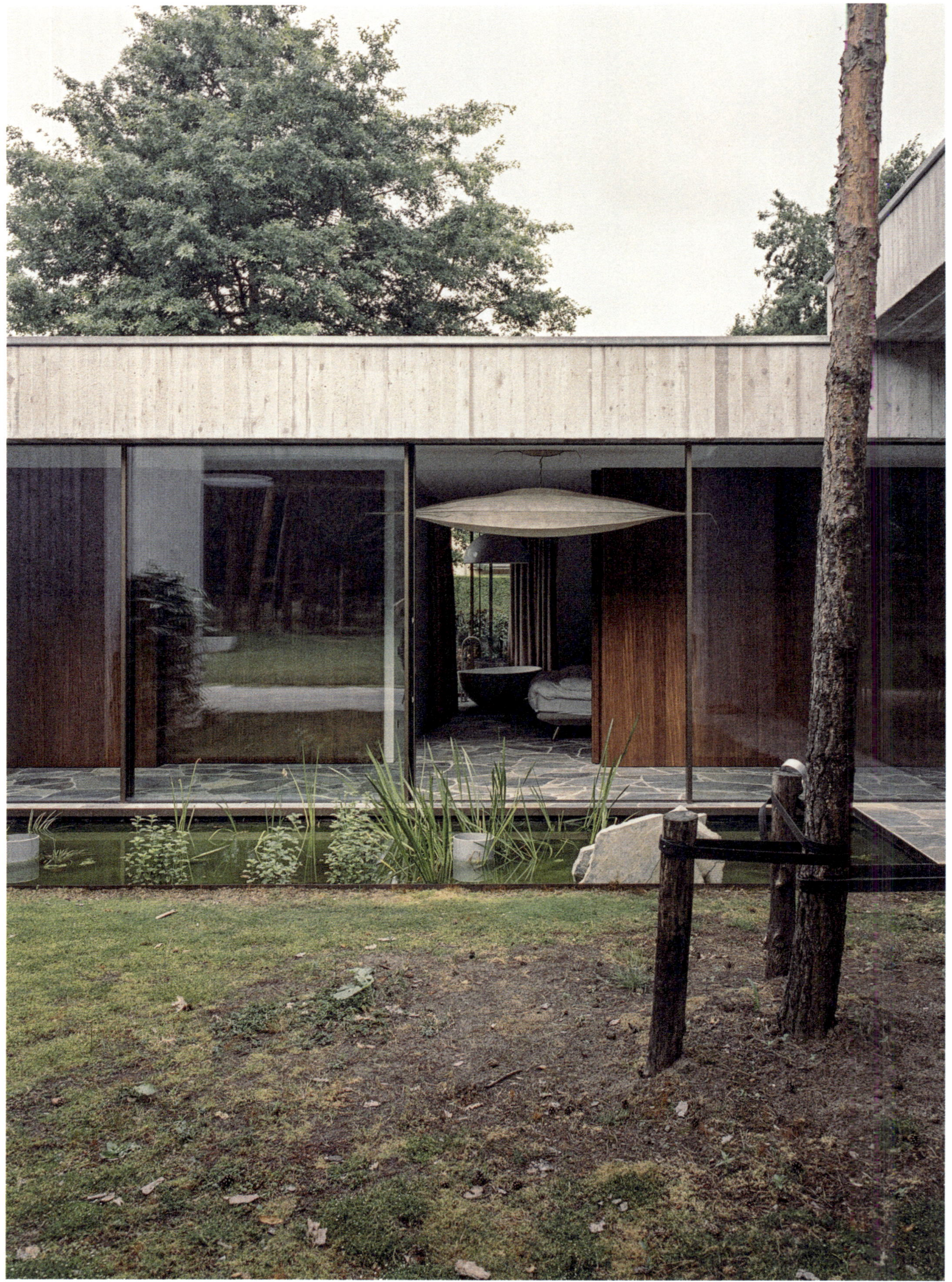

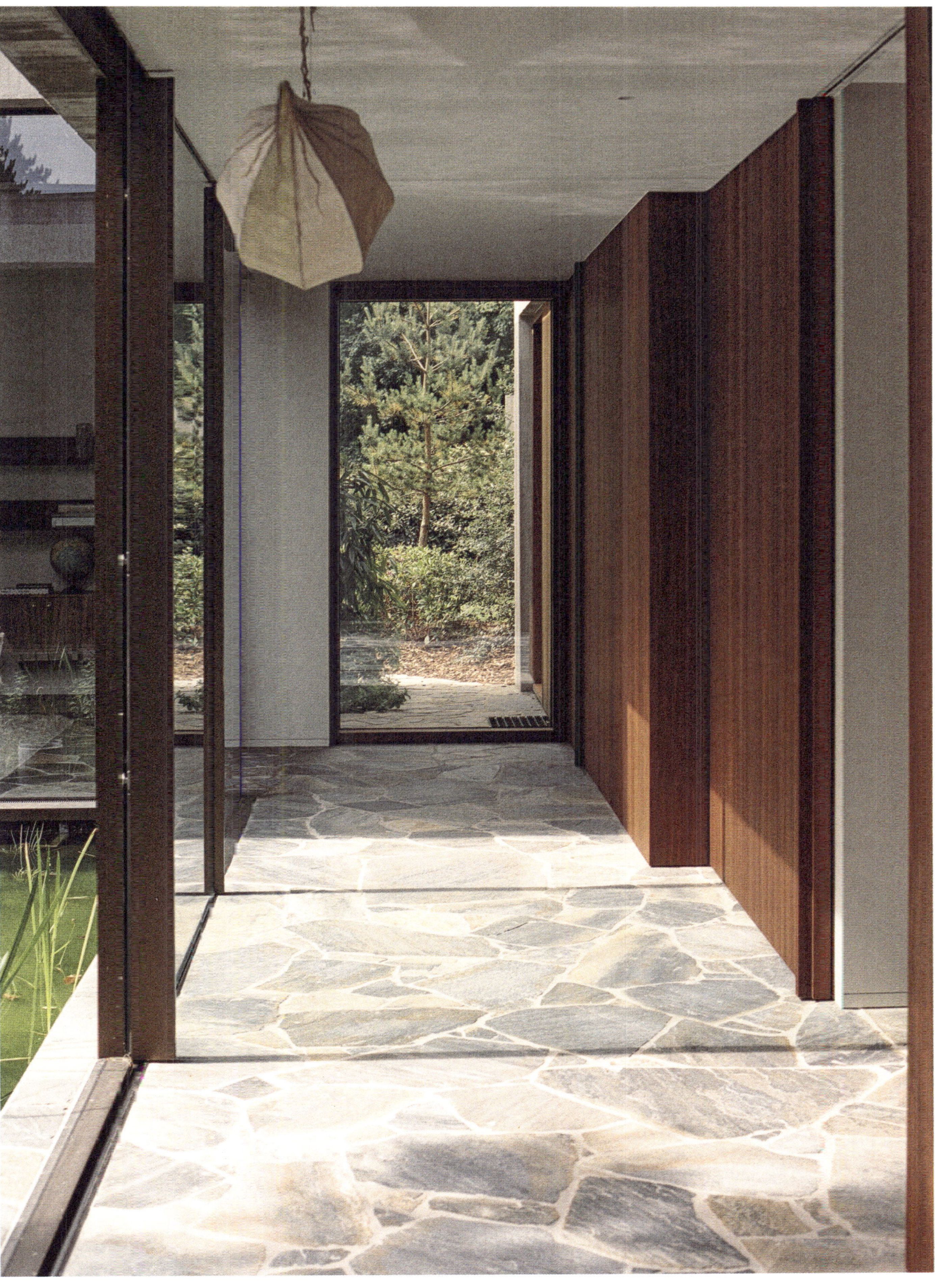

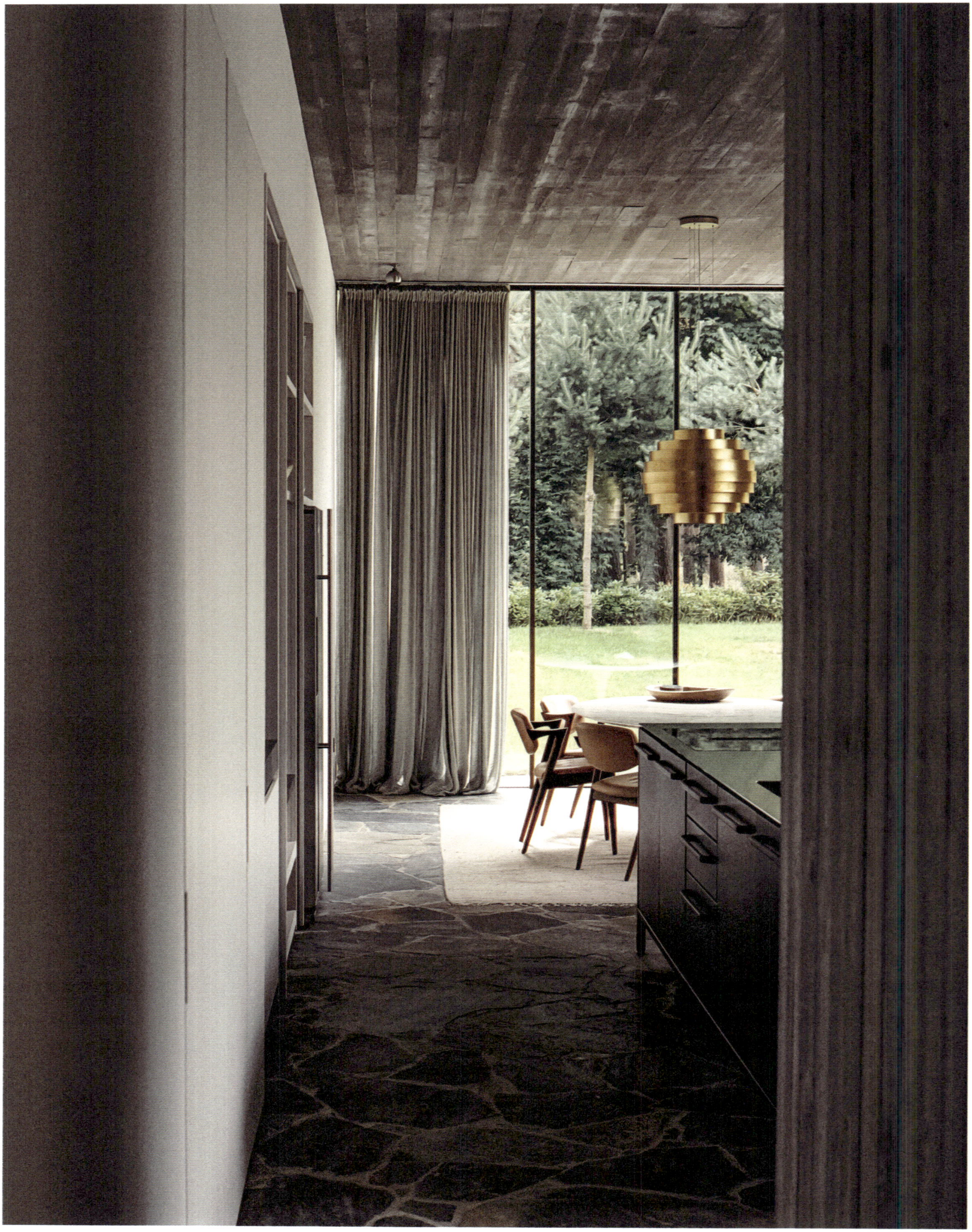

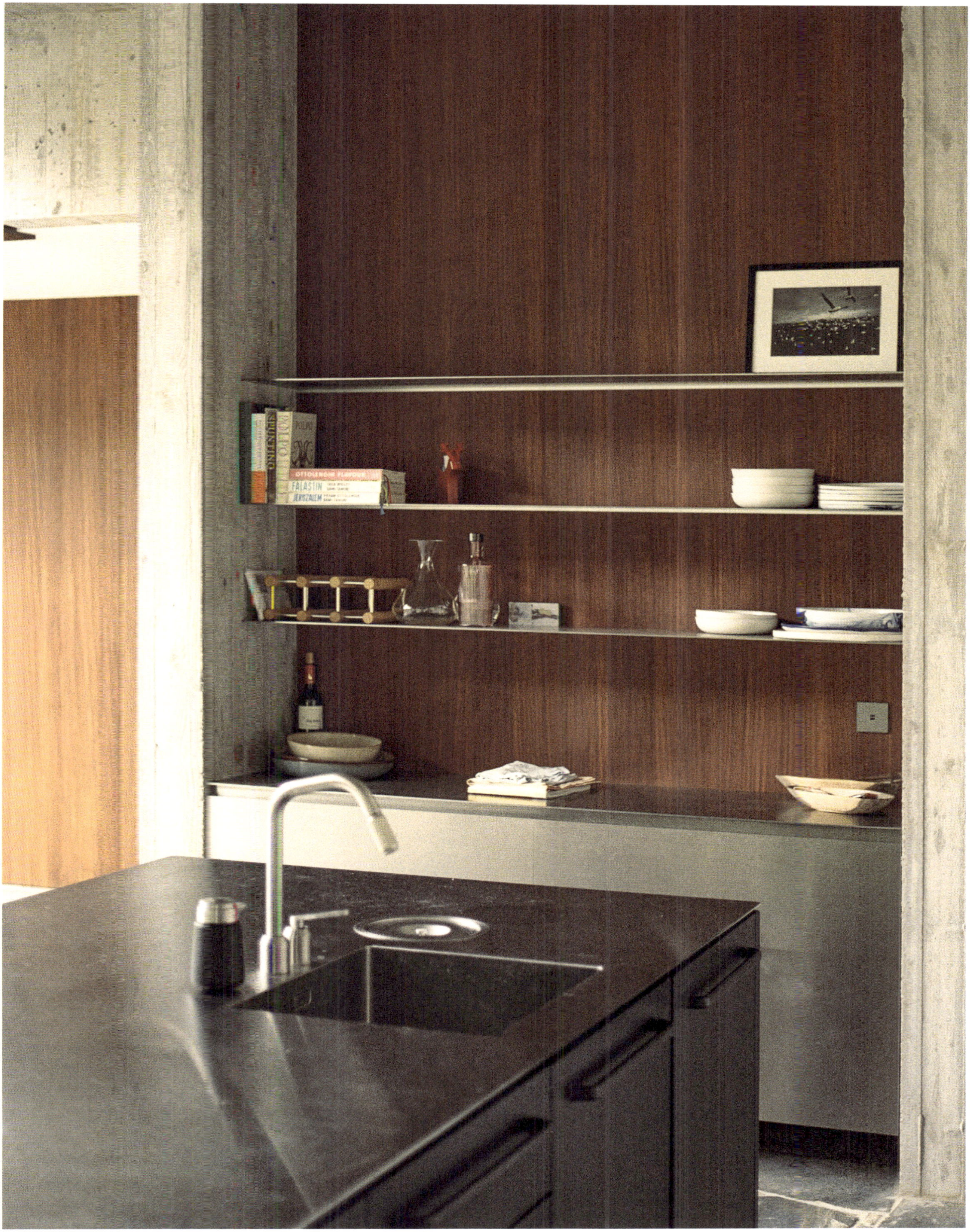

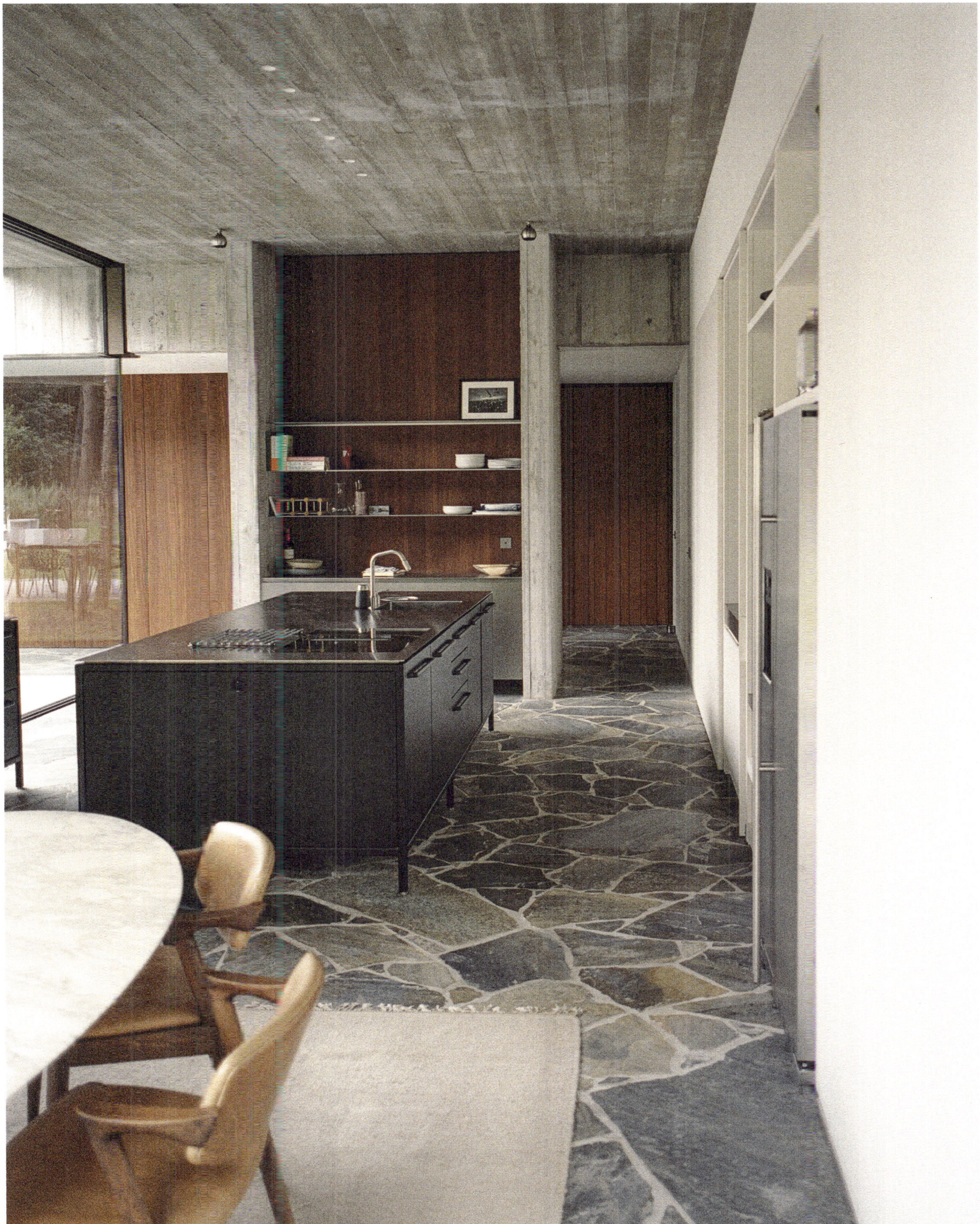

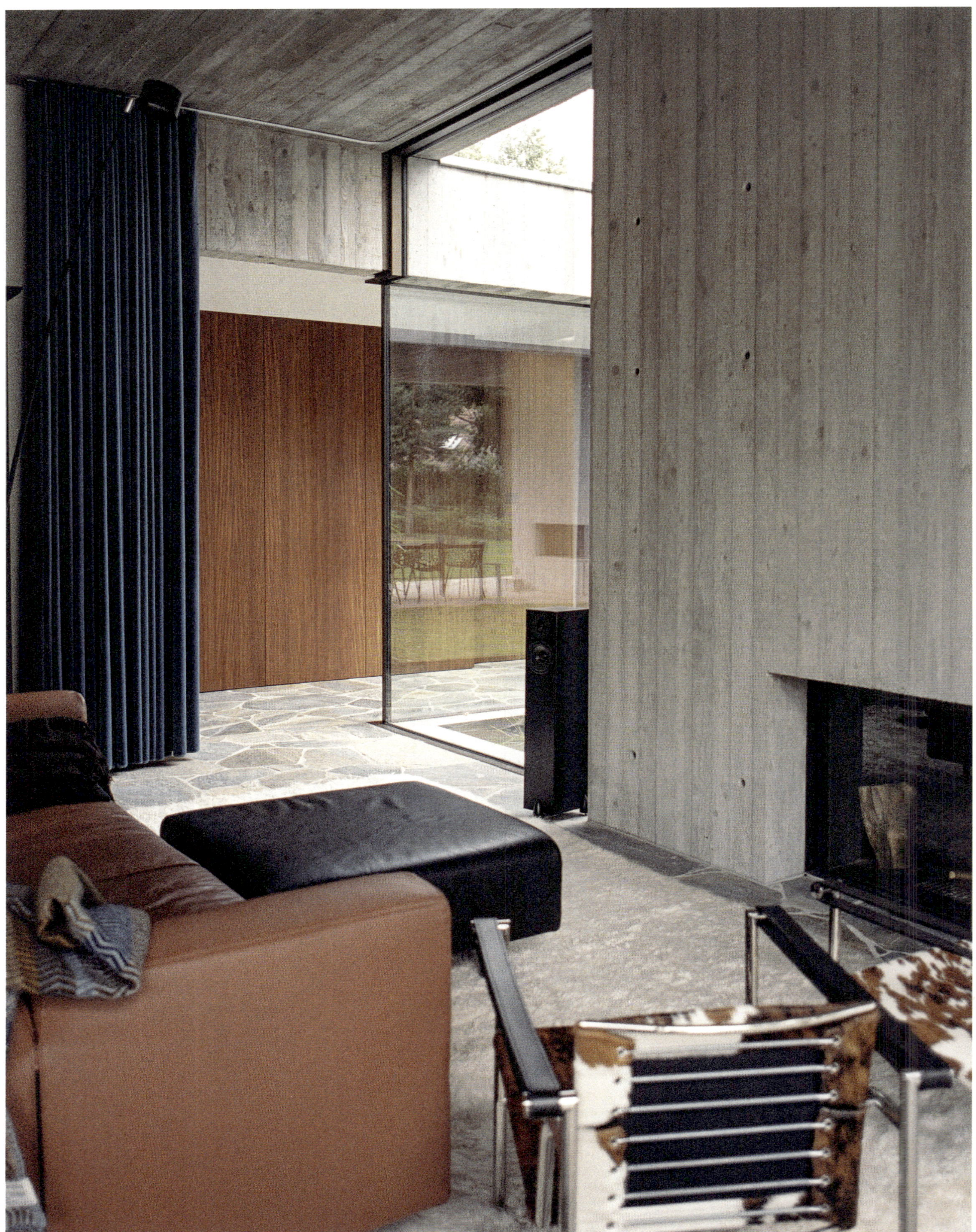

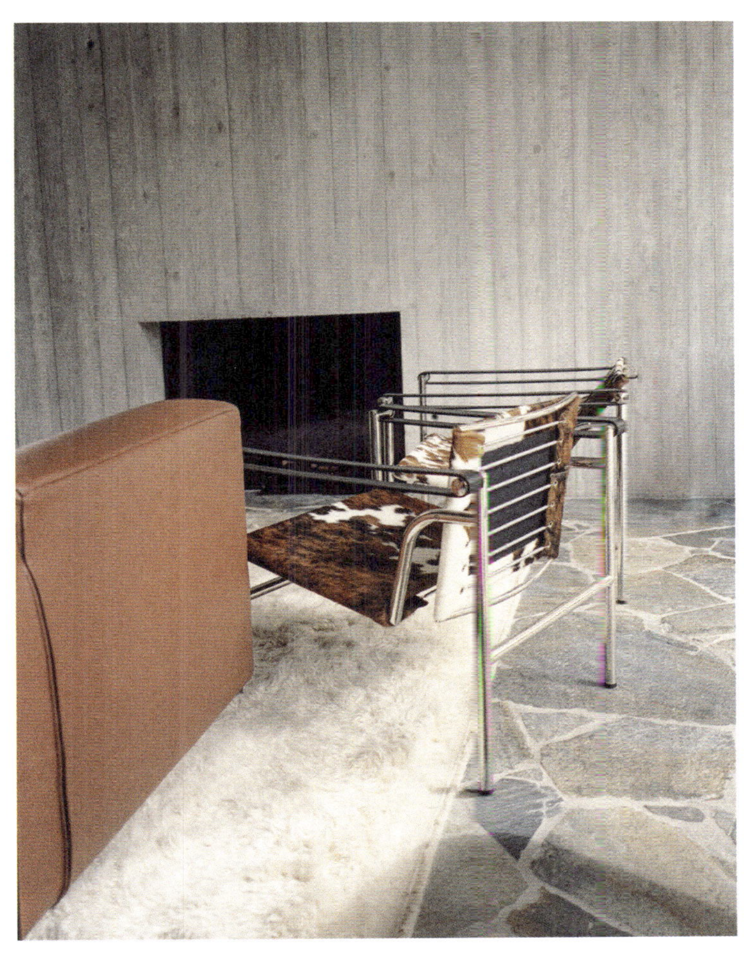

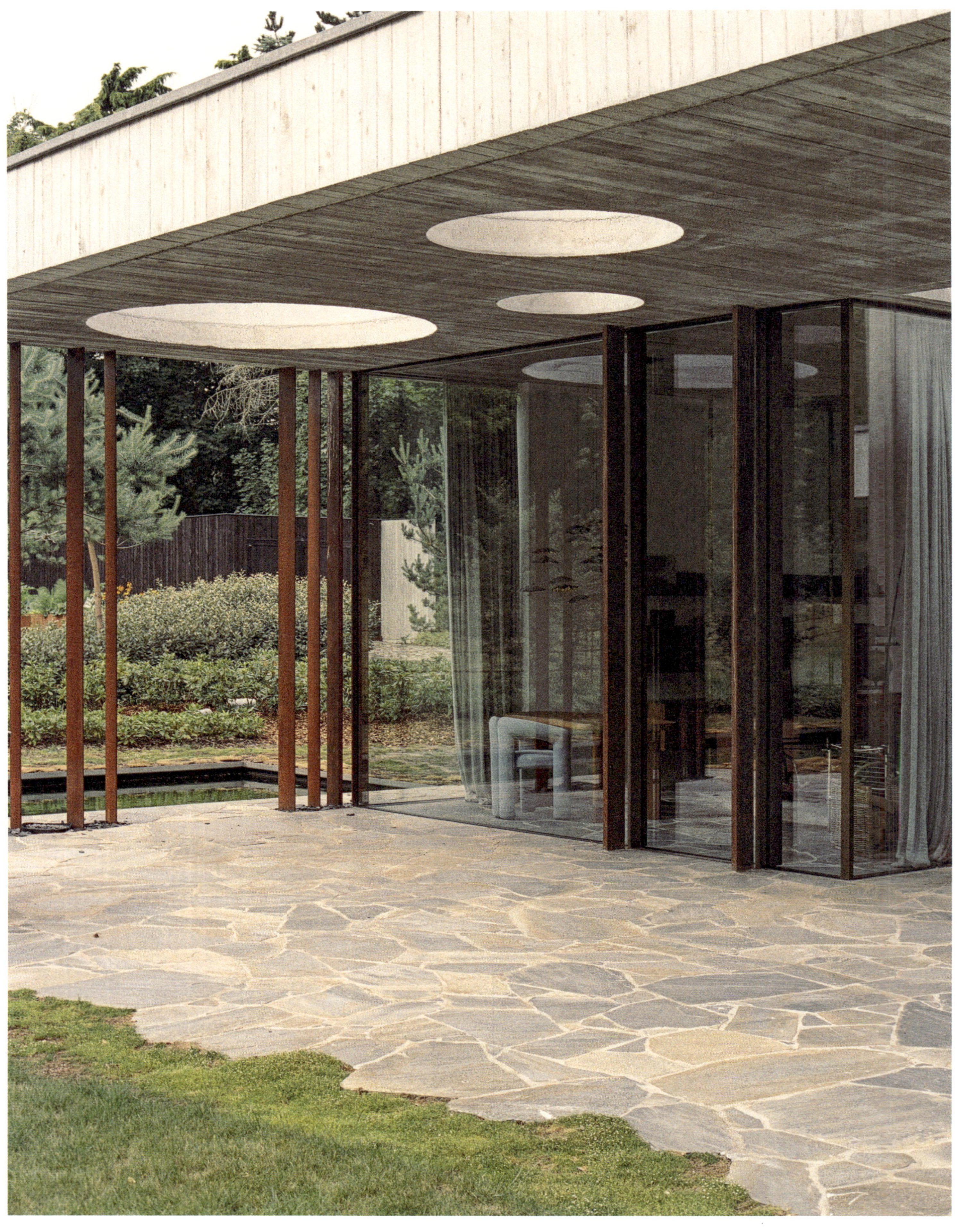

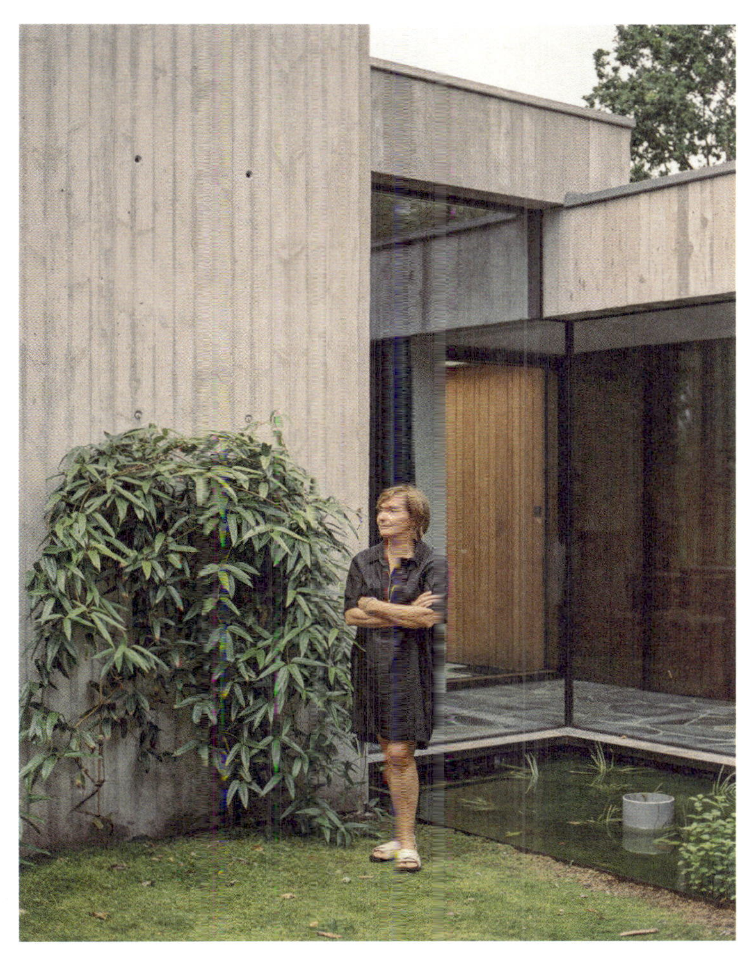

"This concrete home embodies craftsmanship and strength – distinctive yet understated, grey yet never dull – a house that truly stands"

– architect Anne-Mie Noens

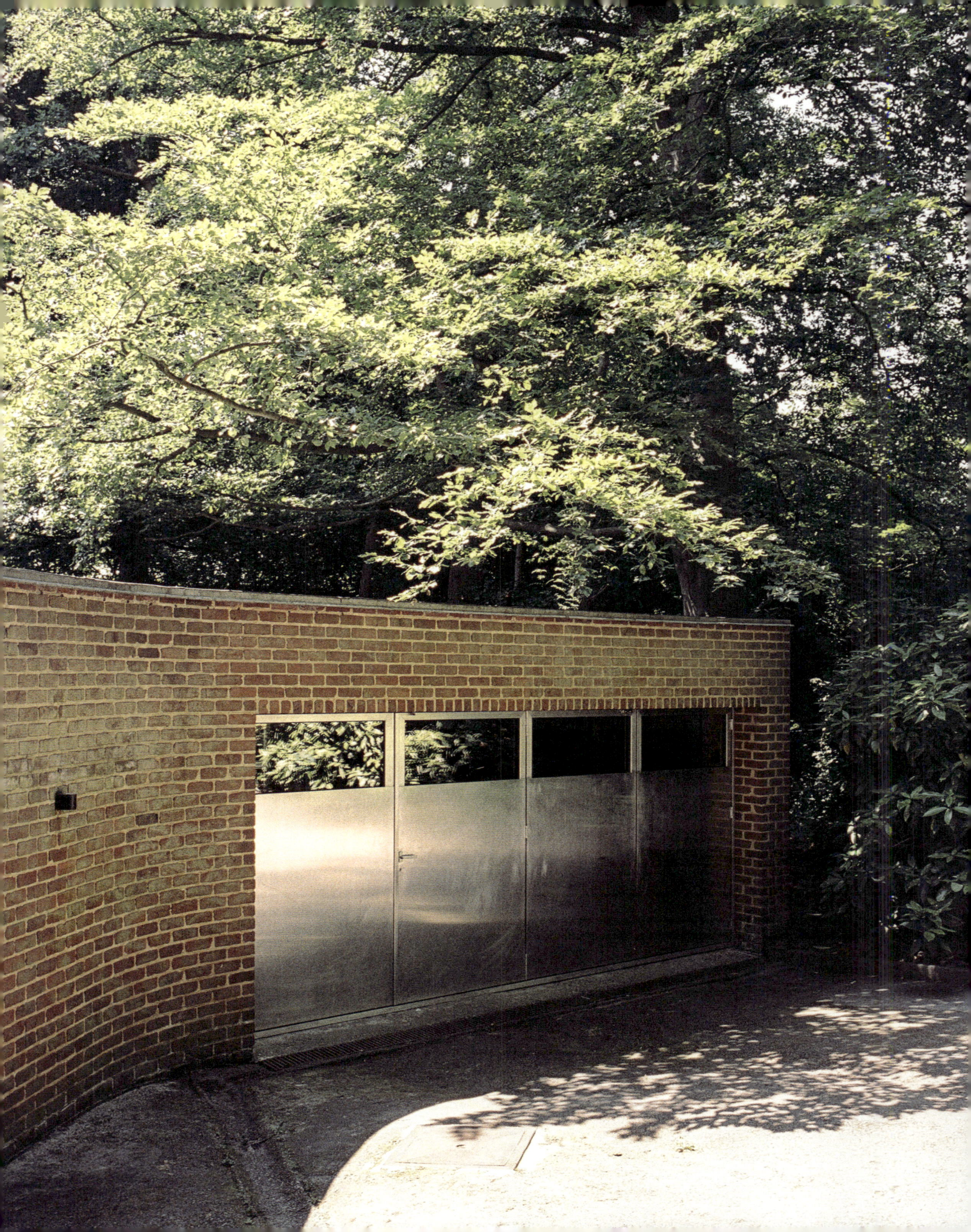

destroyers / builders
Belgium

The house stands on the edge of Brussels, just outside the city, but already surrounded by greenery. From the street, it's almost invisible: low, set back, and tucked behind trees. It looks like a simple 1960s bungalow. But once you step inside, it opens up into something else: a quiet experiment in material, use, and rhythm.

The couple who live here moved from the city in search of space, not just to live, but to work, and to make room for a slower way of doing both. She is a designer and he's a landscape architect. Their house is also their studio, their workshop, and sometimes their showroom. It's a home, but it shifts.

When they bought the house, it hadn't changed much since it was built. The materials were dated, and the layout conventional, but the structure was solid. During demolition, they discovered rough concrete ceilings hidden under plaster – cast in place against wooden formwork. Instead of re-covering them, they kept them exposed. It felt right: raw, honest, and close to the kind of work she does.

The renovation happened in phases. They started with what was essential, then adapted as they went. Rooms were opened up, materials were stripped back, and the interior became quieter, softer. A brick wall was coated in cement plaster to tone it down. Old doors and trims were removed. And the steel windows, though flawed, were kept. "It's not finished", she says. "But that's the idea."

The kitchen is open and mobile – built on wheels, like the trolleys in her studio. It can shift depending on what's happening. Sometimes it's used for hosting, sometimes for working. It's part of a larger idea: nothing is fixed unless it needs to be. Function follows rhythm.

Her work studio sits at the back of the house, behind the living spaces. It's not polished. The floor is raw. The furniture is modular. And there are no barriers between tools, materials, and ideas. It's a space that invites mess, trial, repetition. Pieces are made, tested, and photographed in situ. And so the house becomes part of the process.

The garden follows a similar logic. There's no neat lawn or symmetry. Instead: loose clusters of plants, quiet wildness, and a view that stretches. She's reshaping it gradually, using time and growth as design tools, rather than lines or borders. And inside and outside remain close.

The house doesn't separate public from private, or work from life. Visitors walk through the spaces naturally. There's no front room or back office, just areas with different uses, changing as needed. It's not about showing, it's about sharing and leaving things open.

This is not a statement house. It doesn't aim for completeness. It's precise, but not polished; calm, but not static; a place that evolves slowly, by doing.

Project: destroyers / builders
Location: Belgium
Architect: Jozef Lietaert
Year of construction: 1967
Year of purchase: 2022
Floor area: 192 m²
Resident: Linde Freya Tangelder
Resident's profession: artist, designer

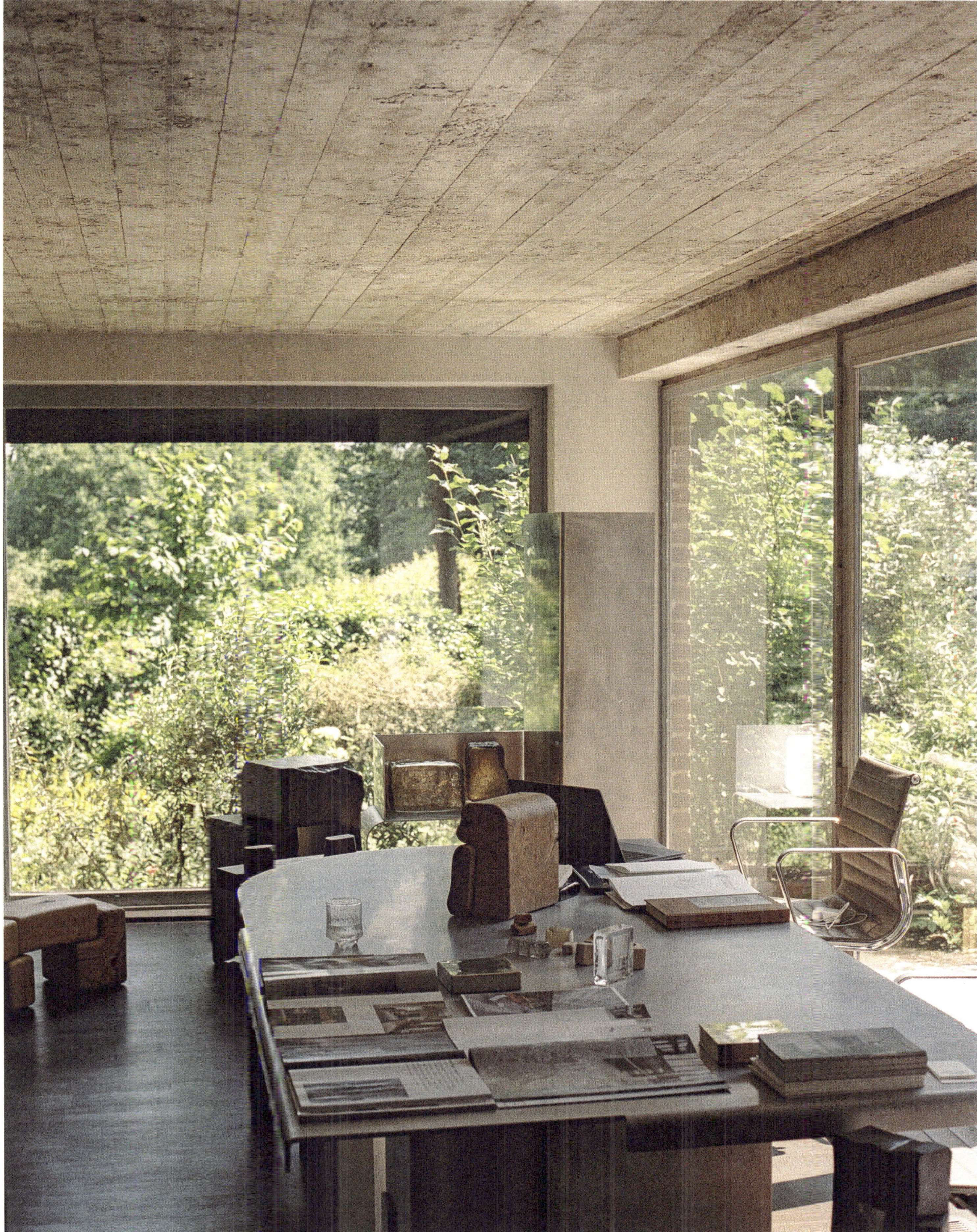

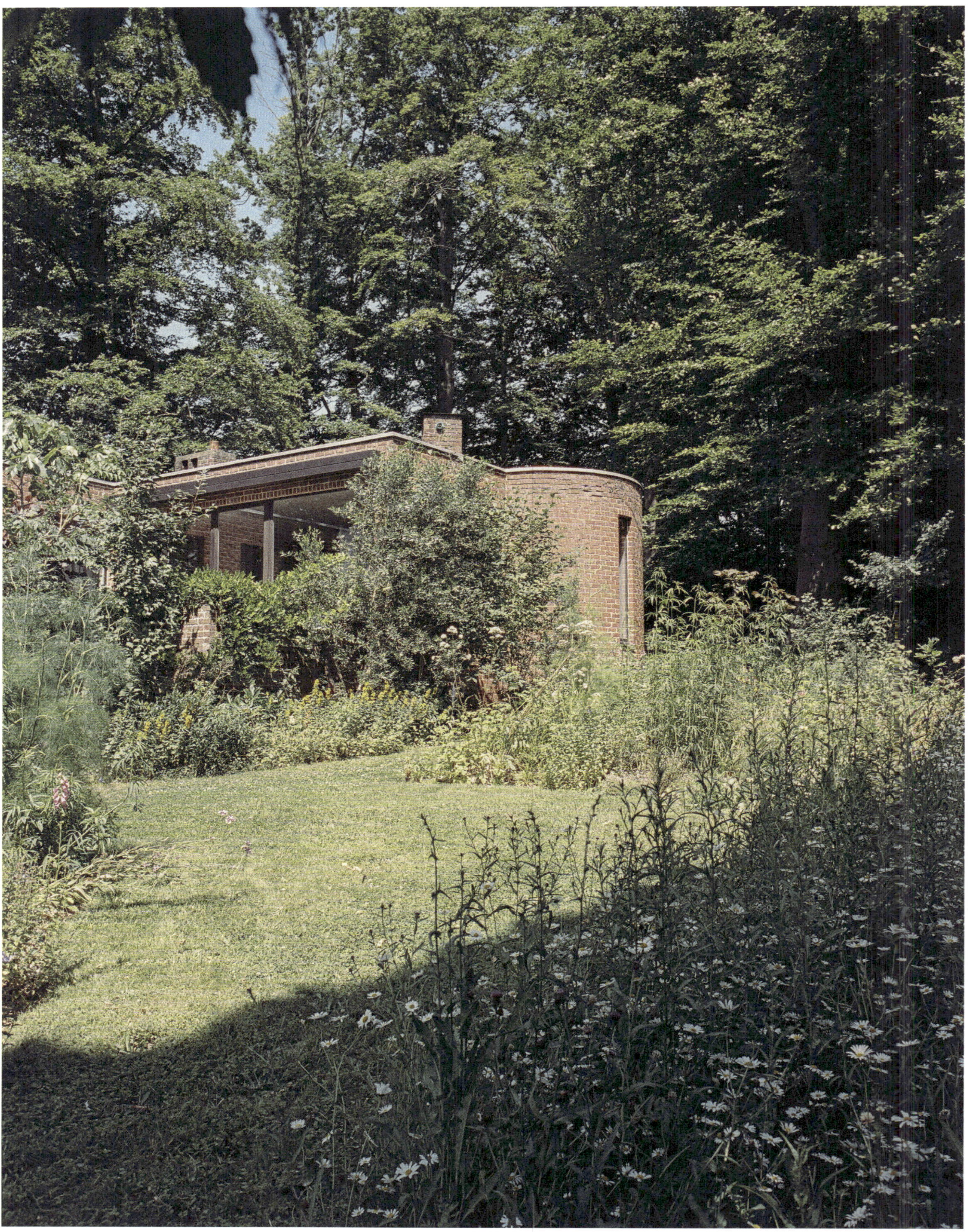

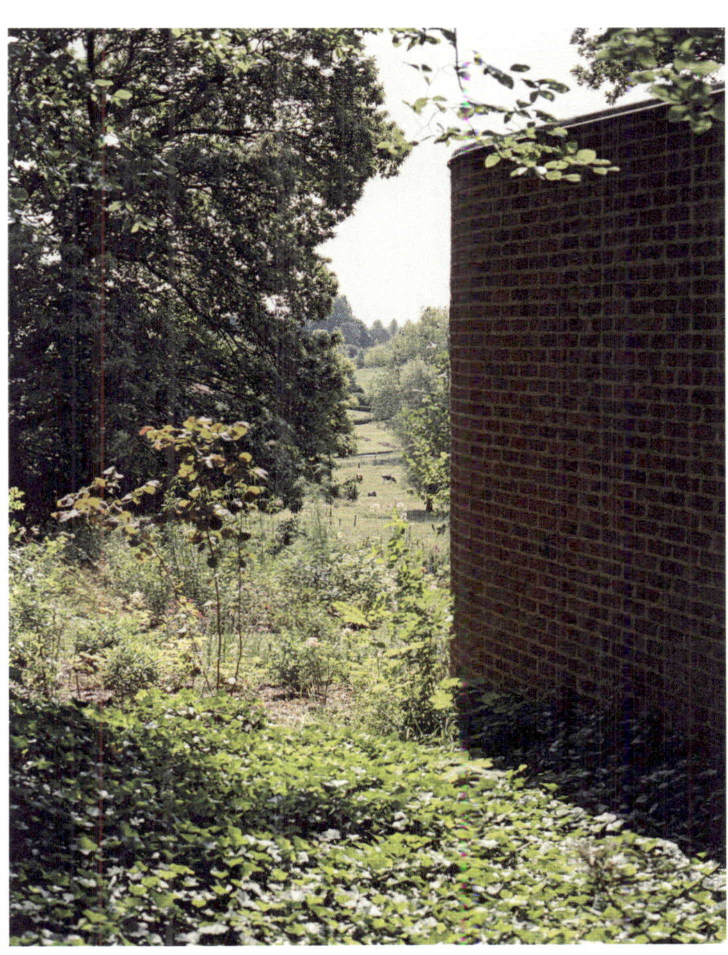

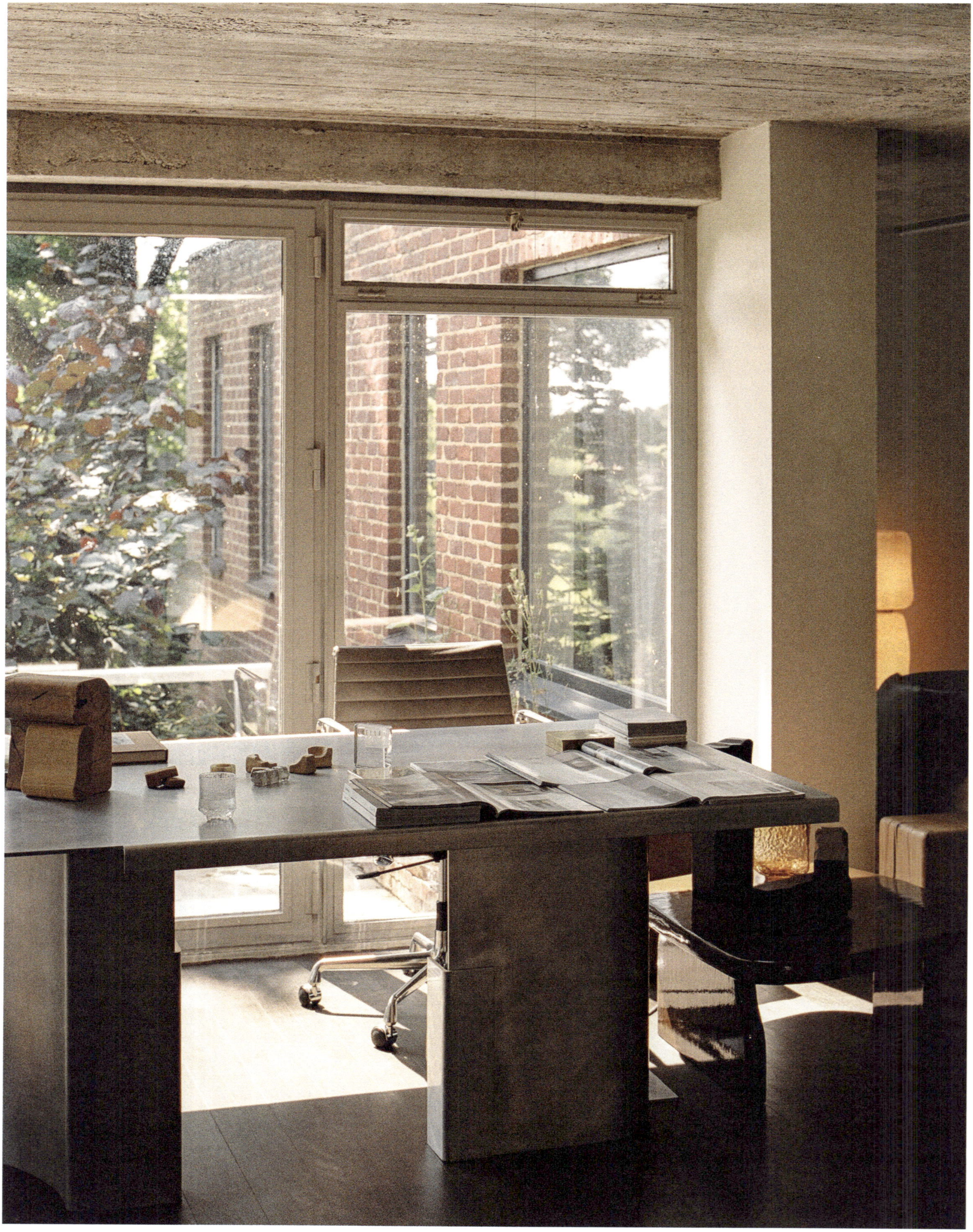

59

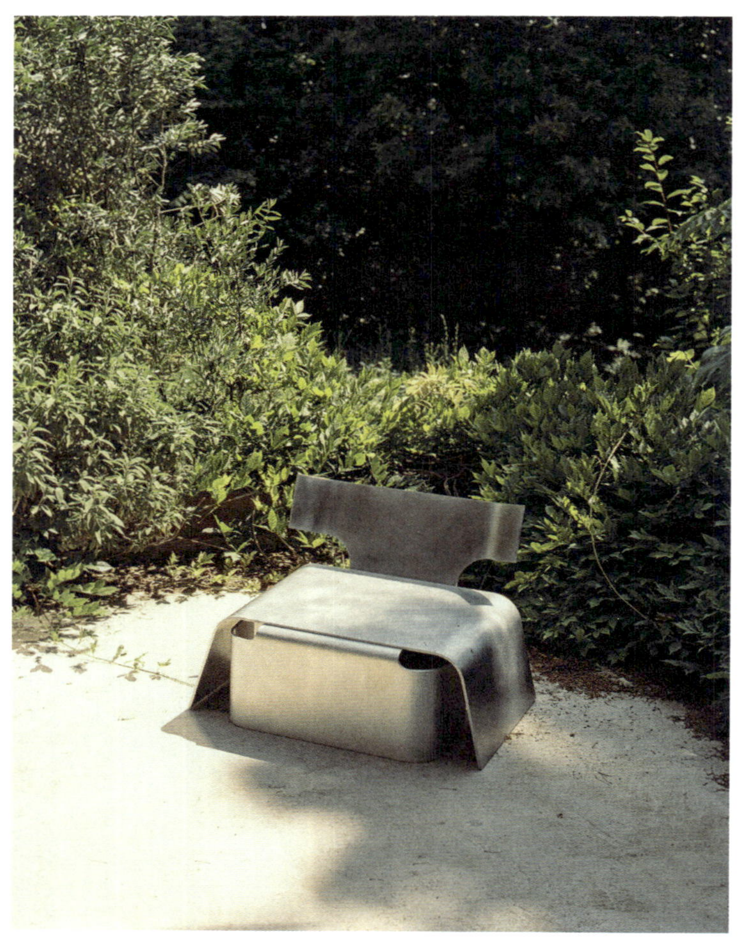

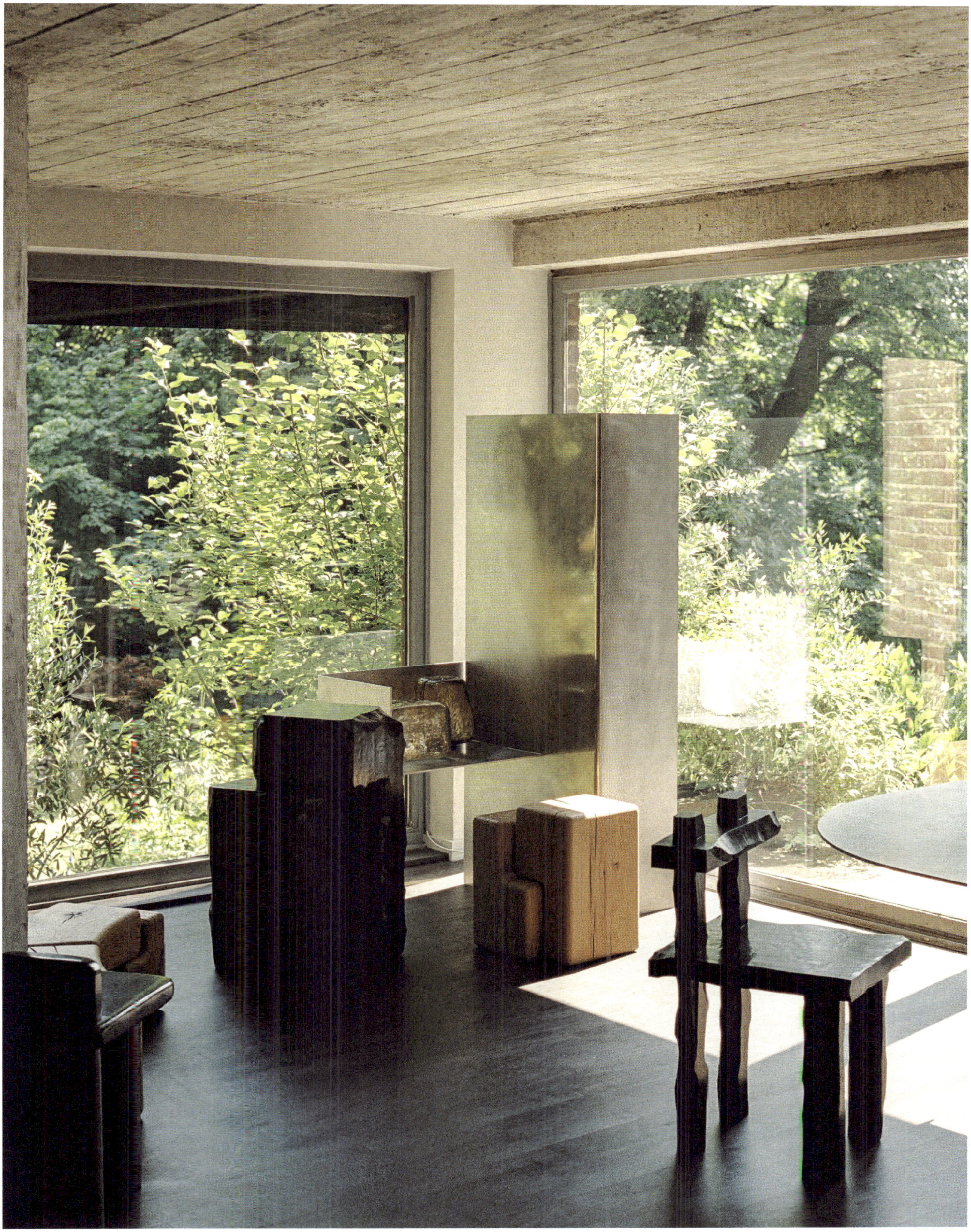

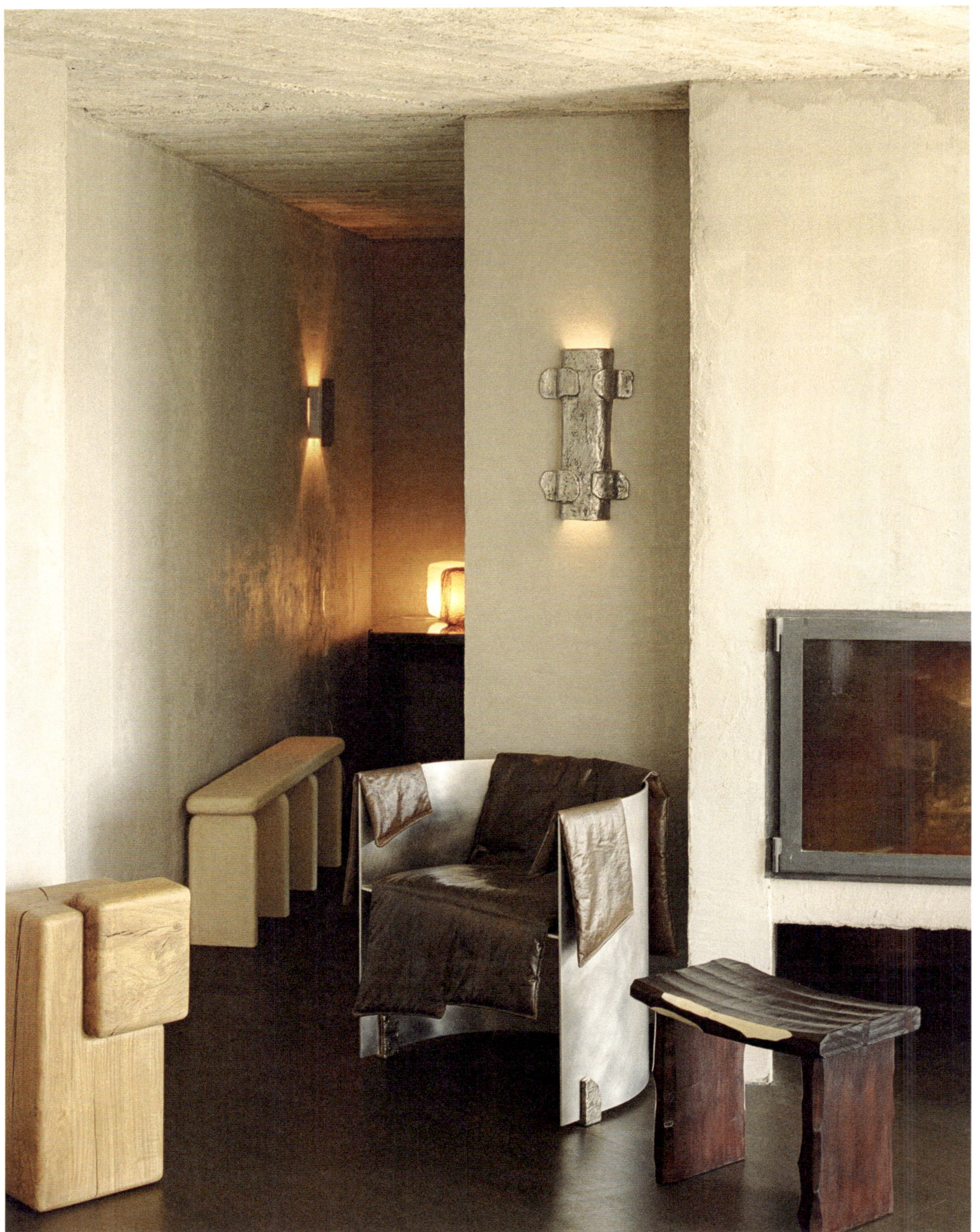

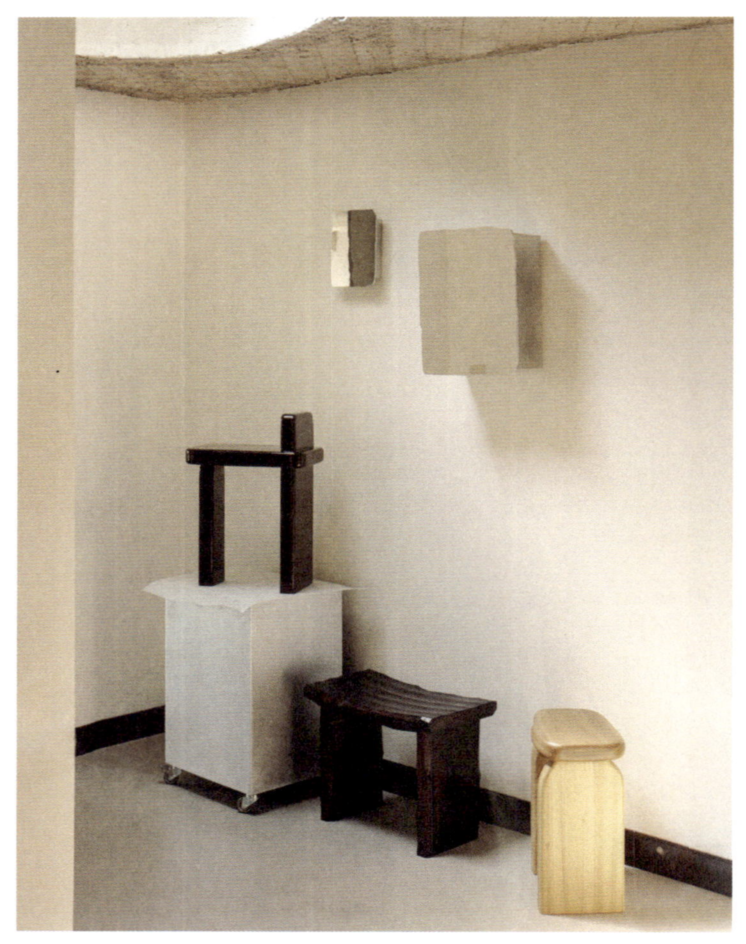

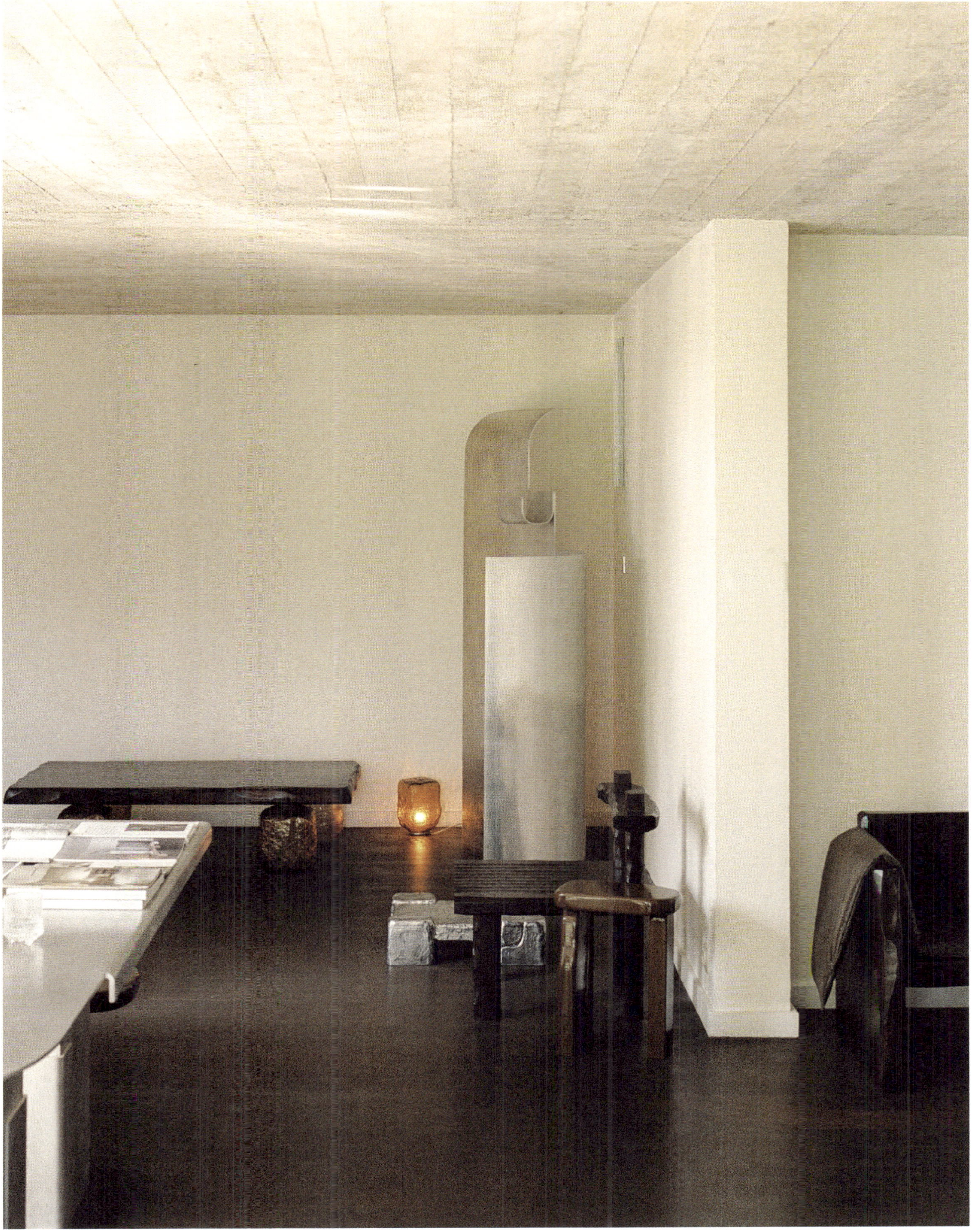

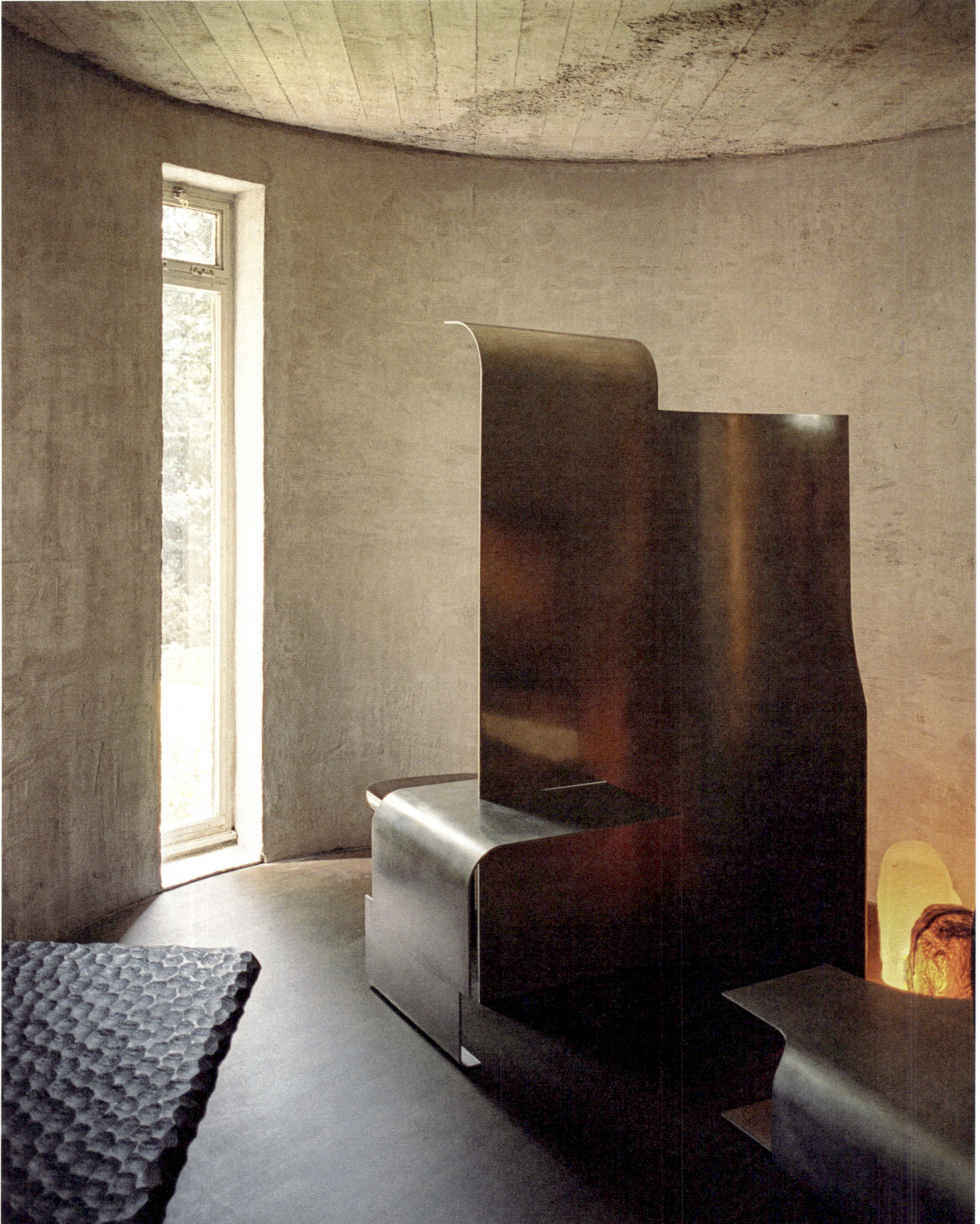

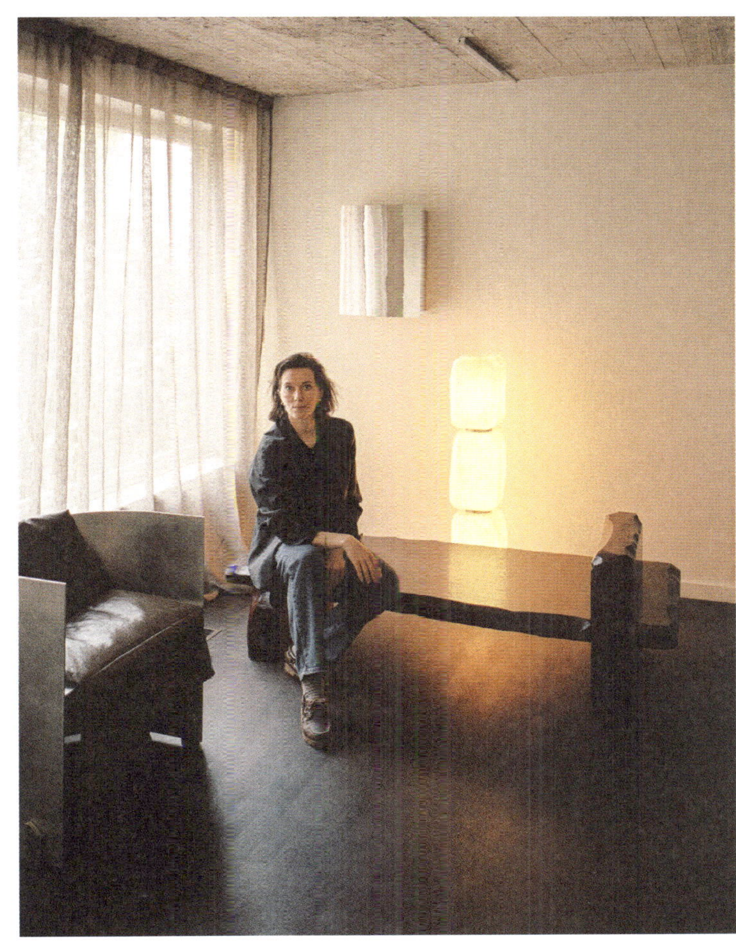

"It is the rawness, the unhidden structure of the house that makes the concrete connect to my work. It connects with the materials I care about: wood, metal, glass. The concrete directs them in space."

– Linde Freya Tangelder

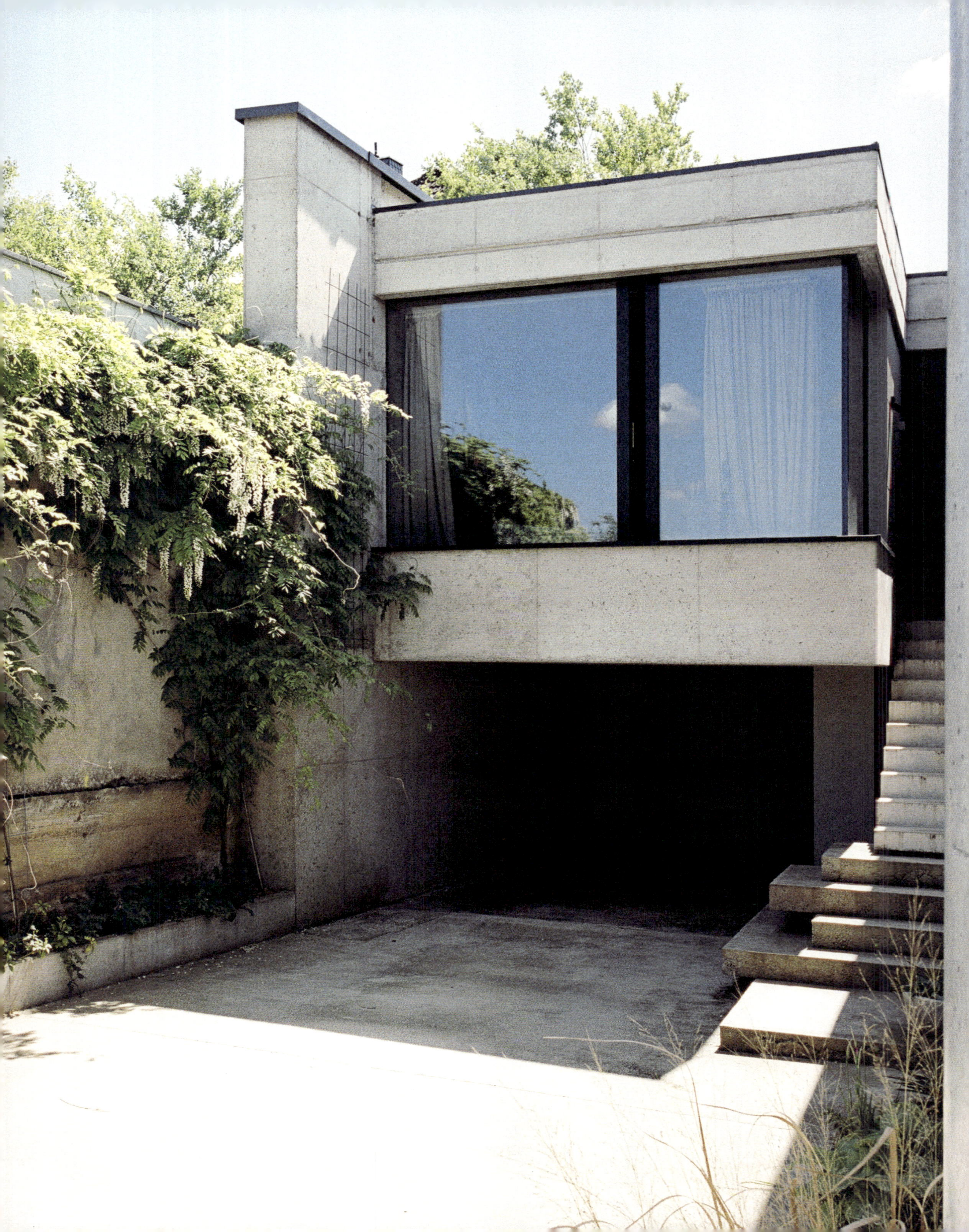

It didn't start with concrete. The original idea was a natural stone wall, something mid-century, textured, and a little softer. But that proved too expensive. Over time, a different idea took hold: a growing interest in the kind of brutalism you can find in Brazilian architecture – raw, honest, tactile. The kind you want to touch, not cover.

The house was already there. A modest 1960s volume with standard brick walls, small windows, and limited light. The plan was to add an extension and do it well. The concrete was poured on site, not prefabricated, and the structure slowly took shape over the course of five years. It was not always easy. The builders kept trying to smooth the surface, to fill the pores, and to make the concrete perfect. The owners kept insisting on the opposite. They wanted it raw and textured, not corrected. "We were always screaming", they say with a laugh.

The extension connects with the old volume but doesn't hide its difference. The original house was insulated and painted to blend in better with the new part. The windows, however, were kept intentionally distinct. Smaller, lighter wooden frames remain in the original section, and in the new part, black framed openings stretch wide across the façade. "We didn't want to copy", they explain. "We wanted both parts to speak to each other, but stay different."

Inside, the feeling is warm and calm. The new space opens directly into the garden, where greenery meets concrete. And light moves gently across the surfaces. A large sofa faces the wide windows: it is a place for resting, reading, or taking a short nap in the afternoon sun. "It's my Brazilian corner", one of the owners says. "Even though I've never been there."

The interior evolved over time, nothing was rigidly planned, and furniture was collected slowly: design classics, family pieces, and vintage finds. "I see something, I love it, I take it with me. Then I find a place for it." The result is a home that feels personal and coherent. Every wall holds something different, but everything feels connected.

The kitchen remains the centre of the older section. It was updated twelve years ago, using simple elements that fit easily into the space. "We cook here, we host friends, we drink wine", they say. "It is the heart of the house. The holy part."

The garden took shape along with the renovation. A shipping container pool is a strong visual anchor, as trees and hedges create layers and privacy, and a low stone wall defines one side of the garden. "You need something to look at", they explain. "Something with presence. Not just lawn."

Visitors are often surprised. In the beginning, neighbours were not sure what to make of the concrete. "They called it the National Gallery in Berlin", the owners say, referring to Mies van der Rohe's famous museum. "Now they love it." Guests tend to spend time walking through the house, not cing things. It's not a museum, but it feels alive.

The house is not big, but it feels generous. Rooms open and fold in again. Materials are raw but warm. And the spaces shift with the seasons and with the people who live here. 'It keeps changing", they say. "We change, the kids grow, the house grows with us."

And that is what this house is, not a rigid concrete statement, but a home that breathes, a place that invites, adapts, and stays honest.

Project: Schuppen
Location: Germany
Architect: Jung & Klemke Architektur und Innenarchitektur
Year of construction: 1979
Year of renovation: 2024
Floor area: 236 m²
Resident: Pirkko Weise
Resident's profession: doctor

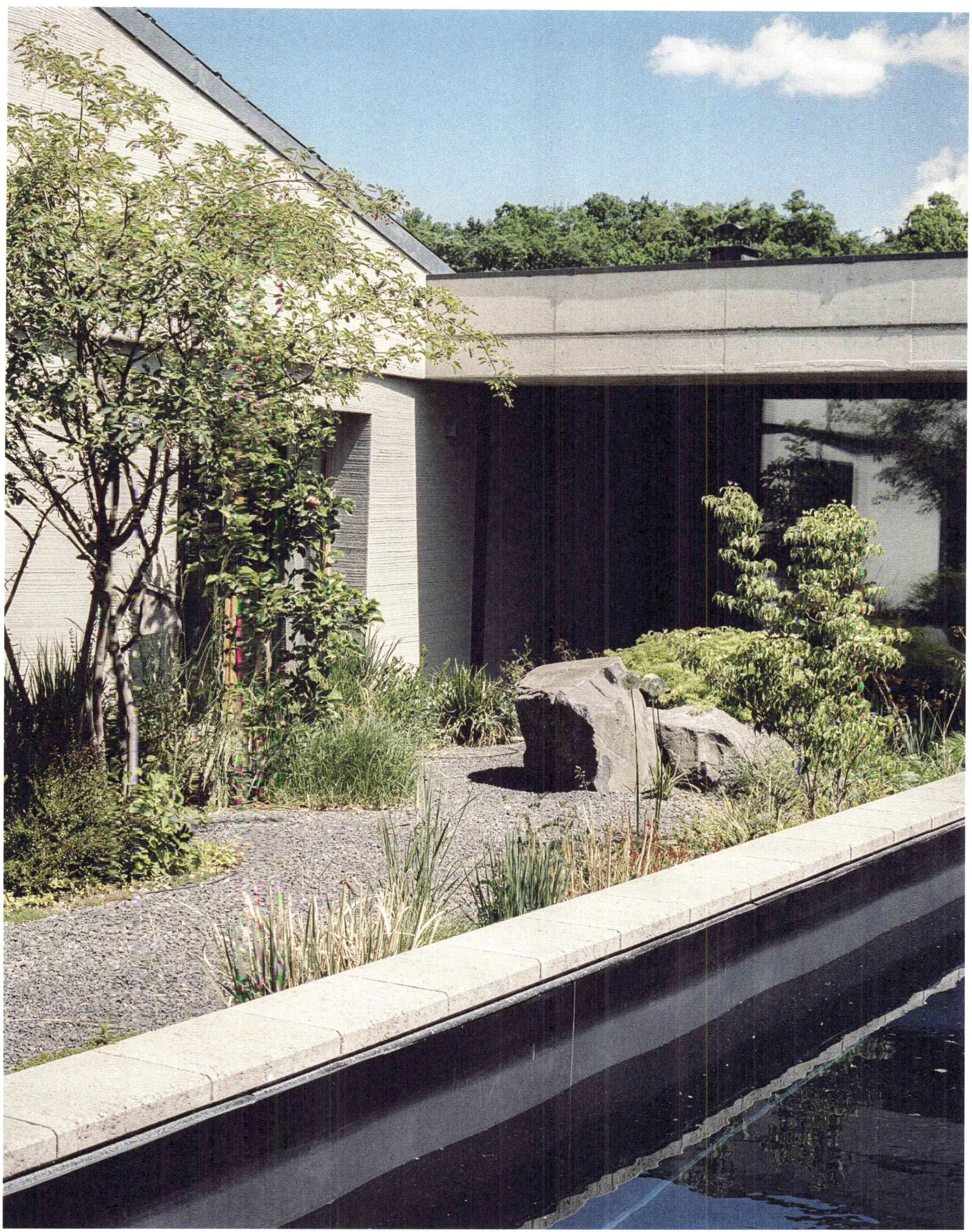

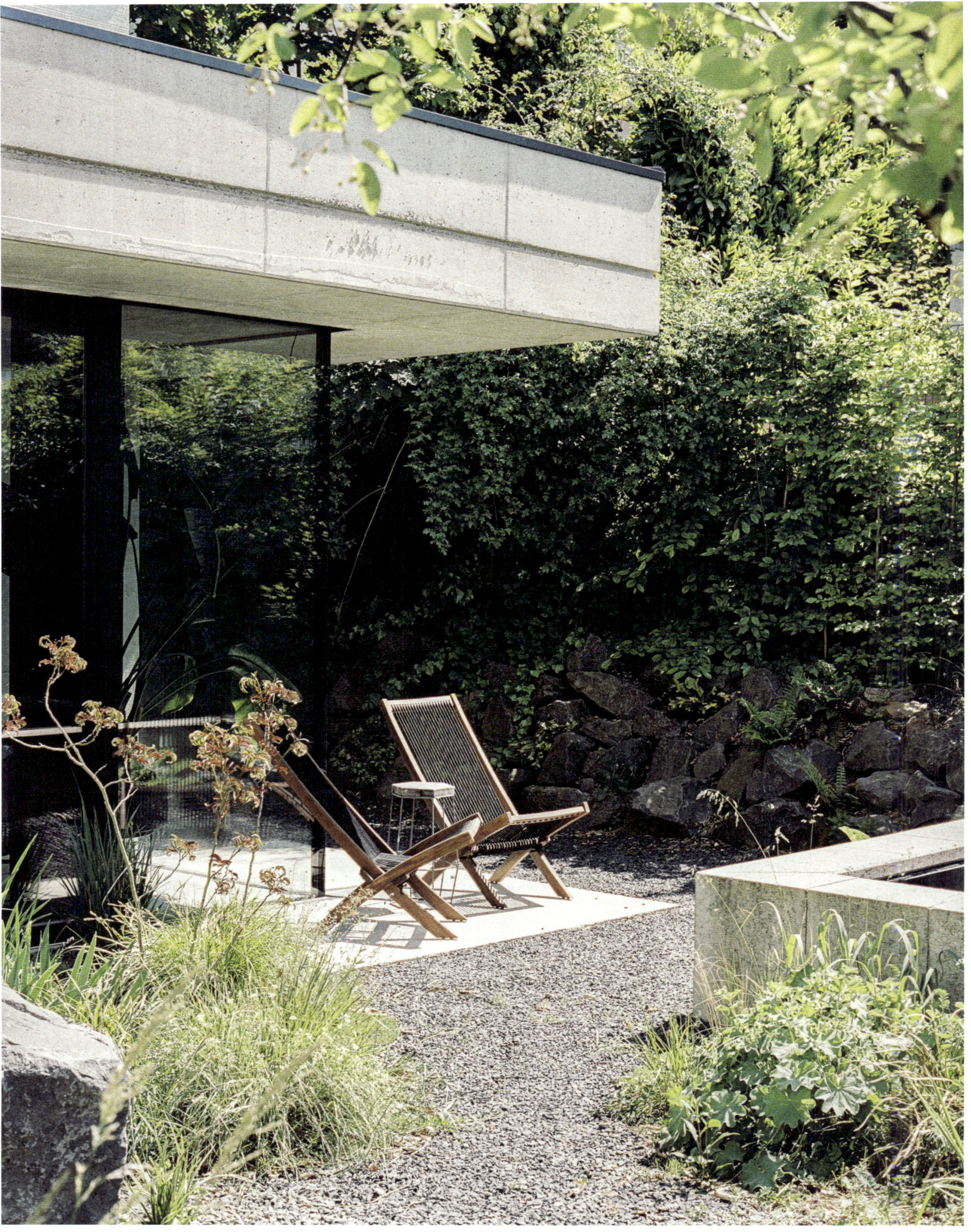

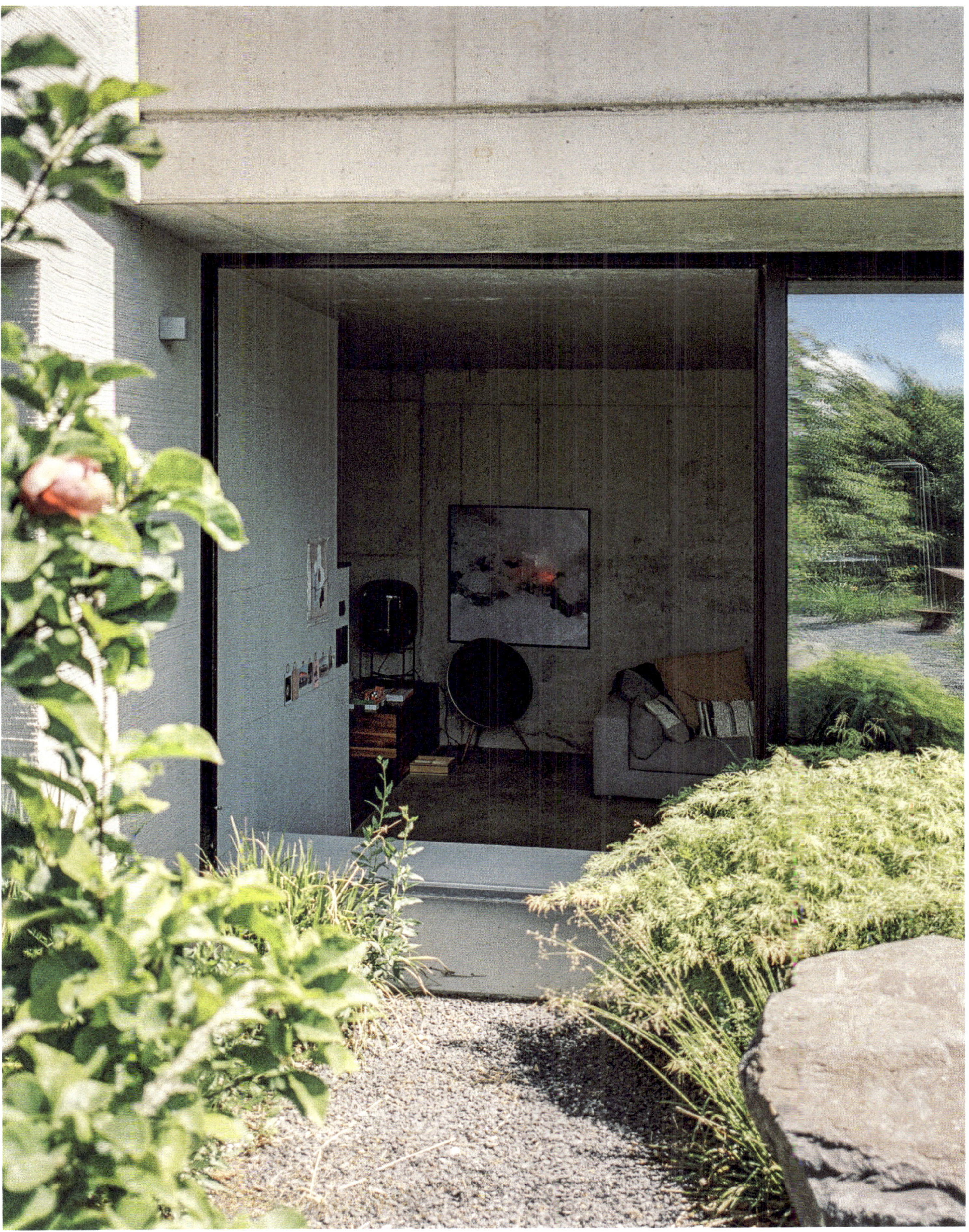

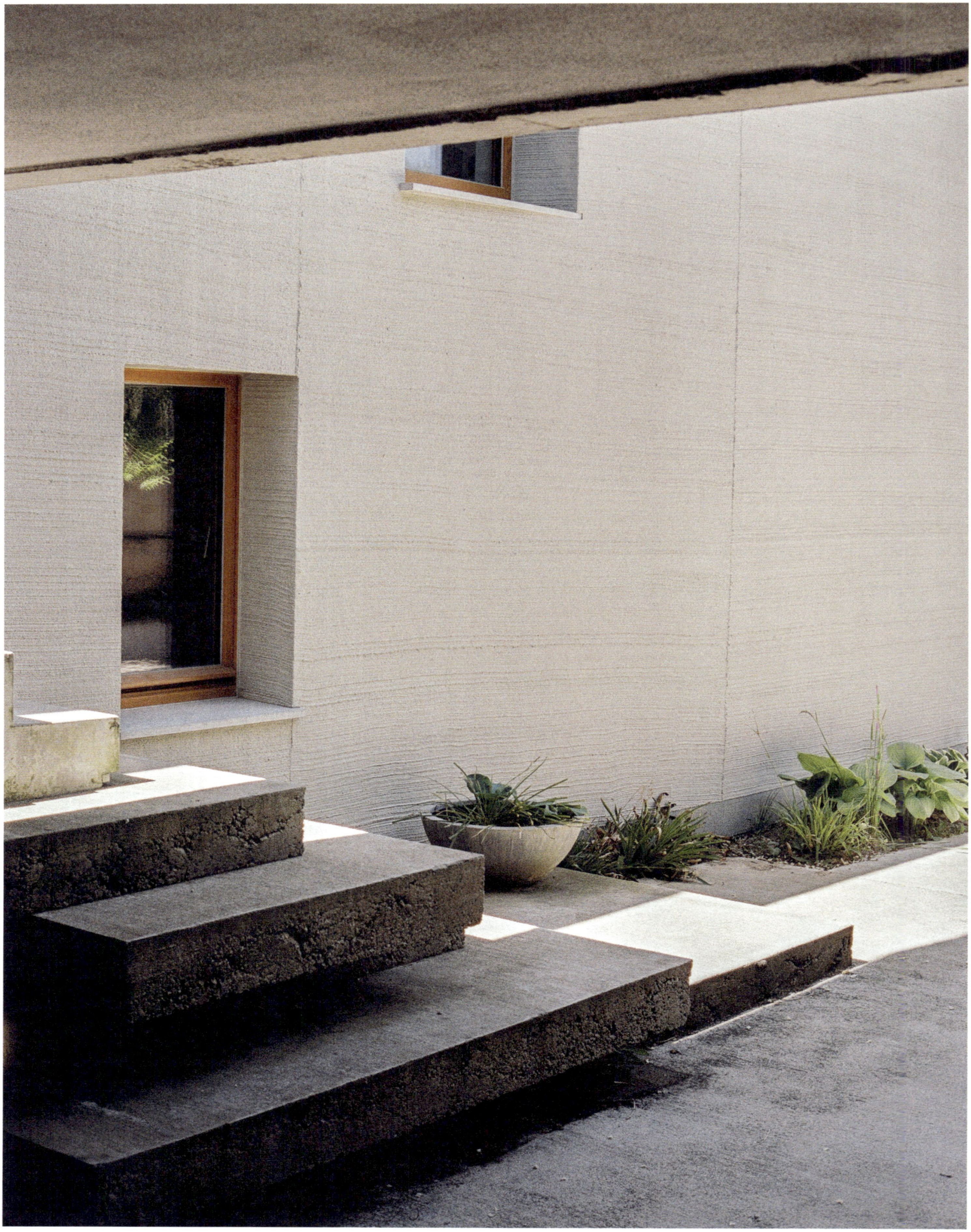

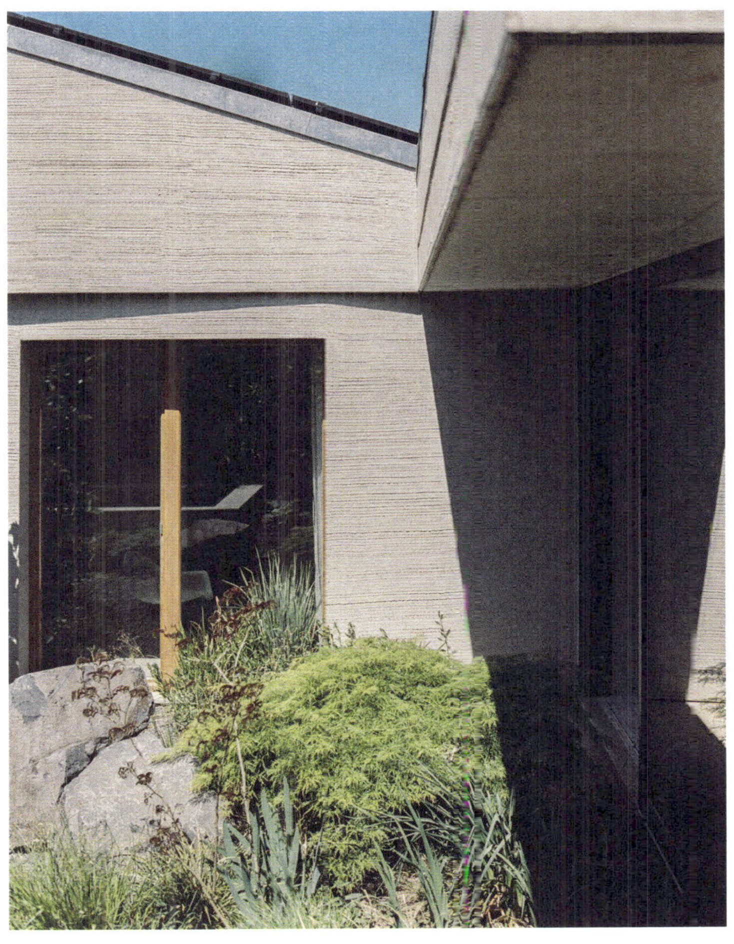

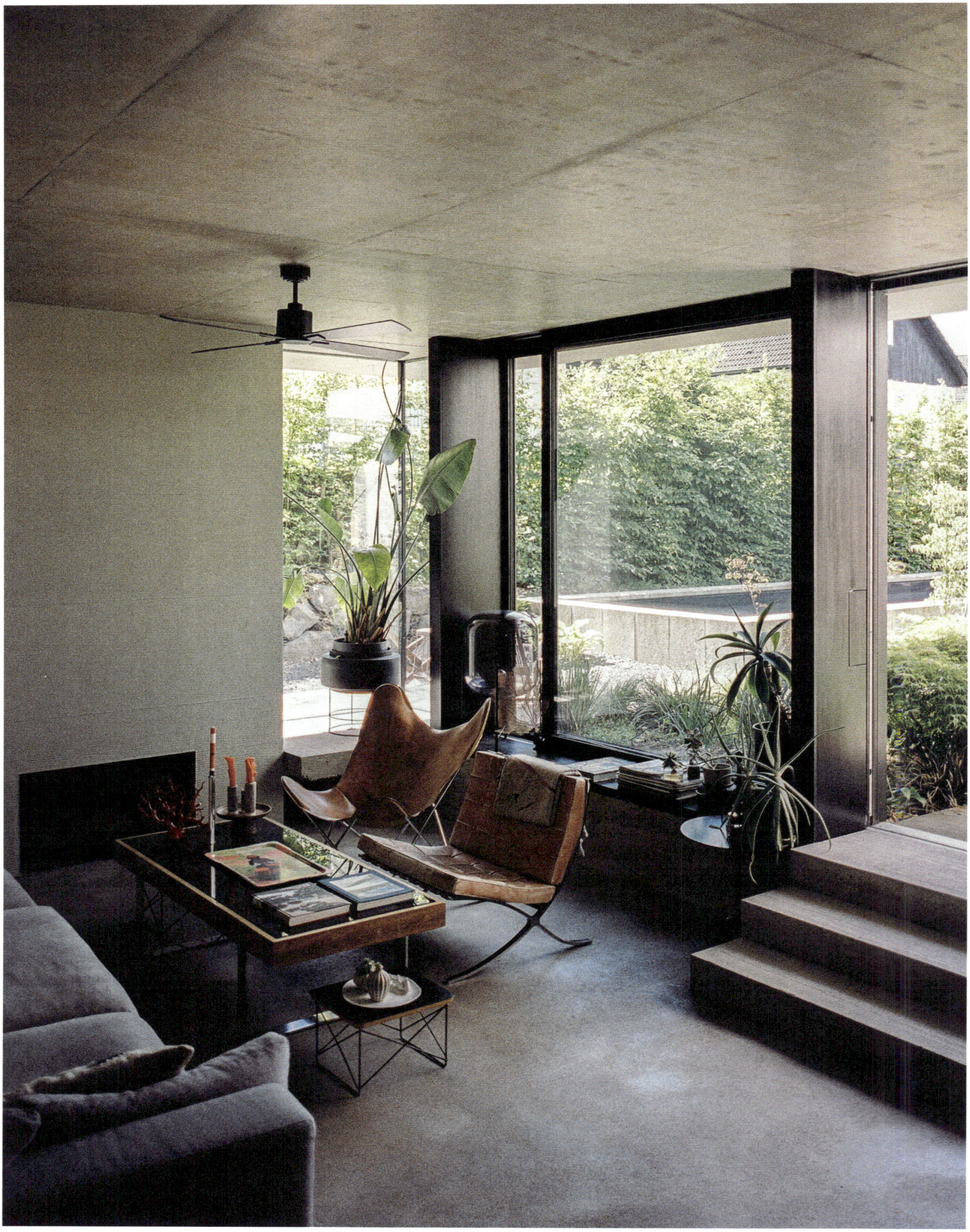

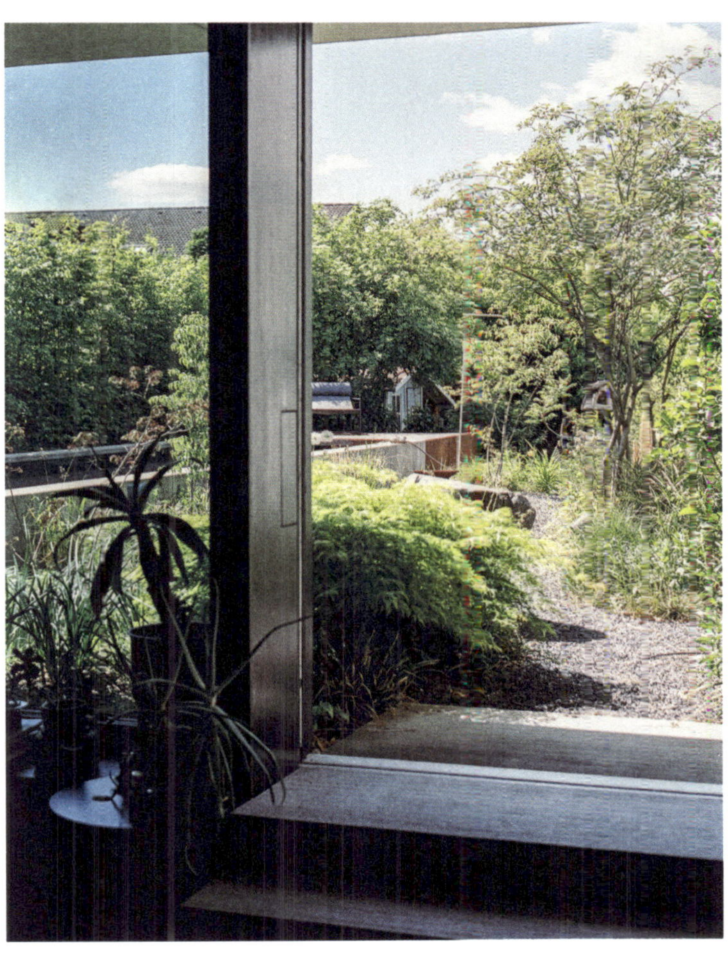

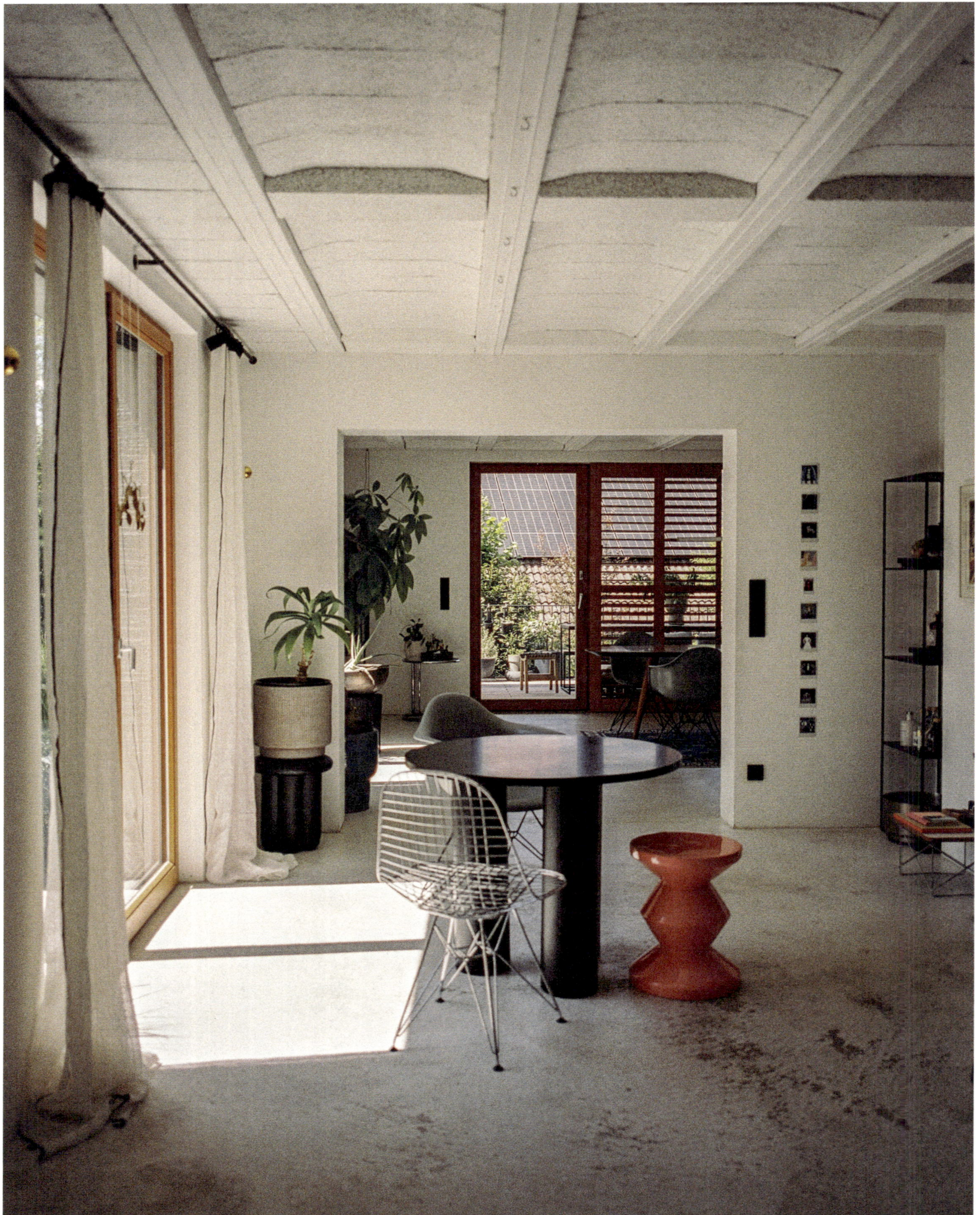

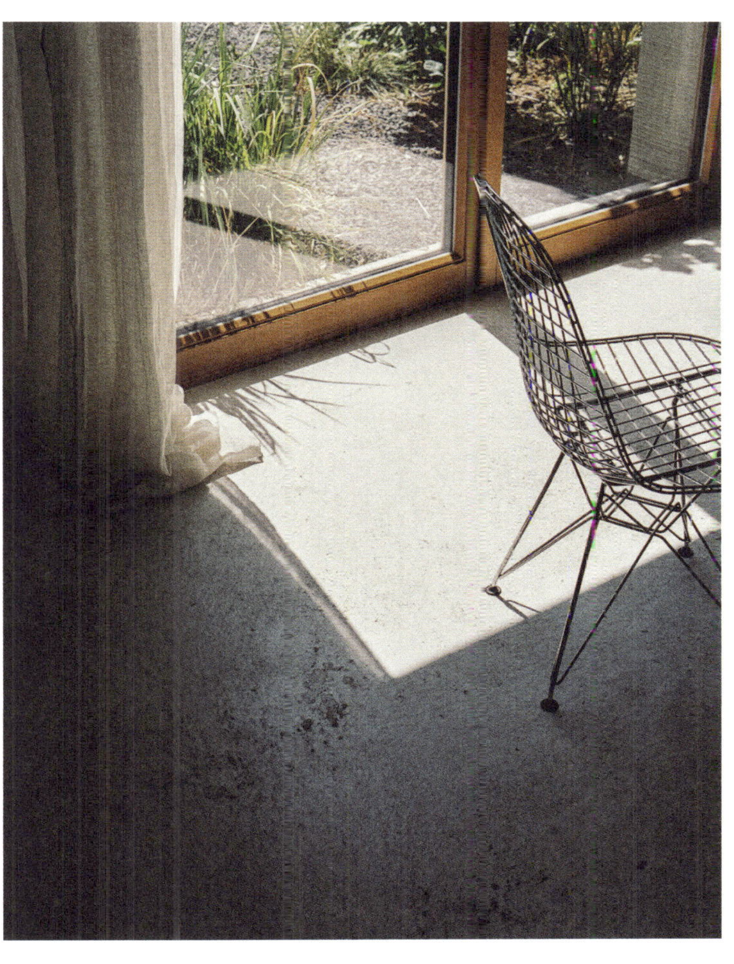

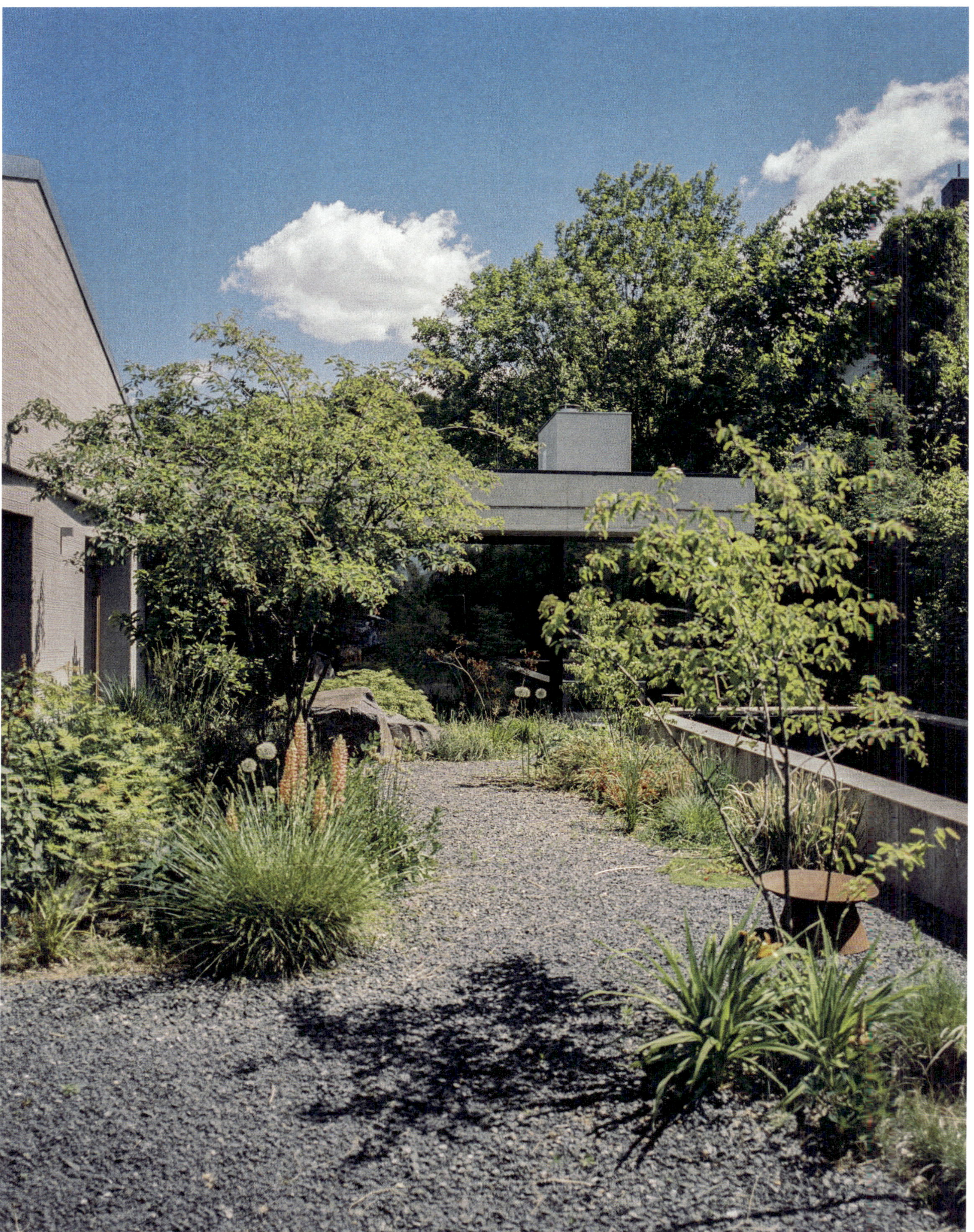

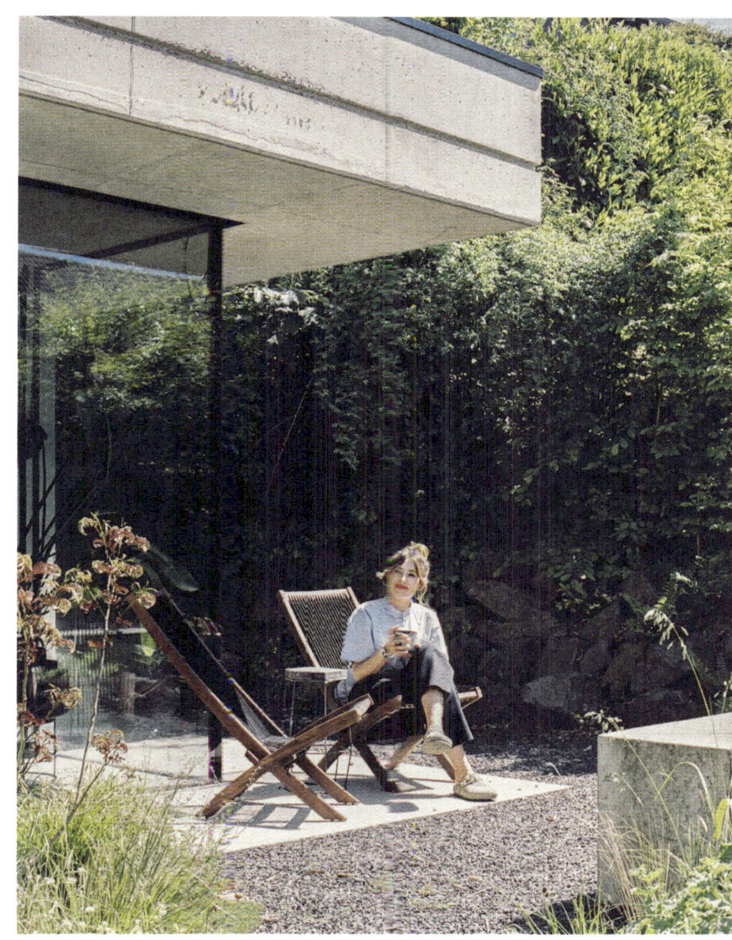

"It grows with us, it ages with us, and it makes space for life to happen in all its rawness and beauty."

– Pirkko Weise

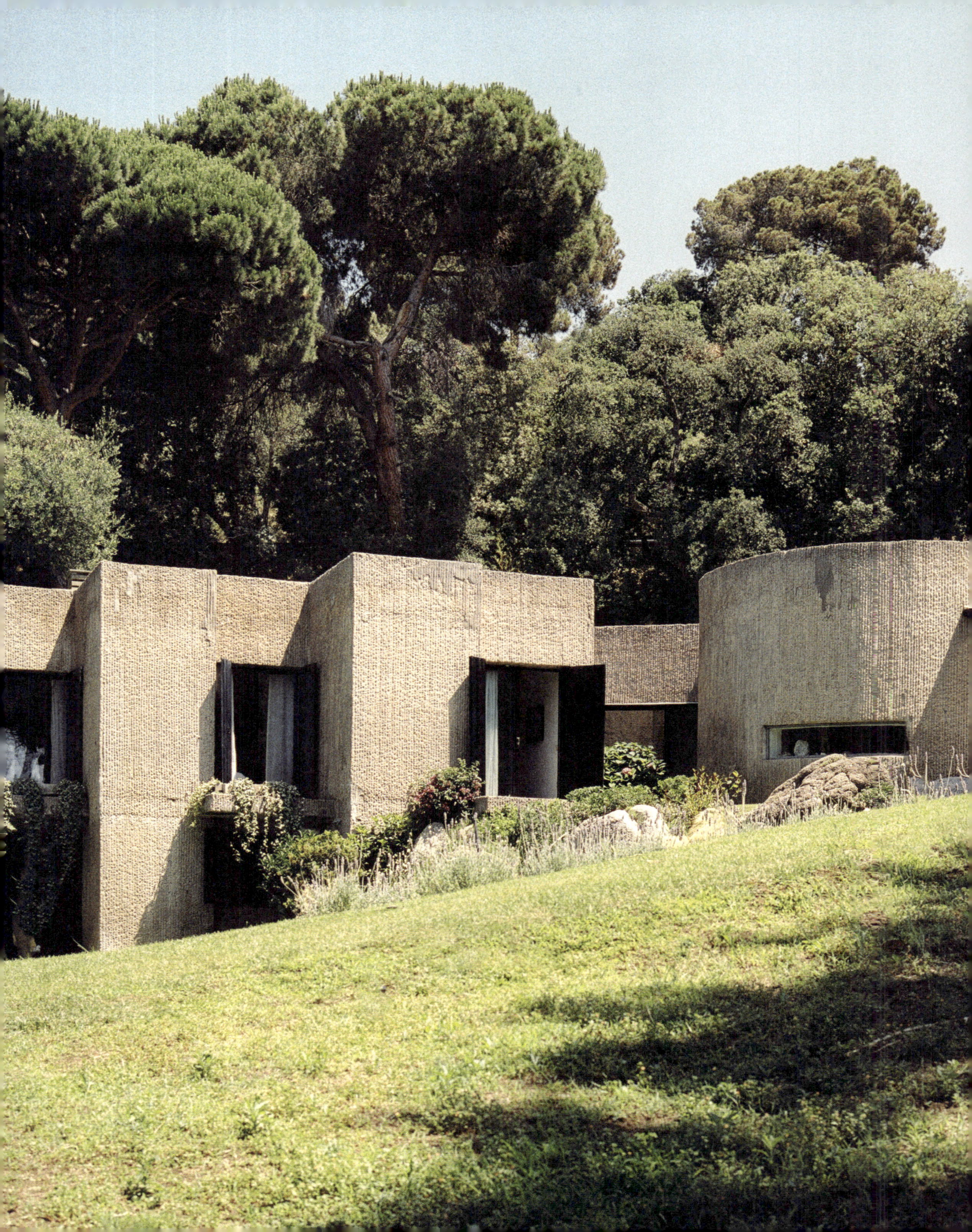

Casa Riera

Spain

Partly embedded in a hillside north of Barcelona, Casa Riera is a house that almost disappears into the land. Only the soft rise of its roof is visible from a distance, the rest is hidden by trees, slopes, and silence. Designed by architect Javier Barba and completed in 1986, the house was an early exploration of bioclimatic principles. It uses passive cooling, thermal mass, and a green roof that blends architecture into its environment rather than placing it on top.

When the current owner, Argentine designer and digital artist Ezequiel Pini – founder of the Barcelona-based studio Six N. Five – first visited, the house had been on the market for years. Many buyers had passed it over. It felt too strange, too still, too separate from the usual image of a home. But something about it made sense. "I didn't expect this to be my first house", he says. "But I grew up in the city, and I needed nature. I fell in love."

Since moving in, he has made very few changes. The house is largely untouched: concrete floors, built-in furniture, and minimal fixtures. Soft light filters in through openings cut into thick, planted walls, and the rooms move from one to the next with quiet continuity. You never feel above ground or fully below it, and the air stays cool even on the hottest days.

The roof is planted with wild grass and native ground cover. It insulates the house and hides it from view. But it does more than that, it shifts with the seasons. In spring and summer, it's green; in autumn it turns gold; in winter it fades to grey. The house moves with it, slowly and without urgency.

The layout is generous but discreet. One side accommodates bedrooms and a guest area. The other contains a large open room used for creative work and occasional hosting. At the edge of the property, a second structure that once held a private sports court is being reimagined as a future studio. But there's no rush. "I'm living in the house before deciding what to do", he says. "Time helps clarify."

The house has aged, but not carelessly. A few surfaces need repair, and some parts will need attention. But nothing is urgent, nothing is being added for the sake of appearance. Even a later addition, an outdoor grill, might be removed to return to the original proportions. "It's not about changing things", Pini says. "It's about listening."

He stays in touch with the architect – not formally, but regularly. They exchange thoughts, reflect on choices, and treat the house not as something finished, but as something alive. The building is still teaching, still adapting.

Casa Riera asks for little. It doesn't seek to stand out, but it rewards close attention. You notice the curve of a wall, the coolness of concrete in the morning, and the way the house holds silence without ever feeling empty. It is not a house that defines how you live; it gives you space to pay attention.

The house is now Ezequiel's canvas of expression, as he gradually takes charge of interior design and subtle modifications. He also plans to create his studio where the current Paddle court is – following the same architectural principles, style, and materials of the current building – and use the landscape as a canvas for his digital and physical sculptures.

Project: Casa Riera
Location: Spain
Architect: Javier Barba
Year of construction: 1986
Year of purchase: 2024
Floor area: 320 m²
Resident: Ezequiel Pini
Resident's profession: visual artist, founder of Six N. Five

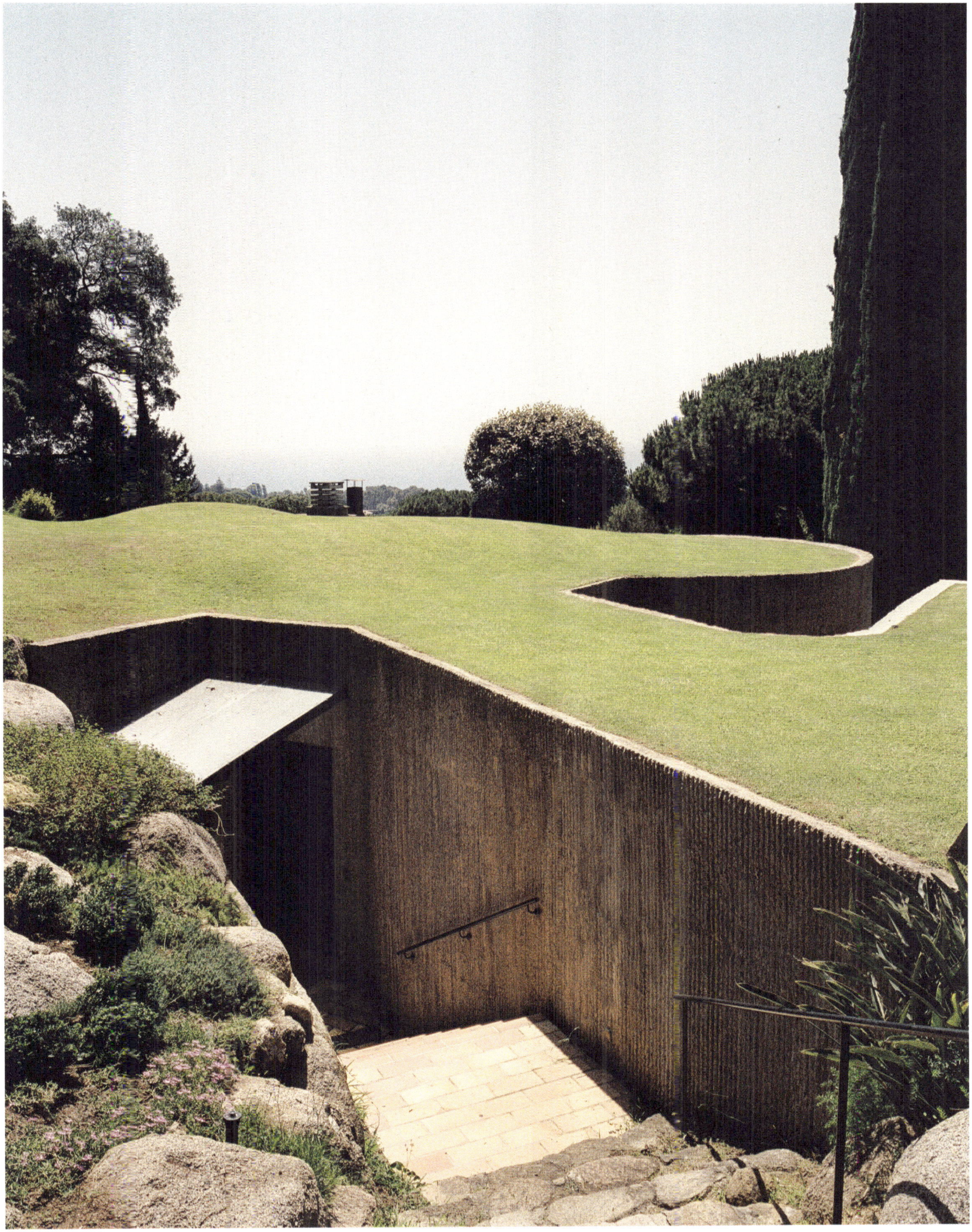

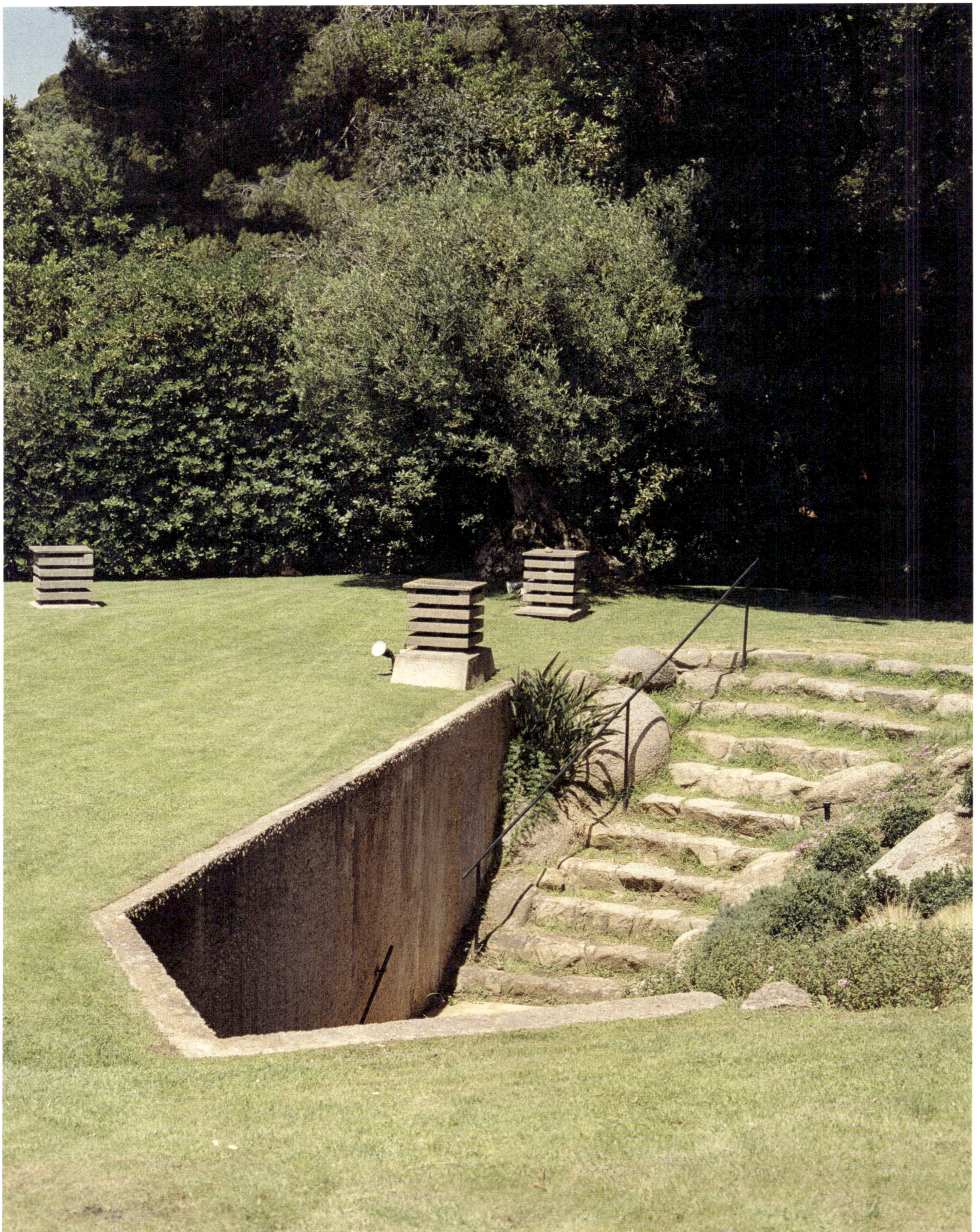

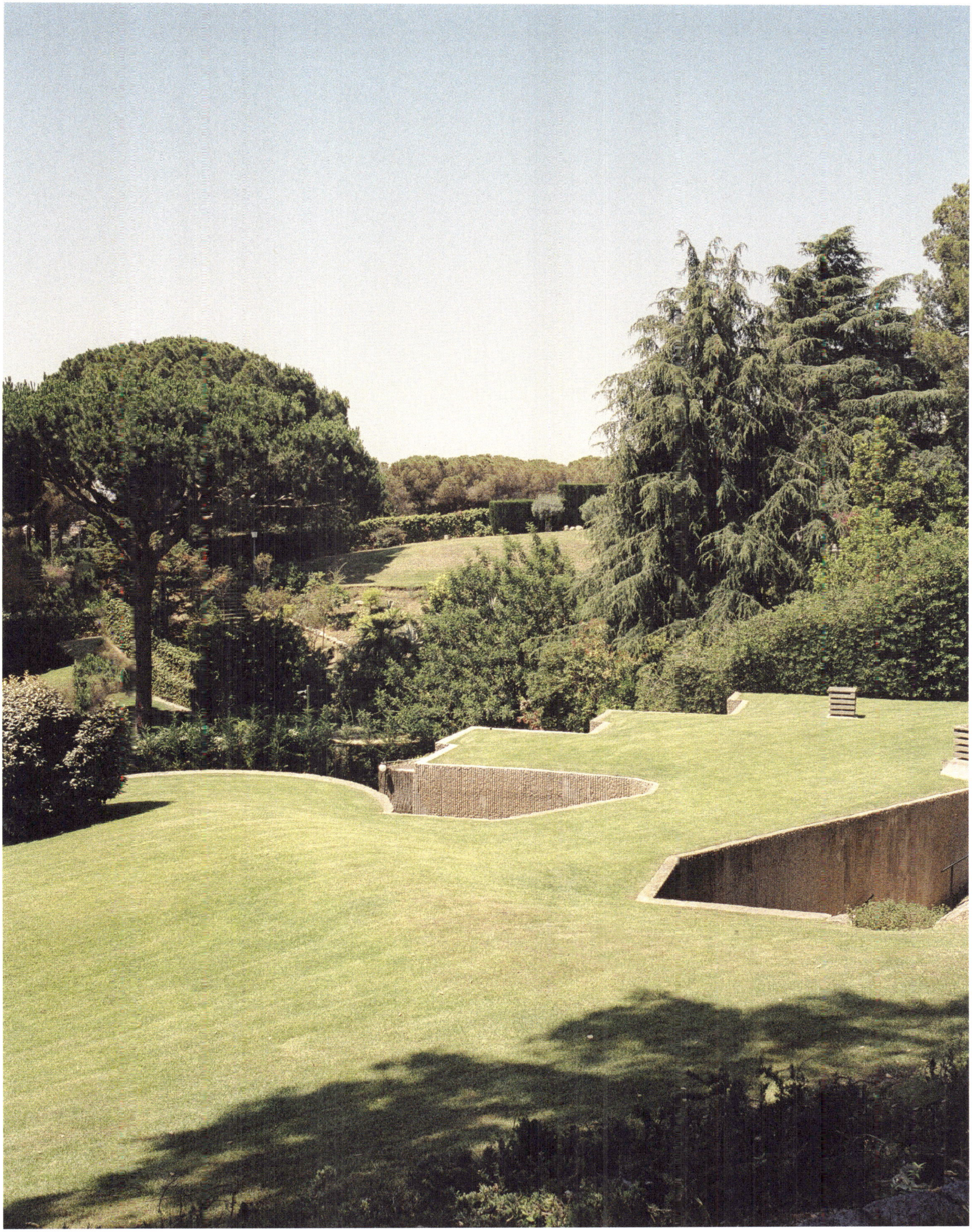

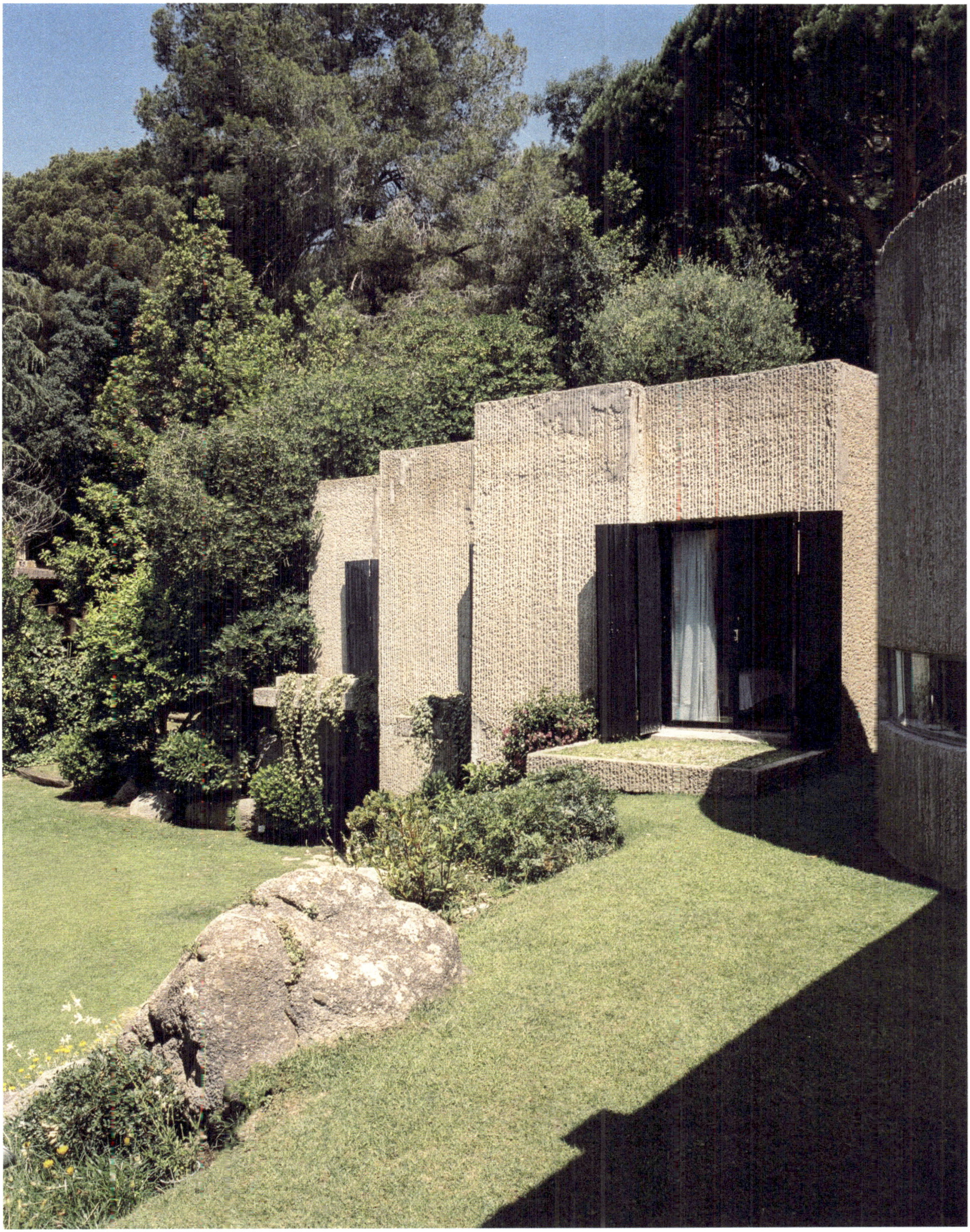

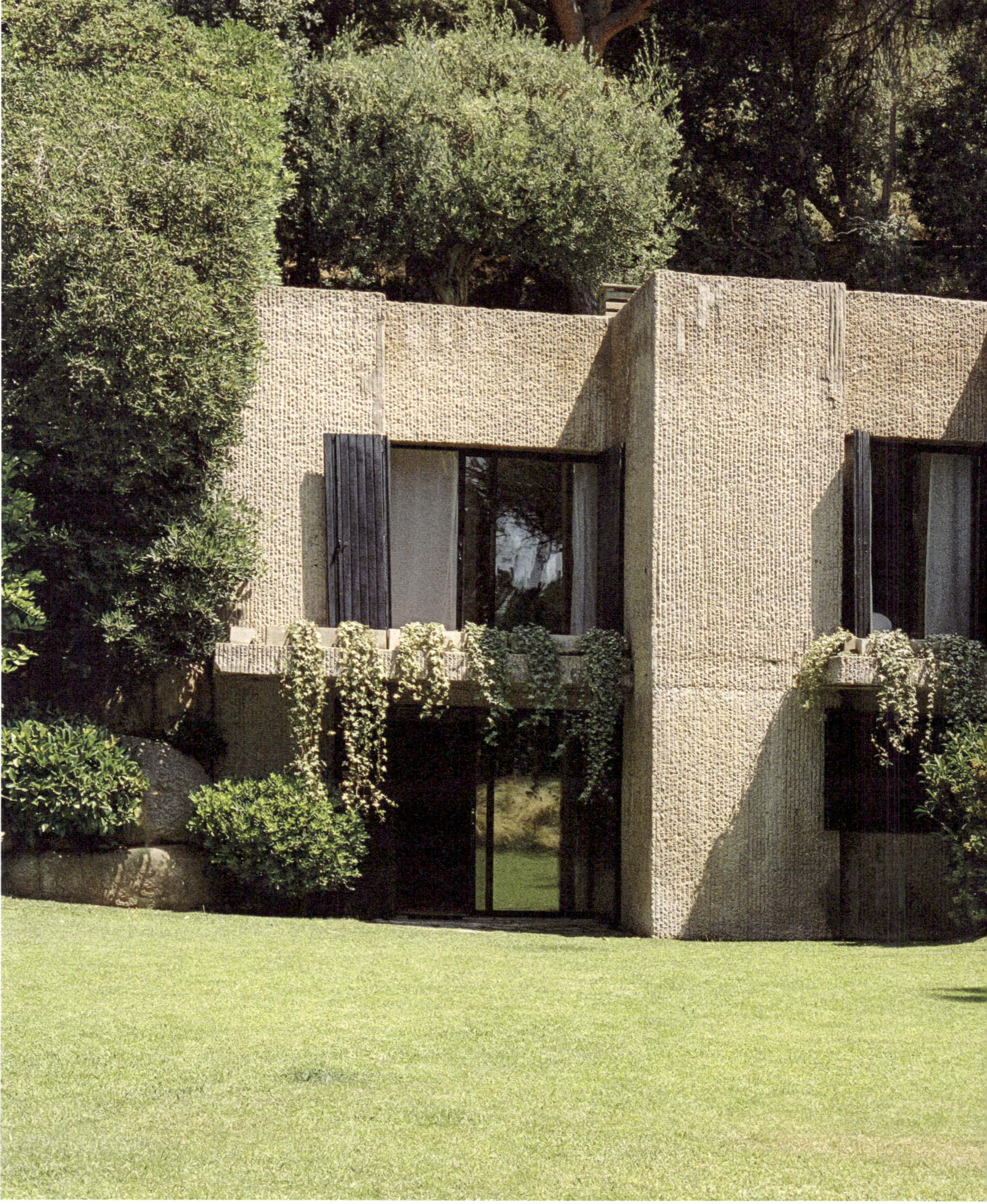

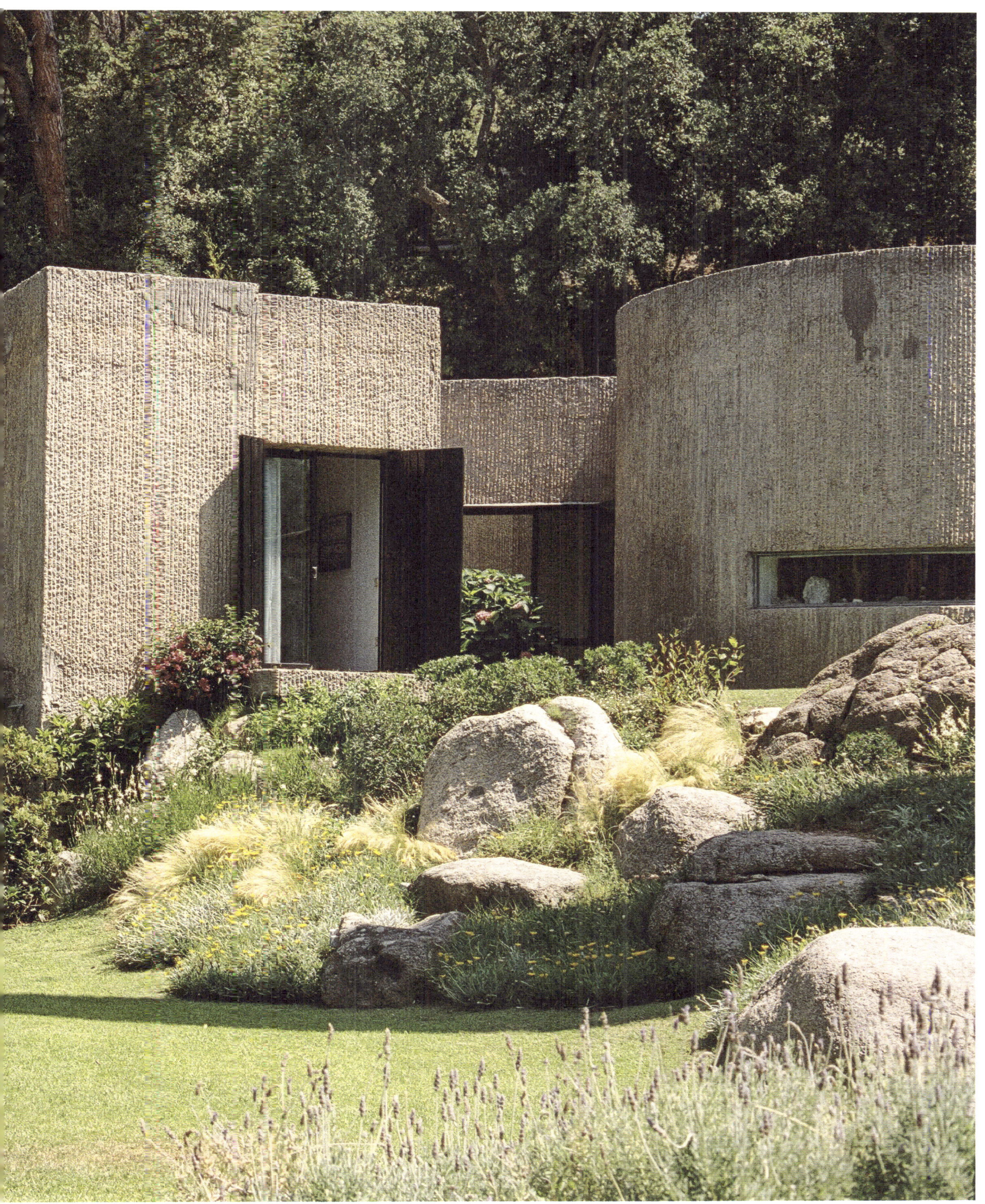

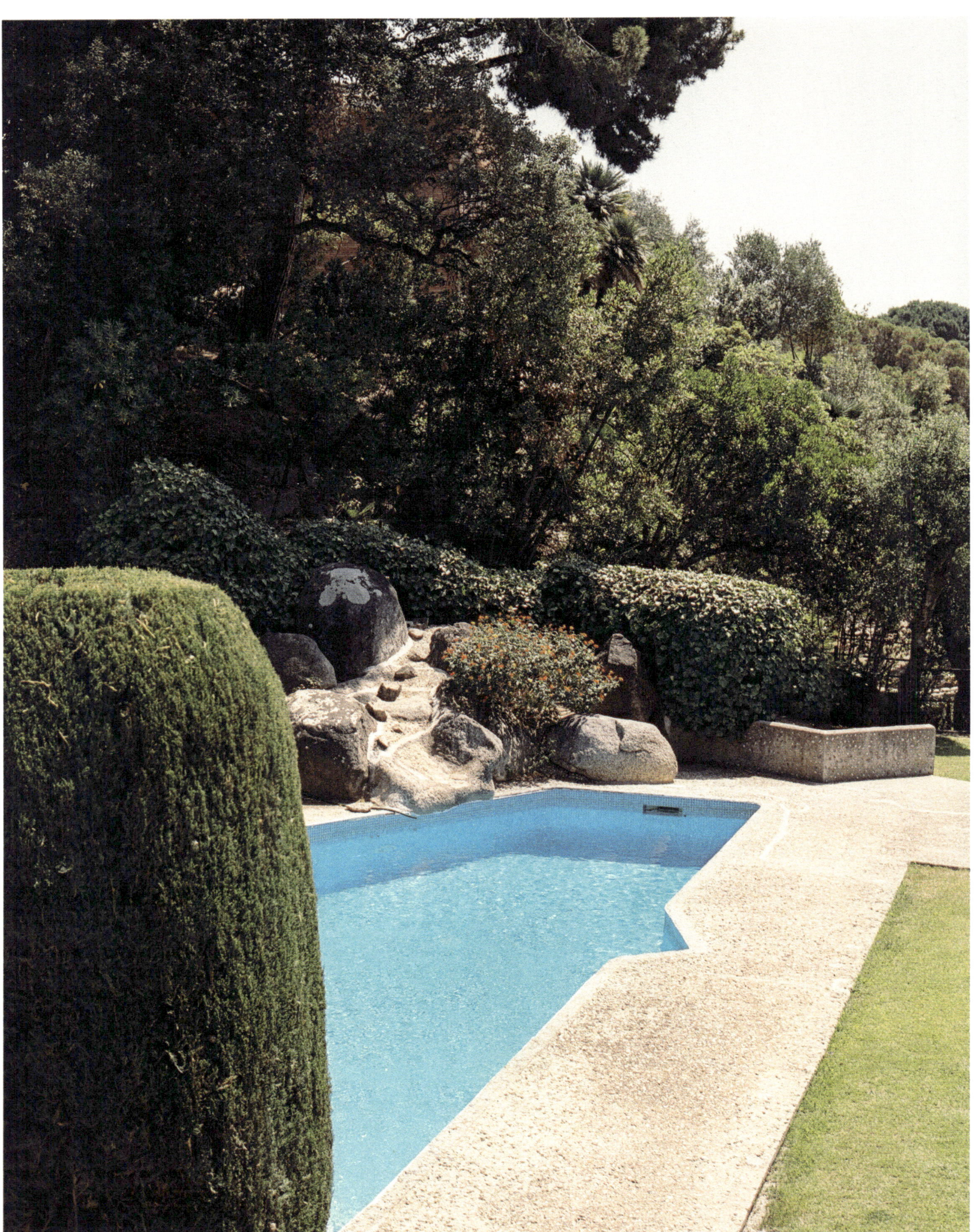

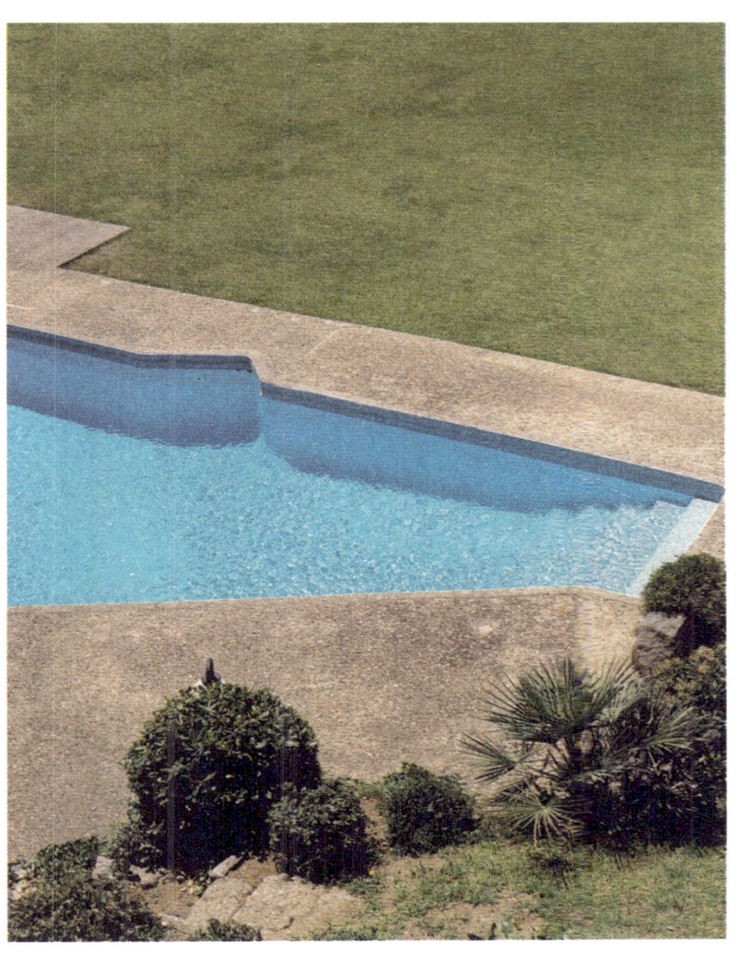

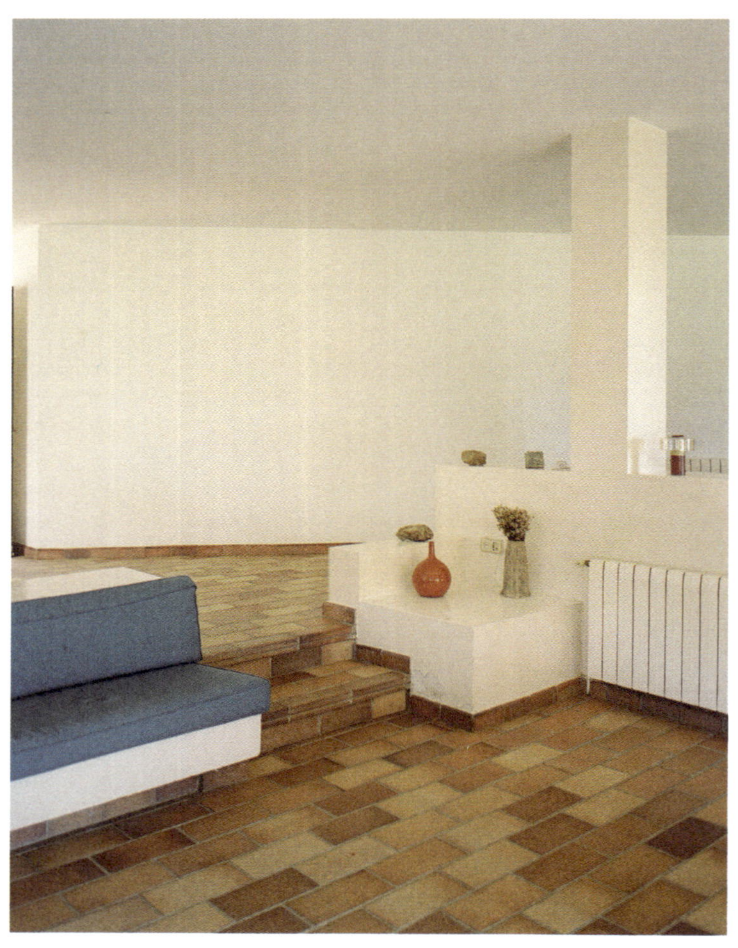

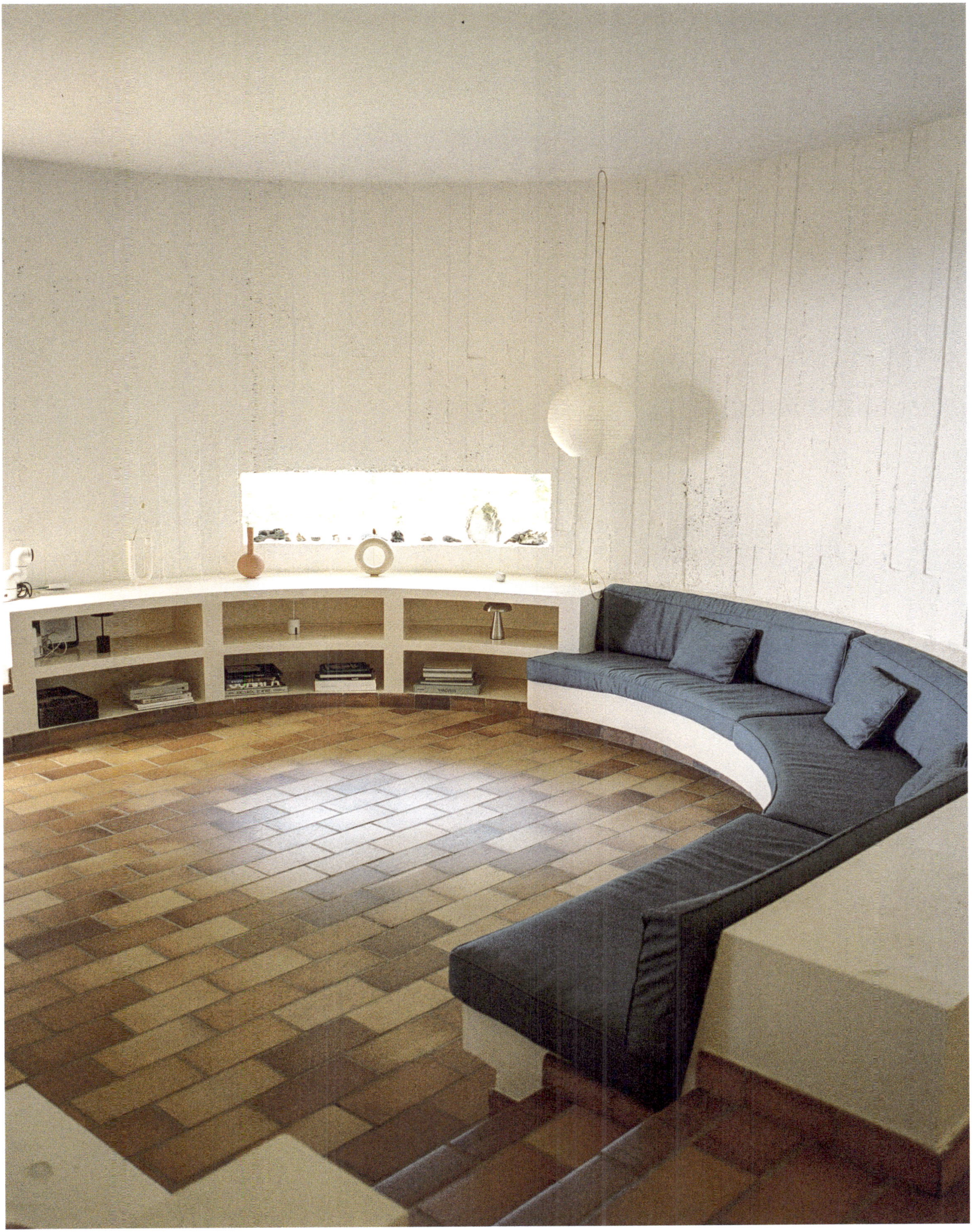

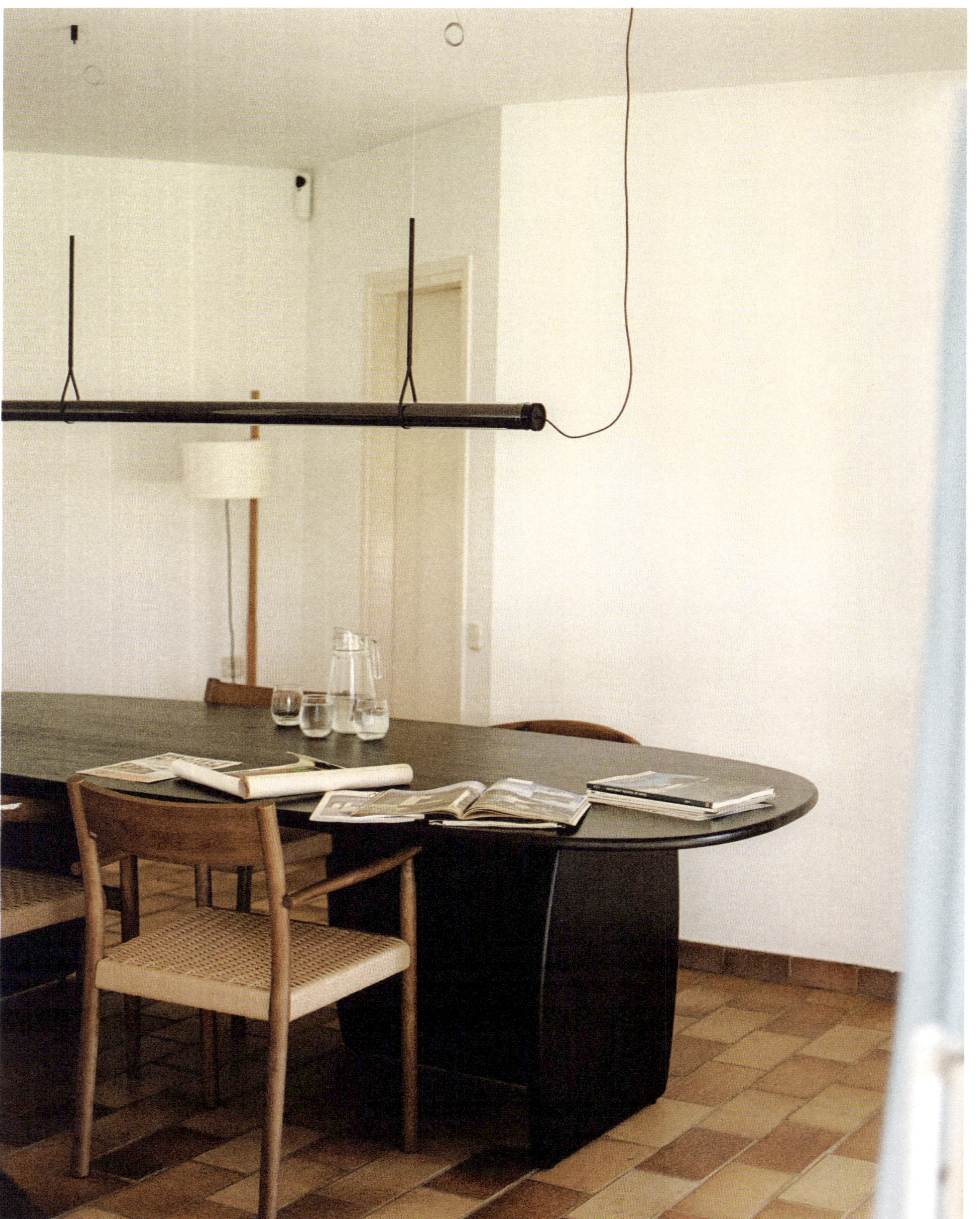

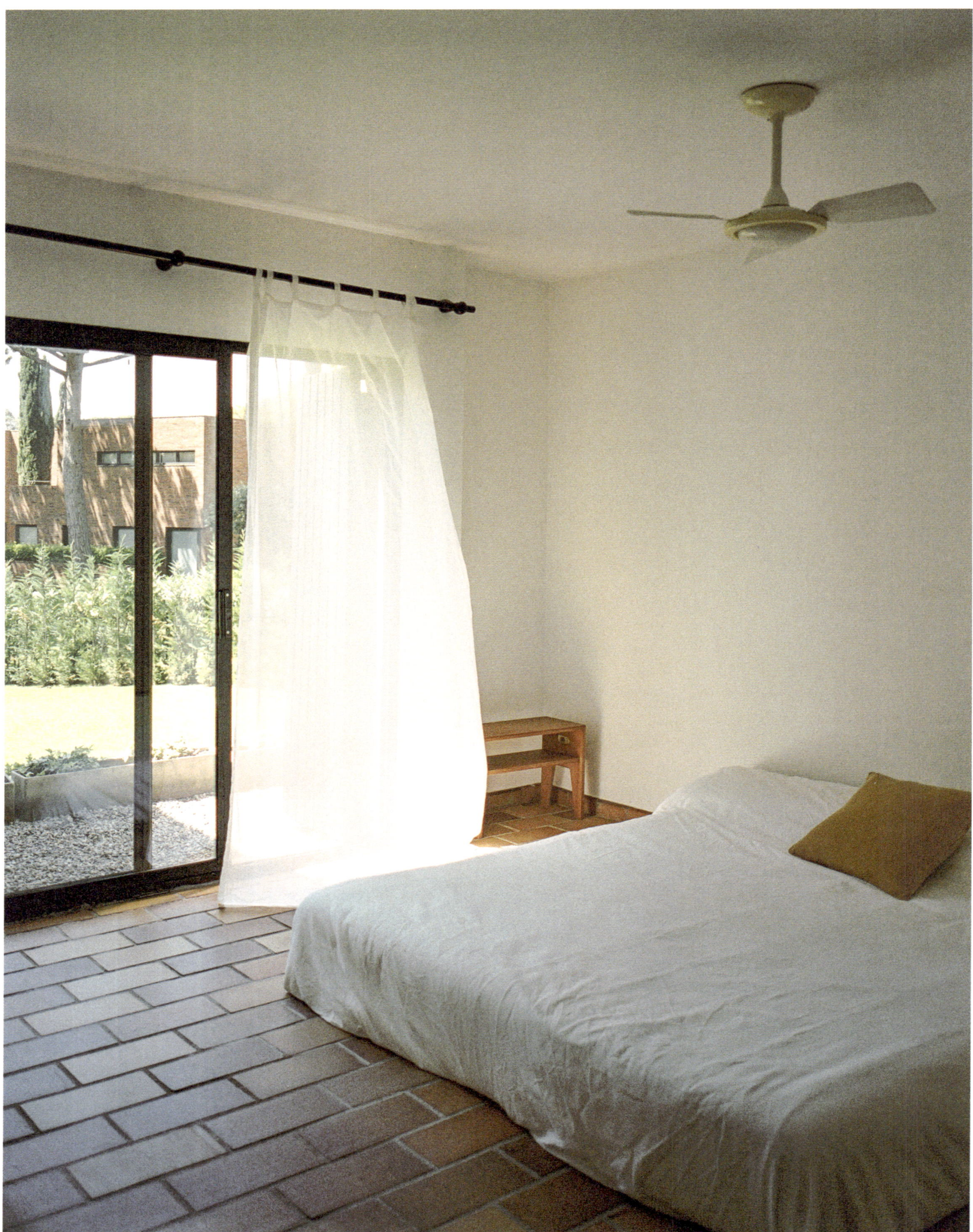

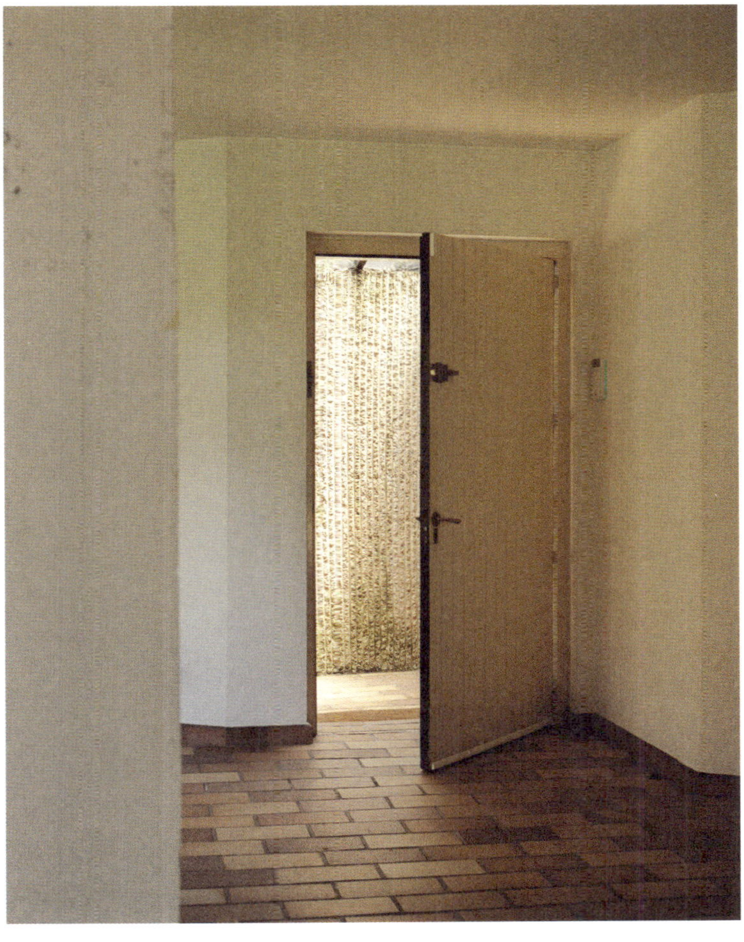

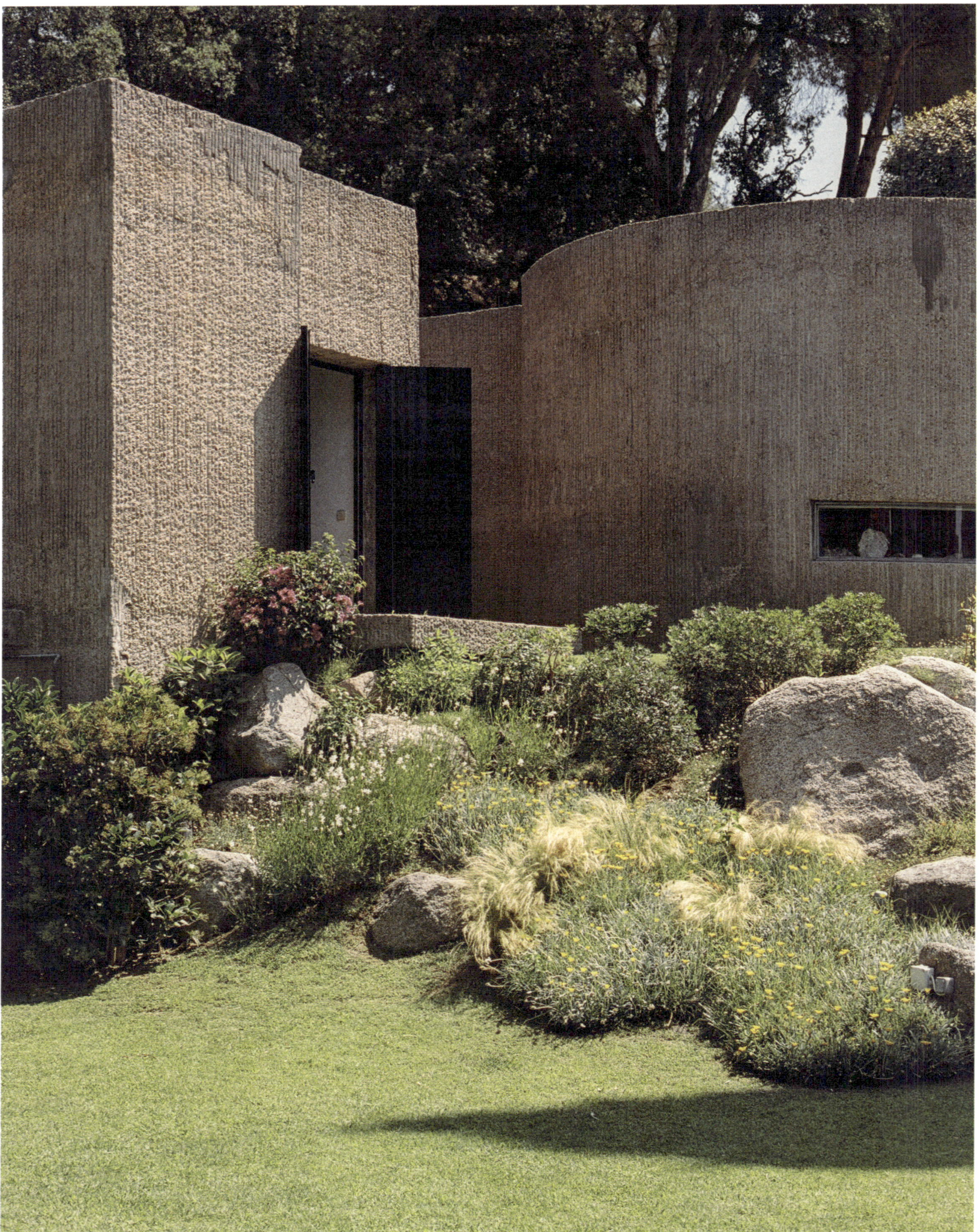

01

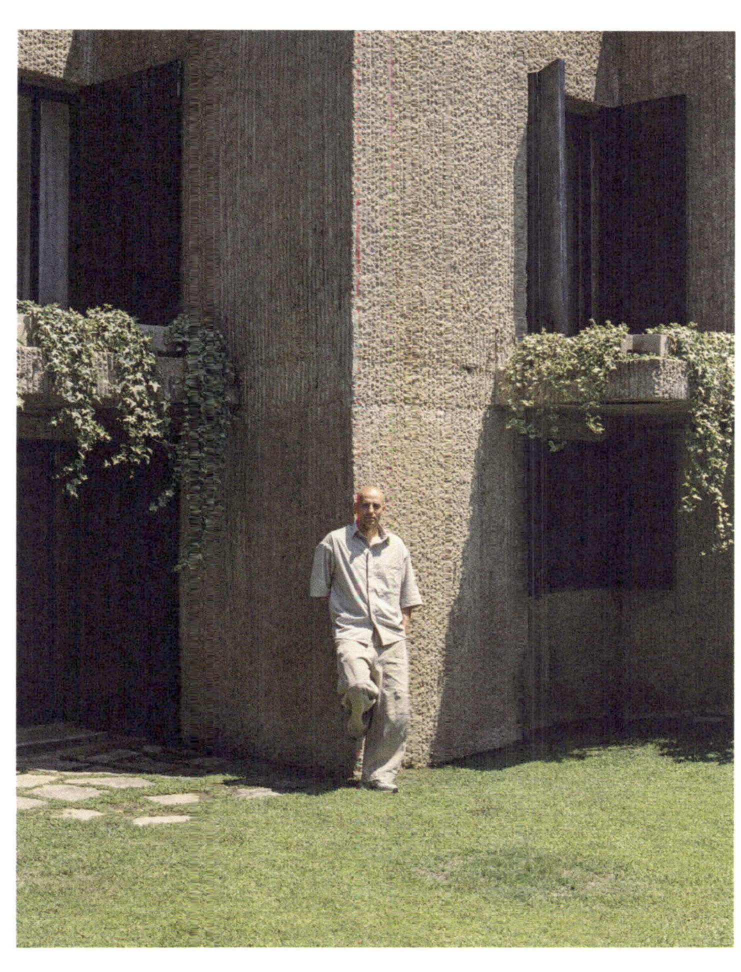

"Living with concrete in this home means embracing the raw, honest nature of the material itself. Here, concrete is not just structural, it's elemental. It speaks to the fusion between nature and the human hand, between permanence and transformation. Living with concrete here is residing within a dialogue, one where material, memory, and the land speak the same language."

– *Ezequiel Pini*

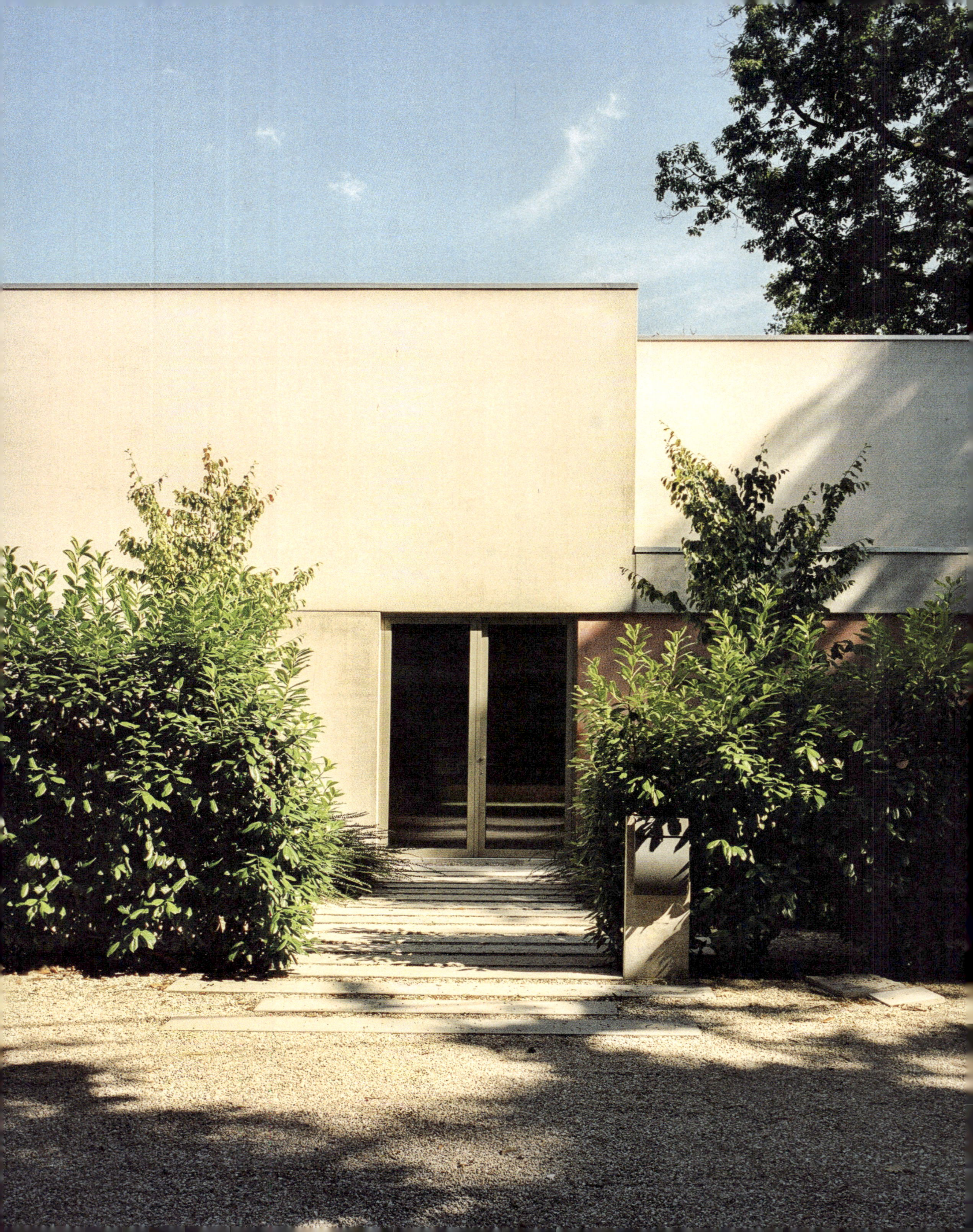

House SS

Belgium

This house doesn't try to hide its structure, it celebrates it. Concrete, glass, wood, each material is allowed to speak clearly. The spaces are wide and open, yet never feel cold. And light moves through the building slowly, across floors, walls, and ceilings. The layout is generous and fluid. From the first step inside, everything feels aligned.

The house was designed by the couple who live here. One of them has roots in the concrete industry, and the couple is expanding the family business to finish the residential building, from concept to completion. Together, they shaped every part of the process themselves, from sketches to structure. "We knew what we wanted", they say. "But it was not always easy to find people who understood it."

Their vision was precise. They were drawn to the calm geometry and generous proportions of American houses from the 1970s. That influence is clear in the warm timber ceilings, the sculptural massing, and the expansive, continuous spaces. They chose concrete not for its harshness, but for its depth and tone. In this case, even the mix was adjusted. A soft pink pigment was added to the concrete, giving the house a warm, muted presence.

From the street, the house reveals little. The front façade is composed, closed, and almost abstract. And openings are minimal and deliberate. It is only after entering that the full scale of the house becomes clear. The rear opens dramatically onto the garden, with a fourteen-metre-wide glass wall spanning the entire back of the house, dissolving the boundary between interior and landscape.

The living spaces are open and connected, designed around flow rather than corridors. The kitchen, dining area, and lounge all follow one continuous gesture. At the heart of the plan stands a grand piano, placed even before the house was drawn. Its presence helped shape the proportions of the main room. It now anchors the space without dominating it.

A concrete swimming pool stretches along the garden side, echoing the material language of the house itself. Large sliding panels open fully, blurring any distinction between inside and outside. The transition is effortless and intentional. This is a house made for movement, for light, and for everyday rituals.

Natural light plays a central role. It enters from above, from the sides, and from the long rear opening. And it moves slowly across surfaces. The timber ceilings add warmth, softening the concrete and extending the tones of the floors and walls. The result is both technical and tactile, minimal yet full of atmosphere.

The building process required precision and patience. Custom concrete blocks were produced for the façade and finishing details had to align perfectly. Because of the highly specific materials and forms, it took time to find the right collaborators. The house was not easy to build, but that was never the goal.

This is not a house that speaks loudly. It reveals itself through rhythm and stillness: in the soft edge of a shadow, in the pink hue of a concrete wall at sunset, in how one space flows naturally into the next. The architecture holds everything in place, quietly and confidently.

Project: House SS
Location: Belgium
Year of construction: 2021
Floor area: 300 m^2
Residents: Katleen Stieglitz and Cynthia Stroomer
Residents' professions: owner of Preton and architecture student

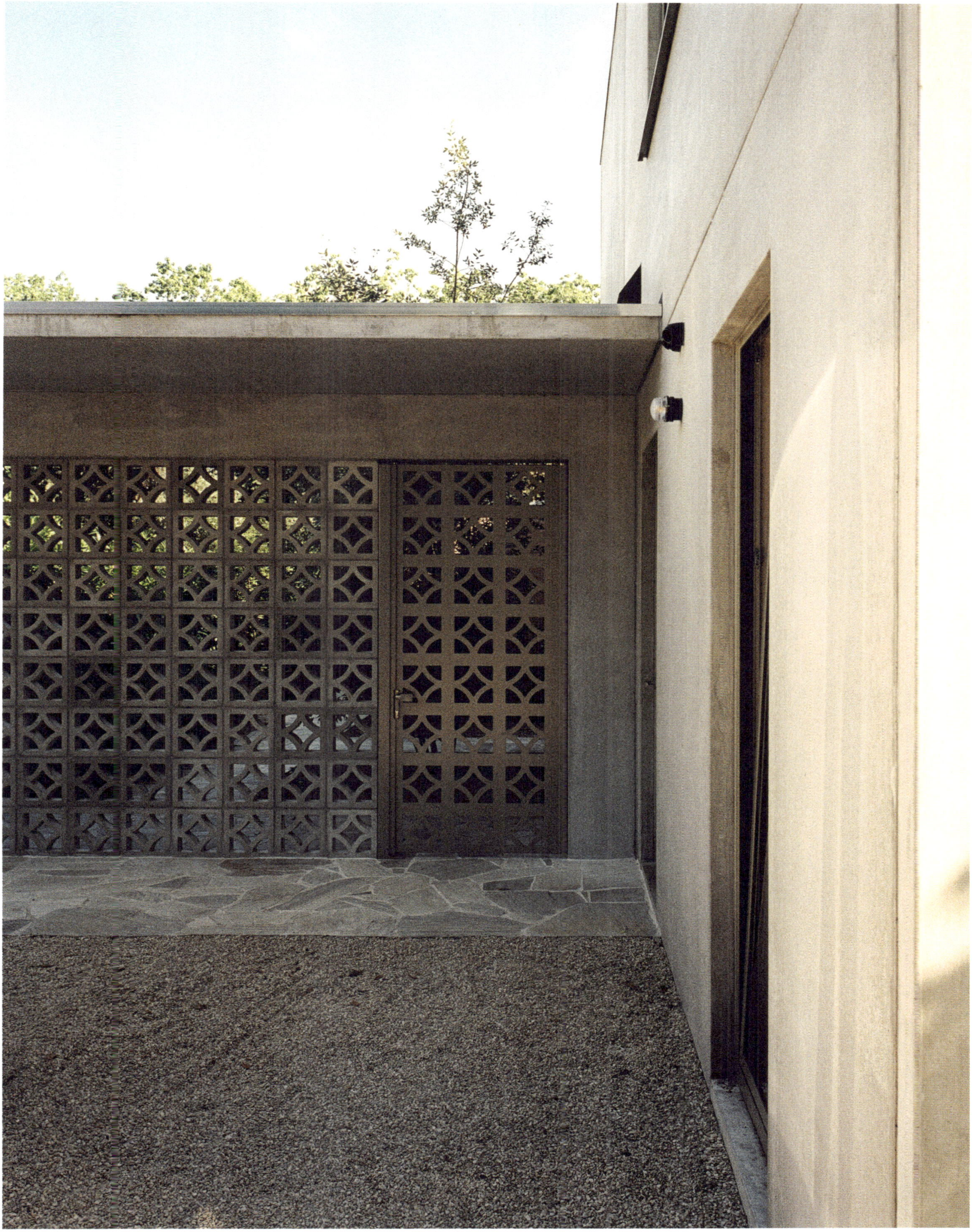

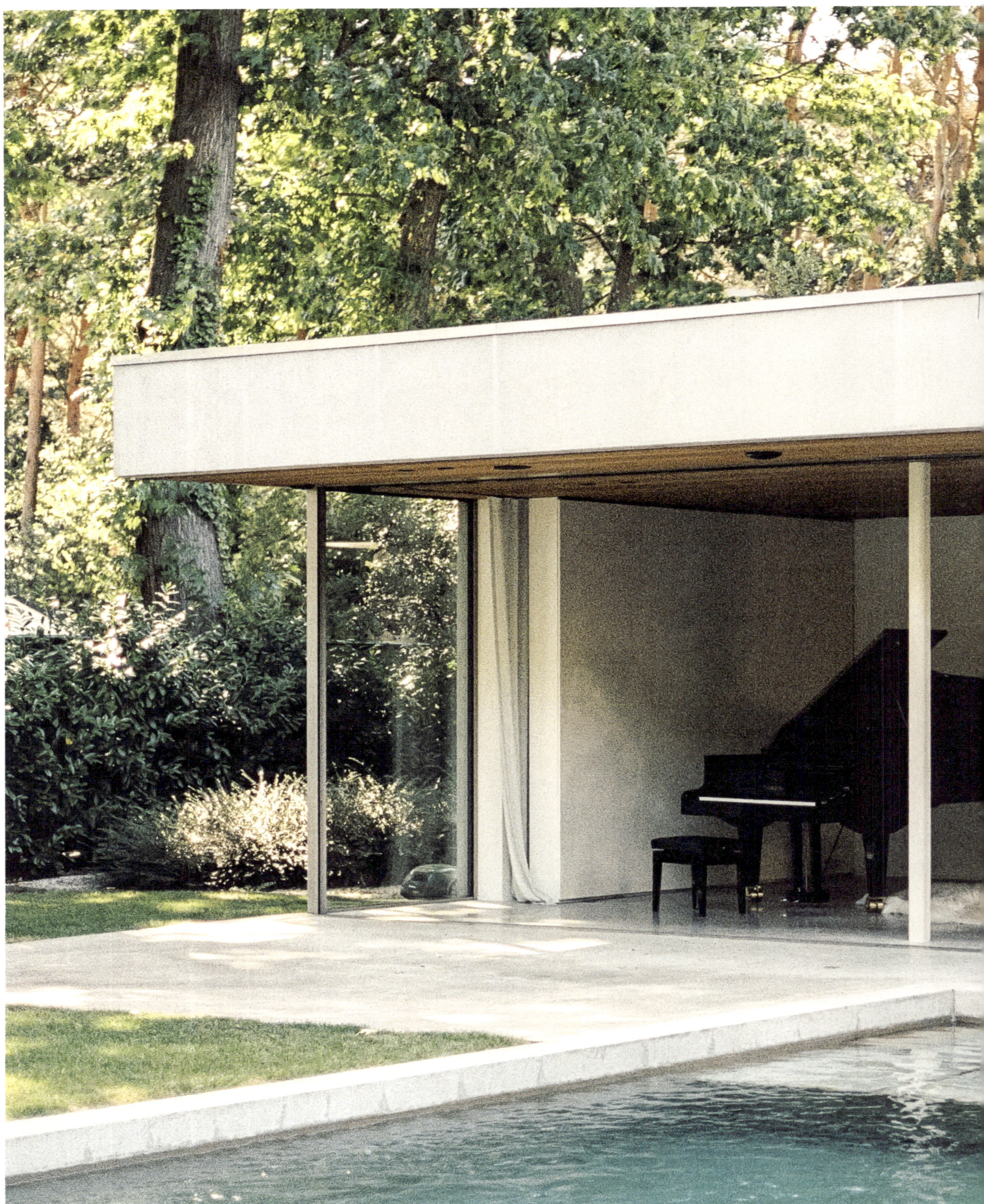

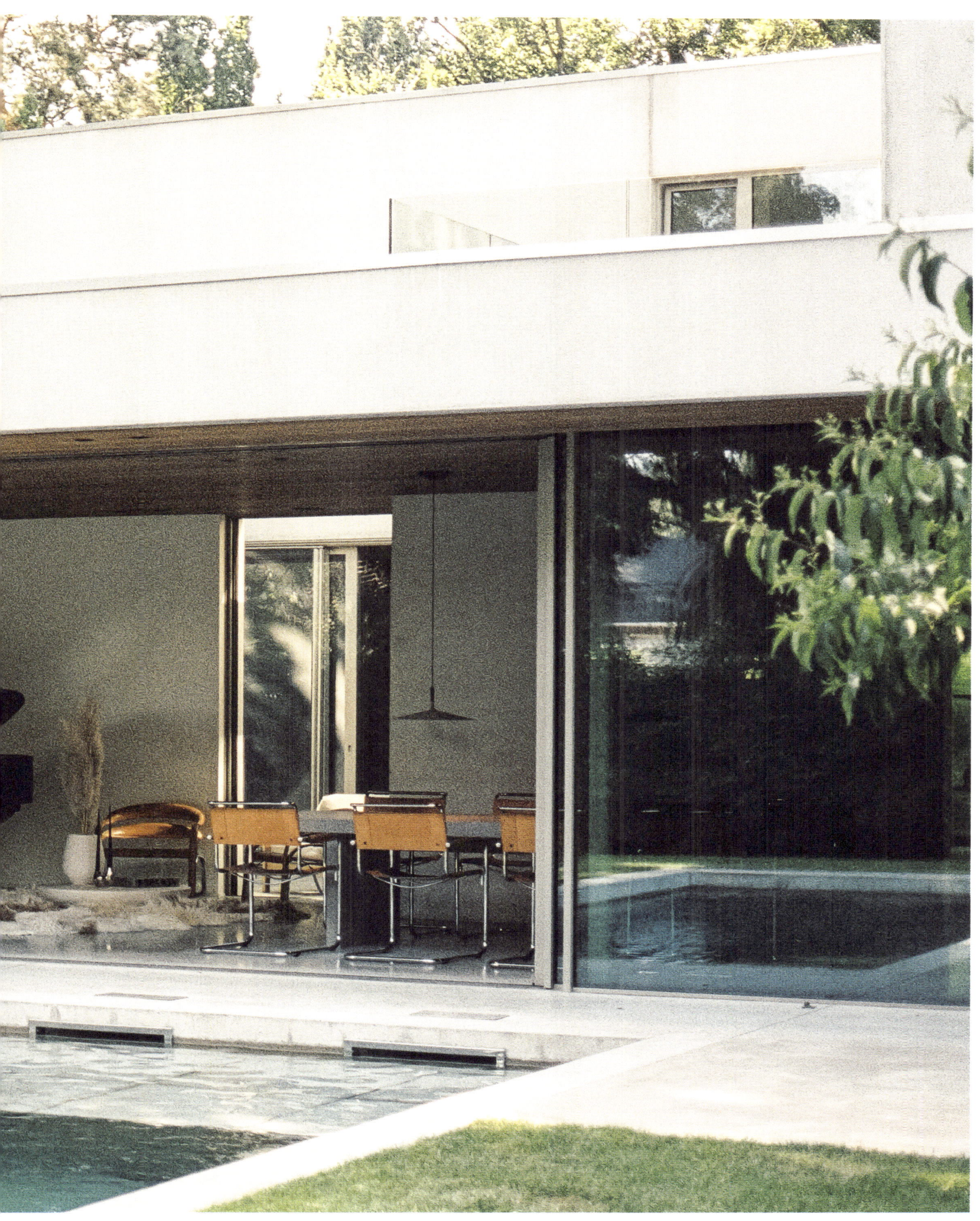

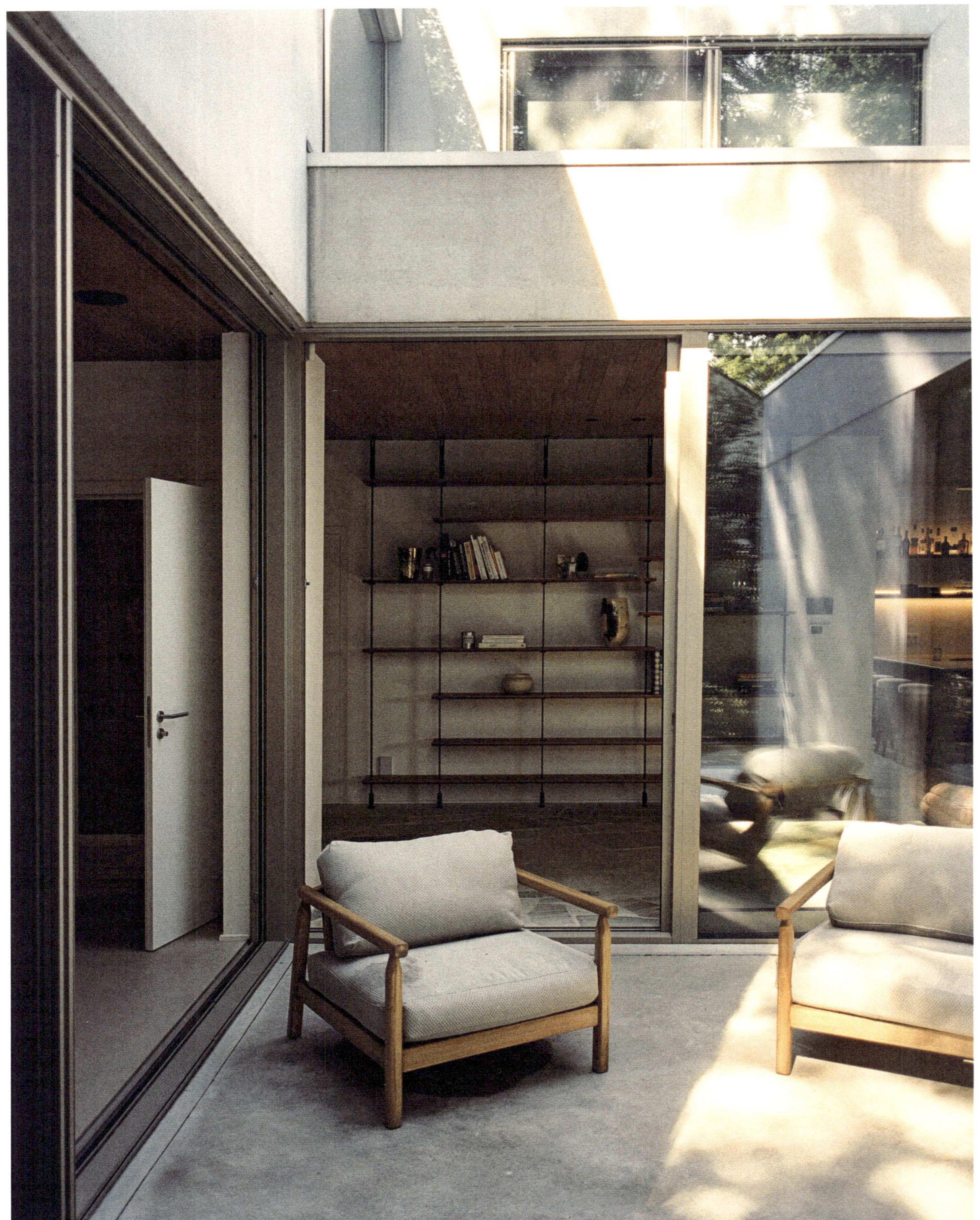

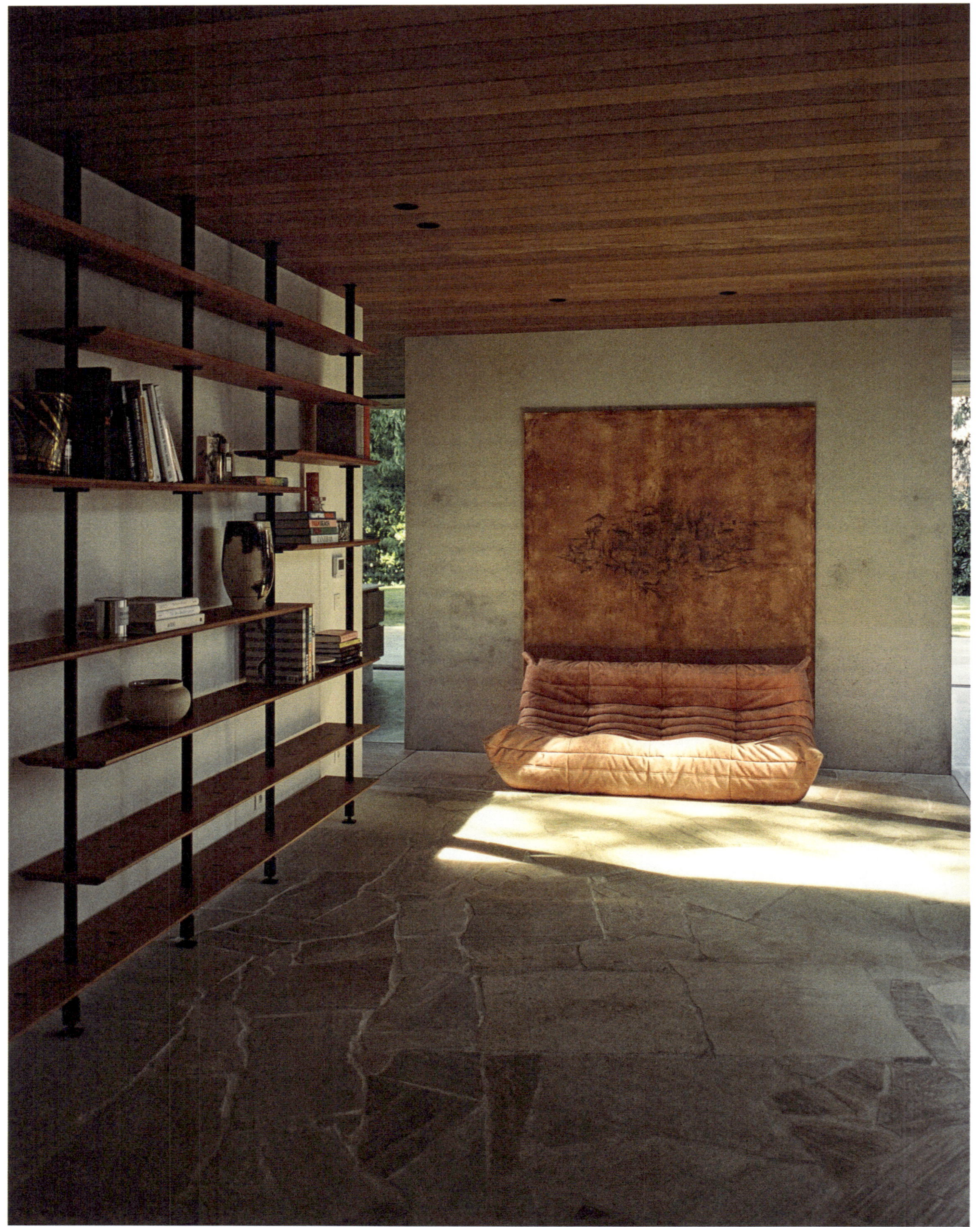

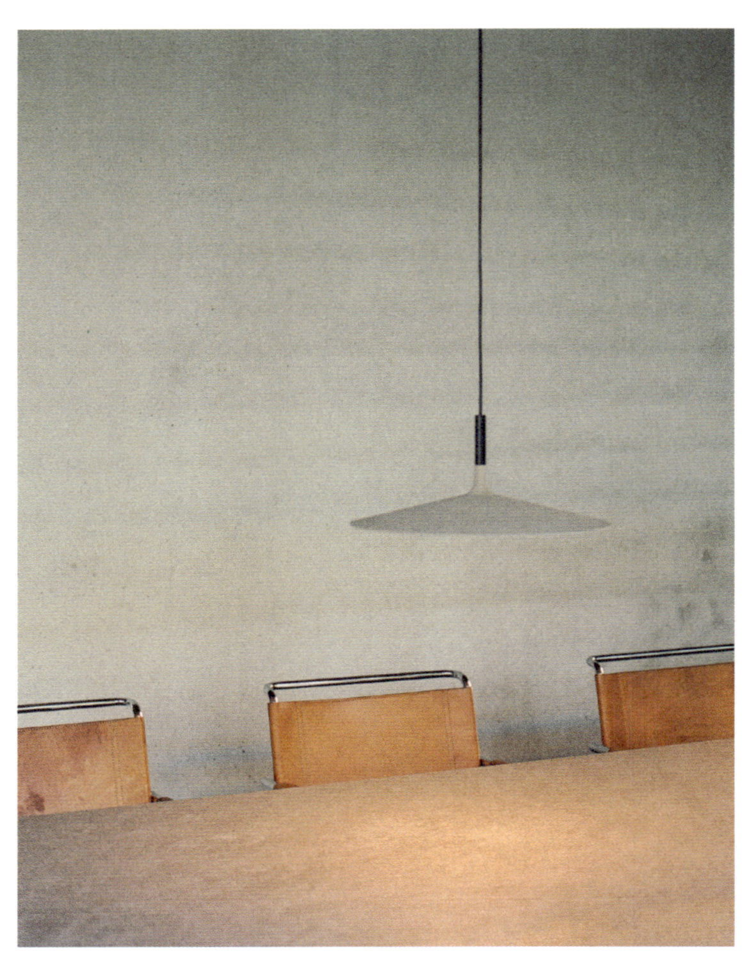

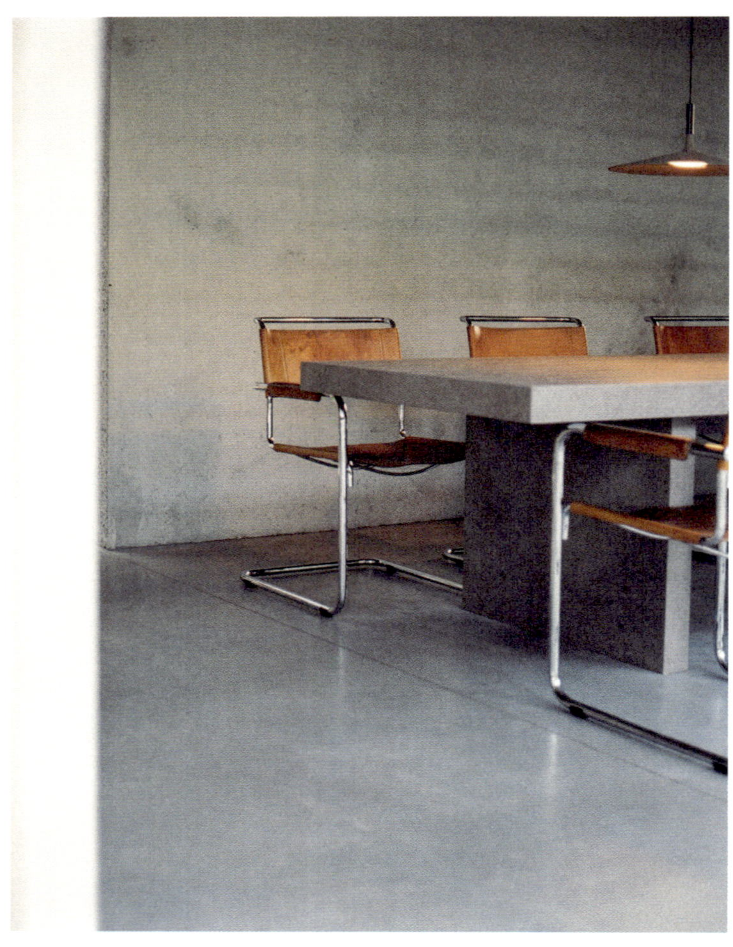

13

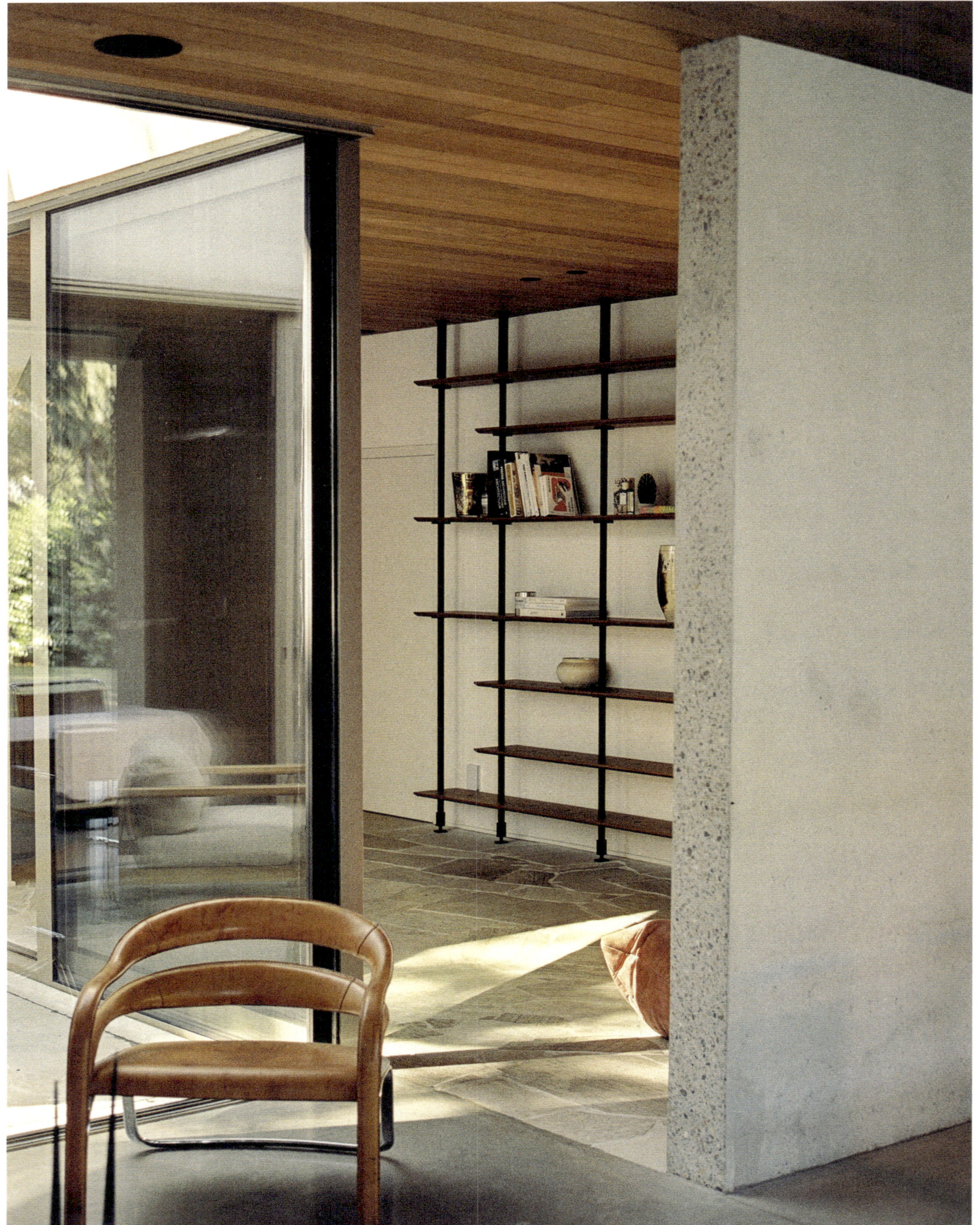

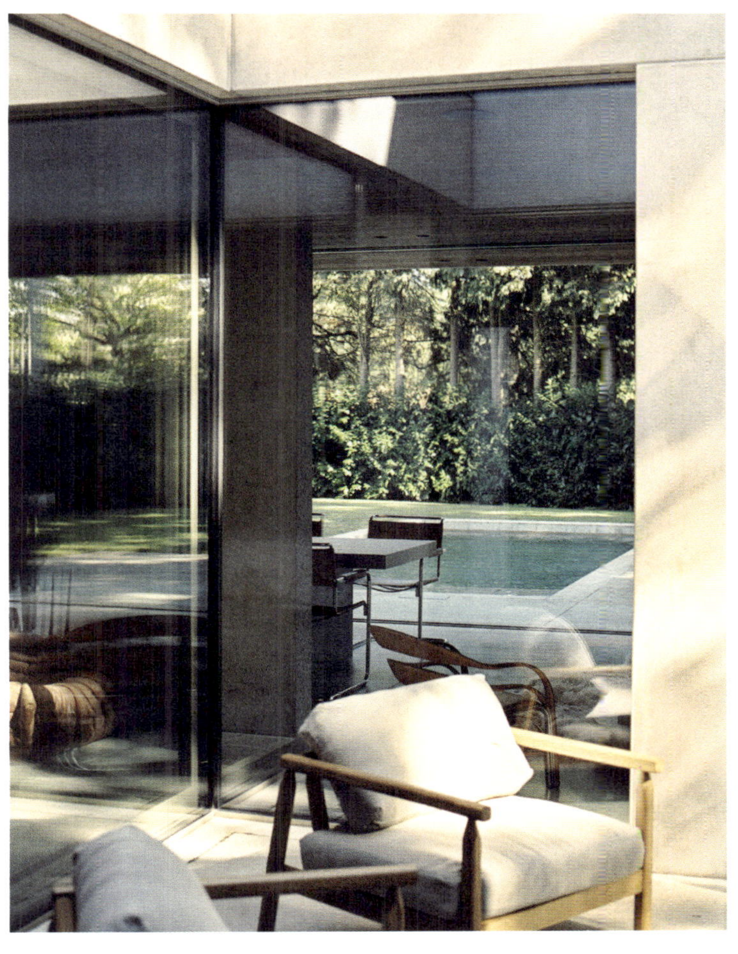

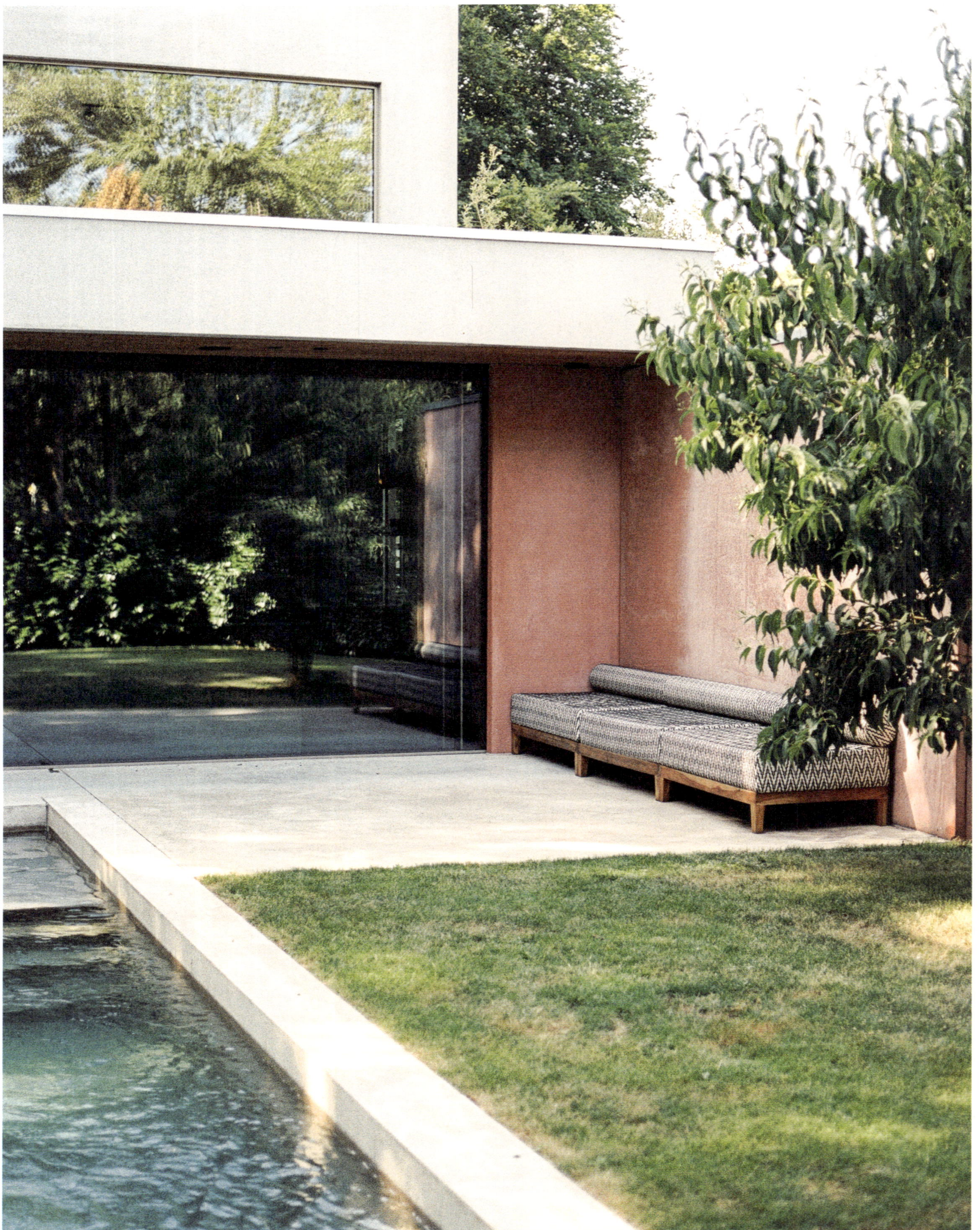

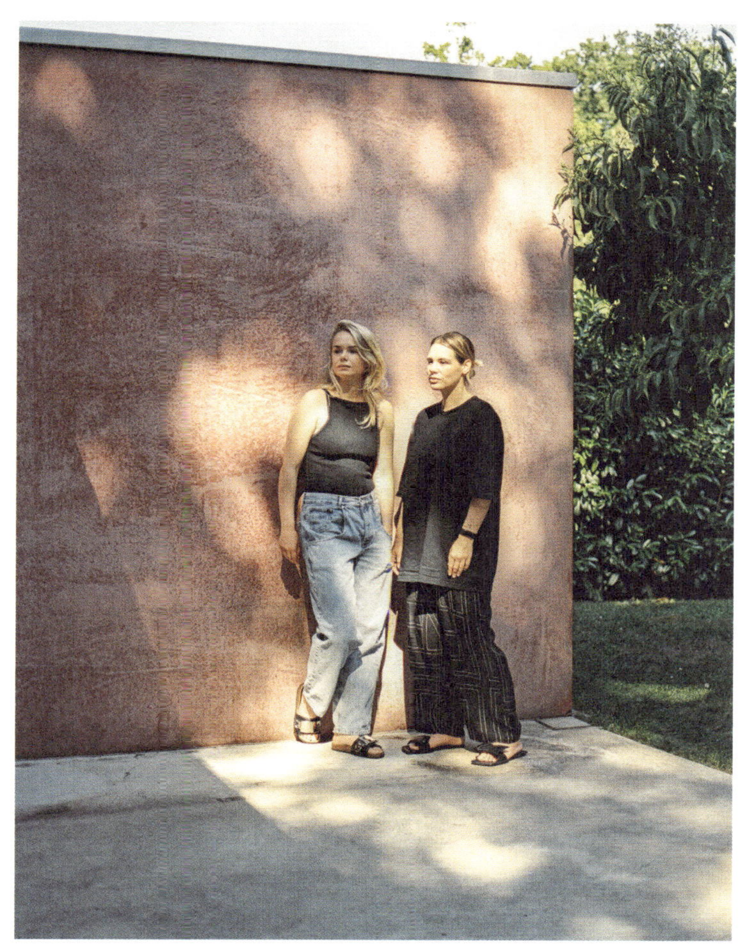

"To live with concrete is to find calm in simplicity. It makes our house feel timeless, yet open to light and life."

– Katleen Stieglitz and Cynthia Stroomer

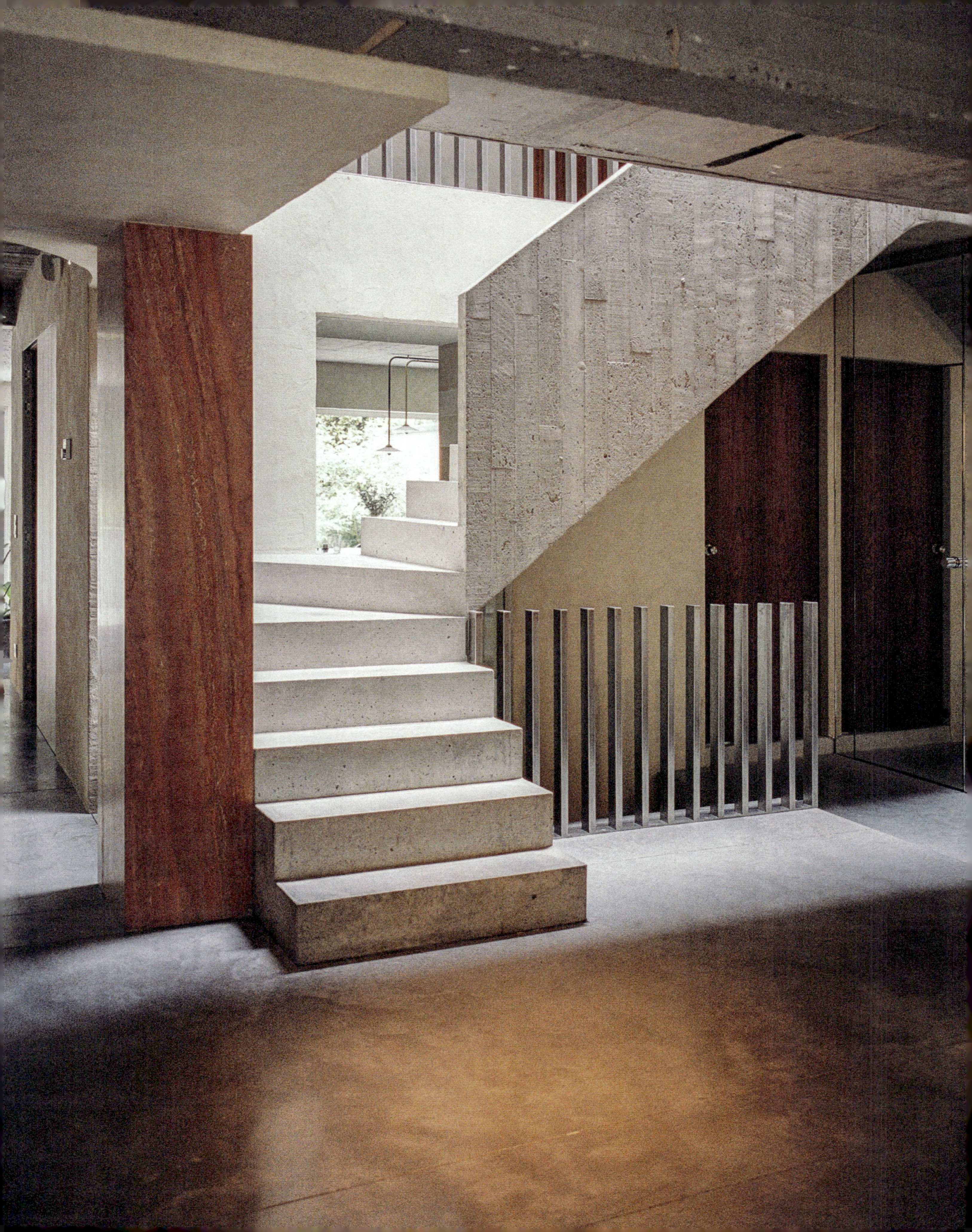

House WESP

Belgium

The new owners weren't looking for concrete, at least not consciously. The goal was to find a horizontal house in Brussels, close to the children's school, with access to outdoor space or the potential to create it. After years in a typical vertical Brussels townhouse, they were looking for something closer to ground level. The idea of a concrete structure was present right from the beginning, not as a requirement, but as part of the architectural language they were drawn to.

They had long admired the deconstructivist work of German architect Arno Brandlhuber, especially his Antivilla, and also the more restrained, structural thinking of Japanese architect Tadao Ando. Brandlhuber's raw approach to material and structure became a guiding reference in their mood board. In architect Arnout De Sutter, they found a partner who shared that sensibility. The renovation became a collaboration, shaped by shared ideas about how to peel back a 1970s home to its core, expose its concrete bones, and add raw interventions while creating a warm, functional space for a family of four.

The house had been designed and lived in by an engineer. Solidly built, recently renovated, and with a clear floor plan, it offered a lot of potential. Demolishing it was never on the table, not financially and certainly not conceptually. The structure was rational and clean. And when the dropped ceilings were removed, the original concrete revealed itself with calm precision. The bones were good. There were no surprises.

The renovation focused on subtraction. Old materials were removed, new openings were introduced, and the concrete frame was left visible. You now see it clearly in the central column, the ceiling lines, and the staircase. It's not polished or decorative, it just is.

A wooden staircase was replaced by a concrete one, bordered by a stainless steel handrail. Above it, a skylight was added to bring natural light deep into the heart of the home. The stair now defines the central hall, connecting the different floors.

The layout avoids corridors. Instead, spaces flow into one another. And from the outside, the house still appears modest and self-contained, but once inside, it opens up in multiple directions. Views extend to the garden and to the canopy of trees above. The materials are restrained: lime plaster, exposed concrete, cellulose ceiling insulation, aluminium details, American oak, and terracotta travertine on the column.

The interior is minimal but not cold. Built-in elements maintain a sense of order. And objects are few and carefully chosen: a chair, a ceramic piece, a table. Each thing has its place, and there is space around it. "It doesn't have to be full", they say. "We want it to breathe."

One resident works in Belgian fashion and design, advocating for creativity and sustainability at the European level. And neither of them has a background in architecture, but decisions were made with clarity and care. Style was never imposed. Every element had to feel right.

Their daughters move freely through the house. The structure is open, allowing space for play, calm, and routine. There is room to move and to rest, and it feels spacious but not distant. Everything is connected, and nothing is sealed off.

This house is not showy; it doesn't push a concept or chase a trend. It is a home that respects its past and makes space for the present. A structure that has been opened, refined, and brought back to life, quietly, thoughtfully, and without force.

Project: House WESP
Location: Belgium
Architect: Arnout De Sutter
Year of construction: 1974
Year of purchase: 2022
Floor area: 370 m²
Resident: Elke Timmerman
Resident's profession: international and business relations

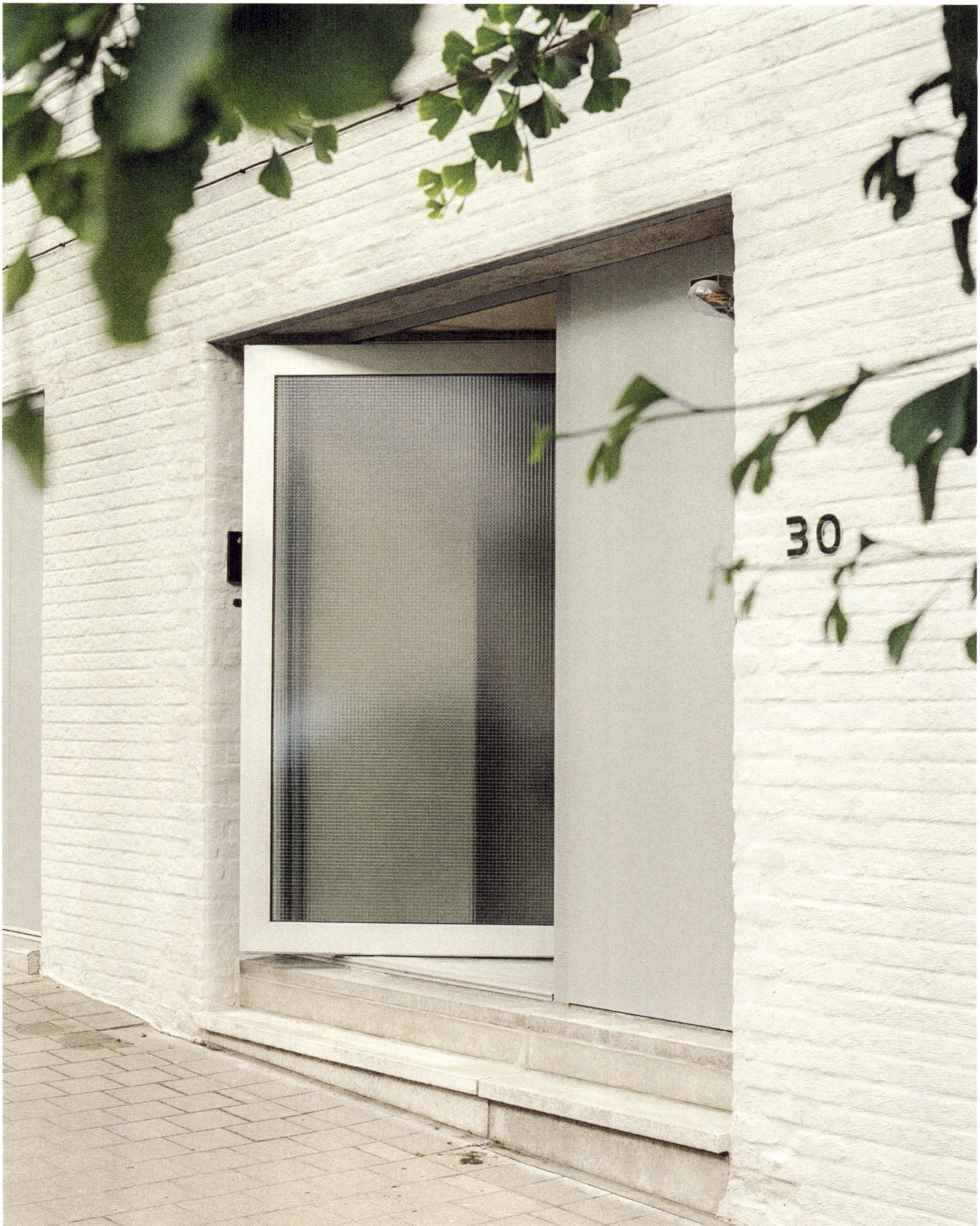

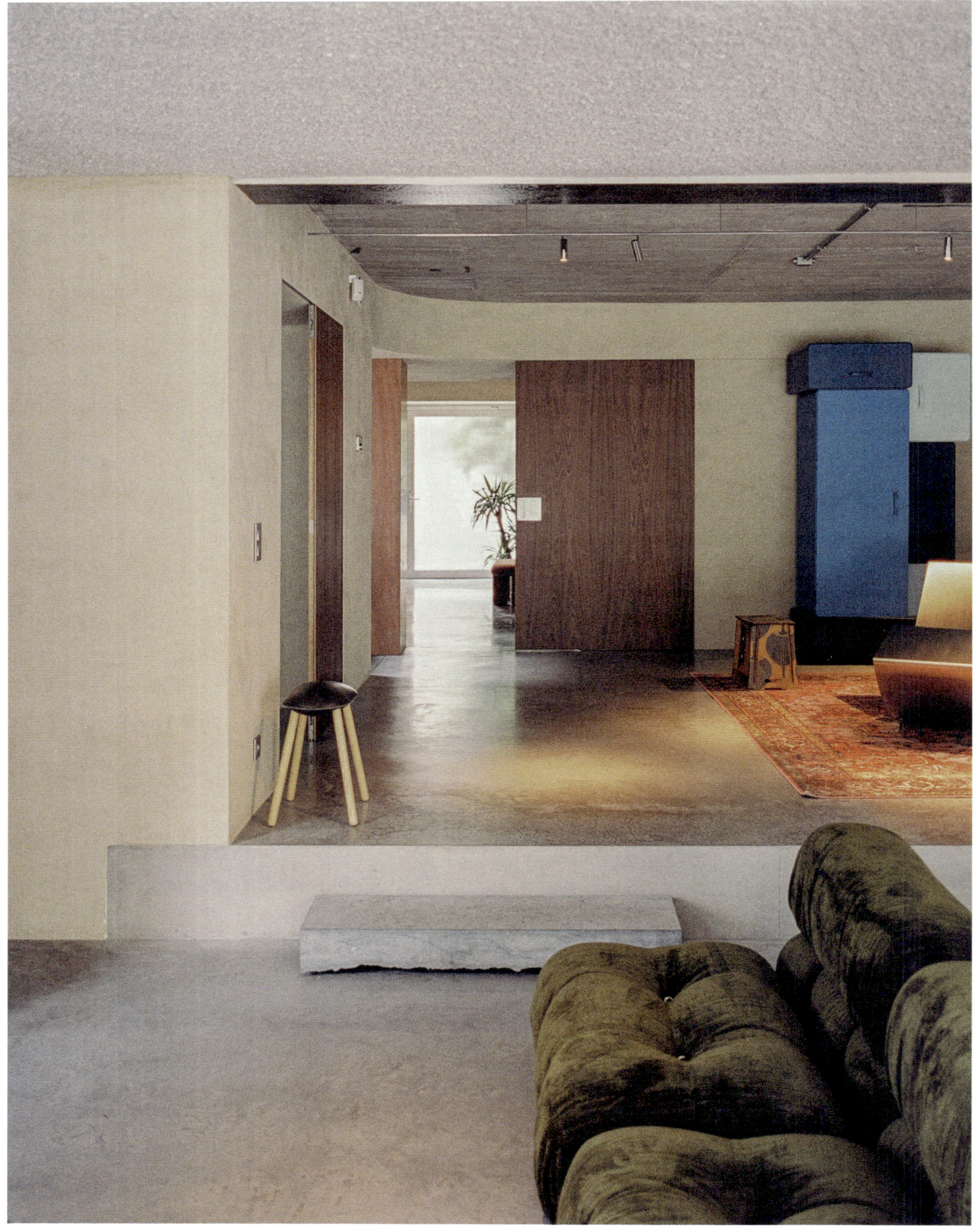

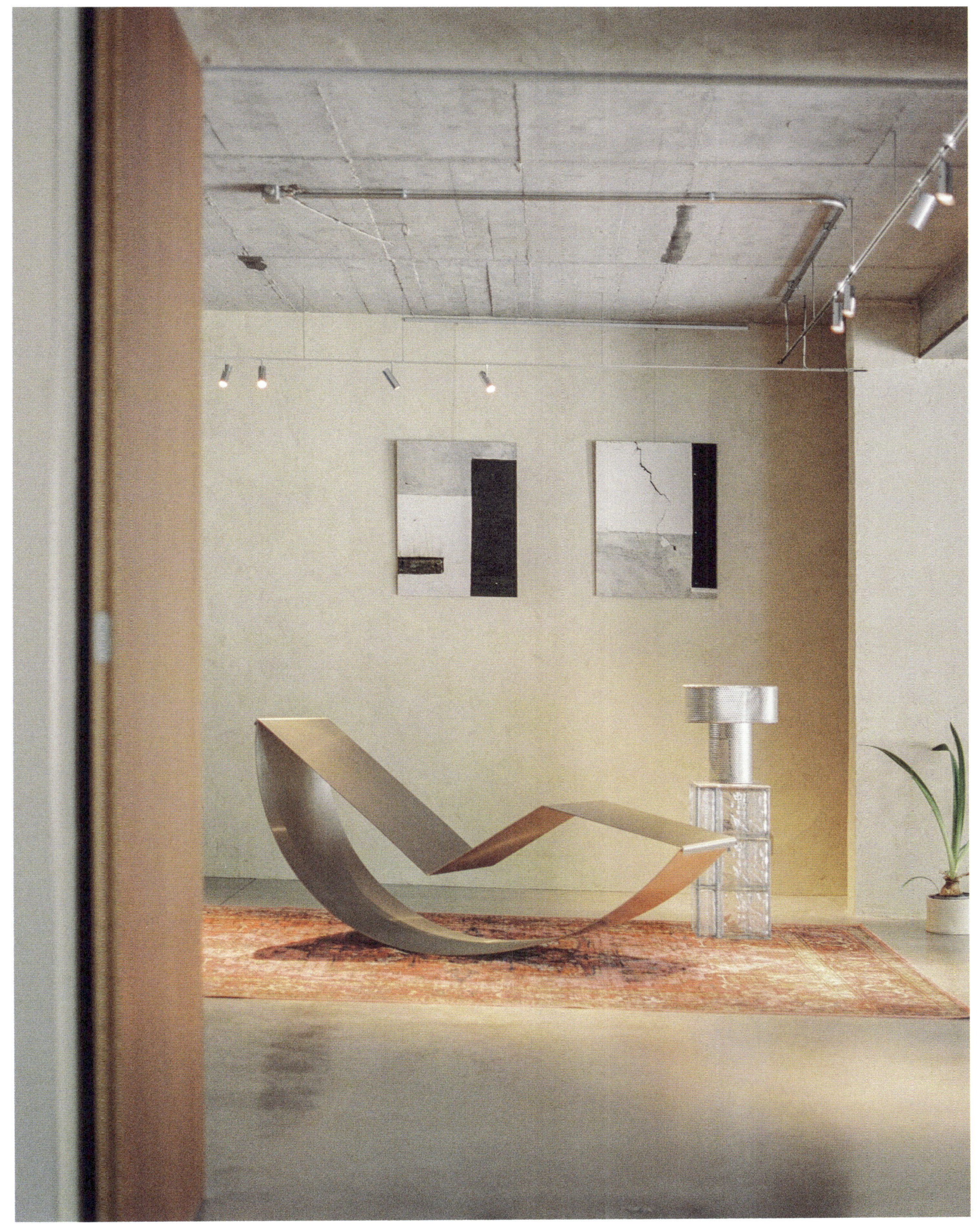

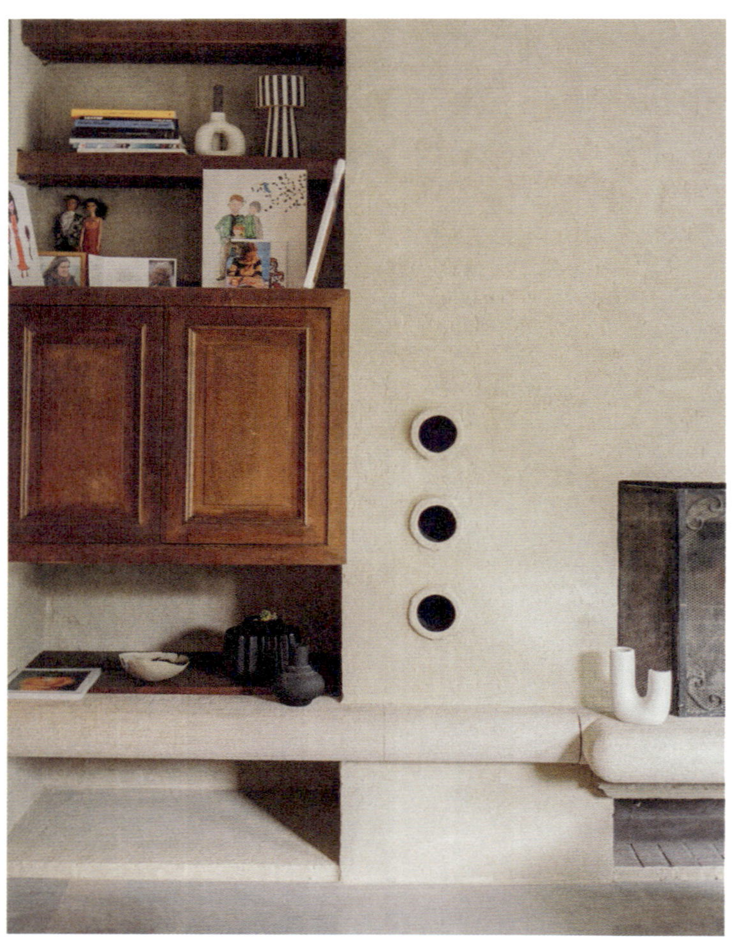

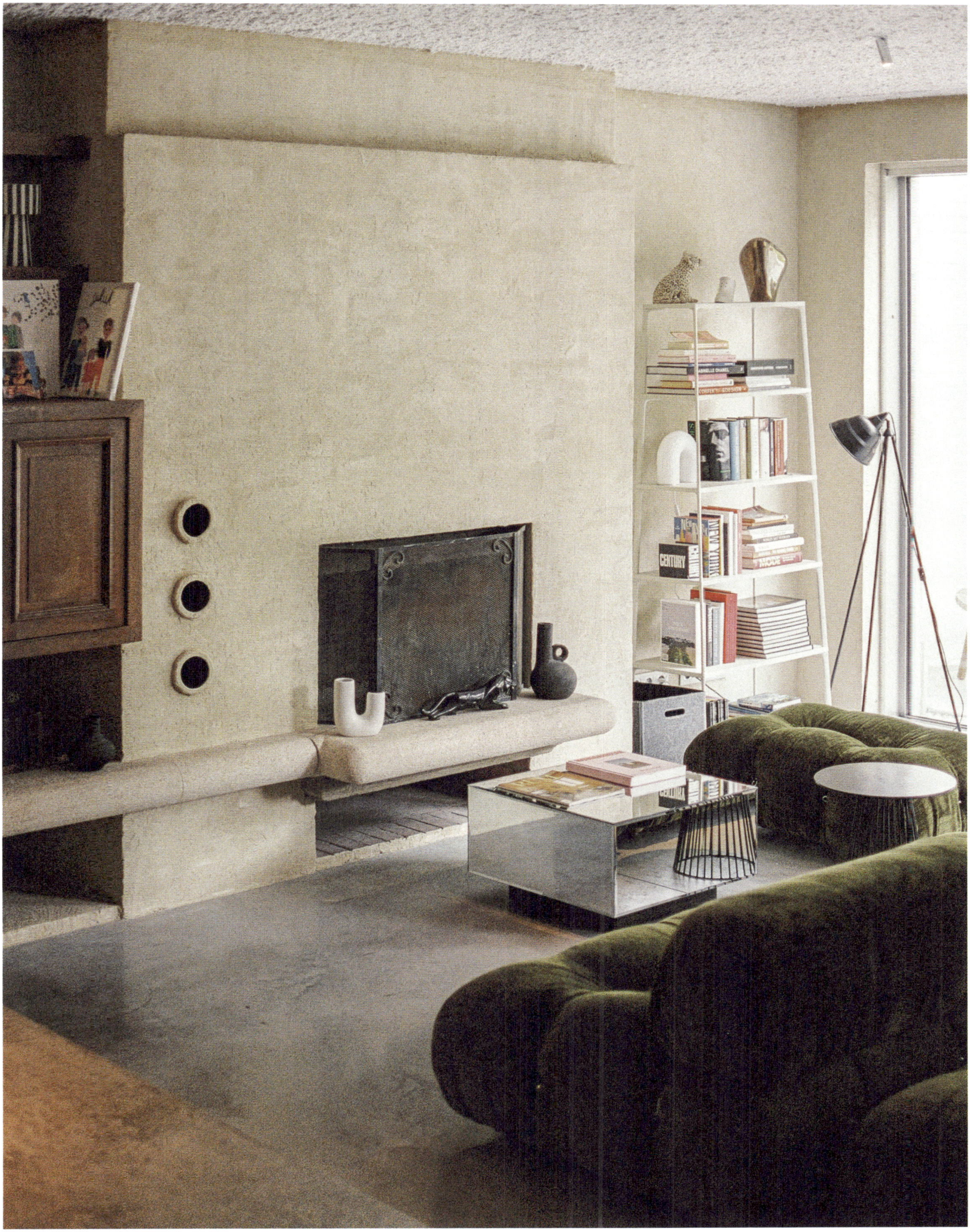

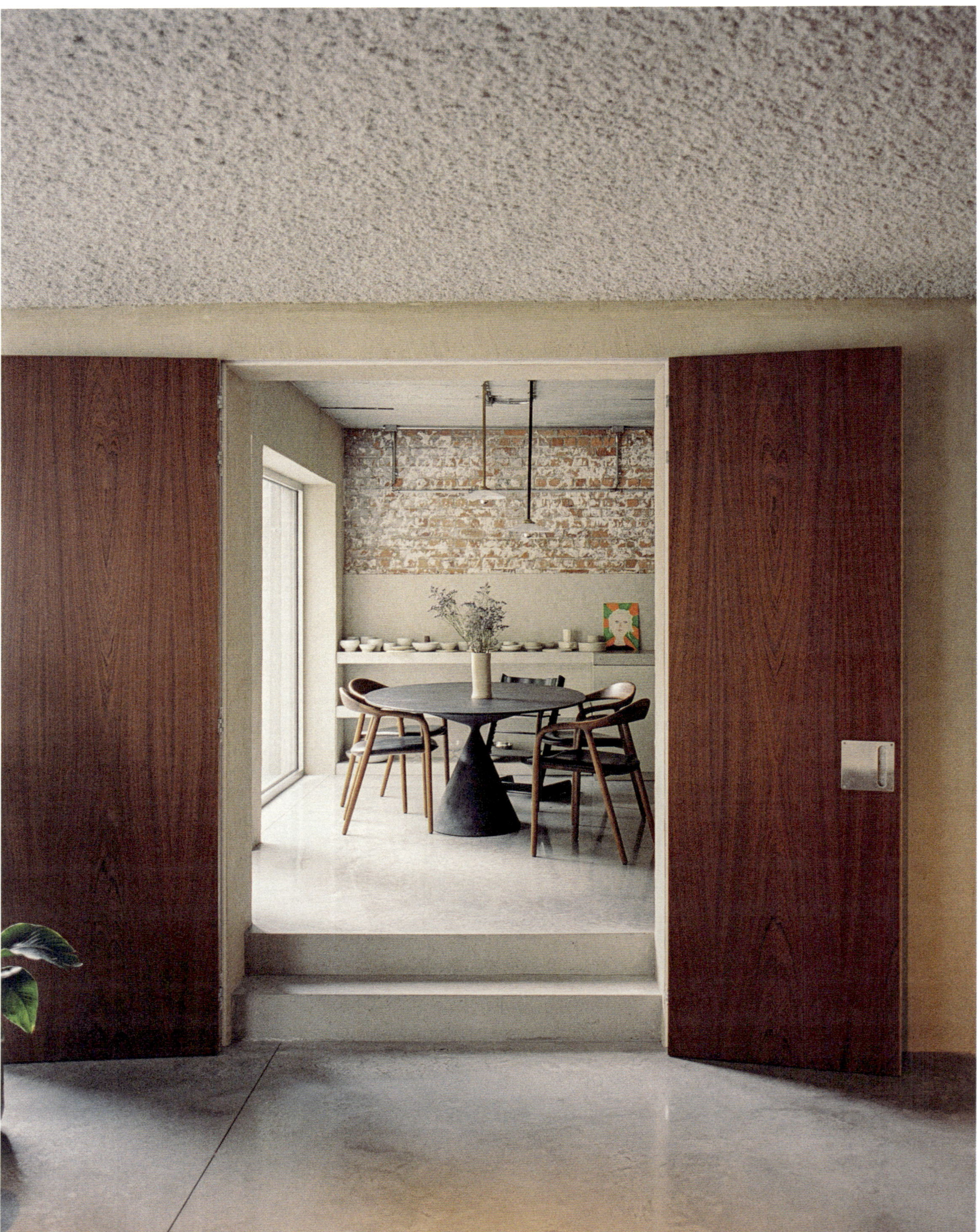

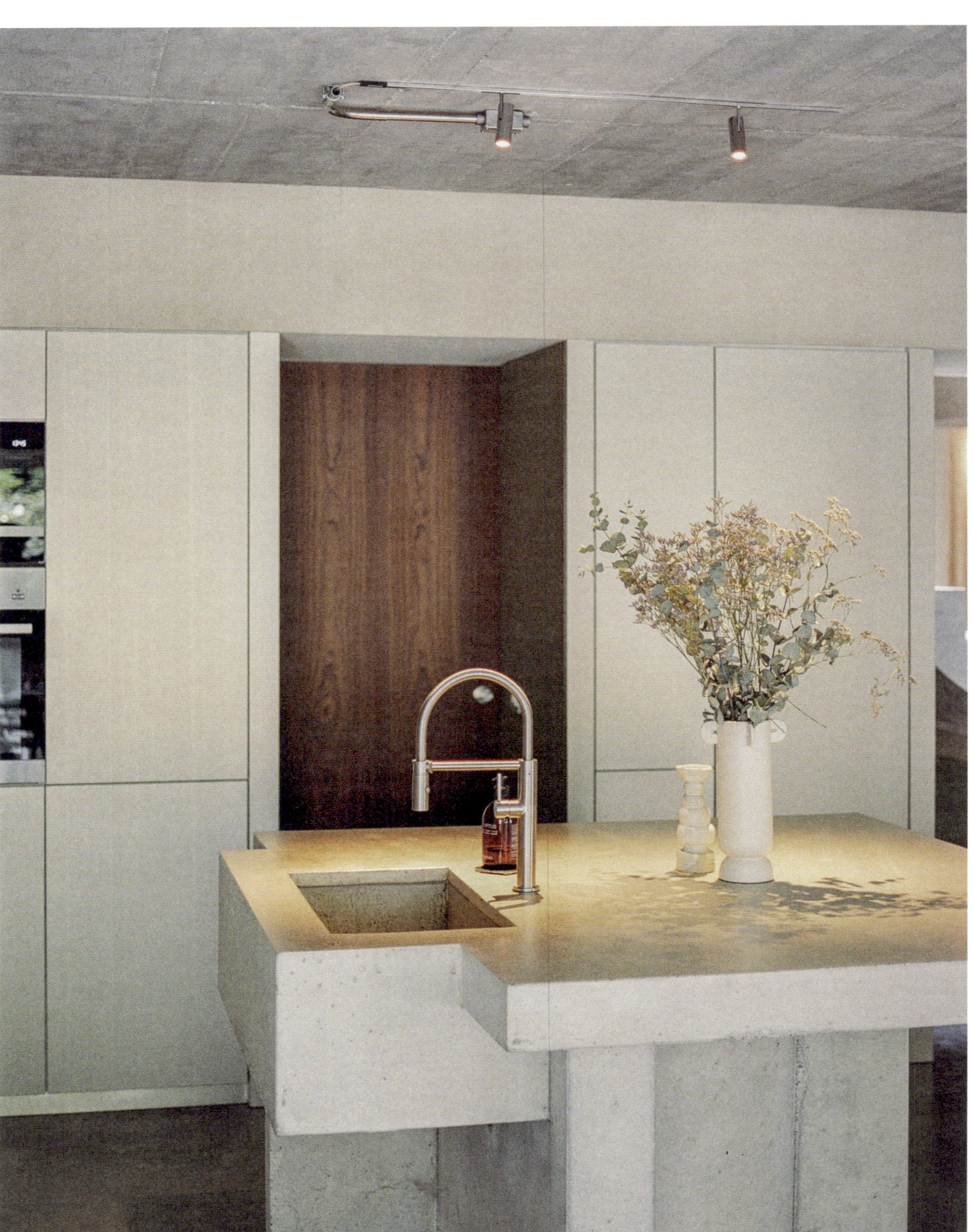

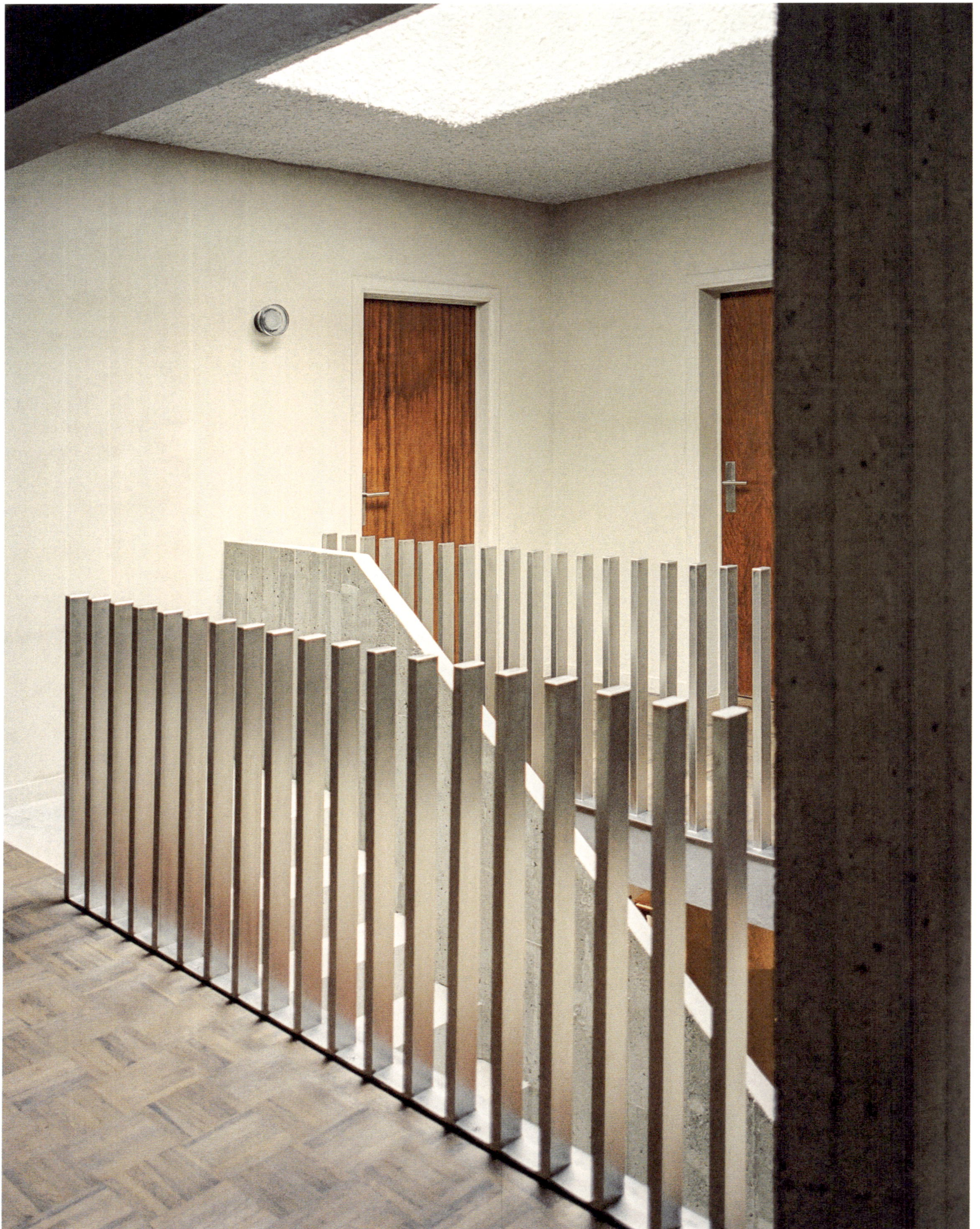

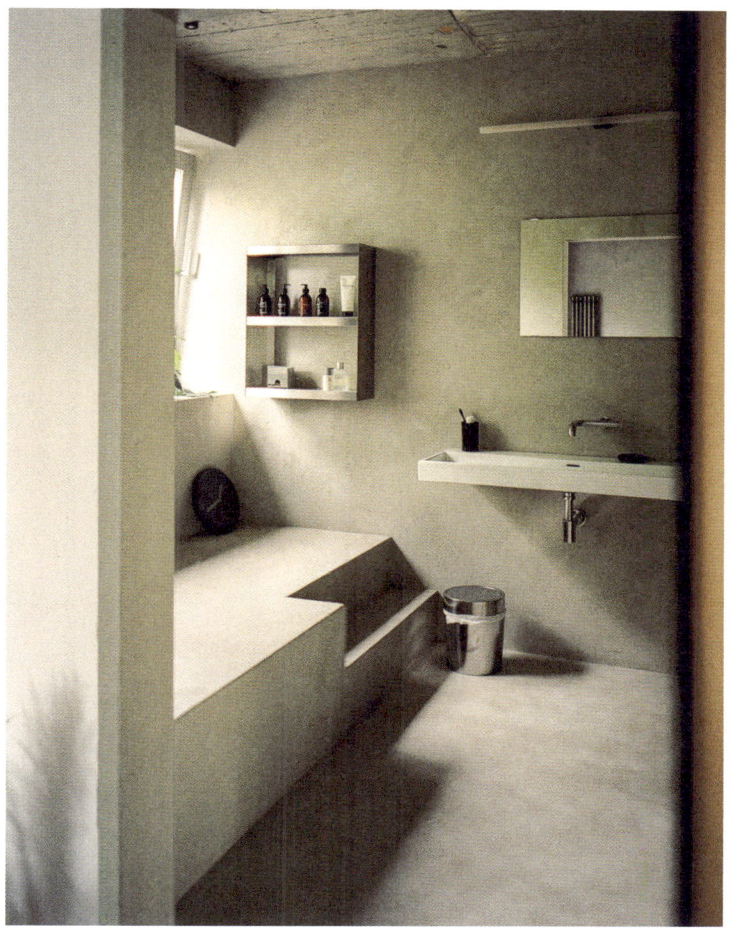

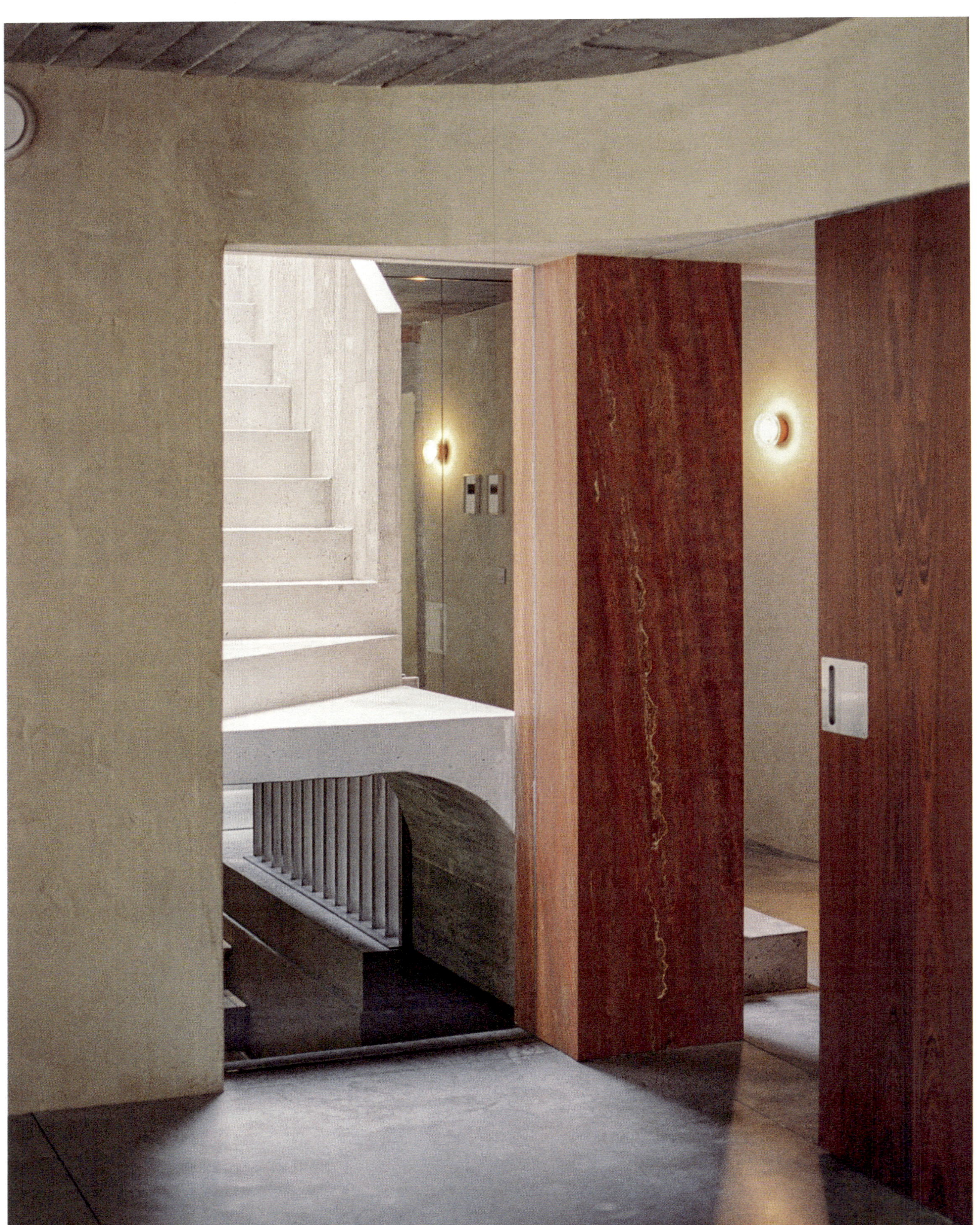

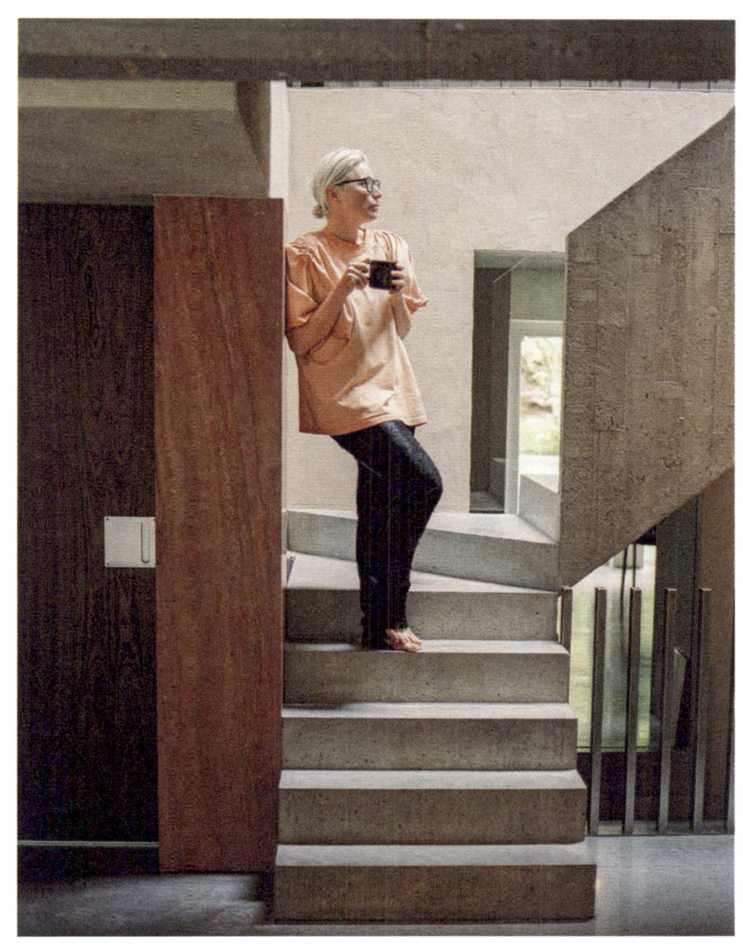

"The strength and beauty of concrete lies in the raw pure dissection of a structure, creating a new aesthetic and language, just as Martin Margiela dissected clothing and Arno Brandlhuber stripped buildings bare."

– Elke Timmerman

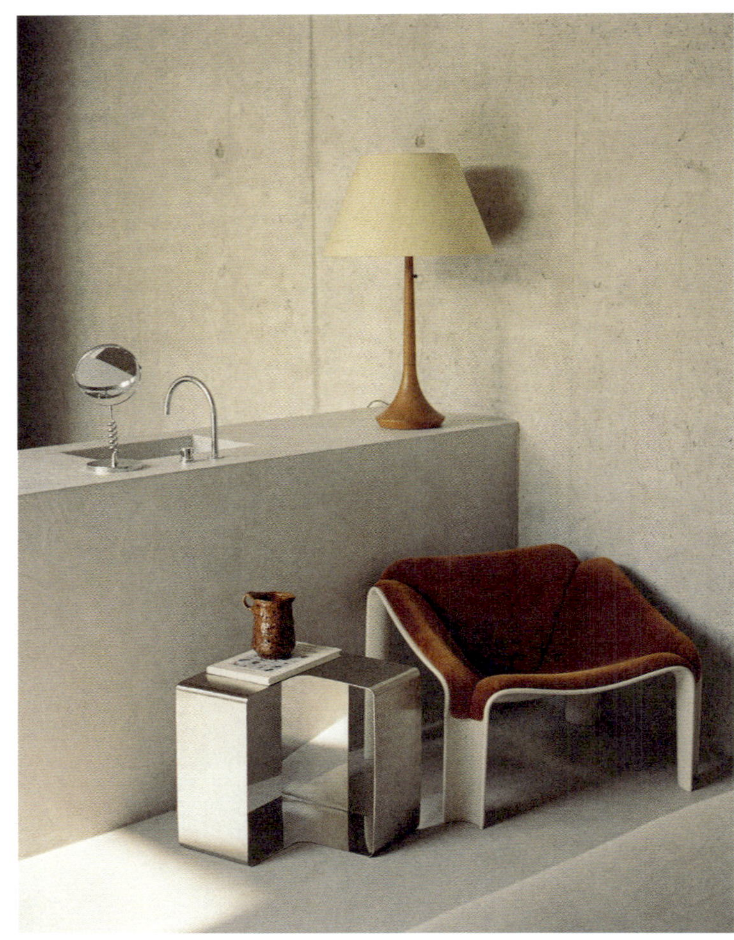

This book started with a quiet idea, a curiosity really. To see how people live with concrete. Not just how it's built, but how it's used, how it ages, how it feels. I didn't know exactly where it would take me. I just knew I wanted to look.

Thirteen houses later, I'm still surprised – by the honesty of the material, by the generosity of the people who live with it, and by how many ways there are to make something feel like home.

Each visit brought something different. Some houses were remote and quiet, while others sat in the heart of a city. Some were designed decades ago, others were only just finished. But all of them had one thing in common: intention. None of these spaces happened by accident, they were shaped, adjusted, thought through. And then lived in, which is something else entirely.

I feel lucky to have been welcomed into these homes, to be shown around, to sit at the kitchen table, and to listen. People spoke openly, not just about materials and light, but about choices, about time, about learning to live differently. That part left an impression.

Travelling to each of these places was a privilege. I saw cities I had never been to, villages I didn't know existed, hills, coasts, forests, and suburbs. Each with its own rhythm and kind of stillness. And in all of them, concrete shaped by hand and holding space.

It is a material that can seem hard or cold from a distance. But when you step closer, it tells a different story, one of care, of texture, of weight and warmth. This book is not just about that material, but about the people who choose to live with it and what that choice says.

Making this book gave me time to pause, to look slowly, to ask questions I don't always ask. And maybe that is what stayed with me most: that architecture, at its best, is not loud. It doesn't have to prove anything, it simply holds things well.

To everyone who opened their doors, thank you, for your time, your trust, and your stories. You made this book what it is.

Pieter Peulen

CONCRETE HOMES

Research, texts, and photography
Pieter Peulen

Final editing
William Loftie

Graphic design
Tina De Souter Bookdesign

D/2025/12.005/15
ISBN 9789460583902
NUR 648, 454

info@lusterpublishing.com
lusterpublishing.com
@lusterbooks

Subscribe to our newsletter for new book alerts
and a look behind the scenes: